# EMERGENCY CARE
## Principles and Practices
## for the EMT-Paramedic

*Editor*
ALAN B. GAZZANIGA, M.D.
Professor of Surgery
University of California
California College of Medicine
Irvine, California

Chief of Surgery
Director, Surgical Emergency Department
Director, Intensive Care Unit
Director, Paramedic Training Program
University of California Irvine Medical Center
Orange, California

*Associate Editors*

LLOYD T. ISERI, M.D.
Professor of Medicine, Division of
  Cardiology
University of California
California College of Medicine
Irvine, California

MARTIN BAREN, M.D.
Assistant Clinical Professor of Pediatrics
University of California
California College of Medicine
Irvine, California

Reston Publishing Company, Inc.
*A Prentice-Hall Company*
Reston, Virginia

To Barbara Parker, R.N.

**Library of Congress Cataloging in Publication Data**
Main entry under title:

Emergency care.

Includes bibliographies and index.
1. Medical emergencies. 2. Allied health
personnel. I. Gazzaniga, Alan B. II. Baren,
Martin. III. Iseri, Lloyd T. [DNLM: 1. Emer-
gency health services. 2. Allied health personnel.
WX215 G291e]
RC86.7.E564     616'.025     78-12463
ISBN 0-8359-1652-9

10  9  8  7  6  5  4  3  2  1

Printed in the United States of America

# CONTENTS

# PREFACE

The boundaries of medical care are constantly and rapidly expanding. The treatment of illness and injury is no longer the sole province of physicians and hospitals. The concept of first aid and Boy Scout handbooks has now grown to the point that almost every medical emergency can be treated by persons other than physicians.

Another concept in medical care that has undergone major rethinking is that of the hospital as the exclusive geographical operational center. It has been shown rather conclusively that many medical emergencies can be cared for quite sufficiently, and most of the time more economically, outside the hospital walls. It has been conclusively established that many problems, such as "heart attacks," are often handled more effectively if treatment is started immediately in the field.

There is currently a gigantic push to correlate the various providers of care from all sectors into a workable union. At the present time this group includes everyone from physicians, nurses, and medical students to hospital corpsmen, medical assistants, and many others. The culmination of the community medical approach has been the development of the Emergency Medical Technician (EMT) or paramedic.

Over the past several years, an increasing number of people have been trained in many aspects of emergency medical care even beyond the traditional models of first-aid providers. These paramedical specialists have become quite proficient and have infused a much-needed booster into the medical lifeblood of many communities. Their popularity has grown to the extent that they are now being fictionalized in the media.

Because of the obvious success of these professionals as well as the real necessity for their existence, the programs continue to grow. A major problem exists in the training area, however. There is a need for people working in this field to have a basic knowledge of anatomy, physiology, and pharmacology, as well as several areas of medical specialty, such as trauma, cardiology, and neurology. Because of the wide diversity of subjects to be studied, the procedure has been to utilize multiple textbooks and pamphlets to try to cover everything necessary in a training program. This has been time-consuming as well as confusing, and has also led to vast differences among the various programs.

Recently there have been some attempts to put all the information thought to be necessary for this type of training program into one volume, but this has usually led to encyclopedic works that are quite impractical. The current need is for a specific textbook and manual that will be comprehensive, practical and, most importantly, field-tested. *Emergency Care: Principles and Practices for the EMT–Paramedic* is meant to answer these needs.

One of the largest and most successful training programs for paramedics has been in existence at the University of California Irvine Medical Center (formerly Orange County Medical Center) for five years. Many people have already been fully trained in this program and are currently in the field. The authors have administered this program during the years of its existence and have had the opportunity to observe their students during training and after graduation. This book is a compilation of the extensive material that has been used for the training of over 350 paramedics, and at the same time objectively tested in patient care by the trainees themselves.

*Emergency Care: Principles and Practices for the EMT-Paramedic* can be easily understood in both theory and practice and contains a large assortment of illustrations. Although this book focuses on material useful for the EMT-Paramedic, it can also be useful to a wide range of persons, such as nurses, physicians' assistants, nurse practitioners, firemen, policemen, lifeguards, medical students, and even most practicing physicians. The material is comprehensively covered, but practical enough for any or all of the above to extract what they need for their own areas of endeavor.

# ACKNOWLEDGMENTS

The editors would like to acknowledge the diligent work of the many people who helped establish the Paramedic Program in Orange County and without whose efforts this book would not have been written. Donna A. Zschoche, R.N. is recognized as a motivating force in establishing postgraduate education for both physicians and nurses, as well as improving emergency medical care. Mobile Intensive Care Unit nurses Colleen Y. Campbell, Pearl L. Crouch, Patricia R. McPherson, Sherrie L. Stevens, and Lillian L. Sundquist are also gratefully recognized. These nurses have contributed to the success of the Paramedic Program by insisting upon high standards of education and training. Acknowledgment is gratefully given to Elaine J. Siner, R.N., Supervisor, Mobile Intensive Care Training Division, who has fought for the current standards of care and teaching.

The editors extend their appreciation to all the contributors for the numerous additions, alterations, and deletions that have been made in order to make each chapter an integrated part of the text. Recognition is also given to the hospital administrators, Mr. Robert W. White, Director of Hospitals and Clinics; and Edward J. Tomsovic, M.D., Medical Director; and to the County Board of Supervisors, who have promoted the Paramedic Program throughout Orange County.

Thanks are given to Janice Stewart and Florence Ellison, who have typed this entire manuscript more than once and dedicated many long, hard hours to its completion. Special thanks are given to Golly Moris, Medical Illustrator, whose attention to detail and accuracy has made the medical illustrations an invaluable teaching aid.

# CONTRIBUTORS

Ragnar N. Amlie, M.D.
Assistant Clinical Professor of Pediatrics
University of California
California College of Medicine
Irvine, California

Martin Baren, M.D.
Assistant Clinical Professor of Pediatrics
University of California
California College of Medicine
Irvine, California

Robert H. Bartlett, M.D.
Professor of Surgery
University of California
California College of Medicine
Irvine, California

Director, Burn Center
University of California, Irvine Medical
Center
Orange, California

W. Benton Boone, M.D.
Assistant Professor of Ophthalmology
University of California
California College of Medicine
Irvine, California

Chief, Ophthalmology Section
Veterans Administration Hospital
Long Beach, California

Milton Brotman, M.D.
Associate Clinical Professor of Anesthe-
siology
University of California
California College of Medicine
Irvine, California


Jay B. Cohn, M.D.
Clinical Professor of Psychiatry and
Director of Graduate Psychiatric Educa-
tion
University of California
California College of Medicine
Irvine, California


Bruce F. Cullen, M.D.
Professor and Chairman, Department of
Anesthesiology
University of California
California College of Medicine
Irvine, California


Audrey T. Day
Clinical Research Nurse
Department of Surgery
University of California
Medical Center
Orange, California

Don R. Defeo, M.D.
  Assistant Professor, Division of Neuro-
    logical Surgery
  University of California
  California College of Medicine
  Irvine, California

Ronald D. Fairshter, M.D.
  Assistant Professor of Medicine
  University of California
  California College of Medicine
  Irvine, California

David W. Furnas, M.D.
  Professor and Chief, Division of Plastic Sur-
    gery
  University of California
  California College of Medicine
  Irvine, California

Alan B. Gazzaniga, M.D.
  Chief of Surgery
  University of California
  California College of Medicine
  Irvine, California

Lloyd T. Iseri, M.D.
  Professor of Medicine, Division of Cardi-
    ology
  University of California
  California College of Medicine
  Irvine, California

Robert I. Kohut, M.D.
  Professor and Chief, Division of Oto-
    laryngology
  University of California
  California College of Medicine
  Irvine, California

Jeffrey R. MacDonald, M.D.
  Director, Department of Emergency Med-
    icine
  St. Mary Medical Center
  Long Beach, California
  Medical Director
  Long Beach Emergency Mobile Care Sys-
    tem
  Long Beach, California

William C. McMaster, M.D.
  Assistant Professor, Division of Orthope-
    dic Surgery
  University of California
  California College of Medicine
  Irvine, California

Dennis L. Ming, Pharm.D.
  Assistant Director of Pharmacy Services
  University of California, Irvine Medical
    Center
  Orange, California

Marjorie A. Mosier, M.D.
  Assistant Professor of Ophthalmology
  University of California
  California College of Medicine
  Irvine, California
  Chief, Retina Service
  Veterans Administration Hospital
  Long Beach, California
    and
  University of California, Irvine Medical
    Center
  Orange, California.

Christine A. Nelson, M.D.
  Assistant Adjunct Professor of Pediatrics
  University of California
  California College of Medicine
  Irvine, California
  Pediatric Education Coordinator
  The Earl and Loraine Miller Children's
    Hospital Medical Center
  Long Beach, California

Victor Passy, M.D.
  Associate Clinical Professor, Division of
    Otolaryngology
  University of California
  California College of Medicine
  Irvine, California
  Chief of Otolaryngology
  Rancho Los Amigos Hospital
  Downey, California

Daniel Pelot, M.D.
Assistant Clinical Professor of Medicine,
Division of Gastroenterology
University of California
California College of Medicine
Irvine, California

Robert I. Pfeffer, M.D.
Assistant Professor of Neurology in Residence
University of California
California College of Medicine
Irvine, California

W. Leslie G. Quinlivan, M.D. (Lond.)
F.R.C.S. (Can.), F.R.C.O.G.
Professor of Gynecology and Obstetrics
University of California
California College of Medicine
Irvine, California

Ralph W. Rucker, M.D.
Assistant Adjunct Professor of Pediatrics
University of California
California College of Medicine
Irvine, California

Director, Intensive Care Unit
Children's Hospital of Orange County
Orange, California

David J. Schapiro, Pharm.D.
Supervisor, Poison Control Center
University of California, Irvine Medical
Center
Orange, California

Elaine J. Siner, R.N.
Supervisor, Mobile Intensive Care Training Division
University of California, Irvine Medical
Center
Orange, California

James N. Thompson, M.D.
Assistant Professor of Otolaryngology
University of California
California College of Medicine
Irvine, California

Consultant Staff
Veterans Administration Hospital
Long Beach, California

Lubomir J. Valenta, M.D.
Professor and Chief, Division of Endocrinology and Metabolism
University of California
California College of Medicine
Irvine, California

N. Dabir Vaziri, M.D.
Assistant Professor of Medicine and Acting Chief, Renal Division
University of California
California College of Medicine
Irvine, California

Director, Hemodialysis Unit
University of California, Irvine Medical
Center
Orange, California

Sidney F. Webb, M.D.
Assistant Clinical Professor of Medicine
University of California
California College of Medicine
Irvine, California

Medical Director, Emergency Room
University of California, Irvine Medical
Center
Orange, California

TECHNICAL ADVISORS

Charles R. Hansen
Emergency Communications Coordinator
Orange County Communications
Orange, California

Neil R. Shocket, B.S.
University of California
Los Angeles, California

MEDICAL ILLUSTRATOR

G. Moris
   Member, Association of Medical Illustra-
      tors

# Chapter 1

# MOBILE INTENSIVE CARE

The police arrived at the scene of a shooting and found two victims; one was dead and the other was severely wounded. An ambulance arrived, and the victim was placed in the vehicle and taken to the Emergency Department. The Emergency Department selected was the closest to the scene. During transport the patient experienced some upper airway obstruction, but the only steps taken to correct this were to reposition his head and administer oxygen by a face mask. Upon arrival at the Emergency Department it was found that the door was locked, and a button had to be pushed to summon a nurse. The nurse arrived at the door and told the ambulance driver that there was no physician on duty in the Emergency Department or in the hospital at that time; it would be better to take the patient to another hospital two miles away. The ambulance took off and drove the additional two miles to a second hospital. This time the Emergency Department was open and there was a doctor available, but he would have to be called from home.

While the patient was in the Emergency Department, vital signs were taken. It was discovered that the patient had no palpable pulse or blood pressure. At the same time, the patient stopped breathing. Cardiac arrest ensued and resuscitation was unsuccessful because the nurse lacked the expertise to do cardiopulmonary resuscitation. When the physican arrived in the Emergency Department, the patient was dead.

The preceding scenario occurred frequently ten years ago. Today, improvement in critical care both outside and inside the hospital makes it a less frequent occurrence. This improvement is the result of the efforts by interested legislators and concerned physicians and nurses, consumer demand, improvement in biomedical technology, and the improved understanding of disease processes.

Mobile Intensive Care is a rapidly growing critical care specialty. Personnel at all levels are being trained to deliver fast, efficient emergency care to the ill and injured at the scene and during transport to an Emergency Receiving Center (ERC). Although field providers of emergency care at all levels, such as police, general fire personnel, lay public, lifeguards, etc., will find some material in this book useful, it is focused primarily at the Advanced Life Support (ALS) team member. In some parts of the country this person is called a Mobile Intensive Care Paramedic (MICP). The prefix "para" literally means next to. Therefore, paramedic means next to the medic or doctor. In actuality, the paramedic is in many ways more capable of handling an emergency medical situation than many physicians. He has now been dubbed the "medic," a term that has been used in the Armed Services for years. Another description of this highly skilled provider of emergency care is the EMT designator. EMT stands for Emergency Medical Technician, and the position has been classified into three categories. The EMTA, EMT-1, or EMT-1A is qualified in basic life support outside the hospital. The EMT-2 is a rural paramedic who is qualified in basic life and advanced life support training. The EMT-T or EMT-3 is qualified in advanced life support for both cardiac and trauma and is under medical control. The EMT-3 or paramedic receives this medical direction from strategically located base hospitals. Additional members of the team include the Mobile Intensive Care Nurse (MICN) and the Emergency Department physician.

Mobile Intensive Care (MIC) has developed extensively in only a short period of time. This new dimension in health care has added hundreds of skilled people to the health care team. As a result of this explosion in prehospital care, many other services have benefited: hospital Emergency Departments are updating their personnel procedures and improved emergency equipment is available; ambulance services are being upgraded and ambulance personnel are being trained to the EMT-1 level; public service agencies are training their personnel to the EMT-1 level; health teaching is improving with the increased MIC manpower pool; and new career opportunities are available through MIC.

MIC means that specially trained people have become available to deal with emergencies outside the hospital irrespective of the patient's age, sex, type of illness, and the location where the emergency occurred. The EMT-paramedic is available for the patient who sustains a myocardial infarction at the top of the football stadium, the farmer who is trapped under a tractor, the scuba diver who has had an air embolism, the infant with airway obstruction, and the psychiatric patient who plans to jump from a building. Also, the Mobile Intensive Care Unit (MICU) has emergency vehicles equipped with sophisticated advanced life support equipment (Chapter 2). The MICU at the scene becomes an extension of the Emergency Department of an acute care hospital. Voice and biomedical telemetry communication provide an exchange of the patient's electrocardiogram (EKG), signs and symptoms, and vital signs between the paramedics and the certified Mobile Intensive Care Nurse or physician at the Base Station Hospital (BSH). These communications are maintained at the scene and during transport to the nearest ERC capable of providing the patient with appropriate critical care.

## EMERGENCY MEDICAL SERVICES SYSTEMS (EMSS)— THE TOTAL CONCEPT

Although the MIC (Advanced Life Support) concept is an essential aspect of an Emergency Medical Services System (EMSS), it should never be considered alone, i.e., as a system in itself. MIC is merely one aspect of a total EMSS. In order to provide emergency medical care competently, all components of the EMSS must be well coordinated because each component plays such an integral part in the total system. A team approach to Emergency Medical Care (EMC) is essential.

Current consensus is that "only a comprehensive EMS program, logically planned and staged, will develop and mature so that all patients in need will receive the most appropriate care in the prehospital, intrahospital, critical care, and rehabilitative phases."[1] Carefully integrated regional planning is necessary in order to develop a functional EMSS. With the passage of the EMSS Act of 1973 (P.L. 93-154),[2] Congress has mandated that EMC must utilize a "systems approach" for the provision of emergency care.

Fifteen component requirements have been identified in the EMSS Act to assist system planners and providers in establishing regional EMS programs.

These components are listed below along with some broad objectives for implementation.

EMSS ACT OF 1973

1. *The Provision of Manpower*
   **Objective:** To develop an EMS Manpower Plan which will insure the public of the 24-hour availability and accessibility of adequate emergency medical manpower resources.
2. *Training of Personnel*
   **Objective:** To insure the provision of adequate educational training programs for all levels of emergency medical care personnel in the region in order to increase their effectiveness in providing emergency medical care.
3. *Communications*
   **Objective:** To complete the present emergency medical commu-

nications system by including basic central access by the public and central dispatch.

4. *Transportation*

    **Objective:** To insure that adequate basic advanced life support and critical care transporting capabilities are available in the region.

5. *Facilities*

    **Objective:** To develop systems of care for specific emergency conditions based on the categorized clinical capabilities of facilities and area planning.

6. *Critical Care Units*

    **Objective:** To provide sufficient critical care facilities to meet the specialized needs of critical emergency patients.

7. *Use of Public Safety Agencies*

    **Objective:** To integrate the public safety agencies into the EMS system.

8. *Consumer Participation*

    **Objective:** To continue the participation of consumers in planning, development, and implementation of the EMS system.

9. *Accessibility to Care*

    **Objective:** To insure the availability of both prehospital and hospital emergency care to all persons regardless of their ability to pay.

10. *Transfer of Patients*

    **Objective:** To provide for the transfer of patients from the initial entry into the EMS System through rehabilitation according to the needs of the emergency patient.

11. *Standard Medical Recordkeeping*

    **Objective:** To develop a compatible recordkeeping system which can be used to assess patient care from initial entry into the system through discharge.

12. *Consumer Information and Education*

    **Objective:** To provide a Public Information/Education program for all the people in the area to enable them access to the EMS system and efficient use of its resources.

13. *Independent Review and Evaluation*

    **Objective:** To evaluate the effectivensss of the EMS system by performing process evaluation studies.

14. *Disaster Linkage*

    **Objective:** To assure system response capability during mass casualties, natural disasters, or national emergencies.

15. *Mutual Aid Agreements*

**Objective:** To develop mutual aid agreements between all areas within the region and between regions for all elements of emergency medical services delivery to assure optimal response for the emergency victim.

## FUNCTIONS AND RESPONSIBILITIES OF THE MIC TEAM

Keeping in mind that quality prehospital care requires the coordinated efforts of many team members in a totally integrated EMSS, we will focus on the Advanced Life Support (ALS) aspect of prehospital Emergency Medical Care (EMC). Each component of EMC in an ALS system has its specific functions and responsibilities. These components include the following:

Base Station Hospital (BSH)

Emergency Receiving Center (ERC)

Mobile Intensive Care Emergency Dept

Mobile Intensive Care Nurse (MICN)

Mobile Intensive Care Paramedic (MICP)—EMT-T or EMT-3

These components must function synchronously, making a supreme effort to maintain standardization and quality control.

To be qualified to function as an MIC team member, specially selected individuals are trained in advanced concepts and techniques of emergency medical care which have been mandated by state law and regional criteria. (In California, the law governing the MICP and MICN is the Wedworth-Townsend Paramedic Act Health and Safety Code.) The role of the MIC team is to deliver fast, efficient emergency medical care to the ill and injured at the scene, during transport to an emergency receiving center, and in the hospital emergency department.

Because only superior quality prehospital and hospital care is acceptable in an ALS system, strict adherence to high standards is essential. Training standards and continuing education requirements for ALS personnel must be well-defined, pertinent, and comprehensive. Selection criteria for BSHs and ERCs must be well-defined, adhering to stringent standards.

## COMPONENTS OF AN ADVANCED LIFE SUPPORT SYSTEM

### BASE STATION HOSPITAL (BSH)

Base Station Hospitals are strategically located acute general care facilities that are equipped with voice and biomedical telemetry equipment, and staffed with MICNs and MIC physicians, or physicians under the direction or supervision of physicians totally versed and committed to emergency medicine. Paramedics in the field transmit patient information to MIC personnel at the Base Station and receive appropriate medical directions from them.

Selection of the Base Station hospital should be made carefully based on the fulfillment of specific criteria. These criteria may vary depending upon the region of the country; nevertheless, an astute team of experts should survey the hospital before the selection is made. Once in operation, the BSH should be reevaluated periodically. Only as many BSHs as are needed for a region should be chosen since standardization, essential in a smooth functioning MIC program, becomes more of a problem with multiple facilities. In addition, duplication of costs for telemetry equipment, staff training and development, paramedic resupply, recordkeeping, data collection, and MIC continuing education is minimized with fewer BSHs.

To function optimally, a BSH should have about five active paramedic units within its jurisdiction. Too many units assigned to a Base Station create a burden for the Emergency Department staff, while too little activity results in a decline of the staff's skills and knowledge.

Ideally, paramedics should be able to communicate with all BSHs within a region. Communications should be coordinated by a central communication center that monitors all paramedic activity and assigns the paramedic unit to the BSH most capable of handling the call at that time (Chapter 2). Should central communications be interrupted, paramedics should have the capability to communicate directly with a BSH.

## PARAMEDIC ADVISORY COMMITTEE

Each BSH must have a Paramedic Advisory Committee that includes a physician chairman, the Emergency Department Director, the BSH MICN Coordinator, paramedics representing all MICUs affiliated with the BSH, and a physician and/or MICN nurse representative from each affiliated Emergency Receiving Center. It is helpful to include specialists on this advisory committee such as pediatricians, cardiologists, surgeons, and pharmacists. A representative from the Office of Emergency Medical Services (OEMS) should also attend to serve as a liaison person between other BSHs. Representatives from law enforcement agencies and ambulance companies may also be involved.

The subregional PAC serves as a monitoring and coordinating group, representing all paramedic service providers within an area contiguous to a BSH.

Functions of the Subregional Paramedic Advisory Committee (PAC) include:

1. Maintain liaison with the regional MIC Program and participating hospitals.

2. Audit paramedic treatment records.

3. Review medical protocol.

4. Resolve complaints involving paramedic service providers.

5. Assure updated continuing education for paramedic service providers.

6. Counsel and remediate providers demonstrating substandard performance in accordance with established criteria.

## EMERGENCY RECEIVING CENTER (ERC)

An ERC must meet the same stringent standards as a BSH in being capable of providing twenty-four-hour acute care to a critically ill patient. An ERC does not, however, have biomedical telemetry equipment within its confines, so the nursing staff need not be MICN certified. ERCs must remain abreast of current changes in regional MIC programs by attending Subregional Paramedic Advisory Committee Meetings and continuing education programs. Again, great efforts to maintain standardization must be put forth.

Paramedics transport patients to the nearest ERC best equipped to handle a patient's particular needs. If the emergency hospital care is regionalized, the patient may go to a Trauma Center, Burn Center, Neonatal ICU, Psychiatric Facility, or General Center. However, in some parts of the country, paramedics transport to the nearest facility, where the patient is stabilized and later transported to another facility if necessary. This type of triage is questionable, since the nearest facility may not be the best for the patient. The main objective of the entire emergency care system is to get the proper medical help to the patient as quickly and safely as possible.

## MIC PHYSICIAN (MIC-MD)

The MIC-MD is a specially trained physician situated in the Emergency Department (ED) of a BSH. He or she is immediately available at all times to provide medical direction to paramedics in the field. Even though MICNs provide medical direction for most paramedic calls, it is often necessary for the MICN to consult with the MIC-MD. In addition, the MIC-MD must totally manage paramedic calls beyond the MICN's jurisdiction. The MIC-MD calls for appropriate specialists when indicated. Based on input from paramedics in the field and sound medical judgment, the MIC-MD decides when, where, and how rapidly the patient is to be transported. The MIC-MD is a vital member of the MIC team.

The MIC-MD is more than an Emergency Department physician since additional responsibilities are included in his role. He or she must have a thorough knowledge of the medical facilities in the area, their capabilities, and their limitations. Frequently the decision must be made whether to transport a patient to the closest ERC, or farther away to a facility that can better provide for a patient's needs. The MIC-MD must know which facilities are designated as Basic Emergencies Care Facilities to handle a variety of problems and which are designated as Critical Care Centers to handle specific problems. Critical Care Centers may be categorized within a region to handle patients with problems in the following areas:

Trauma

Cardiac

Poison

Burn

Neonatal

Spinal Cord

Alcohol

Psychiatric

The MIC-MD also has the responsibility of deciding which procedures must be performed in the field to stabilize the patient and when to transport. For example, the cardiac patient with dysrhythmia should have an intravenous line (IV) established and should perhaps be given drugs before he or she is transported. The patient who is unconscious secondary to hypoglycemia (low blood sugar) needs IV dextrose immediately. On the other hand, the patient with multiple system major trauma needs to be transported to a Critical Care Trauma Center immediately. In this situation, taking the time to start an IV and perform a detailed physical examination may be detrimental and a waste of time.

Responsibility for the patient continues during transport until patient care is assumed by the physician at an Emergency Facility. While the patient is enroute, the MIC-MD or MICN notifies the receiving facility of the patient's chief complaint, status, treatment instituted, vital signs, and estimated time of arrival (ETA). Paramedics continue radio communications with the BSH and, if indicated, the EKG is transmitted by telemetry. Paramedics are usually requested to send updated vital signs, EKG readings, and status reports while enroute to the hospital. Additional orders may be given, for example, to start an IV, draw blood, or give medications. While these requests for information and orders may be indicated, the MIC-MD must set priorities on what is to be done prior to arrival. It must be kept in mind that vital signs are more difficult to obtain, EKGs are distorted with motion artifact, and treatments are more difficult to perform in a rapidly moving vehicle.

The safety of the paramedics, patient, pedestrians, and persons in other vehicles should always be the primary consideration during transport. Establishing an intravenous line or administering a drug in a rapidly moving vehicle is difficult and in some cases impossible. Defibrillation should not be performed in a moving vehicle; if it is necessary during transport, the vehicle must be pulled to the side of the road and must come to a complete stop.

The physician's responsibilities extend beyond issuing orders to paramedics at the scene and enroute to the Base Station Hospital or ERC. If the MIC-MD receives the patient, he will continue the care and call for appropriate help from specialists. The MIC-MD also conducts informal and formal evaluations of the paramedics' and MICNs' performance. The MIC-MD's participation in paramedics' and MICNs' continuing education is also vitally important.

Because of the MIC-MD's extended role, special knowledge and skills are required. A comprehensive course should be successfully completed by the physician prior to accepting this new role. The course should include review of the following:

The Regional EMS System
The Regional MIC System
Roles and Responsibilities of EMC Providers
Legalities Related to the Paramedics
Accepted Treatment Protocols
Local Criteria, Transport, and Dispersal of Patients
Communication System
Facilities in the Community
Monitoring and Quality Control
Emergency Care Review, specifically
    Trauma
    Medical Conditions
    Cardiac Emergencies
    Dysrhythmias
    Pediatric Emergencies
    Obstetric Emergencies
    Environmental Emergencies
    Drugs and IVs Carried by Paramedics

One of the most important aspects of the MIC-MD's preparation is time spent in the field with the paramedics. To be effective medical team members, each must have an understanding of the other's problems. Unless the MIC physician has field experience, it is difficult for him to envision the problems outside of the controlled environment of the hospital. These problems might include extricating a patient trapped in a vehicle on a freeway, resuscitating a cardiac arrest patient in a metal-strewn dump or on a rain-soaked golf course, or starting an IV on a patient covered with mud in a dark ravine at night. The paramedic may often be working under hazardous conditions such as fires, toxic fumes, dangerous gases, downed wires, or radiation. In the field, all equipment and supplies are carried to the patient. Often there are crowd and traffic control problems.

Like all EMC providers, MIC-MDs must attend continuing education programs pertaining to EMC. Actively managing critical patients on a regular basis, of course, promotes clinical competence. Being certified in Advanced Cardiac Life Support (ACLS) according to American Heart Association (AHA) standards is important, since many programs, such as that in Orange County, California, have accepted AHA standards for emergency drugs. In the future there will be certification as well as recertification criteria for MIC-MDs in order to assure standardization and quality control.

## THE MIC NURSE (MICN)

The MICN is a registered nurse who has been certified (in California by the County Health Officer) as qualified in the provision of emergency care and the issuance of emergency instructions to MIC paramedics. The MICN must function within the framework of the state law and protocol established at the local level. Orders issued to paramedics must be within established guidelines, and the latter may vary greatly depending on the community. Some areas allow MICNs to order every approved drug, IV, or treatment, while in other areas MICNs may merely serve as communicators for the physician.

Since the MICN is a highly skilled critical care professional, it is appropriate that his or her skills be utilized. It has been demonstrated repeatedly that MICNs can manage a great many paramedic calls independently and in most other cases can give initial orders until the physician assumes care.

In California, paramedics cannot initiate emergency care (except cardiopulmonary resuscitation and defibrillation) without first receiving orders from an MICN or MIC physician. Thus, the quality of emergency medical care rests heavily on the knowledge and skills of these team members. The MICN must have a broad medical knowledge and must be able to interpret information relayed by paramedics correctly. During the course of a call, it may be necessary to solicit additional information from the paramedics to develop a clear, accurate picture of what is occurring in the field. Assessing the needs of the individual patient, implementing a plan of care in accordance with approved assessment/treatment protocols, and evaluating the effectiveness of care are the MICN's responsibilities.

MICN certification requirements must assure that the candidate possesses the necessary skills and knowledge to perform this sophisticated role. Suggestions for prerequisites to MICN certification include the following. The candidate:

1. Must be a registered nurse currently licensed in the state so certifying.

2. Must have demonstrated proficiency in Emergency Department and/or critical care nursing to the satisfaction of the candidate's employing agency.

3. Must be regularly assigned to the BSH MIC communications console or to other directly related MICN duties.

4. Must possess a current Basic Cardiac Life Support (BCLS) certification.

5. Must have passed the AHA Advanced Cardiac Life Support (ACLS) course.

6. Must have documentation of successful training or experience in:

> The Regional EMS and MIC Systems Role and Responsibilities of EMC Providers
>
> Legalities
>
> Assessment/Treatment Protocols
>
> Local Criteria
>
> Communications
>
> Dysrhythmia Identification
>
> Medical Emergencies
>
> Cardiac Emergencies
>
> Trauma
>
> Pediatric Emergencies
>
> Obstetric Emergencies
>
> Environmental Emergencies
>
> Drugs and IV Solutions
>
> Approved MICN Medical Orders
>
> MICU Rescue and Communication Equipment

When these prerequisites have been verified, the candidate for MICN certification completes a certifying examination process. This should include both comprehensive written and practical exams covering the aforementioned topics. Comprehensive testing is important since the MICN must be able to "wear many hats" and function in all critical care areas.

Additionally, the prospective MICN must spend time in the field responding with paramedics to rescue scenes. The MICN and MICP have uniquely different roles. Each must understand the other's role in the ALS system. Just as paramedics should not be expected to function in the capacity of a critical care nurse, the MICNs should not be expected to perform in the field as paramedics. Field time enables the MICN to see why patience is required when the emergency scene (which she cannot see from behind the Base Station hospital radio console) is highly complex. How the paramedic "paints the picture" to the MICN or

MIC-MD at the BSH can be observed and appreciated from a different perspective.

MICN recertification requirements vary from region to region; however standards must remain high in order to retain quality. Ongoing continuing education in emergency medical care is essential, and continuous service while performing MICN duties is necessary in order to maximize proficiency. Responding with certified paramedics on calls periodically is essential to retain open communications and understanding. The regional EMS office must provide MICNs with updated and new information as it happens. A comprehensive refresher course and pertinent study material should be provided to maintain standardization.

Recertification requirements must be clearly stated and strictly maintained. Clear recordkeeping to document fulfillment of requirements is essential. Once it is documented that an MICN is functioning effectively and has met the necessary recertification requirements, recertification written and practical exams are administered biannually.

The role and responsibilities of the MICN extend beyond providing medical direction to certified paramedics in the field. Since the MIC BSH console is usually located in the Emergency Department, this MIC specialist works in that area. Frequently, she receives patients treated in the field by paramedics and continues their care. Evaluating and constructively criticizing paramedic runs with certified paramedics is an MICN primary responsibility. Conducting formal and informal continuing education classes is another important responsibility. To be maximally effective in these roles, it is helpful if the MICN completes a course in Teaching Techniques.

Ongoing evaluation of prehospital care must not be overlooked. The MICN works with the Paramedic Advisory Committee in areas such as the critique of paramedic calls and patient care audits. Audit criteria for specifically designated conditions such as acute myocardial infarction, blunt abdominal trauma, head injury, etc., should be developed. Prehospital care, Emergency Department care, and in-hospital care are audited. Significant data are extracted from these audits, problems are identified, and remedial plans are implemented. Collection of all types of data is closely coordinated with MIC providers and the regional EMS office.

Many BSHs employ a full-time MIC nurse coordinator. This person coordinates MICN and MICP continuing education and audits activities in order to provide a comprehensive quality control system. MIC records are reviewed daily so that problems can be identified and remedied as they occur. BSH paramedic logs and recordkeeping systems are maintained. Liaison among Paramedic Training, MICU sponsoring agencies, BSHs, ERCs, the Regional EMS Office, and all MIC providers is of utmost importance. A current working knowledge of policies, procedures, legalities, and technicalities is essential to this nurse specialist.

In summary, the MICN is a teacher, a student committed to lifelong learning, a nurse skilled in many critical care areas, a counselor, a statistician, and a comfortably working team member. The MICN maintains a close working relationship with the MIC physician and the paramedic. The MICN must remain flexible in order to keep abreast of changes in emergency care.

## THE MIC PARAMEDIC (MICP)

The MICP is a person who has been trained in the provision of emergency medical care in a certified training program. He or she must pass performance and written exams required for certification. The curriculum for the Paramedic Training Program at the University of California Irvine Medical Center has been developed to meet the requirements of California's Wedworth-Townsend Act. This act gives legal authority for paramedics as well as the Orange County criteria for an ALS System. The curriculum is field-competency based with measurable learning objectives. Paramedic Training is a comprehensive course that includes lecture, laboratory, and hands-on clinical and field experience. This prepares the trainee to become the eyes, ears, and hands of the MIC-MD and the MICN. Training standards must be high because the paramedic has enormous responsibilities. The paramedic himself must be intelligent, decisive, secure, amiable but firm, and a leader. The fire department, because of its personnel screening process, already has many such men available. The fire department has been the most popular resource for potential paramedics. Other persons who become paramedics include ex-medics from the Armed Services and registered nurses.

Course testing is on a criterion-referenced basis relying on various evaluative techniques that include:

Daily Quizzes
Block Exams
Final Exam
Emergency Simulations
Clinical/Laboratory Performance
Field Performance
Oral Evaluation

Simulation of patient management is an essential prelude to field internship. These simulations require the application of previously learned didactic material. Any paramedic training course should emphasize accurate patient assessment and the pathophysiology of life-threatening conditions. Critical differences in the physiology, pathophysiology, signs and symptoms; and reactions to treatments in the neonate, pediatric, adolescent, adult, and geriatric patients are stressed. The DOT National Training Course, Emergency Medical Technician-Paramedic (EMT-P) Curriculum is a model for paramedic trainers to use.

The MIC is a relatively new concept in health care delivery. Consequently, many changes and innovations should be expected and encouraged as more experience is realized. This dynamic situation demands that a paramedic training program shift and change emphasis in response to the lessons of experience. Thus, curriculum method, content, and objectives are continually changing. The training staff must critically review each aspect of training during every class in a constant effort to improve the quality of its graduates.

Basic Paramedic Training is divided into four main sections: (1) didactic, (2) laboratory/practicum, (3) clinical experience, and (4) field internship.

*Didactics.* The didactics portion of Paramedic Training consists of lectures, seminars, and demonstrations. Lecturers and group leaders should be thoroughly familiar with paramedic practice, its capabilities, and limitations. To assure that appropriate material is presented to paramedic trainees, lecturers should be given, well in advance of the lecture, preliminary information such as a Competency-Based Learning Plan. Thus, the objectives, lecture content, and field-related techniques are clearly spelled out. Trainees should also receive a copy of the Learning Plan to be aware of what they need to know, why, and how they will be evaluated.

Lectures during didactic training are given primarily by physicians, pharmacists, and MICN-Paramedic Instructors. Paramedic instructors review every lecture with the trainees to emphasize field-related techniques which require competence. Other categories of instructors include:

Certified Paramedics

Public Service Agencies Personnel

Equipment Experts

Social Workers

An Attorney

The Coroner

Vivarium Staff

Communications Experts

A multimedia approach to learning is used in the classroom.

*Laboratory/Practicum.* In the laboratory, trainees learn the practical application of theory and knowledge by practicing and demonstrating skills. All laboratory procedures are based on techniques that must be performed competently and rapidly in the field. Trainees learn assessment skills by practicing on fellow trainees. Invasive procedures, such as starting an IV, are performed on anesthetized dogs in a licensed animal vivarium. Laboratories include:

*Classroom*

1. Diagnostic Signs
2. Patient Assessment (History and Physical Examination)
3. Sterile Techniques
4. Airway, Suctioning
5. Esophageal Obturator Airway
6. Endotracheal Intubation
7. Nasogastric Tubes
8. Nasopharyngeal Airways
9. Miscellaneous Airway Adjuncts
10. The MAST Suit
11. Bandaging and Splinting
12. Fox Balloon
13. CPR
14. Simulated Emergencies, including communication equipment and techniques

*Vivarium*

1. Intramuscular and Subcutaneous Injections
2. Venipuncture
3. 13-lead EKG
4. Needle Cricothyrotomy
5. Tension Pneumothorax
6. Carotid Sinus Massage
7. Jugular Vein Cannulation
8. Intracardiac Injection
9. Cardiac Arrest Drugs
10. Fist Pacing (Chapter 13).

*Clinical.* Clinical experience correlates didactic theory with laboratory and clinical practice to enable the trainee to develop proficiency in performing those skills essential to the delivery of emergency medical care. Emphasis is placed on quality of patient assessment and care. Trainees must demonstrate proficiency in:

Taking Vital Signs
Performing Neurologic Checks
Starting IVs
Administering IM and Subcutaneous Medications
Administering IV Push (IVP) and IV Piggyback (IVPB) Medications
Performing Venipuncture

Auscultating Heart and Lung Sounds

Managing Cardiac Arrest

Cardiac Monitoring and Dysrhythmia Identification

Running 13-Lead EKGs

Assisting with Positive Pressure Ventilation

Suctioning

Moving and Lifting the Injured Patient

Managing the Airway

Patient Assessment (History and Physical Examination)

Trainees also learn to understand the pathophysiology of various conditions as they accompany physicians on rounds and spend time in various critical care areas, supervised by critical care nurses and paramedic instructors. At the University of California Irvine Medical Center, paramedic trainees receive clinical experience in the following areas:

Psychiatric Emergency Admitting Unit

Anesthesiology

Operating Room

Labor and Delivery

Emergency Department

Pediatric Emergency Department

Pediatric Intensive Care Unit

Neonatal Intensive Care Unit

General Intensive Care Unit

Respiratory Intensive Care Unit

Cardiac Intensive Care Unit

Burn Center

Hemodialysis Unit

IV Teams

Wards

*Field Internship.*   In the field internship, trainees respond to emergencies with certified paramedics in an MICU and perform paramedic skills under direct supervision. Members of the paramedic training staff also spend time in the field with each trainee. When a trainee participates in an emergency run, his performance is formally evaluated by a certified paramedic or a training staff member.

In the field, trainees must transfer previously learned technical knowledge and skills to a new set of circumstances. About 500 hours of field experience are required for the trainee to develop proficiency in communication skills and the assessment and treatment of emergency situations. The trainee must be able to assume the role of a certified paramedic with confidence in his knowledge and ability to deliver advanced emergency medical care to the ill and injured.

## AFTER CERTIFICATION

Like all health care providers, paramedics must be committed to lifelong learning. Lines of communication must be kept open between paramedics and their BSHs. It is essential that the paramedic's knowledge of MIC protocol be current. Also, minimum requirements for continuing education, clinical experience, field experience, and critiques of paramedic runs should be established and strictly enforced.

To assure standardization, each paramedic should complete a Comprehensive Training Course for recertification at least biannually. In Orange County, this course is given by the MIC Training Division (Recertification Course). This course includes didactic information and laboratory review of various procedures. Comprehensive training is followed by written and verbal recertification exams.

Periodic field evaluation of paramedics by specially trained MICNs is also a part of recertification. Paramedics are evaluated in their capacity to be the patient-man (assess and treat the patient), and to be the radioman (transmit information to the Base Station Hospital). The quality and quantity of equipment, supplies, inventory lists, etc., are also reviewed.

Reenactment of the scenario at the beginning of this chapter would be different in 1978.

> The police and the paramedic arrive at the robbery scene at the same time. The paramedic immediately assesses that one patient is dead and the other one has airway obstruction and severe shock due to hemorrhage. The patient's airway is opened and he is placed in a MAST suit after communication with the Base Station Hospital. The Base Station Hospital notifies the paramedic to transport the patient immediately to a nearby receiving center that is able to treat the patient's problems comprehensively. The patient is loaded into the Mobile Intensive Care Unit while his heart rate is monitored. During transport, vital signs are taken and the full extent of his injuries are assessed. This information is transmitted to the Base Station Hospital MICN, who in turn transmits it to the receiving hospital. The receiving hospital Emergency Department physician knows what injuries exist, what the vital signs are, and when the patient will arrive. He calls for additional help, which includes an anesthesiologist and a general surgeon. In the MICU, two paramedics are attending the patient, and an EMT-1 paramedic is driving the vehicle and relaying the information from the treatment paramedics to the Base Station Hospital. Upon arrival at the Emergency Department, the patient is brought into the trauma room where intravenous cutdowns are placed, a chest tube is inserted, and an endotracheal

tube is inserted. Blood is sent for laboratory studies and typing and crossmatching. The patient is immediately taken to the operating room, where it is discovered that the bullet traveled through the left chest, diaphragm, spleen, and stomach. The appropriate surgical therapy is instituted. The patient makes an uneventful convalescence and is discharged from the hospital two weeks later.

*Summary*

Emergency medical care in 1978 has reached a high level of sophistication throughout many areas of the United States. It is clear that this medical system depends upon cooperation, open communication, and understanding among all levels of health care providers.

As a result of legislation, much impetus has been given to the development of an emergency care system. New words have come into usage, as have abbreviations for different components of this critical care area. MIC-nurse, MIC-physician, and MIC-EMT or paramedic have crept into the medical vernacular. Emergency care is no longer considered a strictly hospital phenomenon. It involves the activities of highly skilled professionals in the field linked to the hospital by radio and telemetry communication, and coordination with the Emergency Department physician and his specialist backup. No single part of the system assumes more importance or is isolated from any other. Each phase of emergency medical care must be understood by the various team members. The paramedic must know the problems of the Emergency Department physician and nurse and vice-versa. The magnitude and scope of this system is unparalleled in the world, and lives are salvaged daily.

This chapter has presented the anatomy of the emergency medical care system as an overview for repeated reference while reading later chapters in this book.

*Bibliography*

Boyd, David R. "Emergency Medical Services Systems Development: A National Initiative," *EEE Transactions on Vehicular Technology*, Vol. VT 25, No. 4, Nov. 1976, p. 104.

"Optimal Hospital Resources for Care of the Seriously Injured," *American College of Surgeons Bulletin*, Sept. 1976, p. 15.

# Chapter 2

# INTRODUCTION TO THE MOBILE INTENSIVE CARE UNIT

The concept of prehospital care for patients suffering injury or illness is not new. In Biblical times patients were carried by litter to centers of healing. Horse-drawn vehicles—"ambulances volantes"—were extensively used by Napoleon's armies to transport wounded soldiers to treatment stations near the front lines. The history of the Red Cross is important—it is essentially the outcome of the efforts of organized compassion for wounded soldiers, generated by M. Henri Dunant. The arrival of the internal combustion engine heralded a new era in ambulances, the first one being designed and built in 1906. Since then, the state of the arts of medicine and transportation have dictated the sophistication of the ambulances. The Vietnam War revolutionized the transport of patients again as the helicopter came into vogue; it is now a fact of life in civilian life also, although it has somewhat limited usefulness. Each major armed conflict of the twentieth century saw advances being made in patient transport and field medicine, and by 1959 Russia had evolved a civilian system for prehospital care utilizing physicians and paraphysicians manning ambulances. In 1966 Dr. Frank Pantridge in Belfast, Ireland, introduced Mobile Coronary Care Units utilizing a battery-powered portable monitor-defibrillator he developed. His concept of "Flying Squads" of physician and paraphysician revolutionized the care of prehospital patients and led to a rapid expansion and improvement in community-wide systems for Emergency Medical Services (EMS).

In the United States, communities such as Jacksonville and Miami, Florida, Nassau County, New York, Seattle, Washington, and Long Beach and Los Angeles, California, took the lead in establishing advanced paramedic systems. Pioneers like Cobb, Grace, Nagel, and Lewis became familiar to prehospital care personnel all across the country. Los Angeles County, under Dr. Ron Stewart, became a leader in developing paramedical educational courses and techniques. Orange County, California, developed an advanced paramedic prehospital care system in the early 1970s and has contributed to advancements in extrication, communication, and transportation techniques since that time. In addition, some of the most advanced paramedic mechanical skills such as needle cricothyroid membrane puncture have been pioneered for the prehospital care team in the Orange County system.

This extension of patient care into the prehospital area has become even more important as more and more facts became known. For instance, trauma kills about 150,000 people a year in the U.S. It is estimated that at a minimum 15 percent of accident victims die at the scene from injuries that are potentially reversible by properly trained medical personnel. Many investigators believe the potential "saves" generated by more adequate personnel and equipment is much higher than the oft-quoted 15 percent, perhaps as high as 40 percent. Additionally, the largest single cause of deaths in the U.S. is coronary artery disease (about 700,000 deaths per year) and approximately 60 percent of these patients die in the first two hours following the onset of symptoms. Tragically, most of these patients die before reaching a hospital and in acute ventricular fibrillation, which is potentially reversible with the proper equipment and personnel.

It becomes obvious, then, that the patient's chances for survival will be improved by the following: properly trained mobile intensive care unit personnel arriving quickly; proper equipment for transport of acutely ill or injured patients; and proper direction of this prehospital team, usually by a Base Station physician or a specially trained nurse (Mobile Intensive Care Nurse—MICN).

## COMPOSITION OF THE UNIT

The commonly accepted Mobile Intensive Care Unit (EMT-3, advanced paramedic) today is comprised of the following:

1. Personnel—At least two paramedics are necessary (EMT-3, approximately 1000 hours of training) and a driver.

2. Ambulance—Equipped to carry two paramedics and the driver, 1–2 patients, complete medical and communication equipment, and equipment for "light" rescue and extrication.

3. Field Drug Kit—Carried by the paramedics, containing all medicines, IV equipment, airway equipment, splints and bandages for most acute injuries or illness, including an obstetrical kit.

4. Monitor-defibrillator—Portable, battery powered, capable of monitoring and defibrillating patients in the field. The communications equipment is then capable of voice and telemetry (EKG) communication with a Base Station through a portable transceiver/modulator.

5. Backup Rescue Personnel—Usually fire department personnel, with EMT-1 level medical training and the capability and equipment for difficult extrication ("heavy" rescue).

6. Police Backup for Traffic and Observer Control—In California all police personnel are now also required to have basic first aid and CPR training, the rationale being that they are often the first persons arriving at the scene of an injury or acute illness.

7. Base Station Personnel—Physician or specially trained registered nurses called Mobile Intensive Care Nurses who direct the care of the prehospital patient.

## PARAMEDIC EQUIPMENT

### AMBULANCE

*Equipment.* The most obvious piece of paramedic equipment is the ambulance, which must not be confused with a utility or heavy rescue vehicle. The ambulance is primarily designed to carry one, and hopefully two, patients with the capability and room to fully resuscitate at least one of the patients. The modern paramedic ambulance must additionally meet the following needs: two-way radio communication, storage room for equipment, oxygen and suction devices (installed and portable), and facilities for safeguarding personnel and patients. As originally noted by Dr. John Farrington in Wisconsin, the ambulance must meet these needs by having equipment of five types: basic, safety, access, emergency care, and communications. The basic, safety, access, and emergency care equipment lists modified from Dr. Farrington's lists follow and communication equipment is discussed separately (see below). A complete drug and equipment list from a typical paramedic ambulance (Orange County, California) is listed in Tables 2-6, 2-7, 2-8, 2-9.

The vehicle itself must have a driver compartment and an adequate patient compartment, which means a floor-to-ceiling height of at least 54 inches (with 60 inches the optimum). It is preferable that there be direct access between the driver and patient compartments; lacking this, there must be at least voice communication between the two areas. The minimal interior length of the patient compartment should be 116 inches, and the maximum external vehicle length should not exceed 22 feet. The height of the vehicle, excluding radio antennas, should not exceed 110 inches, including roof-mounted equipment. Cardiopulmonary resuscitation requirements are such that for at least one of the patients there must be 25 inches of space at the head of the litter and 23 inches of kneeling space at the patient's side near the chest. The vehicle must have adequate power to accelerate quickly in traffic and to respond quickly to emergencies, as well as to make evasive turns. It must have adequate brakes (usually disc) for sudden and frequent stops. It should provide a fairly comfortable ride for the patient (i.e., low noise and vibration and good cornering). It must have a bright interior and also exterior illumination. The ambulance must have a heating system adequate for climatic conditions and patient comfort. The suspension must be adequate for sudden evasive moves, and a short turning radius is helpful in congested areas and in narrow streets and alleys. Sufficient storage space must be provided for the recommended equipment. Side windows are not necessary, since they provide an additional hazard should an accident occur during transport. Fuel supplies should provide for a range of at least 150 miles, and four-wheel drive capability may be required in some areas with difficult terrain. The power supply for on-board equipment is extremely critical, both in quality and quantity. A special heavy duty alternator is necessary and the capability for continuous recharging when the vehicle is stationary or moving is mandatory.

The ambulance must be plainly marked and have large flashing lights. It must be painted in highly visible color and should have easily heard horn and sirens. Studies in England indicate the most effective noise is an alternating horn as opposed to a continuous siren. Additionally, some local EMS systems utilize a system whereby the ambulance has a small device that switches traffic lights to favor the emergency vehicle. This system adds approximately 5 percent to the cost of installating the lights.

At present it is commonly recognized that high speed runs with lights and sirens are rarely necessary from the scene of the accident to the hospital—but they do occur with regularity to the scene of the accident when time is often the crucial factor. The above recommendations are designed to get qualified personnel and good equipment to the scene of the accident quickly, to allow paramedics the capability of field stabilization, and then to provide patient transport to the hospital under optimal circumstances.

*Type.*   Many varieties of ambulances are available today. Basically, the types can be divided into four major groups: the automobile, the carryall, the van, and the modular.

1. *Automobile.* The automobile type (hearse or Cadillac type) is still very common in the U.S. Unfortunately, the space standards required now for paramedic care are not met by this style of ambulance; in addition, it is unable to carry enough equipment (Figure 2-1).

2. *Carryall.* The carryall (large station wagon) is usually constructed on a truck chassis, and has difficulty meeting space criteria (Figure 2-2).

3. *Van.* The van ambulance offers a large patient compartment

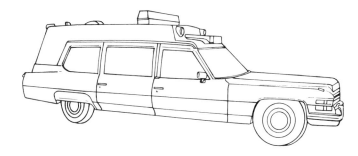

**Figure 2-1.** The automobile-type or hearse-type ambulance.

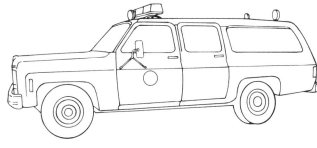

**Figure 2-2.** The carry-all type ambulance.

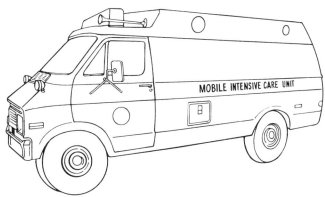

**Figure 2-3.** The van-type ambulance.

combined with a short overall length and wheelbase and is currently a very popular paramedic ambulance (Figure 2-3).

4. *Modular.* The modular unit is essentially a box (patient compartment) mounted on a one-ton truck cab and chassis (Figure 2-4). This decreases replacement costs because the chassis, wearing out first, can be replaced separately by simply fitting the box onto a new chassis. This model, like the van, meets all the space criteria and can carry all the necessary equipment for paramedics. The replacement costs are particularly important in areas of extremely heavy use.

The main complaint regarding the modular unit is that it produces an extremely rough ride, while the chief disadvantage of the van unit

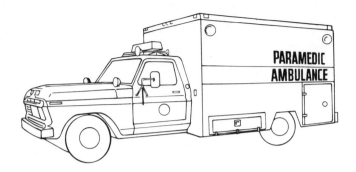

**Figure 2-4.** The modular-type ambulance.

is the extreme forward location of the driver (thought to be a less safe position should an accident occur) and some comments relative to a lack of stability. The four types of ambulances are compared as to cost, advantages, and disadvantages in Table 2-1.

TABLE 2-1.   MOBILE INTENSIVE CARE UNITS AVAILABLE

| Type | Typical Cost (New)* | Advantages | Disadvantages |
|---|---|---|---|
| Automobile<br>Cadillac chassis<br>62″ head room<br>52″ patient compartment | $26,750 | Good Ride | Small patient area, does not meet space criteria, small storage capacity, poor off-highway vehicle, low maneuverability |
| Carryall (Suburban)<br>(Int'l Harv. chassis)<br>54″ head room<br>patient compartment | 14,900 | Good off-road vehicle (4-wheel drive option readily available) | Cannot meet patient area criteria, relatively harsh ride |
| Van<br>Superior<br>(Chevy G-30 chassis<br>or Wayne Carovan) | 16,000 | Large patient area; large storage capacity, good maneuverability | No 4-wheel drive option for off-highway use, relatively harsh ride. Driver exposed in front end accidents |
| Modular Type 1<br>61″ head room | 20,000 | Large patient area, large storage capacity, good off-road vehicle (with special chassis) | Rough ride. Often poor turning radius |

Modified from Carl Jelenko, III, M.D. and Charles F. Frey, M.D. *Emergency Medical Services*. Bowie, Maryland: Robert J. Brady Co., 1976, p. 88.
*Approximate list prices as of 1978.

24

All ambulances must have the basic equipment listed in Table 2-2 simply for patient comfort and safety. The safety equipment for all ambulances as listed in Table 2-3 is necessary to secure an area and make it safe for rescuers and patients until specialized help arrives. The armored vests are becoming increasingly necessary for paramedics in inner city urban areas where violence is an everyday fact of life. The access (light extrication) equipment in Table 2-4 is a list recommended by the American College of Surgeons in 1970 for the ambulance unless the ambulance is routinely accompanied by a true rescue vehicle with extrication equipment aboard. The various access tools utilized to lift, pry, cut, pull, and batter should be located in compartments accessible from outside the ambulance. The Emergency Care List (Table 2-5) is also an original list from the American College of Surgeons 1970. It does not include all of the modern components of the paramedic drug box, discussed separately.

TABLE 2-2.  BASIC EQUIPMENT FOR ANY AMBULANCE

| | |
|---|---|
| Litters—wheeled and adjustable | Urinals |
| Litters—hand-carried | Paper cups |
| Pillows with cases | Wall mounted and portable suction units |
| Sheets | Wall mounted oxygen delivery system |
| Towels | Portable oxygen delivery system |
| Blankets | Sandbags |
| Emesis bags | Blood pressure apparatus |
| Tissues | Stethoscope |
| Bedpans | |

TABLE 2-3.  SAFETY EQUIPMENT

1. Flares, or even better, 12 reflectorized or intermittently flashing warning devices (flares have caused fires at accident scenes)
2. Flashlights—2 standup type, 6V, lantern, battery powered
3. Floodlights—2 portable, each 300 w/120V, with stand, twist-lock type connectors, and 100-foot cords
4. Air masks—2 self-contained (not oxygen-generating), 30 minutes
5. Fire extinguisher—(B:C dry powder type, size 5)
6. Insulated gauntlets—2 pair, foam-insulated, vinyl-coated, fluorescent orange
7. Protective Flak Vests (armored)—2
8. Warning cones or flags for daylight (optional)

TABLE 2-4.   ACCESS AND EXTRICATION EQUIPMENT

One wrench, 12 in, adjustable open end

One screwdriver, 12 in, regular

One screwdriver, 12 in, Phillips

One hacksaw with 12 wire (carbide) blades

One pliers, 10 in, vise grip

One hammer, No. 5, 15 in handle; one fire axe butt, 24 in handle; one wrecking bar, 24 in, separate or as one combination tool

One crowbar, 51 in, pinch point

One bolt cutter, 39 in, jaw opening 1-1/4 in

One portable power jack and spreader tool (minimum 4-ton capacity)

One shovel, 49 in, pointed blade

One double-action tin snips, minimum 8 in

Two ropes, manila 50 ft by 3/4 in diameter

Power winch optional. Front-mounted winch, minimum 2-ton capacity, recommended particularly in areas where not readily available. Chain, 15 ft, with one grab hook and one running hook

Additional suggested items:

   On asbestos blanket

   Two pair goggles

   Two pair gloves (gauntlets, leather)

   Two hardhats

Reprinted from *Bulletin of the American College of Surgeons*, May 1970, p. 13.

The original list of medical equipment (Table 2-5) is a basic list, and most advanced paramedic systems have most, if not all, of the suggested additions (bottom of list). Tables 2-6 to 2-9 have been included to illustrate a complete listing of the equipment utilized daily by the Orange County Mobile Intensive Care program. Costs, whenever possible, are shown to indicate early 1978 costs. Table 2-6 shows the fixed assets of a paramedic ambulance and its miscellaneous supplies. Tables 2-7 and 2-8 show the expendable and nonexpendable medical supplies, some of which are covered in the original American College of Surgeons list (Table 2-5). Table 2-9 is a complete list of drugs and intravenous solutions carried by the Orange County paramedics.

It must be understood that the complete list of equipment illustrated in Tables 2-6 to 2-9 is the response of one locality to its medical and medicolegal needs. Different areas, especially when a different level of training is obtained for the rescue personnel, will demand different equipment lists. The list, however, has been extensively field tested and proven, and a reasonably comparable list should be available wherever advanced paramedics are performing field duties. Figure 2-5 depicts all of the routine equipment utilized daily by an MICU team in Long Beach, California.

1. Portable suction apparatus with wide-bore tubing and rigid pharyngeal suction tip

2. Hand operated bag-mask ventilation unit with adult, child, and infant-size masks. Clear masks are preferable. Valves must operate in cold weather, and unit must be capable of use with oxygen supply

3. Oropharyngeal airways in adult, child, and infant sizes

4. Mouth-to-mouth artificial ventilation airways for adults and children

5. Portable oxygen equipment with adequate tubing and semiopen, valveless, transparent masks in adult, child, and infant sizes

6. Mouth gags, either commercial or made of three tongue blades taped together and padded

7. Sterile intravenous agents, preferably in plastic bags, with administration kits

8. Universal dressings, approximately 10 in by 36 in, compactly folded and packaged in convenient size

9. Sterile gauze pads, 4 in by 4 in

10. Soft roller self-adhering type bandages, 6 in by 5 yards

11. Roll of aluminum foil, 18 in by 25 ft, sterilized and wrapped

12. Two rolls of plain adhesive tape, 3 in wide

13. Two sterile burn sheets

14. Hinged half-ring lower extremity traction splint (ring 9 in in diameter, overall length of splint 43 in) with commercial limb-support slings, padded ankle hitch, and traction strap

15. Two or more padded boards, 4-1/2 ft long by 3 in wide, and two or more similarly padded boards, 3 ft long, of material comparable to four-ply wood for coaptation splinting of leg or thigh

16. Two or more 15 in by 3 in padded wooden splints for fractures of the forearm. (By local option, similar splint of cardboard, plastic, wire ladder, or canvas slotted lace-on may be carried in place of the above 36 in and 15 in boards.)

17. Uncomplicated inflatable splints in addition to Item 16 above or as substitute for the short boards

18. Short and long spine boards with accessories

19. Triangular bandages

20. Large size safety pins

21. Shears for bandages

22. Sterile obstetric kit

23. Poison kit

24. Blood pressure manometer, cuff, and stethoscope

TABLE 2-5.  CONTINUED

The dynamics of the field of emergency medicine are such that this equipment list should be constantly upgraded as newer and more effective equipment becomes available. We believe that additional items to be routinely considered for a more complete list at this time are:

Cervical collars—large, medium, and small

Esophageal obturator airways

Hare traction splints

MAST suit (military antishock trousers)

Needle cricothyroid puncture kit with hi-flow valve

Needle thoracostomy kit with flutter valve

Venous cutdown kit

The contents of the Paramedic Drug Kit (Table 2-9)

Portable monitor-defibrillator (battery powered)

Telemetry and voice communication equipment

Reprinted from *Bulletin of the American College of Surgeons*, May 1970, p. 13.

TABLE 2-6.   ORANGE COUNTY MOBILE INTENSIVE CARE PROGRAM FIXED
ASSETS AND MISCELLANEOUS SUPPLIES

*Fixed Assets*

1. Telemetry and communication equipment as specified by the County Department of Communications
2. Oscilloscope/Defibrillator (about $3,200)
   A. Porta-Pak®, self-contained DC Defibrillator and Monitor—Motorola
   B. Datascope Monitor Defibrillator M/D2—Medtronic
   C. Life/Pak-4®. Portable Defibrillator and Cardioscope with Qwik-Look Paddles. Medical Life Systems
3. Defibrillator Paddles (about $150)
4. Pediatric Defibrillator Paddles (about $200)
5. Extra Batteries, if required (about $250 each)
6. Laerdal Suction Unit, portable (about $195)
7. Hare Traction Splint (about $105)
8. Portable, battery operated EKG Machine or strip recorder—optional (about $500)
9. Stretcher, collapsible scoop, Dynamed (about $150)
10. Oxygen Cart with 3 heads and 2 D $O_2$ Tanks (about $450)
    a. Suggested method of assembling:
       (1) Suction Head
       (2) Humidified $O_2$ with Liter Flow Gauge
       (3) Resuscitator with Robert-Shaw Demand Valve

TABLE 2-6. CONTINUED

*29*

*Paramedic
Equipment*

Oxy-Kart®

b. Oxygen Cart, assemble yourself. Blount Twin-O-Vac #3100, complete unit with same three heads as A, above

*Miscellaneous Supplies*

Trauma and IV Box: (Quantity 2)

1. Craftsman Mechanics Tool Box with double cover, cantilever. 18″ × 10″ × 13-1/4″ (about $23.00) or,
2. Proto 9951 Hip Roof Tool Box. 10″ × 12″ × 18″ (closed). 26″ × 18″ (open). Color: Red. (about $21)

Pediatric Equipment and Drug Box: (Quantity 2)

1. Piano Fishing Tackle Box, or
2. Old Pal Fishing Box 17-1/2″ × 9″ × 9-1/2″, or
3. Adventurer #2013, Vechek Plastics 8-1/2″ × 19″ × 10-1/2″

Backup IV Box:

1. Craftsman Mechanics Tool Box, or
2. Proto 9951

Disaster Box:

Any large suitcase type container for large dressings and IV solutions

*Other*

1. Bandages, triangular (sterile)
2. Bath towel for defibrillating
3. Bottle opener for Glucotol
4. Burn sheets, disposable (sterile)
5. Calipers, (dividers) w/o screw, 5-1/2″ for EKG measurements
6. Container with removable lines for cold sterilization of equipment
7. Disposable pillow case (for gurney)
8. Disposable sheets (for gurney)
9. Lollipops for Pediatric Trauma Box
10. Marking pens
11. Paper bags, #8
12. Paper bags for trash
13. Paper cups, size D
14. Restraints, back board, soft cotton
15. Restraints, wrist, soft
16. Ring cutter, Beaver
17. Toenail or wire cutter
18. Tweezers, blunt
19. Ziplock bags, various sizes

TABLE 2-7.   ORANGE COUNTY MOBILE INTENSIVE CARE PROGRAM EXPENDABLE MEDICAL
SUPPLIES

| Description | Unit of Issue | Planning Unit Price | Quantity Vehicle | Frequency of Use |
|---|---|---|---|---|
| Airway, Oral (Adult) | Each | .65 | 3 | Medium |
| Airway, Oral (Child) | Each | .65 | 3 | Medium |
| Airway, Oral (Infant) | Each | .65 | 3 | Medium |
| Airway, Nasopharyngeal | Each | | 1 | Low |
| Airway Set, Emergency Lifesaver Kit | Set | 11.00 | 1 | Low |
| Airway, Plastic Tongue Depressor (Epistick) | 10 to box | 9.00 | 4 ea. | Low |
| Airway, Resusitube (Adult) 02 Service | Each | 1.44 | 1 | Low |
| Airway, Resusitube (Child) 02 Service | Each | 1.44 | 1 | Low |
| Airway, Resusitube (Infant) 02 Service | Each | 1.44 | 1 | Low |
| Applicators, Cotton, Sterile 6" 2 per package 2000/case | Case | 14.95 | 10 pkgs. | Medium |
| Alcohol Sponges 2000/case 100/box | Case | 17.10 | 100 ea. | High |
| Bandage, Band Aids 1" × 3" Sterile 100/ctn | Carton | 1.74 | 1 ctn. | Medium |
| Bandage, Coban Elastic 4" 12 rolls/box | Box | 9.12 | 4 rolls | Medium |
| Bandage, Steri-Strip 1/2" × 4" 4 boxes/case | Case | 24.65 | 12 ea. | Low |
| Bandage, Steri-Strip 1/4" × 4" 4 boxes/case | Case | 24.65 | 12 ea. | Low |
| Basin, Emesis, Disposable Plastic 250/case | Case | 14.80 | 5 ea. | Low |
| Basin, Round Disposable | Case | | 2 | Low |
| Bedpan, Plastic 20/case | Case | 18.50 | 1 ea. | Low |
| Betadine Solution, Swab Aid 100/box | Box | 4.60 | 1 box | Medium |
| Dextrostix® | Jar | | 1 | Medium |
| Disposa Blanket, KCP | Each | 3.00 | 6 ea. | Medium |
| Boards, Arm, for IVs, Long (Disposable) | Box | 18.00 | 6 ea. | High |
| Boards, Arm, for IVs, Short (Disposable) | Box | 15.00 | 6 ea. | High |
| Catheter, IV placement, 12 Gauge Medicut | Box | 42.50 | 2 ea. | Medium |
| Catheter, IV placement, 14 Gauge Medicut | Box | 42.50 | 2 ea. | Medium |

TABLE 2-7. CONTINUED

| Description | Unit of Issue | Planning Unit Price | Quantity Vehicle | Frequency of Use |
|---|---|---|---|---|
| Catheter, IV Placement, 16 Gauge Medicut | Box | 40.00 | 6. ea. | Medium |
| Catheter, IV Placement, 18 Gauge Medicut | Box | 40.00 | 6 ea. | High |
| Catheter, IV Placement, 20 Gauge Medicut | Box | 40.00 | 6 ea. | High |
| Catheter, IV Placement, 22 Gauge Medicut | Box | 42.50 | 6 ea. | High |
| Catheter, Suction with Mucous Trap 10Fr with 10cc trap 50/case | Case | 29.00 | 2 | Low |
| Catheter, Suction, Plastic 8Fr. 50/case | Case | 8.40 | 4 | Low |
| Catheter, Suction, Whistle Tip, Rubber, Small 12Fr. 12/box | Box | 7.00 | 4 | Low |
| Catheter, Suction, Whistle Tip, Rubber, Medium 16 Fr. 12/box | Box | 7.00 | 4 | Low |
| Catheter, Suction, Whistle Tip, Rubber, Large 18Fr. 12/box | Box | 7.00 | 4 | Low |
| Cleaning Solution, Cidex 4 gal/case | Case | 37.00 | None | Low |
| Dressing, ABD Pads, 7-1/2″ × 8″ Sterile 360/case | Case | 39.56 | 12 ea. | Medium |
| Dressing, Eye Pad, Oval, Sterile 25/box | Box | 1.45 | 25 ea. | Low |
| Dressing, 4″ Kling Nonsterile | Case | 18.93 | 12 rolls | High |
| Dressing, 2″ × 2″ Sponges, Sterile 3000/case | Case | 49.61 | 36 ea. | High |
| Dressing, 4″ × 3″ Sponges, Sterile 2000/case | Case | 31.08 | 36 ea. | High |
| Dressing, Vaseline Gauze, 6″ × 36″ Sterile | Box | 5.23 | 6 ea. | Medium |
| Dressing, 4″ Kerlix Nonsterile | Case | | 12 rolls | High |
| Electrode, Gel, Rudex 6/box | Box | 5.34 | 1 ea. | High |
| Electrode, Monitoring, American 4/pkg 160pkg/case | Case | 20.10 | 10 pkgs. | High |
| Esophageal Airway-Replacement tube & valve | Each | | 4 | High |
| Fox Balloon, Non-Stop, Kerry | Each | 6.95 | 2 | Low |

TABLE 2-7. CONTINUED

| Description | Unit of Issue | Planning Unit Price | Quantity Vehicle | Frequency of Use |
|---|---|---|---|---|
| Gloves, Sterile, Travenol, Large 500/case 100/box | Box | | 4 ea. | Low |
| Lubafax, Individual Packages 144 pkg/box | Box | 9.05 | 144 pkgs. | Medium |
| Needle, Scalp Vein, Butterfly Infusion 19 Gauge 20/box | Box | 7.25 | 6 ea. | Medium |
| Needle, Scalp Vein, Butterfly Infusion 21 Gauge 20/box | Box | 7.25 | 6 ea. | Medium |
| Needle, Scalp Vein, Butterfly Infusion 23 Gauge 20/box | Box | 7.25 | 6 ea. | Medium |
| Needle, Scalp Vein, Butterfly Infusion 25 Gauge 20/box | Box | 7.25 | 6 ea. | Medium |
| Needle, Scalp Vein, Butterfly Infusion 25 Gauge Short 20/box | Box | 7.25 | 6 ea. | Medium |
| Needles, 12 Gauge, 2″ Emergency Tracheal Catheter 25/box Monoject Item 410 (10 Gauge) | 1/5 Box | 3.50 | 2 ea. | Low |
| Needles, 18 Gauge, 1-1/2″ Poly Hub 1000/case | Case | 46.49 | 100 ea. | Medium |
| Needles, 22 Gauge, 1-1/2″ Poly Hub 1000/case | Case | 33.05 | 100 ea. | Medium |
| Needles, 25 Gauge, 5/8″ Poly Hub 1000/case | Case | 46.40 | 100 ea. | Medium |
| Obstetrical Pack DMI Disposable | Kit | 6.50 | 1 | Low |
| Oxygen, Cannula, Nasal Prong, Hudson Plastic, Adult 50/case | Case | 65.00 | 12 ea. | High |
| Oxygen, Cannula, Nasal Prong, Hudson Plastic #33, Pediatric 50/case | Case | 65.00 | 6 ea. | Medium |
| Oxygen, Connecting Tubing, K-25 50/case | Case | 12.49 | 4 ea. | Low |
| Oxygen, Mask, Hudson Plastic Disposable #1040, Adult 72/case | Case | 46.80 | 12 ea. | Medium |
| Oxygen, Mask, Hudson Plastic Disposable #1035, Pediatric 50/case | Case | | 6 ea. | Medium |
| Oxygen, Mask, Hudson Plastic Disposable with Rebreathing Bag 50/box | Box | 26.00 | 2 ea. | Low |
| Pack, Cold, Temp-Aid 40/case | Case | 30.07 | 4 ea. | Medium |
| Pack, Hot, Temp-Aid 40/case | Case | 32.35 | 4 ea. | Low |

TABLE 2-7. CONTINUED

| Description | Unit of Issue | Planning Unit Price | Quantity Vehicle | Frequency of Use |
|---|---|---|---|---|
| Penlight, Examination, Concept Disposable 6/pkg | Package | 5.50 | 6 ea. | High |
| Pins, Safety, Large #3 144/pkg | Package | .75 | 20 ea. | Low |
| Razors, Clarion Disposable 100/case | Case | 21.75 | 4 ea. | Medium |
| Scalpel, Disposable with #10, 15, 20, & 22 Blades | Each | | 2 ea. size | Low |
| Solution, Sterile Water Irrigation 1000 cc 6/case | Case | 2.75 | 2 | Medium |
| Solution, Normal Saline Irrigation 1000 cc 6/case | Case | 2.75 | 2 | Medium |
| Splint, Cardboard, Arm 12/box | Box | 7.00 | 4 ea. | Medium |
| Splint, Cardboard, Leg 12/box | Box | 9.00 | 4 ea. | Medium |
| Sponges, Tri-Ring for Hare Traction Splint 12/box | Box | 9.95 | 2 ea. | Low |
| Syringe, Bulb, 2 oz. 50/case | Case | 17.10 | 1 ea. | Low |
| Syringes, 1 cc TB, w/25 Gauge Needle Monoject 201-TB 500/case | Case | 35.10 | 6 ea. | Medium |
| Syringes, 3 cc Monoject 151991 1000/case | Case | 35.30 | 6 ea. | Medium |
| Syringes, 6 cc Monoject 318108 250/case | Case | 14.50 | 6 ea. | Medium |
| Syringes, 12 cc Monoject 316056 250/case | Case | 15.64 | 6 ea. | Medium |
| Syringes, 35 cc Monoject 315881 100/case | Case | 20.21 | 4 ea. | Medium |
| Syringes, 60 cc, Monoject 151708 with Catheter Tip 100/case | Case | 30.06 | 4 ea. | Low |
| Tape, Transpore, 3M, 2″ 6 rolls/box #1527 | Box | 5.39 | 4 rolls | High |
| Tape, Transpore, 3M, 1/2″ 12 rolls/box | Box | | 1 box | High |
| Tape, Transpore, 3M, 1″ 12 rolls/box | Box | 5.39 | 4 rolls | High |
| Thermometer, Oral TR1735 12/box | Box | 7.65 | 2 ea. | Medium |
| Tubing, Universal Bubble, 5/16″ ID × 1/16″ OD General Suction 205 | Reel | 4.27 | 1 length | Medium |
| Tubing, Latex, Penrose Drainage 1″ 12/box | Box | 5.52 | 1 box | High |

TABLE 2-7. CONTINUED

| Description | Unit of Issue | Planning Unit Price | Quantity Vehicle | Frequency of Use |
|---|---|---|---|---|
| Tubing, Latex 3/16″ ID × 1/16″ OD General 201 Thyrotomy | Reel | | 1 kit | Low |
| Tubing, Latex, Penrose Drainage 1/2″ 12/box | Box | 5.52 | 1 box | Medium |
| Tubes, Feeding, size 5, 50/case | Case | | 2 ea. | Low |
| Tubes, Feeding, size 8, 50/case | Case | 9.83 | 2 ea. | Low |
| Tubes, Salem Sump size 10 Fr. | Each | .77 | 2 ea. | Low |
| Tubes, Salem Sump size 14 Fr. | Each | .77 | 2 ea. | Low |
| Vacutainers, Lavender Top, Oxylated, 100/box | Box | 9.08 | 4 ea. | Medium |
| Vacutainers, Red Top Clotted 100/box | Box | 9.99 | 4 ea. | Medium |
| Valve, Heimlich with 4-way stopcock | Each | | 2 | Low |

TABLE 2-8.   ORANGE COUNTY MOBILE INTENSIVE CARE PROGRAM NONEXPENDABLE MEDICAL SUPPLIES

| Description | Unit of Issue | Planning Unit Price | Quantity Vehicle | Frequency of Use |
|---|---|---|---|---|
| Adapter, Universal Robert-Shaw | Each | .95 | 2 | Low |
| Airway Set, Esophageal | Set | 22.00 | 2 | Medium |
| Airway Set, Esophageal, Replacement Tubes | Each | 10.00 | 2 | Medium |
| Board, Long Back | Each | 64.95 | 1 | Medium |
| Board, Short Spine | Each | 54.95 | 1 | Medium |
| Board, Head & Chin Straps | Set | 9.50 | 1 | Medium |
| Board, Neck Roll | Each | 7.40 | 1 | Medium |
| Board, Torso Straps (set of 4) | Set | 30.00 | 1 | Medium |
| Book, Drug Identification Guide | Each | 4.50 | 1 | Low |
| Book, *Physician's Desk Reference* | Each | | 1 | Low |
| Cervical Collar, Foam, Firm: Sizes: Small, Medium, Large | Each | 6.90 | 1 ea. size | Medium |
| Destruclip, B-D (For destroying needles & syringes) | Each | 6.60 | 1 | High |
| Electrode Wire, American, Red | Pkg of 5 | 5.50 | 1 pkg | High |
| Electrode Wire, American, Green | Pkg of 5 | 5.50 | 1 pkg | High |
| Electrode Wire, American, Black | Pkg of 5 | 5.50 | 1 pkg | High |

TABLE 2-8. CONTINUED

| Description | Unit of Issue | Planning Unit Price | Quantity Vehicle | Frequency of Use |
|---|---|---|---|---|
| Electrode wire, American, White | Pkg of 5 | 5.50 | 1 pkg | High |
| Intubation Set, Laerdal, Complete with Handle, curved & straight: Adult & Ped. Blades | Each | 59.00 | 1 | |
| Mask, Puritan-Bennett, Plastic Benefit #5281, 15mm, Infant Size 1 | Each | 7.90 | 1 | Low |
| Mask, Puritan-Bennett, Plastic Benefit #5282, 15mm, Infant Size 2 | Each | 7.90 | 1 | Low |
| Mask, Puritan-Bennett, Plastic Benefit #5283, 15mm, Infant Size 3 | Each | 7.90 | 1 | Low |
| Mask, Puritan-Bennett, Plastic Benefit #5284, 15mm, Infant Size 4 | Each | 7.90 | 1 | Low |
| Replacement Piece for above Mask sizes: 1, 2, 3, 4 Mask, Puritan-Bennett | Each | .95 | 1 | Low |
| Mask, Puritan-Bennett, Plastic Benefit #5251, 22mm, Adult size | Each | 11.30 | 1 | Low |
| Mask, Puritan-Bennett, Plastic Benefit #5252, 22mm, Adult size | Each | 11.30 | 1 | Low |
| Mask, Puritan-Bennett, Plastic Benefit #5253, 22mm, Adult size | Each | 11.30 | 1 | Low |
| Mask, Fitrite, Nonconductive Robert-Shaw—Adult size | Each | 3.75 | 1 | Medium |
| Mask, Fitrite, Nonconductive Robert-Shaw—Pediatric size | Each | 3.75 | 1 | Medium |
| McGill Forceps Sizes: Pediatric, Adult | Each | 9.50 | 1 | Low |
| Medical Anti Shock Trousers (MAST) Adult size-ST 303: Peds-ST-353 | Each | 330.00 | 1 ea. | Low |
| Oxygen Tank, D-size (for Resuscitator) | Each | | 6 | High |
| Oxygen Tank, Hand Wheel | Each | | 1 | High |
| Resuscitator, Hope, Red. with safety release valve, 2/o carry case | Each | 59.75 | 1 | Medium |
| Resuscitator, Hope, Adult w/safety release valve, carry case & large benefit mask | Each | 59.25 | 1 | Medium |
| Sandbags, #3 & #5 Posie 5163-7503 | Each | 3.95 | 2 of ea. | Medium |
| Scissor and light kit | Each | 17.50 | 1 per man | High |

TABLE 2-8. CONTINUED

| Description | Unit of Issue | Planning Unit Price | Quantity Vehicle | Frequency of Use |
|---|---|---|---|---|
| Sphygmomanometer, Tycos, Complete Adult Arm | Each | 66.00 | 2 | High |
| Sphygmomanometer, Tycos, Complete Adult Leg | Each | 74.50 | 1 | Low |
| Sphygmomanometer, Tycos, Complete Set: Ped. sizes 1″, 2″, & 4″ cuffs (one sphyg. for set) | Set | 66.00 | 1 ea. size | Low |
| Splint, Air Set | Set | 47.95 | 1 | Low |
| Splint, Green, Extrication Back | Each | 70.00 | 1 | Medium |
| Stethoscope, B-D, with 18″ Tubing Red General Duosonic #4270 | Each | 22.65 | 2 | High |
| Tourniquet, Velket, The Velcro Tourniquet Size: Adult Arm, 2″ | Each | 2.25 | 2 | High |
| Tourniquet, Velket, The Velcro Tourniquet, Size: Adult Thigh, 2″ | Each | 3.25 | 1 | Low |
| Tourniquet, Velket, The Velcro Tourniquet Size: Pediatric | Each | 2.50 | 1 | Medium |
| Tourniquet, Rotating Cardiac Emergency Tourniquet Set, Cardiquet, Velcro Sizes: 2-Thigh, 2-Arm | 4 Each | 35.75 | 1 | Low |

TABLE 2-9.   ORANGE COUNTY MOBILE INTENSIVE CARE PROGRAM MOBILE INTENSIVE CARE UNIT DRUG AND IV SOLUTION LIST

*Drugs:*

| | |
|---|---|
| Ammonia Inhalants | Box (10 inhalants) |
| Atropine Sulfate | Prefilled syringe |
| Betadine Ointment | Tube |
| Benzoin Tincture | Bottle |
| Calcium Chloride 1 g/10 ml (10%) | Prefilled syringe |
| Dextrose 25 g/50 ml (50%) | Prefilled syringe |
| Diazepam (Valium) 10 mg/2 ml | Prefilled syringe |
| Diphenhydramine (Benadryl) 50 mg/ml | Prefilled syringe |
| Digoxin 0.5 mg/2 ml | Ampule |
| Dopamine 200 mg/amp | Prefilled syringe |
| Epinephrine 1:1000, 1 ml | Ampule |
| Epinephrine 1:10,000, 10 ml | Prefilled syringe |

TABLE 2-9. CONTINUED

*37*

*Paramedic
Equipment*

| | |
|---|---|
| Epinephrine 1:10,000, 10 ml, cardiac needle | Prefilled syringe |
| Furosemide 20 mg/mg/2 ml | Ampule |
| Instant Glucose Eqv. 25 g | Bottle |
| Glucose Solution (Glucotol) 100 g/12 oz | Tube |
| Ipecac Syrup, 8 oz | Bottle |
| Isoproterenol 1 mg/5 ml | Prefilled syringe |
| Metaproterenol Inhaler | Inhaler |
| Lidocaine 1% 100 mg/10 ml | Prefilled syringe |
| Lidocaine 4% 1 g/25 ml | Prefilled syringe |
| Lidocaine 20% 1 g/5 ml | Prefilled syringe |
| Metaraminol (Aramine) 100 mg/10 ml | Prefilled syringe |
| Metaraminol (Aramine) 10 mg/1 ml IV push | Prefilled syringe |
| Morphine Sulfate 10 mg/ml | Ampule |
| Naloxone (Narcan) 0.4 mg/ml | Ampule |
| Nitroglycerine Tablets 0.4 mg (gr 1/150) 100s | Bottle |
| Normal Saline 10 ml | Vial |
| Normal Saline 100 ml | Vial |
| Pitocin 10 units/ml | Ampule |
| Sodium Bicarbonate 3.75 g (50.0 mEq/50 ml) or (44.6 mEq/v0 ml) | Prefilled Syringe |
| Sodium Bicarbonate 1 mEq/ml 10 ml (Pediatric) | Prefilled Syringe |
| *IV Solutions:* | |
| Dextrose 5% in Water (D5W) | 500 ml |
| Dextrose 5% in Water (D5W) | 250 ml |
| Dextrose 5% in 0.45% Sodium Chloride (D5-1/2NS) | 500 ml |
| Dextrose 10% in Water (D10%) Glass | 250 ml |
| Dextrose 5% in 0.2% Sodium Chloride (D5-1/4NS) | 250 ml |
| Lactated Ringer's Solution | 1000 ml |
| Osmitrol 20% in Water (Mannitol) | 250 ml |
| Solution, Normal Saline Irrigation Glass | 100 ml |

| Description | Unit of Issue | Quantity Vehicle | Frequency of Use |
|---|---|---|---|
| Dextrose 5% in Water (D5W) | 500 ml | 12 | High |
| Dextrose 5% in Water (D5W) | 250 ml | 10 | Low |
| Dextrose 5% in 0.45% Sodium Chloride (D5-1/2NS) | 500 ml | 6 | Medium |

TABLE 2-9.   CONTINUED

| Description | Unit of Issue | Quantity Vehicle | Frequency of Use |
|---|---|---|---|
| Dextrose 10% in Water (D10W) Glass | 250 ml | 4 | Low |
| Dextrose 5% in 0.2 Sodium Chloride (D5-1/4NS) | 250 ml | 4 | Low |
| Lactated Ringer's Solution | 1000 ml | 6 | High |
| Osmitrol 20% in Water (Mannitol) Glass | 250 ml | 6 | Low |
| Solution, Normal Saline Irrigation Glass | 1000 ml | 2 | Medium |
| Blood Administration Set Y-Type 10–15 gtts/ml | Each | 2 | High |
| IV Extension Set with Final Filter for Osmitrol Solution | Each | 6 | Low |
| Solution Administration Set (Macro Drop) 10–15 gtts/ml | Each | 12 | High |
| Solution Administration Set Y-Type (Macro Drop) 10–15 gtts/ml | Each | 4 | High |
| Solution Administration Set (Micro Drip) 60 gtts/ml | Each | 4 | High |
| Solution Administration Set (Micro Drip) | Each | 24 | High |
| Ammonia Inhalants | 10/box | 10 | High |
| Atropine Sulfate 1 mg/10 ml | Prefilled syringe | 2 | Medium |
| Betadine Ointment | Tube | 1 | Low |
| Benzoin Tincture | Bottle | 1 | Low |
| Calcium Chloride 1 g/10 ml (10 g) | Prefilled syringe | 2 | Low |
| Decadron 20 mg/5 ml | Ampule | 2 | Low |
| Dextrose 25g/50 ml | Prefilled syringe | 2 | High |
| Diazepam (Valium) 10 mg/2 ml | Prefilled syringe | 6 | High |
| Diphenhydramine (Benadryl) 50 mg/ml | Prefilled syringe | 4 | Low |
| Dopamine 200 mg/amp | Ampule | 6 | Medium |
| Digoxin 0.5 mg/2 ml | Ampule | 4 | Low |
| Epinephrine 1:1000 1 ml | Ampule | 4 | Low |

TABLE 2-9. CONTINUED

39

Paramedic
Equipment

| Description | Unit of Issue | Quantity Vehicle | Frequency of Use |
|---|---|---|---|
| Epinephrine 1:10,000 10 ml | Prefilled syringe | 4 | High |
| Epinephrine 1:10,000 10 ml (with Cardiac Needle) | Prefilled syringe | 2 | Low |
| Furosemide (Lasix) 20 mg/2 ml | Ampule | 2 | Low |
| Glucose Instant Eqv. 25 g | Tube | 2 | Low |
| Glucose Solution (Glucotol) 100 g/12 oz | Bottle | 1 | Low |
| Ipecac Syrup 8 oz. | Bottle | 2 | Low |
| Isoproterenol (Isuprel) 1 mg/ 5 ml | Prefilled syringe | 2 | Low |
| Lidocaine 1% 100 mg/10 ml | Prefilled syringe | 4 | High |
| Lidocaine 20% 1 g/5 ml | Prefilled syringe | 2 | High |
| Lidocaine 4% 1 g/25 ml | Prefilled syringe | 2 | High |
| Metaproterenol Inhaler | Inhaler | 1 | Low |
| Metaraminol (Aramine) 100 mg/10 ml | Prefilled syringe | 2 | Low |
| Metaraminol (Aramine) IV push 10 mg/1 ml | Ampule | 2 | Low |
| Morphine Sulfate 10 mg/ml | Ampule | 4 | Low |
| Morphine Sulfate 10 mg/10 ml | Prefilled syringe | 1–6 | High |
| Naloxone (Narcan) 0.4 mg/ml, 1 ml/amp | Ampule | 8 | High |
| Naloxone (Narcan) 0.02 mg/ml, 2 ml/amp (Neonatal) | Ampule | 8 | Low |
| Nitroglycerin Tablets 0.4 mg (gr 1/150) 100s | Bottle | 1 | High |
| Normal Saline 10 ml | Vial | 5 | Low |
| Normal Saline 100 ml | Vial | 2 | Low |
| Pitocin 10 units/ml | Ampule | 4 | Low |
| Sodium Bicarbonate 3.75 g (50.0 mEq/50 ml) or (44.6 mEq/50 ml) | Prefilled syringe | 6 | High |
| Sodium Bicarbonate (Pediatric) 1 mEq/ml 10 ml | Prefilled syringe | 4 | Low |

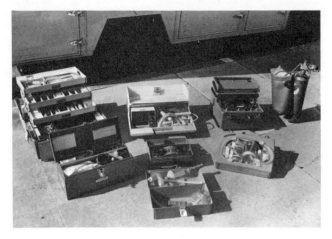

**Figure 2-5.** The portable MICU equipment used by paramedic teams in Long Beach, California. Clockwise from left: drug box, monitor defibrillator (battery-powered), radio transceiver (battery-powered), oxygen equipment, suction equipment (battery powered), esophageal obturator airway equipment and pediatric Ob/Gyn kit. The telephone attached to the radio transceiver is located in the center of the picture.

## MOBILE INTENSIVE CARE UNIT COMMUNICATION AND TELEMETRY

A reliable communication system is essential to the MICU concept. The ability to integrate the prehospital with the hospital phases of care by both voice communication and telemetry has heralded a new era of emergency medicine. The emergency department's capacity to handle an emergency effectively and inpatient bed availability can be determined before a patient arrives at the hospital. Knowledge of a patient's problem before arrival alerts the individual hospital team to marshal necessary resources. The dispersal of patients in multiple casualty situations to various hospitals prevents overloading of one hospital emergency department. Backup units for medical, rescue, or law enforcement personnel can be called quickly to an accident scene. And medicolegally, supervision of the prehospital phase of care by a physician or a specially trained nurse, and allowing the paramedic to intervene quickly in critical situations to salvage life or limb, is made possible only by an intact voice and telemetry communication system between field and hospital. A complete EMS communication and resource setup is diagramed in Figure 2-6.

The paramedic need not have extensive training in the technical details of radio operation; neither must he memorize lengthy radio jargon codes. Rather, the paramedic must become familiar with basic communication concepts, must be familiar with his own equipment, and must understand proper voice communication etiquette and protocol.

### BASIC COMMUNICATION CONCEPTS

The Emergency Medical Services (EMS) system has five major components of the communication system: (1) notification (public call for help), (2) communication center duties (receipt of call for help, dispatch of

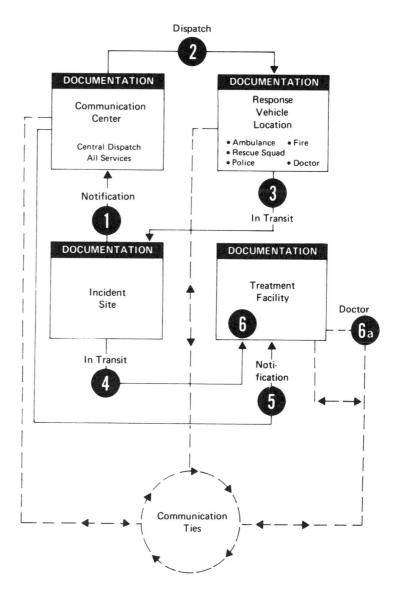

**Figure 2-6.** The Emergency Medical Services Resources and Plan of Operation. (Courtesy of Carl Jelenko III, M.D., and Charles F. Frey, M.D., *Emergency Medical Services*. Bowie, Md.: Robert J. Brady Co., 1976, p. 101.)

rescue units, coordination of team, alerting of medical facility), (3) ambulance, response, and transport units (ambulance, police, fire, light and heavy rescue, and specialty units like neonatal units), (4) fixed facility units for advanced life support (hospital, special care units, doctor's office), (5) the FCC (Federal Communication Commission).

*Notification.* The public telephone is the usual mechanism of activating the EMS system (system entry). A national common emergency telephone number, 911, is being encouraged and has been established in many areas including a "no-coin-required" special feature in pay phones. In other areas it is still possible to dial "O" for operator and ask for police or fire department help and be connected in that manner. Other cities have a special paramedic number, but it is not as effective as a 911 number. Unfortunately, the 911 system is not yet fully operational in many localities, and it appears it will be some time before the 911 system is universal. The major reasons for the delay is that the 911 system requires significant cost input from phone companies, as well as multiple interagency agreements and modern communication command consoles manned by communication experts. Many areas still have multiple possible numbers for the public to call to activate the EMS system; and often the caller is severely taxed as to how to activate the system. Los Angeles County has fifty-four different numbers available for help in a medical emergency. In some areas like Long Beach, California, extensive public education efforts have taken place to make the public aware of the special MICU phone number, and stickers with the paramedic number have been applied to all public phones. Additionally, personnel answering the multiple possible phone listings are being instructed to route the call to the paramedic number whenever possible.

Other means of activating the EMS system are roadside call boxes, citizen band radios (channel 9), and other mobile radio-equipped units such as police cars, fire department vehicles, taxis, trucks, public utility units, etc. Some communication centers now routinely monitor citizen band channel 9 and this is becoming a fairly routine access to the EMS system. No matter what form of citizen access is used, the system must have the capacity to prevent delays in answering calls. In order to accomplish this, the EMS system needs a communication center, or at the very minimum a dispatch office.

*Communication Center.* The communication center, often referred to as "Communication Coordination Center" (CCC), or "Emergency Medical Operation Center" (EMOC), or sometimes simply "Dispatch Office," is perhaps the single most important element in the EMS communication system. The purpose of the CCC is to interface all radio and telephone circuits and to manage the overall emergency response. Thus, the CCC should be capable of monitoring and coordinating all radio frequencies used in a community's EMS response twenty-four hours a day. This necessitates the CCC's having the capability of "cross banding," or allowing a radio on one frequency to communicate with a radio on another frequency. Also, the CCC must have the capability to telephone patch, i.e., to allow someone on a phone to communicate with someone on a radio. The CCC can fulfill its function more effectively if it can control all the frequencies used for communication in that community— that is, the CCC will assign a frequency to an ambulance on a particular run in order that the ambulance may call a hospital without interference from other units that may be utilizing other available frequencies. Additionally, regional CCCs should be tied together by telephone lines, microwave links, and/or radio frequencies to allow for disaster communication, mutual aid, and continuous guidance as an ambulance moves a patient from one EMS region to another. In California, all hospitals are tied together by the HEAR network (Hospital Emergency Administrative Radio), and Los Angeles County Medi-Alert Center (Disaster Response) utilizes this radio to tie together the local EMS regions. Many paramedic vehicles in the county are similarly equipped with HEAR, specifically for disaster responses. HEAR is different from the usual two-way voice communication and telemetry equipment the paramedic ambulances utilize on routine rescues. The CCC should have the capability of recording all conversations.

The dispatcher is important to the EMS system and must have special training, at least to the EMT-1 (A) level, in order that the proper vehicles and backup support may be dispatched as appropriate. The special training should include a thorough knowledge of all EMS resources in the community, the capabilities of the paramedics, all FCC rules and guidelines (see below), and the operational aspects of all public safety and public service agencies in the area.

The dispatcher who answers the original call for help must be trained to ask appropriate questions designed to initiate a proper response by the EMS system (nature of illness, degree of severity, number of patients, etc.). The dispatcher must extract medical data from potential patients, interpret it, and pass it on.

In some EMS systems, the CCC or the dispatcher must be familiar with paging, a technique utilized to alert and call into action personnel not immediately available. Specific frequencies are available for paging in-hospital personnel and personnel outside either the CCC or the hospital. Techniques of paging include public address systems, intercoms, buzzers, beepers, flashing lights, and radios. Paging is used more extensively where personnel are not assigned full-time to EMS duties or where hospital personnel are not always in or near the Emergency Department. Paging is usually a one-way communication system (i.e., dispatcher or CCC to an individual), since two-way communication tends to be time-consuming and in some cases jams frequencies. Two-way communication tends to be more secure, however, since in one-way communication the pager is never sure the person being paged has responded.

*Ambulance Communication.* The absolute minimal communication equipment for any ambulance includes a radio on a medical frequency that enables the ambulance to have two-way communication with the hospital and with the CCC (and with the dispatcher, if the dispatch office is not identical with the CCC). Many ambulances have selective signaling capability so that an ambulance can communicate with specific hospitals without disturbing other radio units on the same frequency.

Often walkie-talkies or portable units are part of ambulance communication. These may be useful for the EMT to communicate with the ambulance itself or directly with the hospital, repeating through the ambulance radio when the EMT is outside the vehicle. The walkie-talkie or portable unit is especially useful in large-scale natural disasters, multiple casualty incidents like train wrecks, and wherever a paramedic has to leave his vehicle and treat a patient remote from the vehicle. (This occurs fairly frequently in large apartment complexes in cities.) Paramedic communication setups utilize the ability of the portable field unit to "repeat" through the ambulance unit, thus magnifying the signal from the field unit in order that the CCC and hospital may receive a clear communication. Most advanced paramedic communication set-ups utilize a portable transceiver that is physically larger and more effective than older style handheld walkie-talkies. These transceivers usually weigh about twenty pounds and are used for both voice and ECG transmission.

Additional communication devices are often needed by ambulances. These include a public address system, intercom between the driver and the patient compartment, and hand-held visual aids for traffic control or helicopter signaling.

The institution of paramedic care in the field is dependent on additional communication links not already covered. In addition to the two-way voice radio communication between the MICU (paramedic) and the hospital and CCC, telemetry is necessary to adequately assess and treat patients. Telemetry is the capability of transmitting vital signs (usually an electrocardiogram pattern) directly from the field to a hospital where it can be monitored by a physician or MICNs, and from where guidance can be given to the paramedic regarding treatment. The biomedical information transmitted by telemetry can be via telephone or radio on appropriate UHF frequencies. This objective data, when correlated with a clinical history and the observations as relayed by the paramedic in the field to the hospital, allows appropriate medical care to be delivered. The telemetered information, as well as the two-way voice communication, is usually tape-recorded at the hospital end and/or at the CCC end of the transmission. The telemetered information may also pass through the ambulance radio, to be "repeated," just as the voice communication is repeated by the ambulance unit.

*Hospital Communication.*   The hospital must, minimally, maintain basic constantly monitored radio equipment that allows two-way voice communication with the ambulance twenty-four hours a day. Many hospitals have decoders on their equipment in order that only calls designated for that hospital will be heard, a feature that reduces the natural tendency of emergency department personnel to turn down a radio that is noisy with calls for other hospitals. Many hospitals in advanced EMS systems have direct-line telephone links or intercoms with paramedic units, the CCC, and private ambulance companies. Hospitals providing support for advanced paramedics have, additionally, telemetry equipment monitored twenty-four hours a day by specially trained nurses or physicians. The two-way voice communication on paramedic calls may be by radio or telephone, and is usually by both, and the telemetered information (EKG) may also arrive via radio or telephone lines. This information is recorded, often by a voice-activated tape recorder, in order that a permanent medical record may be kept on each patient treated by the EMS system. The voice-activation technique is useful because it lessens the amount of actual taping that must be stored as a medical record.

In addition to two-way communication with the MICU, the hospital usually maintains two-way communication with the CCC and / or dispatch office. This may be by radio, phone, or intercom. Interhospital communication is maintained via telephone on a day-to-day basis and by radio for disasters. In California, HEAR for disaster alerts and communication has proven extremely effective. The hospital must also have the capability of paging personnel not immediately available. Again, this is done routinely by intercoms, buzzers, beepers, light call systems, public address systems, and radios, and the paging system may be one-way or two-way communication. The communication equipment for St. Mary Medical Center, the base hospital for Long Beach, California, is illustrated in Figure 2-7.

*Federal Communications Commission.* The use of medical communications is directly responsible for the increased quality of patient care by paramedic units. The veritable explosion of communication systems, however, has created multiple problems in establishing and maintaining effective systems, especially in congested urban areas.

The Federal Communications Commission (FCC) is the regulatory

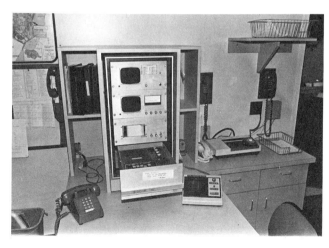

Figure 2-7. The base station hospital. From center: display console containing EKG demodulator, cassette tape recorder, strip chart recorder and EKG oscilloscope, short wave telephone (one outside line and one paramedic line), HEAR radio for disaster, radio control intercom unit, and extension of paramedic telephone.

agency which governs all radio operations in the U.S. At the local level, the FCC allocates bands of frequencies to each EMS system, issues licenses to individual stations, assigns call letters, sets standards of operation for equipment, and sets power limitations. The intention of the guidelines and rules of the FCC is to provide for the orderly use of radio frequencies by qualified and licensed individuals.

In order to more effectively coordinate medical communications, the FCC in 1974 created a new allocation structure specifically for EMS communication. The FCC provides now for a system of frequencies for EMS communication between vehicles and fixed facilities such as hospitals or communication centers, with additional frequencies available for transmission from a portable unit to a rescue vehicle for "repeating" (retransmission). The FCC is now encouraging the use of newer equipment that has this multichannel capability to provide for the simultaneous use of separate channels when several emergencies occur at one time. The multichannel capability allows each incident to be handled without conflict with another incident.

The new FCC rules provide that all channels be shared on a common basis throughout the country. The objective of the rules is to provide a common communication structure and to maximize the usefulness of the limited number of channels available. Obviously, sharing of the limited channels nationwide mandates close coordination between EMS systems. All types of EMS communication, including telemetry, are now confined to the 450–470 megahertz (MHz) UHF frequency band. The rules also permit radio interface with systems operating in other bands through the technique called crossbanding. All locations include two frequency pairs (462.950/467.950 and 462.975/467.975). Table 2-10 lists the currently available frequencies and their primary and secondary roles as determined by the FCC. In addition, the FCC has designated four frequencies in the 458 MHz band for transmission from portable units to associated mobile units (repeating).

COMMUNICATION EQUIPMENT

The objective of the communication system in EMS systems is to minimize the time lapse between the onset of the accident or illness and the rendering of appropriate emergency care. As already discussed, the communication system can be divided into the notification (call for help), the communication center, the ambulance and paramedic communication, and the hospital communication. This section will briefly discuss the actual communication and telemetry equipment carried by modern MICU personnel.

The paramedics must carry (in addition to their drug box, IV solutions, obstetric-gynecology kit, oxygen and suction units, splints, and bandages) a radio transceiver (battery powered) with modulator for telemetry, and a defibrillator and oscilloscope (battery powered). A listing

| Channel Name | Frequency Pair | Primary Role | Secondary Role |
|---|---|---|---|
| Med One | 463.000/468.000* | Paramedic Telemetry | General EMS Requirements |
| Med Two | 463.025/468.025 | Paramedic Telemetry | General EMS Requirements |
| Med Three | 463.050/468.050 | Paramedic Telemetry | General EMS Requirements |
| Med Four | 463.075/468.075 | General EMS Requirements | Paramedic Telemetry |
| Med Five | 463.100/468.100 | General EMS Requirements | Paramedic Telemetry |
| Med Six | 463.125/468.125 | General EMS Requirements | Paramedic Telemetry |
| Med Seven | 463.150/468.150 | General EMS Requirements | Paramedic Telemetry |
| Med Eight | 463.175/468.175 | General EMS Requirements | Paramedic Telemetry |

*The lower frequency must be used for base transmitters and may be used for mobile transmitters. The higher is the designated mobile frequency.

of Los Angeles County MICU portable equipment is found in Table 2-11 (Portable Unit). The oscilloscope allows the paramedic to gather pertinent biological data (an electrocardiogram—EKG) and transmit that data via telemetry to the hospital base station. The hospital base station receives that data via a transceiver, and the voice data is recorded by a cassette tape recorder. A console at the hospital containing an

TABLE 2-11.  LOS ANGELES COUNTY MICU EQUIPMENT

*Portable Unit*

One Cardiac Telemetry Unit—per spec. (includes battery, spare battery, charger, antenna, handset, cable acoustic coupler)

One Physiological Monitor

Defibrillator (with extra paddles and one extra battery pack)

"Fishing Tackle" Drug Box

One IPPB (Elder Valve) or Robert-Shaw Valve inhalation metered flow with Twin-O-Vac suction on E-Cylinder

Six Instaform Splints (assorted sizes) deflatable

One Hare Traction Splint

Datascope Model MD-2

TABLE 2-12.   LOS ANGELES COUNTY MICU EQUIPMENT FOR HOSPITAL
BASE STATION

One Antenna—Phelps Dodge No. 201-509 cut for 465.575 MHz

One Receiver—single frequency, 465.575 MHz with carrier operated relay, with 117 V ac power supply without channel guard General Electric as follows:

Receiver 4ER42G11

Crystal

Top Cover w/metering 19C30367G2

Carrier operated relay

One Remote Control Unit—with handset, General Electric Deskon Mc31ABS11 (with option 5196)

One Demodulator per spec. for 117 V ac operation

One Amplifier—two channel, including power supply for 117 V ac

One Tape Deck—stereo, cassette, Sony Model TC 160

One Strip Chart Recorder—25 and 50 mm/Sec

One Physiological Monitor—Datascope Model 850

One Telephone Coupler for recorder

One Telephone Instrument with push-to-talk handset

EKG demodulator and EKG oscilloscope with a strip chart recorder (Figure 2-7, Table 2-12) allows hospital personnel to see and record EKG telemetry immediately.

## REQUIREMENTS FOR MICU AND HOSPITAL COMMUNICATION

The MICU personnel (paramedics) must have equipment that is portable, sturdy, light enough to carry (for instance, up many flights of stairs), dependable, and reasonably easy to operate. The radio transceiver/modulator typically weighs about 25 pounds. The monitor-defibrillator must, of course, have the ability to be interfaced quickly with the communication system for purposes of telemetry, as well as being dependable and lightweight (15–30 pounds). The radio transceiver should ideally have several channels to enable the MICU and the hospital to switch to an unused frequency when there is radio traffic on other frequencies. Some hospital band systems and some CCCs have a "channel guard" on their radio units to provide for full monitoring of all channels that are available for potential use. The use of multiple channels within the EMS system provides for maximum efficiency and flexibility in managing simultaneous incidents. The CCC routinely should provide guidelines for channel use and should assign channels during periods of high activity.

The alternative solution of adding more equipment to one frequency (often just increasing the strength of the signal, thus blocking out "competing" units) appears, at first, to be an easier solution, but actually it is a less desirable alternative. Multiple channels greatly expand the EMS system capability, and many, if not most, paramedic systems are converting to this technique as the multichannel radio equipment is made available to them. It should be noted that the portable radio equipment carried in the field by the paramedic, as well as the ambulance-based radio equipment, can be equipped with multiple channels.

The principle of MICU communication is quite simple: the field team utilizes a radio transceiver for two-way voice communication, and the modulator unit on its equipment converts the electrical impulse from the EKG into an undulating FM tone, also transmitted by radio on a predetermined frequency or by telephone. The transmission is then received at the hospital base station, again either by radio or telephone. The EKG transmission from the field is passed through a demodulator at the hospital base station in order that the undulating FM tone can be converted back into electrical EKG recordings. It is important to note that the paramedic has the capability of transmitting initially by radio, and that the radio signal may be "patched" to a telephone by the CCC so the hospital base station receives it by land line. The MICU in the field cannot hear other paramedic units, so it will be unaware of multiple incidents unless informed by the hospital or CCC. Other base stations transmitting on other frequencies also cannot be heard by the paramedics in the field. The MICU in the field usually has the option of listening to the transmission from the hospital over a speaker, or on a telephone handset, in which case the conversation will be more private. The hospital base station will override the field unit's transmission when the base is transmitting, since it is occasionally necessary to cut off one unit to talk to another unit on a more critical incident. As an example, the EMS communication system for Miami, Florida, is illustrated in Figure 2-8.

## RADIO PROCEDURES AND PROTOCOLS

The EMS systems are facing a crisis of overloaded radio telemetry frequencies—thus the MICU must determine which incidents must be called in, and then the MICU must learn to transmit pertinent data in an accurate and concise manner. It is not necessary to memorize lengthy radio codes, but it is helpful to know a few commonly accepted terms (Table 2-13) and techniques of communication.

*When to Call the Hospital Base Station.* All MICU teams recognize the need to call the hospital base station for guidance during a full cardiac arrest and most, if not all, MICU teams realize the needless waste of air time to call the hospital for a true nonemergency patient,

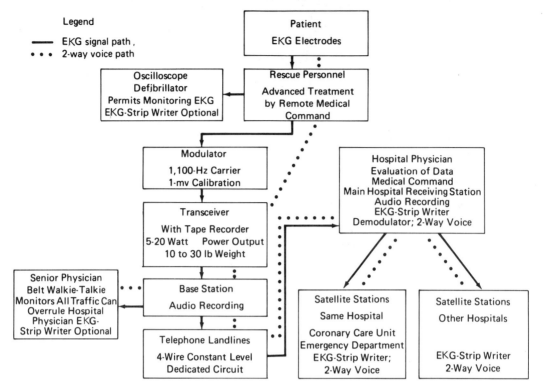

**Figure 2-8.** Emergency medical communication pathways. (Courtesy of J. C. Hirschman, M.D., S. R. Nussenfeld, J. D., MS. (Ad. Med), E. L. Nagel, "Mobile Physician Command," *JAMA*, Vol. 230, Oct. 14, 1974, p. 258)

such as a patient with a two-day-old dog bite on the hand. However, many patients are truly in the gray zone—they may benefit by a call to the hospital base station, but the call may also be an exercise in futility for the paramedic. The hospital may simply order transport for the patient or, more onerously, reply with the stock reply, "Start an IV of D5W and transport."

Which patients to call in on is a vexing problem to most EMS systems. Within Los Angeles County, which has twenty-six hospital base stations, the call-in rate on paramedic runs varies from 5 percent by one MICU team to over 90 percent for other MICU teams. Long Beach, California, consistently has a call-in rate of 25 percent of its 1700 runs per month handled by seven MICU teams. Other localities report figures of 10–70 percent call-in rates.

It must be understood that there are several considerations regarding when to call in:

1. The major concern obviously is for the welfare of the patient. The physician may recognize a need for treatment not recognized by the paramedic.

| *Term* | *Meaning* |
| --- | --- |
| 10-1 | Received poorly |
| 10-2 | Received well |
| 10-4 | Acknowledgment |
| 10-8 | In service |
| 10-9 | Repeat message |
| 10-19 | Return to station |
| 10-20 | Your location |
| 10-22 | Cancel |
| 10-23 | Stand-by |
| Go | Proceed with message |
| Roger | Yes |
| Affirmative | Yes |
| Negative | No |
| Copy | Receive, i.e., "we do not copy" |
| Over | Sentence over, expect answer |
| Cut | Transmission complete |

2. Another concern is to notify the receiving hospital that it will be receiving casualties (that hospital may wish to reroute the patient).

3. Another factor, not to be overlooked, is the medicolegal issue. In most localities, the paramedics are legally able to render field medical care because statutes have been enacted allowing them to do so, usually with the provision that the paramedic is acting under the guidance of a physician. Unless written protocols or statutes provide otherwise, the paramedic rendering medical care or, for that matter, opinions on whether medical care is needed, should be cognizant of the lapse of this statute-based protection if he chooses not to consult the physician on a particular run.

From a matter of practicality, it is clear that the MICU team should utilize the communication system for all patients in moderate or severe distress from any life- or limb-threatening injury or illness. In addition, most areas request the paramedic contact the base station for the following types of incidents:

1. Multiple casualty incidents
2. Penetrating trauma of head, neck, chest, abdomen
3. Chest pain
4. Shortness of breath
5. Unconsciousness or change in mental status
6. Vehicular accidents with injuries

7. Burns over 5 percent or involving the face
8. Suicide attempts or overdoses
9. Patients with distal neurologic loss
10. Seizure patients
11. Patients with suspected major loss of blood
12. Syncope patients
13. Suspected major fracture patients (e.g., pelvis)
14. Violent or dangerous patients

*How to Call.* The actual techniques of radio communication are relatively simple. The paramedic team must assemble pertinent data, then contact the base hospital and report in a succinct manner. The usual opening burst of communication includes the following data regarding the patient: age, sex, chief complaint, vital signs, level of consciousness, and estimate of severity. This information is acknowledged by the base station, and then the base either requests more information or gives the MICU team orders to carry out. For instance, for a patient whose chief complaint is chest pain, the base station may ask pertinent questions not covered in the opening burst, or it may request the MICU team to draw a blood sample, establish an IV, and transmit an EKG while delivering oxygen to the patient.

Several rules must always be followed by the entire team in radio communication (Table 2-14). Following these simple rules will allow the radio airways to be kept as clear as possible, but will minimize errors, usually attributed to a misunderstanding on drug orders.

TABLE 2-14.  RULES OF RADIO COMMUNICATION

1. Be as concise as possible.
2. Utilize medical terms whenever appropriate.
3. Utilize strict identification codes, i.e., always acknowledge who is speaking, and who is being spoken to (i.e., "Orange County Base to Rescue Four").
4. Respond to all transmissions immediately. Utilize the term "stand-by" if you need time before replying.
5. The field unit must repeat all orders given to them by the base, especially drug orders.
6. The opening burst from the MICU team must include age, sex, chief complaint, and vital signs. Additional information may be given and is required in some areas.
7. Each call is ended with the designation of the Base Station. This conforms to FCC regulations.

## PATIENT HANDLING

Routinely, patient handling should be orderly, planned, and unhurried, so as not to further injure the patient. The patient is usually moved from his original position to a new position on a stretcher, positioned properly, covered, secured in place, and then transported to a vehicle. This type of patient movement normally takes at least two personnel, and often more are helpful.

If certain hazards are present, such as fire, the patient may have to be moved suddenly, sometimes by one rescuer. The paramedic must be familiar with such emergency one-person carries as the blanket drag, clothes drag, and the fireman's drag. In the first two of these techniques, the head and neck of the patient are supported, but the fireman's drag leaves the patient's head and neck unsupported.

If more than one rescuer is available, the routine well-known patient lifts may be employed for emergency movement of a patient. Lifting a person onto a stretcher requires at least two and preferably three or four rescuers. Spinal cord immobilization is difficult when multiple rescuers are lifting a patient, but often that is the only mechanism whereby a patient may be moved. Every effort should be made to allow minimal spinal cord and body movement during lifts. If four persons are available, the four-man log roll is one effective technique to position a patient on a spinal board.

During extrication, a short spinal board is often utilized before the patient is removed from a vehicle. In addition, most paramedics are familiar with the "stair-chair" method of putting a patient into a kitchen-style chair or a foldup litter which converts to a chair. The long spinal board should be utilized if the patient can be placed on it and if the situation indicates the patient may have suffered a back injury.

In the ambulance, most patients are secured to the stretcher in the supine position. Velcro straps or some type of belt (abdominal, chest, knee, extremity, or any combination) are utilized to help immobilize the patient to the stretcher during transport. The stretcher must also be secured in position to the patient compartment frame. The MICU must have the capability to put the patient in a Trendelenburg position (i.e., 10–20 percent head of stretcher down) to prevent aspiration should vomiting occur. In some situations, it may be possible to allow the patient to lie on his side to help prevent aspiration. The neck should be protected with a cervical collar, and the back protected by placing the patient on a spinal board in most trauma cases. Aspiration may be prevented by utilizing available suction equipment, manual clearing of the airway, the Trendelenburg position, or putting the patient in the lateral position as needed. If the lateral position is utilized, great care and often extra personnel are needed to safeguard the neck and back.

Some patients have a real need to sit up, especially patients with asthma, congestive heart failure, or chronic lung disease. These patients should be allowed to sit as needed, and should not be forced to a supine position. Shock patients should routinely be kept supine or in the shock position (foot of stretcher elevated slightly).

## EXTRICATION

Patient handling at the scene of injury or illness generally falls into two categories: (1) The routine patient (critical or noncritical) who is easily accessible and who may be routinely treated and transported and (2) the occasional patient who needs extrication. The location of the patient may be dangerous to both patient and rescuer, and the injuries or illness of the patient prompting the call may be critical or noncritical. These extrication runs tax the personnel, equipment, and ingenuity of the MICU team; and certain extrication techniques must be part of the MICU armamentarium. It is understood that most heavy rescues are left to heavy rescue rigs and teams; but the MICU team is often the first on the scene, and its medical expertise becomes part of the total extrication.

In extrication, the following principles must be borne in mind at all times: save the life, prevent further injury, and move the patient only after immobilization and stabilization whenever possible. Extrication is a skill and a field of its own, but the general principles can be covered here. These general principles of extrication are well documented as a result of publications by the U.S. Department of Transportation, and work done by many persons, among them J. D. Farrington, M.D.

The actual emergency care rendered and the degree of effectiveness of the rescue are dependent upon the five stages of extrication, the available equipment, the degree of training and expertise of the rescuer, and the medical condition of the patient. Preliminary to the actual extrication, as the MICU team approaches the accident site, they should survey the entire scene to estimate any potential hazards to either the patient or to the team. If hazards are encountered, an attempt should next be made to correct those hazards, unless lifesaving measures must be instituted immediately (such as airway management or control of severe hemorrhage).

The only major exception to instituting lifesaving measures at this point would be if the hazard itself was a severe threat to the life of the patient and/or rescuers (such as a fire, threat of explosion, threatened collapse of a weakened bridge, etc.). Such a severe threat calls for immediate removal of the patient and the MICU team from the dangerous hazard, before instituting lifesaving measures and without utilizing proper extrication techniques. Obviously it does no good to perform mouth-to-mouth resuscitation in a burning car with a full gas tank ready to explode.

Following the assessment of hazards and the institution of lifesaving measures, the victim should be immobilized as much as possible in place before proceeding with total extrication.

*Stages of Extrication.*   There are five stages to extrication: (1) gaining access, (2) emergency medical care, (3) disentanglement, (4) preparation for removal of the patient, and (5) removal of the patient. The first stage, gaining access, depends on the location and position of the patient, and access frequently is simply through the rear window of a vehicle. However, access may require extensive cutting through the vehicle itself, and typical techniques utilize prying and spreading tools of various types. Most rescue units have cutting tools also, the preferred types of course being those that do not create sparks, which may ignite spilled fuel. Safety must be kept foremost in the minds of the MICU and rescue team as they approach the situation, analyze it, and prepare to gain access. The safety of both the MICU team and the patient must always be considered. The second stage, emergency medical care, would depend solely upon the particular situation encountered by the MICU.

The third stage of extrication is disentanglement. This is accomplished after access has been gained and medical care has been rendered. The principle to be followed is that the vehicle or debris should be "peeled" from the patient, rather than pulling the patient from the debris. The danger during disentanglement is great—the patient may suffer further injury by being pulled or pushed inappropriately, and often cutting or prying tools are in close proximity to the patient. Medical care (stage 2) should continue during the third stage. The disentanglement phase, like the access phase, demands expertise and ingenuity, and familiarity with rescue equipment. The use of safety goggles, hard hats, and gloves is mandatory during access and disentanglement. Often the patient must be covered with an asbestos blanket during cutting operations for disentanglement in order to prevent burns.

The fourth stage of extrication is preparation for removal. This includes continuing the previously instituted medical care, adding of more splints as the patient comes free of the wreckage, and dressing wounds. Thus the patient is "packaged" prior to lifting or moving to the vehicle. Life support, of course, continues during this phase. In this phase, the patient is usually put on the stretcher for the first time, often utilizing a spinal board, or a "scoop" stretcher. The scoop stretcher must be applied from both sides of the patient.

The fifth and last stage of extrication is removal. Here decisions have to be made as to who will move the patient, and how the patient will be moved. This stage demands some planning and usually some teamwork. Usually in this phase of extrication tools and equipment are less important than in the access and disentanglement phases.

*Summary of Extrication.* The most significant points to be cognizant of in extrication are that patient care usually precedes actual extrication and that life support is possible during access, removal, and then transportation. The patient should not be harmed by the extrication process, and some equipment is necessary and standard for routine extrication (Table 2-4) teams. Heavier equipment is usually found on special heavy rescue rigs or other fire department equipment acting as backup to the original units.

## TRANSPORTATION

*Ground Transportation.* Very few medical conditions require high speed runs from the accident scene to the emergency facility, assuming qualified MICU paramedics are caring for the patient at the scene and en route. Conversely, it is often necessary to minimize time lapses to the scene of the accident or illness once the call for help is received, since the paramedic must often institute lifesaving measures within minutes to save a life. The few medical conditions that do require high speed runs to the hospital include: cardiac arrests due to trauma, penetrating chest wounds, some blunt chest trauma, head injuries with deteriorating level of consciousness, some poisonings, and massive trauma with shock. Some cardiac conditions and other medical conditions require high speed runs only if the paramedic is unable to establish an IV line to give adequate drug or fluid therapy. By far the bulk of paramedic runs, including most full cardiac arrests; most trauma cases; seizure patients; cardiac patients; and most obstetric, gynecologic, and pediatric cases are not helped by a high speed run. Studies performed in England indicate adverse changes in the cardiovascular status of many patients while undergoing high speed runs to hospitals. Additionally, and more dramatically, the patient and the crew of the rescue vehicle are being subjected to the serious risk of an accident by a high speed run. The sudden swerves, starts and stops, and the high speed rate all seem to contribute to both an increased risk of worsening the patient's condition by the ride itself, as well as increasing the chances for an accident en route.

The safe speed for an emergency run can only be established while the run is being made. Consideration must be given to the patient's condition, weather, traffic, visibility, and capability of the rescue vehicle, as well as the street surface condition. The use of lights and siren, especially the alternating noise type of siren, does increase the public awareness of the run but by no means guarantees safe passage or the right-of-way. The highest risk an ambulance usually faces is, of course, at intersections. Special care should be taken at every intersection, especially if the vehicle is making a high speed run and is operating against the flow of lights.

Statistics on ambulance accidents are frightening. An average of 10 percent of ambulances nationally are involved in accidents yearly;

but it is estimated that only 3–5 percent of all ambulance runs are true life-or-death emergencies. The statistics on life-or-death runs for MICU would be even less, since the paramedic has the capability of stabilizing many situations in the field and changing them from life-or-death situations to ones of less urgent priority.

There are multiple factors that contribute to unsafe driving practices on ambulance runs, but without any question the biggest factor is unnecessary high speed. Among the other factors are (1) a lack of expertise at the dispatch office, usually making nonurgent calls sound more urgent, (2) inadequate ambulance equipment (not a problem to MICU teams in most areas), (3) inadequate EMT training (again, not usually a problem for MICU teams), and (4) poor driving ability (usually using speed to try to compensate for common sense and/or planning). A good driver on any ambulance, including MICU units, must have a working knowledge of the following factors: (1) road conditions, (2) routes to the patient and to the hospital, (3) availability of police escort, (4) steering and cornering characteristics of the ambulance, (5) the hydroplaning effect of wet roads, (6) proper use of the lights and siren, (7) thorough knowledge of traffic rules and laws, and (8) the actual patient care situation.

The patient must be properly splinted or immobilized for transportation to the hospital. This is of increasing importance due to the acknowledged rougher ride the MICUs have relative to the older Cadillac-style ambulance. The stretcher should be strapped or locked in place, and the patient should be secured to the stretcher as much as possible.

Provision must be made to allow certain patients to assume the sitting position (especially patients with obstructive lung disease), while other patients must be kept in a head-down position due to the possibility of aspiration. At least two rescuers, preferably two EMT-3 trained individuals, must be in the patient compartment with any seriously ill or injured patient. Finally, the MICU should notify the hospital of its estimated time of arrival and, of course, report any major change in the patient's status that may require further intervention.

*Air Transportation.* The Korean and Vietnam conflicts dramatized the utility of helicopter transport, and it has now become an everyday fact of life for many EMS systems. The Maryland Trauma Center and Air-Med EVAC program is immensely successful and is currently the civilian role model to be followed. The capability of the helicopter is best utilized to avoid traffic congestion, to provide care in remote and inaccessible areas, and to provide high speed medical runs for distances of 40–150 miles.

The total picture of EMS must be kept in mind, however, during the current rush to helicopter transport of patients. The helicopter is extremely expensive, and ground transportation is usually just as quick and more comfortable for under a 40-mile radius providing there are good roads. Transport of a patient for more than 150 miles is better suited to fixed wing aircraft and such transports are normally transfers to specialized units, not emergency rescues. The helicopter is noisy, has a very high vibration level, and the ride is often rough due to air turbulence. The helicopter cannot fly in poor visibility or weather. In addition, the treatment area on the usual small civilian helicopter is cramped for patient care, especially in cardiac arrest cases. It is also difficult to land the helicopter in many urban areas due to wires, poles, buildings, or other obstructions.

The most useful helicopter situation is when those helicopters used primarily for other jobs (e.g., law enforcement) can be diverted to med-evac missions as needed, as in Maryland, where state police helicopters are utilized. Much mention is made of the MATS (military) aircraft, but they are not routinely available on an emergency basis because of a lack of aircraft or crew.

At present, then, with few exceptions, helicopters should be low priority for civilian EMS systems. The cost of their purchase and maintenance does not usually justify the benefits of having a helicopter totally dedicated to medical missions in civilian practice. If a helicopter used primarily for other work is available, with a pilot, helicopter transport is extremely helpful in some medical emergencies.

## TRAFFIC AND OBSERVER CONTROL

The primary job for the EMT-3 (paramedic) and entire MICU team is to give medical treatment to the patient. In order to do so, valid emergency extrication and transportation techniques as already discussed must be practiced by the MICU team. Additionally, the team must be able to utilize proper traffic and crowd control procedures if the need arises. Ideally, the MICU team will find it necessary to utilize these techniques infrequently and for short periods of time, since the arrival of additional police and fire department personnel at the scene allows the additional personnel to assume this function.

### TRAFFIC CONTROL

The paramedic, after instituting the medical care of the patient, may decide the situation demands traffic control. The purpose of traffic control is to insure an orderly flow of traffic, which sometimes adds to the safety of the original patient and the rescue team. Traffic control under ordinary circumstances is a difficult task and the conditions existing at an accident will pose serious additional problems. The paramedic should first establish a mechanism to warn oncoming motorists. The techniques utilized will depend on the available light, climatic and visibility conditions, and the traffic situation. The possible warning devices include reflection or flashing devices, flares, cones, or flagmen (obviously utilizing additional personnel).

After establishment of warning signals at appropriate intervals to warn traffic on both sides of the accident, traffic may be redirected as needed. In most accident situations, traffic can be regulated by the use of one of three methods: (1) lane control, (2) total blockade, and (3) detour. Lane control is possible only if there are uninvolved lanes free of debris and/or stalled vehicles. Total blockade is less rarely used, but is necessary if the entire road is covered with debris, wreckage, or patients, and there is no possibility of detour. Detours are useful for accidents in which a long delay is probable and they usually require additional warning devices and/or personnel and signs. The traffic must be redirected safely onto cross streets.

The techniques of directing traffic are critical to smooth and safe traffic flow. Shouting directions at drivers is usually useless; indefinite hand signals often increase the confusion and hazard. Personnel directing traffic should wear distinctive clothing, be highly visible (e.g., in the intersection, not on the curb), and use easily understood hand signals. In addition, the intangible quality of demeanor is important—the attitude and visible conduct of personnel regulating traffic flow allows the motorist to understand traffic is being regulated. The person signaling traffic should stand sideways to traffic authorized to move. Additional hazards, such as downed electrical wires, fire, unstable wrecked vehicles, and debris, must be recognized and allowed for by traffic control personnel. Passing traffic must be encouraged to continue on and not to stop and help, as that usually results in increased traffic and crowd control problems. If passerby vehicles do stop to help, the traffic controller must insure that the cars do not hinder traffic flow and do not block the warning devices.

## CROWD CONTROL

Spectators usually add to control problems at the accident scene. Often, the spectators are persons who have abandoned their vehicles near the accident site and have walked back to offer aid or simply to watch. This, of course, adds to both the traffic and the crowd control problem. Crowd control is usually a police problem; but the MICU team must be able to institute crowd control measures to insure the safety of the patient and rescue team until police help arrives. The spectator can cause monumental traffic jams, cause additional hazards like fire (a cigarette dropped on spilled gasoline), compound the victim's injuries by attempting to help in extrication or medical care, destroy or scatter evidence, increase the theft or looting problems, and increase the noise to levels preventing good patient or base station communication with the rescue team.

The first priority in crowd control is establishing a perimeter beyond which no spectator should pass. This may be a curb, one side of the road, or a more distant line if additional hazards are present. Downed electrical wires must be allowed for, as they pose serious additional hazards to spectators. The perimeter may be established by warning devices, signs, rope, or personnel (usually fire department personnel, but volunteers may be used).

Once the perimeter is established, the main job becomes maintenance of this perimeter. Plainly marked perimeters are usually honored by crowds at accident scenes, especially if manned by courteous but firm personnel. Tact is required, as verbal shouting matches can easily lead to a breakdown in the already instituted crowd control measures. A calm firm demeanor often does much to keep the crowd in check behind the perimeter.

Such major problems as theft prevention, riot control, or suppression of sniper fire rightfully fall to police personnel. Fire department or rescue personnel often help prevent these situations from occurring by the institution of good crowd control measures as soon as possible at the scene of an accident or disaster.

In certain rescue situations it is necessary to begin evacuating spectators and nearby residents due to additional hazards such as fire or dangerous spilled cargoes. This major chore is usually accomplished jointly by police and rescue personnel. In 1973, the U.S. Department of Transportation printed and distributed its "Emergency Services Guide for Selected Hazardous Materials." This extremely useful document gives guidelines to help rescue personnel determine the distance that people should be evacuated from selected health and safety hazards. The guide also includes first aid suggestions, and suggests certain immediate actions when there is a fire, spill, or leak.

## DISASTERS AND TRIAGE

### MEDICAL DISASTERS

A medical disaster may be defined as any situation where the number of casualties overwhelms the existing medical facilities. Thus, a multiple vehicle accident with five to ten major casualties may overwhelm one MICU team and one local community hospital, but would be considered routine to a large county hospital in an urban setting near major highways. Planning for possible disaster situations, especially larger-scale disasters, is extremely difficult; but each MICU team should be familiar with the local disaster response plan and with disaster medicine concepts, including triage.

This plan is, hopefully, at least a citywide disaster plan that involves the mobilization of available EMS resources to cope with disasters. The ideal situation is when the local response can be graded according

to the severity of the disaster (e.g., five to twenty casualties, twenty to fifty casualties, greater than fifty, etc). Additionally, the local citywide plan should be integrated with regional, county, or state-wide plans for severe major disasters (e.g., earthquakes). Local hospital internal disaster plans must also be integrated into the citywide and area-wide plans, and all components of the system must be tested frequently (at least once a year, preferably oftener). It is common knowledge and fact that the most usual breakdown in disaster drills and in actual disasters is in the area of communication. Secure, workable, easy-to-understand communications are the key to the successful handling of disasters, real or practice.

to the severity of the disaster (e.g., five to twenty casualties, twenty to fifty casualties, greater than fifty, etc). Additionally, the local citywide plan should be integrated with regional, county, or state-wide plans for severe major disasters (e.g., earthquakes). Local hospital internal disaster plans must also be integrated into the citywide and area-wide plans, and all components of the system must be tested frequently (at least once a year, preferably oftener). It is common knowledge and fact that the most usual breakdown in disaster drills and in actual disasters is in the area of communication. Secure, workable, easy-to-understand communications are the key to the successful handling of disasters, real or practice.

The role of the MICU in a disaster setting will usually be patient treatment. However, real-life disasters in areas with paramedic systems have proven that the first paramedic team to the scene often becomes the "triage team" for that disaster. It may be replaced later by a hastily-organized physician-led triage team, but for all practical purposes MICUs are perfectly capable of handling field triage. Many areas of the country are discovering that the paramedic team is at least as effective as physician triage teams in patient disposition and, in addition, has more knowledge about traffic and crowd control, hazards, medical resources in the community, and transportation and communications.

Perhaps the ideal triage team would begin with the initial paramedic unit on the scene, utilizing their ambulance or rescue vehicle to set up communications and a triage station. The MICU team must obviously and completely assume medical command at the site, and this triage team would direct additional rescue units as they arrive, concentrating not only on the initial triage of patients but also on the estimate of the total number of casualties. This number is necessary to gauge the proper level of disaster response necessary by the EMS system.

Initially and until relieved by an overall disaster officer (nonmedical), the MICU team would coordinate the various response units. This first paramedic team may later come under the guidance of a physician acting as triage officer, a civil defense administrator, or police or fire department personnel (especially a battalion chief, fire captain, or paramedic coordinator); but at the onset of the disaster it would direct all medical care given at the disaster site, all triage, and all patient disposition. In some areas, the hospital base station directs the actual disposition after communications have been established with the MICU team. This technique, utilizing field triage and base dispositions, allows the paramedics to concentrate on triage and field medicine, while the base station checks area hospitals for bed, manpower, and equipment availability.

## TRIAGE IN DISASTERS

"Triage," a word which originated on World War I battlefields, comes from the French work "trier," to pick out. Triage originally was the term applied to the process of sorting out which casualties could be returned to the front by concentrating the limited medical resources available on their ailments. Now triage has come to mean the process whereby the patients are sorted according to medical need, the idea being that critically ill patients with reversible injuries or illnesses are treated first. Less ill, terminally ill, or fatally injured patients are consigned to lower priorities of care. This system serves to obtain maximum salvage rates with whatever medical resources are available to that particular community. The critical feature of real triage is that it is field oriented. The least critical and the terminally ill patients are not transported immediately but rather are held in the field. This prevents overloading of emergency departments and allows more efficient use of available resources to save lives. Historically, the largest number of patients in most large disasters are ambulatory or less severely injured, and the paramedic can usually triage these patients to a holding area rather than transporting them immediately. This saves the valuable transportation and medical resources for the more severely injured who can be salvaged with prompt treatment. If all injured patients are sent to emergency departments in a large disaster, mass confusion is usually the result and some salvageable patients will die because the facility is unable to cope with the huge influx of patients.

Triage is most useful in a true disaster setting, i.e., when the medical facilities are truly overwhelmed as in an earthquake or aircraft disaster. In this setting, persons who would survive without help are virtually ignored after triage, as are patients who will probably die despite massive medical intervention. The middle group of patients who will benefit most are the patients who receive treatment after categorization by the triage team.

Triage has additional value of some usefulness in the typical large understaffed metropolitan hospital with daily massive case loads usually resulting in waits of six to twelve hours for care. In this situation, the more critical patients are sorted and diverted to high priority treatment areas, while more ambulatory patients wait or are referred to clinics. Triage has its least impact in the routine operation of a small or medium-sized, well-staffed and designed emergency department that usually has a short wait for patient care. In this situation, triage usually means sending the critical cases to a special trauma room.

PRINCIPLES OF TRIAGE

There are several principles that must be learned by paramedics to effectively triage and to deliver disaster style medicine.

1. The magnitude of the disaster and the available resources must be known. Clearly, what may be appropriate in one area would not be correct in another (i.e., in a ten-patient casualty situation, a single

MICU team that has one small hospital for definitive medical care may not be able to institute CPR for one victim because the other nine victims urgently need help. However, in some urban areas, three or four MICU teams may be only minutes away for backup help, and CPR can be instituted and maintained). The initial impact of the destruction at the scene must not cloud the decision-making process of the paramedic—depending on resources, all, some, or only a few of the victims of a disaster may be adequately treated. Only with a thorough knowledge of available resources and a knowledge of the total number of casualties can the appropriate medical response be made.

2. In a large scale disaster (usually a natural disaster like a hurricane, earthquake, or a high speed transportation disaster), total patient care is impossible. The slightly injured patients may get very little treatment or none and may have to wait considerable time, even days. Also, the very critically ill patient with little chance for survival may receive little or no care since that would waste resources that could save many other lives if applied properly.

3. The triage team that does the actual sorting or classifying of patients does no patient care because the institution of treatment slows down the triage capability to an intolerable pace. The triage team classifies and treatment teams then take over, instituting treatment as needed and transporting when appropriate. The one exception to this is airway management, since very often the first person evaluating the patient can and must intervene quickly in airway problems to save a life. Patients with shock and hemorrhage problems should be passed on to treatment teams, unless none are immediately available. Routinely in real disasters a good triage officer, assuming he or she has treatment teams for backup, can triage effectively at the rate of about thirty patients per hour. Most patients take less than two minutes to triage, but an occasional patient takes longer due to emotional difficulties, language barriers, vital signs, or the institution of treatment.

4. The triage team needs to have the capability of taking vital signs, at least pulse, respiration, and blood pressure. A twenty-year-old girl who fainted and has a pulse of 116 and blood pressure (BP) of 88/50 mm Hg should be considered much more urgent than another twenty-year-old girl who fainted and now has a pulse of 72 and a BP of 110/60 mm Hg. Vital signs will not be necessary in the majority of patients, but occasionally they are invaluable.

5. The triage officer in true disaster settings should be an experienced medical person, whether he be paramedic, nurse, or physician. It is a trying role, emotionally and physically draining, and there is no good substitute for field experience when selecting this person.

6. The triage team must tag the patients with initial impression, vital signs if taken, treatment rendered if any, and classification. It is a time-consuming and often fatal mistake to triage in the field but

not to tag the patient, since he must then be retriaged at the medical facility to which he is transported. Often not tagging also delays transportation.

7. The patients must be rated, or categorized. The usual (originally) military system involves five categories of patients and appears the easiest to understand:

    a. Dead or will die

    b. Life-threatened—immediate

    c. Urgent (one to two hours)

    d. Delayed—or noncritical—or ambulatory

    e. No injury

It is important to note that many civilian triage teams only categorize to three levels:

    a. Life-threatened

    b. Urgent

    c. Delayed

The reason, apparently, for the usual civilian mechanism is a natural reluctance to assign patients to categories where they will receive no treatment, i.e., "dead or will die," or "no injury." We believe it is a mistake to utilize only three tiers, since it perpetuates the idea that all patients can be treated in a disaster. It is imperative that the triage team, the transportation personnel, and the receiving hospital not waste time on categories one and five, in order to save lives in categories two and three of the five-tiered system. The critical decision, then, becomes when to declare a multiple casualty incident a disaster, since under normal conditions all patients are offered as much medical care as needed to attempt to resuscitate them.

8. Certain injuries or illnesses can be immediately categorized into one of the five categories. Again, it is imperative for the MICU team to know the available resources and when they are overwhelmed, because consigning patients to a category where no treatment or transport will be offered is correct in a disaster, but may not be appropriate if the EMS system could have responded to all casualties as under normal conditions. Some examples of categorization of patients in a disaster setting follow:

    a. Category 1—Dead or Will Die:
       Full cardiac arrest, neurologic deaths (e.g., through-and-through gunshot wound to the head with no neurologic functions), D.O.A. (Dead on Arrival), burns greater than 80 percent of the body surface third degree (no pain).

    b. Category 2—Life-Threatened—Immediate Treatment Needed (within minutes):
       Airway problems of any type, chest wounds—all penetrating

and some blunt, neck wounds, some severe abdominal wounds, shock, uncontrolled or suspected severe bleeding, head injuries with deteriorating mental status or vital signs, dysrhythmias, chest pain, some poisonings, some diabetic complications (e.g., diabetic coma), and status epilepticus.

   c. Category 3—Urgent (one to two hours to review patient and institute treatment):

Major burns (greater than 20–30 percent body surface), major or multiple fractures, back injuries with or without spinal cord damage, abdominal pain chief complaint with stable vital signs, and most pediatric fever patients.

   d. Category 4—Ambulatory, Noncritical:

Lacerations, minor fractures, most fever patients (except for pediatrics or adults with meningeal signs), and minor soft tissue injuries.

The MICU team can recategorize patients at any time, i.e., a fracture patient may go into shock and then be moved from category three to category two.

The MICU teams and emergency departments active in triage have discovered that most mistakes in triage (mistriaging the patient) arise for one of three reasons: (1) vital signs were not taken or were not taken into account, (2) the presence of drugs or alcohol in the patient severely confuses the capability of the triage officer to decide quickly and accurately, (3) and patients with abdominal pain as a chief complaint are notoriously difficult to assess in large-scale field disasters. However, in-hospital emergency department triage in busy inner city hospital emergency departments is routinely accurate over 80 percent of the time, with another 15–17 percent triaged too high (i.e., categorized more urgent than the patient eventually proves to be), and only 3 percent triaged too low (more urgent cases triaged to less urgent category).

The usefulness of this categorization of patients is most clearly seen in three areas: (1) an institution of medical care in the field (usually reserved for category two), (2) transportation (category two goes first, category three goes second), and (3) at the Emergency Department (category two gets top priority—also the hospital can arrange holding areas away from the public for category one if transportation is available for these patients).

9. A totally separate category of triage is necessary for radiation accidents and certain biological and chemical poison cases. This is a specialized situation that demands decontamination, often in the field, not only of the initial patients, but often of the rescuers and the rescue vehicle itself. Disaster medicine concepts, such as radiation decontamination, are specialized areas of expertise; but the MICU team will hopefully develop basic familiarity with provisions for such care as is found in its city- or area-wide disaster plan.

*Summary*        This chapter has covered the very practical and day-to-day realities of the work of the paramedic. We have seen who the paramedic is and how he is to function. We will now begin to explore the actual knowledge the paramedic must obtain in order to put to use the principles covered in this chapter.

*Bibliography*   American Academy of Orthopaedic Surgeons. *Emergency Care and Transportation of the Sick and Injured*, Second Edition, 1977.

Cowley, R. Adams, and others. "An Economical and Proved Helicopter Program for Transporting the Emergency Critically Ill and Injured Patient in Maryland," *The Journal of Trauma*, Vol. 13, No. 12, (Dec. 1973), pp. 1029–1038.

"Essential Equipment for Ambulances," *Bulletin American College of Surgeons*, 55:7-13 (1970).

Farrington, J. D., M.D. "Transportation of the Injured," *Postgraduate Medicine*, (Sept. 1970), pp. 139–144.

Grant, Harvey. *Vehicle Rescue*, Bowie, Maryland: Robert J. Brady Co., 1975.

Hirschman, J. C., Nussenfeld, S. R., Nagel, E. L. "Mobile Physician Command," *JAMA*, Vol. 230, No. 2, Oct. 14, 1974.

Jalenko, III, Carl, M.D., Frey, Charles, M.D. *Emergency Medical Services, An Overview*, Bowie, Maryland: Robert J. Brady Co., 1976.

Jenkins, A. L. *Emergency Department Organization and Management*, St. Louis, Mo.: The C. V. Mosby Co., 1975.

Kimball, Kenneth F. "Communications," *EMT*, Vol. 1, No. 1, (March 1977), pp. 50–51.

"Medical Requirements for Ambulance Design and Equipment," *U.S. Department of Health Publication No. (HSM) 73-2035*. Washington, D.C.: U.S. Government Printing Office, 1973.

The Ohio State University. *Emergency Victim Care*, Columbus, Ohio: The Ohio State University, 1973.

Snook, R. "Transport of the Injured Patient," *British Journal of Anaesthesia*, (1977), 49, 651, pp. 651–658.

Stephenson, Hugh. *Immediate Care of the Acutely Ill and Injured*, St. Louis, Mo.: The C. V. Mosby Co., 1974.

Stewart, R. E. "The Training of Paramedical Personnel," *British Journal of Anaesthesia*, (1977). 49,659, pp. 659–671.

U.S. Department of Transportation. *Emergency Medical Technician*, 1973–1974.

Warren, James V., M.D. and others. *Saving Lives with Pre-Hospital Emergency Care*, Basking Ridge, New Jersey: ACT Foundation, 1977.

Wasserberger, Jonathan, Eubanks, David H. *Advanced Paramedic Procedures*, St. Louis, Mo.: The C. V. Mosby Co., 1977.

# Chapter 3

# BASIC BIOCHEMISTRY AND PHYSIOLOGY

Studies in college to prepare for entrance into medical school are centered around basic science. These studies include chemistry, physics, and mathematics. In medical school the basic science curriculum continues in the form of biochemistry and physiology. As a physician continues in his medical training and subsequent practice, he constantly is called upon to explain phenomena that are new to him. All disease and drug responses can be explained on the basis of biochemical and physiologic mechanisms. Therefore, knowledge and understanding in this area is never sufficient and is constantly changing. Basic facts, however, are available and should be known by all individuals involved in the care of patients. The paramedic in the field is not going to sit down, scratch his head, and attempt to determine why a patient's blood pressure is low while his tissues seem well-perfused. He will deal with the problems confronting him in a quick and efficient manner, and later attempt to think out explanations for what he has observed. It is the explanation of events that makes biochemistry and physiology so important. The purpose of this chapter is to touch on these subjects and furnish an adequate background to help explain phenomena that are seen daily by paramedic personnel.

## BIOCHEMISTRY

Biochemistry is the study of chemical reactions in biologic systems. All body functions from thinking to vigorous physical exercise can be traced back to chemical reactions in individual cells. Most of these chemical reactions take place in a salt water solution in the body (Chapter 5).

## THE CELL

The cell is the smallest unit of structure in the body. All organs and tissues are made up of these microscopic units. Cells range from five to fifty microns in diameter. About 1000 cells of average size would fit inside a letter of this word. Each cell is surrounded by an outer membrane, contains a nucleus which controls the function and reproduction of the cell, and is filled with a gelatinous fluid called cytoplasm. Most of the biochemical reactions in the body take place within the cytoplasm of individual cells. All cells share the general chemical reactions of keeping the cell alive, creating energy from nutrients to fuel the biochemical reactions, and repairing damage and aging in the cell itself. In addition, each cell has the capability to perform some specific chemical reaction which serves a purpose. For example, a muscle cell can contract, a nerve cell generates and conducts electricity, a liver cell makes bile, etc. Most of these chemical reactions are mediated by special proteins called enzymes. Enzymes are programmed to carry out a single step in a sequence of chemical events, somewhat analogous to robots in an automated assembly line. The rate at which raw materials are brought to these enzymes for processing and the power for doing the chemical reactions are controlled by other proteins called hormones which circulate in the blood.

In an automobile engine, the organic hydrocarbon compound gasoline is combined with oxygen in a process called oxidation (combustion or burning). Oxidation produces carbon dioxide ($CO_2$), water, heat, and energy. The energy may be used directly to turn the crank shaft, or indirectly to drive the fan that cools the radiator which dissipates the heat, or converted to electrical energy to power the radio and the headlights. Excess energy is stored in the battery to help start the car the next morning.

Oxidation is the basic reaction in biochemistry also. Molecules derived from food are "burned" by combination with oxygen which has been inhaled through the lungs. Water, carbon dioxide, and energy are produced by this reaction. Energy is stored as high energy phosphate (analogous to charging the battery) and also as fat. Raw materials which serve as nutrients or fuel for the metabolic machinery are known as carbohydrates and fats. Both are types of chemical molecules made up entirely of carbon and hydrogen atoms. A third category of nutrient chemicals—proteins—serve as the functional and structural materials of the body. Protein molecules contain carbon, hydrogen, and nitrogen. The entire process of breaking down foodstuffs into individual molecules and absorbing these molecules is called digestion. The process of oxidizing molecules, creating energy, and using this energy to run other enzyme systems is called metabolism. The combination of metabolic pathways that make protein and build tissue is called anabolism. The combination of metabolic pathways that break down protein (also fat and carbohydrate) is referred to as catabolism. Anabolism occurs when the food intake provides enough heat and energy (measured in calories) to run the entire metabolic process. Catabolism occurs when the energy intake is less than required and stored reserve energy from the body itself must be used.

During periods in which oxygen is not in sufficient supply for cell metabolism, the cell will continue to function. It does this through a specific metabolic pathway which converts glucose to lactic acid. This type of metabolism is called anaerobic (without oxygen) metabolism. Anaerobic metabolism occurs during shock, occlusion of blood vessels, different types of infections, and hypoxemia. Anaerobic metabolism produces lactic acid which collects within and outside the cell and eventually in the blood. This produces a change in the acid content of the blood that has a profound effect on the peripheral vasculature as well as the heart.

The $CO_2$, water, and bits of soot produced by gasoline oxidation are eliminated through the exhaust system. The $CO_2$ and water produced during metabolism are eliminated through the lung and kidney. Nitrogen-containing molecules resulting from protein breakdown are soluble in water, and are excreted in urine by the kidney.

## PHYSIOLOGY

Physiology is a term used to describe the interrelated functions of organ systems under normal conditions. Organs are body structures that serve at least one specific purpose. The heart, urinary bladder, uterus, and eye are individual organs that serve a single purpose; the liver, pancreas, and brain are individual organs that serve more than one purpose. There are ten organ systems, each including several individual organs which function in a coordinated fashion. These organ systems are the nervous, cardiovascular, respiratory, gastrointestinal, renal, reproductive, musculoskeletal, endocrine-metabolic, hematologic (blood), and host-defense system (including reticuloendothelial and immunologic functions). In this chapter we will deal primarily with the "life support" systems:

Cardiac
Vascular
Hematologic
Respiratory
Endocrine

## CARDIAC SYSTEM

The heart is a single muscular organ with four chambers; but it is best thought of as two separate organs—the "right" heart, consisting of a reservoir (right atrium) and pumping chamber (right ventricle); and the "left" heart, consisting of a reservoir (left atrium) and pumping chamber (left ventricle). The right heart receives venous blood from the body and pumps it into the lungs. The resistance to blood flow in the lung (pulmonary vascular resistance) is low, and the right ventricle does not have to develop much pressure (less than 30 mm Hg). The left heart receives blood from the lungs and pumps it throughout the body. The systemic vascular resistance is four to five times greater than pulmonary vascular resistance, and the left ventricle must generate higher pressures (100 mm Hg) to pump blood into the arteries.

Both the right and left hearts are very special pumps. Through a unique self-regulating system, the ventricle will pump all the blood that is collected in the atrium, regardless of the amount. If the reservoir fills rapidly with a large volume, a higher filling pressure develops in the atrium, filling the ventricle promptly. If the filling pressure is high, the ventricle accepts more blood and pumps harder and faster, pumping the total filling volume with each beat (stroke volume), thereby increasing the amount pumped each minute (cardiac output). This self-regulating system works extremely well with progressively increasing filling pressures, until a level of three to four times normal is reached. Beyond that point the ventricle will be overstretched and will be unable to empty completely with each beat. Blood and pressure backs up in the system and the pump becomes less efficient. This condition is referred to as cardiac failure. Around the turn of the century, an English physiologist named Starling described all of these phenomena that are so important in clinical medicine today. Starling's observations are summarized in Figure 3-1.

The pumping and filling cycles are caused by regular coordinated muscular contractions. The heart muscle requires nutrient energy sources and oxygen continuously. These are not drawn from the blood in the chambers, but rather from a conventional system of arteries, capillaries,

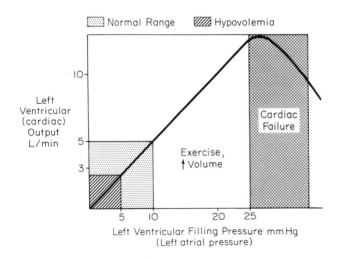

**Figure 3-1.** Left ventricle filling pressure (left atrial pressure) is compared to left ventricular (cardiac) output. In the normal heart, as left atrial pressure increases (by exercise or transfusion), so does left ventricular output until cardiac failure occurs.

and veins which serve the heart muscle (Chapter 4). As with any muscle contraction, electrical impulses are generated with each beat, and these can be recorded from the body surface (electrocardiogram). From the electrocardiogram, we can learn a lot about the heart rhythm (regularity of contractions), rate, and status of the heart muscle in the various chambers (Chapter 12).

The flow of blood through the heart is controlled by a series of four one-way valves. There is a valve between the atrium and the ventricle (tricuspid on the right, mitral on the left), and a valve at the outlet of each ventricle (pulmonic valve on the right, aortic valve on the left). These are one-way flap valves that open whenever the inlet pressure is higher than the outlet pressure, and close whenever the outlet pressure is higher than the inlet pressure. When the ventricles contract, the atrioventricular (AV) valves snap shut in response to the rising pressure in the ventricle. When the pressure in the ventricle is greater than that in the outflow arteries, the outflow valves open and the blood in the ventricle is pumped out through the aortic or pulmonic valve. After full contraction, the ventricle relaxes and the pressure in the ventricle falls. As soon as the intraventricular pressure falls below that in the outflow arteries, the outflow valves snap shut. The intraventricular pressure then continues to fall, and the cardiac muscle relaxes. Since the AV valves open when the ventricular pressure is lower than the atrial pressure, the ventricles fill with blood which has been collected in the reservoir atria during ventricular contraction. This series of events in the cardiac cycle is diagrammed in Figure 3-2. The relationships are shown for the left atrium, left ventricle, and aorta. The same events take place (at lower pressures) in the right heart. Normal valves make no sound when opening, but the closing snaps of the valves are audible through the chest as the familiar paired "lub-dub" of the heart beat. The first sound is caused by the closing of the atrioventricular valves, and the second sound is caused by the closing of the ventricular outflow valves.

## VASCULAR SYSTEM

The stroke volume of blood is pumped by the left ventricle into a branching system of elastic tubes called arteries. The pulse wave from each heartbeat is transmitted throughout the arterial system, and can be felt wherever an artery is close to the skin. Because the arteries are elastic and muscular, they stretch while the ventricle is contracting and rebound to their normal size when the aortic valve is closed, smoothing out the flow of blood. The smallest branches in the arterial tree are called arterioles. Arterioles have muscular walls that are under the control of both nerves and hormones. These muscular walls are normally moderately contracted, forming the resistors to blood flow which determine pressure in the

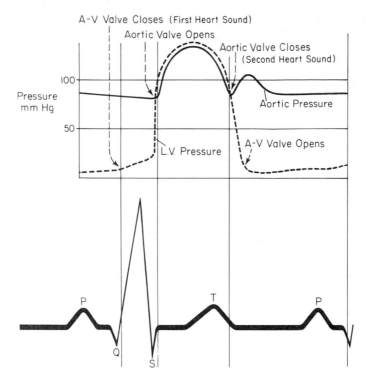

A-V Valve Closes (First Heart Sound)

Aortic Valve Opens

Aortic Valve Closes
(Second Heart Sound)

100

Pressure
mm Hg

Aortic Pressure

50

L.V. Pressure

A-V Valve Opens

P

T

P

Q

S

**Figure 3-2.** The electrocardiogram, left ventricular pressure contour, and aortic pressure are correlated in this diagram. It is noted that the electrocardiographic changes occur before changes in pressure.

arteries. When the left ventricle is pumping into the aorta, the arterial pressure is very slightly less than that in the ventricle itself (normally 120 mm Hg). As the ventricle relaxes, the aortic valve closes at the level of the normal pressure in the aorta (about 80 mm Hg). These relationships are shown in Figure 3-2.

The phase of ventricular contraction is called systole, and the highest pressure during systole is called systolic pressure. The ventricular relaxation phase is called diastole and the pressure at which the aortic valve closes is called diastolic pressure. Systolic and diastolic pressures can be measured directly by attaching a pressure measuring device directly to an artery, but it is easier to measure the blood pressure using a sphygmomanometer. This device is simply a pressure meter (manometer) attached to a pressurized tourniquet which goes around the arm. The tourniquet is inflated to a pressure higher than the expected arterial pressure and then the tourniquet is gradually released while the observer listens with a stethoscope over an artery downstream from the tourniquet. The pressure in the tourniquet at the first flow of blood is noted (systolic pressure), and the blood flowing through the artery makes an audible sound until the diastolic pressure is reached. The pressure is then recorded, listing systolic pressure over diastolic (e.g., 120 mm Hg systolic/80 mm Hg diastolic).

It is useful to know the average or mean pressure in the arterial system (mostly for use in calculations), and this can be measured by damping out the pulse contour or estimated by adding one-third of the pulse pressure (the difference between the systolic and diastolic pressures) to the diastolic pressure. For example, if the blood pressure is 120 systolic and 80 diastolic, the pulse pressure is 40 mm Hg. One-third of 40 is approximately 13; hence, the mean arterial pressure would be 80 plus 13, or 93 mm Hg.

The relationship among flow, pressure, and resistance is important to consider. Flow is the amount of blood flowing in an artery, and resistance is the amount of restriction to that blood flow. Flow and resistance combine to produce a pressure in the artery that can be recorded. If the blood pressure falls and flow remains the same, then the resistance is decreased (vasodilatation). Similarly, if the resistance increases while flow remains the same, then the pressure must increase (vasoconstriction). These important relationships are necessary in evaluating clinical problems, since often a normal blood pressure may be present when the arteriolar resistance is high and the blood flow is low.

The perfusion, or blood flow, to various organs is controlled by the resistance of the arterioles in those organs, which, in turn, is controlled by nerves and hormones. The section of the nervous system that controls arterial or muscle tone (and other vegetative involuntary functions of the body) is called the autonomic nervous system (Chapter 4). The sensitive sites on arterioles can be stimulated by nerve impulses or certain hormones circulating in the blood. These receptor sites can be grouped into those which respond to adrenalin, called sympathetic (adrenergic) and those which respond to acetylcholine, called parasympathetic (cholinergic). To make matters more confusing, the adrenergic receptors are subdivided into two types that have opposite responses. Alpha adrenergic receptors cause arterial or muscle constriction when exposed to adrenalin, and beta adrenergic receptors cause arterial or muscle relaxation. Constriction of arteries is known as vasoconstriction, and relaxation is known as vasodilatation. Finally, since this system was developed, the name of adrenalin has been changed to epinephrine. It is important for emergency medical personnel to learn this terminology because many important drugs are classified by their ability to stimulate or block autonomic receptors (Chapter 6).

Control of perfusion to specific organs is usually caused by vasoconstriction and an increase in vascular resistance in other organs, thereby shunting blood to the desired organ. For example, in response to pain, stress, or blood loss, there is a generalized stimulation of alpha adrenergic receptors (a "sympathetic" response) which causes vasoconstriction and decreased blood flow in skin and muscles. This has the effect of increasing perfusion to the kidneys, heart, and brain.

From the arterioles blood passes into the capillaries. These are short narrow blood vessels with walls that are only one cell thick. Nutrients and oxygen pass freely from the blood through the capillary wall into the interstitial fluid (Chapter 5) and from there directly to the cells. Water, electrolytes, and other crystallized molecules pass through capillary walls almost as if they were not there; but larger molecules, particularly the many proteins found in blood plasma, cannot pass through the capillaries under normal conditions. Since there is much more protein in the plasma (6 g/100 ml) than in the interstitial fluid (1 g/100 ml), an osmotic pressure gradient is set up with the capilla.ies acting as semipermeable membranes and extracellular fluid being "pulled into" the vascular space with a force equivalent to approximately 25 mm Hg. This force, caused by plasma proteins and the ions attached electrically to those proteins, is called the colloid osmotic pressure (Chapter 5). The blood pressure in the arteries is stepped down at the arteriolar level, leaving pressure of approximately 30 mm Hg inside the capillaries. The balance between this hydrostatic pressure that "pushes fluid out" of the capillaries and the colloid osmotic pressure that "pulls fluid into" the capillaries results in the slow continuous filtration of extracellular fluid from the plasma into the interstitial space. This fluid is collected and returned to the blood through a system of thin-walled valved conduits called lymphatics. The amount of extracellular fluid recycled in this fashion is very small (approximately 1 liter per day) compared to the total amount that flows through the capillaries (approximately 7000 liters per day). If the balance of forces controlling capillary filtration changes and excess fluid is filtered through the capillaries, the lymphatic flow can increase by a factor of three. Beyond this point, lymphatic clearance is incomplete, fluid collects in the interstitial space, and swelling of the involved part or organ will occur. This swelling of the involved part or organ secondary to an increase in tissue fluid is called edema. Edema occurs whenever lymphatic outflow is blocked, when hydrostatic pressure increases (caused by blockage of venous outflow), when colloid osmotic pressure is low (low serum proteins), or when extracellular fluid or total body water is grossly increased.

Veins are blood vessels that conduct blood from the capillaries back to the heart. The driving pressure in the venous system is low, dropping from 30 mm Hg at the capillaries to 10 mm Hg in the right atrium. Veins in the extremities have a series of one-way valves that prevent the backflow of blood. Veins have much less muscle than arteries, and show less response to autonomic stimuli.

## HEMATOLOGIC (BLOOD) SYSTEM

The blood volume is approximately 7 percent of the total body weight (Chapter 5). Almost half of the blood is composed of individually circulating cells. The other half, plasma, is an isotonic solution in which sodium and chloride are the major electrolytes. Blood plasma is part of the extracellular fluid, and is the transport medium of the body. The basic building blocks of tissue (amino acids) and energy sources (carbohydrates and fatty acids) are transported to the cells in the plasma. Metabolic breakdown products are transported to the excretory organs. Special molecules (usually proteins) manufactured in specialized cells are carried in the blood plasma. Some of these special proteins are a series of enzymes that cause the blood to clot once stimulated by contact with a foreign surface such as air. When the blood clots, these specific proteins disappear from the plasma and the resulting liquid is called serum.

Blood is a suspension of red cells, white cells, and platelets in plasma. Red blood cells (erythrocytes) constitute about 45 percent of the blood. The percentage of red cells is called the hematocrit (Figure 3-3). Red blood cells are made in the bone marrow, circulate for 120 days, and are then destroyed in the spleen and liver (Figure 3-4). Oxygen transport is the major function of red blood cells. They are filled with an iron-containing molecule called hemoglobin which has the unique capability to bind and release oxygen molecules. When the amount of red cells or hemoglobin is below normal, the situation is called anemia, even though that term literally means no blood.

The hematocrit and hemoglobin concentrations in whole blood are determined by a laboratory test. It must be remembered that both of

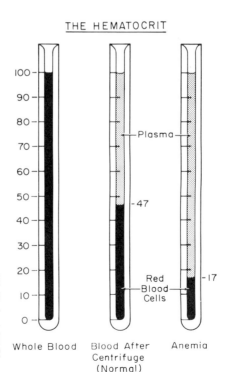

THE HEMATOCRIT

**Figure 3-3.** The hematocrit is measured by taking whole blood and spinning it in a centrifuge. It is a qualitative measurement and determines what percentage of the blood is composed of red blood cells. In anemia, the hematocrit is low.

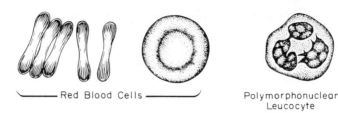

———— Red Blood Cells ————  Polymorphonuclear
Leucocyte

**Figure 3-4.** Red blood cells and polymorphonuclear leukocytes are major components of whole blood. Red and white blood cells can only be seen through the
microscope.

these determinations report concentration (qualitative), and not volume
(quantitative). Simply stated, they measure the concentration of red cells
(hematocrit or hemoglobin) in a sample of blood drawn from the patient.
Blood volume is measured in an entirely different fashion and is not
done as a routine laboratory procedure.

The hematocrit measures the concentration of red blood cells in
whole blood. When the hematocrit falls below normal, it indicates that
the patient has a reduced concentration of red blood cells in a sample
of blood drawn from him. This does not necessarily mean that the patient
is hypovolemic. The patient may have been overtransfused with plasma
or some other solution which has diluted the red blood cells in his
body, but the total quantity of red blood cells has not changed. The
hematocrit rises when plasma is lost, as occurs in burns.

Hemoglobin determination is made by measuring the concentration
of hemoglobin within a sample of red blood cells drawn from a patient.
It has limited usefulness in acute medicine because hemoglobin concentrations do not offer any more information than the hematocrit. It
is simpler to remember hematocrit values and their changes. For example,
a fall in hematocrit from 40 to 30 percent over six hours usually indicates
the patient is bleeding. Hemoglobin is used to assess chronic anemias
such as iron deficiency anemia. Elevation in the hematocrit can occur
due to chronic diseases such as pulmonary emphysema or certain kidney
disorders.

White blood cells make up about 1 percent of the circulating blood.
There are several species of white blood cells, which are categorized
into two types. Polymorphonuclear leukocytes (PMNs), which are made
in the bone marrow, live for 24 to 48 hours and are then destroyed
in the reticuloendothelial system (spleen and lymph nodes) (Figure 3-4).
PMNs are active in acute inflammation, engulfing (by phagocytosis)
and killing bacteria and removing debris; finding an abnormally large
number of PMNs in circulating blood is usually a sign of acute infection.
The other family of white blood cells is called lymphocytes. These cells
are made in lymph nodes and circulate for weeks. They are the mediators
of the immunologic system.

Blood platelets are small particles formed by the breaking of larger cells in the bone marrow. These small particles contain a variety of chemicals that are active in inflammation and blood clotting. Platelets are the hardening agents for blood clots. When platelets are missing, blood can clot, but the clots are flimsy and bleeding is difficult to stop. In fact, if the platelets are very low, spontaneous bleeding occurs in pinpoint areas (petechiae).

Blood serves as a passive transport medium. Arterial blood is delivered to all areas of the body and molecules are removed or added in the capillary beds, going from an area of greater to lesser concentration. Other materials are active only where there are specific receptor sites. Antidiuretic hormone (ADH), for example, circulates throughout the body but exerts its effect only in the kidney.

One of the many plasma proteins is a substance called fibrinogen. When stimulated, this protein converts to a stringy, sticky substance called fibrin which is the glue of blood clots. Fibrinogen becomes activated as a result of a chain reaction of enzymes in the blood plasma. Each one stimulates the next until fibrin is formed. The entire sequence is stimulated by exposure of blood plasma to a surface that is different than the normal lining of blood vessels, for example, air, fat, bacteria, skin, collagen, etc. These same stimuli act on platelets, causing them to stick to each other and to the foreign surface. The platelet aggregates, along with red and white blood cells, become enmeshed as the fibrin forms, forming a blood clot. This process takes about five minutes and is called thrombosis. Thrombus is another term for a blood clot. Among the plasma proteins trapped in the fibrin meshwork in a thrombus is an enzyme called plasminogen or fibrinolysin. As the clot forms, this enzyme is activated and begins to destroy the fibrin. Thus each clot contains the mechanism for its own destruction. This process takes hours in a test tube and days in the body. Normally a clot at the end of a disrupted blood vessel "organizes" (is replaced by a small amount of scar tissue) before the fibrin disappears, so that bleeding does not start again when the clot dissolves (lysis).

# RESPIRATORY SYSTEM

## FUNCTION

The lungs have one major function—to add oxygen and remove $CO_2$ from the blood. Air is inhaled and passed through a series of conducting airways (trachea and bronchi) into small air spaces called alveoli. The alveolar walls are only one cell thick and are in contact with the lung capillaries, so that only two cells and a small amount of interstitial fluid separate the air and the circulating blood (Figure 9-1).

## BLOOD GASES

The air we breathe contains oxygen, nitrogen, water vapor, and small quantities of other gases. It has become common to describe these gases in terms of pressure. The term *partial pressure* is a convenient way to describe the amount of gas in a mixture, since it can apply to single gases or combinations in solution or in the gaseous state. The reference point for partial pressure measurements is normal barometric pressure at sea level, which can be expressed as one atmosphere, 14.7 lb/sq in, or 760 mm Hg. The total pressure of a mixture of gases at sea level must be 760 mm Hg. Each gas in the mixture contributes a portion of the total pressure in proportion to its concentration. For example, air is 20 percent oxygen. The $PO_2$ of air is $760 \times 20\% = 152$ mm Hg. Carbon dioxide in expired gas is three percent. $PCO_2$ is $760 \times 3\% = 22.8$ mm Hg. The amount of nitrogen in expired air is 75 percent, so that partial pressure is $0.75 \times 760 = 560$ mm Hg. When a liquid (such as blood plasma) is exposed to a mixture of gases, gas molecules will move in or out of the liquid, going from an area of higher to lower partial pressure (also depending upon the solubility characteristics of that specific gas and liquid). When blood is exposed to air through the alveoli, $O_2$ moves into blood because the $PO_2$ in the alveoli (150 mm Hg) is higher than the $PO_2$ in venous blood (40 mm Hg). Carbon dioxide moves from the blood to the air because the $PCO_2$ in venous blood (45 mm Hg) is higher than the $PCO_2$ in air (0).

Oxygen is then transferred from the alveoli to the blood. Arterial blood contains 20 ml of oxygen per 100 ml of blood. One percent of this is dissolved in the plasma and the other 99 percent is bound to hemoglobin in the red blood cells. The distribution and amount of oxygen in blood is described in three ways. The actual amount of oxygen is called the oxygen content, expressed in ml per 100 ml of blood (also called volumes percent). The level of oxygen dissolved in plasma is expressed in partial pressure ($PaO_2$, "a" stands for arterial). Third, the amount of hemoglobin that has oxygen bound to it is expressed as a percentage. For example, venous blood is normally 75 percent saturated, i.e., 75 percent of the hemoglobin has $O_2$ molecules attached. Arterial blood is normally 99 to 100 percent saturated. Hemoglobin saturation is easy to measure since the color changes from blue to red with increasing levels of saturation. Oxygen content is important to know, but difficult to measure. The oxygen content can be calculated quite accurately, since 1 g of hemoglobin binds 1.39 ml of oxygen. Therefore, if one knows the amount of hemoglobin in the blood and the percentage of hemoglobin saturated with oxygen, the oxygen content can be calculated. For example, if a sample of venous blood contains

10 g of hemoglobin per 100 ml, and the hemoglobin is 80 percent saturated, then the oxygen content is $10 \times 0.8 \times 1.39 = 11.12$ ml oxygen per 100 ml of blood. This simplified calculation ignores the small amount of oxygen dissolved in plasma but is accurate enough for clinical usage. The normal arteriovenous difference for oxygen and carbon dioxide is about five volumes percent. That is, 5 ml of oxygen are transferred to the blood and 5 ml of carbon dioxide are removed from the blood, for each 100 ml of flow through the lungs. The opposite exchange takes place in the peripheral tissues.

Most of the carbon dioxide in blood is in the form of bicarbonate ion dissolved in the plasma. One-twentieth of the total amount is present as dissolved carbon dioxide. This dissolved fraction combines with water in the blood to make carbonic acid ($H_2CO_3$). The fractions and amounts of carbon dioxide in the blood are measured and described in four ways: (1) the total amount of carbon dioxide per 100 ml of blood (the carbon dioxide content) expressed in ml per 100 ml or volume percent (this is rarely used); (2) moles per liter, a mole of gas contains one molecular weight and fills 22.4 liters; this can also be expressed as volumes percent using moles or millimoles per liter (this is rarely used); and (3) milliequivalents/liter, by combining with water to form carbonic acid and bicarbonate, $CO_2$ converts into charged ions and can be measured by the equivalent weight system mentioned in Chapter 5. This is the method usually used to describe the total amount of carbon dioxide in the blood. The normal value is 27 mEq/l. Almost all of this is present as bicarbonate (25.5 meq/l), so that this value is often referred to interchangeably as "the $CO_2$" or "the bicarbonate" plasma measurement; and (4) the small dissolved portion of carbon dioxide can be measured as partial pressure ($PCO_2$). The normal value is 40 mm Hg in arterial blood. Since the dissolved carbon dioxide changes immediately with changes in breathing, the measurement of this small fraction is very important when measuring respiratory function.

## BUFFER SYSTEMS

The chemical balance between bicarbonate and carbonic acid ($H_2CO_3$) is one of the major buffer systems of the body. Buffer systems are salt solutions that prevent rapid or extensive shifts in the amount of acid or base by "soaking up" hydrogen ions (acid molecules) or hydroxyl ions (base molecules). For example, when hydrogen ions are added to a bicarbonate solution, they combine with bicarbonate ions to form $H_2CO_3$. This in turn converts to carbon dioxide. Therefore, even though hydrogen ions are added, the acidity of the solution does not change. The buffer systems of the body keep the hydrogen ion concentration within a close range of millimoles or milliequivalents per liter. That number of acidic ions is balanced by basic ions, keeping the body environment at a neutral position between acid and base extremes. The acidity or alkalinity of a solution could be measured and expressed as the number of free or unopposed hydrogen ions or hydroxyl ions in the solution, but the numbers would range from one to several million. An alternative measuring system has been devised (based on the negative logarithm of hydrogen ion concentration), called the pH system. The pH scale ranges from 1 (strongly acid) to 14 (strongly basic) with 7 at the neutral position. On this scale, the pH of blood is normally 7.4. Under abnormal conditions, the pH may range from 6.8 to 7.7, but these extremes are poorly tolerated and usually indicate conditions that are incompatible with life.

When the ratio of carbonic acid to bicarbonate is 1 to 20 in that buffer system, the pH is 7.40. If the ratio changes slightly, the pH changes proportionately and predictably. Therefore, if any two of the three variables (carbonic acid, bicarbonate, and pH) are known, the third can be calculated. We take advantage of this fact, since it is easy to measure pH and $PCO_2$ (as a measure of carbonic acid), but considerably more difficult to measure bicarbonate or total $CO_2$. Machines designed to measure $PO_2$ and $PCO_2$ include a device to measure pH. "Blood gas" measurements from these machines (widely used in emergency and critical care units) include measurement of $PO_2$, $PCO_2$, and pH. The normal $PaO_2$ is 90–100 mm Hg. $PaO_2$ less than 80 mm Hg is referred to as *hypoxemia*. Normal $PaCO_2$ is 40 mm Hg. $PCO_2$ less than 38 mm Hg is called *hypocarbia*, and $PCO_2$ more than 46 mm Hg is *hypercarbia*. Blood pH less than 7.40 is *acidemia* and indicates a general condition of acidosis throughout the body. A pH of more than 7.40 is *alkalemia* and indicates a general body condition of alkalosis. If the bicarbonate/carbonic acid ratio is changed by adding or subtracting carbon dioxide through variations in breathing, the corresponding pH change is referred to as respiratory acidosis (excess carbon dioxide and carbonic acid) or alkalosis. This ratio (diminished carbon dioxide and carbonic acid) can be changed by the addition or subtraction of hydrogen ions (and a corresponding change in bicarbonate). The addition of $H^+$ ion occurs during anaerobic (without oxygen) metabolism and is called metabolic acidosis. Hydrogen ions can be lost from the stomach during vomiting producing a metabolic alkalosis.

It is obvious that a blood gas determination cannot be made in the field. However, as will be described in Chapter 9, the diagnosis of certain blood gas abnormalities can be determined by astute clinical evaluation. The important aspect of blood gas determination for the paramedic is correlation of his clinical findings in the field with the objective findings in the Emergency Department. For example, the patient who appears to be well oxygenated by clinical examination during transport to the hospital may instead be found to have a very low $PO_2$ in the Emergency Department. This indicates that the respiratory system was not properly managed. This information will help the paramedic in evaluating his ventilation techniques. If the patient who sustained a cardiac arrest in the field arrives at the hospital with a $PCO_2$ of 80 mm Hg and a pH of 7.01, the paramedic will know the patient was not ventilated properly and the sodium bicarbonate given did not buffer the hydrogen ion ($H^+$). Conversely, if the patient arrives in the Emergency Department with a normal pH and $PCO_2$, the paramedic will know that his resuscitation in the field was done correctly. Therefore, knowledge of blood gas physiology is important to the paramedic in correlating his treatment in the field with the objective data of blood gas determination at the hospital.

## PULMONARY MECHANICS

The inspiratory force created by contraction of the diaphragm is normally about 20 cm of water, and can be as high as 100 cm of water with a forced inspiration. Air enters the lung in response to this pressure. Breathing out is usually a passive process. The lungs and chest wall recoil to their normal position. At the end of a resting expiration, there is still a large amount of gas in the lungs, referred to as the *functional residual capacity (FRC)*. With a vigorous forced expiration, another liter or two of gas can be squeezed out, but a significant quantity of gas still remains in the lungs (the *residual volume, RV*) (Figure 3-5). These phases of the breathing cycle are referred to as *lung volumes*, and are measured with a spirometer. The interrelations between airway pressure, air flow, and lung volume are called *pulmonary mechanics.*

In an adult, during normal breathing, the functional residual capacity is approximately three liters. A normal size breath is approximately 500 ml, making the volume of gas inside the chest 3500 ml during inspiration and 3000 ml during expiration. This 500 ml is referred to as the *tidal*

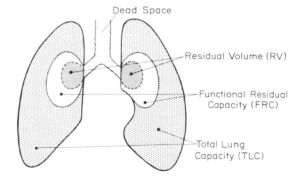

**Figure 3-5.** Lung volumes are divided into residual volume, functional residual capacity, and total lung capacity. The dead space is that space in the pulmonary system that does not actively engage in gas exchange.

Dead Space

Residual Volume (RV)

Functional Residual Capacity (FRC)

Total Lung Capacity (TLC)

TLC - RV = Vital Capacity

volume (TV). With a forced inspiration, a normal man can breathe in three liters, making a total volume in the chest of six liters. This is called the *total lung capacity (TLC)*. Beginning at total lung capacity, the normal individual can forceably exhale about five liters down to the residual volume. This forced exhaled volume is called the *vital capacity*.

The *minute ventilation* is the total amount of air breathed in and out in one minute (the tidal volume × the breaths per minute). Normal minute ventilation is eight to ten liters per minute. The volume of the conduit airways is called the dead space. At the end of expiration this space is filled with gas that had been in the alveoli and hence has a high $PCO_2$ and a low $PO_2$. The inspired air mixes with this gas and displaces it from the airway, but the last 150 ml inhaled occupies the dead space and does not participate in gas exchange. About one-third of the minute ventilation is dead space ventilation. The other two-thirds is fresh air that gets to the alveoli, and is called *minute alveolar ventilation*. The alveolar ventilation must be adequate to support gas exchange. For example, if an adult breathes a tidal volume of 100 ml, 80/min, the minute ventilation would be normal (8 l/min); but all the ventilation would be dead space ventilation, and hypoxia and hypercarbia would result.

Carbon dioxide exchange in the normal lung is directly proportionate to alveolar ventilation. In fact, if the $PCO_2$ is normal (40 mm Hg), the alveolar ventilation must be normal for the patient. If a subject breathes very deeply (hyperpnea), or very rapidly (tachypnea), or both (hyperventilation), carbon dioxide excretion will increase proportionately, and blood $PCO_2$ will decrease, resulting in hypocapnia and respiratory alkalosis. Inadequate alveolar ventilation (hypoventilation) will result in hypercapnia and respiratory acidosis. Hypoventilation will cause hypoxia, since the alveolar $PO_2$ ($PaO_2$) falls without adequate fresh air; but hyperventilation does not cause much of an increase in $PaO_2$ compared to normal, since the $PO_2$ in alveolar gas can never be more than that in air. Of course, if supplemental oxygen is added to the inspired air, the $PO_2$ will rise proportionately in the normal lung. The amount of oxygen in inspired air can be described as the $PO_2$ of inspired air, or the fraction of inspired air which is oxygen ($FIO_2$, pronounced F . . . eye . . . OH . . . two). The latter is the usual method of expression; air has an $FIO_2$ of 0.21; pure oxygen would be 1.0.

When the $FIO_2$ is 1.0, the $PaO_2$ is 550–600 mm Hg. All of the hemoglobin is fully saturated about a $PaO_2$ of 150 mm Hg, so that the large increase in oxygen tension from 150–600 represents a very small amount of oxygen gas dissolved in plasma. We take advantage of this fact in lung function testing by having the patient breathe 100 percent oxygen. Even a small impairment of lung function and inadequate oxygenation can be detected during 100 percent oxygen breathing.

The functions of the body are regulated by two systems, the nervous and the endocrine system. In general, the endocrine system is concerned with metabolic functions such as controlling the rate of chemical reactions. Endocrine glands act by secreting specific proteins called hormones into the blood. The endocrine system includes the pituitary gland (master gland), which resides at the base of the brain. The pituitary gland has an anterior and posterior portion. The anterior portion sends out messenger hormones (trophic hormones) to various other endocrine glands. The posterior portion of the pituitary gland secretes an antidiuretic hormone (ADH) which, in times of shock, will force the kidney to conserve water. The major endocrine glands which respond to stress are the pituitary adrenal glands and the pancreas.

The adrenal glands, which reside above the kidneys, are divided into two portions: the cortex and the medulla. The cortex secretes adrenocortical (cortisol, aldosterone) hormones in response to stimuli from the pituitary gland. Cortisol (hydrocortisone) helps conserve sodium in the kidney, thereby helping maintain extracellular fluid volume in shock, and aids in the breakdown of protein and its conversion to sugar for metabolism during acute illness. It also has multiple other functions. Aldosterone is a salt-retaining hormone that is released from the adrenal gland as a result of stimulus from a hormone called renin, which comes from the kidney. Aldosterone has salt-retaining properties which also aid in the maintenance of extracellular fluid volume.

The medulla of the adrenal gland contains that portion which secretes epinephrine and norepinephrine. These two sympathetic hormones aid in the stress response to shock. Epinephrine produces constriction of certain arterioles and allows for redistribution of blood to critical areas, such as the brain and the heart. It stimulates the heart to increase its output and beat more forcibly. Epinephrine causes inhibition of the gastrointestinal tract and pupil dilatation. Norepinephrine stimulates the heart to beat more strongly and peripheral vasoconstriction.

In times of stress the pancreas secretes insulin. Although this hormone plays a minor role in the initial stress response when compared to the adrenal gland, its function is no less important. Although insulin initially is inhibited by the steroid hormones and epinephrine, it is necessary for the transportation of glucose into the cell for energy metabolism. Other endocrine glands are the thyroid, parathyroids, and ovaries or testicles.

*Summary*

This chapter presented some of the rudimentary details of the biochemistry and physiology of the important body systems. As one makes observations on a patient's disease processes, the changes should be explicable either on a biochemical or a physiologic basis. Disciplining oneself to do this makes care of patients more exciting and allows for a broader and more intelligent interpretation of variations in the presentation of disease processes.

*Important
Points to
Remember*

The cell is the smallest unit of structure in the body; all organs and tissues are composed of these microscopic units.

Each cell performs specific functions, most of which are mediated by enzymes.

The oxidation of food in the body produces water, carbon dioxide, and energy. The nutrients for the metabolic machinery of the body are known as proteins, carbohydrates, and fats.

The breaking down of foodstuffs is known as digestion. Metabolism refers to the oxidation of foodstuff molecules, the creation of energy, the control of enzyme systems, and the building up and breaking down of tissue.

The life support systems include the cardiac, vascular, respiratory, hematologic, and endocrine systems. The cardiac system consists of a single muscular organ with four chambers, which are separated by four one-way valves. The chambers are the right and left atria and ventricles. The valves are the tricuspid (right atrio-vent), mitral (left atrio-vent), pulmonary, and aortic.

The vascular system is comprised of arteries, veins, capillaries, and lymphatics. The flow of blood is from artery to arteriole to capillary to lymphatics (tissues) to venule to vein. The blood volume is approximately 7 percent of total body weight. Half of this is plasma and the other half is comprised of red and white blood cells and platelets.

The major function of the lungs is to add oxygen and remove carbon dioxide from the blood.

The smallest air spaces are called alveoli, which act as an exchange area for gases passing from the lung to the blood and vice versa.

The principal arterial blood gases we are concerned about are oxygen ($PO_2$) and carbon dioxide ($PCO_2$).

The endocrine system is generally concerned with metabolic functions such as the rate of chemical reactions.

*Bibliography*  Berne, R. M. and Levy, M. N. *Cardiovascular Physiology.* St. Louis, Mo.: The C. V. Mosby Co., 1972.

Comroe, J. H. *Physiology of Respiration.* Year Book Medical Publishers, Inc., 1968.

Davenport, H. W. *The ABC of Acid-Base Chemistry,* 2nd ed. Chicago, Illinois: The University of Chicago Press, 1974.

Guyton, A. C. *Basic Human Physiology.* Philadelphia, Pa.: W. B. Saunders Co., 1971.

# Chapter 4

# APPLIED ANATOMY

Anatomy is the term applied to the study of the human body using the method of dissection. Improved scientific techniques such as the electron microscope have made anatomy a very sophisticated discipline. Currently, there are no boundaries for the anatomist since he can travel inside the cell and casually inspect minute intracellular structures. For the purposes of this book, anatomy will be restricted to the portions of the human body that can be seen with the naked eye. Reference may be made to microscopic structures, but only to aid in understanding disease processes. Human anatomy is a vast subject and can only be touched on lightly here. The emphasis will be placed on applied anatomy, or that anatomy which is useful for problems in the field.

## ANATOMIC TERMINOLOGY

The classic anatomic position is erect with the eyes forward and the palms of the hands to the front (Figure 4-1). Although this is not a natural position of the hands, it aids in describing structures in the standard anatomic position. In describing anatomic structures, it is important to be familiar with certain terms:

Anterior (Ventral)—Toward the front of the body

Posterior (Dorsal)—Toward the back of the body

Superior—Above, upper

Inferior—Below, lower

Cranial—Toward the head

Caudad—Toward the tail

Superficial—On or near the surface

Deep—Remote from the surface

Internal—Within, inside

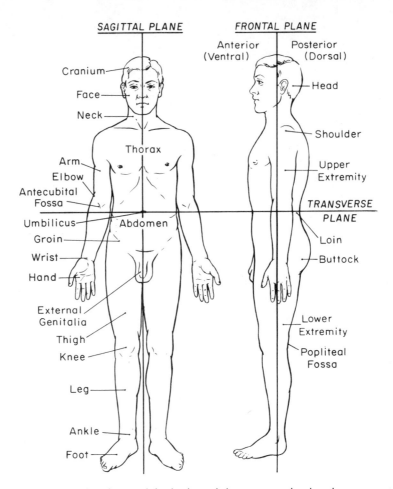

**Figure 4-1.** The planes of the body and the common landmarks.

External—Without, outside

Proximal—Nearest to the body or to some other point regarded as the center of the system, nearest to the point of attachment

Distal—Farthest from the body or from some other central point, farthest from the point of attachment

Medial—Toward the medial plane of the body

Lateral—Away from the medial plane of the body

Infra—Below

Supra—Above

Peri—Around

Para—Next to

Meta—Beyond, farther

The *median plane* is defined as a vertical plane through the body reaching the surface at the midline in the front and back. This is also known as the *midsagittal plane* of the body, and, with the exception of the unpaired viscera in the trunk cavity, divides the body into symmetrical halves (Figure 4-1). Fundamental terms for the front and back of the body are, respectively, *ventral* and *dorsal*. Since man stands erect, ventral is equivalent to the anterior side, and dorsal is the same as posterior. Therefore, the abdominal cavity is anterior, and the back is posterior. *Cranial* and *caudal*, referring to the head and tail regions of the trunk, are also useful terms. It is frequently necessary to stipulate that an object is medial, and thus near or nearer to the median plane of the body; or conversely, lateral, which is further away from the median plane of the body. For example, the heart is medial to the lung, which is thus lateral to the heart. *Proximal* and *distal* describe positions near the root of the limb or blood vessel and further along its length. The proximal humerus is the portion of the humerus near the shoulder, while the distal humerus is that portion near the elbow. *Superficial* and *deep* are terms frequently used to describe a dissection and have their usual meaning, designating positions nearer or further from the surface. An example of this is the location of the veins, which can be superficial (those which can be seen in the forearm and leg), and deep (those which cannot be seen with the naked eye).

In this chapter, pertinent anatomical structures are outlined, and in some cases their relevance to clinical conditions is stressed. The body is divided into various systems which include the following: (1) head and neck, (2) nervous, (3) thoracic, (4) abdominal, (5) musculoskeletal, (6) genitourinary, and (7) vascular. The female gynecologic anatomy will be detailed separately in the chapter dealing with childbirth. While there are many ways to organize the anatomic systems of the body, this appears to be the most practical.

## HEAD AND NECK

### TOPOGRAPHIC ANATOMY

The head is called the cranium and the portions of the skull are named according to the bones that form the skull (Figure 4-2). The top of the head is the vertex. The anterior portion of the head from the eyebrows to the vertex is called the frontal area. The two sides of the skull are composed of the parietal bones and are called the parietal areas. The back of the head is the occipital area, named after the occiput. The temporal regions are those two areas in front of and superior to the

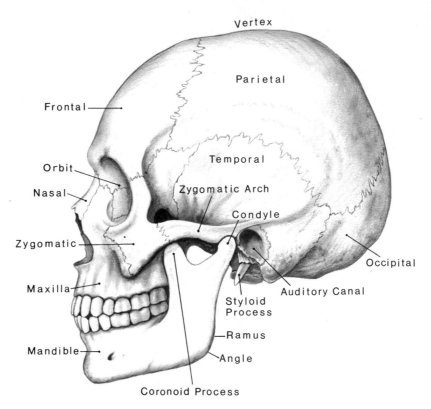

**Figure 4-2.** Lateral view of the skull with the important landmarks. The jagged lines on the skull are the fused connections of the various bones.

ear. There are two bony prominences behind the ear, called the mastoid bones.

There are five orifices (holes) within the facial surface. The two most superior are the orbits containing the eyes. Objects in this region are described in relationship to the orbit: supraorbital (above the orbit), infraorbital (below the orbit), and periorbital (around the orbit). The nose is in the central portion of the face and has two nares which communicate directly posteriorly with the nasopharynx. The mouth makes up the fifth orifice of the face. Beneath the orbit is a bony prominence, the zygomatic bone, commonly called the cheek. This is connected to the zygomatic portion of the temporal bone by the zygomatic arch (Figure 4-2). By palpation of this region, one can appreciate this bridge-like bone between the zygomatic bone prominence and the temporal bone. The jaw bone is called the mandible and contains those teeth which close against the upper teeth, which are imbedded in the maxilla.

The sternocleidomastoid and trapezius muscles are the principal soft tissue landmarks of the neck. The sternocleidomastoids divide the neck into anterior and posterior regions (Figure 4-3). These muscles

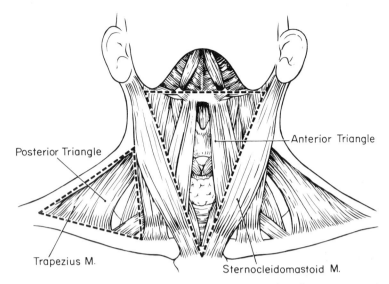

Posterior Triangle

Anterior Triangle

Trapezius M.

Sternocleidomastoid M.

**Figure 4-3.** The neck region has been divided into two triangles: the anterior and posterior triangles.

can be palpated by rotating the head in one direction and the opposite sternocleidomastoid muscle tenses and can be felt between the fingers. The anterior region of the neck is that area anterior to the sternocleidomastoid on both sides and inferior to the mandible (Figure 4-3). The area bounded anteriorly by the sternocleidomastoid muscle, posteriorly by the trapezius, and inferiorly by the clavicle is the posterior triangle of the neck.

In the anterior region of the neck are the hyoid and thyroid cartilages. The thyroid cartilage is the prominent bump one notices upon swallowing and has been termed the "Adam's apple." Below the thyroid cartilage is the cricothyroid membrane and then the cricothyroid cartilage (Figure 4-4). Below this is the trachea, leading inferiorly to the suprasternal notch. By lateral palpation at the top of the thyroid cartilage, the carotid pulse can be appreciated. At the upper border of the thyroid cartilage the carotid artery divides into the external and internal carotid arteries (Figures 4-5, 4-6). All of these landmarks should be palpated and learned. The anterior triangle thus contains the following:

1. Larynx
2. Cricothyroid Membrane
3. Trachea
4. Carotid Artery
5. Internal Jugular Vein

The following structures are located in the posterior triangle:

1. External Jugular Vein

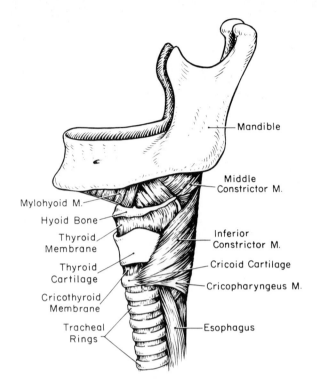

Figure 4-4. The mandible; esophageal constrictor muscles; hyoid bone; and an external view of the larynx, esophagus, and trachea are depicted. Notice that the esophagus is posterior to the trachea.

2. Phrenic Nerve
3. Subclavian Vein arching over the first rib
4. Subclavian Artery
5. Brachial Plexus emerging between the scalene muscles of the neck

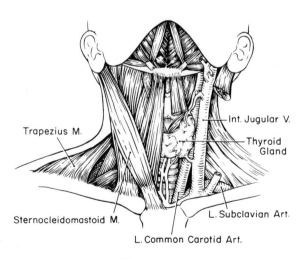

Figure 4-5. The internal jugular vein lies lateral and superficial to the internal carotid artery in the neck.

The scalp or outer covering of the cranium is composed of five layers: the skin, subcutaneous tissue (fatty layer), aponeurosis (fibrous sheet from muscle) or muscle, loose connective tissue, and periosteum. The main blood vessels of the scalp are present within the subcutaneous layer. The scalp's blood supply comes from branches of the external carotid arteries (Figures 4-6, 4-7).

## THE MAXILLOFACIAL COMPLEX

The maxillofacial complex extends anteriorly from the eyebrows to just below the chin, and posteriorly to the base of the skull (floor of the cranium). It contains the eyes and eyelids, the nose and sinuses, the mouth and jaw, the pharynx and nasopharynx, the salivary glands, and the ears.

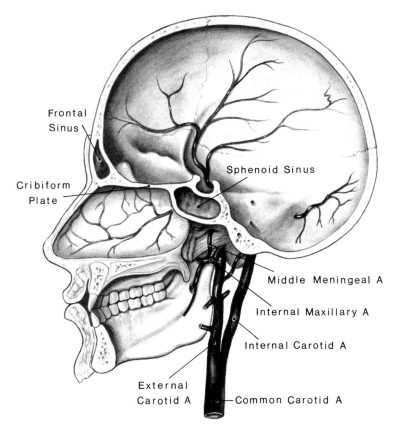

Frontal Sinus

Sphenoid Sinus

Cribiform Plate

Middle Meningeal A

Internal Maxillary A

Internal Carotid A

External Carotid A

Common Carotid A

**Figure 4-6.** A sagittal view of the skull depicting the middle meningeal artery as it arises from the internal maxillary artery and travels inside the skull. The internal maxillary artery is a branch of the external carotid artery.

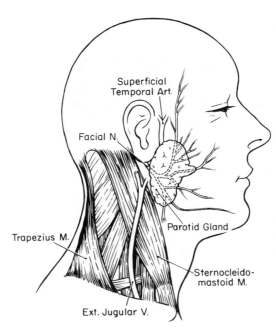

**Figure 4-7.** The facial nerve, which passes in front of the ear and travels through the parotid (salivary) gland. Injuries to the front of the ear can damage the facial nerve, producing facial paralysis.

## THE FACE

The face is a highly vascular area receiving its main blood supply from the branches of the external carotid artery. The three important arteries of the face are the facial, labial, and temporal arteries. When one of these arteries is lacerated, finger pressure may be important. The superficial temporal artery is located just in front of the ear and extends to the forehead (Figure 4-7). The labial artery surrounds the circumference of the mouth. The facial artery crosses the lower border of the mandible (jaw) in its posterior portion. Digital (finger) pressure then may be necessary, in appropriate cases, in front of the ear or against the lower border of the mandible. In lip lacerations, pressure is applied by grasping the inner and outer surfaces of the lip between two fingers.

The facial nerve (cranial nerve VII) extends from the lower portion of the ear anteriorly, branching over the cheek (Figure 4-7). Lacerations in front of the ear, therefore, can cause facial paralysis. The nerve is imbedded in the parotid (salivary) gland, which lies anterior to and inferior to the external ear.

## THE EYE

The orbit is the pyramidal-shaped cavity that contains the eyeball and all accessory structures needed to nourish and move the eyeball. The walls and margins of the cavity are composed of a complex interweaving of various skull bones. The eye moves by a series of six muscles called the extraocular muscles. These include the lateral rectus, medial rectus (Figure 4-8), superior and inferior obliques, and the inferior rectus muscles. These muscles are innervated by three cranial nerves (III, IV, and VI). The eye is protected from the external environment by the two eyelids, upper and lower. The eyelids secret a fluid that lubricates the eye. This fluid, collected by the tear ducts (lacrimal ducts), drains into the nose (lacrimal sac). The white portion of the eye is called the sclera (Figure 4-9). The eyeball itself has a cornea, anterior chamber, and iris. The iris functions as a curtain, opening and closing, and allows beams of light to enter the retina. Posterior to the iris is the lens, and behind that is the aqueous humor (Figure 4-8). The inner portion of the eye consists of the retina and choroid. The cranial nerve bringing light impulses to the brain is the optic nerve (cranial nerve II).

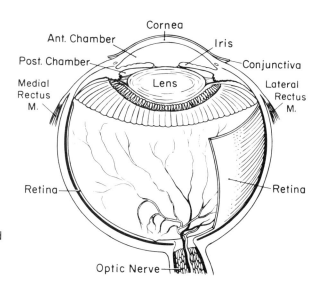

**Figure 4-8.** A horizontal section through the middle portion of the eye. The motion of the eye is controlled by the rectus muscle, and the medial and lateral rectus muscles are identified.

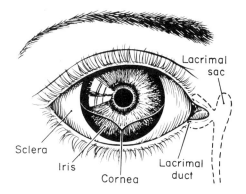

**Figure 4-9.** A frontal view of the eye. Tears wash the eye and are collected in the lacrimal duct to drain into the nose.

THE EAR

The ear is used for hearing and contains the outer ear (pinna) (Figure 4-7) and the inner ear. The outer ear is not as vascular as the other structures of the face. Its framework is cartilage and it is particularly vulnerable to injury. An amputated ear should be placed in an isotonic fluid bath or dressing and transported with the patient. Bleeding can occur between the skin and cartilage in ear injuries. If the collection of blood is not drained and attended to properly, infection can occur and a "cauliflower ear" may result.

The inner ear consists of the ear canal, tympanic membrane, ossicles, cochlea, and semicircular canals. Hearing and balance are provided by the inner ear. The inner ear is connected to the nasopharynx by the eustachian tube (Figure 4-12). This tube allows for equilibrium of the pressure between the inner and outer ears during diving or flying.

THE NOSE

The lower (caudal) portion of the nose is composed of a cartilage septum which divides the right and left sides. Its outer upper third is composed of nasal bones (bridge of the nose) (Figure 4-2). Interiorly, the posterior and posteriosuperior midline components are the ethmoid and vomer bones. The superior limit of the inside of the nose (nasal vault), separating it from the brain, is a thin fragile bone, the cribiform plate (Figures 4-6, 4-12). An upward blow to the nose from below may collapse the weaker portions of the nose, causing fracture and displacement of the cribiform plate into the brain and its vascular structures. No attempt should be made to straighten or unfold the nose because the compressed structures may be acting as a tampon against a bleeding site. The blood supply to the nose can be functionally divided into two groups, anterior and posterior. The anterior blood vessels supply the interior of the nose, having their most exposed vulnerable area at the anterior portion of the nasal septum (Figure 4-10). This is a common bleeding site which

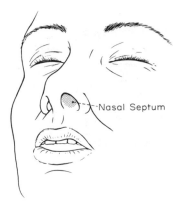

Nasal Septum

**Figure 4-10.** The medial aspect of the nasal septum is a common site for nosebleeds.

can be controlled by compressing or pinching the nose.

The lateral, interior nose is composed of three to four nasal turbinates. These bulbous ridges running from front to back can be mistaken for abnormally herniated tissue or damaged at the time of nasal packing (Figure 4-12).

Midway from the tip of the nose posteriorly to the base of the skull (at the posterior limit of the vomer) the two nostrils (nasal passages) open into a single vault, the posterior nasal space or nasopharynx. Bleeding from this area tends to flow down the throat, possibly causing choking. There is no simple field method to control this bleeding and transport is required. As a temporary measure, leaning the patient forward when other conditions permit will allow the blood to escape the mouth and nose away from the airway.

## THE SINUSES

The sinuses are irregular air cavities that lie adjacent to the nose (Figure 4-6). Theories as to their function have been advanced, but none is supported by sufficient evidence. There are about twelve sinuses on each side; the number is somewhat variable and is not always the same on each side. They are divided into anterior and posterior groups. The anterior includes the frontal, the maxillary, and the anterior ethmoids, while the posterior ethmoids and sphenoids comprise the posterior group. The sinuses all drain into the nose and turbinates. The sinuses are located in bones, the names of which they carry. The frontal sinus lies between the outer inner tables of the frontal bone. The maxillary sinus fills a large part of the maxilla (Figure 4-2). It extends from the orbit where it forms a part of the floor down to the apices of the teeth, some of which may protrude into the cavity. The ethmoidal sinus occupies much of the ethmoidal labyrinth. The sphenoid sinus occupies the sphenoid border extended by the wings of the sphenoid.

## THE MOUTH

The mouth is bounded in front (anteriorly) by the lips, in back (posteriorly) by the posterior wall of the pharynx (throat), superiorly by the hard and soft palates, inferiorly by the floor of the mouth and tongue, and laterally by the cheeks (buccal tissues). Teeth are imbedded in the upper (maxilla) and lower (mandible) jaws within tooth sockets of the alveolar ridges which are covered by gingiva (gums) (Figure 4-2). Examination of the mouth for avulsed teeth is important, as they can lodge in the patient's airway. The tongue is held forward by muscular attachments to the mandible (jaw). The tongue is highly vascular and commonly injured.

The pharynx is divided into the nasopharynx, oropharynx, and hypopharynx (Figure 4-12). The pharynx, in addition to being the inlet to the airway, is bounded laterally by the tonsils and carotid arteries, and posteriorly the pharyngeal wall covers the cervical vertebrae. A potential space exists between these two structures. A laceration of the pharyngeal wall, such as during the insertion of an esophageal airway, can create a false passage into this space. The oropharynx can be seen when one opens his mouth and says, "Ah . . ." The uvula is the appendage that hangs down from the soft palate. The soft palate rises when saying, "Ah . . .," exposing the oropharynx. The nasal part of the pharynx lies behind the nose and above the soft palate. This part of the pharynx is the only part that remains patent at all times. On the lateral wall of the nasopharynx is the opening of the eustachian tube (Figure 4-12). The hypopharynx contains the epiglottis, an opening to the larynx, and the esophagus.

## THE LARYNX

The larynx connects the pharynx with the trachea (Figures 4-4, 4-11, 4-12, and 9-1). It is a tube covered by a movable lid, the epiglottis. Its walls consist of cartilages and ligaments. Attached to these cartilages and ligaments are a complex set of intrinsic and extrinsic laryngeal muscles. The largest cartilages are the thyroid cartilage ("Adam's apple"), and the cricoid cartilage (the only complete cartilaginous ring in the larynx) (Figure 4-4). The other cartilages are the paired arytenoids, the paired corniculates, the paired cuneiforms, and the epiglottis (Figure 4-11). The intrinsic muscles in the larynx are the cricothyroid, the cricoarytenoids (lateral and posterior), the interarytenoids, and the thyroarytenoids (Figure 4-11). The esophagus is located posterior to the larynx. The framework of the larynx, in summary, consists of the hyoid bone superiorly, the thyroid and cricoid cartilages inferiorly, and the epiglottis and arytenoid cartilages posteriorly.

The hyoid bone helps suspend the remainder of the airway to the jaw and tongue (Figure 4-4). Within the thyroid cartilage are the internal parts of the larynx, the vocal cords and attached muscles, ligaments and cartilages (Figure 4-11). The paired true and false vocal cords attach anteriorly near the midportion of the thyroid cartilage. Posteriorly, the vocal cords attach to the arytenoid cartilages which articulate with the cricoid cartilage, allowing for opening and closing of the vocal cords. The larynx serves two main functions: production of sound for speech and protection of the lower airway (trachea and lungs) from aspiration. Below the signet-ring shaped cricoid are the *U*-shaped tracheal cartilages. The membranous posterior wall of the trachea joins the limbs of each *U* and the trachea resides in front of the esophagus.

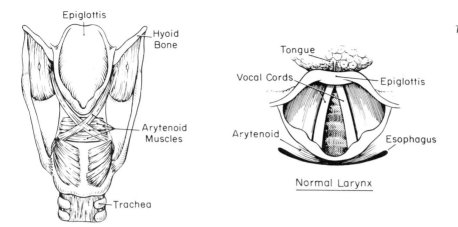

**Figure 4-11.** The anatomy of the larynx. The vocal cords close posteriorly in the midline. The esophagus is posterior to the larynx.

The fibrous membrane joining the hyoid and the thyroid cartilage is the thyrohyoid membrane. The membrane joining the thyroid and cricoid cartilages is called the cricothyroid membrane. The area of the neck overlying the cricothyroid membrane is free of major nerves and blood vessels. The relationships of these structures is important when considering neck wounds or establishing an airway. Penetrating wounds of the thyrohyoid membrane enter the pharynx at the base of the tongue. Wounds of the cricothyroid membrane enter the airway. Also, and most importantly, an emergency cricothyrotomy is performed through the cricothyroid membrane in the midline in a slightly inferior direction. Surgical wounds directed upwards risk injury to the vocal cords, and laterally placed incisions can cause muscle or carotid artery injury with bleeding. The muscles that move the vocal cords receive innervation from the recurrent laryngeal nerves, which pass from the chest to the larynx along the tracheoesophageal grooves. The thyroid gland at the upper extent of the trachea is capable of profuse bleeding in injury to the lower neck.

## THE NERVOUS SYSTEM

The nervous system is composed of the central nervous system (brain and spinal cord), the peripheral nervous system (cranial and peripheral nerves), and the autonomic nervous system. The pertinent anatomy of the central nervous system (CNS) is shown in Figure 4-12. The cerebral hemispheres reside on the diencephalon, which is immediately superior to the midbrain, pons, and medulla oblongata. This area of the brain is called the brainstem. The cerebral hemispheres are generally considered to be that area responsible for speech, memory, and thinking processes.

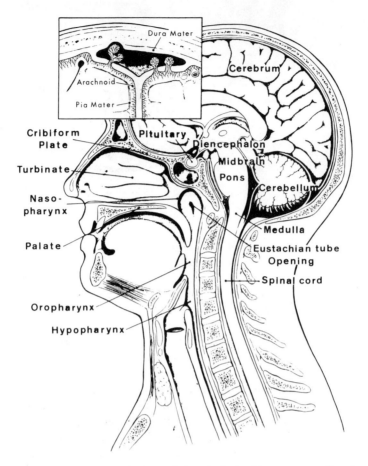

**Figure 4-12.** A sagittal view of the skull, brain, nose, mouth, pharynx, trachea, and spinal cord demonstrates the relationship of the various structures. Notice how close the oropharynx is to the spinal cord. The covering of the brain is shown in the upper left hand box.

The brainstem is considered to have more primitive basic functions such as control over respiration and cardiac function. Minor injuries to the brainstem can cause a loss of consciousness, as well as a change in respiration. Below the medulla oblongata is the spinal cord, which carries afferent and efferent discharges that pass information to and from the rest of the body.

CENTRAL NERVOUS SYSTEM

*The Brain.* The brain and spinal cord are protected by bone. The covering of the brain is called the skull or cranium, and the bones covering the spinal cord are the vertebrae. Beneath the bone is a tissue called the meninges, which encircles the brain and spinal cord tissues. The meninges is composed of three distinct layers: the dura mater, the arachnoid mater, and the pia mater (Figure 4-12). Dura mater is composed of strong white fibrous tissue, which serves as the periosteum for the innermost portion of the skull as well as a covering for the brain. Dura mater is so strong that it has been used to make heart valves. The arachnoid mater is a delicate membrane between the dura and pia maters. Cerebrospinal fluid circulates in this space and acts to cushion the brain and carry nutritive material. The pia mater is the innermost layer overlying the brain and spinal cord tissue.

These three layers make up potential spaces that are important in the management of head trauma. Between the skull and the dura is a potential space, the epidural space. This space can be opened and expanded in head injuries if there is arterial bleeding between the bone and the dura mater. The artery injured in this case is the middle meningeal artery (Figure 4-6). This artery is a branch of the maxillary artery, which is, in turn, a branch of the external carotid artery, supplying the dura mater and surrounding bone. It enters the cranial cavity via a hole, called the foramen spinosum. Bleeding may also occur in the area beneath the dural space (the subdural space), which can compress the brain underneath it. This is called a subdural hematoma. Finally, there may be bleeding underneath the arachnoid tissue, termed a subarachnoid hemorrhage. This occurs in patients with hypertension or aneurysms of the cerebral arteries.

The major arteries supplying the brain are the vertebrals and internal carotids (Figure 4-13). The vertebrals are the first major branches of the subclavian arteries. This artery arises deep within the neck and ascends to the level of the sixth cervical vertebra. At this point the vessels enter the foramen of the transverse processes of the sixth cervical vertebra. They then enter the foramen magnum on each side of the brainstem, and these unite on the undersurface of the pons to form the midline basilar artery. The basilar artery passes forward on the underside of the pons, giving off branches to the brainstem, and then divides on the undersurface of the midbrain to form the posterior cerebral arteries, which form the Circle of Willis (Figure 4-13).

The internal carotid arteries arise at the bifurcation of the common carotid opposite the cranial border of the thyroid cartilage. The internal carotid then travels cranially within the carotid sheath to enter the carotid canal at the base of the skull. The first branch the carotid artery gives off in the brain is the ophthalmic artery to the retina (Figures 4-8, 4-13). The carotid artery then divides into three major branches, which communicate with the posterior branches arising from the vertebral arteries.

The principal venous drainage channels are the large venous sinuses located between the layers of the dura mater. These large channels have no valves and empty into the internal jugular veins (Figure 4-5). The superior sagittal sinus runs convexly over the brain and unites with the straight sinus. Together these sinuses form the transverse sinus,

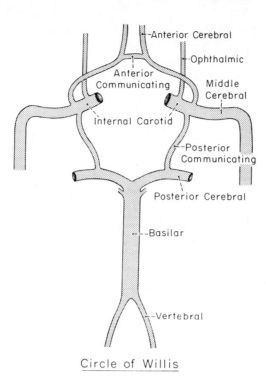

Anterior Cerebral

Ophthalmic

Anterior
Communicating

Middle
Cerebral

Internal Carotid

Posterior
Communicating

Posterior Cerebral

Basilar

Vertebral

Circle of Willis

**Figure 4-13.** The confluence of arteries that reach the brain form a circle called the Circle of Willis. From this circle, branches continue on to supply blood to the brain.

and finally the sigmoid sinus behind the ear, then emerge from the skull as the internal jugular vein. The main point of the venous channels in the head and upper neck is that they contain no valves and are all interconnected. Thus it is possible for infectious material from the face or scalp, for example, to be carried to the skull via the veins in the skull itself to the internal veins in the brain.

*The Spinal Cord.* The spinal cord lies within the spinal cavity from the foramen magnum at the base of the skull to the lower border of the first lumbar vertebra. It is approximately seventeen to eighteen inches long in the average body (Figures 4-12, 4-14). The cord does not completely fill the spinal cavity, and is covered by the meninges as previously described (Figure 4-15). The bony covering of the spinal cord is a series of connected vertebrae. Basic vertebral anatomy should be learned by the paramedic and includes knowledge of the following: (1) the vertebral body (centrum), (2) the pedicles, (3) the spinus processes, (4) the transverse processes, and, (5) the articular facets (Figure 4-16). Bony structures surround the vertebral canal through which the spinal cord travels. The vertebrae are connected to one another by a joint and a ligament that allows for flexion, extension, and rotation of the vertebral column.

The vertebral column is divided into cervical, thoracic, lumbar, sacral, and coccygeal segments (Figure 4-14). On the articulated vertebral

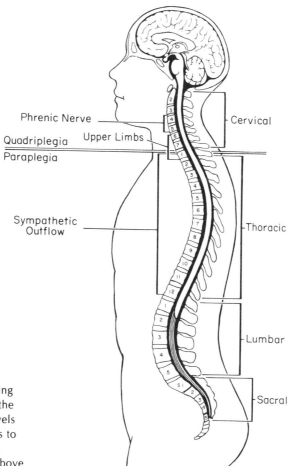

Phrenic Nerve

Quadriplegia    Upper Limbs

Paraplegia

Sympathetic
Outflow

Cervical

Thoracic

Lumbar

Sacral

**Figure 4-14.** Midsagittal section of the body showing the relationship between the brain and the different levels of the spinal cord. Injuries to the spinal cord below T-1 produce paraplegia and above T-1, quadriplegia.

column, notice the primary thoracic and sacral curvatures (concave anteriorly), and the secondary cervical and lumbar curvatures (concave posteriorly). There are seven cervical, twelve thoracic, and five lumbar vertebrae; one sacrum (five fused segments), and one coccyx (four to five fused segments). The spinus process of the seventh cervical vertebra (C7) is especially prominent and is a useful bony landmark in the surface anatomy of the thorax.

The spinal cord performs two general functions: (1) transmission of impulses from the body (afferent impulses) to and through the spinal cord to the brain, and (2) transmission of impulses from the brain (efferent impulses) through the fibers of the white matter of the cord to the peripheral nerves and various systems of the body. Connections between afferent and efferent neurons, which provide the basis for reflex actions, occur in the gray matter of the spinal cord.

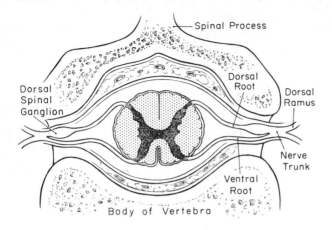

Figure 4-15. The relationship of the spinal cord and bony vertebra. The nerves emanate from the spinal cord anteriorly and posteriorly to form nerve trunks.

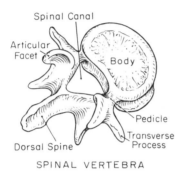

SPINAL VERTEBRA

Figure 4-16. A vertebral bone. The spinal cord resides in the spinal canal.

The spinal cord is divided into three portions: cervical, thoracic, and lumbar. It consists of a series of thirty-one segments, each segment giving rise to paired spinal nerves that are attached to the cord by two roots: a dorsal root containing afferent or sensory fibers, and a ventral root containing efferent or motor fibers (Figure 4-15). These nerves join each other in collection areas in the body to become the peripheral nerves.

Injuries or conditions adversely affecting the spinal cord are more serious the closer to the brainstem they occur. For example, spinal cord lesions above the fifth cervical segment produce a paralyzed patient unable to breathe on his own. The phrenic nerve outflow to the diaphragm takes origin at the C3, C4, and C5 cord segments. Injury to the cord at the C6 level will produce a quadriplegic patient who, although able to breathe on his own with phrenic nerve discharge, will lack control of his thoracic musculature. Any cord injury from the level of the first thoracic segment (T1) distally will produce a paraplegic patient with variable control of the thoracic musculature.

Urinary bladder function is impaired by cord damage above the second sacral segment (S2) because the major discharge from the bladder is from the nerves taking origin at the S2, S3, and S4 levels. The para-

or quadriplegic patient is unable to appreciate a distended bladder and cannot voluntarily empty it.

## PERIPHERAL NERVOUS SYSTEM

The peripheral nervous system is composed of the nerves originating from the head (cranial nerves) and the nerves originating in the spinal cord.

*Cranial Nerves.* Cranial nerves are those nerves whose origins are within the brain and innervate the structures outside of the brain. There are twelve cranial nerves, which are paired on either side. The names and functions of the cranial nerves are as follows:

I. Olfactory—Sense of smell.

II. Optic—The nerve fibers responsible for vision lie in the retina, gathering at the posterior pole of the retina to form the optic nerve. The nerve leaves the orbit in the optic canal, from which it enters the middle of the cranium. The nerves divide and cross so that some fibers of the right optic nerve travel to the left occiput and some fibers of the left optic nerve travel to the right occiput.

III. Oculomotor—The superior and inferior oblique ocular muscles are supplied by this nerve. Traveling along the nerve is the parasympathetic innervation to the iris. Injury or compression of this nerve will cause pupil dilatation.

IV. Trochlear—This nerve innervates the superior oblique muscle of the eyeball.

V. Trigeminal—This is the largest cranial nerve, supplying sensation to the face and innervation of the muscles of mastication (chewing).

VI. Abducens—This nerve supplies the lateral rectus muscle and allows for the lateral and upward gaze of the eye.

VII. Facial—The most important structures innervated by this nerve are the muscles of facial expression and taste to the anterior two-thirds of the tongue. It exits from the brain at the temporal bone and passes through the substance of the parotid gland and distributes to the muscles of facial expression.

VIII. Acoustic—This nerve brings fibers that are responsible for hearing and balance from the inner ear to the brainstem.

IX. Glossopharyngeal—This nerve supplies taste and general somatic sensation to the posterior two-thirds of the tongue. It also gives off the carotid sinus nerve.

X. Vagus—This is an extremely complex nerve. Its two most important parts, from a clinical point of view, are the preganglionic efferent parasympathetic pathways to most of the viscera of the body cavities and the recurrent nerves that supply all the muscles of the larynx (vocal cords) except the cricothyroid.

XI. Accessory—The spinal portion of this nerve innervates the trapezius and sternocleidomastoid muscles.

XII. Hypoglossal—This is the motor nerve of the tongue. It leaves the skull via the hypoglossal canal.

The cranial nerve supply extends from the face and the eye all the way to the gastrointestinal tract via the vagus nerves. It is important to know the cranial nerves and their functions. Loss of function of a cranial nerve may be due to its nucleus, which is its origin in the brain, or due to injuries to the nerve somewhere outside the confines of the brain. For example, a stroke might produce facial paralysis because of damage to the nucleus within the brain substance itself. A contrasting example would be facial paralysis due to laceration of the seventh cranial nerve as it emerges in front of the ear within the substance of the parotid gland (Figure 4-7). One of the disorders most commonly encountered by the paramedic is that of the third cranial nerve, which crosses the base of the brain to supply the internal oblique muscles of the eye. If this nerve is stretched, which occurs during increased intracranial pressure, dilatation of the pupil will result. The twelfth cranial nerve supplies the tongue, and the action of moving the tongue out of the mouth is controlled by constrictors on both sides of the tongue. If one constrictor does not function, the other one will override it and push the tongue to the side of the weak muscle. This deviation of the tongue is often a sign of a stroke, but can occur after a neck injury in which the hypoglossal nerve has been injured.

*Peripheral Nerves.*    All fibers of the peripheral nervous system are either sensory (afferent) or motor (efferent). Second, all fibers belong to either the somatic nervous system or the visceral nervous system. Thus, every fiber (with the exception of some special cranial nerves) falls into one of these four categories: (1) somatic-motor, (2) somatic-sensory, (3) visceral-motor, and (4) visceral-sensory.

The distinction between sensory and motor is obvious. Sensory fibers bring information to the central nervous system and motor fibers carry commands out to effector structures, namely muscles and glands.

The somatic sensory fibers carry sensory information from the periphery into the central nervous system. The main types of somatic sensation are the perceptions of the following: (1) pain, (2) temperature, (3) touch, (4) pressure, and (5) position or muscle sense. These sensations arise in the skin or body wall and are carried via the somatic sensory fibers into the central nervous system. The cell bodies for these fibers are found in the dorsal root ganglia. These impulses travel up the spinal cord and cross at the cervical medullary junction (junction of the cervical spinal cord and medulla) and reach their final destination in the opposite cerebral hemisphere (Figure 4-12).

Somatic motor commands are those carried through striated (skeletal) muscle by somatic motor fibers. These fibers are axons of the somatic motor cells, which are large neurons located in the spinal cord and similar regions in the brainstem. Voluntary control of the limbs by the nervous system is arranged anatomically in such a way that the opposite cerebral hemisphere is the side of origin and control of the contralateral limb and lower face. These fibers cross at the cervical medullary cord junction.

Therefore, disorders in the brain, such as a stroke or injury, may cause a contralateral (opposite side) paralysis; while injury to the spinal cord may cause a paralysis on the same side as the injury (Figure 16-3).

*Visceral Sensory Fibers.* Far less is known about visceral sensation than is known about somatic sensation. Visceral sensation results from afferent impulses coming into the central nervous system from glands and those other structures that contain smooth or cardiac muscle. The major type of information in this category is visceral pain. There are two main differences between visceral and somatic pain. In the somatic system the function of pain is to provide a warning of impending, irreversible damage to tissues; and in this system, all things that cause such damage are attended by pain. This is not true for the viscera. In the intestines, for example, burning, cutting, freezing, or crushing causes no conscious sensation of pain. Pain, however, is caused by distention, forceful contraction of smooth muscle, or traction on the mesentery (membranes which support the gut). The site of origin of somatic pain is accurately localized, and there is usually no difficulty in describing the character of the pain. By contrast, visceral pain is poorly localized and difficult to describe. In the case of a heart attack, for example, some patients feel no pain; others feel a squeezing, constricting pain under the sternum; others describe the pain as a burning sensation with pain radiating to the inner side of the left arm, neck, right arm, or into the back.

Pain felt at all locations not directly related to the site of tissue damage is called referred pain, i.e., referred from the site of the disease to another part of the body.

Nerves that arise from the spinal cord collect in two major areas in the body. The collection point in the upper body is at the posterior triangle of the neck and is called the brachial plexus (Figure 4-17). The brachial plexus supplies the motor and sensory nerves to the shoulder, upper arm, forearm, and hand. The brachial plexus can be injured, for example, in birth deliveries by stretching the shoulder, producing a permanent arm disability. The brachial plexus can also be injured in motorcycle accidents in which the arm is severely stretched, rendering it virtually useless. The three major nerves that emerge from the brachial plexus are the radial, median, and ulnar nerves. The radial nerve courses around the humerus laterally to the proximal forearm and supplies the muscles which dorsiflex or raise the hand. The median nerve continues down the inner aspect of the arm across the elbow and down the forearm into the hand to provide the fine motion of the flexion muscles in the forearm and hand. The ulnar nerve crosses down the inner aspect of the arm and under the medial portion of the elbow (the so-called "crazy bone"), then continues downward to supply the fine muscles of the hand and some of the individual muscles of the thumb and little finger. Traveling with these same nerves are somatic sensory nerves that record position changes, touch, pain, temperature, and pressure, as previously mentioned.

Another set of nerves arise from the lumbar-sacral area supplying one nerve to the back, the sciatic nerve; and one large nerve to the front, the femoral nerve. The sciatic nerve continues down the lateral aspect of the thigh to become the popliteal nerve, which supplies the leg muscles. The sciatic nerve supplies nerves that dorsiflex the foot and flex the knee. The sciatic nerve can be injured either as a result of fracture, stabbing, or injection of a needle with medication into that area. A sciatic nerve injury is noted when the patient cannot flex his knee or lift his foot. The femoral nerve travels next to the femoral artery and is the most lateral structure in the inguinal canal. A femoral nerve injury should be suspected when the individual cannot raise his knee and/or flex his hip (Figure 4-17).

## AUTONOMIC NERVOUS SYSTEM

The autonomic nervous system is that portion of the nervous system which lies beyond our conscious control. These nerves function without our willing them to and, for the most part, without our being conscious of them. The autonomic nervous system conducts impulses from the brainstem or spinal cord to viscera (organs, such as the heart, stomach, blood vessels, and hair), and records and transmits sensory impulses back to the spinal column. The autonomic nervous system functions as a reflex system much as the voluntary nervous system does. This system is divided into two anatomically and physiologically separate divisions, which are termed the sympathetic and parasympathetic divisions.

The sympathetic or adrenergic system will accelerate heart rate, increase strength of cardiac muscle contraction, constrict skin vessels, constrict skeletal muscle vessels, dilate the pupils, produce goose pimples, increase the blood sugar levels, and dilate the bronchioles. The parasympathetic nervous system, on the other hand, will slow heart rate, increase bronchial constriction, contract the urinary bladder, constrict the pupils of the eye, and increase contraction of the intestines.

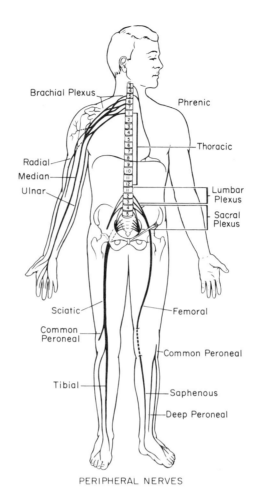

Figure 4-17. Nerves that leave the spinal cord collect in three major places (plexus). The brachial plexus is in the shoulder and the lumbar and sacral plexuses are in the lower abdomen and pelvis.

The sympathetic portion of the autonomic nervous system causes the sweat glands to function and therefore produce a moist, cool skin. The back of the hand can often manifest the difference between the warm, dry skin below the level of a spinal cord lesion and the normally moist, cool skin above the lesion.

THORAX

TOPOGRAPHIC ANATOMY

The thorax (chest) extends from the neck and clavicles to the diaphragm, encompassing all the structures between them (Figure 4-18). The clavicles (collar bones) are two bones extending from the shoulder medially to attach to the sternum (Figure 4-19). The two sternal attachments are

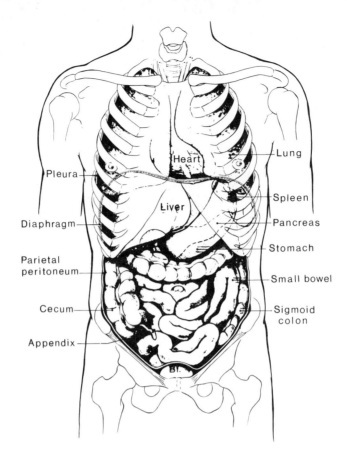

Pleura

Diaphragm

Parietal
peritoneum

Cecum

Appendix

Heart

Lung

Spleen

Liver

Pancreas

Stomach

Small bowel

Sigmoid
colon

**Figure 4-18.** A frontal projection of the thorax and abdomen. The pancreas is dotted and lies behind the stomach in the retroperitoneum. The diaphragm separates the abdomen from the thorax.

prominent and can be easily felt. Medial to both of these prominences is a notch, called the suprasternal notch, a *U*-shaped indentation formed by the sternoclavicular joints. This notch is important to recognize because the trachea can be palpated here in its deep recess (Figure 4-19). Above the clavicles and within the neck region is an area called the supraclavicular fossa. The clavicle forms an anatomic landmark for the location of structures within and on the chest. The midclavicular line is an imaginary vertical line drawn through the clavicle straight down on the chest (Figure 4-19). The line generally crosses in the region of the nipple on the male. Just lateral to this line at the nipple level one can palpate the heart beat. Medial to the midclavicular line and in the midline is the sternum (breastbone). The sternum is composed of three parts: the manubrium, the body, and the xiphoid process (Figure 14-19). As one palpates inferiorly along the sternum beginning at the suprasternal notch, an indentation in the sternum can be felt about two inches below the notch. This

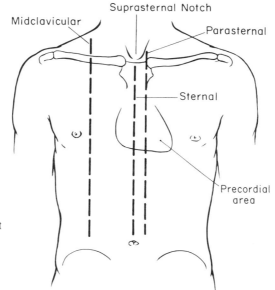

Suprasternal Notch

Midclavicular

Parasternal

Sternal

Precordial area

**Figure 4-19.** Topical landmarks of the chest. The sternal line is directly down the middle of the sternum, and the portion adjacent to it is called the parasternal line. The midclavicular line is directed through the middle portion of the clavicle.

indentation, although slight, is at the level of the articulation with the second rib. This is called the sternal angle. A distinction is also made between the sides of the sternum, called the right and left sternal borders (Figure 4-19). Knowing these locations aids in describing injuries, particularly penetrating injuries to the thorax.

With the shoulder elevated, one gains visualization of the axilla (armpit). Crossing the chest to the axilla is the pectoralis muscle, and the imaginary line formed is called the anterior axillary line (Figure 4-20). The midaxillary line is one drawn straight down from the axilla onto the thorax, and running posterior and parallel to this is the posterior axillary line. These lines are important to know for the insertion of needles into the chest to relieve pneumothorax and also in the description of wounds of entry. The nipple is about the level of the fourth intercostal space (space between the ribs). The location of any wounds of entry above the nipple would be in the first, second, or third intercostal space; any wounds below that would be in the fourth to eleventh intercostal spaces. In the back of the thorax is the scapula, and a line drawn down through the middle of the scapula to the lowest rib would be called the midscapular line (Figure 4-21). Medial to that, one finds the dorsal spines of the thoracic vertebrae. Next to the vertebrae are the paravertebral muscles (para meaning "next to").

In addition to these vertical lines, horizontal lines can be designated by reference to the ribs, intercostal spaces, and/or dorsal spines. Anteriorly, the sternomanubrial angle marks the level of the second rib, and counting downward from there the ribs can be located. On the back, the scapula spans ribs two through seven. Its inferior angle

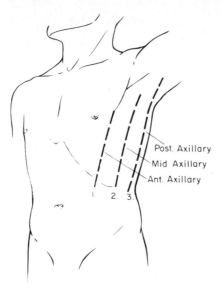

**Figure 4-20.** The left arm is elevated showing the three landmarks of the lateral chest wall.

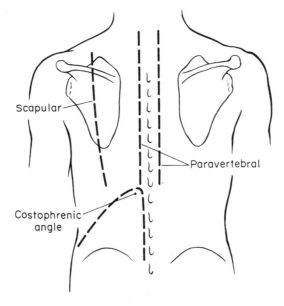

**Figure 4-21.** The common landmarks of the back.

overlies the seventh rib or interspace and is a good reference point for identifying ribs seven, eight, nine, and ten. On the back, horizontal levels can also be related to vertebral levels. The prominent seventh cervical vertebra can be located, and succeeding spinus processes can be counted downward approximately every two inches. In some instances, the spinus process of the twelfth thoracic vertebra can be identified by palpating the course of the twelfth rib. For example, a knife penetrating the back can be described adequately. The knife entered the paravertebral space on the left at the level of the midscapular region, putting it between the second to the seventh space. It would be lateral to the spine but medial to the scapula. This descriptive model is helpful in communication with the base hospital.

The twelfth rib on either side posteriorly continues in an oblique fashion downward and laterally. The angle between these ribs and the paravertebral muscles is called the costovertebral angle. This angle is an area that overlies the kidneys and may be the site of wounds of entry or pain due to infection or kidney stones.

## INTERNAL STRUCTURES

The thorax (chest) extends from the neck and clavicles to the diaphragm and encompasses all of the structures between them. These structures include the ribs, sternum, diaphragm, lungs, esophagus, major blood vessels, and the heart. The diaphragm is an anatomic boundary which separates the thorax from the abdomen. It is a fibromuscular structure consisting of three muscular portions: sternal, costal, and vertebral. The central portion of the diaphragm is made of tendinous tissue and, at the periphery, skeletal muscle which is attached to the chest wall. The diaphragm may function voluntarily, as during a deep inspiration, or involuntarily, as during normal breathing. The diaphragm is innervated by the phrenic nerves, which emerge through the C3, C4, and C5 foramina and pass through the neck down along the heart to the diaphragm. A helpful mnemonic is "C3, C4, and C5 keep the diaphragm alive." At the diaphragm, the phrenic nerve divides into anterior, lateral, and posterior branches. The diaphragm is an important part of the breathing apparatus and, under normal circumstances, contributes 65 to 70 percent of the effective ventilation. Any injury or damage to one or both phrenic nerves (e.g., cervical fracture) can produce severe respiratory problems. The three major structures that penetrate the diaphragm are the inferior vena cava, esophagus, and aorta. Occasionally there may be congenital or acquired (traumatic) defects in the diaphragm which allow viscera in the abdominal cavity to pass into the chest (diaphragmatic hernia).

The ribs and sternum provide a bony cage for protection of the heart and lungs as well as a bellows mechanism for respiration. In each half of the thorax there are twelve ribs, which originate from the thoracic spines posteriorly, travel laterally, and then anteriorly. The first seven ribs are connected to the sternum by costal cartilages. The cartilages of ribs eight, nine, and ten are connected to the costal cartilages of the ribs above. The eleventh and twelfth ribs have no cartilaginous or anterior sternal attachments and are the so-called "floating" ribs. The connection between the ribs and the sternum is called the costochondral junction. The sternum has been described in the section on topography. The most common disorders of the bony thorax are due to trauma, either from penetrating or blunt injury.

Just inside the body structures of the thorax lies the pleura, which is composed of a thin layer of cells that lines both the lung and the chest wall. The pleura is divided into the visceral pleura, which is the lining over the lung and the parietal pleura, which lines the chest wall itself. The pleural space is that space between the two pleural surfaces. This is a potential space since, under normal circumstances, the visceral and parietal pleura are in close proximity without a true space present. When disorders of the lung or chest wall cause fluid or air to collect in this space, a separation of the pleural surfaces occurs.

There are two lungs, each of which is divided into several lobes. The right lung is composed of three lobes and the left lung of two lobes. These lobes are further divided into segments and subsegments. The lung can be compared to a tree with the trunk of the tree being the trachea, and the major bronchi the main branches. The smaller branches are the bronchioles, and more peripherally we find the alveoli (the leaves) (Figure 9-1). Accompanying the bronchi are the arteries and veins. There are usually two veins for every artery in the lung and they travel in proximity to each other. The purpose of the veins is to carry blood that has undergone gas exchange from the lung back to the heart, which then pumps it into the systemic circulation. The lung is an organ with a dual blood supply. That is, it has both the pulmonary arteries, which arise from the heart and deliver unoxygenated blood to the lung, and the bronchial arteries, which originate in the aorta and deliver oxygenated blood to the lung. The only other organ with a similar arterial and venous perfusion arrangement is the liver. Arteries of the lung and the bronchi of the lung respond to neural changes that are usually innervated through the vagus nerves. They also respond to various humoral agents either by dilation or constriction.

Located in the center of the thorax is the esophagus, which travels posteriorly to the trachea and conducts solids and/or liquids from the mouth to the stomach. The esophagus is composed of smooth muscle tissue and swallowing is an automatic action. The muscles of the esophagus are divided into two layers, and the inside lining of the esophagus is made of a column of cells that are very sensitive to heat or caustic substances. There are three potential places where constriction of the esophagus may cause food or objects to stick. These are:

1. The upper end of the esophagus at the cricopharyngeal constrictor (Figure 4-4)

2. The area where the aortic arch crosses in front of the esophagus

3. The junction of the esophagus with the stomach.

The heart is in the mediastinum (middle of the thorax) with the right ventricle positioned just posterior to the sternum. The heart is wrapped in a pericardial sac (Figure 4-22). The space between the epicardium or tissue lining the muscle of the heart and the pericardium

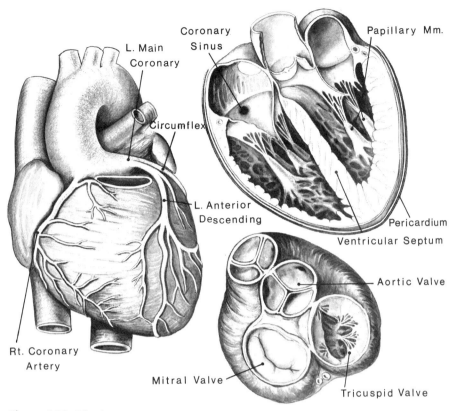

Coronary Sinus

L. Main Coronary

Papillary Mm.

Circumflex

L. Anterior Descending

Pericardium

Ventricular Septum

Rt. Coronary Artery

Aortic Valve

Mitral Valve

Tricuspid Valve

**Figure 4-22.** The heart consists of four chambers and four valves. There are two major arteries to the heart, the left and right coronary arteries. These arteries supply blood primarily to the left ventricle.

is a potential space, and normally there are only a few ounces of fluid in the pericardial sac. Abnormal fluid collection in this space, secondary to injury or inflammation, can compress the heart (tamponade). The heart is divided into four chambers consisting of two atria and two ventricles (Chapter 3). Two arteries supply the atria and ventricles (coronary arteries). The right coronary artery supplies blood primarily to the left ventricle. The right coronary passes around between the right atrium and the right ventricle to the posterior portion of the heart, connecting, in most people, to the posterior descending coronary artery (Chapter 10). The left coronary artery divides quickly into the left anterior descending and circumflex branches. The left ventricle, which has to pump blood against systemic blood pressure, requires the bulk of the blood supply and oxygen for functional purposes. The left anterior descending coronary artery often has been called the "widow-maker" because its occlusion can cause sudden death. Each of the chambers is separated by valves. Between the right atrium and right ventricle is the tricuspid valve (three leaflets) (Figure 4-22). As blood is ejected from the right ventricle, it passes through the pulmonary artery valve and into the pulmonary arteries, pulmonary veins, and pulmonary capillaries, and then into the left atrium. Blood then passes through the mitral valve (two leaflets) to the left ventricle, and then is ejected into the aorta. The heart muscle is thicker on the left side of the heart because it pumps blood against the systemic blood pressure. The aortic and pulmonary valves are similar and are composed of three leaflets. In the normal anatomic relationship, the pulmonary valve is anterior and to the left of the midline of the aortic valve, which is more posterior and to the right of the midline.

The proximal aorta, which connects to the heart, gives off three major arteries to the upper body. These are the right innominate artery, the right common carotid, and the left subclavian arteries (Figure 4-32). It then turns posteriorly and descends in the thorax through the posterior mediastinum to penetrate the diaphragm and subsequently to supply the lower abdomen and legs. As the aorta passes through the thorax from the left subclavian artery to the diaphragm, it is encompassed by pleura and anchored to the posterior mediastinum by the intercostal blood vessels which supply the chest wall.

# ABDOMEN

## TOPOGRAPHIC ANATOMY

The abdomen extends from the costal arches to the pelvis. It is helpful to divide the abdomen into four quadrants (Figure 8-1):

1. Right upper quadrant (RUQ)
2. Left upper quadrant (LUQ)
3. Right lower quadrant (RLQ)
4. Left lower quadrant (LLQ)

Each quadrant contains certain anatomic structures that are helpful in localizing injuries. The epigastrium is that portion of the abdomen just below the xiphoid process including both the right and left upper quadrants. This is often the site of pain or injury. Therefore, pain and injury occurring in this area is referred to as epigastric pain and epigastric injury. Regions around the umbilicus are called periumbilical. Injuries to the lower abdomen just above the pubic bone are called suprapubic injuries. The two flanks, right and left, are areas that reflect disorders in structures behind the peritoneal cavity, including the kidneys, ureters, and abdominal aorta.

The abdominal cavity extends from the diaphragm to the pelvis and includes the liver, gallbladder, spleen, pancreas, stomach, small and large bowel, and appendix (Figure 4-18). The abdominal wall consists of a series of muscles that are used primarily to aid in respiration and protect the abdominal contents from sharp blows. Two flat muscles, lying on either side of the midline of the abdomen, are called the rectus abdomini, and are encased in fascia which arises from three lateral muscles on either side. These lateral muscles are called the external oblique, the internal oblique, and the transversus abdominis muscles (Figure 4-30). Traveling inward, there is usually a fat layer between the abdominal muscles and finally the peritoneum, which is called the parietal peritoneum because it is connected to the abdominal wall (Figure 4-18). In discussing structures within this peritoneal lining the term intraperitoneal is used. Within the abdominal cavity are the structures as previously described with the exception of the pancreas, which resides on top of the spine but is covered by the peritoneum. The kidneys, ureters, female organs, urinary bladder, and adrenal glands are in the region of the peritoneal cavity but also are outside of the peritoneal lining (extraperitoneal). The esophagus travels through the diaphragm or crura and connects to the stomach. The stomach resides in the upper abdomen and is approximately twelve to eighteen inches long. It has a large capacity and can contain as much as a quart of water. It joins the duodenum and the two are separated by a structure called the pylorus, a muscular constricting band. The duodenum is approximately one foot long and joins the jejunum, which subsequently joins the ileum. The purpose of the duodenum and small bowel is absorption of ingested food substances. The total length of these structures in an adult may be as much as twenty-eight feet. The small bowel joins the cecum and ascending colon. The appendix is attached to the cecum and usually is three to four inches long. The colon continues on to become the transverse, descending, and sigmoid colons, which then join the rectum and finally the anus.

The spleen resides in the posterior portion of the left upper quadrant and is involved in destruction of old red and white blood cells (Figure 4-18). It also functions in the immune process to make antibodies from proteins. The spleen is vulnerable to injury and is only protected laterally where the rib cage covers it. It is an extremely vascular organ and is surrounded by a thin capsule that can be easily torn. The liver is situated in the right upper quadrant and is approximately four times the size of the spleen. The spleen weighs approximately five ounces, whereas the liver weighs forty ounces (approximately 2½ lb). The liver's function is to make proteins including albumin and globulin as well as to detoxify substances that enter the body along with a myriad of other complex tasks. It can be damaged by a multitude of drugs and is quite vulnerable to injury. It resides high in the abdomen and is protected by ribs anteriorly, laterally, and posteriorly. However, because of its size, it is often struck by bullets or knives. During an auto accident a forceful chest blow might drive the liver down into the abdominal cavity, making it susceptible to injury. Next to the liver is the gallbladder, which stores bile before it travels to the duodenum through the common duct. The common duct is connected to the pancreas through a pancreatic duct. The pancreas sits behind the stomach and within the curve of the duodenum (Figure 4-18). Its purpose is to secrete insulin for the regulation of sugar metabolism as well as to excrete hormones that aid in digestion. Pancreatic injuries often present the most severe in-hospital problems, whereas in the field the initial injury may not have seemed severe. All of the organs that function in the peritoneal cavity do so automatically, but are under hormonal and autonomic control. These control processes are regulated by the sympathetic and parasympathetic nervous systems. Disorders or conditions involving intraperitoneal organs produce pain and discomfort that is often different from the pain of a leg fracture or skin laceration. Understanding the innervation of the bowel and types of abdominal trauma that produce pain are important in making the diagnosis of abdominal conditions.

## MUSCULOSKELETAL SYSTEM

### TOPOGRAPHIC ANATOMY

There are four limbs, two upper and two lower. The upper limb consists of the following:

1. Shoulder
2. Upper arm
3. Forearm
4. Wrist
5. Hand

The arm literally means the upper limb from the shoulder to the hand, but it usually means that area from the shoulder to the elbow. The arm, then is not synonomous with the upper limb. For purposes of communication, the arm refers to that area from the shoulder to the elbow. The bone of the arm is the humerus. The forearm extends from the elbow joint to the wrist. In the forearm are two bones, the radius and the ulna. The back of the forearm, containing the extensor muscles of the wrist, is called the extensor or dorsal surface of the forearm. The flexor muscles of the wrist are located on the flexor surface (volar aspect) of the forearm. The flexor surface of the elbow is called the antecubital fossa.

The classic anatomic position of the hands is with the palms outward facing the viewer (Figure 4-1). This places the thumb lateral to the little finger. Since the hand can assume different positions, it is easier to specify the anatomic position of the thumb and little finger according to its relationship to the bones of the forearm. Therefore, the thumb side of the hand would mean the radial aspect or side, and the little finger area, the ulnar aspect or side of the hand.

The palm of the hand is called the palmar surface and the back of the hand, the dorsal surface. The hand contains five fingers called digits. These are named the thumb, index, middle, ring, and small fingers.

Dividing the arm and forearm into thirds helps in localization of injuries for the purposes of communication. The proximal third of the arm would extend from the shoulder to the upper arm. The middle third would extend from that point two-thirds the distance to the elbow. Finally, the distal third would be from the previous point to the elbow. The forearm is similarly divided into proximal, middle, and distal thirds.

The lower limb consists of seven parts, as follows:

1. Hip
2. Thigh
3. Popliteal fossa
4. Knee
5. Leg
6. Ankle
7. Foot

The thigh is that portion of the leg which extends from the hip to the knee. The hip consists of the pelvic bones articulating with the femur. The femur is divided into the head residing in the hip socket, the neck, and the greater trochanter. The latter can be felt as the prominent area just lateral to the hip on the upper thigh. The bone should be palpated and knowledge of its location determined. The thigh has an anterior and posterior aspect. The anterior aspect contains the quadricep muscles, which extend the knee. The posterior aspect has the hamstring muscles, which flex the knee. The knee joint is covered with a hard bone, the patella, commonly referred to as the kneecap. In back of the knee, where the joint flexes, is the popliteal fossa (Figure 4-1).

The leg from the knee to the ankle contains two bones, the tibia and the fibula. At the ankle there are two prominences of these bones, the medial and lateral malleoli. The medial malleolus is an important landmark because the saphenous vein crosses in front of, or anterior to it, at the ankle. Behind the medial malleolus is the posterior tibial artery, and its pulse is frequently used to assess perfusion of the leg. The ankle is the joint between the leg and foot at the level of the malleoli. The foot begins at the ankle and extends to the toes. There are five toes, numbered one through five. Number one is the great toe and numbers two through five represent the other toes. The bottom of the foot is the plantar surface and the top is the dorsum.

The lower extremity can be divided into thirds like the upper extremity. For example, an injury to the femur may be in the proximal, middle, or distal third of the thigh. Fractures of the tibia can be in the proximal, middle, or distal third of the leg.

## THE SKELETAL SYSTEM

*Normal Development and Structure.* The skeletal system forms early in fetal life from the developing tissues known as the mesoderm. The long bones, of primary interest in orthopedic trauma, originate for the most part from cartilaginous tissues in the fifth embryonic week. Within certain areas of these cartilages, an ossification (bone) process begins about the seventh week and these areas are designated as ossification centers (Figure 4-23). By a process termed endochondral ossification, the cartilaginous structure is calcified. The calcified cartilage then acts as a matrix for the laying down of the initial bone, and eventually the entire cartilagenous structure will be replaced by bone. Once the major ossification process has occurred in long bones, continued longitudinal growth of the bone occurs from growth centers, which are present at either end of the bone. The bone can thus grow in two planes: longitudinally by way of growth from the growth centers, and circumferentially by a process called appositional bone growth, in which increased width of the bone occurs.

The bone itself is divided into several zones which are specifically named. The long, tubular portion of the bone is called the diaphysis (Figure 4-23). The dense, outer bone of the diaphysis is called the cortex; the honeycombed bone within the marrow space or medulla is called cancellous or spongy bone; the trumpeted flare at either extreme of the diaphysis is named the metaphysis; and the growth area at either end of the long bone is the epiphysis. The bone growth center is represented in the immature bone by a transverse plate of cartilage called the physeal plate (Figure 4-23). It is from this plate that longitudinal growth occurs. The entirety of the bone, excepting the areas covered by articular or joint cartilage, is covered by a layer of specialized connective tissue called the periosteum. Within the periosteum are many specialized cells including fibroblasts and osteoblasts that have the potential for initiating repair responses. The periosteum itself is divided into two layers, the inner layer which contains most of the bone-building potential and an outer, more fibrous layer.

Bone is an active, metabolizing tissue requiring a blood supply for nutrition. The blood supply arrives at the bone by multiple sources. One of the major sources is the nutrient arteries and veins, which usually enter through the diaphysis and course through the medullary canal. Approximately two-thirds of the blood supply to the cortex of the diaphysis comes through the medullary circulation.

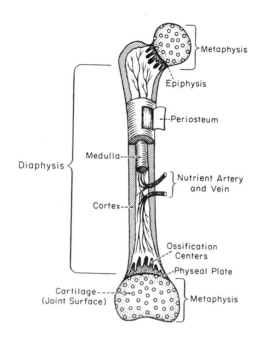

**Figure 4-23.** Early and late stages in the growth and development of the long bones.

A good portion of the outer exposed layer of the epiphysis is actually the cartilaginous surface of the joint. Underneath this lies a spherical miniature-scaled growth plate producing ossification within the center of the epiphysis and affording growth circumferentially. The epiphysis provides a layer of cancellous bone between it and the physeal plate, termed the bone plate. Because it is cartilage, the plate can separate or fracture with trauma, and it becomes the weakest link in the osseous "chain" of the bone. Damage to this plate may partially or totally arrest growth, resulting in a differential growth potential. This may cause angulation of the bone with further growth. Bone growth ceases in most people by the age of seventeen years.

*The Bones of the Body.*   There are approximately 213 functioning bones in the body. While being able to name the bones of the body is important for purposes of communication, a knowledge of the treatment of fractures and the rudiments of bone physiology will aid more in the care of the patient. In this section we will discuss the skeletal system with the exception of the thorax, skull, and the cervical, thoracic, and lumbar spines.

The skeleton of the upper limb is divided into the shoulder girdle and free extremities.

| Shoulder Girdle | Carpus (Wrist)—8 |
|---|---|
| Clavicle | Navicular |
| Scapula | Lunate |
| | Triangular |
| Free Extremities | Pisiform |
| Arm | Multangular |
| Humerus | Greater Multangular |
| Forearm | Capitate |
| Radius | Hamate |
| Ulna | Metacarpals—5 |
| | Phalanges (Digits)—14 |

The clavicle acts largely as a strut to hold the upper limb away from the body (Figure 4-24). The scapula is held to the body wall primarily by muscles and provides a site of articulation for the humerus. The anatomy of the humerus is important since several vital structures pass around it to enter the forearm. The radial nerve, a branch from the brachial plexus, circles on the outside of the midshaft of the humerus and courses down to supply the extensor muscles of the forearm. This nerve can be damaged in fractures of the humerus. It is also the nerve that is damaged when a person has been intoxicated and sleeps with his arm extended over a chair. The same can occur with the person who has undergone a drug overdose. This is commonly called "drunkard's palsy," and leaves the patient with the inability to raise his wrist.

At the distal portion of the humerus is the section of bone called the supracondylar area, which is located just above the condyles (Figure 4-24). The condyles are the two flared portions of the distal humerus that have an articular cartilaginous surface allowing the radius and ulna to form the elbow joint. Fractures to the supracondylar region are very common in children, and, if not properly managed, can produce severe functional and cosmetic disfigurement of the arm. A supracondylar fracture is serious and requires proper splinting and early transport to a medical facility.

The bones of the forearm (radius and ulna) can be fractured at any level and usually produce pain and tenderness over the fracture site. A fracture of the distal radius when one falls on the extended wrist is a common fracture (Colles' fracture). There are eight bones at the wrist, called the carpal bones. The navicular, the most important of these, resides within the "snuff box" space of the wrist. This space can be created by extending the thumb and observing the two tendons that cross on either side at the base of the thumb to form an indentation. Below this space is the navicular bone. It is frequently injured by football

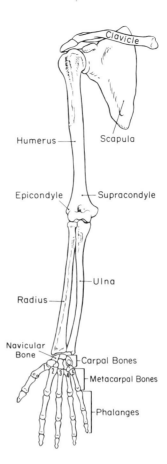

**Figure 4-24.** Bones of the shoulder, arm, forearm, and hand in the anatomic position. There are eight carpal bones.

players and other athletes, but it also can be injured during falls in the snow. It is a very special wrist bone and can produce severe disability if improperly managed.

The word meta means beyond, and it is used to describe those bones beyond the carpus. Therefore, the term metacarpal refers to those bones just beyond the carpus, and there are five of these. These bones, which articulate with the wrist, distally articulate with the first joints of the digits. The metacarpal bones are commonly fractured during fist fights, and the more common fracture is of the fourth or fifth metacarpal. Diagnosis is made easily by feeling over the bone an area of tenderness and swelling. The phalanges are the small bones of the fingers, and there are two phalanges in the thumb and three in the remaining digits. Separation of the bone into smaller parts with joints allows for fine motion of the fingers.

The skeleton of the lower limb consists of the pelvic girdle and free extremity. The pelvic girdle is composed of three fused bones: the ischium, iliac, and pubis bones (Figure 4-25). This bone is called

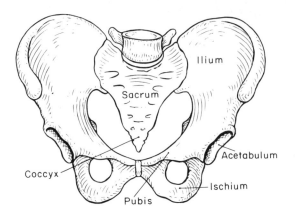

**Figure 4-25.** The pelvis is formed by the fusion of several bones. The acetabulum is the site for articulation with the femur.

the innominate bone; there are two innominate bones, the right and left.

LOWER LIMB

| Pelvic Girdle | | | Free Extremity |
|---|---|---|---|
| Three Fused Bones | | | Thigh |
|   Ischium | ⎫ | |   Femur |
|   Iliac | ⎬ | Innominate Bone | Leg |
| | | |   Tibia |
|   Pubis | ⎭ | |   Fibula |
| | | | Ankle |
| | | |   Talus |
| | | | Foot |
| | | |   Os Calcis |
| | | | Tarsus |
| | | |   Lunate |
| | | |   Hamate |
| | | |   3 Cuneiforms |
| | | | Metatarsals—5 |
| | | | Phalanges—12 |

The two innominate bones together form the pelvis, a highly vascular structure. The pelvis can be compared to a glass bowl. A fracture of one side of the bowl will be associated with fracture on the opposite side. Pelvic fractures are serious and usually are the result of extreme violence. The architecture of the pelvic bone forms the acetabulum, which houses the head of the femur, and together they form the hip joint (Figure 4-26). The hip joint is surrounded by ligamentous tissues that keep the femur in place to facilitate walking. The femur is divided into the head, which sits in the acetabulum; the neck; the greater trochanter; and the body. Fractures of the midshaft of the femur are very common in motorcycle and automobile accidents. These are major traumatic events and massive bleeding into the tissue can occur because of them.

The femur has condyles much like the humerus, and they function as the articular surface for the tibia. This forms the knee joint, which is then covered by the patella (Figures 4-26, 4-27). The tibia and fibula

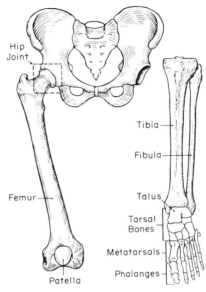

**Figure 4-26.** The pelvis, femur, and bones of the lower leg.

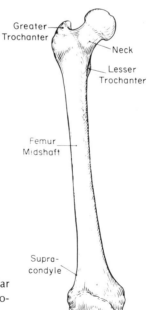

**Figure 4-27.** The femur is a large, heavy, vascular bone commonly injured in automobile and motorcycle accidents.

join to form the ankle joint as they ride on the talus. The bones of the foot include the talus, os calcis, and the five tarsal bones. The names of these bones are navicular, cuboid and the three cuneiforms. Beyond the tarsals are the metatarsal bones, much as in the hand, and finally the phalanges of the toes.

## JOINTS AND LIGAMENTS OF THE BODY

Bones are connected to one another by articulations or joints that allow relative motion between the two structures with a minimum of friction. Joint motion occurs in controlled planes generally designed to position the end organ, either a foot or hand, in a precise manner. Joints have coverings of hyaline cartilage, a specialized cartilage having a sparsity of cell population with a very abundant mucopolysaccharide background substance that is in essence a gel of long chain macromolecules with a large water content. This gel is trapped in a dense meshwork of collagen fibers. These hyaline cartilage surfaces act as the rubbing, bearing surfaces of the joint. The nonarticular portion of the joint is lined by a specialized tissue called synovium, which secretes a slippery, large molecular weight fluid called synovial fluid. This fluid acts as a lubricant for the joint and as a transfer medium for nutritional substances, waste products, and oxygen to and from the articular cartilage cells. This passive motion of material is probably enhanced by the pumping action of the joint during weightbearing. With squeezing of the joint surface, there is a flow of water in and out of the gel. If this delicate balance is upset by trauma, infection, or extrinsic disease processes, it can lead to destruction of the articular surface. Cartilage of the articular variety does have some limited capability of repairing itself; however, large defects are repaired primarily by the deposition of fibrocartilage as a substitute. This substitute material possesses different physical properties than hyaline cartilage, being composed of increased fibrous elements. Its ability to withstand long-term friction and wear seems less adequate and may fail with time. Damaged articular cartilage seems capable of responding by increasing its production of mucopolysaccharide background substance; however, the chemical composition is of a more immature variety that lacks the ability to withstand continued stress, and therefore degenerates more rapidly. Unless accurately repaired, disruptions of the joint cartilage surface will cause discontinuity in the smooth articular surface, and lead to early onset of degenerative changes as a consequence of increased friction.

Joints are intrinsically unstable structures and without additional support they would not function correctly. Each joint has an investing fibrous capsule that maintains the anatomic integrity of the joint, encloses the synovium, and provides the enclosed environment for the joint. However, the capsule itself has little intrinsic strength and the majority of joint stability comes from the surrounding ligamentous investment.

Ligaments are composed primarily of collagen (a multistranded molecule of protein) and are quite strong. Ligaments about joints attach from bone to bone beyond the confines of the joint capsule. This attachment is quite stout.

The joints can be divided into those of the upper limb and those of the lower limb. The shoulder joint of the upper limb is made up of the humerus (ball), which fits into the glenoid cavity of the scapula (socket). Because the glenoid cavity is shallow, the humerus is capable of a wide range of motion. Movements at the shoulder include those occurring between the humerus and the scapula and between the scapula and chest wall. However, in common usage, the movements are referred to the body as a whole. Thus:

1. Flexion—arm forward

2. Extension—arm backward

3. Abduction—arm away from the body

4. Adduction—arm toward the body

5. Circumduction—arm moved in a circle, all of the above movements in sequence

6. Inward Rotation—rotation of arm on its long axis, anterior surface of the arm turned to face the body

7. Outward Rotation—rotation of arm on its long axis, posterior surface of the arm to face the body

*Elbow Joint.*   This is a relatively complex joint because it must allow flexion and extension of the forearm on the arm as well as pronation and supination of the radius and ulna on each other (Figure 4-28). There are two different portions of the elbow joint wrapped in the same synovial membrane: the trochlea of the humerus fits into the semilunar notch of the ulna allowing for flexion and extension and limiting side-to-side motion (hinge joint).

1. Flexion—bringing the forearm forward towards the arm (decreases angle joint)

2. Extension—taking the forearm away from the arm (increases angle of the joint)

There is a joint between the radius and ulna, called the radial-ulnar joint. The head of the radius rotates on the radial notch of the ulna. This part of the joint, in combination with the distal radial-ulnar joint, allows the movements of pronation and supination.

1. Pronation—the radius crosses over the ulna and the palm faces down when the hand is placed on a table

2. Supination—the radius and ulna are parallel and the palm faces up when the hand is placed on a table

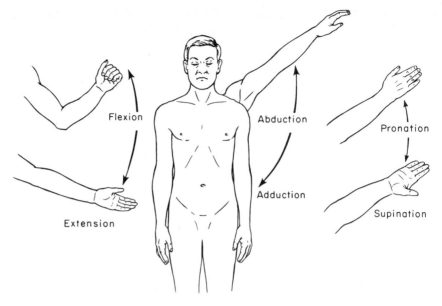

**Figure 4-28.** The common movements of the shoulder, elbow, and forearm.

*Wrist Joint.* The wrist joint (radial-carpal joint) is between the concave distal end of the radius and the convex surfaces of the carpal bones (scaphoid, lunate). This joint allows for the following movements:

1. Flexion—palm of hand toward palmar surface
2. Extension—dorsum (back of hand) toward dorsal forearm
3. Abduction—hand toward the radial side
4. Adduction—hand toward the ulnar side
5. Circumduction—all of the above movements in sequence

There are carpal-metacarpal, metacarpal-phalangeal, and interphalangeal joints. The most important carpal-metacarpal joint is the thumb. The thumb moves in the plane of the palm of the hand:

1. Flexion—thumb toward the hand
2. Extension—thumb away from the hand

The thumb moves at right angles to the palm of the hand:

1. Abduction—thumb away from the palm
2. Adduction—toward the palm
3. Circumduction—all of the above movements in sequence
4. Opposition—rotation of the thumb, and face the palmar surface of the fingers (very important for grasping)

The metacarpal-phalangeal joints can undergo flexion, extension, abduction, adduction, and circumduction. These movements are similar to those of the carpal-metacarpal joints. The thumb is capable of doing all of these motions and is called a hinge joint. The interphalangeal joints, which are between the fingers, allow for flexion and extension.

The joints of the lower limb include the hip joint. The hip joint is a ball and socket joint with the head of the femur fitting into the acetabulum of the innominate bone. The femur is capable of a wide range of motion, but in general the motions are more limited than the corresponding movements of the humerus. These movements are as follows:

1. Flexion—thigh forward
2. Extension—thigh backwards (very restricted; the thigh cannot form much more than a straight line with the trunk)
3. Abduction—thigh pulled laterally to the side
4. Adduction—thigh pulled medially
5. Circumduction—all of the above movements in sequence
6. Medial rotation—knee points medially toward the other leg
7. Lateral rotation—knee points laterally outward

*Knee Joint.* This is basically a hinge joint allowing for flexion and extension of the leg.

1. Flexion—leg up toward the thigh
2. Extension—leg straightened
3. Rotation—10 to 15 degrees of tibial rotation is possible

*Ankle Joint.* The ankle joint is a hinge joint that articulates between the distal end of the tibia, the tibial and fibular malleoli on the one hand, and the talus on the other. The movements permitted include the following (Figure 4-29):

1. Dorsiflexion—the dorsum of the foot drawn up toward the anterior leg
2. Plantar flexion—heel drawn up, toes point downward

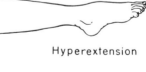

Hyperextension

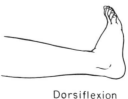

**Figure 4-29.** The foot in hyperextension and dorsiflexion.

Dorsiflexion

*Tarsal Joints.* There are a number of these gliding joints allowing the movement of one or more bones upon one another. The joint allowing most motion is the transverse/oblique tarsal joint, which is between the talus and calcaneus posteriorly, and the navicular and cuboid anteriorly. These joints collectively are responsible for the following movements:

1. Inversion—sole of foot faces medially
2. Eversion—sole of foot faces laterally

The remainder of the joints of the foot are involved primarily with the metatarsal-phalangeal joints. These joints allow for the following movements:

1. Flexion—toes downward
2. Extension—toes upward
3. Abduction—toes away from the midline of the second toe
4. Adduction—toes toward the midline of the second toe

The interphalangeal joints of the toes allow for curling of the toes and extension.

## SKELETAL MUSCLE OF THE BODY

Skeletal muscle is a specialized organ analogous to an accurately regulated controlled motor with attached pulley and cable systems by which joint motion can be made to occur in a precise fashion. The skeletal muscles operating the extremities are composed of a large number of fast twitch muscle fibers that can respond rapidly to voluntary reflex control from the central nervous system. The neuro-control system for muscles is a delicate mechanism at the spinal cord level.

Muscles are composed of bundles of skeletal muscle fibers architecturally aligned in a parallel fashion and surrounded by an enveloping fascia. The muscle mass is called the muscle belly, containing the contractural mechanism that allows the muscle to shorten. Each muscle cell contains specialized contractile protein molecules that are stimulated by chemically mediated nervous impulses (most likely by calcium ions) and link the nerve endplates to the contractural fibers. When stimulated, the contractile molecules (actin and myosin) are able to mechanically shorten relative to one another and thus cause the muscle belly to shorten.

Muscle generally originates on bones or ligaments, the attachment being accomplished by terminal interdigitation of collagen fibers within the muscle tissue directly onto the bone or ligament. At the distal working end of the muscle the interspersed collagen fibers coalesce into a solidified unit of collagen, called a tendon, which courses through a series of pulleys to implant itself distally onto a bone, again by an interdigitation of the distal elements of collagen. Generally the tendon crosses a joint and its action makes that joint operate through a certain range of motion. Muscles work primarily by shortening and, although they are able to relax or lengthen while still maintaining tension, for the most part elongation of a muscle is a passive process. Muscles work as a system of protagonist-antagonist couples in which one muscle designed to move a joint through a given range of motion will be offset by another muscle that can move the joint back through the same range of motion in order to reposition the joint in its starting attitude.

There are 656 muscles (327 pairs, two unpaired) in the body. We will deal here with the muscles of the upper and lower extremities.

## MUSCLES OF THE UPPER EXTREMITY

*Shoulder.* The degree of mobility at the shoulder joint is great and a wide range of movement is possible. The principal movements have been outlined in the section on joints. The primary muscles that move the shoulder joint are: (1) abduction—deltoid, (2) adduction—pectoralis major, (3) flexion—coracobrachialis, (4) extension—teres major, (5) external rotation—infraspinatus, and (6) inward rotation—latissimus dorsi. These muscles act in combination to effect other movements of the shoulder joint. The important muscle to be aware of is the deltoid muscle, which abducts or raises the shoulder laterally (Figure 4-30). Loss of motion of this muscle can occur with brachial plexus injuries to the posterior triangle of the neck or falls in which the back of the arm has been hit and the nerve to the deltoid muscle injured.

*Forearm.* The muscles that bring about flexion and extension at the elbow are: (1) flexion—biceps brachii (biceps muscle group), (2) extension—triceps brachii, (3) pronation—pronator teres, pronator quadratus, and (4) supination—biceps brachii, supinator (Figure 4-30).

The biceps can be appreciated by flexing the biceps muscles. Just posterior to this muscle belly on the medial aspect of the arm is the neurovascular bundle, which contains the brachial artery and median and ulnar nerves. Muscle and vessels are common sites of injury for gunshot and stab wounds of the arm.

*Wrist.* The wrist can be flexed or extended. The flexors are located on the volar aspect of the forearm and the extensors on the dorsal aspect. They are the following: (1) flexion—flexor carpi radialis and flexor carpi ulnaris, (2) extension—extensor carpi ulnaris, extensor carpi radialis longus, and brevis.

Both the flexor and extensor muscles of the fingers are located in these muscle compartments. Loss of flexion or extension of the fingers can be due to infections in these spaces or more proximal nerve injuries.

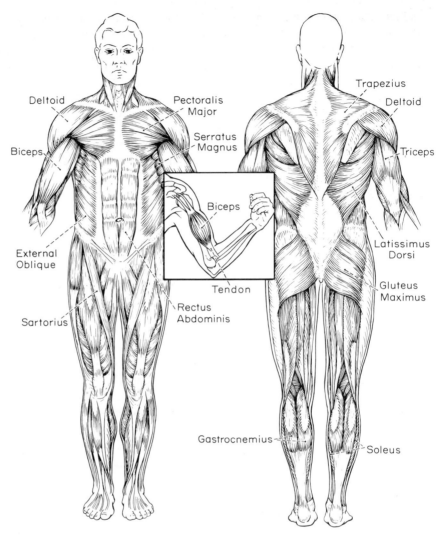

**Figure 4-30.** Skeletal muscles and an example of a tendon (insert).

## MUSCLES OF THE LOWER EXTREMITY

*Hip.* Movements of the joints of the hip have been outlined in the previous section. Muscles of this joint include: (1) flexion—iliopsoas, (2) extension—gluteus (buttocks), (3) adduction—adducti longus, brevis, and magnus (located on the medial aspect of the thigh), and (4) adduction—gluteus minimus and medius.

*Leg.* The principal actions produced at the knee joint are flexion and extension. However, some of the muscles have their insertions on the pelvic bone and consequently may bring about rotation, abduction, and adduction movements as well. These muscles include: (1) extension—femoris, and (2) flexion—sartorius (hamstring muscle).

Quadriceps muscles are the large muscle mass forming the anterior portion of the thigh (Figure 4-30). It is composed of four muscle heads, each of which is considered a separate muscle. All four heads converge into a common tendon and have a single insertion. The quadriceps is one of the largest and most powerful muscles of the body. It is the muscle that is injured during femur fractures. The hamstring muscles are those behind the posterior thigh that flex the knee. These muscles are principally antagonists to the extensors or quadriceps group on the anterior surface of the thigh.

*Foot.* Movements of the foot occur at the ankle and tarsal joints. Extension or plantar flexion (hyperextension) is the downward motion of the foot; flexion or dorsiflexion is the forward motion in which the foot is straightened (Figure 4-29). These movements take place at the ankle joint between the malleoli of the tibia and fibula and the talus. The muscles that act on the foot include: (1) plantar flexion of the foot—gastrocnemius soleus and associated muscles (commonly called the "gastroc" muscles), and (2) dorsiflexion—tibialis anterior and peroneus tertius. The remaining muscles in the leg contribute to fine flexion and extension of the toes and finer movements of the foot. These muscle groups will not be identified here.

## THE GENITOURINARY SYSTEM

### KIDNEY

The kidney is a paired organ located high in the abdomen, posterior (extraperitoneal) to the liver, spleen, and intestine (Figure 4-31). The kidney is protected by the ribs behind and the intra-abdominal organs in front. Each kidney is approximately the size of one's hand. It is a firm organ with a thin investing capsule. The firm consistency makes the kidney vulnerable to fracture from blunt abdominal trauma.

The kidneys together receive almost one-fourth of the total cardiac output. This high rate of blood flow means that an injury to the kidney may be associated with massive blood loss. Each kidney is composed of one million small units called nephrons. Each has a filter, the glomerulus, attached to a long meandering tubule (Figure 16-4). A number of tubules connect to a small duct for the passage of urine to the renal pelvis and ureter. The kidneys perform many complex functions. The most obvious is the regulation of fluid balance by the secretion of urine. However, more important functions are the maintenance of acid-base balance and the elimination of nitrogen waste products of metabolism.

The kidney also plays a role in the maintenance of blood pressure

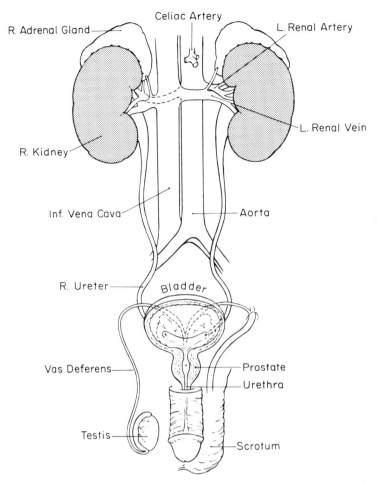

**Figure 4-31.** The adrenal glands reside above both kidneys, which lie in the retroperitoneum. Common sites of injury in the male are the testis, bladder, and urethra.

through secretion of a hormone, renin. It also supports the production of blood cells in the bone marrow by the secretion of a hormone, erythropoietin. Acute injury to the kidney is usually manifested by blood in the urine and/or swelling in the flank (lateral portion of the abdomen).

ADRENAL GLANDS

The adrenal glands are paired endocrine glands that reside on the superior portion of the kidneys. They secrete hormones necessary for metabolism, salt retention, and a general stress response. They can be injured during trauma.

# URETER

The ureter is a slender muscular tube that conducts urine from the kidney to the bladder. The ureter is approximately one centimeter in diameter. It runs along the abdominal wall behind the peritoneal cavity. Urine is propelled by segmental muscular contraction of the ureter. Acute obstruction of a ureter such as by a stone causes severe flank pain.

## BLADDER

The urinary bladder is a strong muscular organ that functions as a reservoir. It is located behind the pubic bone and when empty occupies a space approximately the size of a closed fist. The normal bladder has the capacity to hold a pint of liquid. When full, it may be palpable above the pubic bone and below the umbilicus.

The bladder is vulnerable to injury if blunt abdominal trauma occurs while it is full. It may also be punctured by sharp fragments of bone in a pelvic fracture. Blood in the urine is the usual sign of bladder injury; but in severe damage, the patient may be unable to void as the bladder contents have spilled out into the tissues.

## URETHRA

The urethra is a muscular tube that conducts urine from the bladder to the exterior. In the female, it runs just anterior to the anterior vaginal wall. In the male, it courses through the prostate gland and passes the length of the penis. The urethra is usually empty of fluid since it serves only as a conduit.

## ASSOCIATED URINARY TRACT STRUCTURES

The prostate gland is a small walnut-sized organ surrounding the urethra in the male as it passes from the bladder to the penis. The prostate adds fluid to the semen. The prostate may enlarge in older men to impede bladder emptying.

The testes are the primary organs of reproduction as they are the site of sperm formation. Sperm cells develop in a system of tubules by a series of cell divisions. These are called the seminiferous tubules. All of the tubules end in a series of ducts for the conduction of sperm to the epididymis. Between the seminiferous tubules are cells that produce testosterone, the hormone that determines masculine development including the growth of bone, muscle, penis, and beard.

The epididymis is a small organ immediately behind the testis. It serves as a conduit and a reservoir for sperm cells. The sperm undergo final maturation in the epididymis.

The vas deferens is the small muscular tube for the conduction of sperm from the epididymis to the urethra. The vas conducts sperm by way of muscular contractions. It empties via the ejaculatory ducts into the prostatic urethra, from whence the sperm pass out through the urethra by muscular contractions. Interruption of the vas deferens blocks the passage of sperm and produces sterility in the male.

The seminal vesicles are glands located behind the base of the bladder. They drain into the distal portion of the vas deferens, adding fluid and nutrients to the sperm.

## THE VASCULAR SYSTEM

The vascular system is divided into arteries, veins, and capillaries.

### ARTERIAL SYSTEM

Arteries are substantial structures that conduct oxygenated blood from the heart to the peripheral tissues. Arteries include the major arteries, such as the aorta, its branches, smaller arteries, arterioles, and finally the arteriolar portion of the capillary. Knowledge of the anatomy of the arteries is important in dealing with trauma, strokes, acute abdominal catastrophes, and the palpation of pulses in shock or cardiac arrest. Arteries begin at the base of the aorta where the aortic valve originates, and the first two arteries from the aorta are the right and the left coronary arteries (Figure 4-22). The aorta ascends in the mediastinum and gives off three major branches to the upper trunk (Figure 4-32). The first branch is the right innominate artery, which divides into the right common carotid and right subclavian arteries. The right subclavian artery travels under the clavicle through the axilla (armpits) to become the axillary artery. The axillary artery becomes the brachial artery as it travels down the inner aspect of the arm. The brachial artery divides at the elbow into the radial and ulnar arteries. The radial artery is palpable on the volar, radial aspect of the wrist. The ulnar and radial arteries divide into smaller branches to supply the hand.

The right common carotid artery divides into an external carotid artery and an internal carotid artery. The point at which one artery divides into two is called a *bifurcation*. At points of bifurcation atherosclerosis tends to occur, and the carotid artery is one of the more common places that this develops. This may lead to stroke syndromes, either transient or complete. Knowledge of the anatomy of the carotid artery is necessary for purposes of palpation during cardiac arrest (witnessed or nonwitnessed), as well as the possibility of stimulating the carotid body to enhance vagal response in the diagnosis and treatment of cardiac dysrhythmias. The carotid body resides outside of the artery at the bifurcation of the common carotid artery. Its function is to sense pulse

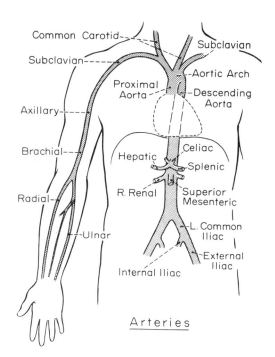

Figure 4-32. The arteries of the arm, neck, thorax, and abdomen.

pressure and regulate systemic blood pressure. The common carotid artery bifurcation occurs at the cranial portion of the thyroid cartilage ("Adam's apple") or at the angle of the mandible. The left carotid artery is the next branch of the aorta and supplies the left side of the brain, and the third branch is the left subclavian artery. The subclavian arteries on either side give off two smaller arteries, called vertebral arteries, which travel up the cervical spine to nourish the brain. The brain, therefore, receives its blood supply from four sources and these join at the base of the brain forming a circle called the Circle of Willis (Figures 4-2, 4-13). From this circle the various arterial branches are given off to the appropriate portions of the brain.

One of the most common sites of injury to the aorta is that portion just distal to the left subclavian artery. At this point the aorta may fracture during deceleration injuries, such as occur in automobile or airplane accidents. The energy that is absorbed in this sudden deceleration very often will be directed at that portion of the aorta just beyond the left subclavian artery. In some patients the pleura over the aorta prevents rupture into the left chest and will keep the patient from exsanguinating (Chapter 14).

The aorta gives off intercostal blood vessels that supply the chest wall; then it passes through the diaphragm to successively give off the celiac artery (liver, stomach and spleen), the superior mesenteric artery (small and large intestines), two arteries to the kidney (renal arteries), and the inferior mesenteric artery which supplies the left colon (Figure 4-32).

Distally the aorta bifurcates into the right and left common iliac arteries. Again, at this point of bifurcation atherosclerosis and occlusion often develop. The common iliac artery divides into the external and internal iliacs. The latter supplies blood to portions of the bowel, bladder, and pelvic structures. The internal iliac (hypogastric) artery and its branches are often torn in pelvic fractures and can produce serious bleeding. The external iliac passes under the inguinal ligament to become the femoral artery. The femoral artery and its relationship to other structures in the groin is shown in Figure 4-33. It is important to remember these relationships for the palpation of pulses, the drawing of blood, and the occlusion of blood vessels following injury. A helpful mnemonic is Nerve–Artery–Vein–Empty space, or NAVE. The femoral artery divides into the superficial and deep femoral arteries, which travel down the leg. The superficial femoral artery becomes the popliteal artery, which is behind the knee and divides into the anterior and posterior tibial branches to become the dorsalis pedis artery on the top of the foot and the posterior tibial artery behind the medial malleolus (Figure 4-34).

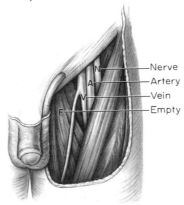

**Figure 4-33.** The vascular anatomy of the groin. The structures from the lateral to medial aspects are the nerve, artery, vein, and an empty space. The first letters spell NAVE, a useful way of remembering the location of these structures.

## VENOUS SYSTEM

Veins accompany arteries and their purpose is to return blood from the peripheral tissues to the heart. A handy rule is that veins above the diaphragm run in front of arteries and veins below the diaphragm run posterior to the arteries, except for the left renal vein, which must cross the aorta to enter the vena cava. An illustration of this is the course of the subclavian vein (often used for venipuncture in cardiac arrest), which runs anterior or superficial to the subclavian artery. The same can be said for the internal jugular vein and other veins that reside above the diaphragm. The confluence of veins from the head and face forms the internal and external jugular veins, which join

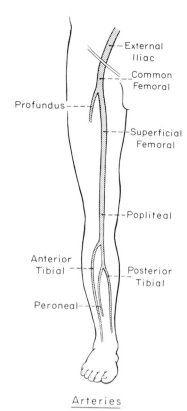

External
Iliac

Common
Femoral

Profundus

Superficial
Femoral

Popliteal

Anterior
Tibial

Posterior
Tibial

Peroneal

Arteries

**Figure 4-34.** The arteries of the leg beginning with the common femoral artery at the groin. The posterior tibial artery resides behind the medial malleolus, and the dorsalis pedis artery (not shown) is on the dorsum of the foot.

the veins from the arms to become the superior vena cava and enter the right atrium. Veins from the arm are important in terms of administration of intravenous fluids (Figure 4-35).

The major veins on the dorsum of the hand should be noted. The cephalic vein begins at the wrist over the head of the radius and is an important vein for the infusion of intravenous fluids in emergency situations. This vein travels up the lateral aspect of the forearm and is joined to the medially placed basilic vein by the median cubital vein. The cephalic vein continues up the lateral aspect of the forearm to empty into the subclavian vein at the shoulder. The basilic vein travels up the inner aspect of the arm to connect with the deep veins of the arm to join and form the axillary vein and then the subclavian vein.

The veins from the lower extremities can be divided into superficial and deep veins. The superficial vein network is called the saphenous vein system and that drains into the femoral vein at the groin (Figure 4-36). The saphenous vein system begins at the foot and travels over the anterior portion of the medial malleolus and is an important landmark. This is the area in which intravenous solutions may need to be given in shock, trauma, or cardiac arrest. The vein then travels up the inner aspect of the leg and becomes too deep for the usual venipuncture

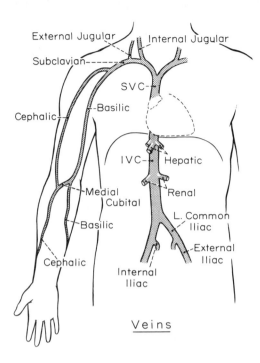

External Jugular    Internal Jugular
Subclavian
SVC
Cephalic    Basilic
IVC    Hepatic
Medial
Cubital    Renal
Basilic    L. Common
Iliac
Cephalic    External
Iliac
Internal
Iliac

Veins

**Figure 4-35.** Veins of the arm, neck, thorax, and abdomen. The cephalic vein begins at the wrist and travels up the lateral aspect of the arm. The median cubital vein connects the basilic vein with the cephalic vein.

techniques. It joins the femoral vein at the groin (inguinal region).

The deep vein system is divided into the smaller branches of the calf called the anterior, posterior, and peroneal veins, which join to become the popliteal vein and then the deep femoral vein. The veins from the leg become the iliac and finally the inferior vena cava. The two-caval system includes the major veins returning to and joining the heart at the right atrium.

Veins are thin-walled structures whose purpose is to conduct blood back to the heart from the peripheral tissues. They have a filling capacity, which means they can be dilated quite extensively. At any given time, 80 percent of the blood volume is located within veins. During over-transfusion and overhydration, these veins can dilate considerably; therefore, they have a much greater capacity for storing blood than do arteries. Knowledge of venous anatomy, especially superficial venous anatomy, is extremely important in terms of initiation of intravenous therapy and administration of drugs and blood during a cardiac arrest situation, as well as when vessel occlusion is necessary after a penetrating injury.

*Summary*     This chapter is an extremely important and basic one. The basic anatomy of the entire body is presented, along with a glossary of terms used in anatomic descriptions. Many diagrams and figures further elucidate these important subjects.

Because of the total necessity for the paramedic to become

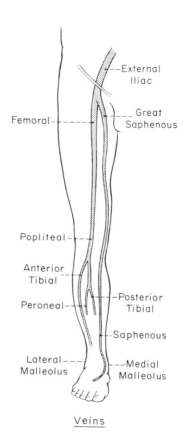

External
Iliac

Great
Saphenous

Femoral

Popliteal

Anterior
Tibial

Posterior
Tibial

Peroneal

Saphenous

Lateral
Malleolus

Medial
Malleolus

Veins

**Figure 4-36.** Superficial and deep veins of the leg. The superficial vein is called the great saphenous vein, and it passes in front of the medial malleolus. This is an important landmark for starting intravenous fluids.

thoroughly acquainted with this material in its entirety, we do not list important summary points here. It is urgent for this entire chapter to become a total part of the daily routine of the experience and work of the paramedic.

Anthony, C. P. and Kolthoff, N. J. *Textbook of Anatomy and Physiology.* St. Louis, Mo: C. V. Mosby Co., 1971.

Steen, E. B. and Montagu, A. *Anatomy and Physiology.* New York, N.Y.: Barnes and Noble, Inc., 1959.

Warwick, Roger and Williams, Peter L. (editors). *Gray's Anatomy,* 35th ed. Philadelphia, Pa: W. B. Saunders Co., 1973.

*Bibliography*

# Chapter 5

# BODY COMPOSITION, FLUIDS, AND ELECTROLYTES

To understand fluid and electrolyte changes in the human being requires repetitive study and frequent exposure to clinical problems. Fluid and electrolyte physiology cannot be learned solely by reading or by dealing with problems in the field. Nowhere in medicine is the study of basic science and physiology more applicable to clinical problems at the bedside than in the area of fluid and electrolyte disturbances. Every physician has his own comprehension of fluid and electrolyte problems, but often cannot express them in understandable fashion. This lack of communication usually confuses the reader because the subject is abstract, while the problems facing doctors and paramedical personnel are not. The understanding of the body composition, interaction among the various body spaces, and the electrochemical physiology involved in ion transport are all necessary parts of understanding fluid and electrolyte disturbances.

## BODY COMPOSITION AND COMPARTMENTS

When one steps on the scale and determines his weight, he is determining the total weight of a body composed of many different substances and divisions of tissue. Body weight and build vary greatly from individual to individual and are determined by genetic factors, sex, dietary habits, age, and exercise. The adult female body, for example, contains a higher percentage of body fat than the male who has more lean (muscular and cellular) tissue. Before puberty, the male and female body compositions are nearly identical. A baby has more fat than lean tissue. The individual, male or female, who eats abundantly has more fat than is needed, and his body composition is thus rich in fat.

Body weight is composed of the following divisions: (1) body fat, largely neutral storage fat that is anhydrous (without water); (2) lean body solids, consisting chiefly of skeletal solids (bone) and soft tissue solids, the heaviest of which are the structured proteins in the body protoplasm; (3) electrolytes: while of crucial importance in determining water distribution in the body, their weight is negligible, consisting of only a few grams; and (4) body water: intracellular and extracellular water (interstitial water and plasma), which constitute 60 percent of the body weight.

Our body weight fluctuates throughout the day as a function of ingestion and excretion of food and water. The weight is at its peak in the late afternoon or early evening. Overnight, from one to two kg disappear by the insensible loss of water through the lungs; and as food is oxidized to carbon dioxide and water, the former is exhaled and the latter is excreted in the urine. Over short periods of time, appreciable gains in weight are due largely to an increase in body water. The synthesis of new protoplasm or the deposition of fat takes days to weeks to affect changes in the total body weight.

Weight loss due to dissolution of tissue (fat and skeletal muscle) occurs more rapidly than weight gain, particularly after injury or acute illness, when fat oxidation rates are accelerated and tissue loss may be as much as 500 g (1 lb) per day. Rapid weight loss may also occur when there is massive loss of water from the body, such as with diarrhea.

As stated previously, the body is composed primarily of fat, water, and lean tissue mass. In normal individuals, the amount of water in the body varies according to the amount of lean tissue present. The lean tissues (cellular tissue) containing the oxidizing and energy exchanging protoplasm are composed largely of skeletal muscle and organs such as the liver, kidney, intestines, lung, heart, and brain. The soft lean tissues are constant in their water content, containing approximately 73 percent water by weight. The rest of the body, other than the skeleton, consists of fat. This nonaqueous neutral fat, therefore, varies inversely to the proportion occupied by water. (The more fat, the less water is a rule that holds for any age.) An obese female whose body composition is 45 percent fat has the same total body water as her thinner counterpart (Figure 5-1). Small losses of water in a fat person will induce more marked changes than equal losses in a muscular man whose total body water is much greater.

Total body water has been determined accurately by laboratory and clinical studies. The concept of using radioactive isotopes to measure total body water is sound and the principle is simple. The measurement is analogous to determining the volume of water in a large tub using a marking dye. When a known volume and concentration of dye is instilled into the tub, the dye then distributes itself evenly. After mixing, a second known quantity of the tub water is used to measure the new dye concentrate. A simple ratio of the concentrations will allow determination of the quantity of water in the tub (Figure 5-2). The same principle applies to total body water measurements. A measured volume of isotope is injected intravenously with a known concentration. It is allowed to

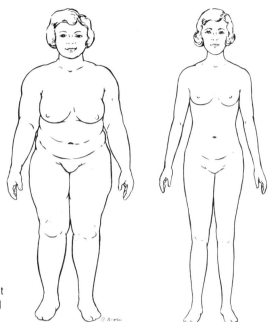

**Figure 5-1.** The two females pictured here have the same extracellular fluid volume, but they differ in their weight and body fat.

equilibrate with the tissues over a given period of time. A second series of blood samples will measure the decay of radioactive isotope in the serum and from that total body water can be determined. These tests have been proven in the laboratory and clinical situations by measuring the total body water just before death. After death, the body is desiccated (dried). The dried weight is subtracted from the wet weight to determine the total water.

In the normal adult male, total body water is 55 percent of body weight with an overall range of 50 to 60 percent depending upon body build. For example, a 70 kg male has a total body water of 42,000 ml (70 kg × 60% = 42 kg × 1000 = 42,000 ml). In calculating body spaces, 1.0 kg is equivalent to 1000 ml of water. The more obese man has smaller body water relative to weight, whereas the lean well-trained athlete has a somewhat higher value. The normal total body water in

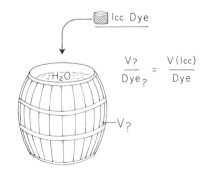

**Figure 5-2.** A simple formula for calculating the amount of water in a barrel. This principle applies to the measurement of fluid spaces in the human.

the female is in the range of 50 percent of body weight with an overall range of 45 to 55 percent. As mentioned previously, the sex differential in body water appears at about puberty when the female grows more subcutaneous fat as a part of her normal body composition and the male puts on more skeletal muscle as a secondary sex characteristic. In the infant (less than one year of age), total body water is somewhat higher, and measures up to 75 percent of the body weight.

## EXTRACELLULAR AND INTRACELLULAR WATER: BLOOD VOLUME

A portion of the body water is not contained within the cells (Figure 5-3). This extracellular space has been divided into interstitial water and blood volume water. These spaces have also been measured by isotopes. Various studies have shown that the extracellular volume of water is about 20 percent of body weight. This 20 percent includes the interstitial water (16 percent) and the plasma volume (4 percent). Extracellular fluid is that portion of body water engaged in transporting substances back and forth between the outside world and the body cells. It is the area in which body tonicity is determined largely by sodium content.

Intracellular water is the difference between total body water and extracellular water. Body intracellular water cannot be accurately measured, so the difference between total body water and extracellular water approximates cell water. Cell water is approximately 40 percent of body weight.

The blood volume is the sum of the plasma and red cell volumes varying between 5 to 8 percent of body weight. In the male, a blood volume of 7 percent of body weight, and in the female 6 percent of

## WATER DISTRIBUTION

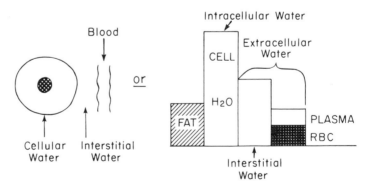

**Figure 5-3.** Distribution of water in the body includes the blood, interstitial space, and cells. Fat is anhydrous; i.e., it does not contain water.

body weight, are good clinical estimates. It is important to know this value and its use for assessing blood loss due to hemorrhage. As in the other compartments of the body, the total blood volume varies inversely with obesity. An extremely obese man has a blood volume closer to the range of 5 to 6 percent of body weight, whereas an athlete in top condition with little fat has a blood volume which may approach 8 percent of his body weight. These factors must all be considered when evaluating a person's blood volume and using his weight as a guide to blood replacement.

The blood volume is divided into plasma volume and red cell volume. In a normal healthy man the plasma volume is about 3 to 5 percent of body weight. Red cell volume, on the other hand, is from 2 to 4 percent of body weight. The concentration of red blood cells in the peripheral blood is called the *hematocrit*. This is measured by collecting blood from a vein in a thin tube. The tube is then spun in a centrifuge so that the red cells settle. The total content of the test tube is 100 percent, and the hematocrit is that percent of the tube occupied by red cells (Chapter 3). The hematocrit only reflects concentration and does not reflect blood volume. Any disorder that causes selective loss of plasma (burns) in preference to red blood cells will raise the hematocrit. Although the concentration of red blood cells increases in burns, total blood volume is reduced. The normal hematocrit for males is 40 to 47 percent, and 35 to 42 percent for females.

The solid proteins are those proteins which exist in the extracellular phase, and which reside in the interstitial fluid and in the blood volume. The most important of these proteins is albumin. In addition, there are other specialized proteins that are responsible for immune responses, coagulation, enzyme production, and many other functions. The solid proteins are referred to as the *plasma proteins*. Proteins are concentrated in the plasma and in the extracellular fluid and may also be located in the lymphatic system. The normal concentration of solid protein in the plasma is 6–7 g/100 ml. The albumin fraction is 4–5 g/100 ml, and the globulin concentration is 2–3 g/100 ml. Albumin is a large molecule (mol wt 60,000) that resides in the blood and maintains colloid osmotic pressure (see below).

## ELECTROLYTES

Inorganic salts are dissolved in the body water spaces. These salts include potassium phosphate (found mostly inside cells) and sodium chloride (the predominant salt in extracellular fluid). Calcium chloride, magnesium chloride, sodium bicarbonate, and a variety of other salts are present in smaller amounts. When these molecules dissolve in water, each salt crystal splits into millions of tiny particles called ions (Figure 5-4). There is an equal number of positively charged ions (cations) and negatively charged ions (anions). Any water solution that contains charged particles conducts electricity, and can be called an electrolyte solution. The variety of salts present in body fluids are often lumped together under the term electrolytes. The important positively charged electrolytes include sodium, potassium, calcium, and magnesium. The important negatively charged electrolytes are chloride, bicarbonate, and phosphorus.

PARTICLES and SOLUTIONS

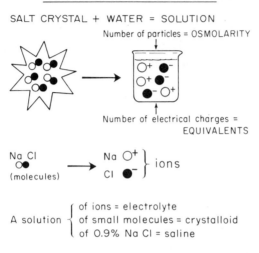

**Figure 5-4.** Salt crystals dissolved in water produce a solution. Solutions can be characterized by their osmolarity, milliequivalents, and type of solute. Solutions with salts produce positively and negatively charged ions.

Because the atoms of the chemicals mentioned above have different molecular weights, the number of ions formed when one gram of sodium chloride is dissolved is different from the number of ions formed when one gram of potassium phosphate is dissolved, which, in turn, is different from a gram of calcium chloride, etc. Because chemical reactions depend more on the number of charged particles than the weight of each particle, the concept of *equivalent weight* was developed to facilitate calculations. One equivalent weight of sodium chloride (NaCl), for example, is 58.5 g. This contains the same number of particles as one equivalent weight of potassium chloride (KCl), which is 74.5 g. How many equivalents of sodium ($Na^+$) are there in a solution containing 0.85 g of NaCl/100 ml? This solution is equal to 8.5 g NaCl/1000 ml. Divide the 8.5 g by the equivalent weight (the molecular weight divided by the charges on the ion) of NaCl, which is 58.5. This gives 0.155 mEq/l. All body fluids contain approximately 0.3 equivalents per liter. Extracellular fluid, for example, contains 0.14 equivalents of sodium, 0.005 equivalents of potassium, 0.1 equivalent of chloride, 0.028 equivalents of bicarbonate, and smaller amounts of other electrolytes. To make the numbers easier to deal with, these values are expressed as thousandths of an equivalent, or milliequivalents. Hence, the values for extracellular fluid become sodium, 140 mEq/l, potassium, 5 mEq/l, etc.

The principal function of sodium chloride is its water-holding capacity. For example, if table salt is left out in humid air, the salt will take up the water. If the humidity is high it becomes a moist mass, taking up and holding water out of the surrounding air. Salt essentially does the same thing in the body, holding water in the extracellular and vascular space. Sodium is an extracellular cation, and, although it may penetrate into the cell, it is actively removed by "sodium pumps" (Figure 5-5). Sodium leaking inside the cell is a pathological condition and can lead to heart, brain, and other organ abnormalities. Since sodium is freely equilibrated in the extracellular fluid space and the blood volume space, its concentration can easily be measured. A blood sample measurement for sodium concentration would give a normal result of 135 to 145 mEq/l. When the serum sodium concentration falls (hyponatremia), it is usually the result of injudicious fluid administration, or, rarely, severe vomiting and hormone imbalance. The converse, hypernatremia or increased sodium concentration, is a result of selective water loss and/or the administration of concentrated sodium solutions to the patient.

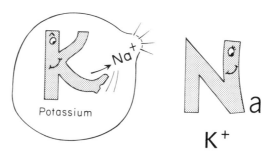

**Figure 5-5.** Sodium is an extracellular ion and potassium is an intracellular ion. This relationship must be protected for the normal functioning of all types of body tissues.

Potassium ($K^+$), on the other hand, is located primarily within cells and is found in low concentration outside of the cell. Ninety-eight percent of potassium in the body is located intracellularly and only two percent is located outside of the cell. The normal serum concentration of potassium is 3.5 to 4.5 mEq/l. This serum concentration is the same as the extracellular fluid concentration because they are in equilibrium. The intracellular concentration of potassium, however, may range from 130 to 150 mEq/l. Potassium and sodium are cations and therefore reside on either side of cell membranes, giving a balance of electrical neutrality. Some clinical illnesses can change the extracellular concentration of potassium and may produce profound changes in the patient. For example, a serum potassium of 7.0 mEq/l will cause cardiac dysrhythmias or even cardiac standstill. On the other hand, a serum potassium of 1.5 mEq/l may also produce cardiac dysrhythmias or occasionally intestinal obstruction. Therefore, even though the concentration of potassium is small outside of the cell, the absolute extracellular level is critical for proper body function.

The remaining cations (calcium and magnesium) are important to the normal function of nerves and muscles including the cardiac muscle.

These ions, although important in specific situations, are not a common cause of clinical disorders. Hypocalcemia (a reduction in serum-ionized calcium) produces muscle spasm and facial twitching.

The anions (chloride, bicarbonate, and phosphorus) are not generally the primary cause of clinical diseases. Abnormalities in their concentration are usually the result of disorders in sodium or potassium balance.

## OSMOTIC AND ONCOTIC PRESSURE

Another way of describing the number of particles in a solution is to describe the amount of osmotic pressure that would be exerted by the particles in solution (osmolality) compared to water alone (Figure 5-4). The number of particles in one equivalent weight of salt is referred to as one milliosmole (mOsm). For the convenience reasons outlined above, particles in biologic fluids are measured in milliosmoles. The reason for developing this system is to have a convenient way to describe the numbers of particles that have no electrical charge (such as glucose) and the particles that have more than one electrical charge on one particle, such as phosphate ions.

Osmotic properties are determined by the number of particles in solution, not by their weight or molecular charges. For example, one molecule of glucose (mol wt 180) has the same osmotic potential as one molecule of albumin (mol wt 60,000). In general, the more molecules of salt or sugar in a solution, the greater the osmotic pressure. Osmotic pressure is a pressure that a solution must possess in order to keep it in equilibrium with the pure solvent when the two are separated by a membrane permeable only to the solvent (Figure 5-6). This is similar to a cell wall where the membrane is semipermeable, and the osmotic pressure produced by the total number of molecules on either side must be equal. Osmotic pressure will change the boiling points and freezing points of solutions. This is analogous to antifreeze, a solution which when added to water will lower the freezing point or raise the boiling point. The smaller the molecular weight of the substance in solution, the more the osmolar effect per unit of solution. For example, sodium chloride is a small molecule and exerts a greater osmotic pressure because it produces more particles per unit weight than a larger molecule. The osmolality of a solution is measured clinically by recording the freezing point of the solute (for example plasma) as compared to water. The results are expressed as mOsm/liter of solutes.

Unlike the total electrolyte concentration, which is exactly the same in all body fluids, the osmolality (or number of milliosmoles) is slightly different in different body fluids. Plasma contains approximately 300 milliosmoles per liter (mOsm/l). Any water solution that contains 300 milliosmoles of particles is said to be isotonic with plasma. A solution of 5 g of glucose in 100 ml of water will contain 252 milliosmoles per

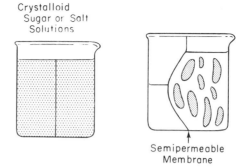

Crystalloid
Sugar or Salt
Solutions

**Figure 5-6.** Osmotic pressure is equally distributed on both sides of a semipermeable membrane. Oncotic pressure is higher on one side since large molecules cannot pass through the membrane. Oncotic pressure is produced primarily by proteins (albumin).

Semipermeable
Membrane

liter, hence is not isotonic with plasma. In contrast, 0.85 g of sodium chloride dissolved in 100 ml of water makes the isotonic fluid called normal saline. The latter solution's osmolality is 308 mOsm/l, or nearly identical to plasma. Solutions that contain more particles than blood are called *hypertonic*; solutions that contain fewer particles are called *hypotonic*.

Colloid osmotic pressure (oncotic pressure) is that very tiny fraction of total osmotic pressure exerted by colloids. Colloids are primarily protein molecules that do not readily cross capillary walls or cell membranes (Figure 5-6). Although the total number of protein molecules is small in comparison to ions, the colloid osmotic pressure is immensely important in maintaining fluid within the vascular compartment. The total osmotic pressure is the same on both sides of a cell membrane, but the effective colloid osmotic pressure is greater in the plasma than in the rest of the interstitial extracellular fluid. Were this not true, fluid would leak from the capillary into the interstitial space and produce edema.

## ACUTE CHANGES IN BODY FLUID SPACES

### FLUID LOSSES INSIDE THE BODY

*Third spacing* is a term used when solutions are lost in the area of tissue injury, but not from the body itself (Figure 5-7). For example, the patient who has sustained a major burn loses plasma-rich fluid into the burn area, which is outside of the circulation but still contained within the body. This third space phenomenon can occur in conditions such as burns, crush injuries, inflammation such as peritonitis or cellulitis of the leg, and intestinal obstruction. The fluid that enters the third space is usually a protein-rich fluid if the phenomenon is a result of trauma or inflammation. This robbing of the other fluid spaces causes

"THIRD" SPACE

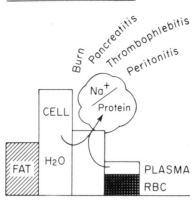

**Figure 5-7.** When damage occurs to body tissues, fluid that is generally rich in protein and sodium is lost into the injury site. This phenomenon is called "third spacing."

a loss of water and protein from the effective body spaces. Understanding this is important, since the replacement solution used to treat these various clinical entities must match the solution that is lost. For example, it would be incorrect to give a patient who has had a burn a glucose solution when it is known that salt and proteins are being lost into the area of injury.

*Dehydration (External Losses of Fluids) and "Desalting."* External losses differ from internal losses in that the fluids are lost to the body system completely. This differs from the preceding discussion (third spacing) where there is maldistribution within a new space in the body. Changes in plasma concentrations are rarely due to the external loss of fluid alone, but are usually the result of losses and dislocations of fluid, various treatments, inward movement of cell water, fat oxidation, and lung and kidney compensation mechanisms. It is appropriate, therefore, to scrutinize the term "dehydration" to find out just what this term means.

*True Dehydration.* If an orange were allowed to lay in the sun, it would lose water and shrivel. The concentration of its solute would rise abruptly and it would become dehydrated. When human plasma is placed in a vacuum distillation apparatus, water is removed and the plasma becomes dehydrated. If a man lies in the desert sun or if he floats on the tropic seas in a life raft without water, he becomes dehydrated. In all these situations of true dehydration, concentrations of solute rise because of the removal of water from the body. True dehydration, therefore, is desiccation. This is a relatively rare occurrence in clinical practice, and the term, therefore, is misleading. The term really should be used for the specific clinical situation in which water is lost and the solute concentration rises, such as with drying out or desiccation.

*Dehydration (Common Usage).* For the more common loss of water with salt, there is no good single word. Dehydration is also used for this situation, but *desalting water loss* appears to be more precise since there is loss of water, salt, and solutes from the body. An example would be massive diarrhea or vomiting. When a patient vomits, he loses water as well as hydrogen ions, sodium, potassium, and chloride. When diarrhea occurs, there are great losses in water as well as in sodium and potassium. Other sources of water loss from the body can occur from pathologic losses through the kidney, as when a patient is given diuretics or has a kidney problem that causes losses of sodium and water from the body. Despite the misuse of the word dehydration for these conditions, it has become so ingrained that it has come to mean both water loss and water plus solute loss.

Additional losses of water can also occur through the skin by sweating. Sweat contains sodium, but the concentration is not the same as in plasma. Therefore, as one sweats he loses more water relative to sodium, which tends to desiccate his tissues, and this causes a rising solute concentration at the same time he has also lost sodium from his body environment. A common problem is to sweat and replace the lost water but not the lost salt. For example, a man who sweats heavily working in the sun and then drinks a large quantity of ice-cold water will, minutes later, find that he feels waterlogged. Most individuals will compensate for large sweat losses by the intake of sodium-free water. If this situation is allowed to progress, hyponatremia occurs. This can lead to muscular cramps, prostration, coma, and possibly death.

The loss of water from the lungs is a normal continuing process of water loss. Although this may not be a factor in the initial onset of an illness, it becomes critically important as the patient's illness progresses. Pulmonary water losses are strictly water and do not include electrolytes. The most common cause of pulmonary water loss outside of the hospital is the patient with a permanent tracheostomy. He may lose large amounts of water through his lungs and become severely dehydrated.

## BODY COMPENSATION FOR FLUID LOSSES

The body has a set of regulatory systems that take effect when fluid is lost from the system, either within a third space contained in the body or outside of the body itself. The most protected function in the body is maintenance of a normal blood volume. This takes precedence over all other regulatory mechanisms, and the body's compensation for fluid loss is predominant. If a person loses fluid that is rich in sodium and has a reduction in his plasma blood volume, the compensation mechanisms are regulated by hormonal influences. Sodium is retained in the kidney as a result of a sodium-retaining hormone secreted by the adrenal gland. Water is retained in the kidney by a hormone called antidiuretic hormone which is created by the pituitary gland. This hormone prevents further losses of water through the kidney. The water located in the extracellular fluid space, in particular the lymphatic system, is immediately called on to respond to the fluid loss by transporting its water into the vascular space. This water loss from the extracellular fluid space is compensated for by cellular water that moves into the extracellular fluid space, then subsequently moves into the vascular space. The water that is being used to compensate for losses elsewhere is low in sodium since it comes from inside the cells, and the patient soon tends to become hypotonic. That is, his osmotic pressure falls as he loses sodium from his system and it is replaced by sodium-free water from cells. The phenomenon of water returning to the system via the capillaries or through the lymphatic system is commonly termed *"transcapillary refilling."* This mechanism will allow the patient to survive sudden losses in fluid in time to be transported to receive specific therapy.

During hemorrhage or shock, an additional compensation mechanism for fluid loss is replacement by ingestion of water through the mouth. Although this is not practical in the field, it is a means of restoring fluid loss under ordinary conditions (exercise with sweating). Thirst is a result of impulses from osmoreceptors in the neck to the brain (hypothalamus). These osmoreceptors recognize a reduction in blood volume as well as an increase in solutes in the blood. The increase in solutes occurs after trauma since metabolites are entering the bloodstream raising plasma osmolality. This sensation of thirst is extremely common and fiercely noted by patients in hemorrhagic shock and fluid loss. It is another body compensation mechanism for reduction in blood volume and/or extracellular fluid volume.

This discussion emphasizes that when dealing with fluid and electrolyte problems, one must understand the rate of fluid loss, the type of fluid loss, and the space from which the fluid is being lost. Table 5-1 shows the clinical stages of different levels of dehydration (or desalting). Multiplying the percent of dehydration by the body weight will give a good estimate of the amount of water loss.

*Summary*

The subject of fluid and electrolytes as related to body composition is important to understand. As the paramedic is asked to become more and more involved in the diagnosis and treatment of various illnesses, he will be expected to utilize this type of information in his daily activities.

*Important
Points to
Remember*

Body weight is composed of body fat, lean solids (bone and soft tissues), electrolytes (minor), and body water (60 percent of body weight).

The more fat present in the body, the less water there is; thus small losses of water are more dangerous in fat people.

Total body water in the adult male is 50 to 60 percent of body weight, and in the female it approximates 45 to 55 percent. Infants

TABLE 5-1. DEHYDRATION AND CLINICAL MANIFESTATION          *155*

| Percentage of Body Weight in Kilograms | Degree of Dehydration | Clinical Manifestations |
|---|---|---|
| 5% | Mild | Detectable from a history such as vomiting. May appear to have a dry mouth or rapid breathing. A clinical guess. |
| 10% | Moderate | The skin turgor is poor (estimated by pinching the skin). The patient's eyes are sunken and he is irritable. However, the peripheral circulation is adequate, i.e., normal pulse, blood pressure, and warm skin. |
| 20% | Severe | The patient is moribund; the eyes are sunken and dry; the skin turgor is poor; the mucus membranes are parched; and the extremities are cold, dry, and mottled. Blood pressure and pulse changes are also sometimes noted, i.e., lower blood pressure and more rapid pulse. |

and small children may have up to 75 percent total body water. Total body water is comprised of intra- and extracellular spaces. The extracellular volume is 20 percent of body weight, of which 16 percent is interstitial and 4 percent is intravascular (plasma volume).

Blood volume is the sum of plasma and red cell volumes; it varies from to 5 to 8 percent of body weight. Plasma volume is 3 to 5 percent and red cell volume is 2 to 4 percent.

A water solution that contains charged particles conducts electricity and is called an electrolyte solution.

Salts that dissolve in water split into positively and negatively charged particles called ions (positive = cation; negative = anion).

The salts dissolved in our body solutions are called electrolytes. The positive ones include sodium, potassium, calcium, and magnesium. The negatives are chloride, bicarbonate, and phosphorus. The concentration of electrolytes in body fluids is expressed as milliequivalents (mEq). All body fluids contain approximately 300 mEq/liter (150 of cations and 150 of anions).

The principal function of sodium chloride is its water-holding capacity. (Sodium is an extracellular cation and measures 135–145 mEq/l.)

Potassium is located primarily within cells and is found in low concentration outside of cells. Serum levels are 3.5 to 4.5 mEq/l. Calcium and magnesium are important for nerve and muscle function.

The amount of pressure that particles in solution exert is called osmotic pressure and is measured in milliosmoles. The more particles of molecules the greater the osmotic pressure.

Plasma contains approximately 300 milliosmoles/liter. Any water solution containing this same amount is isotonic with plasma. Isotonic sodium chloride (saline) contains 0.85 grams (hence 300 mOsm) in 100 ml water. Five percent glucose contains 252 mOsm and is not quite isotonic.

Solutions containing more particles than blood are hypertonic; those with fewer are hypotonic. Colloid osmotic pressure is that pressure exerted by protein molecules, and is important in maintaining fluid in the vascular department.

Losses of fluid from the body can be external or internal.

Dehydration usually refers to the loss of fluids and electrolytes from the body.

Fluid and electrolyte losses may occur secondary to vomiting, diarrhea, extreme sweating, and burns.

Various types of fluid and electrolyte losses produce various clinical states. It is important to understand the rate, type, and locale of loss in order to fully assess the patient's condition.

*Bibliography*    Guyton, A. C. *Basic Human Physiology*. Baltimore, Md.: W. B. Saunders Co., 1971.

Moore, F. D. *Metabolic Care of the Surgical Patient*. Baltimore, Md.: W. B. Saunders Company, 1959.

# Chapter 6

# PHARMACOLOGY

The study of pharmacology in its entirety encompasses the complete study of drugs, including the knowledge of the history; source; physical and chemical properties; compounding; biochemical and physiologic effects; mechanisms of action, absorption, distribution, biotransformation and excretion; therapeutic and other properties; and uses of drugs. Since a drug is broadly defined as any chemical agent that affects living processes, the subject of pharmacology is obviously quite extensive.

For the paramedic, the scope of pharmacology is less expansive than the above definition implies. The practicing paramedic will be primarily interested in the use of drugs to treat a prescribed set of symptoms during a particular emergency situation. He should be able to relate the symptoms observed to a mental anticipation that a drug(s) will soon be ordered; and he should have the ability to predict the onset and duration of actions, primary and side effects, and factors that may alter the patient's response to a given dose of a particular drug. The paramedic should also have an understanding of the basic effects of certain drugs most commonly "abused" and consequently be able to diagnose from physical symptoms the presence of a drug overdose and its appropriate antidote.

## MECHANISMS OF DRUG ACTIONS

The study of biochemical and physiologic effects of drugs and their mechanisms of action is termed *pharmacodynamics*. This term deals with the absorption, distribution, biotransformation, and excretion of drugs.

The term absorption refers to the processes involved in transferring the drug molecules from the place where they are deposited in the body to the circulating fluids. Drugs can be absorbed from the oral route via the gastric mucosa, topically through skin and mucous membrane surfaces, and by injection (parenteral).

*Oral Absorption.*   The most common route of administration is by mouth (orally) because it is the most convenient, the safest, and the cheapest way to get a drug into the patient's system. Most drug molecules are readily absorbed from the mucosal surface of the gastrointestinal tract.

Since the stomach empties more slowly when filled with food, orally administered drugs are usually more rapidly absorbed when taken between meals. Food also binds the drug molecules to its protein component, thereby creating drug complexes that cannot readily pass through the mucosal lining of the intestine. Also during digestion, the increased acidity and peptic activity may destroy some of the drug and thus reduce the amount that is finally absorbed.

Other factors that may limit the amount of drug absorption are the lipid solubility and degree of ionization. Substances (such as alcohol) that are lipid-soluble readily pass through the mucosal surface of the stomach and intestine, while other drugs (sulfas) which are not very lipid-soluble are not likely to be absorbed when taken orally. Drugs that are highly ionized, that is in a form mostly of electrically charged particles, tend to be poorly absorbed due to being repelled by the cell membrane of the intestinal mucosa and by other cell walls.

*Topical Absorption.*   Drugs can be absorbed through various surface tissues of the body. These include the skin, mucous membranes of the mouth, tracheal mucosa, and rectal mucosa. Significant absorption of a steroid can occur if a steroid cream is used for inflamed skin. Oral mucosal absorption of such drugs as nitroglycerine, Isuprel®, epinephrine, and glucose are also common examples. Many drugs can be placed in the rectum for absorption. These include aspirin compounds, bronchodilators (such as aminophylline), and anti-emetic drugs. The most commonly used site for topical absorption in the field is through the oral mucosa. Here, Isuprel®, cardiac vasodilator drugs, epinephrine, and glucose are frequently used for the treatment of certain clinical illnesses.

*Parenteral Absorption.*   This may include administration by intravenous, intramuscular, or subcutaneous routes. The absorption of drugs from parenteral administration is dependent on the blood supply to and from the injection site. Therefore, drugs are more rapidly absorbed from muscles, which are abundantly supplied with blood vessels, than from subcutaneous tissues, which have a relatively poor blood supply. Obviously in patients with circulatory collapse, administering drugs by the intramuscular route would not be beneficial. Patients who require epinephrine subcutaneously for asthma may have enhanced absorption by massaging the injection site.

When a drug is injected intravenously, its absorption is instantaneous and its onset of action is all but immediate (Figure 6-1). This can be an advantage as well as a disadvantage depending upon the drug and the condition of the patient.

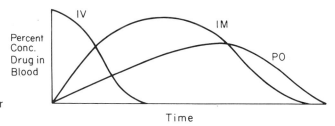

**Figure 6-1.** Blood level curves after three various routes of administration.

Drugs administered in high concentrations or dosages are more rapidly absorbed than drugs administered in lower concentrations and dosages. In certain situations, drugs are administered in very large doses that temporarily exceed the body's capacity for excretion of the drug. This provides for rapid drug arrival at the receptor site. Once an active drug level is established by rapid overloading, smaller daily doses of the drug can be administered. The initial and temporary overloading doses of the drug are priming doses, while the smaller daily doses are maintenance doses.

*Sublingual Absorption.*   Drugs administered under the tongue are absorbed very rapidly. The formulation of the tablet leads to rapid dissolving when it comes into contact with the saliva in this area which is so rich in blood vessels.

DISTRIBUTION

The term distribution refers to the manner in which a drug is transported by the bloodstream to various areas of the body (Figure 6-2). It also includes the factors involved in the drug's ability to accumulate in some tissues, or in its failure to enter other regions in significant amounts. The pattern of the distribution of any given drug often determines how rapidly it acts and how long its effects last, or even whether it will act at all. The rate of entry of a drug into the various tissues of the body depends upon the relative rate of perfusion and the permeability of the capillaries for the particular drug molecules.

The binding of a drug to plasma proteins and unequal passage of a drug across biological membranes may account for differential

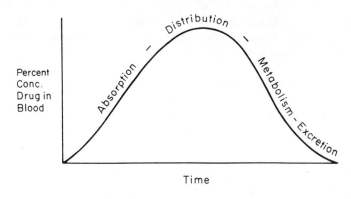

Percent
Conc.
Drug in
Blood

Time

**Figure 6-2.** Blood level curve illustrating the metabolic fate of drugs.

distribution of drugs. Binding of drugs can occur at the sites of absorption, in plasma, or at extravascular sites; but the proteins of plasma appear to be the most common site of drug binding. Drugs combine for the most part with albumin, one of the plasma proteins. Drugs that are bound have a decreased concentration of free drug in circulation, which prevents the drug from reaching its site of action in full concentrations. Once free drug is eliminated from the body, more drug is released from the protein bind to replace that which is lost. This equilibrium condition continues until the drug is totally eliminated from protein and other storage sites, such as body fat.

The ability of a drug to pass into the central nervous system is dependent on its ability to penetrate the "blood-brain" barrier. Drugs whose onset of action on the central nervous system is rapid have a greater affinity for penetrating the barrier than drugs with a slower onset of action and, consequently, poorer penetration.

Drugs such as steroids, narcotics, anesthetics, various teratogenic agents, and antibiotics can cross from the maternal blood supply through the placenta into the fetus. The rate of maternal blood flow to the placenta limits the availability of the drug to the fetus. Chronic administration of drugs to the mother, however, may produce adverse effects on the fetus.

METABOLISM

After drugs are absorbed and distributed, most of them undergo metabolic changes (Figure 6-2). This biotransformation occurs primarily in the liver, although most types of biotransformation result in inactivation of a drug, occasionally the result of the metabolic process is a more active compound that requires further metabolism before being excreted.

The actual site of the metabolism is in the hepatic endoplasmic reticulum, where the hepatic enzyme system is responsible for the process of changing drug molecular structure.

Individuals with impaired liver function may be expected to have prolonged drug action because of a delay in drug metabolism. In this situation, cumulative drug effects may be expected and may be manifested as excessive and prolonged responses to ordinary doses of drugs. On the other hand, stimulation of drug metabolism may produce a state of drug tolerance.

Metabolism is not solely limited to the liver. Other tissues such as the kidneys, intestinal mucosa, and plasma can function to metabolize drugs, although to a lesser degree.

## EXCRETION

Despite the fact that some drugs are metabolized while others remain intact, they all must ultimately be removed from the body. A drug will continue to act in the body until it is changed or excreted. The principal organ of excretion is the kidney, although the lungs will excrete gaseous substances and alcohol. Some drugs will also be excreted via the feces, saliva, breast milk, tears, or perspiration, but excretion via the kidneys remains the most important route of elimination. Thus, patients with impaired renal function may have drug accumulation leading to prolonged activity. Patients with both renal and hepatic dysfunction may be jeopardized through the cumulative effect of drugs. The rate at which drugs will be excreted depends on the rate of glomerular filtration and the half-life of the particular drug. (The half-life of a drug is the time it takes to reach 50 percent of the initial concentration of the drug in the plasma.)

## FACTORS MODIFYING DRUG EFFECTS AND DOSAGES

A number of factors should be considered when drugs are to be administered. These factors have the ability to alter the response of a patient to a given dosage as well as to modify the activity and effect of the drug.

### AGE

A patient's age will make a difference in the way he responds to drugs. Infants have immature liver and kidney systems, thereby requiring reduced dosages usually calculated as a fraction of the adult dose on the basis of body weight or surface area. Elderly patients can be extremely sensitive to central nervous system depressants and may require reduced doses or increased dosing intervals.

### BODY WEIGHT

The greater the body weight or mass, the greater the volume of distribution. Therefore, in order to maintain a desired drug concentration in individuals of various sizes, the dosage must be adjusted in relation to body weight. For a given dose of drug, the greater the volume of distribution, the lower the concentration of drug reached in various body compartments. Therefore, for children, the very lean, and the very obese patient, drug dosage is usually determined on the basis of the amount of drug per kilogram of body weight or surface area.

## SEX

The differences in drug effects between males and females are dependent in part on size differences and relative differences in the proportion of fat and water. Differential drug effects are most pronounced in pregnant women where certain drugs must be avoided.

## TIME OF ADMINISTRATION

Drugs are absorbed more rapidly if the gastrointestinal tract is free of food, while irritating drugs are more readily tolerated if there is food in the stomach.

## ROUTE OF ADMINISTRATION

Although discussed elsewhere in this chapter, the different routes of administration play a very large role in the final effect and dosage of a particular drug. The route will affect the rate and extent of absorption. Thus, if more of a drug is absorbed, the dose may have to be decreased, and vice versa.

## RATE OF METABOLISM AND EXCRETION

If the functions of the organs involved in metabolism and excretion are impaired, the intensity and duration of the drug will be prolonged. Effects of the drug will then be increased and toxic effects may occur. Genetic deficiencies in drug metabolism or in receptor sensitivity may also evoke differences in response.

## MISCELLANEOUS FACTORS

A patient's attitude and the impressions created at the time of drug administration may influence the therapeutic result. A placebo effect is an outstanding example of how strong motivation can influence the emergence of desired drug effects.

1. Onset of Action—The length of time necessary for a drug to start exerting its action.

2. Peak Time—The time when a drug exerts its maximal effect. It can also refer to the peak concentration reached in the serum.

3. Duration of Action—The length of time that a drug exerts its action (Figure 6-3).

4. Half-life (T-12)—The time required to drop to 50 percent of the peak concentration in the serum (Figure 6-4). Many drug dosage intervals are based on the half-life or multiple of the half-life in order to achieve blood levels that will produce continuity of desired effect.

5. Tolerance—Tolerance occurs when the effect of a drug in an individual is decreased after having taken the drug over a period of time, and the dose must be increased to maintain a given therapeutic effect. It may also be a reaction that necessitates an excessive increase in dosage to maintain a given therapeutic effect. The actual mechanism of tolerance is unknown. Recent studies have shown an increase in drug-metabolizing enzymes in the liver that may account for this phenom-

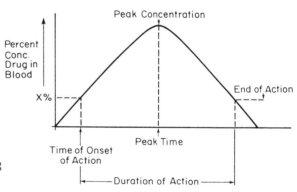

**Figure 6-3.** Blood level curve illustrating drug effects.

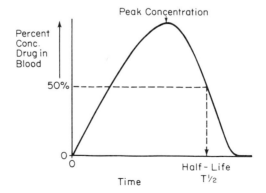

**Figure 6-4.** Blood level curve illustrating the relationship of half-life to the concentration of the drug in the blood.

enon. Cross tolerance between drugs with the same action is known to exist.

6. Tachyphylaxis—A quickly developing tolerance to the rapid, repeated administration of a drug. It is usually quick in onset and the patient's initial response to the drug cannot be reproduced even with larger doses of the drug.

7. Receptor Sites—Many drugs are theorized to act by combining with chemical groups on the cell surface or within the cell for which they possess a specific affinity. The site that the drug fits onto is called a *receptor site.* If the drug molecule fits the receptor perfectly, a particular action is produced. Drugs that share a chemical affinity for a receptor and initiate a reaction are called agonists; drugs that block the receptor site and reverse a specific effect are called antagonists. A competitive antagonist will have an affinity for the same receptor site as an agonist; the competition with the agonist for the site inhibits the action of the antagonist. The effect can be overcome by increasing the amount of agonist and is, therefore, considered reversible. Noncompetitive antagonists combine with different parts of the receptor mechanism and inactivate the receptor regardless of the concentration of the agonist and, therefore, are irreversible.

8. Drug Toxicity—With most drugs, the desired pharmacologic effect is often followed by less desirable effects from those that can produce mild discomfort to those that can be harmful and necessitate cessation of therapy or treatment with antidotes. No drug is completely free of these effects, which include mild side effects that may not require discontinuing the drug, but may call for decreasing the dosage. Occasionally, serious toxic effects may bring about damage or decreased function of vital organs of the body and occasionally death or permanent tissue damage.

*Table of Undesired Effects*

1. Predictability
2. Hypersensitivity (allergies)
3. Drug Addiction
4. Drug Poisoning
5. Idiosyncrasy

  a. *Predictable toxic effects* are effects that are predictable from the knowledge of the action of the drug. Side effects from primary drug action are undesired effects that are due to an extension of the desired action of the drug, often due to excessive dosage. Side effects from secondary drug action are any undesired effects from a drug that are not directly related to the effect for which the drug is intended. Many of these effects may be useful for treating different conditions. Often these side effects may be decreased by decreasing the dose, but the desirable effect of the drug may also be decreased.

b. *Hypersensitivity* or drug allergy is a reaction to a drug resulting from prior exposure and development of an immunologic mechanism into an antigen-antibody reaction. This antigen-antibody complex then reacts with various tissues and cells of the body to produce a release of histamine which is then responsible for provoking the symptom of allergy. Allergic reactions can be classified into two types: mild and anaphylactic (immediate).

The mild reactions are minor skin irritations, angioneurotic edema, rhinitis, fever, asthma, and pruritus. They may occur within several days after the initiation of therapy and individuals who have had prior mild allergic reaction to a particular drug should avoid re-exposure to that drug. Antihistamines may be helpful in the treatment of these reactions. Challenging the patient with another dose may risk an anaphylactoid reaction.

Anaphylactic reactions are sudden reactions occurring within a few minutes of exposure to the drug. They are manifested by shock, bronchospasm, and if not rapidly treated, death. The main mechanism responsible for these effects is a massive release of histamine. Epinephrine and bronchodilators are indispensable in the treatment of anaphylactic shock. The use of antihistamines at this point is of questionable value.

c. *Drug addiction* or dependence are terms used to describe habituation. The dependence or addiction can be physical or psychological. Physical dependence refers to a physiological state produced by a drug which, when the drug is withdrawn, manifests itself as a severe physical disturbance commonly referred to as withdrawal. Psychological dependence is defined as an emotional dependence in order to maintain a state of well-being.

d. *Drug poisoning* is an overdose of a drug that may greatly intensify the toxic effects of the drug leading, in many instances, to severe effects and death. Drugs such as aspirin, barbiturates, other central nervous system depressants, and stimulants are among the leading causes of drug overdose, either through accidental ingestion (such as with children) or in suicide attempts.

e. *Idiosyncrasy* refers to those types of reactions that are totally unpredictable, and may be due to an inherited inability to handle chemicals of certain types, perhaps through a genetic predisposition. This term is generally used to characterize different reactions to drugs which a majority of the patients do not manifest and which cannot be attributed to drug allergy.

9. Drug Interaction—The number of drugs currently available for use in the United States has produced a new field of intense study called drug interaction. Many patients are on multiple drug therapy, and each category of drugs has the ability to interact with drugs within the same category or other categories to alter the final drug effect.

10. Antagonism—Drug antagonism is a decrease in the effect of one drug by the presence of another drug. For example, the anticoagulant effects of warfarin are diminished due to enzymatic stimulation in the liver by the presence of phenobarbital, resulting in the enhanced metabolism of warfarin.

11. Synergism—Synergism occurs when the effect of one drug is increased by the presence of another drug. For example, probenecid, when added to penicillin therapy, will prolong blood levels of penicillin, thereby enhancing its antibacterial effects.

12. Additive Effects—This is the combined effect of two drugs that have similar effects. For example, the combination of alcohol and barbiturates will greatly enhance each drug's ability to depress the central nervous system.

## DOSAGES

One of the prime responsibilities of the paramedic or anyone engaged in the administration of medication is to be able to verify mathematically the dose prescribed versus the dose to be administered.

The following principles are discussed briefly for review in basic mathematics.

### PRINCIPLES OF MATHEMATICS

1. Changing common fractions to decimals: Divide numerator by denominator and place the decimal point in the correct position.

$$\frac{3}{4} = 4\overline{)3.00} = 0.75$$

2. Changing common fractions to percent: Use the above principle except move the decimal point two places to the right and add the percent sign.

$$0.75 = 75\%$$

3. Changing fractions to ratios: Write the terms of the fraction with a colon between the numerator and denominator.

$$\frac{1}{2} = 1{:}2$$

4. Changing decimals to common fractions: Place the number over the proper number of zeros with a number 1 to the left and omit the decimal point. Reduce the fraction if indicated.

$$6.125 = \frac{6125}{1000} = 6\,\frac{125}{1000} = 6\,\frac{1}{8}$$

5. Changing decimal to percent. Multiply the number by 100 and add the percent.

$$0.15 = (0.15)(100) = 15\%$$

6. Changing percent to decimal: Divide the number by 100.

$$66\% = \frac{66}{100} = 0.66$$

7. Changing percent to common fraction: Proceed as outlined in #6 above and reduce the fraction if possible.

$$25\% = \frac{25}{100} = \frac{1}{4}$$

8. Changing ratio to decimal: Divide the first number by the second.

$$1{:}20 = \frac{1}{20} = 0.05$$

9. Changing ratio to percent: Proceed as outlined in #8 and multiply by 100.

$$\frac{1}{50} = 0.02 \times 100 = 2\%$$

## PERCENTAGE, RATIO AND PROPORTION

*Percentage.* Percentage means the number of parts in 100. The term percent is usually indicated by the symbol %. A percentage number is a fraction where the numerator is expressed and where the denominator is understood to be 100. The numerical quantity expressed tells how many parts of a possible 100 parts are being considered. For example:

a. 1/3% means 1/3 of 1 part of 100 parts is being considered.

b. 8% means 8 parts of 100 parts are being considered.

Percentage can also be expressed as a fraction, decimal, or ratio. For example:

$$5\% = \frac{5}{100} = 0.05 = 5{:}100.$$

*Ratio.* This refers to the relative magnitude of two like quantities. These two quantities are being compared and expressed as a fraction, and the fraction is interpreted as indicating the operation of dividing the numerator by the denominator. Thus, a ratio represents the concept of a common fraction as expressing the relation of its two numbers. For example, the ratio of 20 and 10 is not expressed as 2, but as the fraction 20/10 (twenty to ten). If the two numbers of a ratio are multiplied or are divided by the same number, the value is unchanged, the value being the quotient of the first term divided by the second. For example, 20:4 or 20/4 has a value of 5. If both numbers are multiplied by 3, the ratio becomes 60:12 or 60/12, still with a value of 5. One important fact to remember is that the terms of the ratio must be the same, such as grains/grains, mg/mg, and so forth.

*Proportion.* A proportion is the expression of the equality of two ratios, and may be written in any one of three standard forms:

1. $a{:}b = c{:}d$
2. $a{:}b :: c{:}d$
3. $\dfrac{a}{b} = \dfrac{c}{d}.$

Each of these expressions is read as follows: *a* is to *b* as *c* is to *d*; If $a/b = c/d$, then

$$a = \frac{bc}{d}, \quad b = \frac{ad}{c}, \quad c = \frac{ad}{b}, \quad \text{and} \quad d = \frac{bc}{a}.$$

The above series shows how missing terms of any proportion can be determined when the other three terms are known. This is particularly important since most pharmacy-drug dosage calculations are based upon ratio and proportion, and once the principles are learned, the calculations become routine.

WEIGHTS AND MEASURES

*Metric System.* The metric units of measurement are the meter for linear measurement, the liter for capacity of volume, and the gram for weight. The meter tables are simple, for they are based upon the decimal system of notation; tables of length, volume, and weight are conveniently correlated, for the meter is the fundamental unit of the system.

*Apothecary System.* The apothecary system was the system used in England at the time of colonization of the United States. However, it has been replaced by the metric system in terms of medication nomenclature. The basic unit of weight in the apothecary system is the grain, which originally meant a grain of wheat. The other units of weight are the scruple, the dram, the ounce, and the pound. The scruple is seldom used and will not be mentioned. The unit of fluid measure is a minim.

The metric system and the apothecary system have different sized units and subdivisions. The denomination of one system is incompatible with the denomination of the other. The following table gives conversions and their appropriate equivalents:

| Household | Apothecary | Metric |
|-----------|-----------|--------|
| 60 drops or 1 teaspoonful | 60 minim or 1 fluid dram | 4 ml |
| 2 tablespoonfuls | 1 fluid ounce | 30 ml |
| 1 measuring cupful | 8 fluid ounces | 240 ml |
| 1 pint | 1 pint | 500 ml |
| 1 quart | 1 quart | 1000 ml |
| 1 gallon | 1 gallon | 4000 ml |
| | 1/60 grain | 1 mg |
| | 1 grain | 60 mg |
| | 15 or 16 grains | 1 gram |
| | 1 dram | 4 grams |
| | 1 ounce | 30 grams |
| | 2.2 pounds (avoirdupois) | 1 kg |

NOTE: 1 ml of water weighs 1 gram.

Or, simply written, to change:

1. Grains to grams, divide by 15.
   For example, 30 grain = 30 ÷ 15 = 2 grams.
2. Grams to grains, multiply by 15.
   For example, 6 grams = 6 × 15 = 90 grains.
3. Grams to ounces (weight), divide by 30.
   For example, 120 grams = 120 ÷ 30 = 4 ounces.
4. Ounces to grams, multiply by 30.
   For example, 6 ounces = 6 × 30 = 180 grams.
5. Milligrams to grains, divide by 60.
   For example, 120 mg = 120 ÷ 60 = 2 grains.
6. Grains to milligrams, multiply by 60.
   For example, 8 grains = 8 × 60 = 480 mg.

*Calculating Doses.* In calculating dosages, there are a few basic rules to remember before beginning the mathematical process.

1. Determine what is wanted and what is available.

2. Make certain all of the items are in the same standard of measurement and are comparable. That is, do not attempt to calculate without having the units of measurement all in mgs, grains, etc.

3. When three values are known and the fourth value is unknown, the proportion is the simplest method of reaching the answer.

4. Unless otherwise required, it is easier to perform the calculation in the metric system.

5. Perform the mathematical manipulations when the above criteria are completed.

*Calculating Doses for Children.* Most physicians believe that doses for children should be based upon the weight in kilograms. In many cases, however, the correct dosage of drugs seems more nearly proportional to the body surface area than any other variable. (Since most drugs are categorized in terms of weight in kilograms by the manufacturers, surface area is not used very much in practice except for fluid and electrolyte administration.)

A table of the approximate relation of surface area and weights of individuals of average body dimensions follows:

| Kilograms | Pounds | Square Meters (Surface Area) |
|:---:|:---:|:---:|
| 2 | 4.4 | 0.12 |
| 3 | 6.6 | 0.20 |
| 4 | 8.8 | 0.23 |
| 5 | 11.0 | 0.25 |
| 6 | 13.0 | 0.29 |
| 7 | 15.0 | 0.33 |
| 8 | 18.0 | 0.36 |
| 9 | 20.0 | 0.40 |
| 10 | 22.0 | 0.44 |
| 15 | 33.0 | 0.62 |
| 20 | 44.0 | 0.79 |
| 25 | 55.0 | 0.93 |
| 30 | 66.0 | 1.07 |
| 35 | 77.0 | 1.20 |
| 40 | 88.0 | 1.32 |
| 45 | 99.0 | 1.43 |
| 50 | 110.0 | 1.53 |
| 55 | 121.0 | 1.62 |
| 60 | 132.0 | 1.70 |

| Kilograms | Pounds | Square Meters (Surface Area) |
|---|---|---|
| 65 | 143.0 | 1.78 |
| 70 | 154.0 | 1.84 |
| 75 | 165.0 | 1.95 |
| 80 | 176.0 | 2.00 |

**Sample Problem.** The order is to give a patient 35 mg of meperidine. The label on the ampule shows 50 mg/ml. How many milliliters would be given? Answer: A simple proportion would be used here. Obviously, the dose will be less than 1 ml.

$$\frac{50 \text{ mg}}{1 \text{ ml}} = \frac{35 \text{ mg}}{x \text{ ml}}$$ Cross multiply and divide to determine $x$.

$$(50 \text{ mg})(x \text{ ml}) = (35 \text{ mg})(1 \text{ ml})$$

$$x \text{ ml} = \frac{(35 \text{ mg})(1 \text{ ml})}{50 \text{ mg}} = \frac{35}{50} = 0.7 \text{ ml}.$$

## TECHNIQUES OF ADMINISTERING DRUGS

### ROUTE

*Parenteral Administration.* Drugs administered parenterally must be sterile, readily soluble, absorbable and nonirritating. Since parenteral administration of drugs can be dangerous, certain precautions are necessary: (1) sterile aseptic techniques are needed in order to avoid infection; (2) accurate drug dosage, proper route of injection and proper site of injection must be followed in order to avoid tissue injury or nerve damage. An important factor to consider is that an injected drug is irretrievable and a mistake in dosage, method, or site of injection is not easily corrected. When drugs are given parenterally, the onset of action is more rapid and of shorter duration, the dose is often smaller, and the cost may be greater than with other routes of administration.

*Subcutaneous Administration.* When drugs are administered by the subcutaneous route, the needle should preferably be 25 gauge and 5/8 inches long. The site of injection is cleansed with an alcohol swab and the skin pinched between two fingers of the opposite hand, while the needle is inserted into the skin at a 45 to 60 degree angle with a quick movement. The injection of contents is made slowly and steadily. The plunger should be withdrawn slightly before injecting the drug to make sure that a blood vessel has not been entered. When the needle has entered the skin, the tissue of the arm or leg is released and the solution steadily injected. The volume of the solution injected should be limited to 0.5 to 2.0 ml. Larger volumes and irritating solutions can cause the formation of sterile abscesses.

*Intramuscular Injection.* The injection of solution into the skin through the subcutaneous tissue and into the muscular mass is done when a more rapid absorption of the drug is desired and larger volumes are needed than can be achieved with subcutaneous injection. The irritation caused by some solutions may be less noticeable with intramuscular (IM) injection. Volumes of 1 to 10 ml are suitable and can be injected into the buttocks, lateral aspect of the thigh, and deltoid portion of the arm. The drug can be an aqueous suspension or perhaps an oil, which tends to cause slower absorption of the medication.

Needle sizes are preferably 19 to 22 gauge and 1½ inches long, depending on the site of injection and the material to be injected. Once the injection is made, the plunger should be withdrawn to make certain that a blood vessel was not punctured. This is especially important when drugs in oil or suspensions are being administered. After the injection, the area can be massaged gently to help relieve the pain and dispense the drug. Excess scar formation can be avoided by rotating the injection sites during the course of treatment.

*Intravenous Injection.* This route of administering parenteral medications is especially important when an immediate effect is desired and the drug cannot be injected into other tissues, or during a shock situation when the circulation is poor and intramuscular injection would not be sufficient to insure adequate absorption of the drug due to a decreased blood supply. This route requires skill and aseptic technique and the drug must be soluble and sterile. Oily suspensions or solutions should not be administered by the intravenous route.

There are two methods for intravenous injection of drugs: the intravenous bolus and the intravenous infusion.

The intravenous bolus or intravenous push method is used to administer a small dose by means of a syringe into a suitable and accessible vein. The drug is usually dissolved in normal saline or dextrose 5 percent in water and, depending on the type of drug and volume, quickly pushed into the vein. Care must be taken with a large volume (such as 50 ml of sodium bicarbonate) that the rate of injection does not damage the injection site and vein. Blood aspirated into the syringe will indicate that a vein has been entered.

The intravenous infusion route is used to deliver very large volumes of fluid over long periods of time via a catheter or needle inserted into a vein. This method will be useful to enable the patient to receive fluids, relieve tissue dehydration, restore blood volume, replace depleted electrolytes, administer drugs, and utilize hyperalimentation therapy.

The rate of infusion is calculated according to the amount of dehydration, and the rate should be set to prevent a tissue overload, which may impair cardiac and pulmonary functions.

A wide variety of commercial solutions are used for intravenous fluid replacement. Vitamins can be added if warranted.

*Oral.* (See previous discussion under Absorption of Drugs.)

*Sublingual Administration.* Drugs administered under the tongue have a very rapid absorption time. The tablet formation is designed to dissolve quickly when it comes into contact with saliva in order to allow absorption through the thin epithelium and rich network of capillaries in this area. The patient must understand that the drug should not be chewed nor should he drink fluids until the tablet is dissolved. The use of nitroglycerin sublingually for angina attacks has proven very effective. Drugs may also be applied to the buccal mucosa for buccal absorption as well.

*Rectal Administration.* The rectal route of administration may be more convenient for little children or for patients undergoing episodes of nausea and vomiting. It is a reasonably safe method and many medications (such as aminophylline) are available in this form. The use of this route avoids gastric irritation due to local contact with the stomach mucosa.

## STERILE TECHNIQUES

The principles of sterile techniques are relatively easy to follow once the concepts are learned. The following guidelines should be followed prior to administering any intravenous drug:

1. Accurately compare the label of the medication with what is ordered by the physician.

2. Accurately calculate the dose and, if possible, have your calculation verified.

3. Select the appropriate needle and syringe size.

4. Before withdrawing or adding diluent to a vial, swab the top of the rubber stopper with an alcohol swab.

5. Enter the vial with a sterile needle, with the bevel side up to minimize a "coring" effect on the rubber stopper.

6. It is sometimes helpful to inject a small amount of air into the vial to make it easier to withdraw the medication.

7. Swab the injection site on the patient with an alcohol or iodine swab and let it dry.

8. Inject the medication quickly and push the plunger at a rate according to established guidelines for the drug. Monitor the patient for any adverse effects.

9. If the needle becomes contaminated before entering the patient (for instance by touching the bed, patient, yourself, or the side of the vial), discard it and select a new needle. The cost of a single needle is considerably less than the cost involved in treating sepsis in a patient!

10. Expel all air bubbles prior to injection, especially if the medication is given by intravenous push.

The following list of medications are the drugs most commonly used by the paramedics:

## AMINOPHYLLINE

*Action.* Aminophylline is the ethylenediamine salt of theophylline. It can relax the smooth muscle of the respiratory tract, producing relief of bronchospasm and increasing flow rates and vital capacity. Aminophylline can also dilate the pulmonary arterioles, which reduces pulmonary hypertension and alveolar carbon dioxide tension, and this increases the pulmonary blood flow. In large doses, aminophylline can produce a positive inotropic effect on the myocardium and a positive chronotropic effect on the SA node (Chapter 11).

*Uses.* Aminophylline is used as a bronchodilator in the symptomatic treatment of mild bronchial asthma and reversible bronchospasm that may occur in association with chronic bronchitis, emphysema, and other obstructive pulmonary diseases. It is usually effective in treating status asthmaticus after treatment failures with SQ epinephrine.

*Precautions.* Intravenous injection should be done slowly over a period of 15 to 20 minutes to avoid peripheral vascular collapse. Deaths have occurred after IV administration, probably due to cardiac standstill or ventricular fibrillation. Excessive cerebral stimulation, wakefulness, vertigo, nausea, acute hypotension, and convulsions have occurred.

*Preparation.* 250 mg/10 ml ampule; 500 mg/20 ml ampule.

*Dose.* Adult—250–500 mg IV (push slowly), or diluted in IV fluids such as dextrose 5% in water 500 ml and infused over a longer period of time.
Pediatric—10–12 mg/kg/day IV.

## AMMONIA, AROMATIC SPIRIT (AMMONIA INHALANTS)

*Action.* Aromatic ammonia is an aromatic hydroalcoholic solution containing approximately 4 percent of ammonium carbonate. It is a reflex respiratory stimulant that works by peripheral irritation of the sensory receptors of the nasal membranes.

*Uses.* Stimulates respiratory and vasomotor centers. It is useful in treating patients who have fainted or feel quite faint.

*Precautions.* The drug should be used cautiously in patients who have had prolonged exposure to respiratory irritants and in chronic asthmatics, since ammonia can induce bronchospasm. Prolonged inhalation can cause pulmonary irritation and possibly pulmonary edema.

*Preparation.* Marketed in a single dose glass ampule wrapped in a soft cotton envelope. The vial is easily broken; the cotton acts as a sponge for the ammonia.

*Dose.* After breaking the glass ampule, the medication is passed under the nostrils a few times. If the patient regains consciousness, the passes are discontinued. Avoid holding the ampule directly under the nostrils for prolonged intervals.

## ATROPINE (ANTICHOLINERGIC)

*Action.* The primary effect of atropine on the heart is to alter the rate. Large doses cause progressively increasing tachycardia by blocking the vagal effects on the sinoatrial (SA) node. The influence of atropine is most noticeable in healthy young adults. In infancy and old age, even large doses may fail to accelerate the heart.

*EKG Effects.* AV conduction time is decreased, the P-R interval is shortened, the idioventricular rate may be accelerated, and it may lower the T wave.

*Uses.* For treating bradycardia and asystole, atropine often improves the clinical condition of patients with early myocardial infarction by relieving a severe sinus or nodal bradycardia or an AV block. It is not recommended for routine use in postinfarction bradycardia in the absence of hypotension, heart failure, or escape PVCs.

*Precautions.* If atropine fails to correct the bradycardia or asystole, use isoproterenol by intravenous piggyback (IVPB). Atropine will cause dryness of the mouth, blurred vision, increased body surface temperature, and delirium. It can also worsen glaucoma (although it may be given even though the patient has glaucoma), and can cause a flushing of the skin due to the dilation of the cutaneous blood vessels (atropine flush).

*Preparation.* 1 mg/10 ml, 10 ml prefilled syringe.

*Dose.* Adult—0.5 mg IV push, repeated at five-minute intervals until the desired rate is achieved (usually around 60 beats/minute). Maximum: 2 mg.

Pediatric—0.01 mg/kg to 0.2 mg/kg by IV push (maximum of 2 mg).

## CALCIUM CHLORIDE ($CaCl_2$)

*Action.* Calcium chloride is a cardiotonic agent. Calcium is necessary for myocardial contraction.

*Uses.* Calcium can be given during cardiac arrest to increase contractility by increasing the strength of cardiac contraction, especially if a pulse is present. It can be used to convert fine ventricular fibrillation to coarse ventricular fibrillation where there is no response after epinephrine administration.

*Precautions.* Calcium can precipitate digitalis toxicity in patients on this medication. Calcium is very irritating and can cause tissue sloughing; therefore, avoid intramuscular and intracardiac administration. Calcium should never be mixed in the same line, bottle, or syringe with sodium bicarbonate because of the formation of a precipitate (calcium carbonate).

*Preparation.* 10 percent—1 g/10 ml, 10 ml prefilled syringe.

*Dose.* Adult—2.5 to 5.0 ml IV push, inject slowly and repeat in ten minutes if needed.
Pediatric—1 ml/kg body (20 mg/kg) weight IV push (slowly) (maximum 5 ml).

## DEXAMETHASONE (DECADRON®)

*Action.* Dexamethasone is a glucocorticoid (steroid) utilized for its anti-inflammatory effects and as an adjunct in the treatment of shock and cerebral edema. Steroids are made naturally in the adrenal gland (cortisone, hydrocortisone) or synthetically (dexamethasone). The exact mechanism of action of steroids is still unclear. However, it is possible that they can preserve the integrity of small blood vessels from shock, increase cardiac output, and stabilize cellular membranes.

*Uses.* There is strong evidence that shows that steroids are of some benefit when used early and in very large doses in shock and acute cerebral edema. The onset of action in the latter situation is four to six hours and it appears that steroids would not be useful in the treatment of head trauma in the field.

*Precautions.* Steroids have no acute toxicity and no chronic toxicity, even when large doses are given for several days. However, many adverse reactions can occur when they are given for longer periods of time.

*Preparation.* 4 mg/ml. 10 ml vial.

*Dose.* 10–20 mg IV push.

## DEXTROSE INJECTION 50 PERCENT

*Action.* 50 percent dextrose solution is a hypertonic solution of dextrose. Its main action is to replace glucose, which is needed as the principal energy source for body cells. Because of its hypertonicity, it will also pull fluid into the intravascular space.

*Uses.* Dextrose is given as a readily available source of concentrated sugar solution, especially in diabetics who have taken an excessive amount of insulin or oral hypoglycemic drugs and are unconscious. It may also be useful in other comatose patients where hypoglycemia may be present.

*Precautions.* It may be more useful to give oral sugar solutions to conscious patients rather than injecting dextrose, due to its sclerosing effects on veins and possible damage if pushed into the interstitial tissue. Always draw a preglucose blood sample first and label "preglucose."

*Preparation.* 50 percent—25 g/50 ml, 50 ml prefilled syringe.

*Dose.* Adult—50 ml (50 percent solution) IV push.
Pediatric—1 ml/kg IV push.

## DIAZEPAM (VALIUM®)

*Action.* Diazepam is a sedative-hypnotic agent that causes depression of the central nervous system.

*Uses.* The field use for diazepam is primarily as an IV push for use as an anticonvulsant to treat grand mal or generalized prolonged seizures. It can also be used as a tranquilizer to relieve acute anxiety reactions (IM). The onset of action of diazepam is rapid and may last for three hours.

*Precautions.* When used as an anticonvulsant, the drug is to be given by slow IV push. Monitor the respiration and blood pressure, especially if other central nervous system (CNS) depressants, such as phenobarbital, have been administered previously. Have resuscitation equipment available to assist ventilation if needed. Use cautiously in pediatric patients, especially infants. Do not mix with other drugs or in IV solutions, since diazepam will precipitate when mixed. To minimize this problem, inject the drug either directly into the vein, or into the flash ball of the IV set as close to the cannula as possible. The dose should be injected intravenously and slowly at a rate of 5 mg/minute, and titrated until the desired effect is reached.

*Preparation.* 10 mg/2 ml, 2 ml prefilled syringe. 10 mg/2 ml, 2 ml ampule.

*Dose.* Adult—5–10 mg IV push or IM.
Pediatric—0.25–0.5 mg/kg IV (maximum 10 mg). Give 1–2 mg every five minutes until seizures stop, and stop at 10 mg. Use the 2 ml ampule and 1 ml TB syringe; draw up 1 ml; each 0.2 ml = 2 mg.

DIGOXIN (LANOXIN®)

*Action.* Digoxin is a cardiac glycoside that can increase the force of myocardial contraction by a direct action on the myocardium. It will increase the force of contraction, stroke volume, and cardiac output. As a result of these positive inotropic effects, the cardiac size is reduced in patients with congestive heart failure. This is a result of conduction being impaired at the SA and AV nodes. Improved circulation to the kidney produces diuresis in 24 to 48 hours.

*Uses.* Primarily used to treat congestive heart failure by improving myocardial contractility. It can also be used to treat acute pulmonary edema via its positive inotropic action. Digoxin is used to control the ventricular rate in patients with atrial fibrillation and atrial flutter. Also, it is useful in preventing attacks of PAT or nodal tachycardia refractory to other antiarrhythmic agents.

*Precautions.* Digoxin dosages should be monitored very carefully since there is very little difference between the therapeutic and potentially toxic doses. Side effects are mainly cardiac, gastrointestinal, and neurological in nature. EKG changes in patients exhibiting toxic effects are as follows: extrasystoles, bigeminal pulse, coupled rhythm, ectopic beats or other dysrhythmias indicating impending heart block, PVC, ventricular tachycardia, ventricular fibrillation, P-R prolongation, widening of QRS, negative T wave, and depressed S-T segments. Gastrointestinal symptoms usually occur before EKG changes and are related to complaints such as nausea, vomiting, and anorexia. Patients may also complain of visual disturbances such as yellow/green lights, blurred vision, white halos, or borders on dark objects. Digoxin should not be administered to patients who have a ventricular (pulse) rate of less than 60 in adults or 70 in pediatric patients. Avoid its use with calcium, since the two drugs administered together precipitate digitoxicity.

*Preparation.* 0.5 mg/2 ml, 2 ml ampule.

*Dose.* Adults—0.25 to 0.5 mg IV push (slowly over five minutes) initially. Ventricular rate of 60 to 80 beats/minute is an acceptable range after digoxin administration. The effects may occur in five to thirty minutes.
Pediatric—Premature—0.022 to 0.04 mg/kg. 2 weeks to 2 years—0.044 to 0.066 mg/kg. 2 years to 10 years—same as above.

DIPHENHYDRAMINE (BENADRYL®)

*Action.* Diphenhydramine is an antihistamine that competitively antagonizes most of the pharmacological actions of histamine. It appears to act by occupying histamine receptor sites, thereby preventing the action of histamine on the cell. It is most effective by antagonizing

the increased capillary permeability and formation of edema due to
histamine release.

*179*
*Paramedic Drug List*

*Uses.* Diphenhydramine is most useful in relieving severe allergic reactions such as urticaria (hives) and pruritus (itching), as from bee stings. It can be used as an adjunct in treating an anaphylactic reaction, but only after epinephrine has been tried. Diphenhydramine is also useful as a mild sedative.

*Precautions.* Diphenhydramine should not be given to asthmatics because of the "drying" effect on the bronchial mucosa, which may precipitate an asthmatic attack. Be aware of CNS depression, which can be potentiated by the previous injection of alcohol or other sedative hypnotic drugs. Overdosage can lead to convulsions, nervousness, and death. Cardiac effects include shortened diastole, atrial tachycardia, and changes in the T waves. Single parenteral doses greater than 100 mg should be avoided in patients with cardiac disease or hypertension. Avoid subcutaneous administration due to tissue irritability.

*Preparation.* 50 mg/ml, 1 ml prefilled syringe.

*Dose.* Adult—50 to 100 mg IV push or deep IM.
Pediatric—2 mg/kg/dose IV push or deep IM.

## DOPAMINE HYDROCHLORIDE (INTROPIN®)

*Action.* Dopamine is a precursor to norepinephrine and epinephrine. It acts as an alpha and beta receptor stimulant, thereby increasing cardiac output by increasing the stroke volume. The systolic blood pressure is increased; the diastolic may not change or may increase; and renal blood flow is increased, resulting in increased sodium excretion.

*Uses.* Dopamine is indicated for the correction of the hemodynamic imbalance that is present in the shock syndrome due to myocardial infarction and endotoxin septicemia. Increased cardiac output is related to the direct inotropic effects on the myocardium and is seen primarily at low to moderate doses. At high doses, predominant alpha effects are seen and a rise in blood pressure becomes more pronounced.

*Precautions.* Observe closely for tachydysrhythmias and discontinue if they remain uncorrected. Because of deactivation, dopamine should not be added to alkaline (sodium bicarbonate) solution either in the tubing or IV container. Use a small flush of the main IV in between each agent. Where appropriate, the administration of IV fluids to restore blood volume should be instituted. This will allow for an expansion of blood volume and enhance the cardiac output as a result of dopamine. Overtitration of dopamine will result in a disproportionate rise in blood pressure. If this occurs (1) decrease titration rate; (2) if unsuccessful, discontinue titration until the patient's condition stabilizes.

Dopamine should be infused into a large vein wherever possible to prevent the possibility of infiltration, which will result in necrosis and tissue sloughing. The preferred site of administration is a large antecubital vein. If infiltration does occur, immediately discontinue the IV, notify the base station, and restart the IV in another site. Side effects include ectopic beats, nausea, vomiting, and tachycardia.

*Preparation.* 200 mg/ml ampule.

*Dose.* Dopamine must be diluted before administration to the patient.

Adult—2 amp (10 ml = 400 mg) in 250 ml $D_5W$. This will give a concentration of 1600 μg/ml (1.6 mg/ml). Begin the drip rate at 10 to 20 microdrops/min, or 5 μg/kg/min. Titrate closely to the patient's blood pressure and other signs of perfusion.

## EPINEPHRINE (ADRENALIN)

*Action.* Epinephrine is an adrenergic agent with alpha (vasoconstrictor) and beta (cardiac stimulating, peripheral vasodilating, and smooth muscle relaxing) effects. In cardiopulmonary arrest, epinephrine stimulates an asystolic heart to contract and increases the amplitude of fibrillating ventricular waves. This latter effect may increase the success rate of defibrillation, but it may also increase the tendency toward ventricular fibrillation. Its smooth muscle relaxing effect is pronounced in the bronchioles, which results in bronchodilation. Epinephrine can be given IV or intracardiac. It also is rapidly absorbed through the tracheal mucosa and can be administered down an endotracheal tube.

*Uses.* Epinephrine has three main uses. (1) As a cardiac stimulant—in a cardiac arrest situation, epinephrine will increase the force of contraction and cardiac output. It will stimulate an asystolic heart to improve cardiac function. It will also convert fine ventricular fibrillation to coarse fibrillation, thereby improving chances for defibrillation. (2) In bronchoconstriction—Because of its smooth muscle relaxing characteristics, epinephrine will dilate constricted bronchioles during an asthmatic attack and in other chronic lung diseases that induce narrow air passages. (3) For anaphylactic shock—In this severe allergic condition, epinephrine will reverse bronchospasm and increase perfusion if the shock syndrome is present.

*Precautions.* Due to rapid degradation, epinephrine should not be mixed with alkaline (sodium bicarbonate) solutions. Use a small flush of the IV tubing with the main IV solution in between each agent. Repeated doses can cause ventricular fibrillation due to its cardiac irritability effects. Watch for tachydysrhythmias. Avoid use in pregnant women whenever possible.

*Preparation.* 1:10,000—10 ml prefilled syringe (regular needle). 1:10,000—10 ml prefilled syringe (intracardiac needle). 1:1,000—1 ml ampule.

*181*
*Paramedic Drug List*

*Dose.*

1. Cardiac arrest—Adults—Establish an IV line and give 5–10 ml of a 1:10,000 solution IV push initially—if there is no response in three to five minutes, another dose of 5 to 10 ml IV or intracardiac (IC) can be given and repeated every five minutes if needed. If an IV cannot be started, begin with an IC dose (Chapter 13).

Pediatric—1:10,000—0.1 ml/kg body weight IV (maximum 5 ml).

2. Bronchospasm—Use the 1:1000 ampule.

Adult—0.3 ml SQ.
Pediatric—0.01 ml/kg/dose SQ, q15min (up to 0.3 ml dose).

3. Anaphylactic shock.

Adult—5 to 10 ml (1:10,000) IV push.
Pediatric—1:10,000—0.1 ml/kg body weight, IV push, OR 1:1000 SQ in same dose as for bronchospasm.

## FUROSEMIDE (LASIX®)

*Action.* Furosemide is a potent diuretic designed to produce an increased urine output. It acts by blocking the reabsorption of sodium, which results in an increased flow of water, thereby producing increased urine production. There is a rapid onset of action (five to ten minutes) with a maximal effect in thirty minutes and a duration of two hours. Furosemide causes venous pooling and vasodilatation, thereby reducing the preload and afterload of the heart (Chapter 10).

*Uses.* In the field, furosemide is used to promote diuresis in patients with severe acute pulmonary edema to decrease the right heart load. When taken orally, it is most commonly used to relieve congestive heart failure in addition to digoxin.

*Precautions.* Because furosemide causes a massive diuresis, dehydration and a decrease in blood pressure may occur. Prolonged use can lead to potassium depletion and, if the patient is also taking digoxin, it may lead to digitoxicity. Use cautiously in patients with urinary retention, and only if the patient will reach the hospital within thirty minutes. Otherwise, a ruptured bladder may occur because of increased fluid content and the lack of relief.

*Preparation.* 20 mg/2 ml, 2 ml ampule.

*Dose.* Adult—40–200 mg/day, IV push or IM.
Pediatric—1–2 mg/kg IV q2h.

GLUCOSE GEL, INSTANT GLUCOSE

*Action.*   Oral source of glucose replacement.

*Uses.*   High concentration of glucose for the treatment of conscious or semiconscious diabetic patients in a hypoglycemic state. It is useful if an IV cannot be established or is not necessary.

*Precautions.*   Draw a blood sample first and label "preglucose." Be prepared for possible aspiration in the semiconscious patient.

*Preparation.*   Each tube contains 25 grams of glucose in a corn syrup base.

*Dose.*   The contents of one tube can be used as needed and should be administered into the buccal area. Record the amount given.

GLUCOSE SOLUTION (GLUCOTAL®, GLUCOLA®)

*Action.*   Oral source of glucose replacement.

*Uses.*   To be used in a conscious diabetic patient with hypoglycemia.

*Precautions.*   Draw a blood sample before administering the dose and label "preglucose." This solution should only be given to conscious patients in order to avoid aspiration problems that may occur with the semiconscious patient.

*Preparation.*   Each 12 oz bottle contains 100 grams of glucose.

*Dose.*   Administer as needed and record the amount given.

IPECAC SYRUP

*Action.*   Ipecac is a peripherally (gastric irritant) and centrally (brainstem) acting emetic. Its emetic action may be slow, sometimes requiring up to thirty to sixty minutes. In children it often may act in fifteen to twenty minutes.

*Uses.*   It is used in the field to induce vomiting in a conscious patient who has overdosed on drugs or ingested a harmful material.

*Precautions.*   Ipecac should not be administered in the following circumstances: (a) semiconscious or comatose patients, (b) ingestions of caustic agents, (c) ingestions of hydrocarbons (gasoline, etc.). Aspiration of vomitus may occur if the patient becomes comatose and vomits. Large amounts of poison that have not been vomited should be treated with lavage when the patient is admitted to the Emergency Department. Do not confuse syrup of Ipecac with the fluid extract, which is more toxic than the syrup.

*Preparation.* 30 ml unit dose container and 15 ml unit dose container.

*Dose.* Adult—30 ml p.o. followed with a minimum of 8 oz of water. May repeat in twenty minutes if needed.

Pediatric—Under 2 years—5–10 ml. Over 2 years—15 ml. Follow with a minimum of 4 ounces of water. If no results are obtained the dose may be repeated one time in twenty minutes. If there is no response from the second dose, lavage is necessary to remove the stomach contents.

## ISOPROTERENOL (ISUPREL®)

*Action.* Isoproterenol acts predominantly on beta receptors of the sympathetic nervous system and has little or no effect on alpha receptors. The main effects of isoproterenol are cardiac excitation, relaxation of smooth muscle of the bronchial tree and alimentary tract, and dilation of skeletal muscle vasculature. As a cardiac stimulant, isoproterenol has a positive chronotropic effect through the SA node and a positive inotropic action on the myocardium. A therapeutic dose of isoproterenol has the combined effect of increasing cardiac output and stroke volume, maintaining or increasing systolic blood pressure, and decreasing diastolic and central venous pressures. The onset of action following IV administration is a few minutes and the duration of action is one to two hours.

*Uses.* (1) As a cardiotonic to increase cardiac output and heart rate; (2) for treating heart blocks, bradycardia, and asystole; (3) in the treatment of cardiogenic shock to increase tissue perfusion and blood pressure.

*Precautions.* The principal side effects include tachycardia, headache, palpitation, and increased cardiac excitability which can produce extrasystoles and dysrhythmias, such as PVCs. Use with caution in patients with cardiac disease, hypertension, or other cardiovascular disorders. Epinephrine and isoproterenol are both direct cardiac stimulants and, if used together, can cause cumulative effects on the heart. In treating heart block, isoproterenol will usually be ordered if atropine is unsuccessful. Do not use without adequate fluid replacement in treating shock. Avoid its use in hemorrhagic shock.

*Preparation.* 1 mg/5 ml, 5 ml prefilled syringe.

*Dose.* Isoproterenol should always be given in a dilute form and never by IV push.

Adult—1 mg (5 ml) in 250 ml $D_5W$ and give by IV drip. (This concentration is then 4 µg/ml.) The heart rate should be titrated at 60 to 120 beats/min.

Pediatric—0.1 to 0.5 µg/kg/min.

*Action.*  Lidocaine is an antidysrhythmic agent that controls ventricular dysrhythmias by suppressing automaticity in the His-Purkinje system (Chapter 11), and by elevating the electrical stimulation threshold of the ventricle during diastole. Lidocaine is also a central nervous system depressant and can produce sedative, central analgesic, and anticonvulsant effects. (In toxic doses, however, lidocaine can cause seizures.) Lidocaine is rapidly cleared from the blood following IV administration. Following an IV push, the drug has an onset of action within ten seconds to three minutes and a duration of action up to twenty minutes. The onset of action of an IV drip dose (without initial IV push) can occur within ten to twenty minutes.

*Uses.*  To treat ventricular dysrhythmias following acute myocardial infarction (that is, to control PVCs and ventricular tachycardia).

*Precautions.*  The infusion should be discontinued if the following symptoms occur: CNS excitation, convulsions, decreased blood pressure, CV collapse, bradycardia, cardiac arrest, increased P-R interval, or if the QRS complexes become prolonged or the rhythm becomes aggravated. Do not use if the patient has idioventricular rhythm, or heart block. Intramuscular administration is not recommended at this time.

*Preparation.*  1% 100 mg/10 ml, 10 ml prefilled syringe. 20% 1 g/5 ml, 5 ml prefilled syringe.

*Dose.*  Adult—50 to 100 mg IV push up to 200 mg if needed (may be calculated as 1 mg/kg of body weight) followed by an IV drip of 1 gram in 250 ml $D_5W$. Infuse at 2 to 4 mg/min (15 to 60 microdrops per minute).

Pediatric—Prepare an IV drip dose the same as above. However, begin the titration very slowly and monitor the effects. (Run at 1 mg/kg/min).

Infants—0.5 mg/kg IV push, q5–10 min.

Children—1 mg/kg IV push, q5–10 min.

MEPERIDINE (DEMEROL®)

*Action.*  Meperidine, like morphine, is a narcotic analgesic. It can produce the same types of action, such as respiratory depression, sedative and euphoric effects, and, to a lesser extent, suppression of the cough reflex. Meperidine appears to have a more rapid onset and shorter duration of action than does morphine. Peak analgesia occurs thirty to fifty minutes after IM administration and may be maintained for two to four hours.

*Uses.*  Meperidine is a strong analgesic used in the relief of severe pain. The drug has been used to relieve the pain of myocardial infarction, although morphine is found to be more effective. It has also been used to allay anxiety in patients with acute pulmonary edema.

*Precautions.* Since meperidine shares the toxic potentials of other narcotic analgesics, the same precautions regarding the observance of respiratory rates, blood pressure, etc., should be followed. Meperidine may increase the ventricular response rate through a vagolytic action, and therefore should be used with caution in patients with atrial flutter and other supraventricular tachycardias. Avoid its use in patients with head and/or abdominal injuries.

*Preparation.* 25 mg/1 ml, 50 mg/1 ml, 75 mg/1 ml, 100 mg/1 ml.

*Dose.* Adult—IV push, given slowly as a 10 mg/1 ml dilution. Use 100 mg/1 ml ampule and dilute in a syringe with 9 ml of normal saline. Resultant concentration will be 100 mg/10 ml = 10 mg/1 ml. Patient should be lying down when given intravenously. IM—give undiluted.

Pediatric—1.0 to 1.8 mg/kg/dose. Single pediatric doses should not exceed 100 mg.

## METAPROTERENOL (ALUPENT®)

*Action.* Metaproterenol is a beta-2 stimulator with minimal beta-1 effects on the heart. Its beta-2 stimulating effects produce relaxation of the bronchioles.

*Uses.* It is most useful as a bronchodilator for patients having an asthmatic attack, and in other forms of bronchospasm. Its primary beta-2 effect accents its usefulness in patients with preexisting cardiac dysrhythmias during the use of metaproterenol.

*Precautions.* Metaproterenol can cause PVCs, tachycardia, and palpitations, and should not be used in patients with cardiac dysrhythmias associated with tachycardia. Repeated excessive administration may produce paradoxical bronchospasm. It is important to obtain a history of recent use by the patient of his own inhalation drugs. This will aid in preventing the onset of any cardiac effects if further inhalation therapy is warranted.

*Preparation.* 15 ml metered dose inhaler with mouthpiece.

*Dose.* 2 to 3 deep inhalations, not repeated more often than every three to four hours. Total per day should not exceed 12 inhalations. The patient should prolong the inhalation for a few seconds before exhaling.

## METARAMINOL (ARAMINE®)

*Action.*  Metaraminol is a vasopressor drug that causes an increase in blood pressure through stimulation of alpha receptors located in the sympathetic nervous system. Therefore, its actions are similar to norepinephrine, but it is not as intense a vasopressor. The resultant effect is an increase in diastolic and systolic blood pressures and it may also increase cardiac output. Pressor effects occur within one to two minutes after an IV infusion.

*Uses.*  Metaraminol is used in patients with cardiopulmonary arrest, and may be used when hypotension persists and renal and cerebral perfusion remains inadequate after an effective heartbeat, palpable pulse, and ventilation have been established by other means. This drug has been used less in recent years with the availability of dopamine.

*Precautions.*  Pressor therapy is not a substitute for replacement of blood, plasma fluids, or electrolytes. Blood volume depletion should be corrected and vasoconstrictors have no place in the treatment of hypovolemic shock (Chapter 15), since it will cause further decrease in organ perfusion. Overdosage may result in severe hypertension, cerebral hemorrhage, convulsions, acute pulmonary edema, and bradycardia. Therefore, the blood pressure should not be allowed to rise too quickly. Monitoring the blood pressure every five to ten minutes will aid in determining the correct rate of infusion. The base station should be asked what blood pressure reading is to be maintained during metaraminol administration.

*Preparation.*  10 mg/ml, 10 ml vial (100 mg/vial). 100 mg/10 ml, 10 ml prefilled syringe.

*Dose.*  Adult—For IV push dose, draw 1 ml of metaraminol from the 10 ml vial into a 1 ml TB syringe (0.1 ml = 1 mg). Then draw into the same syringe 0.9 ml of NS. This resultant mixture will give a concentration of 1 mg/1 ml. Push IV 0.5 ml (0.5 mg) and monitor the blood pressure. Repeat in fifteen minutes with the rest of syringe if ordered by the base station. For an IV drip, add 100 mg of metaraminol to 250 ml $D_5W$ and titrate the infusion with blood pressure.

Pediatric—Add 25 mg to a buretol (Chapter 20) and add 100 ml D5¼NS. Titrate the infusion to the desired effect.

## METHYLERGONOVINE (METHERGINE®)

*Action.*  Methylergonovine acts directly on the smooth muscle of the uterus to increase the tone, rate, and amplitude of contractions. Contractions may begin thirty to sixty seconds after an IV push dose. The effect on the uterus is to produce a total uterine contraction rather than one of a rhythmic nature.

*Uses.* For the control of uterine bleeding after the delivery of the placenta.

*Precautions.* This drug should not be given before the delivery of the placenta, since the contraction may actually trap the placenta. Hypertension and bradycardia have occurred due to smooth muscle contraction. The blood pressure should be monitored before administration and if it rises above 140/90, notify the base station. Watch for discoloration of the contents in the ampule after prolonged storage.

*Preparation.* 0.2 mg/ml, 1 ml ampule.

*Dose.* 0.2 mg IM.

## MORPHINE SULFATE (M.S.)

*Action.* Morphine is a narcotic analgesic. It exerts its primary effect on the central nervous system (CNS) by interfering with pain conduction and the patient's emotional response to pain. It can also cause a depression of the cough reflex and respiratory center. Its effect on the respiratory center is still unclear. Morphine has been shown to cause a rise in the cerebral blood flow and a resultant increase in CSF pressure, as well as hypotension.

*Uses.* For the control of moderate to severe pain and for use in allaying anxiety and apprehension in patients with acute pulmonary edema. It also causes venous pooling, which decreases the return to the right heart, thus helping to relieve acute pulmonary edema. It is a valuable adjunct for treatment of chest pain due to myocardial ischemia or infarction (Chapter 10).

*Precautions.* Because of its effect on increasing the cerebral blood flow, morphine should not be given to patients with head trauma. It should also be avoided in patients with an acute abdomen, and used cautiously in patients with chronic liver disease. Overdosage can cause respiratory depression, hypotension, pinpoint pupils, and coma, which can be treated with naloxone. Morphine is a narcotic and must be signed out on the narcotic record sheets.

*Preparation.* 10 mg/ml, 1 ml ampule. 1 mg/1 ml, 10 ml prefilled syringe.

*Dose.* Adult—8–10 mg (1/8–1/6 gr) IM undiluted for pain. For IV push use; draw up the contents of one ampule (1 ml) into a 10 ml syringe. Then into the same syringe draw 9 ml of M.S. This resultant mixture will provide a 1 mg/ml concentration. During an acute MI for acute pulmonary edema, initially 4 mg can be given more rapidly than over four minutes, but the remaining doses should be 1 mg/minute.

Pediatric—0.1 mg/kg IV push slowly. Pediatric patients react very quickly to morphine, so monitor the blood pressure and respirations carefully.

## NALOXONE (NARCAN®)

*Actions.* Naloxone is a narcotic antagonist. It reverses the respiratory depression, coma, and hypotensive effects of medically administered narcotics and heroin. It is different from other narcotic antagonists in that it will not produce the additional respiratory depression associated with nalorphine (Nalline®). The onset of action is one to two minutes with a duration of thirty to ninety minutes. The duration of action is shorter than the narcotic it is antagonizing and the effect of the narcotic may return as the effects of naloxone disappear.

*Uses.* For reversing the effects of all narcotic agents including Talwin®, Darvon®, and Lomotil®.

*Precautions.* The duration of action is shorter than that of the narcotics. Therefore, watch for repeated respiratory depression and coma. It may precipitate withdrawal symptoms in patients addicted to but not overdosed with narcotics. It is not effective against sedative-hypnotic or other non-narcotic central nervous system depressants.

*Preparation.* 0.4 mg/1 ml, 1 ml ampule.

*Dose.* Adult—0.4 mg IV push, IM, SQ. The dose may be repeated every two to three minutes for 2 to 3 doses. The initial dose of naloxone may be followed with one to two amp of bicarbonate to control acidosis.
Pediatric—0.01 mg/kg IV push, IM, or SQ.

## NITROGLYCERINE (N.T.G.)

*Action.* Nitroglycerine (Nitrate) is a smooth muscle relaxant (vasodilator) that produces a rapid direct vasodilating effect on arterioles and venules. An effective sublingual dose acts within two minutes and lasts for thirty minutes.

*Uses.* Given to relieve the pain of angina pectoris.

*Precautions.* Blood pressure readings should be recorded prior to the administration of N.T.G. and should not be administered if the blood pressure is too low. N.T.G. should be used with caution in patients with a suspected MI. The most common side effects are headache and flushing due to the vasodilatation effects. Since N.T.G. tablets readily absorb water, they should be kept in an airtight container and protected from light. Because of this, you should avoid the use of the patient's own N.T.G. The bottle should be dated when opened and traded for a fresh bottle every thirty days.

*Preparation.* 1/150 grain (0.4 mg) sublingual tablets in an airtight, amber bottle of 100 tablets.

*Dose.* 1 tablet sublingually every five minutes up to 3 tablets within one hour.

## MANNITOL (OSMITROL®)

*Action.* Mannitol is an osmotic diuretic when administered intravenously. Approximately 90 percent of the dose appears in the urine in three hours. It induces diuresis by elevating the osmolarity of the glomerular filtrate, thereby hindering tubular reabsorption of water. Excretion of sodium and chloride is also enhanced. It is contraindicated in patients with anuria, severe pulmonary congestion or edema, and severe dehydration.

*Uses.* Mannitol is used in treating patients with acute cerebral edema following trauma or stroke, and for patients who have overdosed on long-acting barbiturates, such as phenobarbital. The diuresis invoked by mannitol dehydrates the brain, making it smaller.

*Precautions.* The cardiovascular status of the patient should be evaluated to prevent congestive heart failure due to sudden expansion of the extracellular fluid. Mannitol does this by remaining in the vascular compartment and drawing in fluid. When exposed to low temperatures, solutions may crystalize in concentrations greater than 15 percent. Therefore, when infusing a 20 percent mannitol solution, an in-line filter should be used to filter out crystal particles. If a large number of crystals are visible, the solution should not be used. Crystals can be resolubilized by placing the bottle in a 50°C. warm water bath. Paramedics have stored mannitol solute in a compartment under the hood of the MICU to warm the solute with heat from the engine. Adverse reactions include symptoms such as electrolyte loss and imbalance, dehydration, blurred vision, edema, headache, chills, dizziness, tachycardia, fever, and angina-like chest pains.

*Preparation.* 10 and 20 percent solution container (500 ml); 25 percent prefilled syringe (50 ml).

*Dose.* Mannitol is administered intravenously. The usual adult dosage ranges from 50 to 200 grams in a twenty-four hour period, but in most instances, an adequate response will be achieved at a dosage of approximately 100 grams per twenty-four hours (30 to 50 ml/hr). For the treatment of the head-injured patient who has signs of increased intracranial pressure, 12.5 to 25 grams can be given rapidly intravenously in the field.

## OXYTOCIN (PITOCIN®, SYNTOCINON®)

*Action.* Oxytocin is a hormone that is responsible for contracting the smooth muscle of the uterus (oxytocic). Its effects appear within one minute and persist for thirty minutes once the infusion is discontinued.

*Uses.* To be used to deliver the placenta if it does not spontaneously appear within ten minutes after the delivery of the infant. It has also previously been used to control postpartum bleeding; however, Methergine® is now used for this purpose.

*Precautions.* Oxytocin should not be used in the field to induce labor. Monitor the blood pressure carefully before administering the IV drip preparation. Hypotension and tachycardia have been observed following the IV administration of concentrated solutions. Severe water intoxication (hyponatremia) has also been reported following the prolonged intravenous infusion of oxytocin.

*Preparation.* 10 units / 1 ml, 1 ml ampules.

*Dose.* 10–20 units (1–2 amp) in 1000 ml $D_5W$ or Lactated Ringer's solution. Infuse at a rate of 20 drops per minute and watch the fundus for contraction. Increase the rate slightly if no contractions occur.

## PHENOBARBITAL (PHENOBARB, LUMINAL®)

*Action.* Phenobarbital produces all levels of CNS depression from mild sedation to hypnosis to deep coma. The degree of depression depends on the dosage, route of administration, metabolism, and excretion of the drug. Given by IV push, the onset of action is about five minutes for sedation and fifteen minutes for anticonvulsant activity. The duration of action is four to six hours.

*Uses.* As a sedative/hypnotic and anticonvulsant.

*Precautions.* Overdosage with phenobarbital can cause pinpoint pupils, respiratory arrest, and coma. Be prepared to support respiration during its use. Avoid mixing it with other drugs and flush the IV line to prevent the precipitation of phenobarbital. In pediatric patients, watch for paradoxical effects, which are characterized by CNS stimulation.

*Preparation.* 130 mg/ml, 1 ml ampule.

*Dose.* Adult—130 to 180 mg IM or IV push. IV push at 30 mg/minute.

Pediatric—3 to 5 mg/kg IM or 3 to 10 mg/kg, IV push, slowly. Draw into a 1 ml TB syringe one ampule (130 mg) of phenobarbital. Each 0.23 ml = 30 mg.

*Action.* Physostigmine is an acetyl-cholinesterase inhibitor that can cross into the CNS and reverse both the central and peripheral anticholinergic actions.

*Uses.* The anticholinergic syndrome that physostigmine would be useful against includes central signs such as anxiety, delirium, disorientation, hallucinations, hyperactivity, and seizures. Severe poisoning may produce coma, medullary paralysis, and death. Peripheral signs are characterized by tachycardia, hyperpyrexia, mydriasis, vasodilation, urinary retention, and loss of secretions in the pharynx, bronchi, and nasal passages. Dramatic reversal within minutes of coma, hallucinations, and other signs can be expected if the diagnosis is correct. Since physostigmine is metabolized rapidly, therapeutic doses may be necessary at thirty to sixty minute intervals as life-threatening signs such as dysrhythmias, convulsions, and coma recur. Drugs that can cause anticholinergic symptoms are: tricyclic antidepressants, antispasmodics, antihistamines, antipsychotic drugs, and anti-Parkinsonism drugs. Plants that are noted for their anticholinergic properties when ingested are: aminita, solanum, atropa, dotura, and lantana (Chapter 17).

*Precautions.* Toxic symptoms seen secondary to physostigmine use are cholinergic and include salivation, emesis, urination, and defecation. Relative contraindications to the use of physostigmine include asthma, gangrene, cardiovascular disease, and mechanical obstruction of the GI or urogenital tract. Definite diagnosis as to whether the patient actually ingested large quantities of an anticholinergic drug should be made prior to administering physostigmine to comatose patients.

*Preparation.* 2 mg/2 ml ampule.

*Dose.* 0.5–2.0 mg IV or IM. IV administration should be at 1 mg/min.

## PROPRANOLOL (INDERAL®)

*Action.* Propranolol is a beta-adrenergic receptor blocking drug. It specifically competes for beta receptor sites, which results in decreased chronotropic, inotropic, and vasodilator responses to beta-adrenergic stimulation. It also decreases conduction velocity through the SA and AV nodes and decreases myocardial automaticity via beta-adrenergic blockade. It appears to decrease blood pressure by decreasing cardiac output and by a complex effect on vasoconstrictor mechanisms. The drug usually causes decreased myocardial oxygen consumption and, secondarily, a decrease in coronary blood flow. Following IV administration, the action is almost immediate. The half life of a single dose is two to three hours.

*Uses.* Useful in the treatment of (1) moderate to severe hypertension, especially when combined with diuretics; (2) management of angina pectoris; and (3) prophylactic management of supraventricular dysrhythmias such as atrial tachycardia, persistent sinus tachycardia, persistent atrial extrasystoles, atrial flutter, and fibrillation. Ventricular dysrhythmias do not respond to propranolol as predictably as to the supraventricular dysrhythmias.

*Precautions.* Propranolol should not be used in patients with (1) bronchial asthma, (2) sinus bradycardia and greater than first degree heart block, (3) cardiogenic shock, (4) right ventricular failure secondary to pulmonary hypertension, (5) congestive heart failure, and (6) patients on psychotropic drugs such as MAO inhibitors. Side effects include bradycardia, intensification of AV block, congestive heart failure, lightheadedness, mental depression, nausea, vomiting, and bronchospasm.

*Preparation.* Injection—1 mg/1 ml; 1 ml ampule or tablets.

*Dose.* Adult—Orally, 10 to 30 mg, three to four times/day. IV—1.0 to 2.0 mg and repeat in ten minutes if necessary.
Pediatric—IV—0.025 to 0.1 mg/kg/dose q5min. Maximum 3 mg total.

## SODIUM BICARBONATE (Na HCO₃)

*Action.* Sodium bicarbonate is an alkalinizing agent and exerts its action by altering the plasma pH from acid toward alkaline. It is used if the plasma pH falls below 7.35, at which point acidosis occurs. Each 50 ml supplies 44 mEq of bicarbonate.

*Uses.* During a cardiac arrest, severe metabolic acidosis occurs rapidly because of anaerobic metabolism (Chapter 4). During resuscitation, the acidosis must first be corrected since it depresses the effects of norepinephrine, epinephrine, and alpha and beta receptor stimulating drugs. Sodium bicarbonate can also be given after naloxone administration to relieve the acidosis and resultant combativeness of people who have overdosed on heroin. For sodium bicarbonate to be effective the patient must be adequately ventilated to eliminate carbon dioxide.

*Precautions.* It should not be mixed with calcium chloride or epinephrine in the same bottle or IV tubing. The overadministration of bicarbonate can lead to metabolic alkalosis and the sodium content can lead to fluid retention, hyperosmolality, and congestive heart failure.

*Preparation.* Adult—3.75 gram (44 mEq)/50 ml, 50 ml prefilled syringe.
Pediatric—1 mEq/ml, 10 ml prefilled syringe.

*Dose.* Adult—1 mEq/kg body weight, IV push, which may be repeated; subsequent doses of half the initial dose every ten minutes. For heroin overdose, give 2 ampules after naloxone administration in an IV push.

Pediatric—0.5 to 1.0 mEq/kg/dose, IV push. Repeat the dose every five to ten minutes as needed.

The paramedic will be interested primarily in the use of drugs to treat a prescribed set of symptoms. The ability to anticipate the effects of the drug and the patient's response becomes a necessity!

*Important Points to Remember*

*Absorption* refers to the transfer of drug molecules from the place they are deposited to the circulated fluids. Methods of absorption include:

1. Oral
2. Topical (skin, mucous membranes, rectum, lungs)
3. Parenteral (IV, subcutaneous, IM)
4. Sublingual

*Distribution* refers to the manner in which a drug is transported. This determines rapidity of onset, length of effects, and action in general.

*Metabolism* refers to the changes drugs undergo after absorption and distribution. This is usually biotransformation and usually occurs in the liver.

*Excretion* refers to the removal of drugs from the body. This takes place mostly in the kidney and to some degree in the lungs. Occasionally excretion is via saliva, feces, tears, or perspiration.

Factors modifying the administration and effect of drugs include:

Age

Body weight

Sex

Time of administration

Route of administration

Rate of metabolism and excretion

Miscellaneous factors (attitude, psychological)

Undesired drug effects include:

Predictable (known toxic effects or side effects)

Hypersensitivity (allergies or immunologic reactions)

Addiction or dependence (physical or psychological)

Poisoning (overdose that intensifies toxic effects)

Idiosyncrasy (unpredictable—inherited and individual).

Important points to know for technique of parenteral administration (SQ, IM, IV):

1. Drugs must be sterile, readily soluble, absorbable, and nonirritating.

2. Intramuscular (IM) administration is for more rapid absorption, and larger amounts are needed than is possible with subcutaneous administration.

3. Intravenous (IV) administration is for immediate and rapid effect, when the drug cannot be injected into other tissues, or when shock is present.

4. The steps to follow include:

    1. Check label
    2. Calculate dose
    3. Select appropriate syringe and needle
    4. Swab top of vial with alcohol
    5. Inject air before withdrawal from vial
    6. Prepare patient site
    7. Expel air bubbles
    8. Inject at prescribed rate
    9. Monitor adverse effect

The drug list included in this chapter is not intended to be a complete list of all drugs used; it includes only the most common ones in current usage along with background material and dosage. The paramedic is referred to one of the drug handbooks for a more comprehensive list.

*Bibliography*     American Society of Hospital Pharmacy Formulary, Vol I and II. Washington, D.C., Rev. 1977.

Goodman and Gilman. *The Pharmacologic Basis of Therapeutics*, 5th ed. New York: MacMillan Publishing Co., 1975.

Hansten, Philip. *Drug Interactions*, 3rd ed. Philadelphia, Pa.: Lea and Febiger, 1976.

Martin, Ruth. *Hazards of Medications*. Philadelphia, Pa.: J.B. Lippincott Co., 1971.

*Remington's Pharmaceutical Science*, 15th ed. Boston, Mass.: Mack Publishing Co., 1975.

# Chapter 7

# INTRAVENOUS FLUID THERAPY

Whenever an acutely ill patient is admitted to the hospital, an intravenous solution of some type is started either in the emergency department, coronary care unit, intensive care unit, or on the floor. With the advent of highly trained paramedics in the field, fluid administration in many instances begins prior to hospital admission. Intravenous fluids are a double-edged sword, and can produce harm as well as good. It becomes important, therefore, for the paramedic to have a complete understanding of why solutions are used, what solutions are used, where they are administered, and the potential harmful effects these solutions can have.

## TYPES OF SOLUTIONS

### COLLOID AND CRYSTALLOID SOLUTIONS

Intravenous solutions have been divided in medical slang into "colloid" or "crystalloid" solutions. Colloid solutions, as outlined in Chapters 4 and 5, are those that contain molecules too large to cross the capillary membranes. A colloid solution has oncotic pressure, and remains within the vascular compartment for a considerable period of time. Common colloid solutions used in the United States are plasma, reconstituted plasma, and dextran solutions. Although there is controversy among hospital physicians as to the type of solution which is useful in resuscitation during hemorrhagic shock, the controversy does not exist in the field. In most field situations, prolonged fluid resuscitation will not be undertaken and it makes little difference if the initial fluids are colloid or crystalloid solutions. The expense and storage problems make colloid solutions impractical.

Crystalloid solutions are created by dissolving crystals, such as salt (NaCl) or sugar (dextrose), in water. These solutions do not have oncotic pressure, but do have osmotic pressure (Chapter 5). They will stay in the vascular compartment only transiently and will soon equilibrate with the extravascular fluid spaces. Crystalloid salt solutions are used for fluid resuscitation in hypovolemia and can be sustained within the vascular space for at least one hour. Dextrose crystalloid solutions are used to treat hypoglycemia and as a vehicle to establish an intravenous pathway for drug administration and rehydration.

## SPECIFIC SOLUTIONS AND INGREDIENTS

Intravenous solutions are identified by their solute and its concentration. For example, 5 percent dextrose and water is called $D_5W$ or 5 percent glucose. This means there are 5 grams of glucose per 100 ml of water. Solution concentrates are labeled in bold type, but other information regarding the pH (acidity) of the solution and its osmolality (tonicity) are often overlooked. Five percent dextrose and water has a pH of 4.5 (a range of 4.0 to 4.5) and contains 252 milliosmoles/liter, which is less than the tonicity of plasma.

Intravenous solutions are also packaged in different quantities, which can range from 250 ml to 1000 ml (1 liter). Some intravenous solutions are packaged in bottles that are hazardous for field use since they may be broken, can cause bodily harm if they fall on a patient, may cause air emboli, and cannot be easily stored. Intravenous solutions stored in plastic bags are ideal because they can be easily stored, will not break or shatter, collapse when emptying preventing air emboli, and allow for rapid administration.

*Salt Solutions.* The most commonly used crystalloid solution is Hartmann's solution or Lactated Ringer's solution. Sydney Ringer was a British physiologist who in 1873 discovered by an empirical method an optimal electrolyte solution that contained sodium, potassium, calcium, bicarbonate, and other ions. This solution, although ideal, was not practical for intravenous use because it could not be bottled. Hartmann, following a study of the electrolyte content of diarrhea in children, devised a similar solution to Ringer's in 1922, but used lactate ion as an anion (negative ion) rather than bicarbonate. His solution is therefore called Lactated Ringer's solution or Hartmann's solution. This solution contains the following: 130 milliequivalents (mEq) of sodium per liter, 28 mEq/l of lactate, 109 mEq/l of chloride, 3 mEq/l of calcium, and 4 mEq/l of potassium. The pH is 6.5 and the osmolality is 275 milliosmoles (mOsm) per liter. It has a tonicity slightly less than that of normal plasma. Lactated Ringer's solution is immensely practical for field use since it provides restoration of intravascular volume; it remains within the vascular space; it is relatively inexpensive; and it can be packaged and stored in plastic bags.

Normal saline contains 154 mEq/l of sodium, and has a more limited use. Although it is an effective replacement solution, it has not gained as wide an acceptance as Lactated Ringer's solution. The sodium content is greater than Lactated Ringer's, and for that reason introduces more sodium than is usually needed. In spite of this, it is an adequate temporary solution for resuscitation during hemorrhage or fluid loss due to burns, peritonitis, or massive diarrhea.

Sodium solutions containing half normal or quarter normal saline are used in a situation where sugar should not be given and the quantity of sodium is restricted. An example of this is diabetic ketoacidosis in a patient with congestive heart failure. In this situation, the patient already has an elevated blood sugar, but needs fluid resuscitation without excessive sodium. These solutions are also useful in the treatment of dehydrated infants and children.

*Sugar Solutions.* The pure sugar solutions are useful as a vehicle for maintaining an intravenous route in transport. The most commonly used solution is dextrose 5 percent in water. This solution gives the patient small amounts of sugar. This solution is often given with a microdrip chamber, especially in patients with a myocardial infarction, when dysrhythmias may occur.

*Combination Solutions.* The crystalloid salt and sugar solution combinations are useful when some sugar and saline are needed. An example of this would be in hypoglycemia combined with shock or hemorrhage. The dextrose will elevate the blood sugar and the salt solution will restore the blood volume. The dextrose 5 percent and 0.2 percent sodium chloride solutions are necessary for fluid hydration in infants and small children as stated above. The additional salt prevents hyponatremia, which might occur if too much fluid is administered.

*Colloid Solutions.* The colloid solution most commonly used is reconstituted plasma or a 5 percent albumin solution with normal saline. There are other types of colloid solutions, such as dextran and hydroxyethyl starch, but they have not gained wide acceptance in this country for field use. Dextran solutions might interfere with subsequent blood typing and crossmatch in the hospital. Plasma or albumin solutions are excellent plasma expanders for the in-hospital situation, but their need in the field when transportation to a medical facility is imminent is questionable. They may be useful if transport is to be delayed for more than one hour, or longer.

Table 7-1 is a list of commonly used IV solutions and their indications for use. They are classified as crystalloid sugar solutions, crystalloid salt solutions, crystalloid salt and sugar solutions, and colloid-containing solutions.

TABLE 7-1. COMMONLY USED INTRAVENOUS SOLUTIONS

| | Volume in ml | Concentration of Solutes | pH/ Osmolality | Indications |
|---|---|---|---|---|
| **CRYSTALLOID SUGAR SOLUTIONS** | | | | |
| Dextrose 5% in Water (D$_5$W) | 250 500 | $\dfrac{5 \text{ g Dextrose}}{100 \text{ ml}}$ | pH = 4.5 252 mOsm/1 | Used in transport for possible route to administer drugs, also in cardiac arrest and pulmonary failure. |
| Dextrose 10% in Water (D$_{10}$W) | 250 | $\dfrac{10 \text{ g Dextrose}}{100 \text{ ml}}$ | pH = 4.0 505 mOsm/1 | Hypoglycemia (low blood sugar). |
| **CRYSTALLOID SALT SOLUTIONS** | | | | |
| Lactated Ringer's (Hartmann's) | 500 1000 | $\dfrac{\begin{array}{l}28 \text{ mEq Lactate}\\109 \text{ mEq Cl}\\3 \text{ mEq Ca}\\4 \text{ mEq K}\\130 \text{ mEq Na}\end{array}}{1000 \text{ ml}}$ | pH = 6.5 275 mOsm/1 | Fluid resuscitation in shock, heat prostration, massive fluid loss due to burns, diarrhea. |
| Normal Saline (NS) | 500 1000 | $\dfrac{\begin{array}{l}154 \text{ mEq Na}\\154 \text{ mEq Cl}\end{array}}{1000 \text{ ml}}$ | pH = 5.0 308 mOsm/1 | Same as above. |
| 0.45 Normal Saline (1/2 NS) | 500 1000 | $\dfrac{\begin{array}{l}77 \text{ mEq Na}\\77 \text{ mEq Cl}\end{array}}{1000 \text{ ml}}$ | pH = 5.0 154 mOsm/1 | Diabetic acidosis, ketoacidosis, heat prostration. |
| **CRYSTALLOID SALT AND SUGAR SOLUTIONS** | | | | |
| Dextrose 5% in 0.9 Sodium Chloride (D$_5$NS) | 500 1000 | $\dfrac{5 \text{ g Dextrose}}{100 \text{ ml}}$ $\dfrac{\begin{array}{l}154 \text{ mEq Na}\\154 \text{ mEq Cl}\end{array}}{1000 \text{ ml}}$ | pH = 4.0 559 mOsm/1 | Hemorrhage, burns, peritonitis, massive diarrhea. |
| Dextrose 5% in Lactated Ringer's (D$_5$LR) | 1000 | $\dfrac{5 \text{ g Dextrose}}{100 \text{ ml}}$ $\dfrac{\begin{array}{l}130 \text{ mEq Na}\\4 \text{ mEq K}\\3 \text{ mEq Ca}\\109 \text{ mEq Cl}\\28 \text{ mEq Lactate}\end{array}}{1000 \text{ ml}}$ | pH = 5.0 524 mOsm/1 | Hemorrhage, hypoglycemia, and hypotension. |

TABLE 7-1. CONTINUED

| | Volume in ml | Concentration of Solutes | pH/ Osmolality | Indications |
|---|---|---|---|---|
| Dextrose 5% in 0.2% Sodium Chloride (D₅/0.2% NaCl) | 250 | $\dfrac{5\ \text{g Dextrose}}{100\ \text{ml}}$  $\dfrac{34\ \text{mEq Na}\quad 34\ \text{mEq Cl}}{1000\ \text{ml}}$ | pH = 4.0 320 mOsm/l | Pediatric emergencies, obstetrics. |

## COLLOID–CONTAINING SOLUTIONS

| | Volume in ml | Concentration of Solutes | pH/ Osmolality | Indications |
|---|---|---|---|---|
| Normal Serum Albumin 5% | 500 | $\dfrac{5\ \text{g Albumin}}{100\ \text{ml}}$  $\dfrac{140\ \text{mEq Na}\quad 120\ \text{mEq Cl}\quad \text{Less than 1 mEq K}}{1000\ \text{ml}}$ | pH = 6.8 Equal to plasma osmolality | Hemorrhagic shock, burns, etc. |

## ADMINISTRATION OF FLUIDS

### EQUIPMENT

*Tubing.* Intravenous solutions are given almost exclusively through clear plastic tubing. This allows for direct eye contact of the solution to check for air in the tubing and for possible precipitation of drugs administered through the tube. The intravenous tubing should be packaged sterilely so that at least the connections to the solution vial and patient are sterile as well as the interval lumen. The tubing must contain a drip chamber so that drops can be counted and the size of the drops estimated (Figure 7-1). The drip chambers are filled by either microdrop (small) or macrodrop (large) regulators. The microdrip chamber receives such a tiny drop that if the solution was inadvertently opened, rapid overhydration of the patient would not occur. Usually 60 microdrops is equivalent to one milliliter. The drop size varies depending upon the manufacturer, and this difference should be known when using the microdrip chamber. The macrodrip regulator delivers 1 ml for every 10 drops. The intravenous solution travels by gravity down the tube and connects to a needle at the infusion site. Microdrip chambers are used in infants or small children, and in adults for maintaining an intravenous access without the concern of overhydration. The macrodrip chambers are always used in adults whenever rapid fluid administration is necessary. Every intra-

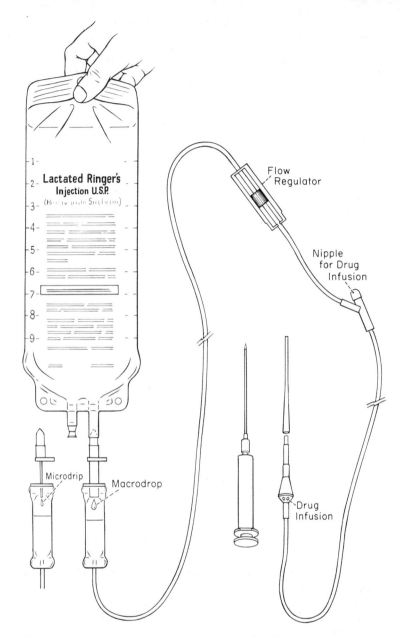

**Figure 7-1.** Intravenous fluids can be administered through a microdrip or macrodrip chamber.

venous tubing has a partial occlusive mechanism to aid in regulating the flow.

There are two commonly used methods for administering drugs to patients through the tubing. One consists of a latex rubber bulb with puncture sites where the needle and intravenous tubing join. A second type consists of latex plugged nipples along the course of the tube. In either case, the important consideration is that potential puncture sites be as close to the vein as possible so that administered drugs are not diluted in a long tube.

Some intravenous tubings have ballooned out plastic portions (which contain a one-way valve) along the course of the tubing. Squeezing the bulb will rapidly deliver a bolus of fluid, and the subsequent release allows for rapid filling of the bulb by negative suction. These devices are very safe and can be quite useful in situations where fluids need to be delivered at a rapid rate. Fluid administration in pediatric patients may be administered from a separate chamber before the microdrip chamber. The advantage of this is that it allows for administration of a specific amount of fluid. Such chambers are called burettes, or more commonly, buretrol chambers (Chapter 20).

Most fluids are administered by gravity drip and the higher the distance from the patient, the more rapidly the solution flows. If there is need to give fluid rapidly and gravity or squeezing the tubing is not possible, the plastic bag containing the fluid can be placed under the patient and his weight will squeeze in the fluid rapidly.

*Needles and Cannulas.*  The needle or cannula that punctures the patient's skin and allows entry into the vein can be made of either plastic or metal. The sizes of needles vary from 12 gauge to 23 gauge. The gauge number is confusing and is the reverse of what it appears to be. For example, a 12 gauge needle implies that the needle is smaller than a 23 gauge needle. Because 23 is a larger number, one would assume the 23 gauge would be a large needle. However, a 23 gauge needle is a fine needle, whereas a 12 gauge needle is a large bore needle. For most field work, a 14 or 16 gauge needle appears to be adequate. The 23 gauge needle may be useful for pediatric problems.

There are different types of needles available for intravenous fluid administration. The traditional needle is a straight metal one with a hub. This needle is inserted directly into the vein. The metal needle may be short with plastic wings (butterfly needle) (Chapter 20). These needles are ideal for infants or adults with small veins. Metal needles are inflexible and can easily poke through the vein and cause infiltration of the fluid into the tissue.

A more desirable cannula for field use is the plastic needle. The most commonly accepted ones are those that have a central metal shaft needle with an outer plastic shaft (Figure 7-1). The metal needle is introduced into the vein with the plastic sheath in place, and the steel needle is then removed. The plastic needle, which is blunt, is allowed to advance along the course of the vein with the IV solution running. The obvious advantage of this type of cannula is that it is flexible, not sharp, and can withstand movement without infiltration. Experience and the clinical situation dictate the size and type of needle to be used. It would make very little sense to put a 21 scalp vein needle into a 200 pound person who has just fractured a femur and ruptured his spleen for fluid administration on the way to the hospital. It would be equally important not to place a steel needle into a vein during cardiac arrest where the patient may be bounced around and the needle might be dislodged. Infiltration into the tissue of drugs, such as sodium bicarbonate, or calcium-containing medications, can cause severe tissue damage with necrosis and loss of skin and muscle.

## SELECTION OF VEINS

*Location.*    The most popularly used veins, either during cardiopulmonary resuscitation or simply to transport a patient who has a dysrhythmia, are the antecubital veins in the forearm. The median antecubital vein is easily distended by a tourniquet placed above it and a cannula can be inserted (Figure 7-2). The next veins of choice are the wrist or hand veins. The cephalic veins that run over the radial head can be distended by a tourniquet at the forearm (Figure 7-3). If these are collapsed and totally inaccessible during cardiopulmonary resuscitation or shock, the external jugular vein (neck) or veins of the foot, such as the saphenous vein or dorsal veins, can be used. Regardless of which vein is selected,

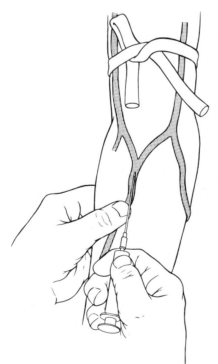

**Figure 7-2.** The median antecubital (cubital vein) is one of the most common sites to start an intravenous. The vein is distended with a tourniquet.

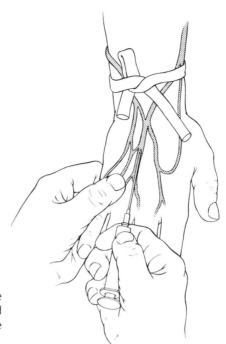

**Figure 7-3.** Veins of the dorsum of the wrist are useful. The skin is stretched with the thumb before inserting the needle.

familiarity with the anatomic location of veins, how best to distend them, proper selection of the intravenous catheter, and repeated practice make the starting of intravenous fluids a highly successful field procedure.

When paramedics are gaining field experience it is helpful to keep the batting average of the number of times an intravenous line can be started successfully in the field. In most experienced units, the batting average is approximately 95 percent. There is a certain percentage of venipunctures that cannot be started and these usually occur in obese patients during shock and cardiac arrest, and in small children where structures are not easy to find. There are no simple solutions to these latter problems, and individual expertise and training are necessary to gain skill.

*Procedures for Starting Intravenous Solutions.* The steps in starting an intravenous line once a vein has been selected are the same no matter which vein is used.

1. The tourniquet is applied and the vein palpated with the finger.

2. When the vein has been identified and distended, the needle with the plastic shaft and syringe are introduced into the skin.

3. When introducing the needle, it is best to grasp the skin around it and pull the skin in the opposite direction the needle is being inserted to make the skin taut and easy to puncture. This prevents pain and

discomfort. The alternative method is to grasp the skin with the other hand behind the vein and pull it tight.

4. The needle should be introduced through the skin and then the vein punctured after the needle has entered the skin. Once there is a flash of blood into the syringe, the needle can gradually be withdrawn from the plastic hub as the hub is pushed inward.

5. The intravenous connector is then attached to the plastic hub and fluid will run in as the plastic portion is introduced farther. Be certain that it is locked in a good distance up the vein from the venipuncture site to prevent back extravasation of solution or blood.

6. Once the cannula is in place and fluid flow noted, the cannula is best secured with tape.

7. The use of antibiotic ointments or other ointments in the field is a waste of time and is of no benefit to the patient. The application of ointments may cause poor sticking of the tape and subsequent dislodgement during transport.

When the external jugular vein is used, the following steps should be taken, if feasible:

1. The patient's head should be turned in the opposite direction of the intended venipuncture and the head positioned down 15°.

2. "Tourniquet" the vein with one finger slightly above the clavicle (Figure 7-4).

3. Align the needle in the direction of the shoulder. Introduce the needle and cannula at a point midway between the jaw and clavicle.

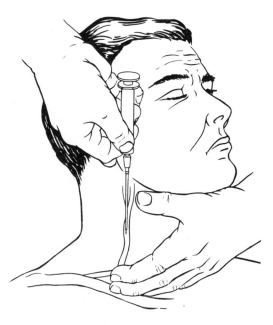

**Figure 7-4.** The external jugular vein can be used. It is distended by compression at the clavicle with the index finger and the skin is stretched with the thumb.

4. Enter the vein and when a blood return is observed, advance slightly to be sure the slanted plastic cannula is entirely within the vein. Withdraw the needle as the cannula is pushed inward.

5. Secure the needle with tape.

If an intravenous line cannot be started readily in the field, it is better to transport the patient rapidly and use whatever resuscitation measures are available. This is especially true in trauma cases. Even in the best of circumstances, with proper lighting, assistance, and positioning, insertion of intravenous lines can be difficult and demanding of one's patience. Nowhere in medicine does the adage "practice makes perfect" better apply than in the area of venipuncture. An outstanding method for learning the proper technique is observing and assisting laboratory technicians drawing the daily blood work in hospitals. Paramedic personnel can soon learn how to enter a vein properly without hurting the patient.

## INDICATIONS FOR THE USE OF INTRAVENOUS FLUIDS

Intravenous fluids are used in a multitude of clinical situations. The list of disorders in which fluids are administered is too long to elaborate on and only general principles need to be known. Fluid is administered to restore blood volume or extracellular fluid deficits, to correct electrolyte abnormalities, to restore the blood sugar to normal, to correct metabolic disturbances (acidosis), for the administration of drugs during cardiopulmonary arrest, for rehydration of the dehydrated patient, and as a route for drugs. The fluid of choice for all types of hypotension, whether the result of fluid loss, hemorrhage, or cardiogenic shock, is either a crystalloid salt or colloid solution. As previously mentioned, the argument over which is indicated is not pertinent in most field situations since rapid transportation is usually the case, and massive amounts of crystalloid solutions are not usually given.

Intravenous solutions for use in comatose patients or patients who have altered mental status without trauma should include glucose, since hypoglycemia may be the underlying cause of the coma. In many portions of the country (before the intravenous solution is started), a blood sample is drawn when the intravenous needle is inserted and preserved in a container ("red top tube") for glucose determination. This is not necessarily useful in treatment, but the baseline glucose level may be helpful in the subsequent hospital diagnosis of the patient's problem (Chapter 16). If glucose is administered to the hypoglycemic patient, this will correct the hypoglycemia, and by the time the patient arrives at the hospital the blood glucose may be normal and the diagnosis never made. Glucose solutions are useful in cardiopulmonary arrest where pulmonary edema may be a problem and salt solutions would not be indicated.

The glucose solution is compatible with most medications and will not produce precipitation of drugs or side effects.

Intravenous solutions are indicated in any situation where drug administration may be necessary. This would include cardiopulmonary arrest, suspected myocardial infarction with dysrhythmia, asthma, congestive heart failure, seizures, and acute pulmonary failure. Since patients in this category are not depleted of intravascular or extracellular fluid, they need not be given large amounts of fluid. (Actually, they may sometimes be overhydrated as part of their clinical problem.) In this situation, dextrose and water in a 5 percent solution with a microdrip chamber is indicated.

Other indications for fluid administration are during obstetric emergencies and in many pediatric problems. These indications and the choice of solution will be dealt with in the chapters dealing with these specific problems.

## PRACTICAL PROBLEMS

Fluid and electrolyte abnormalities in the field include rapid or chronic losses of fluid from body spaces, either by internal shifts or external losses. These can be broken down into salt/water loss, colloid loss, pure water loss, or a combination of these.

### EXTERNAL LOSSES

*Vomiting.* External water losses, in general, are due to vomiting, diarrhea, sweating, or diuresis (increased urination). Fluid loss from the upper gastrointestinal tract has a different electrolyte composition than fluid loss through the lower gastrointestinal tract. Upper gastrointestinal losses will include primarily potassium, hydrogen ion, and some sodium. Losses from vomiting can be so severe as to induce a metabolic alkalosis because of the loss of hydrogen ions. In these patients, the serum potassium and chloride levels are low. When vomiting has been prolonged, the patient may present with evidence of dehydration. This can be evaluated in the field by the pulse rate, the dryness of the tongue, the compressibility of the eyeballs, and the skin turgor (Chapter 5, Table 5-1).

> **Case Study.** A 59-year-old male with a known history of duodenal ulcer disease had collapsed in the bathroom after two days of vomiting. The paramedics were called to the home and discovered the patient to be cold and disoriented, with a rapid pulse rate and sunken eyes. Following communication with the base hospital, it was elected to start an intravenous solution for stabilization and transport.
>
> How much solution and what type should be given?

**Comment:** If the patient has vomited enough to produce dehydration and a history as described, he obviously has lost a significant amount of water and electrolytes. Since the loss is from the upper gastrointestinal tract, it can be assumed that sodium, potassium, and hydrogen ions have been lost from the body. Since the patient's clinical condition is consistent with a 10 to 20 percent loss of body water, an approximate estimation of his fluid requirements can be made. The patient appeared to weigh 140 pounds or approximately 70 kilograms. Seventy kilograms times 10 to 20 percent equals 7000 to 14,000 ml. Restoration of the intracellular and extracellular fluid deficits would be impossible, and is not advised in a short period of time. It is necessary to give a solution that will provide temporary and rapid restoration of the intravascular blood volume. A solution such as Lactated Ringer's should be given rapidly (500 to 1000 ml) and the patient transported for hospitalization and subsequent proper and complete rehydration. It would be a mistake to give a pure glucose-containing solution since the patient already has lost electrolytes, and giving him a solution without salt will dilute his serum sodium (hyponatremia).

*Diarrhea.* Losses through the lower gastrointestinal tract in the form of diarrhea contain more sodium and bicarbonate than upper gastrointestinal losses. This type of loss is seen in acute gastroenteritis (bowel infections). Some examples are viral infection, salmonella infection, staphylococcal enteritis, or, in some parts of the world, cholera. There are medical conditions of the colon called ulcerative colitis or regional enteritis in which dehydration may be so severe that it produces signs of shock and dehydration. People with massive diarrhea will present with shock and metabolic acidosis due to the loss of the bicarbonate ion and sodium. Since the fluid loss may be so rapid as to deplete the intravascular blood volume and cause shock, restoration with a salt solution is necessary. Rapid administration of a balanced salt solution such as Lactated Ringer's will stabilize the patient and allow for transport.

*Perspiration.* External losses due to sweating or dehydration from long hikes and forced marches, such as occur in the Armed Services, produce mixed electrolyte and water losses. Because the skin glands can respond to mineral corticoids and conserve sodium under these circumstances, more water is lost relative to sodium. The consequence of this is heat prostration and the individual will have a high serum sodium (hypernatremia). Rehydration of the patient requires the use of water and smaller amounts of salt solution. An ideal solution for this would be $D_5W$ with 1/2 NS, or $D_5W$ with Lactated Ringer's. An example of this condition is illustrated in the following case.

> **Case Study.** An 18-year-old male was riding in a marathon bicycle race on a hot summer day. Approximately 12 miles into the race

he collapsed and fell from his bicycle. The paramedics were summoned. Observation revealed a pulse rate of 180, blood pressure of 60/0 mm Hg, and cool, clammy skin. The patient appeared to weigh 70 kg.

**Comment:** This patient appeared to be obviously hypovolemic as well as dehydrated. Because he had lost such a large amount of fluid in the form of sweat, he had dehydrated himself. An intravenous solution that contained only sugar would drop his serum sodium precipitously and might produce seizures. The solution of choice is a sugar solution with one-half normal saline or even Lactated Ringer's solution. This will give slightly more water in relation to salt and allow for the appropriate rehydration of his intravascular and extravascular fluid compartments.

*Diuresis.* Diuresis can occur either by taking a diuretic, as in a patient with cardiac problems, in the course of treatment of pulmonary edema, or as a result of diabetic ketoacidosis. In the latter situation, diuresis is caused by the high glucose level and water loss, which produce an osmotic diuresis in the kidney. Water lost through the urinary tract can be severe enough to produce dehydration, hypovolemia, and shock. In these circumstances, stabilization of the blood volume is necessary with a water and salt solution. In the case of the diabetic, a salt solution without dextrose should be used. One-half normal saline (0.45%) would be ideal.

## INTERNAL LOSSES

Burns, peritonitis, blunt trauma (fractures), intestinal obstruction, and inflammation of the pancreas are common clinical syndromes that result in shock and dehydration without external losses of fluid from the body. Since the inciting event usually is inflammation or trauma, there is loss of salt, water, and protein. These losses are termed "third space" losses, and since they do not consist of external losses from the body, their onset may be insidious.

> **Case Study.** A 20-year-old white male involved in an auto accident sustained 40 percent burns over his back and trunk. During the rescue time the patient was trapped in the automobile for nearly an hour. Upon removal from the automobile, his pulse was 120 and the blood pressure was 80/60 mm Hg. He was slightly confused and transport was carried out immediately. Which type of fluid should be given in transport?

**Comment:** A 20-year-old who is involved in a fire causing third degree burns throughout portions of his body begins to lose colloid and electrolyte solution immediately after the burn. These losses can occur rapidly and may produce changes in the blood pressure and pulse early. Since the losses consist of both salt and protein, the use of a colloid solution is ideal but not necessary despite the delay in transport. A salt solution such as Lactated Ringer's is the solution of choice.

*Summary*

Fluid and electrolyte problems encountered in the field require rapid clinical assessment and the judicious use of fluid and electrolyte solutions. The doctor in the hospital has the luxury of obtaining blood tests and serial follow-ups of the patient in order to evaluate the proper amount of solutions to be given. In the field, these are not available. Consequently, the body habitus of the patient, clinical signs of fluid loss, and type of and source of fluid loss are vitally important. The primary purpose of fluid administration in the field is to stabilize the patient's cardiovascular system for transport and prevention of hypovolemia and cardiac arrest. Following transport the patient can be hydrated and full reevaluation of the disease process carried out. Overhydration should also be avoided, and with rapid clinical estimates, one can keep the fluid replacement on the conservative side, yet administer enough to maintain intravascular volume until arriving at the emergency center.

*Important Points to Remember*

Intravenous fluids have been arbitrarily divided into colloid or crystalloid.

Colloid solutions contain molecules too large to cross capillary membranes and remain within the vascular compartment.

Crystalloid solutions are made by dissolving salt or sugar (dextrose) in water. They equilibrate with other fluid spaces.

In most field situations, crystalloid solutions are the most practical to use.

One of the common intravenous solutions is 5 percent dextrose and water ($D_5W$ or 5 percent glucose). This contains 5 grams of glucose (dextrose) per 100 ml water.

The other common crystalloid solutions contain both dextrose and salts of varying concentrations. One of the most popular solutions is Lactated Ringer's solution which contains: 130 mEq sodium/l, 28 mEq lactate/l, 109 mEq chloride/l, 3 mEq calcium/l, and 4 mEq potassium/l. Normal saline (NS) contains 154 mEq of sodium/l.

Intravenous fluids are given through clear plastic tubing.

Needles are either plastic or metal. The sizes vary from 12 to 23 gauge (the 12 is the largest and 23 is the smallest). For most field work a 14 or 16 is adequate (a 23 is used for pediatric patients).

The most popularly used vein in the field is the antecubital. Experienced units usually have a 95 percent rate of success starting intravenous solutions in the field. Failures usually occur in infants, children, obese patients, and during the treatment of shock or cardiac arrest.

Indications for the use of intravenous fluids include:

Restore blood volume or extracellular deficits

Correct electrolyte abnormality

Correct metabolic disturbances (acidosis)

Restore normal blood sugar

Administer drugs

Hydration

Intravenous solutions are indicated in the following conditions for drug administration:

Myocardial infarction

Dysrhythmia

Asthma

Congestive heart failure

Seizures

Pulmonary failure

Obstetric emergency (Chapter 19)

Pediatric emergencies (Chapter 20).

Fluid and electrolyte abnormalities in the field may include:

1. External losses (vomiting, diarrhea, perspiration—heat prostration, diuresis)

2. Internal losses (shock and dehydration without external losses)—burns, peritonitis, fractures, blunt trauma, intestinal obstruction.

*Bibliography*   American Heart Association, Committee on Emergency Cardiac Care. *Advanced Cardiac Life Support Manual.* 1975.

Kurdi, W. J. "Learning Correct IV Therapy," *Emergency*, Vol. 10:28, 1978.

# Chapter 8

# THE HISTORY AND PHYSICAL EXAMINATION

When a person is admitted to the hospital, evaluation of his or her problem depends mostly on the history and physical examination. In terms of making a diagnosis, a properly done history and physical examination supersedes in importance laboratory studies. In most cases the history is more revealing than the physical examination. For example, a doctor called in the middle of the night concerning a complaint can usually make a correct diagnosis over the telephone without a physical examination.

In order to obtain a proper history, rapport must be established between the person taking the history and the patient, relatives, friends, or observers of the patient. A person who conducts himself in a professional manner, keeps the proper distance, yet is friendly and able to break down communication or hostility barriers, will succeed in obtaining a proper history. The individual who, while asking questions, seems rushed, is irritated by the situation, lacks self-confidence, or moralizes about the patient's situation, will often not obtain a proper history and may miss many important clues.

The parts of the history and physical examination include:

Chief complaint
History of the present illness
Physical examination
Diagnosis
Differential diagnosis

The above list can be summarized in one word—assessment. The paramedic in the field will assess the patient by following the preceding outline. Assessment of the patient is the single most important thing the paramedic does. Proper treatment of the patient depends upon accurate assessment. It is of little use to know how to start an IV or administer a drug when the assessment of the patient's disease has been inaccurate.

Remember, the mobile intensive care unit nurse or the physician at the Base Station Hospital is making a decision based on the paramedic's assessment. In order to gain skills in assessment, the paramedic must learn how to take a history and do a physical examination on normal people. These techniques are applied to ill or injured patients. In practice the paramedic must obtain a followup of the patients he sees and treats in order to judge the quality of his assessment skills.

## CHIEF COMPLAINT

The chief complaint is the statement by the patient that initiated the call for help. The chief complaint may be chest discomfort, dizziness, sore ankle, cough, etc. The chief complaint will lead the paramedic in the direction of the patient's history. The patient will be asked questions concerning his condition related to his chief complaint. The chief complaint is why the paramedic was summoned and it is important not to digress from it into other problems the patient might have. This occurs frequently in hospitals when a patient is admitted with one chief complaint and ends up receiving therapy for a totally unrelated illness. He may be discharged from the hospital sometimes without the chief complaint having been investigated. The individual who summons help from the paramedic because of chest pain and at the same time has a black eye should not be questioned about the eye first. Questions about the black eye can be dealt with later in the history. When communicating to the Base Station Hospital, the chief complaint should always be included in the initial transmission.

## HISTORY

In the field, the paramedic who initially sees the patient may simultaneously take a history, do the physical examination, and start treatment. However, for the purposes of this discussion, these entities are separated and discussion will begin with the history.

The importance of the history is to discover as rapidly, concisely, and thoroughly as possible the factors that led to the chief complaint. It is easy to become trapped into discussing irrelevant details that are not pertinent to the present problem. The events surrounding an accident, for example, are extremely important to the physician taking care of the patient at the hospital. In the case of an automobile accident, the mechanism and pattern of injury (Chapter 14) are most important, and the paramedic should ask himself the following questions:

1. Was the patient wearing a seatbelt?
2. Had he been drinking prior to the accident?

3. How much had he been drinking?
4. What had he eaten?
5. Was he thrown from the car or did someone drag him out before police or fire personnel arrived?
6. Was he the driver or the passenger?
7. Was he in the back or front seat?
8. At what time did the accident occur?

In the case of a penetrating injury, the questions to be asked include:

1. What position was the victim in when the injury occurred?
2. What type of object produced the penetrating injury?
3. At approximately what time did the injury occur?

The paramedic will also evaluate problems in the field not related to trauma. These will include such problems as drug overdose, psychiatric emergencies, acute chest pain, complications of diabetes mellitus, coma, strokes, poisoning, and acute respiratory failure. The history of the present illness taken outside the hospital cannot be as thorough as that taken in the hospital because of time and surrounding circumstances.

Medical students when learning how to take a history soon realize that most patients are not familiar with medical terminology. For example, it would be inappropriate to ask a patient if he or she is having dyspnea. It is better to ask, "Are you having trouble getting your breath?" It is also tempting to place words in the patient's mouth and thereby interpret his symptoms based on his yes or no response to your questions. If the individual is complaining of chest pain and the interviewer's first question is, "Does the pain give you a crushing sensation?" this will lead the patient and make his further descriptions unclear. It is better to have the patient describe his pain and have the examiner make his own interpretation of the patient's complaints. As experience is gained, history taking becomes more astute, and questions become more pertinent.

It is important when taking a history not to moralize or criticize the individual giving the history, since rapport will be diminished and the subsequent care of the patient will be more difficult. This is never more evident than in the situation in which the paramedics have been summoned because a child has "swallowed a bottle of pills." The mother is often guilt-ridden because she left the pills where the child could reach them, and is on the defensive. If the paramedic arrives and makes a comment such as, "That was really a dumb move to leave those pills around," subsequent information could be difficult to obtain. The most important information in this situation is to know how many pills were left in the container, how long ago they were taken, what was the medication, and what symptoms has the child experienced? It will become apparent to the paramedic as he gains experience that the history will give most of the information that he needs to interpret a patient's problem and aid in his treatment.

Two of the most common chief complaints will now be discussed in more detail.

CHIEF COMPLAINT: "CHEST PAIN"

One of the most common causes for fright and urgency is the sudden development of chest pain. Questioning of the patient or his immediate relatives or friends about the chest pain should be as detailed as possible. Pain is a subjective phenomenon; it cannot be felt on physical examination and it cannot be expressed by anyone but the individual who is experiencing it. People differ in terms of their pain thresholds and may exaggerate their response depending upon their age, sex, and ethnic or social backgrounds. The important aspects of pain include the following:

1. Time of origin
2. Duration
3. Previous occurrence
4. Radiation
5. Persistence
6. Quality (i.e., sharp, dull)
7. What relieves the pain

*Myocardial Infarction (Heart Attack).* One of the most common causes of chest pain in the United States is that resulting from an acute myocardial infarction. This can occur suddenly following mild or moderate exertion in individuals with no previous cardiac history. It may also occur while sitting quietly reading or watching television. The chest pain of myocardial infarction ranges from mild to extremely severe. Patients will describe the pain as if someone had stepped on their chest, is squeezing their chest, stuck a knife between their ribs, or struck them in the "stomach."

Pain of acute myocardial infarction will often radiate to the neck, jaw, or down the left arm. It can also radiate down the inner aspect of the left arm into the fingertips, more commonly on the left, but also in the right arm or both arms simultaneously. This type of pain, crushing in nature, usually exists for more than five minutes and is not relieved by any of the common measures such as deep breathing, position changes, etc.

When physicians see patients with chest pain, they take a thorough history of the pain syndrome itself and then ask other questions related to the patient's problem. These would include age, weight, height, the level of general physical activity, and current emotional or family problems. The past history is extremely important since many disease processes, particularly myocardial infarction, tend to run in families. Knowing that brothers, sisters, mothers, and fathers have similar disorders helps to narrow down the diagnosis. It is important to know whether the patient has had any prior medical condition for which he is undergoing treatment, including high blood pressure, chronic infection, arthritis, diabetes, kidney disorders, or any other underlying disease process requiring medication.

After the paramedics arrive, the patient may try to deny symptoms or even exaggerate them. When taking a history of chest pain, the patient's wife's, husband's or friend's statement about the patient's chest pain may be more accurate in terms of severity and frequency.

When evaluating problems in the field, time usually is of the essence and treatment is often occurring while the diagnosis is being determined. When the physician deals with the patient at the hospital, the diagnosis must be as precise as possible. To make it so, he must consider other diagnoses as well as the principally suspected diagnosis.

The other diagnoses are called the *differential diagnoses*. Differential diagnoses are the other diagnoses that may produce the symptoms the patient is experiencing. As experience is gained, the person taking the history will soon think about the differential diagnoses during the history. He will then tend to ask the patient questions that will help eliminate other diagnostic possibilities.

Differential diagnoses for chest pain include the following: (1) angina pectoris, (2) acute myocardial infarction, (3) pericarditis, (4) pneumonitis, (5) pulmonary embolism, (6) dissecting aortic aneurysm, (7) pneumothorax, (8) ruptured esophagus, (9) hiatus hernia, (10) cervical arthritis, (11) costochondritis (inflammation of rib cartilage), (12) acute pancreatitis, (13) acute cholecystitis, and (14) perforated duodenal ulcer.

In terms of chest pain, all of the above diagnoses are possible. However each, upon careful questioning, can be eliminated. For example, pneumonitis and pulmonary embolism produce chest pain, but the pain is usually worse on deep inspiration; may be localized to one side of the chest or the other; and does not radiate into the neck, jaw, or arm. A pneumothorax can produce chest pain that varies with respiration and the patient will complain of difficulty in breathing. Disorders of the esophagus, such as hiatus hernia or esophagitis (inflammation of the esophagus), prove to be the most common source of pain that is confused with cardiac pain. Chest pain relieved by belching can be due to a hiatus hernia or gastric distress, but may also represent cardiac pain. It is also noted that upper abdominal conditions can produce chest pain. Acute pancreatitis or a perforated duodenal ulcer can produce pain high in the epigastrium that simulates a myocardial infarction. In like manner, upper abdominal disorders may also present as chest pain. Patients with a perforated duodenal ulcer have been treated for pneumonia or myocardial infarction.

Based on the preceding remarks, it is clear that chest pain is not always related to disorders of the heart. Despite this, the conservative approach to chest pain dictates that all patients with chest pain be assumed to have a myocardial infarction or at least some cardiac disorder. The reason for this is that, despite our best clinical judgment and diagnostic techniques, the etiology of chest pain is not always clear. Close examination of coronary care unit admissions shows that approximately 50 percent of the admissions are subsequently found to have something other than a cardiac disorder as an explanation for their chest pain.

## CHIEF COMPLAINT: "STOMACH PAINS"

Abdominal pain is a prominent symptom that heralds the onset of many disease processes. Patients will refer to the abdomen as their stomach. The stomach is an organ within the abdomen. Patients will not say they are complaining of "abdominal pain," however. Abdominal pain should be analyzed by considering a thorough history in the same fashion as for chest pain. The primary difference between abdominal pain and chest pain is that often the location of the pain and the location of the disease process are not anatomically related. Disorders in an organ producing pain may refer the pain to other parts of the abdominal cavity or chest. Disorders that have spread from the organ to the surrounding peritoneum will produce pain at the site of the disease process. It is important to remember that pain pathways in the abdominal cavity travel along either the parasympathetic or sympathetic nervous system to the spinal cord, or via peripheral nerves, such as those which innervate the parietal peritoneum (Chapter 4). The onset of pain, its duration, quality, radiation, and previous history are of utmost importance.

*Appendicitis.* One of the common diseases that presents with abdominal pain is acute appendicitis. It is important to detail the mechanism for the pain of acute appendicitis since it will help in understanding the importance of a proper history.

Appendicitis is due to infection of the appendix, which is attached to the cecum. The appendix generally resides in the right lower quadrant, but occasionally it may be in a different location inside the peritoneal cavity or, uncommonly, behind the cecum outside of the peritoneal cavity. It is for this reason that appendicitis may present with different types of pain syndromes that can confuse the examiner. For the most part, however, appendicitis usually presents with a typical history that initially includes epigastric pain. This is pain above the umbilicus in the "pit of the stomach" experienced as nausea, a dull ache, or a "funny feeling." The reason for this is that appendicitis begins as an obstruction within the lumen of the appendix, followed by infection; it stimulates nerve fibers of the parasympathetic nervous system, which travel to the ninth and tenth thoracic vertebra. These fibers then transmit referred pain signals to the epigastrium; this pain is termed *visceral pain.*

Abdominal organs produce violent pain when they contract against an obstruction or are dilated due to infection or the lack of oxygen. The epigastric pain in appendicitis will persist for about twelve hours and will gradually disappear as the appendix becomes more inflamed and the infection spreads to the outer layer of the appendix. At this time, inflammatory fluid exudes from it. This irritates the parietal peritoneum and the pain then moves to the area of the organ, or the right lower quadrant. This two-point change in pain over a period of time is almost always diagnostic of acute appendicitis. If a detailed history were not taken and the events leading up to the pain were not recorded, the diagnosis would not be so apparent.

*Abdominal Conditions Described by an Observer.*   The patient may not be able to give a history about his or her abdominal complaint, as is the case with chest pain or neurologic disorders. For that reason it is important to get as much information as possible from friends or bystanders. The following case is an example.

**Case Study.**   A sixty-one-year-old white male was square dancing on a Friday evening and suddenly experienced pain in the abdomen, felt dizzy, and collapsed to the floor. He had been at the square dance with a friend who knew him quite well. The paramedics were called and found the patient pale, unable to respond to questions, with a blood pressure of 60/0 mmHg and a rapid heart rate. The friend stated that he knew the patient had an abdominal aortic aneurysm and that he was to have surgery the following week. The abdomen was found to be tense upon physical examination. The paramedics radioed this history ahead to the Base Station Hospital Emergency Department personnel, who alerted the surgical team. At the same time they started an intravenous solution of Lactated Ringer's, applied the MAST suit (Chapter 15), and immediately transported the patient.

**Comment:**   An early history was of great help since it avoided a delay in the Emergency Department to ascertain the patient's problem and prevented a delay in care. Had the proper history not been taken and the diagnosis not made prior to admission to the hospital, this would have delayed the patient's treatment.

*Trauma.*   Pain following abdominal trauma (e.g., that due to a ruptured spleen) may be entirely different from that encountered in a chronic illness or an acute inflammatory illness. In abdominal trauma the initial abdominal pain is most often related to the spilling of blood, intestinal contents, or air into the peritoneal cavity producing irritation. As the patient breathes, he creates negative intra-abdominal pressure and blood, fluid, or air tend to collect under the diaphragm. This irritates the diaphragm and the sensation is transmitted via the phrenic nerve to the C3, C4, and C5 portions of the spinal cord. This pain is then referred to the shoulder tips, which is the somatic sensory area supplied by the fifth cervical vertebra. Patients with abdominal pain following trauma will usually experience pain in their left or right shoulder tip depending upon the site of injury. This is an important sign that there has been injury to some organ that has exuded fluid or air into the peritoneal cavity. This information would be helpful to transmit to the physicians since this pain often disappears quickly and may not be a complaint when the patient is seen in the Emergency Department.

*Visceral and Parietal Pain.* *Visceral pain* (Chapter 4) has been defined as pain that originates within organs such as the heart, stomach, gallbladder, etc. *Parietal pain* is pain that originates in the parietal peritoneum and receives its innervation in the same manner as skin or muscle. For example, pain in the gallbladder is often referred to the right shoulder; but once there has been inflammation of the gallbladder to the point that the parietal peritoneum next to it is irritated, the pain will be at the site of the gallbladder in the right upper quadrant. Therefore, visceral pain may be referred to parts distant or away from the organ itself, whereas parietal pain occurs at the site of the inflammation or injury. It is important in determining the diagnosis of abdominal pain to know that these two types of pain mechanisms occur.

*Classification of Abdominal Pain by Illness.* Figure 8-1 is a diagram of the abdominal cavity. The abdominal cavity is divided into four quadrants as well as the epigastric, the two flanks, the suprapubic, and the periumbilical regions. For the purposes of acute medicine, abdominal illnesses can be classified as either acute traumatic or nontraumatic and further categorized by the region.

     1. Acute nontraumatic illness of the right upper quadrant and epigastrium would include the following conditions:

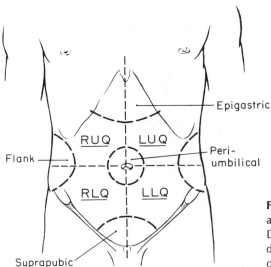

**Figure 8-1.** The topographic anatomy of the abdomen. Different locations can be described using the terms outlined in this diagram.

     a. Acute cholecystitis

     b. Acute pancreatitis

     c. Perforated duodenal ulcer

     d. Duodenal ulcer without perforation

     e. Gastric ulcer

2. Acute traumatic conditions producing right upper quadrant and/or epigastric pain are:

     a. Acute traumatic pancreatitis

     b. Rupture of the duodenum

     c. Penetrating injury to any of the organs of the right upper quadrant

     d. Rupture of the liver or gallbladder

3. Right lower quadrant acute nontraumatic illnesses are:

     a. Acute appendicitis

     b. Regional ileitis

     c. Carcinoma of the colon

     d. Ischemia or infarction of the bowel

4. Acute trauma of the right lower quadrant includes:

     a. Small bowel rupture, blunt or penetrating injury

     b. Colon rupture due to penetrating injury

     c. Injury to the iliac artery or vein

     d. Injury to the ureter

5. Acute nontraumatic illnesses in the left upper quadrant and/or epigastrium include:

     a. Perforated duodenal or gastric ulcer

     b. Spontaneous rupture of the spleen (patients with leukemia or infectious mononucleosis)

     c. Perforated esophagus due to vomiting

6. Acute traumatic conditions of the left upper quadrant and/or epigastrium include:

     a. Ruptured spleen

     b. Ruptured stomach

     c. Injury to the pancreas or liver

     d. Kidney injury

     e. Diaphragmatic rupture

7. Acute nontraumatic conditions of the left lower quadrant encompass:

     a. Acute diverticulitis

     b. Perforation of the sigmoid due to a foreign body

     c. Carcinoma of the sigmoid with perforation

     d. Ulcerative colitis

8. Acute traumatic illnesses in the left lower quadrant are:
   a. Perforation of the sigmoid due to a penetrating or gunshot wound
   b. Rupture of the small bowel
   c. Injury to the ureter
   d. Injury to the iliac vessels
9. Right or left flank nontraumatic illnesses include:
   a. Acute pyelonephritis
   b. Kidney or ureter stone
   c. Abdominal aortic aneurysm, sudden expansion, or rupture
10. Right or left flank traumatic illnesses include:
    a. Kidney injury
    b. Ruptured duodenum with right flank tenderness
    c. Traumatic pancreatitis with left flank tenderness
    d. Retroperitoneal bleeding
11. Suprapubic discomfort includes:
    a. Bladder distention
    b. Bladder stone or bleeding into the bladder
    c. Infection of the bladder (acute cystitis)
12. Traumatic suprapubic tenderness encompasses:
    a. Pelvic fracture
    b. Ruptured bladder

Conditions of the visceral retroperitoneum (those structures behind the peritoneum) will often present with abdominal or flank pain. Pain in either the right or left flank is consistent with a kidney stone or some genitourinary problem. However, pain in either the right or left flank can also be due to a ruptured or expanding abdominal aortic aneurysm. It is important to know if the pain is abdominal or flank in nature, since the diagnosis will often be entirely different.

There are certain other parts of the history that can be organized into direct questions concerning the present illness. These are:

1. Medications
2. Allergies
3. Past medical illnesses
4. Previous operations
5. Review of systems

MEDICATIONS

It is important to learn what medication the patient might have been receiving. If the patient is a diabetic, it is important to know when he last took his insulin and how much he took. The hypertensive patient may have forgotten to take his medication for the past two or three days, accounting for a sudden elevation in blood pressure and a severe headache. Often a patient is found unconscious and has a Medi-alert bracelet indicating that he is a diabetic or cardiac patient. If the patient cannot remember the medication he or she is taking, but has a sample bottle of pills, these pills can be compared to drug identification charts. These charts are printed in color and are in the central portion of the *Physician's Desk Reference* (PDR). This book can be found in every Base Station or Receiving Hospital Emergency Department.

Medications not known by the patient and not identified on the label should be brought with the individual to the hospital. Information concerning the use of cardiac drugs in anyone experiencing chest pain is important. A number of different drugs are used to alleviate chest pain and treat conditions of the heart. These include: propranolol (Inderal), nitroglycerine, digoxin, quinidine, Pronestyl$_®$, Isordil$_®$, etc. The number of antihypertensive agents is extensive and information concerning use of these drugs is important for treatment at the hospital.

## ALLERGIES

Allergies to drugs are common; penicillin is an obvious example. A paramedic would not be administering penicillin in the field, but knowledge of the patient's allergy would be important at the hospital. This would be especially true if the patient was unconscious and the information was received from a friend or relative.

## PAST MEDICAL ILLNESSES

Prior medical illnesses are an important part of the history. For example, it would be important for the paramedic to know that the patient had recently recovered from a bout with hepatitis before he starts an IV, since hepatitis can be transmitted by a needle stick. In a patient who is suffering from an acute myocardial infarction, it would be relevant to know that he has been treated for a seizure disorder.

## PREVIOUS OPERATIONS

The frequency of heart surgery for coronary artery disease in this country makes knowledge of previous operations an important part of the history. Patients who have had coronary bypass surgery can experience chest pain, and information about previous heart surgery should be relayed to the Base Station Hospital. Patients who have had heart valve replacement may be on anticoagulant drugs and the present illness might be related to bleeding.

Previous operations on the abdomen, including duodenal ulcer surgery, gallbladder surgery, and surgery for cancer, are important parts of the history. The patient who recently underwent a removal of the stomach for cancer and appears to have a stroke might instead have a cerebral metastasis.

It is important to attempt to learn about previous operations only as to how they might relate to the chief complaint or the history of the present illness. In a patient with chest pain related to coronary artery disease, it is not important to know that the patient had a hemorrhoidectomy thirty years ago.

REVIEW OF SYSTEMS

Review of systems is a systematic check of the various body organ systems. In the field it cannot be complete and will not compare to an in-hospital review of systems.

1. HEENT (Head, Eyes, Ears, Nose, Throat)
   a. Eyes: Does the patient have diplopia? Blurred vision? Does he wear contact lenses?
   b. Ears: Does he have ringing in the ears? Difficulty in hearing? Pain in the ears?
   c. Nose: Does the patient experience frequent nosebleeds?
   d. Mouth: Is the tongue sore? Does the patient have false teeth?
   e. Throat: Is there hoarseness? Is the throat sore?
   f. Neck: Is there pain on motion of the neck? Is the neck stiff?

2. Respiratory System

   Does the patient have chest pain? Shortness of breath? Wheezing? Nocturnal dyspnea? Cough? Hemoptysis? Pleuritic chest pain? Previous chest illness?

3. Cardiovascular System

   Are there palpitations? Irregularities of the heart rate? Pain in the chest? Shortness of breath on exercise? Shortness of breath at night? Cough? Cyanosis? Pain in the legs on ambulation? Previous history of phlebitis?

4. Gastrointestinal System

   Are there changes in digestion? Changes in weight? Difficulty in swallowing? Abdominal pain? Blood in the stools? Previous jaundice?

5. Neurologic System
   a. Review of the Cranial Nerves

      Is there difficulty in swallowing? Smelling? Facial weakness? Disturbances in taste? Difficulty in opening and closing of the eyelids?
   b. Motor System

      Has there been previous paralysis? Previous strokes? Tremors? Convulsions? Weakness?

c. Central Nervous System
  Is there difficulty in speech? Difficulty in naming objects? Headaches? Loss of memory?

It is obvious that all of the preceding questions could not be asked of every patient. As experience is gained in assessment, those questions in the review of systems which are pertinent to the history of the present illness will be asked. The purpose of the systems review is to organize the history so that important details about the patient's illness are not overlooked.

## PHYSICAL EXAMINATION

### GENERAL REMARKS

It is one thing to question an individual about his or her illness, but it is another to have the individual allow you to examine him. This is especially true when the patient is female and there are people watching. It is important to be discreet and not to expose portions of the body that will embarrass the patient. Having respect for the patient's privacy and yet carrying out a physical examination will mean a great deal in terms of rapport and confidence. In describing physical findings, it is important for those who are interpreting your findings to have careful details and proper terminology. The four procedures that a physical examination involves are inspection, palpation, percussion, and auscultation.

*Inspection.* The physical exam involves the use of the fingers, hands, eyes, ears, and nose. The physical exam begins with inspection. This means that the site to be examined is looked at initially. When inspecting areas to be examined, it is important to look at normal landmarks, observe asymmetry, and investigate for swelling and changes in normal body contours. Observe changes in skin color and the presence of blood or discharges from orifices such as the nose, ear, mouth, etc.

*Palpation.* The second step in the physical examination is palpation, which is done with the fingers. Palpation is feeling for swellings, tenderness, instability of body structures (such as bones), pulses, subcutaneous air, and normal landmarks. Figure 8-2 shows an example of abdominal palpation.

*Percussion.* Percussion can be done by tapping with the fingers of one hand over the fingers of the other, or by directly striking the body cavity involved (Figure 8-3). Percussion is immensely important in evaluating chest and abdominal conditions. Since air in a cavity will produce a hollow sound, and blood or other fluid will produce a solid

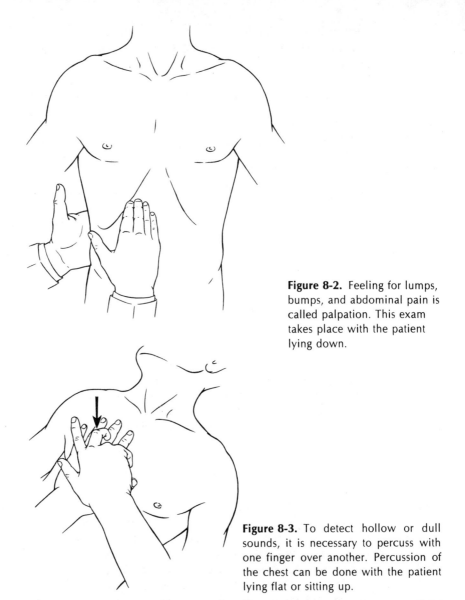

**Figure 8-2.** Feeling for lumps, bumps, and abdominal pain is called palpation. This exam takes place with the patient lying down.

**Figure 8-3.** To detect hollow or dull sounds, it is necessary to percuss with one finger over another. Percussion of the chest can be done with the patient lying flat or sitting up.

sound, percussion may give a great deal of information. Percussion is absolutely essential in determining whether the chest cavity is filled with air or filled with a dense fluid.

*Auscultation.* The final step in the physical examination is auscultation, which is done with a stethoscope (Figure 8-4). The stethoscope magnifies the sound and transmits it to the examiner. Stethoscopes can be used to evaluate sounds of the heart, lung, blood vessels, and bowel sounds in the abdominal cavity.

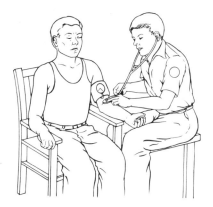

**Figure 8-4.** Blood pressure is recorded using a sphygmomanometer and stethoscope. Blood pressure is determined by listening (auscultation) for a sound with the stethoscope.

## APPROACH TO THE PHYSICAL EXAMINATION

The physical examination begins by observing the general appearance of the patient. The paramedic reports this information to the Base Station Hospital during the initial transmission. For example, statements that the patient appears shocky, cyanotic, clammy, anxious, and/or diaphoretic are helpful in giving the MICN or MIC-MD a picture of the patient. On the other hand, the paramedic might report that the patient appears to be in no acute distress and is sitting comfortably watching television. The statement of the general appearance does more in terms of describing the overall condition of the patient than anything else. If the general appearance is that of an elderly woman who is disheveled, unable to answer questions coherently, yet not in distress, this information will aid the Base Station Hospital personnel in understanding the patient's problem. The general appearance must be objective and accurate.

*Vital Signs.* The physical examination usually begins with the recording of the vital signs. (In cases of acute injury, the evaluation may begin entirely differently, as outlined in Chapter 14.) This would include pulse, blood pressure, and respiration. The pulse is usually determined at the wrist, but under circumstances of acute illness, such as shock or suspicion of a cardiac arrest, the carotid pulse is palpated. The blood pressure is taken using the arm while listening over the brachial artery. Under certain conditions it may be necessary to place a blood pressure cuff on the thigh and listen over the popliteal artery to record a blood pressure.

> **Case Study.** A twenty-six-year-old female had her left arm severed at the shoulder. The right arm was used for the infusion of intravenous fluids in the field, and it was not practical to interrupt this flow while blood pressures were taken. A blood pressure cuff was placed on the right thigh and pressures were recorded by auscultation in the popliteal fossa.

**Comment:** Under normal circumstances, the blood pressure recorded in the leg using the blood pressure cuff on the thigh and listening over the popliteal artery is 20–30 mm Hg greater than the arm. Respirations should also be counted and recorded. The type of breathing pattern should be appreciated (Chapter 9).

*Examination of the Head, Eyes, Ears, Nose, and Throat.* Look at the position of the head on the shoulder, particularly in the unconscious patient where the head may be in an exaggerated position indicating a cervical fracture. Observe the ears for discharge, including clear fluid, which may indicate a spinal fluid discharge. Look at the nose for its contour and shape. Open the eyelids and look for differences between the pupils as well as the presence of contact lenses, which should be removed if present. If the patient is conscious, have him open his mouth and inspect for any foreign bodies (broken teeth, etc.). Observe the neck for any abnormal swellings and tugs, which may indicate an airway obstruction.

Palpation during the head and neck examination should include the nose and supra and infraorbital rims to be familiar with their normal contours. Palpate over the cheek bones and the zygomatic arch. The angle of the mandible should be noted and palpated. Place both index fingers in the ear and have the patient open and close his mouth to get an appreciation of the normal movement of the temporomandibular joint, which is just in front of the ear canal. Palpate the thyroid cartilage and continue down and feel the depression between the thyroid cartilage and cricoid cartilage. This is the cricothyroid membrane. Then move the fingers laterally at the angle of the mandible or top of the thyroid cartilage and feel the pulse in the carotid artery. This is the level of the bifurcation of the common carotid. Palpate the trachea in the suprasternal notch to become familiar with its location. Run the fingers up and down the cervical spines and note the bony prominence of the seventh cervical spine. Learn how rubbing in this area will produce discomfort.

With a flashlight and throat stick, have the patient open his mouth and examine the oropharynx. Look at the tonsils and soft palate and watch it move up and down as the patient says, "Ah . . . ." Examine the uvula. See what the normal oropharynx looks like and see how much you can visualize in the hypopharynx with just a throat stick and flashlight. Practice striking the teeth with a throat stick to become familiar with what normal teeth feel like. A loose or partially avulsed tooth should be looked for in any case with serious facial trauma.

Examination of the eye in a suspected head injury is an important part of the evaluation. It is important in examining the eyes to be familiar with pupil reactions and the sizes and diameters of the pupils. This should be practiced using a flashlight in broad daylight by cupping over the eye to see what sort of response occurs. Familiarity with pupil reaction to light will help in the early detection of intracranial problems.

The important aspects of palpation are to become familiar with normal landmarks and to practice feeling them over and over again. Once the normal becomes second nature, then quick assessments will pick up abnormalities automatically.

*Examination of the Thorax.* The physical examination of the chest begins by watching the patient breathe. Determine if the breathing is done by the diaphragm and thoracic muscles or by the abdominal muscles. Is the abdomen moving up and down or is the chest moving up and down? Determine asymmetry in the breathing pattern (one side of the chest is moving and the other is not), which will indicate splinting due to pain or fluid or air in one side of the chest. Look for alterations in the normal bony landmarks of the chest such as indentation or protrusion of the sternum or swellings or alterations in the normal rib contours. Look at the clavicles and be certain they are in the normal position and that there is no swelling over them. One of the commonly missed fractures following automobile accidents is that of the clavicle, since immediate swelling may not occur and the differences between sides are not appreciated. Look at the precordial area to see if the heartbeat can be appreciated by visual inspection.

Palpation begins by feeling the trachea in the midline in the suprasternal notch. The fingers should then run along the clavicles looking for any deformity or swelling. Then the fingers are run down the sternum with inward pressure to be certain the sternum is stable and this maneuver does not produce pain. Next the ribs are palpated along the costochondral arch, running the fingers up and down and laterally. This type of palpation can pick up subcutaneous air, areas of localized pain that indicate a fracture, and even an appreciation of the breathing pattern can be made by this maneuver. If the airway is partially obstructed, rhonchus (noisy) sounds can be palpated by the fingers during respiration. The hands should travel around the back as far as possible, palpating the ribs posteriorly and even the thoracic spines posteriorly by partially tilting the patient. When this is completed, the chest can be barrel-hooped by placing the hands anteriorly and pushing inward. Palpation should then continue, feeling the precordial impulse. If the precordial impulse is absent, one should suspect pericardial effusion; however, it will often be absent in extremely obese patients or in patients with chronic pulmonary emphysema. If the point of maximal impulse is greater than the midclavicular line, which is approximately the nipple line, the possibility of cardiac enlargement or a heart disorder should be suspected.

Percussion can be performed by tapping with one finger or on the fingers of the other hand, which are spread out evenly over the chest cavity. Percussion in the normal physical examination in the hospital situation is done while the patient is sitting up by tapping the posterior portion of the thorax. This type of percussion will allow blood and air to settle. Air will rise to the top of the cavity and blood or fluid will settle to the lower portion of the cavity. The difference in the percussion sound will allow the level of the fluid to be ascertained. In the field situation, however, often the patient cannot sit up because of injury or discomfort. In that case, opening the shirt and percussing anteriorly and laterally on either side will give some information. Obvious marked differences in sound may suggest a pneumothorax, hemothorax, or fluid in the chest. Fluid produces a dull sound, whereas air produces a hyperresonance or a sound such as striking a drum. Since the chest has bilateral compartments, one side can be compared to the other.

Listening to the heart sounds needs to be practiced over and over. The heart ordinarily makes a sound that has been mimicked as "lub-dub," "lub-dub," "lub-dub." One can become familiar with heart sounds by listening to other people's hearts as well as to recordings of heart sounds. The important thing for the paramedic to learn is the presence or absence of heart sounds, and to see whether this changes with time. Friction rubs are sounds made when there is fluid between the heart and the pericardial sac. This sound is a scratching sound and there is no other sound that can mimic it. Of less importance for the paramedic are heart murmurs, since the use of this information in the field is of questionable value. When listening to the heart it is important to learn what normal heart sounds are like and to have a feeling for heart sounds that are distant, muffled, or changing from beat to beat.

Auscultation of the chest in the hospital situation begins by listening at the base of the lungs posteriorly. Again, this may not often be possible in the field situation, but patients in pulmonary edema will feel more comfortable sitting up, and in that situation listening at the base of the lungs is important. When listening at the base of the lungs in normal people, be certain that they breathe deeply in and out through the mouth. If the patient were to breathe through his nose, this would alter the sounds and make the interpretation difficult. Deep inspiration with the mouth open is the standard maneuver for breath sounds. Once normal breath sounds are learned, abnormal sounds can be appreciated. These include rales (air rushing through water), rhonchi (air rushing through fluid or mucus in the larger bronchial tubes) and wheezes (due to air whistling through airway obstructions either in the smaller bronchioles of the lung or higher up in the bronchus or trachea). Rales are present in pulmonary edema and once heard will not be mistaken.

The first question to ask is are there breath sounds at all? If they are not heard at the base, then the auscultation should be carried out higher or even moved to the front of the chest. If there is fluid in the chest, no breath sounds will be heard at the bases, and until the stethoscope is placed higher and higher to the point where air is entering the lungs, sounds may often be muffled or absent. Again, the symmetry of the bilateral nature of the chest allows comparison of sounds from one side to another. Diminished sounds on one side as compared to the other is a very important physical finding. It may mean that there is fluid or air trapped in one pleural cavity versus the other. Constant practice in listening to normal chest sounds and the sounds of patients with respiratory problems or other chest discomforts will vastly increase the paramedic's ability to make diagnoses in the field. However, do not be discouraged if your stethoscope gives totally false information and subsequent chest X-rays at the hospital minimize your diagnosis. This is a problem that the physician faces all the time, and only because X-rays are available to him is the physician able to modify diagnoses based on physical findings. In the management of patients who cannot sit at all, breath sounds should be listened to anteriorly and laterally. In this situation, the presence of differences between the two sides can be of great importance.

*Examination of the Abdomen.* Observe the abdomen for contour. Is the abdomen distended or is it scaphoid? (Scaphoid means flat or even indented.) If on initial observation of a trauma patient the abdomen is scaphoid and five minutes later it is markedly distended, this constitutes a serious change in the physical examination. Observe the abdominal musculature and see if it is being tensed during expiration or inspiration because of peritoneal irritation. Inspect the umbilicus and see if it is flat or protuberant. In children, blood in the peritoneal cavity can often be seen through an umbilical hernia or thin umbilical skin.

Abdominal palpation should begin in the area that does not hurt so the patient is not made uncomfortable by the first encounter with the examiner. For example, if the pain is in the right lower quadrant, palpation might start in the left upper quadrant.

Auscultation is the last portion of the examination in the field and does not have much practical use. Bowel sounds are often absent after trauma due to the sympathetic response and therefore do not have meaning. Often noise at the roadside or other situations make listening to bowel sounds difficult at best.

*Neurologic Examination.* A neurologic examination done in the hospital by a neurologist is an extremely tedious, lengthy, and involved procedure. For the paramedic the examination need not be so detailed. The important things the paramedic must know are the patient's level of consciousness, degree of orientation, response to stimuli (painful and verbal), and motor function. Although not strictly a part of the neurologic examination, it is also important to be aware of the patient's pupil size and equality as well as types of breathing patterns. A thorough discussion of the neurologic examination in the trauma patient is presented in Chapter 14. The type of neurologic examination presented there differs little from the neurologic exam without trauma. For example, the patient with a stroke can be equally well assessed with the same neurologic examination that is used for the trauma patient. In conducting the examination, be constantly alert to neurologic signs that are present on one side of the body and not the other. This will help localize lesions and will reveal valuable information to be transmitted to the Base Station Hospital. A single neurologic examination and evaluation is not nearly as important as sequential examinations. That is, changes in neurologic findings are quite important to the Emergency Department physician, neurosurgeon, or neurologist who will be dealing with the patient in the hospital. It is important for them to know these changes, and the paramedic will often be the first one to observe them. Written records of the findings at the scene are often not·kept, but in the ideal situation the status of the person at the time he was first checked is of utmost importance to the patient's subsequent treatment at the hospital.

*Cranial Nerves.* The cranial nerves are shown in Table 8-1. Examination of each nerve cannot be made in the neurologic evaluation of every patient. However some signs should be known.

The fifth cranial nerve is tested by noting the corneal reflex. This is usually done on the unconscious patient. The cornea is touched lightly with a cotton applicator tip in order to elicit an eye blink. Loss of the corneal reflex indicates severe central nervous system depression.

Injury to the seventh cranial nerve (facial nerve) will present with sagging and loss of the facial contours on one side (Chapter 16). This may indicate a stroke. The eyelids are also controlled by the facial nerves. Patients who are malingering will often present with eyes closed and refuse to open them on command. Running a cotton applicator over the eyelashes and eyelid will elicit a fluttering of the eyelids. This indicates that the patient is not ill and is taking advantage of the attention derived from the paramedic.

The oculomotor or third cranial nerve carries with it fibers that dilate the pupil. Compression of this nerve will result in an enlarged pupil unreactive to light. The light reflex (pupil response to light) is an important part of the neurologic evaluation and is discussed more thoroughly in Chapter 14.

*Motor System.* Examination of the motor system can be performed by having the patient grip the examiner's hand. Comparing one hand's strength with the other will detect weakness. It is important to have the patient make voluntary movements of all four extremities. If he cannot move his legs, the indication is that he has injured his spinal cord and is paraplegic. If the patient can move one side of his body but not the other, then a stroke can be suspected.

*Verbal Patterns.* The quality of the patient's speech may indicate neurologic difficulties or, possibly, drug overdose. Slurred speech can occur as a result of a stroke, alcohol, or drug abuse. If during an interview the patient's speech becomes slurred, a progressing disorder is indicated (e.g., evolving stroke).

TABLE 8-1.  CRANIAL NERVES

*231*

Physical
Examination

| Cranial Nerve | Dysfunction |
|---|---|
| Olfactory (CN I) | Loss of olfaction (smell) |
| Optic (CN II) | Loss of vision |
| Oculomotor (CN III) | Poor medial, upward and downward gaze, large unreactive pupil |
| Trochlear (CN IV) | Poor downward gaze when the eye is medially located; loss of intorsion in the laterally placed eye |
| Trigeminal (CN V) | Loss of facial sensation and corneal reflex; weak pterygoids, masseter, and temporal muscles (poor bite) |
| Abducens (CN VI) | Unable to move eye laterally |
| Facial (CN VII) | Weak facial muscles, loss of taste on anterior two-thirds of the tongue; dry eye, hyperacusis (painful sensation of sounds) |
| Auditory (CN VIII) | Loss of hearing, nystagmus, vertigo (dizziness) |
| Glossopharyngeal (CN IX) | Decreased sensation in back of the throat; loss of taste on the posterior third of the tongue |
| Vagus (CN X) | Poor gag reflex, poor speech |
| Accessory (CN XI) | Weak sternocleidomastoid muscle; weak shoulder shrug |
| Hypoglossal (CN XII) | Poor protrusion of the tongue forward and to opposite side (i.e., tongue deviates to paretic side) |

*Deep Tendon Reflexes.*  The knee jerk reflex is tested by striking the tendon just below the patella. This tendon is easily palpated below the knee. When testing for this deep tendon reflex, the leg will extend. Knee reflexes are important in the evaluation of spinal cord injuries, strokes, and metabolic disorders. Reflexes are important if they are generally decreased, or if one side is more decreased or exaggerated as compared to the other.

Constant practice and repeated application of the neurologic examination and attention to details will aid greatly in the patient's care.

*Orthopedic Examination.*  The orthopedic examination begins with the inspection of the upper and lower limbs. Since the limbs are symmetrical, one limb can be compared to the other. The limbs are best examined with all clothes off, but this is clearly impossible in the field situation.

Acute angulation of bones can be appreciated through clothing and with portions of the clothing cut off if a fracture is suspected. Look for swelling, deformities, angulation, and skin injuries. These should alert the examiner to the possibility that a fracture exists.

The best way to diagnose a fracture is by palpation. A thorough orthopedic examination would begin by placing every joint through a range of motion and assessing limitation or pain. The normal range of motion for joint examination should be practiced by the paramedic on himself or fellow students. The shoulder, elbow, wrist, fingers, hip, knee, ankle, and foot should be examined in order to determine the normal limits of motion. This type of training also helps one use the proper terminology in terms of the correct motion of the joints. Following the range of motion joint examination, the long bones should be palpated with the hand, looking for breaks in the skin, instability, swelling, or tenderness. It is the rare fracture that does not produce local tenderness over the fracture site. Local tenderness is not diagnostic of a fracture, but certainly makes one suspicious. Instability of a fracture can be assessed by grasping the limb on either side of the fracture and stressing it mildly. If there is instability, it can be appreciated by a crunching sound under the stress, or by frank instability of the bone. The circulation must be assessed distal to any fracture or dislocation of the joint. This is particularly true of the elbow, knee, and ankle. The pulses and color of the skin should be evaluated as part of the orthopedic examination whenever fractures or dislocations are suspected.

*Examination of the Vascular System.* It is difficult to inspect the vascular system visually, but changes produced by the vascular system are often visible. These would include a difference in skin color between one extremity and another. The person with acute thrombosis of the popliteal artery may have a cold leg and foot. The difference in color can be appreciated by comparing one leg to the other. Vascular injuries may produce pulsatile masses that can be seen upon inspection. Venous thrombosis of a major deep vein of the calf will produce swelling of one leg in contrast to the other. Therefore, inspection for the vascular system includes skin color differences, swellings, and abnormal pulsations.

The paramedic should learn how to palpate the following pulses:

1. Carotid pulse in the neck
2. Axillary pulse in the axilla
3. Brachial pulse in the antecubital fossa
4. Radial pulse at the wrist
5. Femoral artery pulse
6. Dorsalis pedis pulse at the dorsum of the foot
7. Posterior tibial pulse (behind the medial malleolus).

Constant practice for palpation of these pulses on another individual will allow one to determine the normal anatomic location of the pulses. Whenever a pulse is absent it can be due to cessation of the circulation or obstruction of a pulse proximal to the point of palpation. It also may be due to severe shock in which the circulation is intact but the cardiac output is very low. The presence of pulses in an extremity following a fracture is very important to note. A pulse that initially was present and is subsequently lost should be recorded. This may indicate that the vessel has been damaged near the fracture site or that swelling in the fracture area has occluded the vessel. Knowledge of the location of arteries will help in controlling the hemorrhage due to injury of blood vessels. Skill in palpating arteries will give the paramedic experience, and the following information can be ascertained from a pulse:

1. Presence of an intact circulation
2. Rate of heartbeat
3. Amplitude of the heartbeat (i.e., cardiac output)
4. Regularity of the heart rhythm.

*Summary*

The efficiency and quality of the history and physical examination will improve as the paramedic gains field experience. This chapter is meant to be a guide in the proper conduct of the ideal assessment. In the field, however, the paramedic will look immediately for shock, hemorrhage, and/or respiratory distress. The paramedic in many cases will not have the time to do a thorough history and physical examination, and this is where his assessment differs from the physician's in most cases. An orderly approach to the patient will more often result in the right diagnosis and treatment rather than random stabs at diagnoses based on brief impressions. The paramedic's assessment skills must be practiced and must be very accurate so that useful and believable information is relayed to the MIC-nurse and MIC-physician at the Base Station Hospital.

*Important
Points to
Remember*

The history and physical examination are urgent in making a diagnosis; the history is the more important of the two. The paramedic must determine as rapidly, concisely, and thoroughly as possible as many details as possible about what led to the problem. History may be obtained from the patient, family, or bystander.

Important points of history include:

1. Chief complaint
2. Past medical history
3. Allergies to drugs
4. Medication history
5. Review of systems.

Always use terms the patient can understand. Do not moralize, criticize, or cast guilt.

Chest pain history is often associated with myocardial infarction (heart attack). The pain is usually squeezing or gripping, substernal, and may radiate to the left arm or jaw.

Other cases of chest pain may include:

1. Angina pectoris
2. Pericarditis
3. Hiatus hernia
4. Pulmonary embolism
5. Dissecting aneurysm
6. Costochondritis
7. Ruptured esophagus
8. Pneumonitis
9. Gallbladder disease
10. Duodenal ulcer.

A conservative approach dictates that all patients with chest pain be assumed to have a myocardial infarction.

Abdominal pain is a common complaint and often the site of the pain and illness differ.

The pain associated with appendicitis usually begins in the epigastrium and travels to the right lower quadrant. Abdominal pain following trauma is often localized to the shoulder tips.

The physical examination includes four procedures: inspection, palpation, percussion, and auscultation. An examination of the general appearance of the patient is important.

The physical usually begins with recording of vital signs including pulse, blood pressure, and respirations.

The technique of examination of the body depends upon the type of injury or illness present. The usual sequence is as follows:

1. Head, eyes, ears, nose, and throat
2. Neck
3. Chest
4. Abdomen
5. Neurologic system
6. Orthopedic system
7. Vascular system.

*Important Systemic Checks*

*Head*—Position, ear discharge, nose shape, pupil size, foreign body in mouth, teeth, neck swelling.

*Neck*—Pulses, subcutaneous air.

*Chest*—Breathing, symmetry, bony landmarks, swelling, noises, lung and heart sounds (have patient breathe through mouth).

*Abdomen*—Contour, distention, musculature, tenderness, masses.

*Neurologic*—Level of consciousness, orientation, response to stimuli, motor function. Also unilaterality of signs and changing signs.

*Orthopedic*—Symmetry, swelling, function, pain, tenderness, motion, instability, gait.

*Vascular*—Skin color, temperature changes, pulses, swellings, heart beat.

*Bibliography*

Harvey, Abner McGehee and Bordley III, James. *Differential Diagnosis: The Interpretation of Clinical Evidence*, 2nd ed. Philadelphia, Pa: W. B. Saunders Co., 1970.

Prior, John A. and Silberstein, Jack S. *Physical Diagnosis: The History and Examination of the Patient*, 4th ed. St. Louis, Mo.: The C. V. Mosby Co., 1973.

Stern, Thomas N. *Clinical Examination: A Textbook of Physical Diagnosis*. Chicago, Ill.: Year Book Medical Publishers, Inc., 1964.

# ACUTE RESPIRATORY FAILURE

Respiratory failure occurs frequently and is one of the most common problems encountered by paramedic personnel. The physician in the hospital environment has the ability to adequately define the degree of respiratory failure with the use of such aids as chest X-rays, arterial blood gas analyses, and other laboratory work. In the field, however, respiratory emergencies often have to be assessed, diagnosed, and treated simultaneously without laboratory backup. Knowledge of the anatomy, physiology, and function of the upper and lower airways is mandatory in the assessment and treatment of respiratory failure.

DEFINITIONS

RESPIRATION

The function of respiration is to supply the cells of the body with adequate oxygen ($O_2$) and to remove carbon dioxide ($CO_2$). Respiration includes the following:

1. Ventilation—delivery of fresh atmospheric air (inspiration) to the alveoli, where it is exposed to the blood and removed (expiration) after giving up oxygen and receiving carbon dioxide

2. Diffusion—the movement of oxygen across the alveolar lining capillary walls into the blood and the reverse for carbon dioxide

3. Circulation—the method of carrying oxygen to the cells of the body, removing the carbon dioxide from them.

In general, "respiratory failure" may be said to be present when the tension of the respiratory gases in the blood is no longer within physiologic limits. This may occur when the lungs are normal because of inadequate overall ventilation, or in association with lung disease. Respiratory failure can be acute (recent onset) or chronic (long-standing).

HYPOXIA, HYPOXEMIA, AND HYPERCARBIA

Hypoxia is defined as a state in which insufficient oxygen is available to meet the oxygen requirements of the cell of a particular tissue. Obviously if the artery to the leg is clamped, the leg is suffering from hypoxia. Hypoxemia, on the other hand, is reduced oxygen or reduction in the partial pressure of oxygen in the arterial blood below normal limits (<75 mm Hg). Hypoxemia, in a strict sense, is a measure of the adequacy of alveolar ventilation, diffusion, and inspired oxygen concentration. Hypercarbia (hypercapnea) is defined as too much carbon dioxide in the blood ($PCO_2$ > 46 mm Hg). It produces a set of responses in the patient that should be diagnosed without the use of arterial blood gases.

CYANOSIS

Cyanosis is a bluish discoloration observable on the lips, nail beds, or conjunctivae. Cyanosis may be due to a reduction in the arterial oxygen saturation, or it may occur as a result of the reduced perfusion of tissue or slow flow through the tissues. Detecting cyanosis requires a concentration of unsaturated hemoglobin of approximately 5 grams percent of the circulating blood. If the hemoglobin concentration is normal, the arterial saturation must be reduced below 70 percent and the arterial oxygen tension ($PO_2$) must be less than 35 mm Hg. Hence, cyanosis is a late sign of hypoxemia.

BREATHING PATTERNS

The terms used to describe patterns of breathing are confusing and often used incorrectly. The root "-pnea" means breathe and the prefix combined with it describes the type of breathing. *Dyspnea* is a common term applied to respiratory problems and, strictly speaking, means difficult or labored breathing (shortness of breath). Exertional dyspnea, for example, is that difficult, labored breathing produced by exertion. Dyspnea is a subjective phenomenon and is something that the patient experiences. *Tachypnea* is rapid respiration, and *hyperpnea* is deep inhalation. *Orthopnea* is labored breathing lying flat. *Apnea* is a complete cessation of respiration or respiratory arrest. *Hypoventilation* means under-inflation of the lungs, and *hyperventilation* means over-inflation of the lungs. The preceding definitions elaborate the breathing pattern and only help in characterizing the breathing for the purposes of diagnosis.

AIRWAY OBSTRUCTION

The various terms used to describe airway obstruction depend upon the level of the obstruction. Obstruction may occur at the larynx, trachea, bronchi, or bronchioles. The terms used to describe an obstruction are often the same words used to describe its manifestation; therefore, clear definitions are hard to find. For example, the word bronchospasm is used to describe wheezes; wheezes are high-pitched sounds that may be due to bronchospasm (asthma). Therefore, the two words are used interchangeably. Wheeze is a commonly used term and it is not a diagnosis. Many conditions not related to asthma (foreign body obstruction, bronchiolitis, compression of the bronchus, etc.) can cause wheezing. Wheezes can occur during inspiration or expiration or both. Stridor is a high-pitched inspiratory sound usually associated with obstruction at the larynx. This is seen with epiglottitis, laryngeal edema, or the presence of a foreign body at the larynx. Nasal flaring occurs with airway obstruction. When the patient breathes, the nasal alae flare out. There may be retraction of the chest, abdomen, or neck as the individual breathes in but does not expand his chest due to the airway obstruction. In children, airway obstruction can be noted by inward tugging of the tissues at the level of the neck.

## SIGNS AND SYMPTOMS OF ACUTE RESPIRATORY FAILURE

The signs and symptoms of respiratory failure are hypoxia (inadequate tissue oxygenation) and hypercarbia. Symptoms of hypoxia resemble those of alcohol intoxication (muscular incoordination, loss of judgment, extreme listlessness, and, sometimes, frankly combative behavior) (Table 9-1). Often the person who has cerebral or brain hypoxia will behave in such a manner, and will be given a sedative or narcotic to quiet him. This may lead to a cessation of all breathing. The diagnosis of hypoxia is often overlooked as a cause of irrational behavior. Tachycardia (bradycardia in children and infants) and hypertension are also frequent

TABLE 9-1. HYPOXIA

SYMPTOMS:
  Symptoms similar to alcohol intoxication
    Confusion
    Loss of judgment
    Paranoia
    Restlessness
    Dizziness
SIGNS:
  Cyanosis
  Sympathetic responses
    Tachycardia
    Mild hypertension
    Peripheral vasoconstriction

TABLE 9-2.  $CO_2$ NARCOSIS (HYPERCARBIA)

SYMPTOMS:

Headache

Mild sedation

Drowsiness

Coma

SIGNS:

Vasodilatation

Redness of the skin, sclera, and conjunctivae secondary to cutaneous blood flow

Sympathetic responses

Hypertension (systolic and diastolic)

Tachycardia

Sweating

signs. Cyanosis is helpful in arousing an index of suspicion, but, as mentioned earlier, it is a late sign in respiratory failure and its presence may be dependent upon factors other than gas exchange.

The symptoms of hypercarbia are basically those that would be produced by an anesthetic. The patient becomes progressively more somnolent, disoriented, and, if untreated, comatose (Table 9-2). Headaches may be present due to cerebral vasodilatation or metabolic toxicity. The signs of hypercarbia are related to the release of epinephrine (sympathetic response) from the adrenal gland and to the direct effect of carbon dioxide on the blood vessels of the skin. These signs include redness of the skin and mucosa, redness of the conjunctivae, and increased sweating. Mild to moderate systemic arterial hypertension is frequent in acute carbon dioxide retention.

## DISORDERS CAUSING RESPIRATORY FAILURE

Respiration in man requires a lung plus an integrated feedback mechanism that involves the central nervous system, respiratory muscles, rib cage, and upper airways. Disease of any portion of this system can cause inadequate ventilation (Figure 9-1). In Table 9-3 the common causes of respiratory failure are outlined. It is helpful to know the diseases that may produce respiratory failure since this aids in the early diagnosis of the problem and helps in the subsequent treatment. Disease and/or trauma of the following systems may be involved.

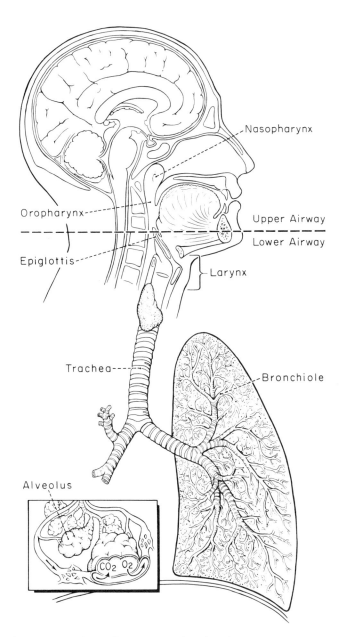

**Figure 9-1.** The respiratory tract from the nose to the alveolus. Gas exchange occurs in the alveolus.

TABLE 9-3.   DISEASES CAUSING RESPIRATORY FAILURE

| Diseases of | Examples |
|---|---|
| 1. Brain | Sedative overdose<br>Cerebrovascular accidents<br>Head trauma |
| 2. Spinal Cord<br>(Neuromuscular System) | Poliomyelitis<br>Spinal cord trauma<br>Cervical vertebral fracture |
| 3. Upper Airway | Tongue obstruction of larynx<br>Foreign body in oropharynx or<br>   hypopharynx<br>Nasal obstruction<br>Jaw fracture<br>Epiglottitis |
| 4. Lower Airway and Lungs | Laryngeal trauma<br>Laryngeal foreign body<br>Laryngospasm or edema<br>Bronchitis<br>Asthma<br>Emphysema<br>Severe pneumonia (particularly viral<br>   pneumonia such as influenza)<br>Pulmonary embolus |
| 5. Heart | Congestive heart failure<br>Cardiac arrest |
| 6. Chest Wall, Diaphragm | Rib fracture with flail chest<br>Burn eschar<br>Diaphragmatic rupture |

BRAIN

Since the brain integrates the reflexes and coordinates the breathing mechanism based on peripheral sources, it is the key to adequate ventilation. Any condition that depresses the central nervous system will directly or indirectly affect the respirations. The most common cause of central nervous system depression is an overdose with a sedative drug (barbiturate). Severe head injuries and strokes can cause marked changes in respiratory function. Hypercarbia causes dilatation of cerebral blood vessels, and may therefore increase intracranial pressure. This, in turn, superimposed on already existing cerebral hypoxia, creates a situation in which immediate provision of a patent airway and adequate ventilation are of utmost urgency.

Injuries to the spinal cord can produce acute respiratory failure. This is discussed in Chapter 14 under Neurological Injuries. Severe damage to the cervical vertebrae may lead to injury of the phrenic nerve, diaphragmatic paralysis, and respiratory failure. This can be recognized quickly as shallow breathing or hypoventilation with a marked change in the patient's color. Acute infections, such as poliomyelitis, can produce muscle weakness and loss of diaphragmatic motion. These respiratory emergencies require maintaining the airway and possible positive pressure ventilation.

## UPPER AIRWAY

The upper airway consists of the mouth, nose, nasopharynx, oropharynx, and hypopharynx. Upper airway obstruction is probably the most common cause of respiratory failure. The airway obstruction can be due to the tongue falling posteriorly and obstructing the airway; foreign bodies lodged in the oropharynx or hypopharynx; injuries to the face, jaw, tongue or nose; and infection of the epiglottis (epiglottitis) (Figure 9-2). Recognition of upper airway obstruction is of prime importance to the paramedic. He must be able to ascertain the anatomic level of the obstruction and be able to deal with it. This often requires positional changes of the jaw or neck, insertion of an airway through the nose or mouth, or removal of a foreign body.

## LOWER AIRWAY AND LUNGS

The lower airway consists of the larynx, trachea, and lungs. Obstruction at the larynx can occur due to injuries to the larynx, foreign bodies,

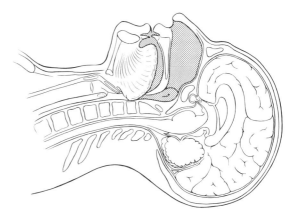

**Figure 9-2.** The shaded area shows the nasopharynx and oropharynx. The tongue has fallen back and is obstructing the airway.

edema of the larynx as a result of an acute anaphylactic reaction, or infection of the larynx. Obstruction at the trachea is most commonly due to aspiration of a foreign body, swelling in the neck or mediastinum compressing the trachea, or to trauma.

Respiratory failure can be based on conditions within the lung itself. The most common type of lung disease in the United States is emphysema. The two general types of emphysema patients are called the "pink puffer" and the "blue bloater." The pink puffer is characteristically a thin man with dyspnea on exertion. His disability is relatively fixed from week to week and from month to month, but gradually progresses from year to year. He hyperventilates markedly and thereby can maintain normal arterial blood gases until late in the disease process. His dyspnea cannot be explained by a blood gas abnormality and must be attributed to other causes, such as stretch receptors in the lungs. His lungs are large, having a 12-liter capacity (Chapter 3). His breath sounds are reduced.

The type B patient, one with chronic bronchitis (blue bloater), is of normal or stout body build, and tends to have repeated attacks of heart failure during acute exacerbations of chronic bronchitis. Unlike the pink puffer, his disability varies widely. At times he may be able to work, while at other times he needs hospitalization for the treatment of heart failure. He often appears surprisingly comfortable and relatively free of dyspnea despite abnormal blood gases. The characteristic feature of both types of emphysema patients is that they can become ill precipitously because of pulmonary infection or heart failure, and over-treatment in the field may worsen their condition. These patients often have a compromised heart, and fluid overload is not well tolerated. Patients with advanced pulmonary disease and chronic hypoxemia have a respiratory drive stimulated through chemoreceptors in their neck. Ordinarily respiratory drive is controlled in the medulla of the brain and works based on the amount of carbon dioxide and the pH of the blood. When carbon dioxide increases or the pH falls, the respiratory rate increases. Since chronic hypercarbia may be present in these patients, the CNS control of breathing is lost and breathing is controlled by the chemoreceptors. Sudden improvement of their chronic hypoxemia by administration of oxygen shuts the chemoreceptors off and can cause apnea. The use of oxygen in these patients is discussed further in this chapter.

The patient with asthma often presents with wheezing, cyanosis, retraction of his neck, and markedly labored breathing. These patients often have a previous history of asthma and may require epinephrine or some other medication to reverse their bronchospasm. Asthma is a frightening condition and may easily lead to death if not properly treated. The use of oxygen is mandatory in these patients either by nasal prongs, mask, or positive pressure ventilation.

Severe infections of the lung, such as pneumonia, can produce respiratory failure and these patients present with dyspnea, cyanosis, and agitation. Treatment of these patients consists of the administration of oxygen and hospitalization.

## CHEST WALL

Injuries to the chest wall, such as massive sternal or rib fractures, can produce flail portions of the chest (Chapter 14). This may lead to uneven ventilation of the lung and acute respiratory failure. Treatment for this may include stabilization of the thorax and positive pressure ventilation if the patient is unconscious. Burns to the chest wall may produce such heavy and restrictive skin that breathing is impossible. These patients need positive pressure ventilation support or even incision of the burn scar to allow for proper ventilation. The different types of pneumothorax are discussed in Chapter 14.

## HEART

The heart can contribute to respiratory failure by sequestration of fluid in the lung tissue. This occurs when left ventricular failure is severe enough to cause high pressure in the pulmonary veins and leakage of fluid into the lung tissue. The lungs become heavy and are not easily moved with deep inspiration. Oxygen cannot readily diffuse across the alveoli because of the amount of fluid in the interstitial space. Such a condition is called pulmonary edema, and oxygen as well as diuretics are the treatment of choice. Spontaneous breathing ceases during cardiac arrest and the need for maintenance of the airway during resuscitation is obvious.

## DIAGNOSIS OF AIRWAY PROBLEMS

The first principle of emergency medical care, in or out of the hospital, is that adequate ventilation of the lungs supersedes all other considerations. Without an open airway, all other therapeutic measures cannot prevent death. In many conditions, such as comatose states associated with head injury, diabetes, stroke, drug poisoning, and other causes, a fatal outcome often is the result of inadequate gas exchange rather than of the effects of the original condition.

The crucial factors in airway management are speed and technical expertise. The paramedic must develop rapid, reliable diagnostic and therapeutic skills, similar to those of trained athletes. The training program should involve study, extensive practice, and repetitive drilling if the necessary skills are to be acquired and maintained. After an airway is established, constant vigilance is necessary in order to guarantee continued patency of the airway. This is true regardless of any devices that may be in use for this purpose.

## BASIC FACTS

In the area of airway management there are no "life and death" situations (they do not mix); the choice is "life or death." In view of this, and the need for speed, the following basic ideas must be kept in mind for instant application:

FACT 1. Noisy breathing always means obstruction (partial).

FACT 2. Obstructed breathing is not always noisy (if the obstruction is complete, no air moves).

FACT 3. The brain can only survive a few minutes of asphyxia.

FACT 4. Breathing efforts are useless if the airway is blocked.

FACT 5. A patent airway is useless if the patient is apneic.

FACT 6. Do not waste time looking for help. Your own skills are the most helpful in an emergency.

While it is true that in the area of airway management diagnosis and treatment can (and usually should) be essentially simultaneous, it is also true that correct identification of the conditions present (and their causes) provides the best basis for rational treatment. Hence, the answers to such questions as the following should be sought as soon as the patient is approached:

## ASSESSMENT OF THE PROBLEM

1. Is the patient apneic? (No chest movement or respiratory effort.) If so, attempt to ventilate. This will initiate treatment and simultaneously demonstrate whether any degree of airway obstruction is present. If the airway is clear it may be advisable to temporarily delay attempts at insertion of artificial airway devices which may produce untoward effects such as vomiting, aspiration, and laryngeal spasm.

2. Is the patient trying to breathe, and is the airway partially obstructed? Obstructed breathing may or may not be noisy. If obstruction is present one may observe chest and/or neck retraction and flaring of the nares.

3. Is the patient breathing, but cyanosis is present? If so, ventilatory volume may be inadequate, or there may be respiratory or circulatory problems, such as pulmonary edema, atelectasis, pneumothorax, severe hypotension, certain poisonings, etc.

4. Does the patient inhale fairly easily, but experience great difficulty during exhalation? If so, think of asthma (bronchospasm), foreign body obstruction, or laryngeal obstruction, and listen to the chest for wheezing sounds during exhalation.

5. Are there bubbling sounds? If so, are they arising in the upper airway, trachea, or lung areas?

6. Is the patient's skin pink despite severe respiratory depression and unconsciousness? If so, think of carbon monoxide poisoning, and start vigorous hyperventilation with 100 percent oxygen.

## EVALUATION OF THE AIRWAY

Initial assessment of the airway can be done without sophisticated diagnostic procedures and devices. Often they are not immediately available, and they are almost always more time-consuming than is the use of your built-in diagnostic kit: the senses of sight, hearing, touch, and smell. Examples of information rapidly available by these means are as follows.

*Sight.* Upon initial encounter of the patient with a possible airway problem, look for: retraction of the chest and/or neck muscles, absence of respiratory movement, flaring of the nares, chin tugs, pupillary dilatation, constriction or inequality, pallor or cyanosis.

*Hearing.* Listen for snoring, which usually means soft tissue obstruction in the mouth or pharynx, crowing or stridor (usually laryngospasm), and bubbling or gurgling (usually foreign material, secretions, or pulmonary edema). Listen closely to determine whether the sounds arise from the mouth, trachea, or lungs. Also listen for wheezing, which is usually associated with bronchiolar obstruction as in asthma, but can also be caused by a small foreign body in a bronchus or at the carina (Table 9-4).

*Touch.* Hot skin usually means that there is a fever due to infection, sunstroke, or a cerebral accident. Cold and/or wet clammy skin may be secondary to shock, exposure, or severe depressant poisoning.

*Smell.* The following can often be noted: alcohol (intoxication); acetone (diabetic coma); and industrial solvents (e.g., benzene, gasoline, carbon tetrachloride, which also often exhibits an ashen-gray cyanosis).

*Taste.* This sense is rarely of value in the context of this chapter. However, in correlating all of the above, the "sixth sense" is paramount, that is, *common sense.*

## TABLE 9-4. SURVEY OF AIRWAY

| Airway Level | Observation | Diagnostic Meaning | Treatment |
|---|---|---|---|
| Oronasopharynx | Snoring, low pitched sounds | Soft tissue obstruction | Tilt head backward; lift mandible forward; use airways, nasal and/or oral |
| | Gurgling or bubbling | Foreign material present | Clear airway, manual removal and/or suction; place head and neck downward and to the side (gravitational positioning) |
| Larynx | Crowing or stridor, High pitched sounds | Laryngospasm (cord adduction) | Positive pressure ventilation; bag and mask with $O_2$; muscle relaxants should be given by qualified personnel only |
| Trachea | Gurgling or bubbling | Foreign material, secretions, edema, fluid | Gravitational positioning; tracheal suction if feasible (may require intubation or bronchoscopy) |
| Lungs | Bubbling (rales or rhonchi) | Aspirated material, as above | As above, stimulate cough; positive pressure ventilation with oxygen |
| | | Pulmonary edema | As above |
| | Wheezing, high pitched sounds (musical rales), especially on expiration, which is prolonged | Bronchiolar spasm, asthma | Bronchodilator drugs by qualified personnel; secretions may require bronchial suction; positive pressure oxygen; use of helium-$O_2$ mixtures |

## TREATMENT

### PRIORITIES

Emergency airway management requires, in addition to speed and vigilance as noted above, a system of priorities. In the case of the unconscious patient, the following should be done in rapid sequence until an open airway is established:

Positioning of the patient

Backward tilt of the head (except when spinal injury is suspected)

Forward displacement of the mandible

Clearing the mouth and oropharynx

Positive pressure inflation (mouth-to-mouth, mouth-to-nose, mouth-to-stoma, mouth-to-Laerdal mask)

Face mask with a snug fit to allow positive pressure to be given

Insertion of an oro- or nasopharyngeal airway, if there is any obstruction to good ventilation

Insertion of an esophageal obturator airway (EOA)

Endotracheal intubation

Cricothyrotomy

Tracheostomy

*Positioning.* The unconscious patient should ordinarily be placed supine if in need of resuscitation. If there is good color and pulmonary exchange, the patient may be put on his side to promote the outflow of foreign material. Regardless of the position, the patient's head should be tilted backward. Avoid the prone position; since the face is inaccessible, there is a tendency for airway obstruction, and thoracic compliance is impaired.

*Backward Tilt of the Head (Extension of the Neck).* This is done to correct the obstruction that results from relaxation of the tongue so that it presses against the posterior pharyngeal wall (often described in lay terms as "swallowing one's tongue") (Figure 9-2). Backward tilt of the head stretches the anterior neck structures between the mandible and the larynx and thus lifts the base of the tongue forward and away from the posterior pharyngeal wall (Figures 9-3, 9-4). The maneuver is also beneficial since, not uncommonly, the mouth will open and further facilitate breathing. If a neck fracture is suspected, the airway is opened

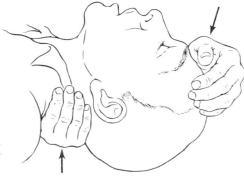

**Figure 9-3.** The airway can be opened by placing one hand behind the neck and extending the neck with the other hand on the forehead.

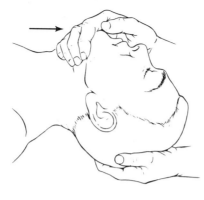

**Figure 9-4.** An alternative way of opening the airway is to place the hand behind the occiput, and extend the neck by pulling the chin upward with the other hand.

by the chin-lift method and the neck is not extended (Figure 9-5). The angle of the mandible is lifted directly upward with the little fingers at the same time the chin is pushed forward (toward the feet) with the thumb. The rescuer can be positioned straddling the patient's head, or at either side of the head. Mouth-to-mouth resuscitation is then instituted if breathing is absent.

*Clearing the Upper Airway.* Before beginning mouth-to-mouth resuscitation, any visible foreign material should quickly be wiped from the lips or removed from the patient's mouth and pharynx. This frees the airway and prevents aspiration of material into the larynx or trachea.

*Positive Pressure Inflation.* There are two ways to inflate a patient's lungs after correct positioning of the head when no other equipment is available. This technique varies with infants and is discussed in Chapter 20.

 *Mouth-to-Mouth.* The nose is pinched shut and the paramedic inhales deeply and expels his air into the patient (Figure 9-6). This implies

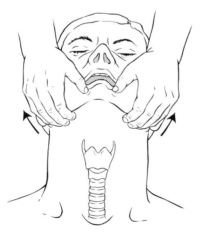

**Figure 9-5.** In cases of neck trauma, the neck cannot be flexed or extended. The mouth can be opened by positioning oneself at the head of the patient. Using the little finger, the jaw can be lifted upward as the thumbs push the mouth open.

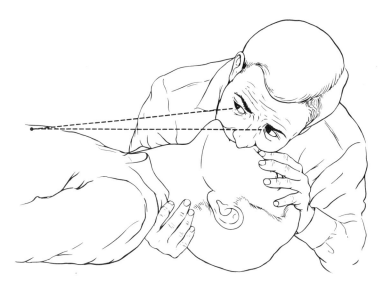

**Figure 9-6.** When doing mouth-to-mouth resuscitation, it is important to watch the chest to be certain that proper expansion of the chest occurs.

that there is a tight seal between the lips. The paramedic should also watch the chest to be certain it is lifting properly. The oxygen concentration of exhaled air is approximately 16 to 18 percent, and is quite adequate for mouth-to-mouth resuscitation. This type of resuscitation provides a tidal volume of approximately 1000 to 1400 ml when the paramedic takes a deep breath. The hyperinflation by the paramedic increases the oxygen concentration of his exhaled breath as well as reducing the carbon dioxide concentration to 2 percent. Although the rescuer normally has a 4 percent carbon dioxide concentration in his expired air, the patient will tolerate this as long as the ventilations are done with a large tidal volume. The respiratory rate should not be more than 12 to 16 per minute.

*Mouth-to-Nose.* This becomes useful if the patient's mouth cannot be opened due to arthritis, a jaw fracture, possible cervical injuries, or other obstructions. The head is positioned in the same manner and, following a deep inspiration, the paramedic exhales into the nose, which is cupped with his lips. The mouth is held shut during this maneuver. It may be necessary to open the mouth during exhalation since the nasal passages may not be large enough to allow the full escape of air rapidly enough to support life. A nasal pharyngeal airway discussed below is quite helpful in this procedure.

*Mouth-to-Stoma.* Many patients are situated outside of the hospital with a permanent tracheostomy with a tube, or with the trachea joined directly to the skin. In a respiratory arrest situation, the mouth can be applied directly to the stoma and the patient ventilated in this manner. All the other conditions regarding mouth-to-mouth and mouth-to-nose

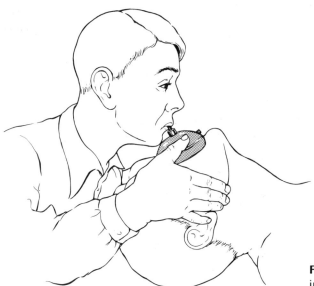

**Figure 9-7.** The pocket mask in use. The inlet near the chin is for oxygen.

resuscitation pertain to the mouth-to-stoma resuscitation. If there is inadequate ventilation, foreign body obstruction may be present, and this will have to be removed by direct extraction or by the indirect methods described later in this chapter.

*Mouth-to-Laerdal Mask.* This mask (pocket mask) is accompanied by an air cushion and fits snugly over the nose (Figure 9-7). It has two ports, one for entry of oxygen and one for the rescuer. With the mask fitting snugly down and held by the thumbs, the fingers grasp the jaw and lift and tilt the head backward. Following inhalation, air is blown into the mask and will inflate the lungs. With oxygen streaming in through the second port, the oxygen concentration mixture the patient receives is greater than can be received from room air. If the rescuer is unable to ventilate the patient, he should reposition the head and try again. If this does not work, foreign body obstruction likely exists and steps to correct this should be taken (see section on Airway Obstruction).

*Airway Adjuncts.* Ventilation can be aided by holding the airway open with a mechanical device during mouth-to-mouth breathing.

*Oropharyngeal Airway.* This is shown in Figure 9-8 and consists of a rigid tube that conforms to the mouth and pharynx. It is inserted with the concave side facing the top of the mouth and then twisted into position as it crosses to the back of the pharynx. This device holds the tongue forward and assists in mouth-to-mouth ventilation or aids in the comatose patient who is breathing, but has soft tissue upper airway obstruction due to relaxation of the jaw muscles.

*252*

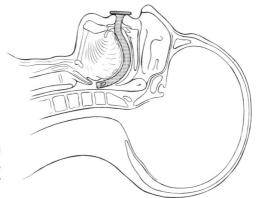

**Figure 9-8.** The airway can be opened using an oropharyngeal airway. This allows air to enter the trachea through the airway or the nasopharynx.

*Nasopharyngeal Airway.* The nasopharyngeal airway is introduced through the nose and advanced to the pharynx to reside near the laryngeal opening (Figure 9-9). Its purpose is to hold the tongue forward and to provide a passage of air from the nose to the larynx. It is a very effective means for maintaining the airway in the partially conscious or unconscious patient who can exchange air, but has a soft tissue obstruction. Its best indication is obstruction with a tight jaw because a nasal airway circumvents the clamped jaw. It can also be used as a passage for mouth-to-nose respiration.

*Face Mask and Positive Pressure Breathing.* During general anesthesia in the operating room, many patients are put to sleep and then manually ventilated using a snug-fitting mask and positive pressure. At times, lengthy operations are performed while using this method of supporting

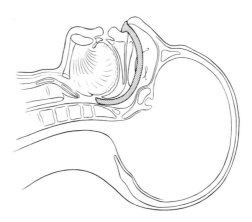

**Figure 9-9.** A nasopharyngeal tube can maintain patency of the airway.

the respirations. A naso- or oropharyngeal airway is used in conjunction with the face mask. When the mask is fitted snugly over the face, the neck is hyperextended, and using one hand to hold the mask in place while grasping the jaw and tilting the head backward, the other hand is used to inflate the patient's lung with a mechanical device. The device most commonly used with a face mask is an AMBU bag, which will be discussed later (Figure 9-10).

The face mask should be made of a clear plastic material so that the paramedic can observe the color of the lips under the mask as well as the presence of vomitus, should it occur. If the patient vomits and the mask is in place, quick reactions are necessary to clear the oropharynx of this material, which may be aspirated into the lung. The Laerdal pocket mask is perfectly suitable for this, since it is made of clear plastic and will adapt to the AMBU bag.

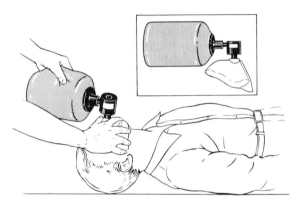

**Figure 9-10.** An AMBU bag and the clear plastic mask allow inspection of the lips.

*Esophageal-Obturator Airway.*   This airway is an outstanding advance in the management of airway support in the field. It was developed by Dr. Archer Gordon and others. The advantages of the esophageal-obturator airway (EOA) are that it is easy to insert, occludes the esophagus preventing aspiration from the stomach, and permits lung ventilation. An additional advantage is the ease of teaching its insertion, which is facilitated by not requiring the use of a laryngoscope. The disadvantages are the possibility of injury to the esophagus by overdistention of the obturator balloon, inability to apply suction to the stomach and empty it, difficulty in maintaining a tight fit of the mask on the face, occasional inability to insert the esophageal airway far enough down the esophagus to allow a face mask fit, accidental insertion into the trachea, and potential aspiration with deflation of the esophageal balloon. The inability to aspirate the stomach has largely been overcome by modification of the EOA as shown in Figure 9-11. The stomach can be aspirated by passing a tube through the center portion of the airway. Insertion of the EOA is shown in Figure 9-12. The rescuer grasps the mandible, pulling it

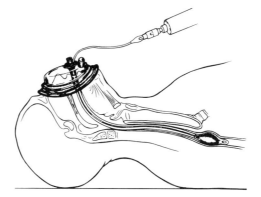

**Figure 9-11.** The esophageal obturator airway with a central lumen allowing passage of a nasogastric tube for decompression of the stomach.

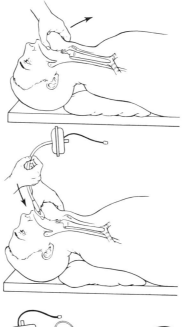

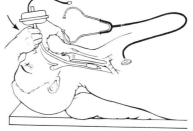

**Figure 9-12.** The steps for insertion of the esophageal obturator airway are shown. The airway must be positioned so that the balloon is distal to the trachea and fits down into position comfortably. It is important to listen to the chest once the airway is inserted to be certain that it is not positioned in the trachea (absent breath sounds).

forward, and introduces the obturator directly along the posterior pharynx and then slides it down into the esophagus. The mask should be positioned to fit down on the face snugly so that when the esophageal balloon is blown up it is distal to the trachea. With the balloon inflated, positive pressure is applied to the port on the mask and ventilation is maintained. The adequacy of ventilation is gauged by listening to the breath sounds on either side of the chest with a stethoscope. If there are no breath sounds, the obturator airway may have entered the trachea. It should be removed immediately and ventilation sustained by mouth-to-mouth or mouth-to-mask, until the airway is reinserted.

An additional disadvantage of the oroesophageal airway is that the tracheobronchial tree cannot be aspirated. It is also mandatory that personnel working in the Emergency Department appreciate the nature of the tube. If the balloon is deflated in the Emergency Department prior to endotracheal intubation, aspiration of gastric contents will usually occur. Once the patient's trachea is intubated, the EOA balloon must be deflated before it is removed. Smaller EOA tubes are not yet available for use in children, and the current adult models should not be used in patients under 16 years of age.

All things considered, the EOA appears to be a useful adjunct in resuscitative management, especially for mobile intensive care unit personnel, police, fire, and volunteer rescue workers. The EOA is used in cases of full cardiac arrest or with patients who are comatose with no gag reflex.

*Endotracheal Intubation.* Endotracheal intubation is the ideal way of managing the airway, but this procedure requires a laryngoscope and suction. In the field, portable suction is not always adequate; and secretions in the hypopharynx may conceal the larynx, making it impossible to accomplish the procedure. Although endotracheal intubation is done by paramedics in certain areas of the country (Denver, Seattle, Hawaii), most of the other regions of the country have favored the use of the EOA. The technique of endotracheal intubation will not be detailed here since it is so adequately described and illustrated in the text by Applebaum and Bruce referenced at the end of this chapter.

*Cricothyrotomy.* Cricothyrotomy is a procedure used to form an opening between the skin and the larynx through the cricothyroid membrane (Chapter 4). The cricothyroid membrane is located between the cricoid and thyroid cartilages, an area just below the vocal cords. The cricothyroid membrane can be palpated easily by feeling the "Adam's apple" in the midline and moving one's finger inferiorly, to encounter a depression. This is the cricothyroid membrane; just below it is the cricoid cartilage.

Cricothyrotomy is a simple and rapid procedure for gaining access to the airway in emergency conditions of upper airway obstruction. These would include impacted foreign bodies, epiglottitis, and massive facial fractures or burns. Paramedics should be familiar with this technique and can practice on the anesthetized dog.

Cricothyrotomy is an emergency lifesaving procedure. When the diagnosis of a severe upper airway obstruction is made and the decision is made to do a cricothyrotomy, the patient's neck should be fully extended on a rolled towel, sheet, or blanket placed under the shoulders. This position brings the larynx and cricothyroid membrane into the extreme anterior position. Using a knife or scalpel, a one-inch transverse incision is made over the skin of the cricothyroid membrane. It is imperative that the skin incision be made wider than the subsequent puncture into the cricothyroid membrane. This will prevent the skin from folding over the opening and will also prevent the entrapment of air from the trachea as it rushes out the membrane. The cricothyroid membrane can then be punctured with a knife or any sharp object. Once it has passed into the membrane, it is twisted to open a space between the cricoid and thyroid cartilages, as depicted in Figure 9-13. It is important not to aim the knife superiorly (toward the head), since injury to the vocal cords may occur. Many instruments, and even kits that can be carried in the pocket, have been developed to facilitate this procedure. They include trochars, knives, cannulas, daggers, dilators, and large bore needles. However, no commonly accepted devices are relatively free of complications for use in the field. The best approach is to incise the skin and cut the cricothyroid membrane directly, maintaining its patency by either twisting the blade as shown, or inserting a rigid tube to maintain the airway.

In an adult, a single #10 or #12 cannula is satisfactory for relieving airway obstruction. This method should be used when a knife is not available, or when the paramedic does not feel confident in that technique. With the patient in the same position, the needle is directed through the cricothyroid membrane and the inner metal needle is removed while

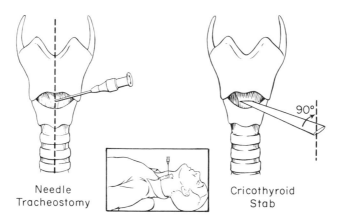

Needle
Tracheostomy

90°

Cricothyroid
Stab

**Figure 9-13.** Cricothyrotomy is used in a life or death situation; when indicated, it must be done quickly and accurately. It is important to have the neck extended so that the cricothyroid membrane is brought anterior and can be palpated easily (see insert).

the outer plastic cannula remains through the cricothyroid membrane. Six liters of oxygen/min. can be insufflated via this cannula, and the cricothyrotomy can be performed in less than one minute. Constant practice and review of the anatomy, and of the indications for this procedure, are necessary.

Cricothyrotomy in the young child is hazardous since the neck structures are so close together. A slip from either side of the cricothyroid membrane may injure the carotid artery or esophagus. Regardless, in a life or death situation, these considerations should be abandoned and the procedure should be done without delay. In children or infants, a large bore needle with a plastic cannula that appears satisfactory for the size of the child will usually suffice.

*Tracheostomy.* Tracheostomy is not a field procedure. Ideally, a tracheostomy should be done in an operating room with lighting and proper assistance. Tracheostomy literally means "hole in the trachea." The trachea is below the cricothyroid membrane and cricoid cartilage. To do a tracheostomy requires either mobilizing or dividing a portion of the thyroid gland to expose the trachea. This makes it hazardous and impractical to do a tracheostomy in the field.

## THE OBSTRUCTED AIRWAY

Airway obstruction can be the result of a foreign body that may occur during eating or as a result of objects placed in the mouth. Large chunks of meat are the most common foreign bodies. The background for such an occurrence is often alcohol intoxication, the use of upper or lower dentures, talking and trying to chew at the same time, and/or large portions of food poorly chewed and swallowed in a hurry.

The following are true incidents of airway obstruction due to foreign bodies:

**Case 1:** A tired 25-year-old intern had completed his thirty-six-hour duty and had returned to his apartment at 12:00 Noon on a Saturday afternoon. He took an apple from the fruit bowl and began eating. While eating he fell asleep with his head forward. He aspirated a portion of the apple and was found dead the following day.

**Case 2:** An 18-year-old high school student was chewing gum while playing basketball. He had just rebounded and was dribbling to the opposite court when he collided with another player. The gum, due to the force of the blow, was driven down into the trachea. He asphyxiated and died on the basketball court.

**Case 3:** A husbands and wives' dinner meeting for the American Heart Association was progressing satisfactorily. The room was filled with cardiologists, internists, and one cardiac surgeon. Suddenly there was a commotion at one end of the dining room where a woman had collapsed on the floor. She had pointed to her neck just before collapsing and quickly became unconscious and blue. The cardiologists at the scene thought she might have had a coronary thrombosis and were considering closed chest massage when the surgeon heard of the problem. He leapt over several tables and immediately made the diagnosis. From his pocket he took a money clip that had a small knife blade attached and jammed it into the cricothyroid membrane, relieving the obstruction. He then milked the meat from the woman's hypopharynx into her mouth and removed it. She made an uneventful recovery.

The above incidents indicate how quickly and tragically, in what seems like pleasant circumstances, foreign body aspiration or obstruction of the airway can lead to devastating results. Some of the accidents seem preventable, but in all cases of an obstructed airway due to a foreign body, the problem is mechanical. Mechanical problems require solutions that involve mechanics.

Individuals who have foreign body obstruction of the upper airway can present in any of three positions: (1) standing, (2) sitting, or (3) lying. The individual at a cocktail party who gulps down a bacon hors d'oeuvre and has it stick in the back of his throat will be standing when he first experiences upper airway obstruction. His first reaction is to grab his throat with one hand and someone else with the other to gain attention and help. If no one were to notice him, he would eventually become hypoxic and collapse to the floor. If he is then discovered and is not breathing, it would be impossible to tell if he had an obstructed airway or had suffered a myocardial infarction or sudden dysrhythmia. Therefore, patients can present with foreign body obstruction in either the conscious or unconscious state.

Once the diagnosis is made, the next consideration is how the foreign body is to be removed. There are two ways to remove a foreign body: (1) direct extraction or (2) indirect extraction.

*Direct Extraction.* The direct extraction of a foreign body involves inserting the fingers into the back of the patient's mouth, grasping the foreign body, and pulling it out. This is nearly impossible because one cannot reach far enough into the hypopharynx with two fingers to grasp a slippery foreign body. Finger probing, which involves insertion of the finger down the side of the cheek deeply into the hypopharynx along the base of the tongue, is a useful procedure (Figure 9-14). The finger is then curled, hopefully under the foreign body, and it is pushed along the opposite lateral pharynx out into the mouth where it can be removed. The purpose of the hooking maneuver is to enable the finger to travel down under the foreign body and either lift it out or push it into the opposite wall of the oropharynx. If one were to probe directly down on the foreign body with the finger, it might become impacted more deeply and make extraction nearly impossible.

California law at one time stipulated that mechanical fingers were

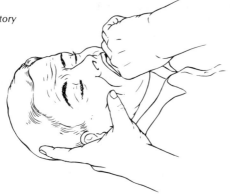

**Figure 9-14.** The finger sweep method is used to clear the oropharynx of foreign material. It is important that the index finger be swept along the lateral pharyngeal wall deep into the oropharynx. The finger is then hooked under the material and brought upward. This avoids impacting the material deep into the oropharynx or into the glottis.

required in all restaurants. This hook-shaped pronged device would fit back in the oropharynx and enable the rescuer to extract the foreign body. The problem with this technique was that it was blind and the epiglottis and/or other oropharyngeal tissues were often grasped and pulled, causing bleeding and making the situation worse. The law has subsequently been changed.

The foreign body can also be visualized by direct inspection with a throat stick and a hemostat (curved clamp) or McGill forceps (curved forceps without teeth). The physician working in an Emergency Department can use either this method or a laryngoscope to expose the hypopharynx and directly remove foreign material.

*Indirect Extraction.* Since the opportunities for direct extraction of a foreign body are limited because of location, equipment, and expertise of personnel, indirect methods are recommended. Indirect methods include maneuvers that cause a forceful impact on either the back, chest, or abdominal cavity. These maneuvers are as follows:

1. Back thrust
2. Chest thrust
3. Abdominal thrust (Heimlich maneuver)

*Back Thrust.* A series of rapid sharp blows is delivered with the hand on the spine between the shoulder blades (Figure 9-15). Back blows may be administered with the patient standing, sitting, or lying. Four back blows should be delivered in rapid succession. It has been shown that back blows produce their effect by sudden forward displacement of the larynx, dislodging the foreign body.

*Chest Thrust.* This procedure consists of placing one fist on top of the other at the distal (lower) end of the sternum and pushing inward four times in rapid succession. This maneuver may dislodge the foreign

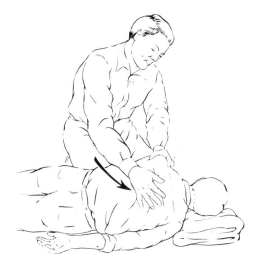

**Figure 9-15.** With the patient on his side, the backslap method is shown; four forceful blows are made between the shoulder blades.

body upwards to the oropharynx, where it can be extracted using the finger probe technique. This procedure produces a sudden artificial cough by forcing out residual air from the lung and moves the foreign body from the hypopharynx into the oropharynx. The chest maneuver is used for obese patients and pregnant females.

*Abdominal Thrust (Heimlich Maneuver).* The abdominal thrust or Heimlich maneuver is done with the patient standing, sitting, or supine. The rescuer stands behind the patient and grasps him with both hands at a point midway between the umbilicus and the xiphoid process. The thumb of one hand should be positioned inward and the opposite hand cupped over the first to form a tight grip (Figure 9-16). A rapid upward

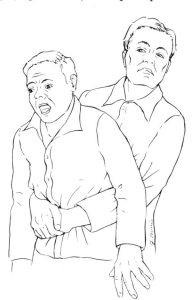

**Figure 9-16.** The abdominal thrust maneuver is four quick thrusts in the epigastrium with the patient as relaxed as possible and leaning forward. This may disimpact a foreign body in the hypopharynx or trachea.

motion forces the abdomen inward and delivers an upper thrust to the diaphragm, which expels air from the trachea. In this maneuver the foreign body may become dislodged and the patient can cough it out.

## SEQUENCE OF MANEUVERS FOR THE OBSTRUCTED AIRWAY

*The Conscious Patient.* The urgency of this situation cannot be overemphasized and immediate recognition with proper action is essential. If the patient has some air exchange and is partially obstructed, he may be able to speak or cough effectively. Do not interfere with his attempt to expel a foreign body. Especially do not attempt to dislodge it with your fingers since the gagging and fear may cause damage to your fingers. If the patient is pointing to his throat and seeking help, ask if he can speak; if there is no reply, follow this sequence:

If conscious:

Position yourself behind the patient.

Do four sharp back blows.

Do four abdominal thrusts.

Continue this sequence until the patient can dislodge and cough out the foreign body, or until he becomes unconscious.

If he becomes unconscious:

Place in the supine position.

Place knees close to the patient's hip or straddle the hip and one leg.

Place the heel of one hand on the abdomen between the umbilicus and xiphoid, and then place the second hand on top of the first. Press into the patient's abdomen with a quick upward thrust.

Do four abdominal thrusts.

Roll patient on his side; do four back blows.

Clear the oral airway with the finger probe technique.

If initially unsuccessful and the patient remains unconscious, do the maneuvers as described in the following section for the unconscious patient.

If the patient is obese or pregnant, substitute chest thrusts for abdominal thrusts.

*The Unconscious Patient.* Sudden collapse and loss of consciousness is a grave emergency. It may be due to fainting, a stroke, or a heart attack, as well as to hypoxia from a foreign body obstruction of the airway. Hypoxia of four to six minutes duration may result in irreversible brain damage.

The following procedures for the unconscious patient should be initiated:

Shake and shout, call for help.

Establish an airway, check for breathing, and attempt to ventilate.

In cases of suspected neck injury, open the airway by modified jaw thrust rather than the head tilt.

If unable to ventilate, reposition the head and attempt to ventilate.

If unsuccessful, do four manual abdominal thrusts, leaning to the side of the patient. Then grasp the patient's arm opposite to you and pull the patient up on his side and do four quick back thrusts.

Following this, return the patient to the supine position and attempt the finger probe to remove the foreign body.

When the foreign body is removed, reposition the head and attempt to ventilate.

If unsuccessful, repeat the four abdominal thrusts followed by four back thrusts and subsequent finger probe.

If the patient is obese or pregnant, use the chest thrust instead of the abdominal thrust.

Persistence is important since, when the patient becomes hypoxic, his muscles relax and recovery of the foreign body may be much easier. Also, when the muscles relax, a previously fully obstructed airway may become only partially obstructed. When ventilating a patient with a partial obstruction, it is best to use slow, full, forceful ventilations rather than short, quick breaths. The latter may aggravate the obstruction. If there is vomitus in the mouth or oropharynx, turn the head to the side and wipe it out quickly and proceed with the sequence.

## THE OBSTRUCTED AIRWAY IN INFANTS AND CHILDREN

If an airway obstruction is diagnosed or suspected in an infant, it is best to place the child in the prone position over the forearm. He can then be held face down with the legs up and the back slaps performed. This should dislodge any foreign body and the oropharynx may need to be aspirated or finger-probed with the small finger. In some cases, turning the baby completely upside down and patting him on the back may dislodge a foreign body. If the child is not breathing, mouth and nose artificial respiration should be started and the back slap sequence repeated.

In the older child the same maneuver can be used by placing the child in the head down position over the thigh (Chapter 20). Back slaps can then be delivered. Remember, when attempting to remove a foreign body from an infant or child, that the head down position with the body elevated is most important. The advantage is that gravity is in favor of the foreign body dropping away from the oropharynx. If it were possible to pick up an adult by the heels and shake him, it would also be a valuable aid in dislodging a foreign body.

Oxygen is a drug and its administration, like that of any other drug, requires evaluation of its response. In the hospital situation, the patient's response to oxygen is evaluated either clinically by observation or by drawing arterial blood gases. In the field, the latter is not possible and clinical signs must be used. These include an improvement in nail bed color, a slowing of the respiratory rate, in an adult a decrease in the heart rate, and in a child an increase in the heart rate. Other changes include improvement in mental status and relief of anxiety.

OXYGEN DELIVERY

In the patient who is breathing adequately without airway obstruction and needs an increase in his oxygen concentration, there are four routes for delivery:

1. Nasal prongs
2. Vented face masks
3. Venturi masks
4. Non-rebreathing masks

*Nasal Prongs.*    Nasal prongs are plastic and conform to the nose with an adjustable head strap (Figure 9-17a). Two prongs fit into the nostrils and oxygen can be delivered at different flow rates. If low concentrations of inspired oxygen are desired, such as in the patient with chronic obstructive pulmonary disease, 1 to 2 liter flow rates will suffice. Nasal prongs are also indicated in patients who have shortness of breath but do not demonstrate marked hypoxemia. They may be used in asthma, myocardial infarction, pneumothorax, pneumonia, and trauma. Table 9-5 shows the approximate oxygen concentrations depending upon the different flow rates from the oxygen tank valve.

TABLE 9-5.   APPROXIMATE $FIO_2$ OBTAINED WITH NASAL PRONGS

| Oxygen Flow Rate | $FIO_2$ |
|---|---|
| 1 l/min | 24% |
| 2 l/min | 28% |
| 3 l/min | 32% |
| 4 l/min | 36% |
| 5 l/min | 40% |
| 6 l/min | 44% |

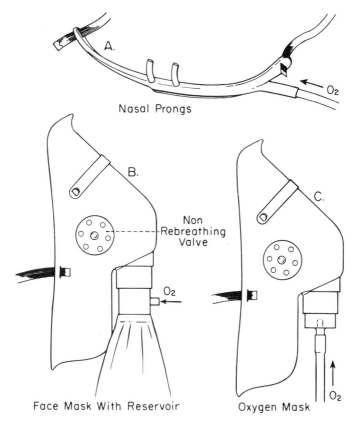

Nasal Prongs

Non-Rebreathing Valve

O₂

Face Mask With Reservoir          Oxygen Mask

O₂

**Figure 9-17.** Three commonly used devices for the delivery of oxygen: A. nasal prongs; B. face mask with reservoir; and C. oxygen mask.

*Vented Face Masks.* This is a clear plastic mask that fits over the nose and mouth and has an adjustable elastic strap. Oxygen is generally introduced into the mask through an inferior or anterior port (Figure 9-17c). There are holes in the mask so that exhalation can be vented to outside air, thus reducing rebreathing. Oxygen concentration can be varied with this mask by adjusting the flow rate to produce an alveolar oxygen concentration between 35 and 55 percent. These masks are useful for patients with acute myocardial infarction, trauma, stroke, pneumonia, pulmonary embolism, and head injury. They should not be used in patients with chronic obstructive pulmonary disease because the oxygen concentration may be so great as to eliminate the hypoxemic stimulus for breathing.

*Venturi Masks.* The Venturi mask is based on the principle that a great flow of gas through a small opening will react with partial amounts

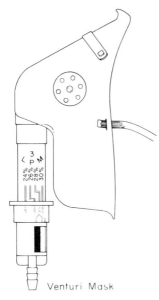

Venturi Mask

**Figure 9-18.** With the Venturi mask, the FIO$_2$ can be altered by adjusting the size of the port near the oxygen inlet. At a 3 l/min oxygen flow rate, the dial is on 28% and this opening will entrain enough air to mix with the oxygen to give a 28% oxygen concentration in the mask.

of the surrounding gases (Figure 9-18). The Venturi mask has a fixed narrow valve through which oxygen is introduced into the mask. The amount of air that will pass through the air entry ports depends on the liter flow rate through the fixed orifice valve. This type of mask can deliver fairly precise oxygen concentrations of 24, 28, 35 and 40 percent. Venturi masks are indicated for use on patients with acute respiratory failure secondary to obstructive lung disease. The concentration of oxygen is therapeutic, yet it will not remove the all-important hypoxemic drive. These masks have been used in the hospital, but have not been generally accepted for field use.

*Non-rebreathing Masks.* These masks are made with non-rebreathing valves and a reservoir bag to assure a high oxygen concentration without the introduction of air into the mask (Figure 9-17b). A properly fitted non-rebreathing mask used with sufficient oxygen flow can deliver an inspired oxygen concentration of nearly 100 percent. The one-way valve on the side of the mask allows for the escape of carbon dioxide during exhalation. Oxygen flow rates used with this device range from 6 to 12 liters per minute, and can best be adjusted by observing the reservoir bag and being certain that it does not become overdistended. This type of high oxygen concentration is indicated for people with myocardial infarction, pulmonary edema, near drownings, smoke inhalation, massive pulmonary embolism, and severe pulmonary insufficiency due to pneumonia. This mask is obviously not useful for patients with chronic obstructive pulmonary disease because of the high oxygen concentrations that are delivered.

Mouth-to-mouth resuscitation is positive pressure ventilation without the use of a mechanical device. Since this is exhausting to the rescuer and cannot deliver a high concentration of oxygen to the patient, mechanical devices come into play during the course of resuscitation, or during the course of treatment of the patient with acute respiratory failure. Positive pressure ventilation is necessary in patients who cannot sustain an adequate inspiratory effort. This would be true for patients in a coma who are apneic or ventilating inadequately, or during cardiopulmonary arrest, neuromuscular disorder, severe flail chest, respiratory failure due to severely damaged lungs that are noncompliant, and respiratory failure due to severe pneumonia. Positive pressure devices that are used in the field are pneumatically driven; that is, they are powered by gas under pressure. The gas source may be compressed oxygen or air. These devices aid in giving positive pressure ventilation to the apneic patient or in assisting spontaneously breathing patients who are hypoventilating. There are essentially two types of pneumatically powered resuscitators:

1. Pressure cycled
2. Manually cycled

## PRESSURE-CYCLED RESUSCITATORS

Pressure cycled resuscitators include the Emerson, E&J, and Stephenson resuscitators, among others. These devices provide a flow of gas until a preset pressure between the patient and machine is met. Suction is then exerted to evacuate the gas until a preset negative pressure is reached. High pressure can be used by a manual override.

Pressure-cycled oxygen-powered resuscitators have been disapproved by the American Heart Association Committee on Cardiopulmonary Resuscitation and Emergency Cardiac Care. These devices were found to be inadequate during cardiopulmonary resuscitation, since the devices respond to changes in airway pressure. Therefore, during cardiac compression, the device may trigger prematurely. These devices are also complex, difficult to use, and more costly than oxygen-powered ventilation devices that are manually triggered.

## MANUALLY CYCLED RESUSCITATORS

The manually operated oxygen-powered resuscitators are simple to operate and are quite effective when used in conjunction with cardiac compression. The two common types of devices are the Elder valve

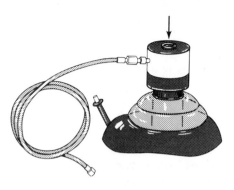

**Figure 9-19.** The arrow indicates the button for delivering oxygen to the face mask or esophageal obturator airway. This is a manually operated oxygen-powered pressure device. It will deliver at least 100 l/min with an inspiratory force up to 40 mm Hg.

and the Robert-Shaw valve (Figure 9-19). These positive pressure devices are pneumatically driven from an oxygen tank with a high liter flow gauge. The device connects directly to an oroesophageal airway, a face mask, or an endotracheal tube or tracheostomy tube. When it is triggered, it has the potential of delivering at least 100 liters of oxygen per minute with an inspiratory force up to 40 mm Hg. When used in conjunction with an EOA, the device is triggered manually and the inspiratory result is evaluated by watching the patient's chest. Care must be taken not to overinflate the lung or distend the stomach. Some of the newer devices have a demand valve and will inflate when triggered by a voluntary inspiration of the patient.

There are mechanical devices that are pressure-cycled ventilators which are not manually operated. These ventilators are commonly used in the hospital situation, but may be used in the transport of critically ill patients. Ventilators can be either pressure-cycled or volume-cycled. In the pressure-cycled ventilator, a certain inspiratory pressure is reached, and the ventilator stops and then recycles. The rate of respiration as well as the amount of pressure can be varied before the ventilator shuts off. Although these ventilators are very accurate, any rise in airway pressure whether by clamping down on an endotracheal tube, mucus obstruction, or breath holding will raise the pressure in the airway and cause the ventilator to shut off before an adequate tidal volume has been delivered to the patient. Such pressure-cycled ventilators are adequate, but a concise understanding of the principles of how they work is necessary in patient management.

Volume-cycled ventilators, on the other hand, deliver a specific volume regardless of airway pressure up to certain limits. A volume ventilator, such as a Mark I Bennett respirator, the Engstrom, or the Ohio, deliver a volume of gas mixture that has been prescribed. When the volume is reached, the ventilator shuts off and recycles. Volume ventilators are extremely important in the ventilation of patients with severe pulmonary failure. Again, their use is limited in the field, but they may be necessary in the transportation of critically ill patients.

These devices allow for the insufflation of air into a face mask, Laerdal pocket mask, EOA, endotracheal tube, or tracheostomy tube. Various bags are available for use and include the AMBU, Laerdal resusci-folding bag, Puritan-Bennett and other devices. The important factors are that these bags have a standard fitting to accommodate the endotracheal or EOA tubes. The manually operated resuscitation device must consist of a self-refueling bag, a one-way valve to prevent rebreathing, and a mask. The bag should be easy to grip and compress and capable of re-expanding quickly. There should be an inlet for supplemental oxygen, and slow release and refilling of the bag should allow the oxygen rather than ambient air into the bag. Valves should be one-way, non-sticking, and constructed of durable material. It is important that the face mask that accompanies these valves be made of clear plastic so the resuscitator can evaluate the patient's lips and investigate for any foreign bodies that may occur under the mask, including vomitus.

## MANAGEMENT OF SECRETIONS

Although portable suction devices are available for airway management outside of the hospital, there is not yet a really adequate device available. Although several vacuum-operated devices are available and able to generate negative pressures of 200 and 300 mm Hg, they still are not a good substitute for in-hospital suction devices. Along with the suction device, there must be a catheter that will reach into the oropharynx and aspirate large amounts of material. A tonsil tip suction catheter is ideal for this, since it will take out large chunks of material and it is rigid so that it can be forced into the oropharynx if there is involuntary biting by the patient (Figure 9-20).

The entire question of respiratory failure, airway problems, obstruction, and resuscitation is a very urgent one. It is imperative that the paramedic become intimately acquainted with the material presented in this chapter, since almost all of his work in the field will deal with some aspect of respiratory and ventilatory diagnoses and management. — *Summary*

The function of respiration is to supply oxygen and to remove carbon dioxide from the body cells. — *Important Points to Remember*

Respiration includes:

Ventilation—delivery to and removal of air from lungs

Diffusion—movement of oxygen and carbon dioxide from respiratory cell to blood

Tonsil Sucker

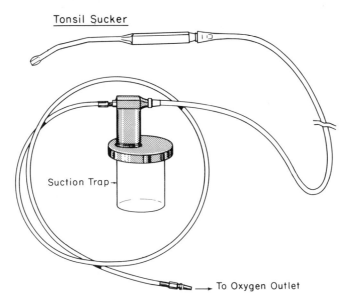

Suction Trap →

→ To Oxygen Outlet

**Figure 9-20.** An oxygen suction device is shown. The suction device works from the oxygen outlet. The tip of the suction device is called a tonsil sucker, and it is important that it be made of clear plastic in order to be able to evaluate the type of materials suctioned from the oropharynx, and strong enough to be jammed between the teeth and suck out large particles from the back of the mouth.

Circulation—method of carrying oxygen and carbon dioxide to and from cells of body.

Respiratory failure occurs when the tension of the respiratory gases in the blood is not within physiologic limits (may be acute or chronic).

*Hypoxia* is an insufficient supply of oxygen to meet cellular oxygen requirements of a particular tissue.

*Hypoxemia* is reduced oxygen in arterial blood.

*Hypercarbia* (hypercapnea) is too much carbon dioxide in the blood.

*Cyanosis* is a bluish discoloration of the lips or nail beds.

*Dyspnea* is labored breathing (short of breath). It is subjective.

*Apnea* is complete cessation of respiration.

*Tachypnea* is rapid respiration.

*Orthopnea* is labored breathing while lying flat.

*Hyperpnea* is deep inhalation.

Hypo- and hyperventilation mean under- and overinflation of the lungs.

Signs and symptoms of respiratory failure are hypoxia (inadequate tissue oxygenation) and hypercapnia. Respiratory failure can be caused by disorders of the following: brain, spinal cord, upper airway, lower airway and lungs, chest wall, and heart.

The first principle of emergency medical care is that adequate ventilation of the lungs supersedes all other considerations.

The crucial factors in airway management are speed and technical expertise. In airway management the choice is life *or* death.

Assessment of the problem includes answering the following questions:

Is apnea present?

Is obstruction full or partial?

Is cyanosis present?

Are there expiratory problems?

Are there bubbling sounds?

Is the skin color abnormal?

Evaluation of the airway includes:

Sight (absent movement, flaring, retraction, cyanosis, pallor, pupil changes)

Hearing (snoring, stridor, bubbling, wheezing)

Touch (skin temperature)

Smell (alcohol, acetone, chemicals).

Priorities of treatment include:

Positioning patient

Backward tilt of head (except spinal injury)

Clearing mouth and oropharynx

Positive pressure (mouth–mouth, etc.)

Face mask with positive pressure device

Airway (oral or nasopharyngeal)

Esophageal obturator airway (EOA)

Cricothyrotomy

Tracheostomy.

Maneuvers for obstructed airway:

In the conscious patient—

Four sharp back blows

Four abdominal thrusts

In the unconscious patient—

While supine—four abdominal thrusts
                four back slaps

Clear airway; ventilate

Call for help

Finger probe

May need to repeat above and also use chest thrusts.

When attempting to remove a foreign body in an infant or child, the head down position is important.

Oxygen therapy can be delivered by four methods: nasal prongs (for low concentration of oxygen), vented face masks (for infarction, trauma, stroke), Venturi masks (acute respiratory failure secondary to obstructive lung disease), and non-rebreathing masks (myocardial infarction, pulmonary edema, near-drowning, smoke inhalation, pneumonia).

Positive pressure ventilation is necessary for comatose patients who are apneic or ventilating inadequately or those experiencing cardiopulmonary arrest, neuromuscular disorder, flail chest, damaged lungs, or severe pneumonia.

Devices used in the field include:

Pressure-cycled (Emerson, E&J, Stephenson)
Manual-cycled (Elder and Robert-Shaw).

*Bibliography*   Applebaum, E. L. and Bruce, D. L. *Tracheal Intubation.* Baltimore, Md.: W. B. Saunders Co., 1976.

Cervenak, M. M., Garavaghia, M. M., and Fields, L. J. *Principles of Emergency Respiratory Care.* Sarasota, Florida: Glenn Educational Medical Services, Inc., 1976.

King, T. K. C. and Briscoe, W. A. "Abnormalities of Blood Gas Exchange in COPD," *Postgraduate Med.* 54:10, 1973.

Chapter 10

# CARDIAC FUNCTION

With the advent of telemetry, radio communication, and the use of intravenous drugs, the paramedic has been placed in the important position of managing emergency cardiac problems in the field. In dealing with those problems, it is necessary for him to be familiar with normal as well as abnormal cardiac function. He should be able to anticipate development of abnormal function and take appropriate steps, since so often when abnormalities occur they are catastrophic and too late for corrective action. Mechanical, electrical, and metabolic functions of the heart are all interrelated, and the paramedic must understand these relationships to treat heart problems intelligently. The importance of cardiac problems is evident since approximately one-fifth of this book is devoted to problems dealing directly or indirectly with the heart.

## BASIC PRINCIPLES OF CARDIAC FUNCTION AND PHYSIOLOGY

The basic principles that govern the function of the heart as a pump can be discussed under the following headings:

Cardiac output
Systemic and pulmonary blood pressures
Coronary circulation
Myocardial blood flow and metabolism
Electrical activity of the heart beat (Chapter 11)

### CARDIAC OUTPUT

Normally at rest the heart pumps 5000 to 6000 ml of blood per minute. Cardiac output can increase by increasing the heart rate or the stroke volume or both. Sympathetic nervous stimulation has a profound, positive

273

effect (inotropic) on both heart rate and stroke volume. Parasympathetic nervous stimulation (vagus nerve), on the other hand, has a marked slowing effect on the rate, but very little effect on stroke volume.

The stroke volume is also determined by the filling pressure of the ventricle and consequently the distention of the ventricles during diastole. Up to a certain point, the greater the distention of the ventricles, the greater the cardiac output (Frank Starling concept, Chapter 3).

Peripheral blood vessels can also modify cardiac output. The large venous capacitance vessels can constrict and increase venous return to the heart. This in turn will increase the filling pressure of the right ventricle (preload), and consequently will increase the output of the right ventricle. Vasodilation of arteries will decrease peripheral vascular resistance and diastolic arterial pressure (afterload), thereby permitting an increase in cardiac output. Vasoconstriction of arteries and the smaller arterioles, on the other hand, will increase the total peripheral vascular resistance and will tend to decrease the cardiac output. The left ventricular muscle, however, responds to the increased amount of blood remaining after each beat by contracting more forcefully to maintain normal cardiac output. The blood pressure consequently rises, since this is a function of the cardiac output and peripheral arterial resistance.

## THE SYSTEMIC AND PULMONIC BLOOD PRESSURES

The arterial blood pressure (BP) is governed by the cardiac output (CO) and peripheral vascular resistance (BP = CO × PVR). A drop in either component without a compensatory increase in the other will cause a drop in the blood pressure. Peripheral vascular resistance is influenced mostly by the autonomic nervous system and the circulating hormones (Chapter 3). In addition, certain metabolites such as carbon dioxide and lactic acid can cause vasodilation and a tendency toward a drop in arterial pressure.

Systolic blood pressure is determined largely by the left ventricular stroke volume, the rapidity of ejection, and the distensibility of the proximal aortic wall. Diastolic pressure is determined primarily by the rapidity with which blood in the aorta flows forward through the small arteries and arterioles after ejection ceases and the aortic valve closes (Chapter 3).

Normal systemic arterial pressure is about 120/70 mm Hg, and pulmonary arterial pressure is much lower (around 25/10 mm Hg) because of the low resistance in the pulmonary vessels. The systolic blood pressure increases with age so that at age fifty it is normally around 150 mm Hg. It usually increases 1 mm Hg every year after 50 so that at age 60 it is approximately 160 mm Hg.

The heart cannot use the blood within its chambers for oxygen and it must first pump the blood into the aorta. The blood then circulates (approximately 5 percent of the cardiac output) through the myocardium via the coronary arteries. The right coronary arises from the right anterior sinus of Valsalva near the base of the aorta and circles around the right atrioventricular groove to reach the posterior inferior aspect of the heart (Chapter 4). The left main coronary artery arises from the left anterior sinus of Valsalva and divides almost immediately into the left anterior descending and the circumflex arteries. Other major branches arise from the right coronary, the circumflex, and the left anterior descending arteries (Chapter 4).

It is important to note that the right coronary artery supplies the posterior surface of the heart in 95 percent of the cases. In only 5 percent of the cases does the left circumflex artery system dominate and supply the posterior portion of the heart. Whichever artery supplies the posterior wall also supplies the AV node (Chapter 11).

Intramyocardial branches then penetrate down into the muscle wall and divide into a dense capillary network to supply the myocardial cells. Anastomosis of the arteries is also found in the muscle wall connecting the branches of the parent vessel as well as the branches of the three major coronary arteries.

Venous blood from the left ventricle drains into the right atrium via the coronary sinus. Blood from the right ventricle, on the other hand, empties into the right atrium via the anterior cardiac veins or directly into the right ventricle via small endocardial (thebesian) veins.

## MYOCARDIAL BLOOD FLOW AND METABOLISM

As might be expected, myocardial blood flow occurs mostly during diastole when cardiac muscle fibers are relaxed (Chapter 3). Under normal conditions the heart is able to restore its chemical and metabolic balance after every beat by complete oxidation of fatty acids, fat, carbohydrate, and amino acids. The heart is even able to utilize lactate ions entering the cells provided enough oxygen is available. Glucose is not absolutely essential to the heart except during ischemia when anaerobic glycolysis of glycogen stores assumes a very important role.

Extraction of oxygen from blood by the myocardium is near the maximum and almost complete even in the resting state so that any increase in demand for oxygen by the myocardium, such as during exercise or stress, is accomplished by marked vasodilation of the coronary arteries and arterioles to allow for additional flow and delivery of oxygen.

A large percentage of paramedic calls deal with abnormalities of cardio-vascular function. These calls come over the air very pointedly as "man down," "chest pain," "heart attack," "short of breath," "fainted," "dizzy," "passed out," "choking," "pounding in the heart," "stroke," etc. Although these initial complaints received by the dispatcher and transmitted to the paramedics provide certain clues, they are often misleading and not fully reliable. When the paramedic arrives at the scene, he should quickly confirm or revise the story. He should also obtain a brief history noting especially the time of onset of each symptom and the drugs taken by the patient.

Physical signs usually recognized by paramedics as suggesting an acute cardiovascular disorder include such findings as abnormal cardiac rhythm, abnormal breathing, marked drop or elevation of blood pressure, changes in skin color and moisture, edema, rales, asymmetry of the face, and unilateral loss of motor power. The electrocardiogram on the cardioscope, of course, provides the information necessary to determine the cardiac rhythm. It may also indicate the presence of ischemia or hyperacute infarction (Chapter 11).

## CLASSIFICATION OF HEART DISEASE

Many different types of diseases affect the heart to produce acute or chronic illnesses. Conditions of the heart that occur as a result of an illness are called *acquired diseases* of the heart. This is in contrast to *congenital heart diseases,* which are anatomic disorders present at birth (Chapter 20). The following classification of acquired heart diseases is presented to allow the paramedic to become familiar with various terms and to provide a brief explanation of the effects the disease produces.

## CLASSIFICATION OF ACQUIRED DISORDERS OF THE HEART

### DISORDERS OF THE CORONARY ARTERIES

|  | *Pathophysiology* |
| --- | --- |
| Coronary artery arteriosclerosis | Narrowing of the coronary arteries due to arteriosclerotic plaques produces diminished blood flow to the myocardium. This diminished blood flow may be aggravated during periods of exercise, after eating, or at rest with emotional stress. |

Conditions directly related to coronary artery disease are as follows:

|  | *Explanation* |
|---|---|
| 1. Angina pectoris | Chest pain from transient myocardial ischemia brought on by physical or emotional stress. Usually lasts 5 to 15 minutes. |
| 2. Myocardial ischemia | Prolonged chest pain due to severe ischemia of the heart muscle. May occur spontaneously at rest or after stress. Usually lasts 15 to 60 minutes. |
| 3. Myocardial infarction | Acute occlusion of the coronary artery or diminished blood flow to certain parts of the heart which produces death of heart muscle. Pain usually lasts 1 to over 4 hours. |
| 4. Ventricular aneurysm | A ballooning out of the left ventricle after a myocardial infarction. The aneurysm is composed of scar tissue and acts as a reservoir for blood, making the left ventricular ejection inefficient. |

## DISORDERS OF THE CARDIAC VALVE TISSUE

|  | *Pathophysiology* |
|---|---|
| Heart valve inflammation | Heart valve inflammation due to rheumatic fever (rheumatic endocarditis)—the most common disorder that damages heart valves—produces scarring and stiffening of the heart valve. During the aging process the heart valve becomes calcified. Bacterial and fungal infections can also damage heart valves. |

Conditions directly related to rheumatic endocarditis:

|  | *Explanation* |
|---|---|
| 1. Mitral stenosis | Narrowing of the mitral valve opening to produce elevations in left atrial pressure. This causes pulmonary venous congestion and shortness of |

breath. This may also produce high pressure in the pulmonary capillaries of the lungs and pulmonary edema. Hemoptysis may also occur due to rupture of bronchial varices.

2. Mitral insufficiency

The mitral valve leaks and during ejection of the left ventricle a certain portion of the stroke volume returns back into the left atrium. This exerts an additional workload for the heart, and, if acute, may raise left atrial pressure and also cause pulmonary congestion or pulmonary edema.

3. Aortic stenosis

Thickening and narrowing of the aortic valve requires the left ventricle to force blood out with high pressure. This causes the left ventricular muscle to become thick and subject to ischemia. Failure to pump blood out effectively may result acutely in syncope or chronically in congestive heart failure. Because of the ischemia, certain dysrhythmias and angina may also occur.

4. Aortic insufficiency

The aortic valve may become dilated or retracted and fail to meet in the middle. Blood in the aorta may then leak back into the ventricle during diastole. This causes the left ventricle to enlarge and produce symptoms of shortness of breath and congestive heart failure. It may also produce ischemic chest pain because of the insufficient amount of blood entering the coronary artery during diastole.

## HEART VALVE BACTERIAL INFECTION

*Bacterial Endocarditis.* Infections of the heart valve can be caused by many types of bacteria. The most common bacterial organisms are *Streptococcus viridans, Staphylococcus aureus,* and *Pseudomonas aeruginosa.* Heart valve infection produces destruction of the valve and may lead to acute congestive heart failure and disturbances of the cardiac rhythm.

Conditions directly related to bacterial infection of the heart valve:

| 1. Aortic insufficiency | Occurs when the heart valve has been so destroyed by bacteria that there may be acute leakage of the valve during diastole. This produces a strain and overload of the left ventricle. |
| 2. Mitral insufficiency | Rupture of the chordae tendinae or damage of the valve leaflets may occur with endocarditis, producing severe leakage of the mitral valve. This may then produce acute congestive heart failure. |

DEGENERATION OF HEART VALVES

*Explanation*

| 1. Mitral valve prolapse | Myxomatous degeneration (idiopathic, may be congenital) of the valve and chordae causes the valve to herniate into the atrium or to leak during systole. The chordae may also rupture spontaneously. These changes put a great strain on the left ventricle and cause dysrhythmia and chest pains. |
| 2. Calcific aortic stenosis | Degenerative changes, fibrosis, and calcification may slowly cause a congenitally deformed valve to become stenotic. |

DISORDERS OF THE PERICARDIUM

*Explanation*

| 1. Pericarditis | Pericarditis is a nonspecific term used to describe inflammation of the sac surrounding the heart. The inflammation may be due to a bacterial, viral, or tubercular organism. This produces chest pain and accumulation of fluid in the pericardial sac, which may lead to cardiac tamponade. |
| 2. Cardiac tamponade | Any condition that causes fluid to accumulate in the pericardial sac may embarrass the diastolic filling of the |

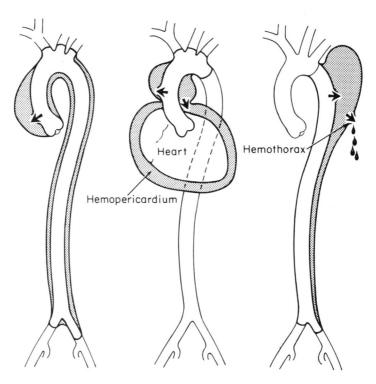

**Figure 10-1.** There are two types of aortic dissection. The dissection occurs between the intima and the adventitia of the artery. This layer of the aorta can rupture into the left thorax or back into the pericardium, producing cardiac tamponade.

heart. This will produce impedance to venous return to the heart and consequently decreased cardiac output and hypotension. Cardiac tamponade is a clinical condition caused by pericarditis and other conditions, such as acute injury with bleeding into the pericardium, rupture of the aorta back into the pericardium, and/or rupture of the heart after myocardial infarction (Figure 10-1).

## DISORDERS OF THE LUNG AFFECTING THE HEART

| | *Pathophysiology* |
|---|---|
| 1. Disease of the lung | When fibrotic lung disease has progressed, especially chronic |

obstructive pulmonary disease, pressure in the pulmonary artery may increase, placing a strain on the right ventricle. This causes ventricular hypertrophy and heart failure. Such a condition is commonly called *cor pulmonale.*

2. Pulmonary embolism

A sudden large blood clot or a series of small clots released from the veins or from the right heart may increase pulmonary vascular resistance and cause acute cor pulmonale.

## DISEASES OF SYSTEMIC BLOOD PRESSURE

*Pathophysiology*

1. Hypertension

High blood pressure causes a tremendous increase in the work of the heart. The heart has to eject blood against elevated systolic blood pressures, leading to thickening of the left ventricle. Hypertension also aggravates coronary artery disease and may accelerate its progression. Hypertension is a common cause of left ventricular problems, including cardiac failure and pulmonary edema.

## CARDIOVASCULAR PROBLEMS SEEN IN THE FIELD

Acute cardiovascular problems that frequently confront the paramedics can be classified as follows:

Acute Myocardial Ischemia or Infarction
Acute Cardiac Failure
    Acute left side failure
    Cardiogenic shock
    Acute cor pulmonale
    Acute tamponade
Acute Dysrhythmias (Chapter 12)
Sudden Cardiac Arrest (Chapter 13)
Acute Dissection or Rupture of Aorta

In over 95 percent of the cases, the etiology of acute myocardial ischemia or infarction is coronary arteriosclerosis with a critical narrowing of the lumen in one or more major vessels. Although the development of arteriosclerosis is a slow, chronic process, myocardial ischemia or infarction can occur acutely when the oxygen demand suddenly exceeds the oxygen supply. Exertion, emotional stimulation, acute systemic pressure overload, and acute volume overload (such as recumbency at bedtime) may suddenly increase the myocardial oxygen demand. On the other hand, a drop in blood (perfusion) pressure, acute blood loss, acute respiratory failure, and acute hypoxemia (carbon monoxide poisoning, etc.) can suddenly decrease the blood flow and oxygen supply to the myocardium. Fibrin thrombus (clot) formation appears to play a minor role in the development of an acute ischemic episode or infarction. Even in the late stages of hospitalized patients with cardiogenic shock, it is questionable whether primary clot formation is responsible for the infarction, although it is obvious that formation and extension of a clot can certainly cause greater myocardial damage.

In a small percentage of cases, coronary arteriosclerosis may not be grossly evident to explain the acute event. In these situations, arteritis (inflammation) of the coronary vessels, emboli to the coronary arteries, or severe protracted coronary spasm (acute narrowing) may be responsible.

## COMMON CLINICAL SYNDROMES PRODUCED BY CORONARY ARTERY DISEASE

*Angina Pectoris.* Angina pectoris, or pain in the chest, is usually brought on acutely by exertion and, after cessation of the exertion, the pain subsides within five minutes. Occasionally, it may be brought on by emotional stress, in which case the pain may persist for fifteen minutes since it is more difficult to shut off emotion. There is also a tendency for this type of angina to recur for an hour or so as the individual smolders in his or her emotional turmoil.

Angina pectoris due to coronary artery disease is usually described by the patient as a heavy squeezing pressure over the lower half of the sternum with radiation of an aching type pain to the left shoulder and left arm (Figure 10-2). During the attack of pain, the patient may appear anxious, diaphoretic, clammy, and short of breath. The pain usually lasts five to fifteen minutes and then subsides.

*Myocardial Ischemia.* Ischemic myocardial pain may occur anytime and usually lasts unabated for thirty to sixty minutes. The myocardium is not permanently damaged, but during this period of ischemia, it may fail acutely or it may fibrillate.

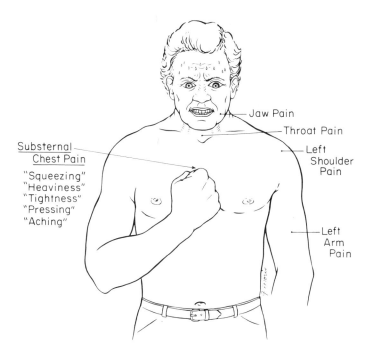

**Figure 10-2.** Angina pectoris can range from very mild pain with only minimal discomfort to very severe pain with a critically ill appearing patient. The pain of myocardial infarction can be very severe and usually lasts longer than the pain due to angina pectoris.

A recent onset (within two weeks) or worsening of angina pectoris or the development of prolonged myocardial ischemic pains should be considered as a prodromal manifestation of an impending myocardial infarction, and should be managed as such with a period of observation in the hospital. Furthermore, every effort should be made to prevent development of infarction. These measures include removing aggravating factors, giving oxygen, correcting hypovolemia and hypotension, and reassuring the patient with or without use of sedatives and analgesics. Ventricular dysrhythmias should also be anticipated and treated vigorously if they occur.

*Myocardial Infarction.* Myocardial infarction pain is usually more severe than angina or ischemia; lasts unabated over hours; and is often associated with sweating, nausea, faintness, shortness of breath, and an irregular heart beat.

The chest pain in all three forms of coronary insufficiency is usually located near the lower half of the sternum and often radiates upward to the neck, jaw, left shoulder, and down the inner aspect of the left arm. This radiation of the pain and ache (called *referred pain*) is explained by the fact that the sensory fibers from the heart enter the cervical cord at the same level that also receives fibers from the left neck, shoulder, and arm (C4-T1, Chapter 4). It is thought that ischemic myocardial cells release substances that stimulate the cardiac pain fibers.

Unfortunately, the electrocardiogram taken in the field or telemetered to the base hospital is not all that helpful in making the diagnosis. It must be remembered that electrocardiograms may appear perfectly normal in myocardial ischemia or infarction.

## MANAGEMENT OF THE PATIENT WITH CHEST PAIN

The preceding clinical syndromes all have one basic characteristic: they all present with chest pain. The paramedic should consider severe anterior chest pains in any adult over 40 years of age to be due to myocardial infarction or impending myocardial infarction until proven otherwise. Even transient angina pectoris necessitating a paramedic call should be considered preinfarction angina since it would be unlikely that a call would be made by someone with chronically recurring exertional angina. Angina pectoris, if it is of recent origin, occurs with less exertion, happens more frequently and with more intensity, requires more nitroglycerine, or lasts longer than usual, should be considered unstable and preinfarction in type.

Other conditions that may mimic acute myocardial infarction should not alter the emergency management by the paramedic; these conditions include such disorders as pericarditis, dissecting aortic aneurysm, pancreatitis, gallbladder disease, pleurisy, pneumonia, simple pneumothorax, and pulmonary embolism. Remember, if errors are to be made, they should be in the direction of under-diagnosing conditions that might not be a myocardial infarction rather than diagnosing something else and subsequently finding out that the patient did have a myocardial infarction.

### MANAGEMENT OF MYOCARDIAL ISCHEMIA OR INFARCTION

Patients suspected of having an acute myocardial infarction, or myocardial ischemia, should receive the following:

Nonspecific Measures

Oxygen therapy should be applied by mask or nasal catheter at 6 l/minute.

An intravenous line using 500 ml of $D_5W$ should be established as soon as possible.

Electrocardiographic electrodes should be applied to the chest and the rhythm examined immediately.

Repeated pulse rate and blood pressure measurements should be made.

When the diagnosis of acute myocardial infarction or impending infarction has been made in the field, more specific management can be instituted. This management can be discussed under the following objectives:

Specific Measures
    Relief of pain and apprehension
    Prevention of serious dysrhythmias
    Prevention of development or extension of the infarct
    Prevention of heart failure
    Prevention of shock

*Relief of Pain and Apprehension.* Individual responses to chest pains vary. About 25 percent of the patients become hyperkinetic, apparently from sympathomimetic discharges with a rise in the blood pressure and heart rate. About 50 percent of the patients become more passive, presumably from parasympathetic vagal responses leading to bradycardia and a tendency for hypotension. The remaining 25 percent remain unchanged with a normal blood pressure and heart rate.

Much of the apprehension can be relieved by verbal assurance and a positive deliberate approach, and excitable relatives should be removed from the scene. The pain of myocardial infarction is best relieved by morphine sulfate intravenously in a dose of 1 mg per minute titrated to the desired effect, up to 10 mg. Overactive and severely anxious patients probably could tolerate and benefit from the full dose but less active patients may be extremely sensitive and lesser amounts should be given. Demerol® (meperidine hydrochloride) may be better in this situation (Chapter 6). Valium® (5 mg intravenously) may be given if the patient is extremely agitated, apprehensive, or anxious, but is having little pain.

Although nitroglycerine sublingually will not alleviate the pain of a myocardial infarction, it may be very effective in myocardial ischemia. It is best to give nitroglycerine gr 1/150 sublingually, repeating once in two minutes if no effect is obtained with the first dose.

*Prevention of Serious Dysrhythmias.* The most feared dysrhythmia associated with myocardial infarction or ischemia is ventricular fibrillation (VF). Since about 10 percent of all cardiac arrests occur after arrival of the paramedics, every effort should be made to prevent this. Hospital coronary care unit experience has taught us that premature ventricular beats occurring frequently at 6 or more per minute, in pairs or triplets, early on top of T waves, in varying coupling intervals, or from more than one foci (multifocal) frequently precede ventricular fibrillation

(Chapter 12). These same prodromal warnings, however, are not often observed during the prehospital phase of acute myocardial infarction. Nevertheless, when they do appear, a lidocaine IV push in doses of 50 to 100 mg should be given. If necessary, this dose may be repeated at five-minute intervals up to a total of 300 mg. This should be followed by an IV drip at 1 to 4 mg/minute.

In our experience a rapidly increasing ventricular rate, whether sinus or supraventricular in origin, often precedes sudden ventricular fibrillation. It is felt that tachycardia predisposes the ischemic myocardium to be depolarized more asynchronously, thus allowing for the greater possibility of an isolated premature ventricular contraction (PVC) to reenter a previously depolarized area and set up a series of chaotic circus movements. Whether propranolol or lidocaine will prevent this type of onset of VF is not known, but it would appear indicated.

On the other side of the scale, sinus bradycardia sometimes leads to premature ventricular beats. In spite of the controversy, it is recommended that atropine be given in an effort to raise the sinus rate to at least 60 per minute. A lidocaine injection in these situations with a sinus rate below 50 per minute will be hazardous because it may suppress an escape mechanism in the event further sinus bradycardia or sinus arrest occur.

During the acute phase of infarction and ischemia, sinus bradycardia and hypotension are found in about half of the cases. This is usually due to increased vagal activity and responds well to atropine. A sinus rate of 50 per minute or less should be treated with 0.5 mg atropine IV every five to ten minutes up to 2.0 mg total in an effort to increase the rate to about 60 per minute. Low blood pressures usually respond to the above regimen. Sinus bradycardia with rates above 50 and with good blood pressures above 120 mm Hg systolic may not have to be treated (Table 10-1).

In certain situations, sinus bradycardia may be a manifestation of ischemia or infarction of the SA node and responds poorly to atropine. Sinus arrest in this situation is a definite possibility and isoproterenol infusion at 1 to 2 microgram/min is recommended.

Atrioventricular block may also be vagal in origin and may respond to atropine, but the AV node may be ischemic due to a right coronary

TABLE 10-1.  USE OF ATROPINE IN ACUTE MYOCARDIAL INFARCTION WITH BRADYCARDIA

| Heart Rate/min | BP mm Hg (Systolic) | | |
| --- | --- | --- | --- |
| | <100 | 100–120 | >120 |
| 60–55 | yes | no | no |
| 54–50 | yes | yes | no |
| <50 | yes | yes | yes |

artery occlusion so that isoproterenol again may be required to maintain an adequate escape rhythm. High grade second degree (3:2, 2:1) with periods of third degree AV blocks not responding to atropine should be treated with an isoproterenol infusion, especially if the overall ventricular rate is below 50 per minute. It is common to have ischemic suppression of both the sinoatrial and atrioventricular nodes due to the anatomic reliance of these structures on the right coronary artery (see below).

*Prevention of Development of Extension of the Infarct.* At the present time, considerable research is underway in hospitals to develop methods for limiting the infarct size by such procedures as after-load reduction, beta-adrenergic blockade, and circulatory assist. There are no proven methods for accomplishing this in the field, even though it is obvious that great inroads could be made during this phase.

Oxygen therapy is recommended to increase the availability of oxygen since there is evidence that arterial $PO_2$ tends to fall during acute myocardial infarction. Alleviation of the pain with morphine will reduce the sympathetic response to pain and thus reduce myocardial oxygen demand. Morphine also reduces the myocardial work load by dilating the veins and decreasing the myocardial preload. Morphine, on the other hand, may depress respiration and cause a further drop in arterial oxygen saturation. Even though nitroglycerine is ineffective in relieving the pain of acute infarction, it may be helpful in reducing the work load on the heart. As long as the blood pressure does not fall to hypotensive levels, nitroglycerine sublingually can be used repeatedly every ten to fifteen minutes. Nitroglycerine is recommended for myocardial ischemia and preinfarction angina. At present, propranolol has not been recommended for use in the field because of its myocardial depressant effect on the failing heart.

*Prevention of Heart Failure in Myocardial Infarction.* Heart failure in acute myocardial infarction will manifest itself as acute pulmonary congestion or a low cardiac output with a tendency to cardiogenic shock. Heart failure can also occur with acute myocardial ischemia.

Symptoms of acute heart failure with orthopnea and dyspnea often may mask the symptoms of acute myocardial infarction. A direct question while events are still fresh in the patient's mind usually reveals the fact that chest pains preceded shortness of breath. Patients with heart disease who develop left ventricular failure and retrograde congestion of the pulmonary veins and capillaries will have sudden onset of dyspnea (especially upon lying down at night—paroxysmal nocturnal dyspnea) and secondarily will feel heaviness in the chest. The presence of a few basal rales is not uncommon in acute myocardial infarction or ischemia. They indicate mild early left ventricular failure.

It is important to keep these patients in the semiupright (Fowler's) position of at least 45° elevation. Occasionally patients may be more comfortable at a higher position. As long as the BP remains above 90 mm Hg systolic, positions of 60° can be tolerated without difficulty. The difference in absolute plasma volume between sitting and supine positions may be as much as 400 ml. This amount may be sufficient to overload a compromised left ventricle. Morphine used judiciously may also help to prevent development of left ventricular failure by pooling blood in the veins. Strong diuretics and digitalization are usually not needed unless delay in hospitalization is anticipated.

Patients who previously have been in chronic congestive heart failure and who suffer an acute myocardial infarction or ischemia pose a different problem. If neck veins are visible at 30° Fowler's position or if peripheral edema is noted and rales are heard in the lungs, the possibility of pulmonary edema developing during transport to the hospital will be so great that furosemide (Lasix$_®$) 40 to 80 mg IV should be given.

*Prevention of Cardiogenic Shock.*   Rapidly falling blood pressure and signs of cutaneous vasoconstriction such as cold extremities indicate the development of cardiogenic shock. (See section on Cardiogenic Shock).

## ACUTE CARDIAC FAILURE

Emergency cardiac failure will be discussed under the following categories:

> Acute left ventricular failure and pulmonary edema
> Cardiogenic shock
> Acute pericardial tamponade
> Acute cor pulmonale
> Acute cardiac dysrhythmias (Chapter 12)
> Cardiac arrest (Chapter 13)

While each of these conditions in its full-blown state requires immediate recognition and specific treatment at the scene, it is also important to recognize the early phases so that preventive measures against progression, especially during transport, can be started. Some of these conditions may also be preceded by a chronic state of failure that can be recognized from a cursory but pointed history and physical examination. For example, patients with a history of severe hypertension, "over 200," may also give a history of minor episodes of nocturnal dyspnea for several nights previously.

### Acute Left Ventricular Failure and Pulmonary Edema

*Common Causes.*   Acute left ventricular failure from various types of heart disease including hypertension is the most common cause of heart failure. Patients with arteriosclerotic coronary artery disease with previous myocardial infarction or with recent infarction and ischemic episodes may suddenly develop left ventricular failure. Frequently, the initial and only manifestation of an acute infarction may be acute left ventricular failure with or without pulmonary edema. The respiratory distress consequent to the heart failure may be so severe as to completely obscure the myocardial infarction. The electrocardiogram in these situations may eventually reveal the true nature of the underlying condition. The other cardiac conditions that may produce acute left ventricular failure are aortic stenosis or insufficiency, mitral insufficiency, or acute overadministration of intravenous fluids.

When left ventricular failure occurs, the cardiac output falls and left atrial pressure rises. This rise in left atrial pressure is transmitted to the pulmonary veins and capillaries. When pulmonary capillary pressure rises to 30 to 35 mm Hg, the serum oncotic pressure is exceeded and fluid diffuses into the interstitial and alveolar spaces. Failure of the lymphatic system to remove the fluid results in acute pulmonary edema. Pulmonary edema can result from conditions other than left ventricular failure. These include cerebral vascular accidents, pulmonary embolism, pulmonary infection, allergy, inhalation of noxious fumes, heroin, and high altitude sickness.

*Signs and Symptoms.*    Shortness of breath and difficulty in breathing (dyspnea), especially on lying down (orthopnea) or with exertion, are the usual complaints of left heart failure. A typical history of paroxysmal nocturnal dyspnea (PND), characterized by dyspnea and discomfort in the chest occurring ten to thirty minutes after lying down at night and relieved after sitting or standing up within five minutes, is almost pathognomonic of left heart failure. Occasionally, especially during the initial episode, shortness of breath may continue and worsen to the point of acute pulmonary edema with extreme dyspnea, wheezing, coughing, frothy white or pink sputum, cyanosis, cold sweats, dizziness, and oppression in the chest. The patient will usually appear very apprehensive and frightened since he is literally drowning in his own fluid. Auscultation will reveal moist rales, rhonchi, and frequently wheezing throughout both lung fields.

*Treatment.*

1. The field treatment of acute pulmonary edema should be directed toward immediate reduction of pulmonary capillary pressure. This can be accomplished by decreasing the inflow of blood into the right ventricle or by increasing the outflow of blood from the left side of the heart.

Patients suspected of actual or impending pulmonary edema will usually be found in an upright sitting position. They should never be laid down even for a brief examination. When patients change from an upright to a supine position, venous return is immediately augmented, and in addition, the plasma volume is rapidly increased by as much as 500 ml. A failing left heart cannot handle this extra volume without the diastolic filling pressure rising still further to levels above 35 mm Hg.

2. Start an IV of D$_5$W with a microdrip chamber and run at a slow rate simply to keep the IV open.

3. Mask oxygen at 6 l/min, will help increase arterial oxygen saturation and make more oxygen available to ischemic tissues. Oxygen will often quiet the patient and reduce his sympathomimetic response, especially when augmented with verbal assurances.

4. Morphine in 1.0 mg doses IV up to 8.0 mg is also very effective in alleviating fright and anxiety, as well as in decreasing the amount of blood returning to the right ventricle.

Diuretics should be used for frank pulmonary edema and are also useful if given early in cases of severe pulmonary congestion. Furosemide (Lasix$_®$) 80 mg IV begins to work within fifteen minutes or even quicker because it promotes venous pooling, decreasing the work load of the heart and subsequent diuresis. It is advisable to administer furosemide as soon as left-sided heart failure is diagnosed in order to prevent frank pulmonary edema during transport.

5. Rotating tourniquets are also helpful. They are managed by releasing one extremity and reapplying to another extremity every ten minutes in a clockwise manner in order to trap sufficient amounts of venous blood and reduce the right ventricular output (Figure 10-3). In

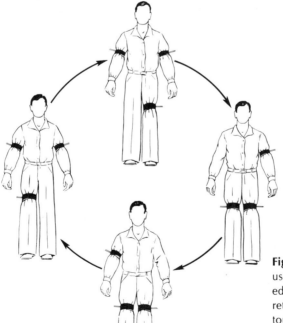

**Figure 10-3.** Tourniquets are used in acute pulmonary edema to reduce venous return or preload. The tourniquets are rotated in a clockwise fashion.

frank shock, with a systolic blood pressure below 80 mm Hg, tourniquets may further reduce the blood pressure and decrease the cardiac output. In these cases, tourniquets should be discontinued.

6. Perhaps the only time digitalis should be given in the field is when pulmonary edema is due to or aggravated by atrial fibrillation with a very rapid ventricular response (>130/min). If the patient is already taking digitalis, the initial dose of digoxin should be no more than 0.25 mg IV. If the patient has not been taking digitalis, the initial dose should not be more than 0.5 mg IV. Subsequent doses are best given after arrival at the receiving hospital.

7. When bronchospasm with audible wheezes is associated with pulmonary edema, aminophylline is indicated. An initial dose of 250 mg IV given slowly over ten minutes is recommended. An alternative is to use 500 mg in 50 ml $D_5W$ over twenty minutes.

8. Patients with actual or threatened pulmonary edema should be transported upright and facing the front of the van (Figure 10-4). This latter recommendation is made because ambulances decelerate more abruptly than they accelerate. If patients are transported in the conventional manner, i.e., head first, each time the ambulance slows down at an intersection, a sudden surge of blood will return to the heart and enter the lungs, worsening the pulmonary edema. Windows should also be covered and sirens avoided if possible, since psychic stimulation will increase circulatory demands.

*Cardiogenic Shock.* Cardiogenic shock occurs when left ventricular function has been so compromised that cardiac output falls and the systolic blood pressure is below 80 mm Hg. Patients are usually semiconscious, have cold and clammy skin, and exhibit mild to moderate cyanosis of their lips and nail beds. By far the most common cause of cardiogenic shock is acute myocardial infarction or diffuse myocardial ischemia.

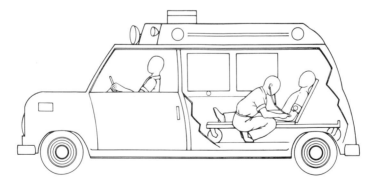

**Figure 10-4.** When transporting the patient in pulmonary edema, the patient's head should be to the back of the vehicle so that during deceleration the centrifugal effect of venous blood on the heart is eliminated.

Other causes include acute myocarditis (infection in the muscle) or severe valvular heart disease. The EKG usually reveals sinus tachycardia. However, cardiogenic shock in the field is occasionally associated with a serious dysrhythmia such as ventricular tachycardia or sinus arrest with a slow escape rhythm. It is frequently difficult to determine whether the dysrhythmia or the shock was the initiating event.

In some cases, cardiogenic shock may be due to unsuspected hypovolemia. If the patient appears dehydrated and the neck veins are collapsed in the recumbent position, this diagnosis is further supported. Hypovolemia is treated entirely different than cardiogenic shock.

### Treatment

1. Pressor drugs are indicated, but prolonged periods of observation in the field to see the effects of these drugs is not recommended. Metaraminol (Aramine$_®$) can be used. The dose is 0.5 to 1.0 mg IV. More recently, dopamine has been used in the field with good results. Mix 400 mg of dopamine in 250 ml of $D_5W$ and infuse at a rate of 2 to 10 $\mu cg/kg/min$.

2. If hypovolemia is suspected, infuse 200 ml of $D_5W$ or Lactated Ringer's over a ten-minute interval. If the blood pressure fails to increase measurably, rapid infusion should not be continued. If the blood pressure does increase by 20 mm Hg or greater, then the diagnosis of hypovolemia is possible, or at least the infusion of fluids will help improve the patient's vital signs.

3. A dysrhythmia is usually present when cardiogenic shock occurs in the field phase of acute myocardial infarction. Since there is an element of increased vagal tone, especially after the use of morphine, atropine in the usual doses should be administered even if the pulse rate is as much as 90 per minute.

4. Oxygen administered by mask at 6 l/min.

5. Monitor the heart and vital signs during transport.

*Acute Cardiac Tamponade.* Recognition of acute cardiac tamponade may be lifesaving since early notification of this possibility can alert the hospital and allow time to prepare for immediate treatment upon arrival. Cardiac tamponade occurs when fluid, pus, or blood accumulates rapidly in the pericardial sac, inhibiting normal diastolic filling of the ventricles. Both systemic and pulmonary venous pressure rise to maintain the inflow of blood into the atria and ventricles. Common conditions that might produce cardiac tamponade include chest trauma, viral and bacterial infections of the pericardium (pericarditis), bleeding into the pericardium (spontaneous or with anticoagulant therapy), dissection of the aorta, ruptured myocardium (following an acute myocardial infarction), uremia, malignancy, and rheumatic fever.

Acute pericarditis, from whatever cause, usually gives rise to anterior chest pains that radiate in a similar manner to those due to acute myocardial infarctions. However, the pain of acute pericarditis is sharper and is often aggravated by respiration.

Auscultation of the heart may reveal a leathery to and fro scratching sound of a pericardial friction rub. Cardiac tamponade should be suspected when the heart rate exceeds 120 per minute, systolic blood pressure falls below 100 mm Hg, neck veins become distended above the clavicle in the 30° upright position, and the heart tones are distant and difficult to hear. An additional sign is "pulsus paradoxicus," an exaggeration of the normal drop in systolic pressure with inspiration. Inspiration causes distention of the right ventricle, which, in turn, further limits the filling of the left ventricle and the stroke volume. A blood pressure cuff measurement of over 15 mm Hg difference in systolic pressure between inspiration and expiration makes the likelihood of pericardial tamponade very high. This sign, although reliable, may be absent when acute bleeding into the pericardial sac has occurred.

### Treatment

1. In the field, management of acute cardiac tamponade will depend on the personnel and facilities available at the scene. Currently, non-physician personnel are restricted from performing a pericardiocentesis (aspirating the pericardial sac with a needle and syringe). This seems justified since a pericardiocentesis under ideal circumstances is a difficult enough procedure.

2. A patient should have a #14 or #16 cannula inserted into an accessible arm vein and Lactated Ringer's started. By giving the patient additional fluid, the elevation of pressures in the right side might force more blood through the lungs and into the left ventricle, improving cardiac output.

3. Perhaps the greatest danger lies in the fact that impending cardiac tamponade is not suspected and drugs that abruptly decrease right ventricular filling pressure such as morphine and Lasix₍ᵣ₎ are administered. This results in sudden cardiovascular collapse, since both drugs tend to decrease venous filling and right ventricular filling pressure. Rotating tourniquets are contraindicated since they also decrease venous return, dropping right ventricular filling pressure and further aggravating hypotension.

4. Drugs such as dopamine or isoproterenol may reduce cardiac size and allow for greater filling and cardiac output.

*Acute Cor Pulmonale.* This condition is virtually synonymous with an acute pulmonary embolism secondary to a blood clot but occasionally due to fat or amniotic fluid emboli. The clot in the pulmonary arterial system produces a sudden increase in pulmonary vascular resistance by obstructing major vessels or by associated vasoconstriction of smaller arterioles due to hypoxia. Humoral substances such as serotonin and histamine may also be released and these will produce pulmonary artery vasoconstriction. The normal right ventricle is not prepared to generate high pressures and is unable to maintain an adequate flow of blood through the lungs. Consequently, there is a decrease in cardiac output and the subsequent circulatory failure produces shock. The patient with chronic cor pulmonale due to lung disease can have sudden deterioration of his condition and present in a similar fashion.

A patient with acute cor pulmonale will usually have a sudden onset of unexplained shortness of breath and difficulty in breathing. The heart rate is elevated and chest pain with cough is present. The dyspnea is not aggravated by lying flat, as would be the case in acute congestive heart failure. The patient will be sitting up, taking deep breaths, almost gasping for air, cold, diaphoretic, and cyanotic. The blood pressure may be diminished. Occasionally a loud systolic murmur can be heard along the left portion of the sternum and the neck veins may be distended. Presence of a venous thrombosis in the leg further suggests a diagnosis of an acute pulmonary embolism. Although EKG changes occur with acute cor pulmonale, they will not be of much help in the field. Frequently secondary tachydysrhythmias such as atrial tachycardia, atrial flutter, and atrial fibrillations occur, and their presence should not detract one from the diagnosis of pulmonary embolism. Although bronchospasm, wheezing, and rales can occur with pulmonary embolism, the incorrect diagnosis of left ventricular failure or asthma is frequently made. These patients are also diagnosed as having a myocardial infarction.

*Treatment*

1. From the standpoint of emergency management, the treatment of acute cor pulmonale is the same as acute left ventricular failure and myocardial ischemia or infarction. Start an IV of $D_5W$ with a microdrip chamber.

2. Administer oxygen by face mask 6 l/min except if chronic obstructive pulmonary disease is present (Chapter 9).

3. If there is hypotension, dopamine might be effective in the same dose schedule as for cardiogenic shock.

4. Pressor agents that might increase pulmonary vascular resistance should not be used. Morphine and diuretics should be used cautiously if at all since both of these drugs will reduce venous return and decrease the filling pressure of the right ventricle.

Acute dissection of the aorta occurs in hypertensive patients or patients with tissue diseases of the aorta. The blood tears into the media (middle wall of the aorta), usually near the aortic valve, and dissects along this path to reenter the aorta distally or retrograde to the pericardium (Figure 10-1). This can close off vessels to the head, arms, kidneys, etc.

Acute dissection of the aorta mimics acute myocardial infarction, but the pain is usually more severe and somewhat tearing in quality. The pain more often radiates directly to the back. The pain is so severe that morphine in the usual dosage for myocardial infarction will not control it. There may be blood pressure discrepancy in the arm, since one of the vessels to the arm may have been occluded by the dissection. Pulses in the peripheral, femoral, and arm regions may vary depending on the degree and extension of the dissection.

*Treatment*

1. The patient with a suspected acute aortic dissection should be treated like any patient with severe anterior chest pain. The use of oxygen is mandatory.

2. The patient should have an IV of Lactated Ringer's started and his heart rate and vital signs should be monitored.

3. Transport to a facility able to deal with these problems if possible.

4. Acute hypertension, if present, can be managed by allaying the patient's fear and controlling the pain with the use of intravenous morphine. If the blood pressure is or remains high (above 170 mm Hg systolic), one injection (300 mg) of Diazoxide can be given intravenously rapidly. The use of Diazoxide in the field is controversial and instead some people would recommend Lasix ®, 40 mg IV.

## USE OF CARDIAC DRUGS

Most cardiac drugs have a therapeutic effect as well as a toxic effect. Despite this, most cardiac drugs are safe when used for the proper indications and in the therapeutic recommended dose range. However, under certain situations, such as severe hypoxia or altered electrolyte balance, toxic effects may be produced even though the drug concentration in the patient is normal or low. It is essential for the base hospital paramedic team to be familiar not only with the drugs approved and carried by the paramedics, but also with certain drugs commonly used by cardiac patients.

DIGOXIN (LANOXIN®)

Digoxin and other digitalis preparations are used primarily to: (1) increase myocardial contractility (inotropic effect), (2) prevent or reverse recurrent supraventricular tachycardia, and (3) increase the degree of AV block in atrial fibrillation and atrial flutter. The inotropic effect to increase the myocardial contractility in congestive heart failure is dependent upon the ability of digitalis to mobilize calcium and make it available to the muscle fibers. This direct action of digitalis presumably occurs through the inhibition of the cell membrane Na-K activated adenosine triphosphatase (an enzyme). By increasing the contractility and decreasing the diastolic pressure in the ventricles, digitalis will also decrease atrial distention and, thus, reverse or protect against atrial tachydysrhythmia. Also, digitalis directly slows conduction through the atrium and directly and indirectly (through the vagus nerve) prolongs the refractory period of the AV node. These actions further help to control supraventricular tachycardias.

The toxic action of digitalis occurs through further inhibition of adenosine triphosphatase (ATP) activity with the excessive loss of cellular potassium. This causes increased automaticity of the AV junction and the His-Purkinje system. At the same time, the uneven prolongation of action potential and the decrease in the effective refractory period of these tissues cause not only ectopic beats but also a tendency for supraventricular and ventricular tachycardias to occur.

In addition to tachydysrhythmias, digitalis toxicity may suppress the sinus node or cause various degrees of AV block. One of the most difficult dysrhythmias to manage is ventricular irritability and heart block, occurring concomitantly in digitalis toxicity. Drugs that suppress ventricular irritability may also suppress an escape rhythm needed for a complete SA or AV block, and drugs that accelerate the slow escape rhythm may induce ventricular tachycardia or ventricular fibrillation.

If digitalis toxicity is suspected from a history of overdose or overuse of the drug, every effort should be made to prevent the sudden deterioration of the rhythm into a state of cardiac arrest with ventricular fibrillation or asystole. Recommendations can be made for the field management of digitalis toxicity dysrhythmias (Table 10-2).

LIDOCAINE

Much of the success of the paramedic program throughout the country probably can be attributed to the use of certain drugs in the field. Notable among these is lidocaine. Because of its general acceptance, it would be difficult to conduct a study to determine how frequently lidocaine can prevent ventricular fibrillation in the field. The evidence that is available suggests that it does this often and is now being used in many areas as a prophylactic drug even though life-threatening dysrhythmias are not present.

TABLE 10-2. DIGITALIS TOXICITY DYSRHYTHMIAS

*297*

*Use of Cardiac
Drugs*

| | Recommended Field Treatment |
|---|---|
| PAC*, PNC, SVT < 140/min, PAT with 2:1 Conduction, PVCs < 6/min, 1° AV Block, SB 50–60/min, or Junctional R > 60/min | Usually require no specific or immediate treatment |
| PVCs > 6/min, multifocal, or in pairs (if no bradycardia) V Tach | Lidocaine, Dilantin®, KCL |
| SVT > 140/min | May require propranolol |
| SB with PVCs. SB < 50/min 2° ABV, Junct R 40–60/min | Atropine |
| Junctional rhythm < 40/min | Atropine and Isoproterenol |

*See Chapter 12 for key to these abbreviations.

Lidocaine very effectively suppresses PVCs and reverses ventricular tachycardia. The drug acts by reducing the rate of spontaneous depolarization (phase 4) in normal and ectopic pacemaker tissues and also by enhancing conduction velocity, shortening the action potential and decreasing the effective refractory period (Chapter 11). Lidocaine, therefore, specifically suppresses ectopic beats and abolishes unidirectional blocks, which propagate a reentry type of tachycardia. At the subcellular level, lidocaine apparently influences the transmembrane flux of sodium and potassium. This action is most evident in the ventricles and less evident in the supraventricular tissue, accounting for its effectiveness in ventricular dysrhythmias.

The toxic effect of lidocaine is usually not seen during the initial field phase of cardiac disorders, presumably because toxic blood and tissue levels are reached after repeated cumulative doses of the drug. However, patients in severe congestive heart failure or in hepatic failure may manifest central nervous symptoms of drowsiness, disorientation, or seizures if intravenous doses exceed 300 mg during the first hour. Intravenous pushes (over a one-min period) of 1 mg per kg body weight repeated twice if necessary, followed by IV drip 2 to 4 mg per minute are recommended. It should be remembered that IV push doses maintain a blood level for only about fifteen minutes.

## ATROPINE

Atropine is a very useful drug with relatively few side effects when one or two doses are used in the field. It is indicated for sinus bradycardia, sinus arrest, sinus block, and atrioventricular intranodal block. Atropine blocks the effect of acetylcholine at its receptor sites, and thus selectively increases the rate of spontaneous depolarization in pacemaker cells and hastens the conduction of impulses through the AV node. In very small doses, atropine may have a short paradoxical effect and will decrease the heart rate and increase AV block. Atropine should be used in doses of 0.5 to 1.0 mg IV repeated in fifteen minutes if necessary to a total of 2.0 mg.

After an IV injection, atropine produces a peak effect in thirty to ninety seconds and disappears rapidly from the bloodstream thereafter. Glaucoma, acute urinary retention, mental aberrations, and dryness of the mouth may be precipitated with large doses of atropine.

## PROPRANOLOL (INDERAL®)

Propranolol is a relatively new drug but it is rapidly becoming very widely used not only for control of dysrhythmia, but also for angina pectoris and hypertension. Intravenous use of propranolol may be recommended for use by the paramedics to control life-threatening dysrhythmias.

Propranolol is a beta-adrenergic receptor blocking agent and thereby inhibits adrenergic stimulation of the heart. It also has a direct effect on the myocardium, reducing spontaneous diastolic depolarization (phase 4), slowing conduction velocity, and shortening the refractory period (Chapter 11). In general, propranolol is more effective in supraventricular than ventricular dysrhythmias, but it may at times be quite effective in controlling the latter when used in combination with other drugs. Propranolol is effective in the treatment of digitalis induced tachydysrhythmias of the supraventricular type, but it should not be used in paroxysmal atrial tachycardia (PAT) with block because of its effect on AV conduction. For emergencies, 1.0 to 2.0 mg of propranolol can be given intravenously and repeated once in ten minutes if necessary.

Propranolol is contraindicated in cardiac failure (unless tachycardia itself is responsible for the failure) because it blocks the compensatory increase of sympathetic activity which attempts to maintain maximal myocardial contraction. This drug is also contraindicated in bronchial asthma, chronic obstructive pulmonary disease, and in those who may develop hypoglycemia.

Overdosage with propranolol results in severe sinus bradycardia or sinus arrest. Ventricular rates below 44 per minute, especially when associated with hypotension or signs of cerebral anoxia, should be treated with an isoproterenol infusion at 1 to 4 micrograms per min.

## QUINIDINE

Quinidine has for years been one of the most widely used antidysrhythmic drugs. Because of its high toxicity, the drug is not recommended for parenteral use. It is rapidly absorbed from the GI tract and its action may be noted within thirty minutes; its peak action occurs at about two hours. Conceivably, in certain situations, quinidine could be given orally in an emergency before hospitalization.

Quinidine is classed as a Group I antidysrhythmic drug and depresses automaticity by decreasing the rate of diastolic depolarization (phase 4), not only in the normally functioning pacemaker cells but also in other cells. It also decreases the rate of rise of the initial depolarization (phase 0) wave and thereby decreases the rate of conduction of the impulse through the atria and ventricles. Quinidine therefore suppresses ectopic beats and prevents reentrant tachycardias by blocking conduction of the impulse around a circuit. It has a mild vagolytic effect and indirectly increases the AV nodal conduction. It also has a myocardial depressant effect and in large doses worsens cardiac failure.

Although quinidine is very effective in controlling ectopic dysrhythmias, the drug, even in therapeutic doses (0.8 to 1.6 g per day), may frequently cause nausea, vomiting, abdominal cramps, diarrhea, blurred vision and tinnitus, and on rare occasions can cause fever, purpura, hypotension, ventricular tachycardia, or ventricular fibrillation presumably on the basis of hypersensitivity. With therapeutic doses and serum levels of 4–6 mg per liter, there is Q-T prolongation; but with toxic doses and levels above 10 mg per liter, there is QRS interval prolongation followed by SA block, AV block, and ventricular standstill. Unfortunately, there is no specific antidote for quinidine toxicity and even cardiac pacing may be ineffective. Calcium may be a good antidote.

## PROCAINAMIDE (PRONESTYL$_{®}$)

Procainamide is electrophysiologically similar to quinidine. It can be used intravenously, but it must be given no faster than 100 mg per minute and no more than 1.0 g at a time because of its hypotensive effect. Oral ingestion in therapeutic doses causes very few side effects, but the drug might produce a lupus erythematous-like syndrome. The effects of procainamide and quinidine are additive therapeutically and toxicologically. Serious toxic effects of procainamide are similar to those of quinidine.

## DIPHENYLHYDANTOIN (DILANTIN$_{®}$)

Dilantin$_{®}$ has been used for many years in seizure disorders and more recently in the treatment of dysrhythmias. The drug acts by depressing diastolic depolarization (phase 4) in common with other antidysrhythmic drugs and thus suppresses premature ectopic beats. Unlike others, however, Dilantin$_{®}$ does not delay AV conduction. Blood levels of 10–20 mg/liter are considered to be in the therapeutic range. This level can be reached by intravenous infusion of 50 to 100 mg given slowly every five minutes until a total of 1000 mg is given. Oral doses of 300–400 mg per day will usually result in therapeutic blood levels in three to five days.

It is felt by many that diphenylhydantoin is the drug of choice in digitalis-induced dysrhythmias. It should not, however, be considered the drug of first choice in other types of tachydysrhythmia.

The intravenous use of Dilantin₍₎ is fraught with serious toxic manifestations in the form of shock and even cardiac arrest, but such reactions are considered to be due to extremely rapid administration of the drug. The oral intake of Dilantin₍₎ is frequently attended with side effects such as ataxia, diffuse skin rash, hepatitis, and blood dyscrasias.

## ISOPROTERENOL (ISUPREL₍₎)

Isoproterenol, an analog of epinephrine, is such a potent drug that it is only administered by a slow intravenous infusion at the rate of 1 to 4 micrograms per minute. Its action is primarily as a beta-adrenergic stimulant and in the heart it increases myocardial contractility (inotropic) and heart rate (chronotropic). The drug may also precipitate ventricular tachycardia and ventricular fibrillation because of its excitatory effect. Isoproterenol also dilates the peripheral arteriolar bed by stimulating the beta-adrenergic receptors.

Isoproterenol is recommended in heart block to increase and maintain an adequate ventricular rate. It may also abolish the heart block and initiate a sinus rhythm. Its infusion rate should be regulated carefully in heart block so as not to allow the blood pressure and heart rate to exceed 110 mm Hg systolic and 70 per minute, respectively.

Isoproterenol can also be used in cardiogenic shock, but a paradoxical fall in blood pressure may occur if hypovolemia or extensive myocardial damage is present. This drug is also potentially helpful in severe mitral regurgitation because of its ability to reduce peripheral vascular resistance.

## DOPAMINE HYDROCHLORIDE (INTROPIN₍₎)

Dopamine, a biological precursor of norepinephrine, has just about replaced isoproterenol for cardiogenic shock. It has much less of a vasodilatory effect than isoproterenol so that a paradoxical drop in blood pressure is less likely to occur. Furthermore, dopamine appears to have a direct non-beta mediated renal vascular dilatation, which promotes diuresis. The initial claim that dopamine does not cause tachycardia should be discounted with the higher doses now being recommended. It is recommended that dopamine be prepared in a concentration of 1.6 mg/ml (400 mg in 250 ml 5 percent dextrose in water) and infused at a rate of 5 μgm per kg body weight per minute. In a 70 kg adult, the rate would be about 10 to 15 microdrops per minute. The infusion rate is then increased every five minutes in increments of 10 microdrops per minute up to 60 microdrops per minute, or until the blood pressure is raised to 90 to 110 mm Hg systolic. When ectopic beats appear, the dosage should be reduced.

FUROSEMIDE (LASIX®)

Furosemide is another very useful cardiac drug in acute pulmonary edema. When given intravenously, it appears to have an almost immediate venous dilatory effect, reducing the inflow of blood into the lungs and thereby reducing the pulmonary capillary pressure. Furosemide is also a potent diuretic and initiates diuresis within fifteen minutes. The reduction in blood volume induced by the diuresis results in decreased venous return and lowering of the diastolic ventricular pressure.

This chapter contains information of utmost importance because of the frequency of cardiac conditions seen in the field. Both physiology and disease of the heart should become familiar to the paramedic in his important role in the early management of these problems. The paramedic will probably find this chapter one of the more frequently reread ones as he works in the field.   *Summary*

Normally at rest the heart pumps about 5 to 6 liters of blood per minute. This can be increased by increasing rate or stroke volume or both. Sympathetic nervous stimulation has a positive (inotropic) effect on rate and stroke volume. Parasympathetic (vagus) stimulation slows the rate of contraction and dilation of peripheral vessels, and also effects cardiac output.   *Important Points to Remember*

Arterial blood pressure is governed by cardiac output and peripheral resistance.

Systolic pressure depends on left ventricular stroke volume, rapidity of ejection, and arterial wall distensibility.

Diastolic pressure depends primarily on peripheral arterial and arteriolar resistance.

Normal systemic arterial pressure is about 120/70 mm Hg, and pulmonary artery pressure runs around 25/10 mm Hg.

Acquired disorders of the heart include:

1. Disorders of coronary arteries
   A. Coronary artery arteriosclerosis
      (1) Angina pectoris
      (2) Myocardial ischemia
      (3) Myocardial infarction
      (4) Ventricular aneurysm
2. Disorders of cardiac valves
   A. Related to rheumatic disease

(1) Mitral stenosis
(2) Mitral insufficiency
(3) Aortic stenosis
(4) Aortic insufficiency

B. Heart valve bacterial infection
(1) Aortic insufficiency
(2) Mitral insufficiency

C. Degenerative diseases
(1) Prolapsing mitral valve
(2) Calcific aortic stenosis

3. Disorders of pericardium
A. Pericarditis
B. Cardiac tamponade

4. Disorders of lung affecting the heart
A. Acute cor pulmonale
B. Chronic cor pulmonale

5. Diseases of systemic blood pressure
A. Hypertension
B. Hypotension

Acute cardiovascular problems confronting the paramedic include: acute myocardial ischemia or infarction, acute cardiac failure, acute dysrhythmias, sudden arrest, and acute dissection or rupture of the aorta.

Physical signs suggesting acute cardiovascular disorders include abnormal rhythm and breathing, blood pressure changes, changes in skin color and moisture, edema, rales, facial asymmetry, and muscle power loss.

Angina pectoris is usually brought on by exertion, and after cessation of exertion the pain subsides within five minutes. Emotional problems can also cause angina, which can last for fifteen minutes and intermittently up to an hour.

Myocardial ischemia presents with pain for fifteen to sixty minutes and may produce dysrhythmia. Myocardial infarction pain is more severe, lasts over an hour, and may be associated with other signs such as sweating, nausea, faintness, shortness of breath, and irregular beats. Chest pain from the above conditions is usually in the lower sternal area and may radiate to the neck, jaw, left shoulder, and arm. An electrocardiogram may initially be normal in myocardial infarction.

The paramedic should consider anterior chest pain in any adult over 40 as due to coronary artery disease with myocardial ischemia or infarction until proven otherwise.

Other conditions that mimic acute ischemia or infarction are: pericarditis, dissecting aneurysm, pancreatitis, gallbladder disease, pleurisy, pneumonia, pneumothorax, and acute pulmonary embolism.

Management of myocardial ischemia includes: oxygen therapy; an intravenous line; placement of EKG electrodes; repeated vital sign measurements; pain relief and prevention of serious dysrhythmias; extension of the infarct, heart failure, or shock.

The pain of myocardial infarction is best relieved by morphine sulfate IV in a dose of 1 mg/min up to 10 mg; Demerol® and/or Valium® may also be useful.

Ventricular fibrillation is the most feared dysrhythmia associated with ischemia or infarction.

Nitroglycerine is recommended for myocardial ischemia and preinfarction angina.

Heart failure may precede or follow myocardial infarction. Rales, neck vein distension, and peripheral edema may help in the diagnosis. Semiupright (Fowler) position and Lasix® injection may be indicated in these cases.

Acute left ventricular failure from various types of heart disease (including hypertension) is the most common cause of heart failure.

Dyspnea and orthopnea are the usual complaints of heart failure. Treatment includes oxygen, IV fluid (for medications), morphine, diuretics, furosemide (Lasix®) tourniquets, digitalis, aminophylline, and upright position. Transport of patients with acute left ventricular failure should be undertaken with the patient facing forward in the ambulance.

Patients with cardiogenic shock are usually mildly stuporous and have a BP below 80 systolic, and show cold, clammy hands and cyanosis. Treatment includes pressor drugs (Aramine®, dopamine), IV fluids, treatment of dysrhythmias, and oxygen.

Cardiac tamponade occurs when fluid accumulates in the pericardial sac. Signs include friction rub, rate over 120/min, falling systolic blood pressure, distended neck veins, distant heart sounds, and "pulsus paradoxicus."

Acute cor pulmonale is usually synonymous with acute pulmonary embolus. Sudden shortness of breath, chest pain, cough, and elevated heart rate are seen. Treatment is similar to that for acute left ventricular failure.

Acute dissection of the aorta mimics infarction but the pain is more severe, tearing in quality, and often radiates to the back. Treatment includes IV fluids, antipressor drugs, rapid transport, and management of pain, but morphine and diuretics should be used cautiously.

Some of the more common drugs and medication follow. This very important subject should be learned and constantly reviewed by the paramedic.

1. Digitalis (increase myocardial contractility, treat supraventricular tachycardia, increase the degree of AV block in atrial fibrillation or flutter).

2. Lidocaine (prevent ventricular fibrillation, suppress PVCs, reverse ventricular tachycardia).

3. Atropine (sinus bradycardia, sinus arrest, sinus block, and AV intranodal block).

4. Propranolol (Inderal ®) (control of dysrhythmia, especially supraventricular; digitalis dysrhythmias; angina; and hypertension).

5. Isoproterenol (Isuprel®) (heart block, cardiogenic shock).

6. Dopamine (most often used drug for cardiogenic shock).

7. Furosemide (Lasix®) (acute pulmonary edema, diuretic).

*Bibliography*    Braunwald, Eugene. *The Myocardium: Failure and Infarction.* New York: H. P. Publishing Co., Inc., 1974.

Gunnar, Rolf M.; Loeb, Henry S.; and Rahimtoola, Shahbudin H. *Shock in Myocardial Infarction.* New York: Grune and Stratton, 1974.

Katz, Arnold M. *Physiology of the Heart.* New York: Raven Press, 1977.

Rushmer, Robert F. *Structure and Function of the Cardiovascular System.* Philadelphia, Pa.: W. B. Saunders Co., 1976.

# Chapter 11

# ELECTROPHYSIOLOGY AND ELECTROCARDIOGRAPHY

It is obvious that a complete understanding of electrical activity of the heart is essential for the proper management of cardiac patients encountered by paramedic personnel. This complex subject cannot be extensively discussed in a single chapter. The bare rudiments of electrophysiology and the principles of electrocardiography will be covered. A more extensive study of this subject can be obtained in the basic textbooks referenced in the bibliography at the end of this chapter.

## ANATOMY AND PHYSIOLOGY OF THE CONDUCTION SYSTEM

### SINOATRIAL NODE

The normal heart beat begins in the sinoatrial (SA) node, which is located at the junction of the superior vena cava and the right atrium (Figure 11-1). The pacing cells in this neuromuscular tissue are electrically unstable and periodically discharge an impulse that spreads through the atria inscribing the "P" wave on the electrocardiogram and activating the atrial muscle into contraction. The activity of the SA node is stimulated by epinephrine, the sympathetic nervous system, thyroid hormone, and temperature elevation, and is depressed by the parasympathetic nervous system, severe anoxia, severe cold, toxic chemicals and drugs.

The blood supply of the SA node is somewhat unique in that the SA nodal artery arises from the very proximal segment of the right coronary artery 55 percent of the time, and from the proximal left circumflex artery, 45 percent of the time. The SA nodal artery passes through the center of the node.

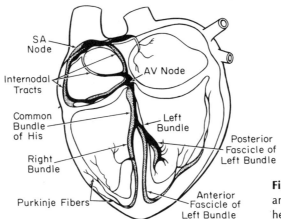

**Figure 11-1.** Pacemaker sites and conduction system of the heart.

## ATRIOVENTRICULAR NODE

After traversing both atria, the electrical impulse arrives at the atrioventricular node (AV) and slowly trickles through this node accounting for the interval between the "P" and the "QRS" (P–R interval). The node is located near the tricuspid valve ring at the inferior medial portion of the right atrium adjacent to the coronary sinus. It receives its blood supply in 95 percent of the cases from the distal right coronary artery just before it gives off the branch to the posterior descending interventricular artery. In 5 percent of the cases, the AV node and the posterior descending artery are supplied by the left circumflex artery.

Adjacent to the AV node are junctional tissues that are capable of initiating an impulse (an escape beat) in the event the SA node is suppressed or conduction through the AV node is halted. Like the SA node, the activities of the AV node and the junctional tissue are suppressed by the vagus nerve and enhanced by the sympathetic nerve and catecholamines, such as epinephrine.

## CONDUCTION SYSTEM BELOW THE AV NODE

The electrical impulse, after a measurable delay, emerges from the AV node and rapidly descends down the Bundle of His. This bundle of specialized conducting tissue is approximately 12 mm long before it branches. It lies in the subendocardium on the right side of the interventricular septum. Normally, the AV node and Bundle of His constitute the only pathways for conduction from atria to ventricles. The bundle then divides into a thin long right bundle and a thick short left bundle. The left bundle then divides immediately into an anterior fascicle and a posterior fascicle. The three fascicles, including the right bundle, then spread out through their respective endocardial surfaces of the ventricles as the Purkinje network (described by Purkinje in 1839). The conduction velocity for propagation of the action potential over the Purkinje fiber system is the fastest of any tissue within the heart; estimates vary from 1 to 4 meter/sec. The two ventricles are then activated almost simultaneously by the electrical impulse giving rise to the QRS complex and to a mechanical systole. Most of the blood supply of the lower conduction system comes from the anterior descending coronary artery.

## THE ELECTRICAL SYSTEM AND THE ELECTROCARDIOGRAM

### QRS–RST SEGMENT—T WAVES

Although a single bipolar lead electrocardiogram (usually Lead II) may be adequate to diagnose most of the significant dysrhythmias in the field, there may be occasions when multiple lead EKGs might be helpful in diagnosing other forms of acute cardiac disorders. For this purpose, we should have some knowledge as to how QRS and T waves are formed.

When the electrical impulse enters a responsive ventricle via the Purkinje network, a wave of electrical current progresses from the endocardial surface outward to the epicardial surface creating a positive potential ahead and a negative potential behind the wave front. The electrical current is propagated from one cell to the next much like a row of dominoes falling after the initial piece is tripped.

The electrical activity of a single cell can be graphically recorded as a transmembrane action potential (Figure 11-2). The inside of a resting cell has a $-90$ mV negative potential when compared to the outside primarily because of differences in concentrations of sodium ($Na^+$) and potassium ($K^+$) inside and outside the cell. When this so-called resting

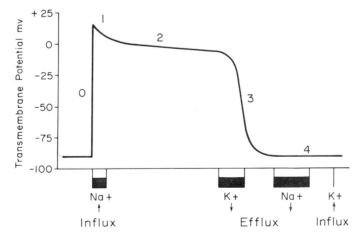

**Figure 11-2.** Single myocardial cell electrogram.

state of the myocardial cell is disturbed with an electrical charge arriving via the Purkinje network, $Na^+$ ions rapidly enter and less $K^+$ ions emerge from the cells, making the cells less negative (or more positive) and inscribing the phase 0 on the transmembrane action potential. This rise in positivity above the threshold then triggers the next cell into a similar action. Very quickly, in about 0.08 sec., the entire heart is activated and the QRS wave is inscribed on the surface electrocardiogram (Figure 11-3). The net direction and intensity of these propagated action potentials will determine the characteristics of the QRS. After a brief overshoot (phase 1) of the action potential, a transient period of stable zero activity (phase 2) occurs in each cell. Since there is no change in action potential occurring at the cell level, the surface electrocardiogram will briefly record an isoelectric interval between the end of the QRS and the onset of the T wave, identified as the RST segment.

Immediately following this RST interval, the myocardial cell begins to repolarize; that is to say, the $K^+$ ions come out of the cells. Phase 3 on the cell electrogram is thus accomplished. During the early part of phase 4 the cell reorganizes itself by pumping $Na^+$ ions out and allowing $K^+$ ions to reenter the cells. Pacemaker cells such as those in the sinus node do not remain stable and depolarize themselves during the later part of phase 4. Repolarization usually begins from the epicardial surface inward to the endocardial surface. The advancing wave is negative and the trailing wave is positive; thus, a positive T wave is usually inscribed on the surface electrocardiogram, which shows a positive QRS deflection.

The typical clinical electrocardiogram strip is shown in Figure 11-3. The tiny squares represent 0.04 seconds when the paper speed is 25 mm/second. From the paper speed and the size of the small boxes, a quick look at the electrocardiogram reveals the difference in the various segments. The normal PR interval is approximately 0.12 to 0.20 seconds. The normal QRS interval is 0.06 to 0.10 seconds. These time intervals will have importance in interpreting dysrhythmias (Chapter 12).

THE ELECTROCARDIOGRAM

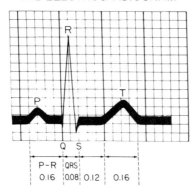

**Figure 11-3.** A sample electrocardiogram is shown. Each small box represents 0.04 seconds. The paper speed is 25 mm/second. The QRS interval is 0.08 seconds.

Cardiac activity associated with depolarization and repolarization of cardiac muscle develops an electrical field in surrounding tissues, which are considered a relatively uniform volume conductor. Electrodes placed on a surface of the trunk or extremities are situated within the electrical field of the heart. When these electrodes are connected to a galvanometer in the electrocardiograph machine, changes in electrical potentials from moment to moment between sites of these electrodes are recorded as a continuous curve, the electrocardiogram (EKG) (Figure 11-3). Time is the abscissa and voltage is the ordinate. The standard limb leads are bipolar leads. *Bipolar* means that one lead is influenced by negative potentials and the other by positive potentials.

The paramedic in the field is always faced with the problem of getting the maximum amount of information within the shortest interval of time. Consequently, the EKG electrodes are usually limited to limb leads only. Precordial leads are possible, but they are time-consuming to apply and are rarely used. It is recommended that right and left arm leads be placed in the upper chest and right and left leg leads in the lower chest or upper abdomen, respectively (Figure 11-4). Lead I will then record the summation of the positive waves coming to the left upper chest and the reciprocal of negative waves coming to the right upper chest. Lead II will record positive waves to the left lower abdomen and the reciprocal of negative waves to the right upper chest (Figure 11-5). Lead III will record positive waves to the left lower abdomen and the reciprocal of negative waves to the left upper chest (Figure 11-6).

By proper switching of the EKG machine, augmented unipolar lead tracings designated as $aV_R$, $aV_L$, and $aV_F$ can be obtained. These leads are considered unipolar and record only the positive waves coming to each of the respective leads because the opposite two negative electrodes are damped out with 5,000 ohms resistance and brought to a central terminal.

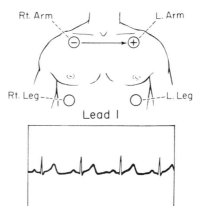

**Figure 11-4.** Placement of EKG lead electrodes and typical Lead I electrocardiogram.

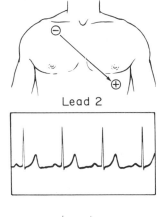

Lead 2

**Figure 11-5.** Lead 2 electrode placement and electrocardiogram. This lead usually gives the most useful tracing in the field.

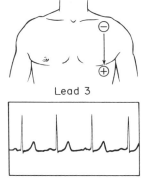

Lead 3

**Figure 11-6.** Lead 3 electrode placement and electrocardiogram.

Because of the placement of the arm leads on the upper chest and lower abdomen, it would be fallacious to interpret the EKGs from a frontal plane vectorial system. It would thus appear more rational for the paramedic to become familiar with certain EKG patterns which might be helpful in prehospital emergency medicine. Pattern recognition would also be much quicker than vector analysis.

## ABNORMAL EKG PATTERNS

### ACUTE MYOCARDIAL INFARCTION

During the first hour of acute myocardial infarction, the electrocardiogram may be perfectly normal. A normal electrocardiogram, therefore, does not rule out the possibility of acute myocardial infarction. The initial changes may be quite subtle and completely overlooked. During the hyperacute phase, there may be a slight elevation of the "j" point and a tall upright T wave (Figure 11-7). Shortly after this phase, the "j" point becomes more elevated and the RST segment becomes curved upward and the T becomes shorter.

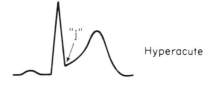

Hyperacute

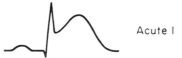

Acute 1

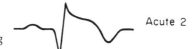

Acute 2

**Figure 11-7.** Various EKG patterns during acute phase of myocardial infarction.

Infarcted muscle fails to generate electrical potentials so that EKG leads facing the infarcted area will inscribe pathologically negative Q waves, which will be at least 25 percent of the succeeding R wave in depth and at least 0.04 seconds in duration. QRS changes of acute myocardial infarction are usually seen after these patients are admitted to the hospital.

These changes may be evident in Leads II, III, and $aV_F$ for inferior wall infarction and in Leads I and $aV_L$ for high lateral wall infarction. Precordial leads will be needed to diagnose anterior and anteroseptal infarctions.

## MYOCARDIAL ISCHEMIA

Prior to infarction, there may be a period of ischemia that would cause certain EKG changes. Since ischemia is usually subendocardial in location, the surface EKG will record an RST segment that is depressed (Figure 11-8). The usual explanation given for this phenomenon is that the negative current of injury in the subendocardial layer compared to the more positive epicardial layer raises the apparent resting isoelectric point on the surface electrocardiogram. Immediately after depolarization, the current of injury is wiped out and the RST segment descends to the true isoelectric point, which is lower than the apparent isoelectric point before depolarization.

Frequently, the direction of repolarization may also become abnormal in acute ischemia so that downward sloping of the RST segment and inversion of T waves may be recorded. Again, the various limb

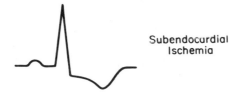

Subendocardial
Ischemia

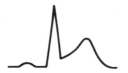

Acute
Pericarditis

**Figure 11-8.** Electrocardiogram showing RST-T changes of ischemia and pericarditis.

leads facing the involved area tend to show the maximum effects of
ischemia.

These ischemic changes do not necessarily lead to infarction but
they may lead to fatal dysrhythmias. If the RST depression is over
2 mm and the T wave is markedly inverted and these changes persist
for over several hours, subendocardial infarction without QRS changes
may be present.

## ACUTE PERICARDITIS

At times, the EKG may be helpful in the field to diagnose acute
pericarditis. The earlier this diagnosis is made, the better, since cardiac
tamponade can occur at anytime. If it should happen, the receiving
hospital could be prepared for such an emergency before the arrival
of the patient.

The hallmark of EKG changes in pericarditis is the elevation of
the RST segment (Figure 11-8). This may be seen in Lead II. Initially,
the T wave may be very tall and upright. RST elevation usually is
most pronounced in those leads with the tallest T waves suggesting
early repolarization as one possible mechanism for RST segment elevation. The T wave rapidly becomes flattened and then inverted as more
of the myocardium becomes involved. RST segments also come down
and become isoelectric.

RST segment elevation in acute pericarditis, whether it be due to
viral infection, purulent infection, free blood in the pericardium, or
trauma, is due to the current of injury in the epicardium. The negativity
artificially lowers the isoelectric point on the surface electrocardiogram.
After depolarization, the stylus returns to the true isoelectric point,
which would be seen on the EKG as an elevated RST segment.

With acute pericardial effusion, the only changes seen may be
markedly diminished voltage of the QRS and T complexes in all three
limb leads.

The EKG changes found in acute pulmonary embolism are nonspecific and unreliable as far as helping in the diagnosis, but if a pulmonary embolus is strongly suspected, the EKG changes may be confirmatory.

A deep S wave in I and a Q wave in III ($S_I Q_{III}$) associated with a depressed RST and upright T in I and elevated RST and inverted T in III are considered to indicate sudden right ventricular pressure overload associated with acute cor pulmonale. The Q wave in III suggests inferior wall infarction, but the absence of Q in II and $aV_F$ favor right ventricular overload.

Precordial leads on the right side ($V_{4R}$ to $V_3$) may show conduction aberrations such as incomplete or complete right bundle branch block or elevated RST segments and inverted Ts without conduction aberrations. Supraventricular tachydysrhythmias are reasonably common in acute pulmonary embolism. Secondary ventricular fibrillation and brady-asystolic cardiac arrest may supervene if shock and/or hypoxia are present.

## ACUTE METABOLIC AND ELECTROLYTE DISTURBANCES AND MEDICATION CHANGES

1. Myxedema coma due to thyroid hormone deficiency usually develops gradually so that patients are brought into hospitals in ample time, but an early field diagnosis may insure an immediate evaluation and treatment. Complications such as circulatory collapse and sinus arrest could thus be avoided. These patients will have dry scaly skin, puffy eyelids, and a low pitched crackling voice. From the electrocardiographic standpoint, the findings are nonspecific. There is generalized flattening of the T waves with a decreased amplitude of the QRS waves. Sinus bradycardia is also often noted.

2. Hypokalemia may be the determinant factor in circulatory collapse as well as the cause for tachydysrhythmias, especially in patients receiving digitalis preparations. Typically, U waves develop immediately following the T wave. The apparent Q–T interval which incorporates the U wave is therefore prolonged (Figure 11-9). With a further loss of potassium, the Ts flatten out, leaving the U wave as the sole positive wave. The RST segment may also sag downward.

3. Hyperkalemia is an important abnormality which should be recognized in the field. Sudden cardiac arrest can occur with advanced hyperkalemia. Initially, T waves become peaked and tall with a narrow base. (Serum $K^+$ above 6 mEq/l) (Figure 11-9). Next, the P waves become flattened and the QRS may become broadened. With the serum $K^+$ above 9 mEq/l, the Ps drop out; the R wave decreases; and the

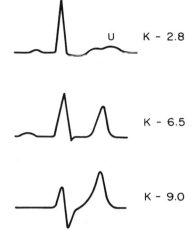

U    K - 2.8

K - 6.5

K - 9.0

**Figure 11-9.** Electrocardiographic changes in hypokalemia and hyperkalemia.

S wave deepens, fusing with the T wave in a sine wave. Asystole or ventricular tachycardia may abruptly terminate life.

4. Hypocalcemia and hypercalcemia affect the length of the RST segment, the former prolonging and the latter shortening the segment. There is no direct effect on the level of the S–T segment or the T wave.

5. Digitalis shortens the Q–T interval, sags the S–T segment, and flattens the T wave.

6. Quinidine toxicity may simulate hypokalemia with flattening of the T waves, development of U waves, prolongation of the true Q–T as well as the apparent Q–T (Q–U) interval and, unlike hypokalemia, eventual widening of the QRS interval.

*Summary*

Since the paramedic often is called upon to help in the diagnosis and management of problems relating to the heart, the use of the electrocardiogram becomes part of his daily routine. A thorough understanding of the electrical system of the heart is therefore useful, so that the electrocardiograph is not a total mystery. This chapter has attempted briefly to present such a background.

*Important
Points to
Remember*

The conduction system of the heart includes the SA (sinoatrial) node, the AV (atrioventricular), the Bundle of His, and the fascicles in the ventricles.

The paramedic in the field usually uses the limb leads of the electrocardiogram. These are usually placed on the upper chest (arm leads) and lower chest (leg leads). Early EKG changes in myocardial infarction include: possibly normal in first hour, slight elevation j point, tall upright T wave, and RST segment curved upward; or development of pathologic Q waves.

Myocardial ischemia usually shows a depressed RST segment and perhaps inverted T waves.

Acute pericarditis shows an elevated RST segment, which may be seen in Lead II.

The electrocardiogram is limited in making the diagnosis of acute cor pulmonale.

Hypokalemia flattens the T waves and elevates the U waves.

Hyperkalemia results in tall, peaked T waves.

*Bibliography*

Goldman, Mervin J. *Principles of Clinical Electrocardiography.* Los Altos, California: Lange Medical Publications, 1970.

Hurst, John W. and Robert J. Myerburg. *Introduction to Electrocardiography.* New York: McGraw-Hill, 1973.

Marriott, Henry J. L. *Practical Electrocardiography.* Baltimore, Md.: Williams and Wilkins, 1977.

# Chapter 12

# DYSRHYTHMIA IDENTIFICATION AND MANAGEMENT IN THE FIELD

There are several reasons for the paramedic and the base hospital personnel monitoring the EKG to establish the precise cardiac rhythm of patients encountered in the field. In the first place, the cardiac rhythm may explain the symptoms for which the distress call was made. Secondly, the dysrhythmia may aid in the diagnosis of an underlying cardiopulmonary disorder. And, most importantly, certain cardiac dysrhythmias that precede cardiac arrest may be recognized and appropriate steps taken to prevent a catastrophic event.

## PRACTICAL POINTS IN IDENTIFICATION OF CARDIAC DYSRHYTHMIA

In order to identify abnormalities of the cardiac rhythm, the paramedic in the field must often rely solely on the oscilloscopic EKG tracings. He will usually not have the luxury of a rhythm strip and calipers to decipher complex dysrhythmias. These are best analyzed at the base hospital through telemetered EKG records. Since time is of the utmost urgency, and since ventricular contractions are crucial, the paramedic should first identify the QRS complexes and determine their rate, character, and regularity. Obviously, rapidly undulating QRS complexes, or markedly retarded or absent QRS beats in an unconscious patient, indicate cardiac arrest and require immediate action. Bizarre QRST complexes with prolonged QRS intervals, whether occurring regularly at a rapid rate (ventricular tachycardia) or intermittently by themselves or in pairs (PVCs), should be identified immediately as prodrome to ventricular fibrillation and appropriate therapy should begin. Marked slowing of QRS beats should also be recognized as potentially dangerous. Frequently used terminology in EKG interpretation is shown in Table 12-1.

After primary ventricular dysrhythmias are ruled out, the P waves should next be identified and their rate, contour, and regularity should

TABLE 12-1.  EKG TERMINOLOGY FREQUENTLY USED IN EMERGENCY MEDICINE

LBBB—Left bundle branch block. Failure of cardiac impulse to descend down the left bundle. Impulse reaches the left ventricle via the right bundle through the interventricular septum.

RBBB—A block through the right bundle.

LAHB—Left anterior hemiblock. The left bundle divides into anterior and posterior fascicles. Anterior fascicle is blocked.

LPHB—Left posterior hemiblock. Posterior fascicle is blocked.

AVB—Atrioventricular block. Failure of impulse to go from atria to ventricles, usually through AV node but may be below AV node.

TFB—Trifascicular block. A block through the right bundle and both left anterior and left posterior fascicles.

BFB—Bifascicular block. A block through two of the three fascicles. (Right bundle is considered as one fascicle.)

Aberrancy—Impulse coming down from the AV node enters the ventricles through an aberrant pathway or at unequal speed through usual pathways, giving rise to QRS patterns that are somewhat bizarre.

AV Dissociation—Atrial and ventricular beats occurring independently without any relationship to each other.

Capture—A supraventricular impulse entering the ventricles and initiating a ventricular beat or a pacer blip initiating a beat. Intermittent capture may occur after a period of AV dissociation.

Accelerated Idiojunctional Rhythm—Rhythm originating in AV junction at rate of 60 to 100 per minute.

Accelerated Idioventricular Rhythm—Rhythm originating in the ventricle at rate of 50 to 100 per minute.

Coupling—An ectopic beat following a normal beat. Coupling interval may be constant or variable.

Brady-tachy Syndrome—Sinus bradycardia alternating intermittently and abruptly with a tachydysrhythmia.

WPW (Wolff–Parkinson–White)—Short PR interval with irregular slurring at onset of QRS wave, which is widened.

SSS—Sick sinus syndrome. Inability of the sinus node to maintain an appropriate sinus rate. Often showing sinus bradycardia, periods of sinus arrest, or supraventricular tachycardia.

FLB (funny looking beats)—Usually premature ventricular beats. May be supraventricular beats with aberrant QRS conduction.

R on T—A premature QRS beat falling on top of T wave from previous beat.

Sawtooth P Waves—Undulating P waves (F, flutter waves) in atrial flutter.

Triphasic QRS—QRS complex that goes above and below base line three times ($rsR^1$ in $V_1$).

High-Grade Second-Degree AVB—2:1 second degree AV block that occasionally shows complete third degree AVB.

be determined. The relationship of P waves to QRS waves should be established. If P waves can be identified one should ask the question, Are the P waves related to the QRS and if so, do they precede or follow the QRS, or do they very subtly distort a segment of the QRS because they are buried in it? Or, are the P waves and QRS unrelated to each other, each going its own merry way? The atrial and ventricular dysrhythmias and time intervals are shown in Table 12-2. Normal and abnormal intervals on the EKG are listed in Table 12-3. For calculation of the heart rate from the EKG strip, see page 680 of the Appendix.

TABLE 12-2.  DYSRHYTHMIA RATES

|  | *Atrial Rate/Minute* | *Ventricular Rate/Minute* |
|---|---|---|
| Sinus Rhythm | 60–100 | 60–100 |
| Sinus Tachycardia | 100–160 | 100–160 |
| Sinus Bradycardia | <60 | <60 |
| Atrial Tachycardia | 150–220 | 150–220 (1:1) |
| Atrial Flutter | 220–350 | 110–175 (2:1) |
| Atrial Fibrillation | 350–600 | 60–180 |
| AV Junctional Rhythm | 40–60 | 40–60 |
| Idioventricular Rhythm | Variable | 20–40 |
| Ventricular Tachycardia | Variable | 110–200 |

TABLE 12-3.  NORMAL AND ABNORMAL INTERVALS

|  | *Seconds* |
|---|---|
| PR Interval | 0.12–0.20 |
| QRS Complex | 0.06–0.10 |
| Aberrancy (QRS) | 0.08–0.14 |
| Incomplete BBB (QRS) | 0.08 through 0.11 |
| Complete BBB (QRS) | 0.12 and greater |
| QT | Depends on heart rate |

### SINUS DYSRHYTHMIAS

Any heart rate over 100 beats per minute may be regarded as a tachycardia. Sinus tachycardia up to 180 beats per minute is possible, but any rate over 140 beats per minute in an adult should be suspect for an ectopic tachycardia (Figure 12-1). At times, the sinus node may be influenced by vagal discharges associated with respiration so that sinus rhythm may slow down during inspiration and speed up during expiration (sinus dysrhythmia). During the slow phase, the pacemaker may shift to the AV junction (shifting pacemaker), so that P waves disappear or become buried in the QRS (Figure 12-2).

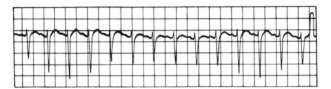

**Figure 12-1.** Sinus tachycardia at 154 per minute.

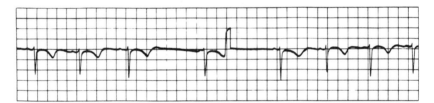

**Figure 12-2.** Sinus dysrhythmia.

### PREMATURE ATRIAL COMPLEXES (PACs)

Premature atrial complexes are frequently seen in normal individuals but they may herald an abrupt onset of atrial tachycardia, atrial flutter, or atrial fibrillation (Figure 12-3). Since PACs originate from an irritable focus remote from the SA node, and the impulse spreads through the atria in an abnormal manner, the configuration of the P wave will be different from the sinus P wave. Usually, the P–R interval will also be slightly shorter. Occasionally, the premature atrial beat will find the AV node refractory so that the P–R interval may be prolonged or even blocked (nonconducted PACs).

At times, conduction through the two ventricles may be partially blocked and unequal resulting in an abnormal QRS configuration (PACs with aberrancy). These complexes are frequently mistaken for premature

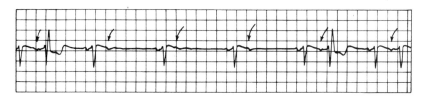

**Figure 12-3.** Premature atrial complexes, several (second to fourth arrows) non-conducted; others (first and fifth arrows) conducted with aberrancy; and one (sixth arrow) conducted normally.

ventricular complexes (PVCs) if the ectopic P waves are overlooked or not recognized (Figure 12-3). PACs will usually reset the SA node so that the compensatory pauses seen with PVCs are not seen with PACs. Occasionally, when PACs occur very early, the SA node may still be refractory to incoming impulses and will maintain its dominant rhythm. In this situation, a compensatory pause will be observed.

Premature beats can also originate from an irritable focus at the junction of the AV node—premature nodal complexes (PNCs). Conduction of the impulse into the ventricles is usually normal but is at times aberrant. Depending on when retrograde conduction into the atria occurs, P waves will appear before, buried in, or after the QRS (Figure 12-4). If retrograde conduction is blocked, no P waves will be found and compensatory pauses should be present.

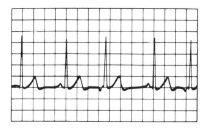

**Figure 12-4.** Premature junctional complexes with early retrograde P waves.

## PAROXYSMAL ATRIAL OR JUNCTIONAL TACHYCARDIA (PAT)

Paroxysmal atrial or junctional tachycardia is a relatively common dysrhythmia and may give rise to symptoms of palpitations in the chest or throat, dizziness, faintness, syncope, shortness of breath, and discomfort or pain in the chest. The onset of palpitations is invariably quite abrupt and the cessation is frequently just as abrupt, much like the faucet being turned on and off. The severity of the symptoms and manifestations will depend on the rate of the tachycardia, the underlying heart disease, and the causal factors for the dysrhythmia. These dysrhythmias may occur without any apparent cause, but are often associated with rheumatic heart disease, hypertensive and arteriosclerotic heart diseases, chronic lung disease, pulmonary embolism, drug overdose (especially tricyclics), and Wolff–Parkinson–White and Lown–Ganong–Levine syndromes. Recently, more and more cases of "sick sinus syndrome" with alternating episodes of sinus bradycardia, atrial tachycardia, and periods of sinus arrest have been recognized. Since atrial and junctional origin of the tachycardia is often difficult to differentiate and since the clinical manifestations, prognosis, and treatment are similar, these two forms of tachycardia are frequently referred to as supraventricular tachycardia (SVT). The ventricular rate may vary from 140 to 250 beats per minute in these conditions.

The mechanism by which these dysrhythmias occur can be explained by a circus movement in and around the SA or the AV nodes (reciprocating or reentry tachycardia) or by an ectopic focus discharging an impulse repetitively.

Electrocardiographically, atrial tachycardia can be definitively diagnosed if abnormal P waves are identified preceding each QRS by an appropriate interval (Figure 12-5). In junctional tachycardia, P waves are usually absent or buried in the QRS and not visible (Figure 12-6). The greatest difficulty occurs when conduction through the ventricles becomes aberrant. In this situation, differentiation from ventricular tachycardia becomes a challenge to all personnel involved in the case. If atrial P waves are found dissociated with the QRS waves, or if fusion beats between normally conducted QRS and ectopic QRS are found, ventricular tachycardia should be diagnosed. If the QRS complexes show a typical triphasic right bundle branch block (RBBB) pattern, SVT with aberrancy should be diagnosed. Carotid sinus massage may establish the diagnosis if the tachycardia could be stopped even for a brief moment.

The necessity for the emergency treatment of paroxysmal supraventricular tachycardia will depend on the severity of the symptoms manifested by the patient. Carotid sinus stimulation (CSS) is not without risk but should be attempted if patients are hypotensive, obviously

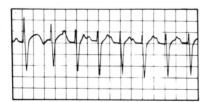

**Figure 12-5.** Paroxysmal atrial tachycardia initiated by the second complex.

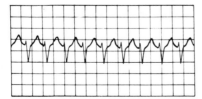

**Figure 12-6.** Junctional or supraventricular tachycardia at 166 per minute.

dyspneic, or mentally clouded. CSS should not be used in patients over 72 years of age or in patients with a carotid bruit. Some patients are extremely sensitive to CSS and it is recommended that the procedure be conducted in three separate steps:

1. Simple location of the carotid artery by palpation of the area between the angle of the jaw and the thyroid cartilage anterior to the sternocleidomastoid muscle.

2. A firm one-second posterior pressure of the carotid sinus against the transverse process of the sixth cervical (C6) vertebra.

3. A firm five-second massage of the carotid sinus. (The EKG monitor should be watched closely during the procedure to avoid prolonged asystole or PVCs.)

The Valsalva maneuver (forced expiration against a closed glottis) can be tried if the patient is able to cooperate. Eyeball pressure is not recommended. Immersion of the face in a pan of ice water while holding the breath has been known to convert PAT when other measures have failed but, here again, the patient must be able to cooperate.

When these measures fail and there is still a need to attempt conversion, parenteral drugs can be used. The number of drugs carried by the paramedics vary from one locale to another, and is determined by the extent of the teaching and training programs extended to the paramedics and by the risk and complications which might be encountered by the use of these drugs in the field. It is best to avoid treatment that might change a tolerable rhythm into an intolerable life-threatening rhythm.

In most cases, mild sedation with intravenous diazepam (Valium®) (5 mg) may be sufficient to control the situation in order to transport the patient to the nearest facility. Morphine in small doses can also be used. Hypotension can be treated with dopamine. Hypertension can be treated with propranolol (Inderal®), 1 to 2 mg IV slowly.

## PAROXYSMAL ATRIAL TACHYCARDIA WITH A 2:1 AV BLOCK

Paroxysmal atrial tachycardia with a 2:1 AV block is usually not an emergency since the ventricular rate is slow and well tolerated (Figure 12-7). The circus movement which propagates this tachycardia may occur

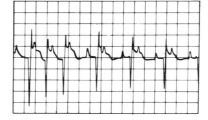

**Figure 12-7.** Paroxysmal atrial tachycardia with 2:1 AV block (last four complexes).

in and around the SA node to explain the fact that P waves appear near normal and that conduction through the AV node is intermittently blocked. The only way PAT with block can occur in and around the AV node would be to interpose a block below the AV node, perhaps in the His bundle. In this situation, the P waves will be negative in Leads II and III. Immediate treatment is not necessary, but the dysrhythmia should be recognized because over half of these cases are due to digitalis toxicity.

## ATRIAL FLUTTER

Atrial flutter is often an exciting dysrhythmia with variable clinical manifestations. Symptomatology of atrial flutter will depend on the underlying heart disease, the condition that precipitated the dysrhythmia, and the ventricular rate determined by the degree of AV conduction. Shortness of breath, chest pains, faintness, and even syncope may occur with atrial flutter, resulting in a rapid ventricular rate.

Although atrial flutter may occur in normal hearts, usually there is underlying pulmonary or cardiac disease. Atrial flutter may follow an acute pulmonary embolus or acute respiratory failure. It is very rarely due to digitoxicity. Bedside diagnosis of this condition is possible when rapid flutter waves are seen in the neck veins.

Atrial flutter is most probably caused by a circus movement of electrical activity within the atria. Electrical impulses are presumably spun off with each revolution in a consistent manner and pathway through the two atria. The P waves, therefore, have a uniform undulating saw-tooth pattern without any isoelectric (inactive) interval (Figure 12-18). This pattern should be seen in at least one EKG lead to distinguish it from atrial tachycardia. The rate of these flutter waves is also faster, ranging from 250 to 350 beats per minute.

Atrial depolarization can occur without a staged ventricular response. If the ratio is two atrial depolarizations to one ventricular, this will give rise to atrial flutter with a 2:1 AV conduction. A 2:1 atrial flutter is frequently overlooked because the nonconducting atrial P wave is invariably buried in the QRS. Any regular tachycardia with a rate around 140 should always be suspected as being due to atrial flutter with 2:1 AV conduction. In these situations, rapid flutter waves may be visible in the neck vein; or carotid sinus stimulation may transiently decrease AV conduction so that flutter P waves are easily seen on

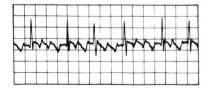

**Figure 12-8.** Atrial flutter with variable ventricular response with atrial rate of 330 per minute.

the EKG; or different EKG leads, especially the $V_1$ lead, may reveal a distorted QRS due to superimposed Ps.

A 4:1 AV conduction is not uncommon but a sustained 3:1 AV conduction is very unusual. Occasionally, AV conduction is variable so that an irregular rhythm resembling atrial fibrillation is produced (Figure 12-8). The term degree of AV conduction is preferred over degree of AV block since the AV node is not organically diseased and blocked, but functionally unable to handle the traffic coming to it. A 1:1 AV conduction, a rare occurrence, with ventricular rates over 200 per minute may result in a state of circulatory standstill. In some cases, however, pulsus alternans (ventricles eject completely on alternate beats) occurs allowing time for ventricular filling and greater cardiac output. Borderline perfusion is maintained despite an electrocardiographic rate of over 200 per minute.

Emergency field treatment of atrial flutter with a 3:1 or 4:1 AV conduction is not required. With a 2:1 conduction, the patient may be on the verge of pulmonary edema or in shock. Immediate treatment is recommended if transport is delayed. In the field, digoxin 0.5 mg/IV to undigitalized and 0.25 mg to digitalized patients given over 1 minute, followed by propranolol 0.5 to 1.0 mg IV is recommended. This decreases AV conduction so that the ventricular rate is slowed. When a patient has a 1:1 atrial flutter with circulatory arrest (no palpable pulse or blood pressure), use of an immediate 100 watt-seconds defibrillation is justified (Chapter 13). In the field the defibrillation may not be synchronized, and it may be necessary to countershock with 400 watt-seconds if ventricular fibrillation follows the initial shock. The patient who is cardioverted and/or defibrillated should receive 0.5 mg digoxin and 1.0 mg propranolol IV before transport to the receiving hospital.

## ATRIAL FIBRILLATION

Atrial fibrillation is one of the most common dysrhythmias seen in the field. It is usually a manifestation of underlying heart disease with atrial enlargement, but it can occur with metabolic (hyperthyroidism) or toxic (alcohol) disorders without apparent cardiac enlargement. The exact mechanism by which atrial fibrillation occurs is disputed, but it is believed that a series of waves are produced by several irritable ectopic foci in the atria. One can also look at the atrium as being activated by a series of chaotic circus movements spewing off impulses irregularly into various sections of the atria.

In the field, atrial fibrillation has its greatest significance from its association with acute cardiac and respiratory failure. Cardiac output is decreased by about 25 percent when atrial fibrillation supplants sinus rhythm. It may also be an important finding in someone who had just sustained a cerebrovascular accident (CVA). Rheumatic mitral stenosis with a recent onset of atrial fibrillation may manifest itself as acute

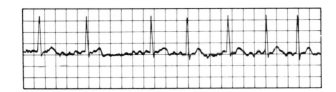

**Figure 12-9.** Atrial fibrillation with a ventricular response of 60–70/minute.

pulmonary congestion, hemoptysis, and pulmonary edema, or as an acute embolic complication to the brain with a sudden CVA.

Electrocardiographic recognition is relatively easy. The occurrence of the ventricular QRS complexes is grossly irregular, and distinct P waves are absent (Figure 12-9). Undulating irregular fibrillatory waves with variable contour and frequency can usually be found in lead $V_2$. The ventricular response in atrial fibrillation is variable, being as slow as 60 beats per minute, to as fast as 180 beats per minute. In the presence of AV nodal disease, the ventricular rate may be as slow as 40 or 50 per minute (Figure 12-10). In the Wolff-Parkinson-White syndrome, (Figure 12-11) the AV node is bypassed and the ventricular rate may be so rapid that circulatory arrest exists.

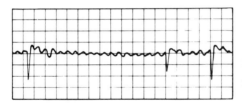

**Figure 12-10.** Atrial fibrillation with slow ventricular response due to high-grade AV block.

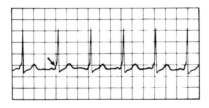

**Figure 12-11.** Wolff–Parkinson–White Syndrome with short P–R interval and "delta" waves.

The field treatment of atrial fibrillation with rapid ventricular rates resulting in acute cardiac failure is largely dependent on digitalization. For this purpose, 0.5 mg digoxin IV over one minute followed by a second dose of 0.25 mg in 15 minutes is recommended. Patients previously on digitalis should be given only a single 0.25 mg IV dose. Other measures to control LV failure, such as IV diuretics, morphine, tourniquets, upright position, and $O_2$ should be instituted (Chapter 10).

## PREMATURE VENTRICULAR COMPLEXES

Perhaps the most important dysrhythmia that should be recognized in the field to prevent further difficulties is the premature ventricular complex (PVC) (Figure 12-12). In the proper clinical setting, PVCs are predictors of ventricular fibrillation in as many as 50 percent of all sudden cardiac deaths. PVCs occur in acute myocardial ischemia or infarction, chronic ischemic heart disease, drug overdose, including digitalis toxicity, the prolonged Q–T interval syndrome, and aortic valve disease. Frequently, PVCs occur in apparently normal hearts. In ischemic or infarcted hearts, PVCs occurring (1) more than five per minute (Figure 12-12), (2) on top of T waves (Figure 12-13), (3) at variable coupling intervals after a regular beat (Figure 12-14), (4) in runs of two or three, and (5) from two or more separate foci (Figure 12-15) are followed by a high incidence of ventricular tachycardia and ventricular fibrillation (Figure 12-16). In other disorders of the heart, PVCs have a lesser degree of prognostic implication, and in normal people, isolated PVCs appear to be quite innocuous although longterm follow up studies tend to indicate a higher incidence of sudden deaths than in the population without PVCs.

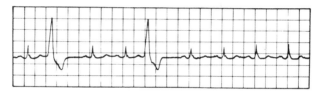

**Figure 12-12.** Premature ventricular contractions showing widened QRS.

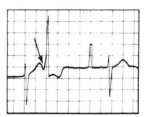

**Figure 12-13.** Premature ventricular complex with R on T (arrow).

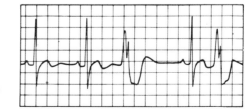

**Figure 12-14.** Premature ventricular complexes with variable coupling intervals.

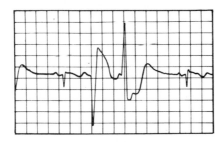

**Figure 12-15.** Two premature ventricular complexes from two different foci.

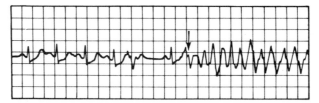

**Figure 12-16.** Premature ventricular complex (second PVC) with R on T initiating ventricular fibrillation.

Electrocardiographic identification of PVCs is usually simple with widened QRS complexes over 0.12 seconds in duration occurring prematurely, not preceded by an ectopic P wave, and followed by a compensatory pause, so that a dominant rhythm is maintained (Figure 12-12). Occasionally, a premature atrial beat is followed by an aberrantly conducted ventricular beat mimicking a PVC. Usually, an ectopic P wave can be identified; the compensatory pause will be absent; and the aberrant conduction may be triphasic like a right bundle branch block (Figure 12-16).

Treatment of PVCs will depend on the clinical setting. Any suspicion of myocardial infarction or ischemia, cardiac failure, respiratory failure, generalized anoxia (asphyxia), cardiac trauma (due to physical, electrical, or chemical injury), digitalis toxicity, drug overdose, or myocarditis should be monitored carefully for PVCs. Should any of the criteria mentioned above be met, a lidocaine IV bolus of 1.0 mg/kgm of body weight followed by an IV infusion of 2 mg per minute should be given. If PVCs cannot be controlled, another bolus can be given in 5 minutes, or the IV infusion can be increased to 4 mg per minute.

In marked sinus or junctional bradycardia (50/min) with PVCs, lidocaine may be dangerous to use because of the possibility of suppression of an escape rhythm in the event of sinus arrest. In this situation, atropine in doses of 0.5 mg IV may be given in an effort to increase the sinus or junctional rate and thereby eliminate the PVCs.

Other drugs are available to control PVCs, but the feasibility of stocking the paramedic units and familiarizing the personnel with their utilization in the field would be difficult and unwarranted. In the case of PVCs due to digitalis toxicity, diphenylhydantoin (Dilantin®) given slowly by the intravenous route (50 to 100 mg over 2 minutes) might be safe and effective.

## VENTRICULAR TACHYCARDIA

Ventricular tachycardia as a prodromal rhythm to ventricular fibrillation has been well established. The ventricular rate is usually anywhere from 120 to 200 beats per minute (Figure 12-17). Hemodynamically, the patient with this rhythm may be well compensated and able to tolerate the tachycardia, but with advanced myocardial or valvular damage, ventricular tachycardia may lead to acute cardiac failure with pulmonary edema or low output shock. Syncopal attacks simulating Stokes-Adams attacks are also common with paroxysmal episodes of ventricular tachycardia.

Ventricular tachycardia is associated with organic heart disease in 90 percent of the cases, and well over 75 percent of these are due to coronary artery disease. Ventricular aneurysms from old myocardial infarctions, acute myocardial infarction or ischemia, aortic stenosis, a prolapsing mitral valve, myocardiopathy, digitalis toxicity, quinidine toxicity, drug overdose, myocardial injury, electrocution, the prolonged Q–T syndrome, and alcohol abuse are some of the underlying causes of ventricular tachycardia. It is suspected that ventricular tachycardia results from a circus movement in the ventricles where asynchronous propagation of electrical impulses is produced by ischemic or injured tissue.

Electrocardiographic confirmation of ventricular tachycardia is not always simple. As mentioned previously, ventricular tachycardia can

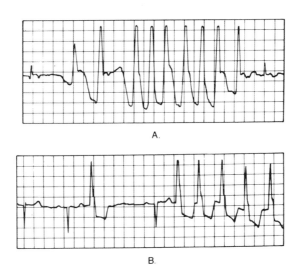

A.

B.

Figure 12-17. (A) Ventricular tachycardia at a rate of 200/minute; (B) ventricular tachycardia at a rate of 125/minute.

be confused with a supraventricular tachycardia with an aberrant ventricular conduction. Atrioventricular dissociation with identifiable P waves running through the tachycardia, fusion beats, captured beats, and PVCs before the onset of tachycardia appearing the same as with tachycardia QRSs all favor ventricular tachycardia. Triphasic QRS complexes (Figure 12-18) and bundle branch block QRS patterns seen before tachycardia and, appearing the same as during tachycardia favor the diagnosis of supraventricular tachycardia with aberration. Accelerated idioventricular rhythm, occasionally up to 110 per minute, should not be confused with paroxysmal ventricular tachycardia even though fusion beats and captured beats are seen. Usually, the higher pacemaker sites are slower than optimal or are arrested.

A witnessed ventricular tachycardia, i.e., ventricular tachycardia beginning while the patient is being attended and monitored electrocardiographically, might be converted with a sharp thump on the chest. This is indicated if the patient is showing signs of inadequate cardiac output (shock) and approaching coma. One must be prepared to defibrillate immediately if a precordial thump fails or if ventricular fibrillation is produced.

If hemodynamic consequences are being tolerated, medical conversion using full doses of lidocaine is advocated in a dose of 1 mg/kg of body weight intravenously followed by a 2 to 4 mg/min IV infusion.

## VENTRICULAR FIBRILLATION

This will be covered in the section on cardiac arrest (Chapter 13).

## BRADYCARDIA AND HEART BLOCK

### ETIOLOGY

Various etiological factors affect the sinus node, giving rise to sinus bradycardia, sinus arrest or block, and the sick sinus syndrome. These factors are as follows:

1. Ischemia due to coronary artery disease or generalized anoxia.
2. Inhibition by reflex vagal effect, blockade of beta-adrenergic fibers (propranolol), depletion of catechols (reserpine), hypothermia, and hypothyroidism.
3. Intoxication by drugs and chemicals such as morphine, heroin, digitalis, quinidine, and fluorinated hydrocarbons.
4. Idiopathic degeneration of the SA node (may be familial).
5. Infarction due to acute coronary artery disease.
6. Inflammation due to acute myocarditis, pericarditis, or myocardiopathy.

7. Invasion by neoplasm and other abnormal cells.

Electrocardiographically, sinus block can be differentiated from sinus arrest when the P-to-P interval during the block is two or three times the P-to-P interval during regular sinus rhythm. The assumption is made that an impulse had originated, but was blocked from emerging out of the SA node. A 2:1 sinus block may be mistaken for simple sinus bradycardia. Probably, the most common cause of sinus pauses is neither sinus block nor sinus arrest, but an unrecognized premature atrial beat without AV conduction (nonconducting PACs). During prolonged periods of sinus arrest or sinus block, regular sinus P waves disappear and escape junctional beats with normal QRS and with or without retrograde Ps (inverted in II) are shown in Figure 12-19. Very frequently, in marked sinus bradycardia, a junctional escape beat may occur immediately after a normally inscribed P wave. In these cases, the P-R interval will be abnormally shortened. Occasionally, regular P waves cannot readily be identified leading to the mistaken diagnosis of sinus arrest when in reality there is sinus bradycardia or AV block. Different EKG leads may clarify these rhythms.

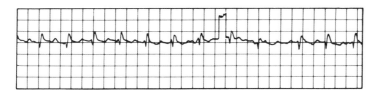

**Figure 12-18.** Flutter waves are revealed after the ninth ventricular complex when 2:1 AV conduction momentarily changes to 3:1 conduction. Note also aberrant triphasic QRS complexes.

## SINUS BRADYCARDIA

Sinus bradycardia refers to a heart beat that originates from the SA node at a rate of less than 60 per minute. In extreme cases, sinus bradycardia may fall below 40 per minute and give rise to dizziness and syncope, although in well-trained athletes, resting rates of 40 per minute are not unusual.

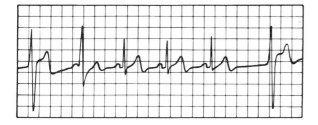

**Figure 12-19.** Sinus pause or arrest with junctional or ventricular escape beat.

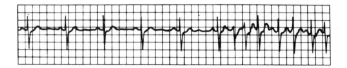

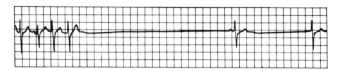

**Figure 12-20.** Sick sinus syndrome with sinus arrest and sinus bradycardia following cessation of atrial fibrillation.

## SICK SINUS SYNDROME

Recently, more patients are being identified as having sick sinus syndrome. These patients may manifest the following: (1) inappropriate sinus bradycardia in which the sinus rate fails to increase appropriately to exercise and other demands placed on the circulation; (2) periods of atrial tachycardia, flutter, or fibrillation interspersed with sinus bradycardia (Figure 12-20); (3) variable periods of sinus arrest, often times following the cessation of tachycardia; and (4) AV junctional escape rhythm usurping the pacemaking function of the SA node.

*Treatment of Bradycardia Syndromes.* The treatment of sinus bradycardia syndromes will depend on whether the symptoms occurred before or after the arrival of the paramedics. Extreme bradycardia with a rate below 45/minute should be treated with at least one dose of 0.5 mg atropine IV regardless of the symptoms. The management of sinus bradycardia in acute myocardial infarction or ischemia has already been discussed in Chapter 10. The same indication and dose schedule for atropine can be applied to other cardiovascular insults resulting in sinus bradycardia and hypotension. Sinus bradycardia with PVCs should be treated if possible only with atropine. Attempts to eliminate the PVCs with lidocaine is attended with some risk, since escape centers may be further depressed. Attempts to speed up the SA node with isoproterenol may induce ventricular tachycardia and ventricular fibrillation. Epinephrine will have the same effect. Morphine frequently will precipitate marked bradycardia and hypotension, but these changes will usually respond to atropine.

In the event that sinus bradycardia is severe and nonresponsive to atropine, an isoproterenol infusion should be started with careful monitoring of the BP, heart rate, and the EKG. A slow IV infusion 1 to 2 μg/min, bringing the pulse rate up only to 60 per minute and raising the BP only up to 100 mm Hg systolic, is recommended. In acute myocardial infarction, it is realized that isoproterenol might increase infarct size, but the possibility of sinus bradycardia progressing to sinus arrest is so ominous that careful use of this drug is recommended in these situations.

Transient sinus pauses and sinus block may also respond to atropine, but if syncope or severe dizziness had been the presenting symptom, isoproterenol IV, 1 mg in 250 ml $D_5W$ should also be piggybacked on an IV infusion and be readied for immediate use. Sinus arrest with good strong accelerated junctional escape rhythm over 60 per minute need not be treated, but an IV line should be established. If the junctional escape rhythm is slow, atropine and isoproterenol should be given.

Prolonged sinus arrest or severe sinus bradycardia with very slow escape or no escape rhythm constitute a state of brady-asystolic cardiac arrest and will be discussed in Chapter 13.

## ATRIOVENTRICULAR BLOCK

Atrioventricular block (AV block) may take place at several locations in the conduction system between the atria and the ventricles: (1) AV nodal block, (2) His bundle block, and (3) trifascicular block. Etiologically, the same factors which cause sinus node dysfunction may also affect the AV node. Parasympathetic vagal action may extend into the His bundle area, but it is doubtful that it extends beyond into the ventricles. Atropine, therefore, may be effective in AV nodal and possibly His bundle block; but most probably will not be helpful in trifascicular blocks.

*First Degree A V Block.* First degree AV block with minimal prolongation of the P–R interval may be due to slowing of the conduction through the His bundle or the fascicles as well as through the AV node. With marked prolongation of the P–R interval, the block is usually through the AV node only (Figure 12-21).

Usually, simple prolongation of the P–R interval requires no treatment, but if severe dizziness or syncope had been the presenting symptom, or if the P–R interval is over 0.28 sec, an IV line should be established immediately and both atropine and isoproterenol be kept in readiness. At times, the P–R prolongation is associated with a rapid sinus tachycardia. In this situation, both atropine and isoproterenol should be withheld until high grade second or third degree AV block supervene.

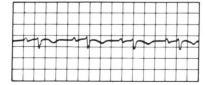

**Figure 12-21.** First degree AV block. P–R interval of 0.22 seconds.

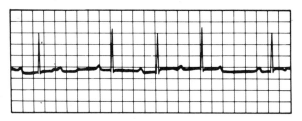

**Figure 12-22.** Second degree AV block, Type I (Wenckebach's Disease).

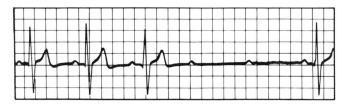

**Figure 12-23.** Second degree AV block, Type II.

*Second Degree A V Block.* Second degree AV block refers to intermittently complete AV block when no QRS response follows the usually occurring P wave. There are two distinct types of second degree AV block. Type I block or the Wenckebach phenomenon is present when P–R intervals progressively lengthen before a complete block takes place. In the Type II block, P–R intervals remain the (Figure 12-22) same before a complete block occurs (Figure 12-23). A common error made even by experts in this field is to call a 2:1 AV block a Type II block. There is no way one can determine a 2:1 block as being Type I or Type II, since there is only one P–R interval to analyze before the next dropped beat. It is most probable that a Type II block is infranodal, and if the QRS complex of the conducted beats is irregular and broad, the block is probably below the His bundle in the fascicles. It is, however, possible to have a conduction aberration such as right bundle branch block and still have an AV nodal block.

A high grade second degree AV block should be recognized since the ventricular rate may be so slow that an aggressive form of treatment will be indicated. Here a partial second degree AV block is interspersed with periods of complete third degree block and junctional escape beats. In overdigitalized patients with atrial fibrillation, a high grade second degree AV block is not an uncommon finding. All atrial fibrillation should be considered to have a partial functional block. When a high grade block occurs, the ventricular response decreases markedly and a good percentage of the longer QRS intervals will be constant in time, due to a complete block and escaped junctional beats.

*Third Degree A V Block (Complete A V Block).* Most forms of third degree AV block are nodal in type and, as such, the escape beat originates

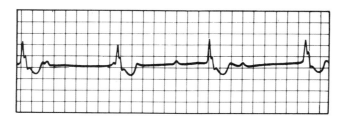

**Figure 12-24.** Complete AV block, probably infranodal with slow ventricular escape beats at 34 per minute.

from tissues adjacent to or just below the AV node. The QRS complexes are, therefore, narrow and normally conducted through the ventricles. The escape rate is also variable around 40 to 60 per minute and influenced by vagolytic drugs such as atropine.

Third degree AV block is usually not permanent except when due to idiopathic degeneration of the AV node, invasion of the node, or actual infarction of the node. Complete AV block is often associated with acute inferior myocardial infarction. The block is transient in 85 percent of the patients who usually develop normal sinus rhythm in one week.

Infranodal AV blocks are usually more permanent and associated with more severe myocardial damage. They also escape more slowly at a rate of about 30 to 40 per minute and are not influenced by atropine (Figure 12-24). The cause of infranodal trifascicular block in many cases is unknown, but extensive fibrosis of the crux of the heart (Lev's disease) is often found at autopsy. Acute anterior wall infarction occasionally causes this type of block.

Prior to the development of complete trifascicular AV block, the electrocardiogram may give evidence of bifascicular block, with the entire heart being activated through the last remaining fascicle. Complete right bundle branch block (RBBB) and left anterior fascicle block is the most common form of bifascicular block. A left anterior fascicular block can be identified on the EKG as marked left axis deviation, with the widened QRS in Lead I predominantly upright, and in Leads II and III predominantly negative. RBBB is recognized by a widened QRS of 0.12 seconds with delayed secondary R' in Lead $V_1$ and $V_2$. The P–R interval may be normal or slightly prolonged, suggesting a delayed conduction through the last fascicle. A Type II second degree AV block may also be noted. A His bundle analysis performed in the hospital will confirm the diagnosis. It is suggested that whenever the single Lead II monitor routinely used in the field reveals a sinus rhythm with widened QRS waves over 0.11 seconds in duration, the possibility of a bifascicular block should be considered.

Usually, atropine will not improve the rate of idioventricular bradycardia in trifascicular block, but it should be given since the block may still be at the AV nodal area. An isoproterenol infusion at 1 to

2 μg/minute should be started if the ventricular rate remains below 44 per minute, or if hypotension is present at a rate below 50 per minute. Any patient experiencing extreme dizziness or syncopal attacks and manifesting bifascicular block should be monitored continuously, and isoproterenol infusion piggybacked on the IV line for immediate use if necessary. The receiving hospital should be alerted and the patient transported as quickly as possible.

A complete AV block with an extremely slow escape or no escape rhythm is a rare cause (10 percent) of sudden cardiac arrest in the field. Emergency treatment for this type of cardiac arrest will be discussed in Chapter 13.

## PACEMAKER FAILURE

More and more patients are given a new lease on life with permanently implanted pacemakers. In spite of sophisticated remote monitoring systems to detect impending pacemaker failures, sudden dislodgement or fracture of electrodes or sudden malfunction of the generator still occur frequently enough to warrant some discussion (Figure 12-25).

Most pacemakers now being implanted are of the "demand" mode. That is to say, the pacemaker is able to sense the patient's own QRS impulse and fire on demand, only after a preset interval of time (usually about 0.8 seconds). Because of this sensing mechanism, these pacemakers may shut off temporarily when they are brought too close to microwave ovens, electric shavers, electric motors, etc. Failure to sense the patient's own QRS on the other hand may result in discharge of an impulse on the vulnerable T wave, with a subsequent ventricular tachycardia. Of equal importance is the possibility that failure to sense may also be associated with failure of the pacemaker to initiate a heart beat. The mere presence of pacemaker blips on the EKG does not guarantee captured heart beats (Figure 12-26). Normally paced beats should reveal blips followed by QRS and T waves.

As the batteries become exhausted, most pacemakers begin to slow down their rate of discharge. A demand mode pacemaker whose rate of discharge has fallen to 64 or 68 per minute from its originally set rate of 72 per minute may begin to behave erratically and cause symptoms of dizziness and syncope or even sudden cardiac arrest. Mercury batteries will have about three to four years of life, whereas the new lithium

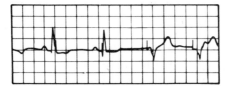

**Figure 12-25.** Two normal beats and two artificially paced beats.

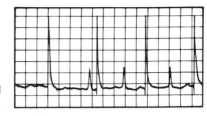

**Figure 12-26.** Pacer blips not pacing and not sensing patient's own QRS complexes.

batteries may have over seven years of life. Runaway pacemakers, due to battery depletion, are no longer seen; but rapid rates due to malfunction of pacemaker circuitry are still occasionally seen.

There are two general ways in which these permanent pacemakers are implanted. The most common type is the endocardial pacer in which either a bipolar or a unipolar catheter electrode is placed near the apex within the right ventricle. The catheter is introduced into the cephalic or the external jugular vein and the battery pulse generator attached to the proximal end of the electrode is implanted subcutaneously in the upper chest wall. The second type gaining prominence is the epicardial electrode which is twisted into the wall of the right ventricle through a surgical dissection of the subxiphoid area. The pulse generator is then implanted subcutaneously in the upper abdominal wall.

*Summary*

The paramedic and base hospital personnel must be able to establish the precise cardiac rhythm of patients encountered in the field. The precise diagnosis of certain disorders, the prediction of cardiac arrest, and the prevention of cardiac catastrophes can all be accomplished through the knowledge of proper diagnosis and treatment of cardiac dysrhythmias. This chapter covers atrial and ventricular dysrhythmias (except for ventricular fibrillation, which is presented in Chapter 13), bradycardias, heart block, and pacemaker failure. The physiology, clinical picture, and therapy of these conditions will become an important part of the EMT-Paramedic's knowledge and as such will be used on a frequent basis. Constant review and updating of this particular material is suggested.

*Important Points to Remember*

Atrial dysrhythmias include:
1. Sinus dysrhythmias
   a. Sinus tachycardia (over 140/min)
   b. Normal sinus dysrhythmia (with respiration)
2. Premature atrial complexes (PAC)
3. Paroxysmal atrial or junctional tachycardia (supraventricular tachycardias) (PAT)

(Supraventricular tachycardias—SVT—are common and may occur without any previous cause, but are often associated with rheumatic, hypertensive or arteriosclerotic heart disease and pulmonary disease. Supraventricular tachycardia is diagnosed if abnormal P waves are not identified preceding each EKG by an appropriate interval.)

4. Paroxysmal atrial tachycardia with a 2:1 block

5. Atrial flutter

6. Atrial fibrillation

Atrial fibrillation is commonly seen in the field. It is seen with underlying heart disease and metabolic or toxic disorders (thyroid, alcohol). EKG recognition of atrial fibrillation includes irregular R–R intervals and the absence of distinct P waves.

Ventricular dysrhythmias include:

1. Premature ventricular complexes (PVC). (These are the most important dysrhythmias to recognize because they are predictors of ventricular fibrillation.)

EKG recognition includes widened QRS (over 0.12 seconds), occurring prematurely, not preceded by an ectopic P wave, and followed by a compensatory pause.

Lidocaine is the drug of choice for PVCs except with sinus bradycardia where atropine is used.

2. Ventricular tachycardia (ventricular tachycardia often preceeds fibrillation and is associated with organic heart disease in 90 percent of cases).

3. Ventricular fibrillation (to be more thoroughly covered later).

Bradycardia and heart block include:

1. Sinus bradycardia: Sinus bradycardia refers to a heart beat from the SA node of less than 60/minute. Treatment of bradycardia below 50/minute with atropine is often indicated.

2. Sick sinus syndrome

3. Atrioventricular block (AV block)

There are many points to remember concerning complete and partial heart blocks (first degree, second degree, third degree, complete). The reader should consult the text for specifics.

*Bibliography*   Cosby, Richard S. and Michael Bilitch. *Heart Block.* New York: McGraw-Hill, 1972.

Dreifus, Leonard S. and William Fikoff. *Cardiac Arrhythmias.* New York: Grune and Stratton, 1973.

Dubin, D. *Rapid Interpretation of EKGs.* Third Ed. Tampa, Fla.: Culver Publishing Co., 1977

Krikler, Dennis M. and J. F. Goodwin. *Cardiac Arrhythmias.* London: W. B. Saunders Co. Ltd., 1975.

Phillips, Raymond E. and Mary K. Feeney. *The Cardiac Rhythms.* Philadelphia, Pa.: W. B. Saunders Co., 1973.

# Chapter 13

# CARDIOPULMONARY RESUSCITATION

Each year in the United States approximately 700,000 people die from the consequences of coronary artery disease, and more than half (350,000) die within the first two hours before arriving at a hospital. Since most of these patients die from acute dysrhythmias, resuscitation with basic and advanced cardiac life support may result in the recovery and return of the individuals as useful members of society. The fact that people have been salvaged after a full cardiac arrest in the field has been documented repeatedly. The conference on Cardiopulmonary Resuscitation (CPR) and Emergency Cardiac Care (ECC), cosponsored by the American Heart Association and the National Academy of Sciences—National Research Council held in Washington in May of 1973, developed and published a set of standards for CPR and ECC. Reference to these articles should be made by anyone who is learning CPR and who may use it in the field, emergency department, or hospital.

## THE MOBILE INTENSIVE CARE UNIT

The concept of the mobile intensive care unit (MICU) evolved from four observations related primarily to cardiac death. The first of these was the discovery that life could be maintained for a reasonable time after cessation of the heartbeat by closed-chest cardiac massage. The second was the discovery that electrical countershock applied across the chest could defibrillate a fibrillating heart. The third observation was that coronary care units in the hospital could not only successfully resuscitate patients who develop cardiac arrest, but that they could also monitor patients and prevent cardiac arrest from taking place. The fourth observation was that more patients were dying suddenly from heart disease outside the hospital than were dying in the hospital. In 1967, Pantridge, a Belfast, Ireland physician, initiated the first ambulance system capable of resuscitating patients who had collapsed from cardiac arrest. As a result of Pantridge's observations, various adaptations of the mobile intensive care unit concept developed rapidly throughout this country. Use was made of existing fire and rescue units and professional and paraprofessional personnel, as well as hospitals that served not only as base stations, but also as training centers for the MICU nurses and paramedics.

It was obvious from the standpoint of resuscitating cardiac arrest cases that the response time of the initial rescue squad had to be less than five minutes. In certain communities this was readily accomplished by having the Fire Station rescue squad trained in basic cardiopulmonary resuscitation (CPR). Since these people were stationed widely throughout the community, they could respond to emergency calls within three minutes. The mobile intensive care (paramedic) units stationed less widely throughout the county could then be dispatched simultaneously from another station slightly farther away and be able to respond to a call within six minutes.

## CAUSES OF CARDIAC ARREST

It has been shown by many studies that about 70 to 80 percent of sudden deaths that occur outside the hospital are due to coronary artery disease and about 20 to 30 percent are due to noncoronary artery disease. In the noncoronary artery disease category, cardiac arrest and sudden death may be secondary to obvious causes such as drug or chemical toxicity, asphyxiation, trauma, electrocution, anaphylaxis, hemorrhage, heroin overdose, and pacemaker failure. Less obvious causes are pulmonary embolism, myocardiopathy, myocarditis, valvular heart disease, pulmonary insufficiency, sick sinus syndrome, fibrosis of the AV conduction system, cerebral hemorrhage, meningitis, ruptured abdominal aortic aneurysm, and internal hemorrhage. In the past, the reasons for cardiac arrest outside of the hospital often remained obscure. Now, however, with trained paramedics responding to calls and making searching inquiries at the scene, the causes of cardiac arrest are better understood.

In people who have died suddenly as a result of coronary artery disease, post mortem studies have shown that in a majority of cases, the three major coronary vessels are diseased and significantly narrowed by more than 75 percent of the cross-sectional area. Only about one-fourth of the cases show a significant single vessel disease. A fresh thrombus (clot) is found in less than one-third of the patients. Similar observations have been made using angiography in patients who have been successfully resuscitated from ventricular fibrillation. Although left main coronary artery lesions are known to be associated with a high incidence of sudden death, autopsy series fail to show this as a common cause of sudden death outside of the hospital.

There are three different, but interrelated mechanisms by which sudden cardiac arrest can occur:

Ventricular Fibrillation
Brady-asystole
Electromechanical Dissociation

All three mechanisms may be operative in a single case, and at times it may be difficult to ascertain which mechanism occurred initially.

The most common mechanism for sudden cardiac arrest is ventricular fibrillation. This fatal dysrhythmia was seen as the initial cause of circulatory failure in 75 percent of the cases seen within 10 minutes after their collapse. Severe bradycardia or ventricular asystole (brady-asystole) was seen in 25 percent of the cases. The third type, electromechanical dissociation (profound cardiovascular collapse with normal electrical activity and an absent pulse and blood pressure) is difficult to identify as the mechanism for cardiac arrest, although some patients with severe bradycardia could be categorized in this group.

## VENTRICULAR FIBRILLATION

In ventricular fibrillation, the electrical activity of the ventricles is chaotic with multiple undulating waves of irregular circuits resulting in a nonejecting wiggling motion of the ventricles (Figure 13-1). It has been generally accepted that the impulse that initiates this dysrhythmia is a premature ventricular contraction (PVC) from an ectopic focus. Such a beat apparently finds a segment of the myocardium resistant to a normal antegrade flow of electrical current, although retrograde flow is preserved. A circuit is thus established for reentry of the impulse and for ventricular tachycardia. As more and more circuits are formed, the ventricle begins to fibrillate. Certain features of the premature ventricular contraction seem to presage the development of ventricular tachycardia and ventricular fibrillation. (These have been discussed in Chapters 11 and 12.) Although premature ventricular contractions serve as a warning for the development of ventricular fibrillation, many patients have no such warnings. In the field, the initial PVC may be all that is needed to trigger ventricular tachycardia and ventricular fibrillation (Figure 13-1).

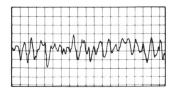

**Figure 13-1.** In ventricular fibrillation there is no organized conducted electrical activity. The heart does not eject blood.

Ventricular Fibrillation (Coarse)

In those cases of ventricular fibrillation occurring after the arrival of the paramedics, sinus tachycardia and supraventricular tachycardia appeared to herald the onset of ventricular fibrillation in over half the cases. Sinus bradycardia was present in about 15 percent of the cases and PVCs in 15 percent of the cases before the onset of ventricular fibrillation.

## BRADY-ASYSTOLIC CARDIAC ARREST

This is a form of arrest in which there is an inadequate circulation of blood due to extremely slow and ineffective cardiac contraction, or to no contraction at all. Close examination of the cardiac rhythm in these cases reveals that in over 90 percent of the time sinus node activity is completely arrested or extremely depressed, and in only 5 or 10 percent of the cases AV conduction is blocked (Chapter 12). The escape mechanism of the AV junctional tissue is also severely depressed or nonfunctioning in these cases, as evidenced by an extremely slow or absent escape rhythm. Even with resuscitative efforts, including the use of atropine and epinephrine, the sinus activity fails to respond in over 90 percent of the cases. About one-third of these patients develop ventricular fibrillation. It is common for these patients to go from brady-asystole to ventricular fibrillation, then back to brady-asystole again after each countershock.

## ELECTROMECHANICAL DISSOCIATION

The heart can continue to beat after myocardial infarction, but not eject enough blood to allow for adequate circulation to the brain or other tissues. Although a normal sinus rhythm may be seen on the monitor, the patient does not have a palpable peripheral pulse or an identifiable blood pressure. Thus he is, in effect, in circulatory collapse and needs immediate assistance. This type of arrest can be considered to be the same as severe cardiogenic shock. Naturally, if these events continue, the heart may develop bradycardia, asystole, or fibrillation. The exact incidence of this condition is not known since it has not always been possible to place monitors on patients in cardiac arrest and determine their basic rhythm. By the time such a patient has been seen and transported to a hospital, electrocardiographic changes have occurred. Treatment in these cases involves immediate transport to the hospital and the use of cardiac stimulants such as dopamine, calcium, or epinephrine.

# BASIC CARDIOPULMONARY RESUSCITATION

Basic CPR can be performed by any adult or youth. In communities where the response time of the initial rescue squad is over six minutes, resuscitation of individuals collapsing with cardiac arrest would not be feasible unless CPR could be initiated by someone before that time. The latest campaign by the American Heart Association to teach the lay public basic CPR is definitely a step in the right direction. Recent studies have shown the efficacy of this approach based on the increased quality and quantity of the surviving patients who had a cardiac arrest outside of the hospital. Of course, if CPR is to be done by anyone, it would be essential that the initial CPR be performed correctly in order for the subsequent efforts by the paramedic units to be successful. If CPR is performed incorrectly, eventual resuscitation may fail, or if heart resuscitation succeeds, a totally inadequate personality may result in all sorts of social, economic, and medical consequences.

The ABCs of basic CPR consist of:

1. Airway
2. Breathing
3. Circulation

## AIRWAY

If the person has collapsed, determine if he is conscious by shaking his shoulder and shouting, "Are you all right?" If he does not respond, the paramedic must open his airway. First, be certain he is lying flat on his back, and if he must be rolled over, do this so his body moves as a single unit.

In an unconscious patient lying supine on his back, the tongue falls back on the posterior pharynx and obstructs the airway. To open the airway, lift up the neck with one hand while pushing down on the forehead with the other to tilt the head back (Chapter 9). This will hyperextend the neck and open the airway. Next, place your ear close to the patient's mouth with your eyes facing the chest in order to:

Look—At his chest and abdomen for movement.

Listen—For sounds of breathing.

Feel—Breathing on your cheek.

If upon opening the airway the patient is not breathing spontaneously, you must provide artificial respiration. The best way to do this is to use the mouth-to-mouth technique. This is explained fully in Chapter 9. It is imperative that the head be extended and the nose pinched off while doing mouth-to-mouth resuscitation. Four quick breaths in rapid succession should be given and the chest observed to be sure air is entering the lungs.

When cardiac arrest occurs in restaurants or in the home while the individual is eating, the possibility always exists that a large bolus of food became lodged in the hypopharynx causing asphyxia. Friends or witnesses can confirm this fact by indicating that the patient could not utter a sound and pointed frantically to his mouth before he became unconscious. It must be remembered that mouth-to-mouth resuscitation will not succeed in the presence of an obstructed airway, and it will do no good to begin full cardiac arrest procedures if the patient cannot be ventilated. If the patient is unconscious and cannot be ventilated, he should be rolled on his side and given four back blows between the scapulas followed by four upward manual thrusts to the upper abdomen (in the obese or pregnant patient the thrusts should be directed to the lower sternum). Following this, the index finger should be inserted into the oropharynx, and a sweep made from top to bottom and from side to side. This maneuver should be repeated three times. When patients become deeply comatosed, artificial respiration may be effective despite a bolus of food in the larynx.

BREATHING

If the airway is found to be open but breathing is not present, artificial breathing must be instituted immediately. The most efficient and quickest way to accomplish this is by mouth-to-mouth breathing with the head fully extended (Chapter 9). In cases of possible trauma to the neck, hyperextension should be avoided; instead, the chin and jaw lift maneuver should be used with mouth-to-mouth or mouth-to-nose ventilation. At this critical stage, time should not be wasted to insert an esophageal obturator or an endotracheal tube. With one hand behind and lifting the neck and the other hand pinching the nose and pushing the forehead back, blow four quick breaths into the lungs and watch for a definite expansion of the chest. This will ensure an open airway and ventilation can be continued. An oropharyngeal airway can be used, but it must be remembered that hyperextension of the neck or forward lifting of the lower jaw is still necessary to keep the airway open.

CIRCULATION

After giving four quick breaths, locate the carotid pulse to determine if the heart is beating. Cardiac arrest can be recognized by the absence of breathing and the absence of a pulse in the neck. The carotid artery can be found by palpating in the groove lateral to the larynx. If a pulse is not palpable, artificial circulation must begin immediately by external cardiac compression. The series of steps for external cardiac compression are as follows:

1. Place the patient supine on the floor or ground. If the patient is in bed, place a firm, wide board under him to obtain maximum compression of the heart.

2. Run the finger up the costochondral margin on the left or the right, depending upon which side of the patient the rescuer is placed. The finger will arrive at the xiphoid process and then travel up the sternum to locate the junction between the middle and lower third of

the sternum. It is imperative that compression be done there, not higher where the heart will not be compressed, or lower where the xiphoid process may be pushed inward and lacerate the liver.

3. Superimpose the heels of both hands on one another and place them exactly in the midline of the sternum at a junction between the middle and lower third of the sternum. It may be easier to grasp one hand on top of the other and lock the fingers. This will give a sturdy and firm ball-like point to the heel of the hand (Figure 13-2).

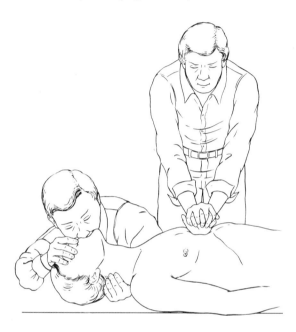

**Figure 13-2.** Two-man resuscitation. In an adult, the heels of the hands should be placed over the lower third of the sternum and the depression should displace the sternum posteriorly 1.5 to 2 inches.

4. Bring the shoulders over the sternum and keep the elbows stiff.

5. The compression begins by a rocking downward motion from the waist upward so that the sternum is pushed vertically downward one and one-half to two inches. For the average adult this may amount to 80 pounds of pressure.

6. Compressions should be at the rate of 80 per minute in a one-man operation and 60 per minute in a two-man operation.

7. During relaxation the negative upward phase allows the heart to fill with blood as the thorax re-expands. The hands should not be taken off of the sternum during relaxation so that subsequent compressions could be continued repeatedly at the exact position over the lower half of the sternum.

8. In a one-man CPR, two quick artificial breaths are given for each fifteen cardiac compressions. In a two-man operation, one breath is given for each five compressions without breaking the rhythm (Table 13-1).

TABLE 13-1

| Rescuers | Ratio of Compressions to Breaths | Rate of Compressions |
|---|---|---|
| One | 15:2 | 80/min |
| Two | 5:1 | 60/min |

This sequence of steps is best practiced and evaluated using an artificial resuscitation manikin, appropriately named "Resusci-Annie." Paramedical, nursing, and fire personnel throughout the United States are now being checked out regularly on the "Resusci-Annie."

In a small child or infant, the volume of air blown into the lungs and the force of cardiac compression is reduced according to body size. For example, in a fifteen pound infant, cardiac compression can be done with two or three fingers, and the rate of compression increased to 80 to 100 per minute (Chapters 19 and 20). The neck of an infant should not be hyperextended, and artificial respiration should be performed by sealing one's mouth over the baby's nose and mouth (Chapter 20).

## PARAMEDIC MANAGEMENT OF CARDIAC ARREST

The initial assessment begins immediately with the first information given by the radio dispatcher. Various descriptions of the initial symptoms are received by the dispatcher and transmitted over the air to the rescue squad and the paramedic unit. "Heart attack," "chest pain," "man (woman) down," "fainted," "unconscious," "seizures," "short of breath," "choking," and "stroke," are all descriptions which might be associated with, or followed by, a cardiac arrest. The paramedic unit quickly learns that these initial descriptions can be misleading but, because cardiac arrest is so frequent, the paramedics learn quickly to prepare for the worst possible situation.

Upon arrival at the scene, CPR may be underway by lay personnel or advanced rescue personnel. The paramedic should assume the responsibility of cardiopulmonary resuscitation and replace the lay personnel. If CPR has not begun, the paramedic begins his approach to the unconscious patient the same as previously described for lay personnel. During this initial response, the paramedic may make a more thorough assessment of the individual and find that the individual may have been dead for some time. This can be determined by the skin color, temperature, and rigidity of the extremities. Fixed and dilated pupils, lack of respiratory effort, and absence of pulses does not necessarily indicate that the patient is dead. While one paramedic is assessing the patient, the second paramedic can be obtaining the history from family, friends, or bystanders.

The important information would consist of when the patient was last seen conscious, any symptoms prior to losing consciousness, past or present illnesses, and the use of medications. When the paramedic assumes or begins CPR he will soon go to advanced cardiac life support.

## ADVANCED CARDIAC LIFE SUPPORT (ACLS)

While basic CPR is being performed, other important procedures are carried out quickly in the following sequence: defibrillation, intravenous line, airway, assessment.

### DEFIBRILLATION

Defibrillator paddles smeared with electrode jelly are applied to the right anterior and left lateral chest walls to determine the underlying cardiac rhythm on the cardioscope (Figure 13-3).

In most communities, a trained paramedic is allowed to identify the dysrhythmia on the scope and defibrillate the patient once, before making radio contact with the base hospital. The amount of watt-seconds for countershock should be adjusted according to Table 13-2. The next section gives the details of correct defibrillation technique.

In the event the scope reveals asystole or extreme bradycardia, without fibrillatory waves or QRS complexes (brady-asystolic arrest), countershock is not recommended. This is because the resumption of cardiac rhythm is unlikely, and massive muscle contractions with countershock in the presence of circulatory arrest can cause profound lactic

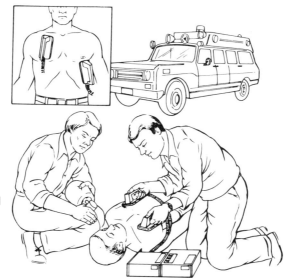

**Figure 13-3.** Placement of paddles for monitoring and defibrillation. The battery-operated defibrillator has made defibrillation in the field possible.

TABLE 13-2.   SCHEDULE FOR DEFIBRILLATION

| Weight | | Initial Watt-Seconds | | Subsequent Watt-Seconds | |
| Pounds | Kilograms | Pounds | Kilograms | Pounds | Kilograms |
| --- | --- | --- | --- | --- | --- |
| 0–50 | 0–23 | 1 W-S/lb | 2 W-S/kg | 2 W-S/lb | 4 W-S/kg |
| 51–150 | 23–70 | 2 W-S/lb | 4 W-S/kg | 2-1/2 W-S/lb | 5 W-S/kg |
| Over 150 | Over 70 | 400 W-S | | 400 W-S | |

acid production (metabolic acidosis). Instead, repetitive "fist pacing" or "thump pacing" can be tried (see below). Epinephrine and atropine should be given as soon as the IV line is established. If the initial rhythm shows ventricular fibrillation and it is unknown how long the patient has been arrested, then defibrillation should await adequate CPR. This is based on animal studies which have shown that after two minutes of ventricular fibrillation without oxygenation the heart cannot be defibrillated. Cardiac surgeons have known this for years. It is futile to attempt defibrillation of the human heart in the operating room if it is anoxic and the tissues and blood are acidotic. Therefore, before attempting to defibrillate the heart, it should be established that the patient has been adequately ventilated and has undergone cardiac compression long enough to restore circulation. If the paramedics arrive and a proper resuscitation effort is underway, then it is feasible to go ahead and attempt to defibrillate the heart without further delay.

As previously stated, the anoxic heart cannot be defibrillated. It must have adequate oxygen and sufficient circulation to allow some respiratory compensation for the metabolic acidosis due to the lack of circulation.

INTRAVENOUS LINE

An intravenous line (Chapter 7) should be established next, using 5% dextrose in water at a rate of 10 to 20 microdrops per minute to keep the line open. Usually the forearm veins or antecubital veins are used. The forearm veins, if they can be entered, are more favorable than the antecubital veins since sudden bending of the arm during countershock defibrillation will often dislodge the cannula. If the antecubital vein is used, then the arm must be securely fastened to an armboard or cardboard splint to prevent kinking at the elbow.

As soon as the IV line is established, two ampules of sodium bicarbonate (44 mEq/ampule) should be infused. This dose may be repeated in ten minutes. Thereafter, one ampule can be given every ten minutes of the arrest. For brady-asystolic arrest, epinephrine 5 ml to 10 ml (1:10,000) and atropine 0.5 mg should be pushed IV and, if necessary, repeated every ten minutes for three additional doses. If

348

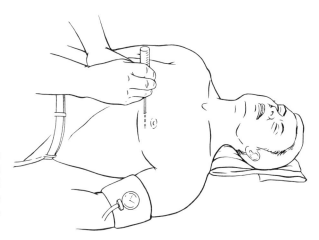

**Figure 13-4.** Epinephrine is injected into the heart through a transthoracic needle puncture. The best location is below and just medial to the left nipple. Injury to the lung and heart can occur with this technique.

an IV line cannot be established, an intracardiac injection of 5 ml of 1:10,000 epinephrine should be tried. This can be accomplished by plunging a prefilled syringe with a three-and-one-half-inch needle straight posteriorly from the left fourth parasternal interspace and then withdrawing the needle with light suction on the syringe until a free flow of blood is obtained. Epinephrine solution is then injected into the cavity of the left ventricle (Figure 13-4). Another approach less likely to injure the coronary arteries is to enter the heart from the subxiphoid area. In this method, the needle is directed at a 45° angle with the frontal and sagittal planes toward the left axilla (Figure 13-5). The needle is then withdrawn slowly until a free flow of blood is obtained. A three-and-one-half-inch needle may be too short to reach the ventricles in tall individuals. A six-inch needle would be more than enough to reach the left ventricle through the right ventricle and the septum by this approach. There is some evidence to indicate that the left ventricular

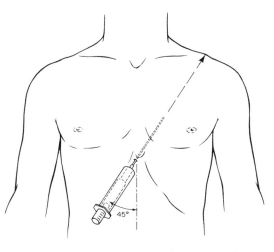

**Figure 13-5.** The subxiphoid approach to intracardiac injection of epinephrine. The needle is inserted just below the xiphoid process and directed toward the left shoulder. The needle is at a 45° angle at the midline and off the chest. This should allow entry of the needle into the left ventricle for injection of epinephrine.

injection of epinephrine is more effective than right ventricular or even venous injection because of the possible inactivation of epinephrine by the lung. Epinephrine may be given by the intracardiac route, but lidocaine, calcium chloride, sodium bicarbonate, and other drugs should not be given in this manner.

AIRWAY

Most paramedic units upon arrival at an arrest situation will forego mouth-to-mouth resuscitation and place an airway in the mouth and begin bag/mask breathing. This is an excellent way to ventilate the patient and allows for the administration of high concentrations of oxygen. When it becomes obvious that cardiac arrest might persist, the preferred treatment is to insert an esophageal obturator airway and use positive pressure ventilation with a bag-mask-valve device (Chapter 9). The reason for this is to prevent further gastric distention by bag/mask or mouth-to-mouth breathing. Also, the esophageal obturator airway will prevent aspiration. The newer esophageal obturator tubes have a separate lumen running down to the distal end making it possible to aspirate gastric contents. Because oxygen is delivered into the pharynx, a tight seal over the nose and mouth is required.

ASSESSMENT

During CPR, constant reassessment is necessary to evaluate the progress of the resuscitation. This includes frequent checking of the pupil size with a flashlight. Naturally, in the daytime this will be difficult, but the eyes can be shaded and the degree of pupil dilation measured. This helps assess the effectiveness of the resuscitation. Whenever normal sinus rhythm is shown on the scope, attempts should be made to feel pulses, since if the heart is beating, further compressions during diastole might interfere with cardiac filling. If the pulse is palpable, attempts to take the blood pressure should be made. This constant reassessment is necessary and must be practiced over and over during the state of arrest. Further definitive treatment would be determined by the course of events that follow.

DEFIBRILLATION

As mentioned previously, ventricular fibrillation is an uncoordinated contraction of the various muscle units of the heart leading to loss of mechanical activity. Electrical defibrillation results in depolarization of these muscle units and hopefully in the return of a normal electrical impulse leading to coordinated muscle contractions.

The apparatus that delivers this electrical impulse is called a defibrillator (Figure 13-6). Defibrillators were originally made for alternating current, but for many reasons they have been abandoned. Direct current (dc) defibrillators are now the accepted standard in the field. Cardioversion is the electrical conversion of one rhythm to another. For example, ventricular tachycardia can be converted with electrical shock to normal sinus rhythm. This technique requires synchronization. That is, the delivery of current is synchronized to the QRS wave on the electrocardiogram so that the countershock does not occur during a vulnerable period of the T waves. Since cardioversion in the field is invariably for ventricular fibrillation, the defibrillators need not be synchronized.

The ideal defibrillator must be light in weight and carry with it an oscilloscopic monitor. The defibrillator must be battery operated, and the paramedic must carry spare recharged batteries in his vehicle. More than once, a paramedic has gone to an arrest only to find that the defibrillator batteries were worn down and that he could not defibrillate. Delay in calling for another defibrillator invariably will ruin the chances for a successful outcome. In most paramedic units, the batteries and defibrillators are checked with each change in shift.

Clearly, there are different types of defibrillators for field use, and the paramedic must become familiar with his own special apparatus. He must know how to turn it on and off, how to change the batteries, how to charge the paddles, and how to discharge the defibrillator. The newer models measure stored as well as delivered energy, and actually deliver as much as 400 watt-seconds. They also have two buttons located on the paddles that must be pressed simultaneously to activate the defibrillator. The paddles also have isolated handles to be held during a quick-look readout of the rhythm on the scope. The paddles act as a monitoring electrode and will monitor the rhythm. A regular protocol should be clearly written for a sequential approach to defibrillation.

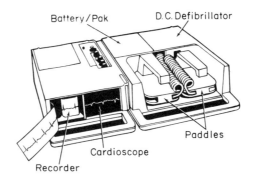

Battery/Pak    D.C. Defibrillator

Paddles

Cardioscope

Recorder

**Figure 13-6.** Portable defibrillators can weigh less than 20 pounds and have direct readout and printout of the electrocardiogram. They are battery operated.

Once it is decided to defibrillate a patient, the process begins by turning on the defibrillator and selecting the desired watt-seconds. This is usually controlled with a single knob, and as the watt-seconds are dialed on the defibrillator, a needle will move into the appropriate range. Once the desired watt-seconds are reached, a second button is pushed to charge the paddles. Conductive electrode paste is then smeared on the surface of the paddles, and they are applied to the chest as shown in Figure 13-3. Commercially available adhesive pads with electro-gel on them can be applied to the skin and left in place. It is important that good skin contact be made; in the hairy individual, while it may not be possible to shave the skin in the field, the use of alcohol may increase conductivity between the paddles and skin. The drying effect of alcohol may allow the application of an electrode pad. At this time, it should be ascertained that the patient is not touching any metal, that all electrical equipment being used on the patient is disconnected, and that the electrode gel is not bridging the two paddles. The paddles should be placed firmly on the chest to prevent dispensation of the electrical current by tilting the metal off of the skin. Before defibrillation, shout loudly, "Stand back, I'm going to defibrillate." Then press the discharge button on the paddles. Following the initial defibrillation, the paddles should be kept in place for direct readout of the cardiac rhythm.

Occasionally, a patient may be so big that anterior-posterior defibrillation may be necessary in the field. The patient is rolled up sideways slightly with a pillow or blanket, and the paddles placed directly over the precordium and directly posterior on the back. However, with the newer units, which can actually deliver 400 watt-seconds, this technique may not be necessary.

An additional consideration in the discussion of the defibrillation procedure is the unusual circumstance of infant defibrillation in the field. Some of the newer defibrillators cannot defibrillate in a range less than 20 watt-seconds. It is probably safe to use 20 watt-seconds as the initial defibrillation dose in an infant. This makes it impossible to adhere to the guideline of 1 watt-second per pound, or 2 watt-seconds per kilogram in very small infants. The data to establish this dose in the infant is based on retrospective studies and is somewhat controversial.

## ERRORS

Mistakes in defibrillation include skin bridging, in which the paddles are too near each other and there is some contact of the electroconductive material. This may cause a spark and burn the patient. It is important not to spill electrode paste on the skin since bridging between the paddle and paste may occur. The paddles sometimes cannot be directly laid on the skin without some sort of conductive material between the paddle and the skin. The paddles must be placed firmly against the chest wall with approximately 25 pounds of pressure to be certain that there will be no electric spark generated. It is probably best to use the lowest amount of watt-seconds to achieve the desired result because myocardial damage is directly related to the energy level of the shock, the frequency of shock, the recovery time between shocks, and the electrode paddle size. Although the paddles in the present defibrillators are isolated from the ground to reduce the probability of inadvertent shock, this danger still exists and should be avoided.

RESULTS

After the initial defibrillation, the heart may:

1. Continue to fibrillate, in which case, if the fibrillatory waves are small, sodium bicarbonate/epinephrine are given and defibrillation with higher energy is repeated. If the fibrillatory waves are adequate, lidocaine is given and defibrillation with a higher force is repeated.

2. Become and remain asystolic or extremely bradycardic, in which case, epinephrine, calcium, and atropine are given. Lidocaine will be contraindicated in this situation.

3. Show sinus rhythm, sinus tachycardia or supraventricular tachycardia. (These patients have the best prognosis.) In this case, lidocaine 1 mg/kg/IV push and 1 to 4 mg per minute IV drip is recommended to prevent the recurrence of ventricular fibrillation. If the blood pressure falls below 80 mm Hg systolic, an intravenous dopamine drip is recommended. Additional IV pushes of lidocaine up to a total of 300 mg may be necessary if PVCs or ventricular tachycardia cannot be controlled.

BRADY-ASYSTOLIC ARREST

If this is indentified and if five minutes of conventional treatment using CPR, epinephrine, and atropine fail to restore an adequate effective heart beat, a trial of fist pacing is recommended. This is accomplished by a sharp rhythmic blow with the ulnar surface of the clenched fist (at a rate of one/second) to the lower half of the sternum or slightly to the left of the sternum. The shock wave in asystolic or markedly bradycardic hearts may initiate an electrical impulse which would spread through the ventricles inscribing QRS and T waves on the EKG monitor and cause the ventricles to contract in a mechanical systole. If QRS and T waves are noted, femoral pulses are felt, and signs of adequate circulation (color, warmth, pupils) are noted, fist pacings should be continued. If shock is present, dopamine could be administered and fist pacing tried again. If none of the above signs of circulation are seen after 30 seconds, fist pacing should be discontinued in favor of the conventional external cardiac compression. If fist pacing and compression can be applied concomitantly, either by coordinated thump-massage motion or by special machine, it would appear that this would be the most physiologic method to maintain life in a brady-asystolic arrest.

Conventional cardiac massage even at its best produces only about 35 percent of the normal resting cardiac output, whereas, if the myocardium is still responsive, the cardiac output should be greater with fist pacing. Furthermore, with any ventricular activity at all, external cardiac massage will be counterproductive since the massage will be applied 50 percent of the time when the heart is trying to fill itself with blood during diastole. In this sense, cardiac massage synchronized to the QRS complexes should be most effective.

## WHEN TO TRANSPORT

When CPR in the field is underway and there has not been an immediate response to therapy, the question of transport is considered. This largely depends upon the nurse or doctor who is handling the communications at the base station hospital. In general, it is accepted that one-half hour is the minimum time needed to begin basic and advanced CPR by the paramedics before transport. The biggest cause for delay in transport from the field is the starting and maintenance of an intravenous line. This can be time-consuming and difficult. Often the line will be placed and come out within seconds because of being improperly taped, the arm not being positioned correctly on the armboard, or other factors. If CPR continues to be necessary and maximum defibrillation (approximately four defibrillations) has been attempted, and an intravenous has been started, it is probably best to transport the patient to the hospital while CPR is underway.

If the patient has responded initially to the resuscitation and has developed a normal sinus rhythm with a good blood pressure, proper time should be spent assuring that a secure IV is in place and that the vital signs and the electrocardiogram are stable. This would include starting a lidocaine drip and assuring that the proper oxygenation is being maintained. This sort of stabilization will prevent subsequent cardiac arrest in transport. It is also helpful to have certain drugs mixed and ready for administration should they become needed during transport. This would include a dopamine drip, as well as sodium bicarbonate, epinephrine, and calcium syringes ready and available.

If the paramedic arrives and decides to begin CPR even though the situation may seem hopeless, it is best not to discontinue CPR in the field. This is because the cessation of CPR means the individual has died, and this can produce much emotional trauma if there are immediate family members around. This is especially true if cardiac arrest resuscitation begins in the home.

Cardiac arrest can occur anywhere and at any time. The paramedic may find himself on the second floor of an apartment house, hotel, or private dwelling. CPR may begin in an airplane, in a stadium, beside a backyard pool, or in a mountain ravine. This raises the question as to when and how to transport the patient who is undergoing CPR. This type of procedure is physically exhausting to the paramedic and requires a great deal of patience and skill. Since during external cardiac compression only about 35 percent of the cardiac output is generated, it is obvious that delays in CPR would not be well tolerated. In some circumstances the addition of less than optimal oxygenation makes delays in CPR even more critical. Although there is no documented evidence as to how long CPR can be interrupted, the recommendation is that it be no longer than five seconds. Paramedics should time themselves to see how far they can travel with a stretcher and a patient on it for five seconds while they are interrupting CPR. This might include one flight of stairs, or a run across the front lawn, or down the ramp of an airplane. It is recommended that when transporting the fully arrested patient down the stairs, it is best to place him on a collapsible gurney (Chapter 14). This has a hard back and it is easier to negotiate the turns in a stairway with this type of apparatus than with a stretcher. At each landing the legs can be dropped and CPR continued for approximately one to two minutes when transport is again resumed. Although five seconds may be impractical, by limiting the team to this time for interruption of CPR, at least something near this time may be achievable. Remember that if during CPR only one-third of the normal cardiac output is being generated, five seconds of interrupted CPR is equivalent to fifteen seconds under normal circumstances. Any normal person whose heart is interrupted for fifteen seconds will become unconscious from cerebral anoxia.

## COMPLICATIONS OF CPR

Complications of cardiopulmonary resuscitation center around the external compression of the heart by the sternum and the use of needles and drug injections.

1. The most common complication is a fracture of the ribs or costochondral arch. These fractures may actually lacerate the lung producing a tension pneumothorax or bleeding into the chest cavity (hemothorax). Fracture of the costochondral arch may be so severe in patients with a rigid thorax and pulmonary emphysema, that ventilator support after resuscitation, if successful, is necessary for ten days. This is the time required for the arch to become stable and eliminate the

flail portion of the sternum. Whenever fractures occur, fat embolization to the lung and actual bone marrow emboli have been observed. These complications must be weighed against effective CPR. Rib fractures should not occur in a younger patient with a flexible sternum and chest, and when they do occur, it indicates that the force of compression was too great.

2. Contusion and rupture of the heart have been reported. This is probably related to over-vigorous compression with a subsequent hydrostatic rupture of the heart. Hemorrhage into the myocardium from compression has been documented on many occasions and may aggravate an already present myocardial infarction.

When compressions are to the lower end of the sternum, the xiphoid has been known to lacerate the liver. Also, the sudden increase in intraabdominal pressure with compression too low on the sternum has caused ruptured spleens and livers. These ruptures may not become apparent until the patient has been successfully resuscitated and doing well, when they suddenly develop severe hypotension, shock, and secondary cardiac arrest. Oftentimes, the second resuscitation is unsuccessful since bleeding is not suspected. At autopsy the peritoneal cavity may be filled with blood, which tells what really happened.

3. A whole host of complications are related to the intracardiac injection of medications. Using the fourth intercostal space and attempting to inject epinephrine directly into the heart will often cause laceration of the left lung. The lingular portion of the left upper lobe passes in front of the heart in many people. When the needle passes through the chest, it lacerates the lung before it enters the heart. This laceration causes air to leak into the pleural space, and subsequently to produce a tension pneumothorax. Whenever intracardiac injection of medication has been attempted through this route, breath sounds should be carefully monitored. On occasion, a tension pneumothorax will have to be relieved while CPR is in progress. This complication has prompted people to use the subxiphoid approach to the insertion of medication into the left ventricle (Figure 13-5).

4. Laceration of the coronary arteries is a well known complication of intracardiac injections. This may produce hemorrhage about the artery with occlusion and/or bleeding within the pericardial sac leading to tamponade.

5. Tears in the myocardium with hemopericardium are well known complications. The individual injecting medication into the heart must satisfy himself that there is a free flow of blood into the syringe. If he does not, he or she will be injecting epinephrine into the myocardial wall. This will produce a very irritable focus, with intractable ventricular fibrillation. Should the patient be resuscitated, it may be a source of recurrent premature ventricular contractions.

6. Insertion of needles into veins and administration of drugs carries

with it many complications. The most severe of these is the infiltration of medications, such as calcium or sodium bicarbonate, into the tissues. These substances are hypertonic and very caustic and may lead to severe damage. On more than one occasion, forearm skin and muscles have been injured.

7. Complications with the insertion of esophageal obturator airways, endotracheal tubes, etc., are numerous. These include dislodgement of teeth with aspiration into the lung, laceration of the posterior pharynx with bleeding, and rupture of the esophagus with the esophageal obturator airway.

The above list of complications is by no means complete, but it gives a general idea of the problems. It should be noted that all of the problems center around careless application of technique.

To avoid the complications of CPR, constant practice of the different procedures that are used is necessary. It is equally important to remember that complications can occur. A life may be saved and a patient may appear to be doing well otherwise, but he may suddenly deteriorate without an immediate explanation.

## WHEN TO STOP CPR

1. If cardiac death persists over thirty minutes in the presence of adequate ventilation, CPR should be discontinued. This will become clear as the heart either is in electrical standstill or persists in ventricular fibrillation, despite the many attempts at defibrillation. Usually all types of drugs and means to resuscitate the heart have been tried, and the rescue team, paramedics, and/or nurse and physician feel that the heart cannot be resuscitated.

2. If there is clear central nervous system death, CPR should be stopped. This question always arises in the hospital situation in which a Code Blue has been called and many physicians arrive to resuscitate a patient. Once CPR is underway, the question is always asked, "What size are the patient's pupils?" This information is helpful if the pupils are normal and respond to light. If the pupils are dilated and do not react to light, CPR should be continued. If the pupils come down in size shortly thereafter, it is worthwhile to continue. Remember, dilated and fixed pupils by themselves are not an indication to stop CPR.

3. When CPR has been initiated by nonphysicians, the American Heart Association has specific guidelines as to what sequence should be followed.

  a. The resuscitator can stop if effective spontaneous ventilation and circulation have been restored.

  b. Arrival of more experienced personnel has occurred (e.g., when the paramedics arrive, the citizen may discontinue his therapy).

c. A physician arrives and assumes the responsibility for transfer of the patient to the hospital.

d. Single efforts at CPR are exhausting, and the individual doing the CPR may become so exhausted he cannot continue.

If one of the above indications is not present, then only a physician can terminate CPR, since it is only the physician who has the legal right to pronounce death.

## CASE EXAMPLES

**Case 1.** A 43-year-old male patient suddenly became ill and requested medical aid. The fire department rescue squad and the paramedic unit were dispatched at 1045 hours. He had become unconscious at 1047 hours and cardiopulmonary resuscitation was initiated by the rescue squad at 1051 hours. The paramedic unit arrived on the scene at 1052 hours and immediately identified the rhythm on the cardioscope and defibrillated with 400 watt-seconds of countershock three times in one minute. This successfully converted the ventricular fibrillation into sinus bradycardia at sixty per minute with frequent premature ventricular beats (Figure 13-7).

An intravenous line was established at 1057 hours and one ampule of sodium bicarbonate (45 mEq) was immediately given. The cardiac rhythm improved into a slow multiformed atrial rhythm at seventy-four per minute. A good carotid pulse was palpable at 1100 hours and the blood pressure at 1106 hours was 90 mm Hg

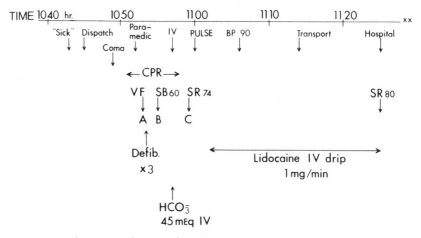

43 yr. male. History of myocardial infarct 1 year ago.
On Digoxin, Nitroglycerine, Quinidine & Isosorbide.
xx Discharged from hospital 22 days later.

**Figure 13-7.** The sequence of events of cardiopulmonary resuscitation in Case 1.

systolic. Respiration was spontaneous and intubation was not necessary.

Lidocaine at 1 mg per minute was infused intravenously and the patient was transported to the nearest receiving hospital ten minutes away under continuous EKG monitoring and radio contact with the base hospital. The patient did well and was discharged from the hospital three weeks later. The patient had a past history of myocardial infarction one year previously, and had been on digoxin, nitroglycerine, quinidine, and Isosorbide₍ᵣ₎.

**Comment:** Early resuscitation correctly done provided a suitable situation for successful defibrillation by the paramedics.

**Case 2.** A 44-year-old male patient with no prior history of heart disease collapsed in the bowling alley at 2207 hours. He was attended by the advance rescue unit and given CPR within five minutes. The MICU paramedic team arrived three minutes later, inserted an esophageal obturator airway, and identified ventricular fibrillation on the cardioscope. The patient was immediately defibrillated with 400 watt-seconds into marked sinus bradycardia and complete heart block (Figure 13-8). Junctional escape rhythm deteriorated rapidly

A   VENTRICULAR FIBRILLATION ON SCOPE

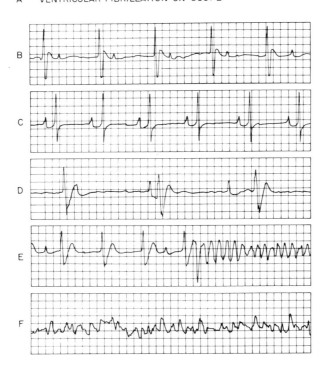

**Figure 13-8.** The cardiac dysrhythmia following initial ventricular fibrillation in Case 2. Panels B, C, D, E, and F correspond to the B, C, D, E, and F shown in Figure 13-9.

to twenty-two per minute, and despite the administration of sodium bicarbonate, atropine, epinephrine, and calcium chloride, the rhythm reverted to intractable ventricular fibrillation (Figure 13-9). Postmortem examination revealed a thrombus occluding both the left anterior descending artery at its origin and the proximal left circumflex artery.

**Comment:** Autopsy follow-up of deaths in the field will help in the critique of CPR. This patient could not have been resuscitated even under ideal circumstances in the hospital based on the autopsy findings.

**Case 3.** A 74-year-old male suddenly became comatose at 2005 hours. Paramedics arrived at 2009 hours and found the patient unconscious, but breathing on his own and with a palpable pulse. The EKG showed a junctional rhythm at 90 per minute. Sinus beats with distinct P waves were only seen infrequently. The rhythm then rapidly deteriorated into a very slow junctional rhythm at 20 per minute despite the administration of sodium bicarbonate, atropine, isoproterenol, and calcium chloride (Figure 13-10). A second dose of atropine restored a junctional rhythm of 80 per minute (Figure 13-11). He was then transferred to the nearest hospital, but was dead on arrival.

Postmortem examination revealed a ruptured aortic aneurysm and a 90 percent occlusion of the left anterior descending artery.

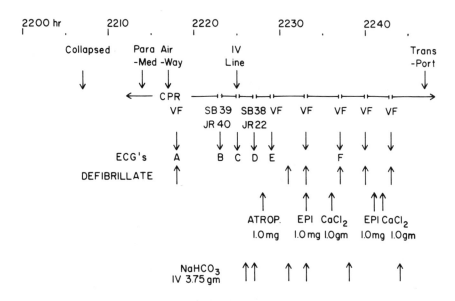

44 yr M. No prior history of heart disease. Collaped in bowling alley. Intractable ventricular fibrillation.

**Figure 13-9.** Reversion of cardiac rhythm to intractable ventricular fibrillation in Case 2.

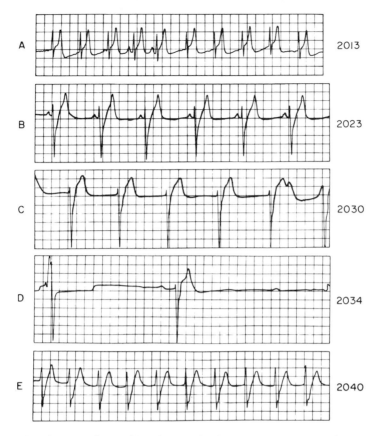

Figure 13-10. The electrocardiographic changes in Case 3. Letters A, B, C, D, and E correspond to the letters A, B, C, D, and E in Figure 13-11.

**Comment:** Ruptured abdominal aortic aneurysms can present with the same clinical findings as an acute myocardial infarction. Initial astute assessment by the paramedic may make the correct diagnosis possible.

> **Case 4.** A 71-year-old male patient without a prior cardiac history suddenly collapsed at 1306 hours and was attended by the paramedics within four minutes (Figure 13-12). The initial rhythm revealed a complete AV block without ventricular escape (Figure 13-13). Atrial P waves were visible. Following the administration of sodium bicarbonate and epinephrine, an idioventricular rhythm was obtained, but this was supplanted by protracted ventricular fibrillation which could not be reversed.

**Comment:** Sudden death is a common occurrence. There may be dysrhythmia without myocardial infarction. Autopsy on this patient would probably show severe coronary artery disease.

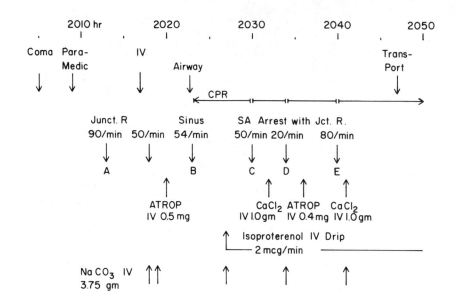

74 yr M.   No past history of cardiac disease. No chest pains.
No medications.

**Figure 13-11.** Restoration of a junctional rhythm in Case 3.

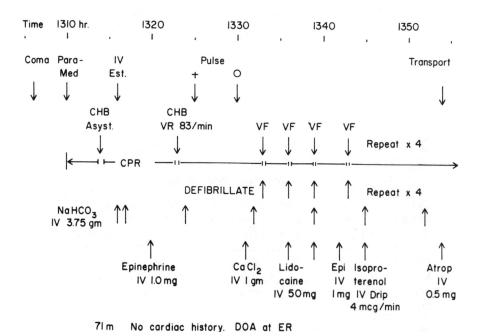

71 m   No cardiac history. DOA at ER

**Figure 13-12.** The events of resuscitation in a 71-year-old male following sudden death (Case 4).

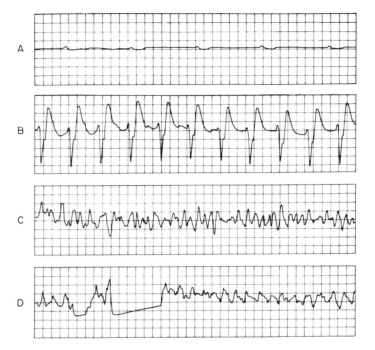

**Figure 13-13.** Upon arrival of the paramedics, the initial rhythm was complete AV block without ventricular escape. An idioventricular rhythm was obtained with drugs, but ventricular fibrillation ensued and the patient was not successfully resuscitated.

*Summary*

This chapter contains some of the most important and, at the same time, familiar material basic to the armamentarium of the paramedic. It is almost a necessity to commit a large part of the information in this chapter to memory, since it will become part of the daily routine of the EMT-Paramedic. It can also be seen that many of the facts included in this chapter must be correlated with material in the other chapters to make it even more useful and meaningful.

*Important Points to Remember*

Seven hundred thousand people in the United States die each year from coronary artery disease. More than 50 percent of these deaths are in the first two hours before hospitalization. Most of these people die from acute dysrhythmias. Therefore, cardiopulmonary resuscitation and advanced cardiac life support in the field may save many of these people.

The concept of the Mobile Intensive Care Unit evolved from the following observations:

1. Life can be maintained for a reasonable amount of time after cessation of heartbeat by closed chest massage.
2. Electrical countershock can counteract fibrillation.

3. Coronary Care Units can successfully monitor patients to both treat and prevent cardiac arrest.

4. More patients die suddenly from heart disease outside the hospital than inside.

The first ambulance system capable of resuscitating patients was established in Belfast, Ireland, in 1967. The response time of the initial rescue squad must be less than five minutes. Seventy to eighty percent of sudden deaths outside of the hospital are due to coronary artery disease.

Non-cardiac causes of sudden death include:

1. Drug or chemical toxicity.
2. Asphyxiation.
3. Trauma.
4. Electrocution.
5. Anaphylaxis.
6. Hemorrhage.
7. Drug overdose.
8. Pacemaker failure.
9. Pulmonary embolism.
10. Myocarditis.
11. Valvular heart disease.
12. Pulmonary insufficiency.
13. Cerebral hemorrhage.
14. Meningitis.
15. Ruptured aneurysm.
16. Internal hemorrhage.

Mechanisms of sudden cardiac arrest include:

1. Ventricular fibrillation (75%).
2. Brady-asystole (25%).
3. Electromechanical dissociation (hard to identify).

Ventricular fibrillation may be presaged by premature ventricular contractions and then ventricular tachycardia; however, in the field sinus and supraventricular tachycardias herald this complication in over 50 percent of cases.

In ventricular fibrillation the electrical activity of the ventricles is chaotic, with multiple undulating waves of irregular circuits resulting in a nonejecting wiggling motion of the ventricles.

Brady-asystolic arrest is one in which there is an inadequate circulation of blood due to extremely slow and ineffective or absent cardiac contractions. Patients with brady-asystole often develop fibrillation.

Electromechanical dissociation is present when the heart continues to beat after myocardial infarction, but does not eject enough blood to allow adequate circulation to vital tissues.

The essential ingredients of basic cardiopulmonary resuscitation are:

1. Airway
2. Breathing
3. Circulation

Some important points concerning these basics include:

1. Determine consciousness.
2. Place the patient on his back.
3. Observe for breathing.
4. Use the mouth-to-mouth technique.
5. If eating, watch for food obstruction.
6. Open airway by hyperextension, except in neck trauma.
7. Establish presence of cardiac arrest (absent neck pulse).
8. External cardiac compression.
   a. 80/min for one person.
   b. 60/min for two persons.
9. In a one-person resuscitation, two breaths are given for each fifteen compressions.
10. In a two-person resuscitation, one breath is given for each five compressions.

Some elements of advanced cardiopulmonary circulation include:

1. While basic CPR is being performed, defibrillator paddles should be prepared and applied.

2. If asystole or extreme bradycardia without fibrillation is present, "fist pacing" or "thump pacing" can be tried. Epinephrine and atropine should also be given intravenously.

3. An intravenous line should be established, using D/W.

4. Sodium bicarbonate (two ampules) is given IV.

5. If an IV line cannot be started, intracardiac epinephrine may be used.

6. Most paramedic units will use an airway with bag and mask breathing instead of mouth-to-mouth ventilation. The esophageal obturator airway is often used here also.

7. During CPR, constant assessment is necessary (includes pulse, respiration, BP, pupil size, and rhythm on scope).

Electrical defibrillation hopefully results in the return of a normal electrical impulse leading to coordinated muscle contractions.

The paramedic must become familiar with his own special type of defibrillator apparatus, how to operate it, change batteries, discharge it, and charge paddles.

The procedure for defibrillation is as follows:

1. Turn unit on.
2. Select desired watt-seconds.
3. Charge paddles.
4. Apply conductive electrode paste.
5. Attach paddles to chest (with good skin contact).
6. Do not allow patient to touch metal.
7. Announce procedure loudly.

Events following defibrillation may include:

1. Continuation of fibrillation (epinephrine given and higher energy repeated, or lidocaine followed by another effort).
2. Asystole or bradycardia (give epinephrine, calcium, and atropine).
3. Sinus rhythm, tachycardia, or supraventricular tachycardia (best prognosis). Give lidocaine and, if blood pressure falls, dopamine.
4. Brady-asystolic arrest. (If CPR, epinephrine, and atropine fail, use "fist pacing." Dopamine may help. If all fails, use conventional closed chest compression.)

Transport: Thirty minutes is the minimum accepted time needed to begin basic and advanced CPR before transport. If CPR continues, maximum defibrillation (4) has been tried, and an IV has been started, it is best to transport. After the patient is stabilized, it is important to have certain drugs mixed should they be needed during transport. These include a dopamine drip, sodium bicarbonate, epinephrine, and calcium. If CPR is started in the field, it should not be terminated because of emotional trauma. External cardiac compression generates only 35 percent of normal cardiac output; therefore, delays of longer than five seconds are not recommended.

Complications of CPR Include:

1. Fracture of the ribs or costochondral arch with lung laceration or hemothorax.
2. Contusion and rupture of the heart.
3. Laceration of the liver.
4. Laceration of the lung by intracardiac injection.
5. Laceration of coronary arteries.
6. Tears of myocardium.
7. Injection of toxic drugs outside of veins and tissue destruction.
8. Complications of insertion of airways (dislodgement of teeth, laceration of pharynx, rupture of the esophagus).

When to Stop CPR:

1. If cardiac death persists over thirty minutes.
2. If there is clear central nervous system death.
3. When spontaneous ventilation and circulation are restored.
4. Upon arrival of more experienced personnel.
5. When physician assumes responsibility.
6. Upon exhaustion of the rescuer.

*Bibliography*

Copley, D. P., Mantle, J. A., Rogers, W. J., Russell, R. O., and Rackley, C. E. "Improved Outcome for Prehospital Cardiopulmonary Collapse with Resuscitation by Bystanders." *Circulation.* 56:901, 1977.

McEnany, M. T., Morgan, R. J., Mundth, E. D., and Austen, W. G. "Circumvention of Detrimental Pulmonary Vasoactivity of Exogenous Catecholamines in Cardiac Resuscitation." *Surgical Forum.* 26:98, 1975.

*Standards for Cardiopulmonary Resuscitation (CPR) and Emergency Cardiac Care (ECC).* Supplement to JAMA, 227:833, 1974.

Chapter 14

# TRAUMA

Trauma is the third leading cause of death in the United States and the most common cause of death in individuals between the ages of twenty and forty years. More hospital beds are used for patients with trauma than for patients with heart disease or pregnancy. More and more emphasis is being placed on the management of trauma and the proper transport and distribution of the trauma patient to facilities able to handle these complex problems. In the United States alone approximately 150,000 people die each year as a result of trauma, and many more are permanently or partially disabled. The cost to our society runs close to thirty billion dollars a year. It makes little sense to spend millions of dollars in equipping and training paramedics to have the patient die or be maimed because some basic step was overlooked or forgotten. The principles and management of trauma patients in the field require common sense and reflex reactions. Constant reminding and practice are the necessary ingredients for effective and useful field treatment. In this chapter, trauma is presented in the following sequence:

1. Head and Facial
2. Neck
3. Eye
4. Nervous System
5. Thorax
6. Abdomen
7. Musculoskeletal System
8. Vascular System

However, in real life situations the diagnosis and management of the trauma patient often occur simultaneously, and may involve different systems at one time. The basic tenet of *primum non nocere* (i.e., first, do no harm) has no more applicable a place than in the management of trauma. Skillful extrication of the patient, airway management,

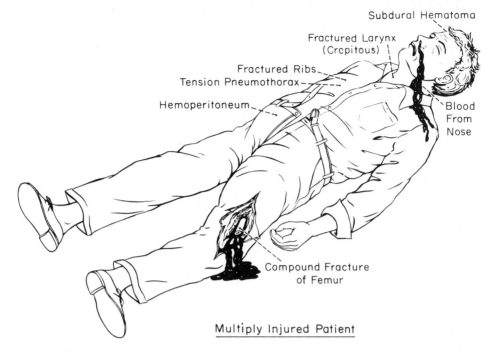

Subdural Hematoma

Fractured Larynx
(Crepitous)

Fractured Ribs

Tension Pneumothorax

Hemoperitoneum

Blood
From
Nose

Compound Fracture
of Femur

Multiply Injured Patient

**Figure 14-1.** A systematic approach to the assessment of the multiply injured patient is necessary so that injuries are not overlooked.

protection of the spinal cord, control of bleeding, splinting of fractures, and rapid transportation to a proper facility are all key factors in a successful outcome.

Obvious signs of illness or injury will often direct the examiner away from the life-threatening condition, such as an obstructed airway. Therefore, a systematic approach to the multiply injured patient is essential (Figure 14-1). In order to establish priorities in providing emergency care, a primary and secondary survey are always done in sequence.

## PRIMARY SURVEY

The primary survey refers to life-threatening situations, and it must be done as soon as the paramedic reaches the patient. The paramedic completes the primary survey within seconds, checking for the following:

Airway and Breathing
Pulse and Circulation
Severe Bleeding
Shock

If breathing is not absolutely obvious, open the airway and feel for air exchange at the patient's nose and mouth and watch the chest for rise and fall. Do not hyperextend the neck if a spinal injury is suspected. If breathing is absent begin mouth-to-mouth ventilation.

## PULSE AND CIRCULATION

The quickest way to assess the circulation is to palpate the carotid pulse, listen for the apical pulse, and apply cardiac monitor electrodes or electrocardiogram read-out paddles to determine cardiac status. Even though cardiac activity may be present, perfusion may be inadequate. This is assessed by looking at the patient's skin color, nail bed color, and general condition. If the pulse is absent, begin cardiopulmonary resuscitation. If the patient is in ventricular fibrillation, the paramedic may defibrillate one time before contacting the base station hospital for additional orders.

## SEVERE BLEEDING

If bleeding is present, determine whether it is superficial or life-threatening. Serious bleeding is controlled (hemostasis) by applying direct pressure with the hand, fingers, or a bulky dressing. Do not attempt to clamp bleeders since this is not a field procedure.

## SHOCK

Signs of shock include clammy skin, dilated pupils, and irrational or anxious behavior. Measurement of the blood pressure will help determine the degree of shock as well as the heart rate. If there is hypoventilation or air hunger, the patient should be ventilated with oxygen.

The preceding survey is called the primary survey and should be done on every ill and injured patient within seconds of arriving at the patient's side.

## SECONDARY SURVEY

The secondary survey occurs after the primary survey has been completed and appropriate action taken. The secondary survey is a complete examination designed to check for specific, although not necessarily life-threatening injuries. This survey may take several minutes to complete, depending upon the nature and extent of the patient's problems, his location, and the experience of the paramedic. After examining the patient, the paramedic must establish priorities and treat problems in the order of their severity. In dealing with trauma, neck injury should always be considered, especially in the presence of head or facial injuries. If a spinal injury is a possibility, stabilize the neck and back immediately to prevent spinal cord damage, using a cervical collar, sandbags, and short or long backboards. This could also be considered as part of the primary survey. Splint the neck in the position found unless the airway is compromised. If necessary, move the head to a neutral position, applying constant slight traction to the head.

## SCALP AND SKULL

Beginning at the back of the neck, palpate the cervical spine looking for pain and deformities. Then work anteriorly to the top of the head, checking the scalp for lacerations, and other signs of trauma.

## EARS AND NOSE

The ears and nose are checked for fluid, blood, and foreign objects, such as glass or metal particles. The presence of a clear draining fluid from the ears or nose indicates a cerebral spinal fluid leak, and is almost always diagnostic of a basal skull fracture. If the fluid is clear, it will form a yellow "halo" around blood on a 4 × 4 dressing.

## EYES

The eye examination should begin by inspection of the cornea to see if contact lenses are in place. Pupillary reaction is noted with light stimulation. Pupil inequality is indicative of intracranial problems. Pupils may not respond to light in the presence of daylight because of the sunlight. If the patient is unconscious close the eyelids.

## MOUTH

Examination of the mouth begins with smelling, and looking for unusual odors such as alcohol. Also look in the mouth for broken teeth, dentures, foreign objects, or signs of local injury.

## NECK

The anterior neck should be palpated beginning with the thyroid cartilage and moving laterally to either side for palpation of the carotid pulse. If the head is fixed in an abnormal position and the patient's airway is patent, immediately stabilize the head in that position. The external jugular veins in the posterior triangle of the neck should be inspected for distention.

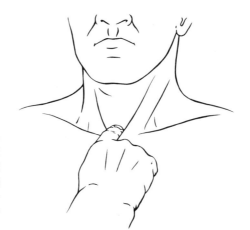

**Figure 14-2.** The trachea resides in the midline above the suprasternal notch and can be easily palpated. It deviates to the right or left following a tension pneumothorax. This deviation is to the side opposite the pneumothorax.

## CHEST

The chest comprises part of the lower airway and therefore must be examined thoroughly. Observe the chest for equal expansion and depth of respiration. If expansion is asymmetrical, this may indicate rib fractures or lung damage. Examination of the bony thorax begins by feeling within the suprasternal notch for the trachea to be certain it is in the midline (Figure 14-2). Deviations to either side indicate a tension pneumothorax. Sternal compression will reveal any instability of the costochondral arch. Palpation of the clavicles will reveal any fractures. Chest fractures can be detected by grabbing the chest on either side of the costal arch and squeezing inwardly (barrel hoop test). Both sides of the chest should be auscultated for breath sounds. Heart sounds should be listened to in order to assess their quality and distance from the stethoscope.

## ABDOMEN

Gently palpate the abdomen to assess guarding or rigidity. Localized tenderness may indicate blood or a ruptured organ, particularly in the left upper quadrant. A distended abdomen is an indication of massive intraperitoneal hemorrhage and requires immediate attention.

## PELVIS

The pelvic girdle can be examined by pressing on the symphysis pubis. If this does not elicit pain, push in on the pelvis by squeezing in laterally on either side (barrel hoop test). Put your hand between the patient's knees and have him squeeze inwardly. If this produces pain, a pelvic fracture should be suspected. Check the leg for outward rotation, which indicates a broken hip or posterior dislocation of the hip.

If the patient can be rolled on his side, the back should be inspected for deformity or injury. Avoid moving the patient unnecessarily to examine the back, particularly if there are no complaints in this region. All four limbs should be examined for deformity, instability, swelling, discoloration, or crepitus. The distal parts of the extremities should be inspected for pulses and skin color. If the patient is conscious, he should be asked to move all four extremities by flexing his toes and fingers.

## SPINAL CORD INJURIES

To assess a spinal cord injury, sensation should be checked in all four extremities. The patient's hand should grip the examiner's hand bilaterally for equality of movement and strength. The same examination should be conducted with the feet, having the patient wiggle his toes and press his feet against the examiner's hands. Any diminished sensation or strength, particularly if bilateral, could indicate spinal cord injury and proper precautions should be taken. If the patient is unconscious, a spinal cord injury can be checked for by pinching the patient below the cervical spine to see if this painful stimulus will produce a response. Scratching the skin of the hands and feet will produce an involuntary muscle reaction if there is no cord damage. If the cord is damaged, this reaction will be absent. The presence of a normal neurologic exam does not rule out a cervical fracture and the patient should still be considered to have a serious neck injury until proven otherwise.

The primary survey is done on all trauma patients. With experience and constant practice, it becomes second nature to the paramedic. In many instances, the secondary survey cannot be done because the patient is so critically injured that time should not be wasted assessing injuries. Instead, the patient should be transported as quickly as possible to the emergency receiving center or base station hospital.

## MECHANISM OF INJURY

Prior to the advent of the paramedic, trauma patients were brought to the hospital by ambulance drivers, police, or fire personnel. Because there usually was no communication with the hospital, patients often arrived on the doorstep without any prior knowledge of what happened or how the patient was injured. It is the details from the scene of the accident radioed ahead or at least brought with the patient to the hospital that makes management of these complex problems easier.

The paramedic must ask himself:

1. What happened before and at the instant of injury?
2. What object or objects caused the injury?
3. How large was the object?
4. What direction was it going?
5. How much force did it have?
6. What was the position of the patient and what were his movements at the instant of injury?

## EXAMPLES

From information available at the scene of the accident, the story of what happened should be obtained. This information can be learned from bystanders, fellow passengers, and even the patient himself. Often the picture of the forces and direction of the victim and the object that struck him can be determined within a few seconds of well directed questions and observation. For example, a motorcycle collision, where the victim is located one hundred feet from his vehicle, presents an entirely different set of possibilities than a dog bite. The patient who sustained his wounds from a motorcycle accident would be more likely to have concomitant injuries than the dog bite victim. Hidden problems can sometimes be solved by careful attention to the mechanisms, e.g., a patient with obvious cerebral trauma was presumed to be the victim of a shooting, but no obvious wounds were present; on analysis of the direction of the trajectory of the bullet, and the position of the victim, the examiner was able to find a wound of entry within one nostril.

## PATTERN OF INJURY

The mechanism of injury and the patient's anatomy will determine the pattern of injury. Patterns are helpful to know, because if one part of a known pattern is recognized, the examiner can seek the other portions. An example of a life-threatening pattern is as follows: A driver of a small car collided with another car and was thrown forward against his seat belt; his chin hit the upper part of the steering wheel causing a large, tearing laceration; the forward movement of his body continued until his neck hit the upper part of the wheel. On examination, the victim was in obvious respiratory distress. A quick reconstruction of events led the examiner to suspect a laryngeal fracture from the blow to the neck and steps were taken to establish an airway. Other possible injuries associated with this pattern are chest injuries from contact with the steering wheel, abdominal injuries from the force of the seat belt, and cervical spine injury secondary to a sudden flexion of the neck.

## CLASSIFICATION OF WOUNDS

### CONTUSION

A contusion is a severe bruise in which the skin is intact, but there is swelling and possibly a hematoma in the area of injury (Figure 14-3). Contusions usually result from a blunt blow, and injuries to tissues deeper than the contusion should be suspected. For example, fractures often hide under contusions; laryngotracheal damage can occur with contusions of the neck; in contusions of the abdomen, a rupture of the spleen or liver may be present.

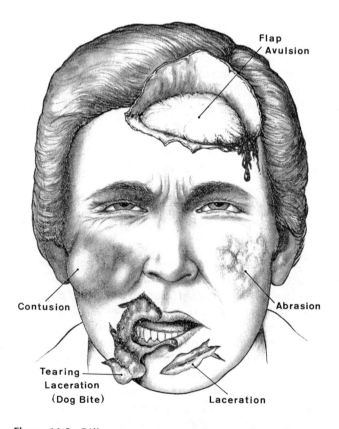

**Figure 14-3.** Different types of wounds are shown. These types of injuries can occur to any part of the body.

In an abrasion the surface layers of the skin are scraped away by friction. Most frequently abrasions are caused by bodily contact with the pavement or sidewalk. The depth of penetration depends on the force and duration of the contact with the damaging surface. A superficial abrasion poses a problem only if dirt or foreign material is embedded in the abraded area or if the wound becomes infected. If dirt is left in any wound, but particularly in an abrasion, it will remain as a permanent, blue-black "traumatic tattoo" or "accidental tattoo." Superficial abrasions should be carefully cleansed, and given surface treatment with an antibacterial agent. If any fragments of dirt are visible these should be removed by a physician. Deep abrasions may scrape right through all the layers of the skin and can even continue right through underlying anatomical features, causing serious skin loss and damage to deep structures. Deep abrasions require surgical cleansing, debridement, and repairs. Again, removal of embedded foreign material is very important.

## LACERATION

Although in the strict sense the term laceration should apply only to a tearing wound, the term has been expanded to include a simple cut. This is referred to as a simple laceration and results from the direct cutting effect of a sharp edge such as glass or metal. A tearing laceration results from the hard impact of a blunter force. Considerable force is needed to tear the human skin. A burst or stellate laceration is caused by a very forceful impact of a blunt object against a confined area of the skin. A penetrating laceration is a wound that extends into the underlying deep anatomical structures. Knife blades, large glass fragments, or a bullet may cause serious injury in the depths of their paths. Although a mere puncture wound may be visible in the skin, a puncture of the abdomen may cause perforation or hemorrhage from a large vessel, and a puncture of the chest may cause a tension pneumothorax. A moment's hesitation should precede the removal of a penetrating knife while one considers whether removal might accelerate the bleeding from injured vessels in the depths of the wound.

## FLAP AVULSION

The attachments between subcutaneous fascia and the investing fascia are much weaker than the skin itself. Often an injury will elevate the skin along this plane from the underlying tissues. The deeper layer of vessels sustaining the overlying skin are detached in the process of a flap avulsion. Whether the flap will survive or not depends upon the amount of blood supply which remains intact to nourish the flap. Avulsion flaps often result from a high impact tangential force. A special type of flap avulsion is called the "degloving flap" where the skin of the hand or leg is pulled partly off, as if it were a glove or stocking. The most common cause of degloving of the hand is industrial machinery, and the most common cause of degloving of the leg is the tire of a vehicle rolling over the lower limb. Once bleeding has been controlled, an avulsion flap should be accurately replaced and lightly dressed so that the blood vessels entering the flap are neither kinked from poor position or compressed from excess pressure.

## COMPLETE AVULSION

In a complete avulsion skin and attached tissues are torn completely away by the force of the injury. A woman's scalp can be avulsed away in its entirety as a result of long hair being caught in industrial machinery. If a large piece of tissue has been avulsed away, it should be preserved in an iced plastic bag in case it can be used to repair the defect. The wound itself is treated by obtaining hemostasis and applying a light dressing.

## AMPUTATION

Amputation refers to any injury that cuts off an appendage or projection of the body. If the amputated part can be recovered, it should be saved for possible replantation. It is placed in a plastic bag which is then placed in a container of crushed ice. The amputated part is then carried to the hospital with the patient. Fingers, toes, feet, hands, penis, and scalp have all been saved by restoring the circulation with microvascular anastomoses.

## ULCER

An ulcer is a punched out area that opens either on the body surface or in a body cavity and is accompanied by tissue necrosis and purulent drainage. It does not occur as an acute wound, but is included here to complete the primary categories of classification.

Wounds can also be classified as to whether they are clean or dirty, referring to the amount of dirt and foreign material in the wound; and they can be classified as to whether they are tidy or untidy, referring to clean incised wounds contrasted to ragged irregular wounds with flaps and nonviable tissue.

# SYSTEM REVIEW OF INJURIES

## HEAD AND FACIAL

The face is a common site of injury and over half of the patients with multiple injuries sustain damage to the face. Injuries to the face assume great importance when it is realized that the brain, spinal cord, and airway are all in close proximity. Facial injuries can occur to either the soft tissue, facial skeleton, or a combination of these.

*How Facial Injuries Occur*

*Falls.* Falls are the most common source of injury to the face since so many toddlers and children are involved in tumbles and strike furniture, the floor, tricycles, or other object surfaces. Usually the wounds are small, ragged lacerations of the forehead, scalp, or chin, which do not penetrate deeper than the scalp or subcutaneous tissue. If exceptional force has occurred during the fall (e.g., a fall down a stairway), a spinal cord intracranial injury must be suspected. High impact falls occur from high places (e.g., electrical linemen, mountain climbers, general aviation, riders of large animals [equestrians or ranchers], and in vehicle/pedestrian accidents).

*Dog Bites.* Dog bites of the face are exceedingly common and range in severity from simple lacerations to widespread multiple wounds with extensive tissue loss and facial fractures. Most frequently, the dog bites the central part of the face, damaging the lips, cheeks, and eyelids (Figure 14-3). Avulsion of the skin and subcutaneous tissues is common. Sometimes, the missing segment can be retrieved for possible use in repair.

*Automobile and Motorcycle Accidents.* Automobile and motorcycle accidents may result in serious face and neck injuries as seen in a high percentage of vehicle accidents. The head is usually in the lead as the body is propelled forward and absorbs the first shock on impact. Cervical spine fractures must be ruled out as well as serious injuries elsewhere in the body. Vehicle injuries commonly are high velocity, high impact injuries with a combination of sharp and blunt forces which inflict tremendous violence to the victim. Low impact injuries can also occur after vehicle accidents and result from low speed "fender benders." In this case, the victim's face may penetrate the windshield and he can have multiple facial lacerations without other serious injury.

*Fist Fights.* Blows to the face from fist fighting are usually low impact, blunt injuries. They are characterized by contusions and fractures of the jaw and facial skeleton. The upper airway is also vulnerable to obstruction. Occasionally, a very hard fist blow or a blow augmented with a club, pipe, or gunstock can cause damage comparable to that seen in vehicle accidents.

*Penetrating Injuries.* In a stabbing, the wound of entry gives little suggestion of the serious injuries that may be inflicted along the line of the penetrating wound tract. A moment's study may show whether the assailant was right- or left-handed, and whether the victim was engaged in face-to-face combat or was trying to escape at the instant of injury. Knowledge about the length and size of the weapon is useful. This information will help in the evaluation of the injury. Usually the assailant's weapon travels a downward path, so that structures lower than the wound of entry are at risk. If a long, sharp knife enters the cheek, the carotid artery, jugular vein, esophagus, larynx, and trachea are all exposed to possible injury. If the victim was in a supine position at the instant of injury, a wound of the orbit might connect with the anterior cranial vault and damage the brain.

The possibilities of lethal damage are highest in firearm wounds, as more often than not, this was the expressed intent of the wound, whether inflicted by an assailant or by the victim himself. The bullet from a handgun or a small bore rifle can sometimes traverse the face without causing obvious extensive injury either to the soft tissues or the facial skeleton. However, the shock wave that accompanies the penetration may cause considerable tissue damage in the depths of the wound; a tract that goes near the eyeball or the large vessels may inflict irreparable injury.

A shotgun fired at close range, particularly if it is a large bore, can inflict extensive soft tissue injury. An unsuccessful suicide attempt with a shotgun can cause calamitous destruction to facial tissues. The victim attempts to cause brain injury by placing the muzzle beneath his chin and directing the barrel toward the vertex of the skull. However, because of the distance between the muzzle and the trigger, the victim's hands pull the gunstock toward his body, and the trajectory goes anterior to the cranial vault; thus only the anterior face and jaw are injured. The facial tissues which are in the path of the pellets are devastated. Instability of the mandible and tongue results from loss of the central block of tissue and airway obstruction is a great risk.

*Fractures of the Facial Skeleton.* Facial fractures are a frequent concomitant of facial injuries. The facial skeleton is made up of the following:

Mandible

Maxilla

Zygoma (cheek)

Zygomatic arch

Nasal bones

*Mandible.* The jaw forms a bony arch which is secured at each end in a condylar fossa. A blow which causes a fracture from a direct force often causes a second fracture due to the transmitted force to the opposite side of the arch. A direct fracture of the mandibular body is often coupled with an indirect fracture of the angle, ramus, or condylar neck on the opposite side (Figure 14-4). A direct fracture of the chin may be accompanied by indirect fractures of the condylar necks. This set of three fractures causes an open bite and instability. A segmental fracture (double fracture) of the anterior mandible may permit dangerous

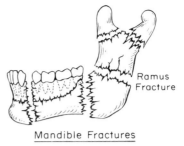

**Figure 14-4.** The mandible can be fractured in many different locations. An alveolar ridge fracture is a linear fracture occurring below the teeth. Mandibular fractures can be diagnosed by palpating the jaw.

Ramus Fracture

Mandible Fractures

mobility of the jaw and tongue. The most common fracture of the jaw and maxilla is a small segmental fracture of the alveolar ridge. These should be identified and protected so that the teeth are not lost and so that the airway is not threatened.

*Maxilla.* The maxilla and adjacent facial bones are extensively hollowed out by the paranasal sinuses, leaving bone that is eggshell thin but buttressed by thick struts. The heaviest bone makes up the maxillary floor, composed of the palatal processes, the nasal floor, and the bone of the alveolar ridge of the maxillary arch.

A direct blow to the lower part of the maxilla detaches the maxillary floor from the rest of the maxilla (Figures 14-5, 14-6). The palate and the maxillary teeth can often be freely moved as a block with finger pressure alone (floating palate). Sometimes the maxillary fragment is impacted posteriorly causing obstruction of the nasal airway and a diminished oral airway.

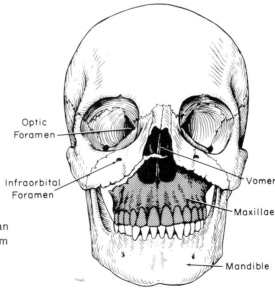

Optic Foramen

Infraorbital Foramen

Vomer

Maxillae

Mandible

**Figure 14-5.** The maxilla can be completely detached from its moorings. A free-floating maxilla can obstruct the airway.

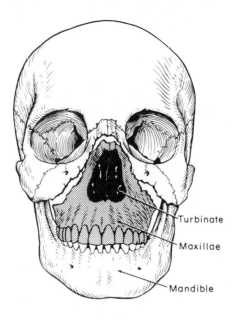

Turbinate

Maxillae

Mandible

**Figure 14-6.** Maxillary fractures can include detachment of portions of the nasal bone.

In some instances the entire maxilla, the nasal bones, and the cheek bones stay together as a block, and are detached from the skull by the force of injury (Figure 14-7). The roofs of the orbits and the roof of the nasal cavity remain with the skull, so the orbits and nose are elongated vertically. The airway implications are the same as with the other maxillary fractures.

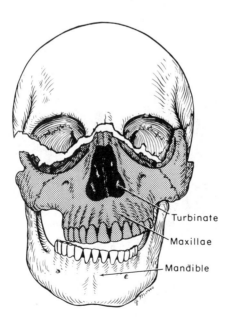

Turbinate

Maxillae

Mandible

**Figure 14-7.** The entire nasal bone, maxilla, zygoma, and floor of the orbit can be detached.

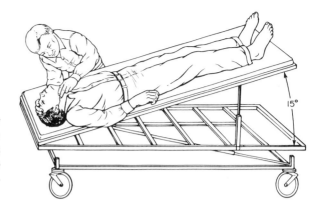

**Figure 14-8.** Patients with a neck injury should be transported with the head down and the feet elevated. This will raise venous pressure and prevent air from entering the veins. The wound must be directly compressed to prevent bleeding.

*Zygoma (Cheek) Body Fracture.* A direct blow to the body of the zygoma causes the thin supporting bone of the maxillary antral wall and the orbital floor to collapse. The zygoma body itself stays intact, but is depressed, causing asymmetry of the face. As an isolated fracture, this most commonly occurs from a fist blow, from contact sports, and from blunt objects. The fracture line goes through the inferior orbital rim near the exit of the infraorbital nerve, and usually numbness of the cheek and upper lip are present.

*Zygomatic Arch Fracture.* The zygomatic arch is a thin arch of bone that connects the body of the zygoma to the root of the zygoma as it arches over the coronoid process (Chapter 4). A direct blow to the posterior cheek or temple can break this arch and cause inward displacement. The depressed segment of the arch can impact against the coronoid process of the mandible, preventing the patient from fully opening his mouth. If quick access is needed to the oral cavity, a firm pull downward and forward on the mandible can effectively dislodge the depressed arch sufficiently to permit free mandibular movement. Pain at the site of the fracture will be experienced during this maneuver.

*Nose.* Nasal fractures are the commonest fractures and they range from a minimal undisplaced crack due to a low force blow to a complete shattering of the nasal bones. Bleeding from the nose and into the airway can sometimes be profuse. In cases of great violence, the medial orbital skeleton is broken in addition to the nasal bones. The medial canthal ligaments that give medial attachment to the eyelids may pull loose from their moorings and cause eyelid deformities. The ethmoid sinuses may be badly disrupted and hemorrhage can result. Cribriform plate fractures with cerebral spinal fluid leak are an extension of this pattern (Chapter 4).

*Injuries to Other Facial Structures.* Facial nerve paralysis can result from injuries within the cranial vault, within the temporal bone (basal skull fracture), or along the peripheral pathway of the facial nerve.

*383*

Deep stab wounds or cuts from glass fragments commonly transect branches of the facial nerve.

The patient should be asked to move the facial muscles group by group starting with the frontalis ("Raise your eyebrows"), and working downward to the depressors of the lower lip ("Pout out your lower lip"). The presence of good function right after an injury is an important finding. If paralysis then comes on a day or two after, it can be attributed to edema, and the return of function can be anticipated.

The infraorbital nerves are the most commonly affected sensory nerves in facial injuries. The nerves are a branch of the fifth trigeminal nerve (Chapter 4). Fractures of the zygoma, the maxilla, or the naso-orbital area all pass through or near the infraorbital foramen, causing contusion to the nerve. The examiner will find numbness of the cheek, the upper lip, the lower eyelid and the side of the nose with this injury. The supraorbital and supratrochlear nerves are often transected in deep lacerations of the forehead, causing sensory loss of the forehead and scalp above the laceration.

*Injuries to the Mouth.* If the patient is conscious and can open his mouth, a jaw fracture is probably not present. If he cannot open his mouth and has difficulty breathing through his nose, a jaw fracture is likely. Palpation along the lower rim of the mandible and the temporomandibular joint may indicate a fracture of the mandible. Pain and swelling over the fracture site would be present. The zygomatic arch should be palpated, since if it has collapsed inwardly, it may impinge on the coronary process of the mandible locking the jaw. Inward and outward traction will unhinge this and allow the patient to open his mouth. If the patient is unconscious, the examination should begin by opening the jaw and pulling downward and outward. The jaw can be opened by grabbing the chin or lower teeth and then grasping the tongue and pulling it forward. This would reveal any mandibular instability and also allow for inspection of the mouth for loose teeth, dentures, food, or foreign bodies. The patient should be placed in the left lateral decubitus position partially forward so that his jaw and tongue hang forward and any blood or debris can pour outward. An oral airway should be inserted if the patient is unconscious and the jaw fracture extensive.

The upper portion of the jaw is the maxilla, and fracture to this can be appreciated by grasping the upper teeth or upper alveolar ridge and rocking it back and forth. If it is unstable, a maxillary fracture in any of the ways previously mentioned can be suspected. Again, protecting the oral airway is of primary importance.

*Injuries to the Forehead.* The forehead is frequently damaged in windshield accidents resulting in multiple upward cuts. Glass fragments are frequently found in the debris of the wound. If the patient has been knocked unconscious during the accident, suspect that the forehead injury may have been caused by a higher impact object than the windshield and be suspicious of a fracture or intracranial bleeding. Forehead lacerations that are bleeding profusely are best treated with a circular compressive dressing.

*Injuries to the Eyelids and Periorbital Region.*   Suspect possible injury to the eyeball, extraocular muscles, or levator of the eyelid and treat the patient accordingly. Avoid pressure to the globe and remove any glass that is still found in the wound. The eye can best be assessed by having the conscious patient open his eyes on command (see section on eye injuries).

*Injuries to the Nose and Lip.*   Suspect nasal fractures in the presence of nasal lacerations. If the nose has been pushed inward, do not attempt to pull back on it, since this may produce profuse bleeding from the base of the brain. If the lip is lacerated, it may be bleeding profusely and is best controlled by digital pressure on the labial artery at the corners of the mouth.

*Injuries to the Chin.*   A wound of the chin from a direct blow or from a fall may be associated with jaw fractures. It may also be associated with laryngeal fractures.

*Injuries to the Ear.*   Preserve detached segments of the ear and lay the flaps out in correct orientation so that the nourishing vessels will not be kinked and the skin will survive.

## NECK INJURIES

The neck is composed of two triangles, the anterior and posterior (Chapter 4). Although the cervical spine is theoretically part of the neck, it will be discussed in a separate section. Neck injuries can be caused from blunt or penetrating objects. The larynx and trachea span the middle of the anterior triangle of the neck. The larynx and trachea can be injured as a result of direct blunt force (most commonly the steering wheel of an automobile), by choking, or by strangulation, as in hanging. The patient may present with only pain to total airway obstruction. The blunt force may be violent enough to completely transect the trachea and separate it from the larynx:

> **Example:** A 26-year-old female driving 40 mph struck a bridge abutment. She was not wearing a seat belt or shoulder strap and struck her forehead on the windshield. Upon examination at the scene, she was found to be bleeding from a forehead laceration and was coughing blood. There was no obvious jaw fracture and the patient appeared to have difficulty on expiration. Palpation revealed a depression between the cricoid and trachea. There was

also crepitus in the area. This information was radioed to the base station and upon arrival at the Emergency Department, the patient was experiencing obvious respiratory difficulty. A diagnosis of a fractured trachea was made. She was taken immediately to the operating room where neck exploration showed the trachea to be completely separated from the larynx. It was resutured and a tracheostomy was placed below. The patient made an uneventful recovery.

Fractures of the trachea and larynx due to blunt injury are often not diagnosed. This diagnosis should be considered with any upper airway obstruction following blunt injury. Physical examination will reveal swelling, crepitus, and depressions or protrusions over the normal landmarks of the larynx. If total laryngeal crush has occurred and airway obstruction is complete, a cricothyrotomy (see Chapter 9) at the scene may be indicated.

Penetrating injuries to the trachea and larynx can occur from knives or bullets. Swelling due to hemorrhage may compress the trachea and cause partial to complete obstruction. The trachea itself may be exposed to the external environment by the loss of skin and tissue over it when the wounding agent is a shotgun. Field treatment of these injuries would include direct compression to stop hemorrhage and rapid transport. In hematomas of the neck, the physician will not do a tracheostomy if there is airway obstruction, but will insert an endotracheal tube upon arrival at the Emergency Department. Incision in the neck may release bleeding that cannot be controlled in the Emergency Department. Also included in the anterior triangle of the neck are the carotid arteries and the jugular vein. Both of these may be lacerated by penetrating injuries to the neck. Direct compression to stop bleeding and transport is the treatment of choice. If lacerations of the jugular vein are suspected, it is imperative that the compression be occlusive to prevent air from entering the vein and causing an air embolism. This can be minimized by having the patient transported with the head down slightly and the feet elevated (Figure 14-8).

Injuries to the posterior triangle of the neck may injure the brachial plexus, the external jugular vein, the subclavian artery or vein, and nick the top of the lung. Injuries to the subclavian artery or vein are best treated by direct compression and pushing the shoulder down to press the clavicle onto the artery or vein. No immediate treatment is necessary for a brachial plexus injury. Any penetrating wound of the posterior triangle should alert the examiner to the possibility of a tension pneumothorax since the apex of the lung often enters this space.

## EYE INJURIES

The three principal types of eye injuries encountered by the paramedic are due to:

Trauma, blunt and penetrating blows

Burns

Foreign bodies, including chemicals

The kind of emergency care that is given depends on the nature of the injury. This makes it essential to determine, by history and by careful observation, what actually occurred. Life or death matters should be cared for first; but after the patient is out of danger, the injured eye should receive immediate attention. Of the three categories of trauma listed above, chemical injury requires the fastest action to avoid permanent damage (see below).

*Physical Examination.* The examination of the injured eye should be performed with the utmost gentleness. In the case of suspected ocular perforation, it is better not to examine the eye than to cause additional damage by improper examination. If the patient can voluntarily open the eyes, so much the better. If not, elevation of the upper lid may be accomplished by either: (1) sliding the lid upward against the superior orbital rim with the thumb, with care to avoid pressure on the globe, or (2) grasping the upper eyelashes between thumb and forefinger. Cotton-tipped applicators may also be used to expose the globe (Figure 14-9).

A penlight or small flashlight is of great assistance in evaluating an injured eye. As the lid is elevated, the light should be directed at the eye from the temporal side, across the anterior chamber toward the nose. A bright light directed at an injured eye from the front can increase discomfort, producing withdrawal. The presence of foreign bodies in the cornea, the state of conjunctiva and cornea, and the presence of blood in the anterior chamber can be satisfactorily determined by this method.

It is wise, whenever possible, to determine and record the approximate visual acuity of each eye separately (with glasses if the patient wears them), using some standard print reading material. Newsprint

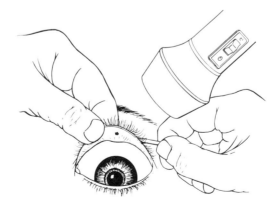

**Figure 14-9.** A foreign body is shown in the upper eyelid. Eversion of the eyelid in this fashion is a very useful procedure for examining the surface of the eyelid.

or a magazine is convenient for this purpose. This information will be of help to the Emergency Department physician. Some injuries will be too severe to allow for this evaluation.

*Trauma.*    Direct trauma to the eye can occur as a result of automobile accidents, fights, athletic activities, and a variety of industrial circumstances. Trauma may be penetrating, causing laceration or tearing of lids and globe; or blunt, producing contusion of the lids and surrounding tissues as well as bleeding or inflammation within the eye.

*Penetrating Trauma.*    If glass, metal, wood, or a gunshot are involved in the circumstances of the accident, the globe may have been ruptured and be in danger of extruding its contents (Figure 14-10). There may or may not be associated lacerations of the eyelids. There may be no external evidence that the globe has been penetrated. The eye is usually painful, although the degree of pain is variable. Even in the presence of a through-and-through laceration of the globe, vision may be surprisingly good.

*Treatment*

1. If it is suspected that the globe has been ruptured, the patient should be kept in a recumbent position if possible, with the head slightly elevated. He will be probably be more comfortable with the eyes gently closed, but active squeezing of the lids or straining should be avoided. These precautions are taken to minimize the possibility that the ocular contents will be forced out through the wound in the globe, with permanent loss of vision. If a foreign body is seen to be penetrating the globe, it is often best to leave it in place, as it may be serving as a plug to prevent loss of ocular contents.

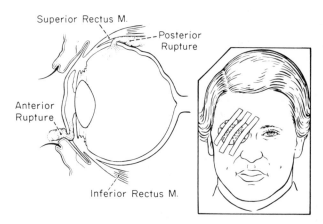

**Figure 14-10.** A ruptured globe is an ophthalmologic emergency. The eye must be patched and the patient kept as quiet as possible during transport.

2. No medications or fluids of any kind should be placed into an eye suspected of having sustained a penetrating injury, as these substances may enter the eye and cause irreparable damage to the retina and other structures. A sterile gauze square, moistened with sterile saline may be laid gently over the eye. No pressure should be placed on the eye, and unnecessary manipulation of the eyelids should be avoided.

3. A metal or plastic shield should be taped over the injured eye for protection (Figure 14-10). If these are not available, a paper cup can be used as a shield. A ruptured globe requires the attention of an ophthalmologist as soon as possible, for it is a true ophthalmic emergency.

4. Lid lacerations simply require light bandaging with a sterile eye pad, after removal of any large foreign bodies. No attempt should be made to stop bleeding of the lids with a pressure bandage, because of possible serious damage to the underlying globe. Bleeding, while copious at first, will generally stop spontaneously. Pressure bandages, in general, should be avoided in the presence of an injured eye, until an ophthalmologist has made certain that all foreign bodies lying beneath the lids (in the conjunctival sac) have been removed.

5. It is best to leave detailed examination and determination of visual acuity, if difficult, to the Emergency Department physician or ophthalmologist. The physician will determine the extent of injury. Possible damage from penetrating blows include laceration of the cornea, conjunctiva, sclera, choroid, and retina, all of which usually require surgical repair. Better visual results are obtained when surgery can be performed as soon as possible after the injury.

*Blunt Trauma.* Tennis, racquetball, squash and golf balls, fists, fingers, bottle corks, and other relatively large objects may cause internal damage to the eye as well as abrasion and bruising of the surrounding tissues. If the cornea has been abraded, there may be severe pain. Vision may be markedly decreased, either because of corneal damage or because of bleeding within the eye. Corneal trauma generally causes severe pain even in the absence of internal damage to the eye. For example, wearing contact lenses for too many hours (generally more than twelve), or falling asleep with them in place, can cause extreme pain because of roughening of the corneal surface. Corneal abrasions often do not cause permanent decrease of vision, but should still be treated by a physician because of the danger of secondary infection. Treatment generally consists of topical antibiotics and firm patching of both eyes for twenty-four hours or so. The dispensing of a topical anesthetic to alleviate pain is a serious error, and should never be done. Chronic use of such an agent can lead to permanent blindness.

Blunt trauma can cause serious internal damage to the eye. This may include hemorrhage into either the anterior chamber (hyphema), or into the vitreous cavity (Figure 14-11). It may rupture the iris, pulling

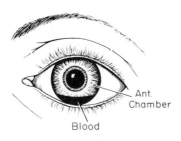

Ant.
Chamber

Blood

**Figure 14-11.** Hyphema is blood in the anterior chamber between the iris and the cornea. This represents a serious intraocular injury and must be evaluated by an ophthalmologist.

it away from its peripheral attachments and causing an irregular pupil. The lens can be dislocated into the anterior or posterior chamber. Bleeding can occur beneath the retina, and there may be edema, or swelling of the retina. Hemorrhage into the vitreous chamber may accompany the tearing of retinal vessels and retinal detachment. A severe enough blow to the eye, even with a blunt object, can cause rupture of the globe.

Blunt force to the eye area may result in contusion to the muscles surrounding the eye, and hemorrhage into loose orbital tissues behind the globe. Both of these may result in decreased movement of the eye in any or all directions. A forceful blow may cause fracture of facial bones, including the orbital rim and the floor of the orbit. A fracture of the orbital rim may be suspected if exquisite point tenderness is present along the bony ridge above or below the eye, or discontinuity in the curve of the rim is felt with the fingertip. A fracture of the orbital floor may cause the eye to appear smaller than the opposite eye, or sunken, or displaced downward. Such fractures may entrap orbital tissues and extraocular muscles (muscles that control movement of the eye), limiting the freedom of movement of the globe. Often, this is manifested by an inability to turn the eye upward.

*Treatment*

1. If blunt injury to the eye occurs in the absence of chemical substances, no immediate measures need be taken other than taping a sterile eye pad in place (Figure 14-10).

2. Although blunt injuries to the eye require evaluation by a physician, they do not require the same urgency of action as does a perforated globe.

*Burns.* Burns caused by flame, electricity, ultraviolet light, and even the so-called "snow burn" are painful because of damage to the corneal surface and in some cases to the conjunctiva as well. The patient will be more comfortable with both eyes closed and, if possible, patched to minimize movement of the lids over the damaged corneas. Even if only one eye is so injured, patching the opposite eye as well tends to decrease movement of both eyes and eyelids, increasing comfort. Leading an ambulatory, bilaterally patched patient must be done with care, lest a broken ankle be added to the list of injuries!

These injuries should be cared for by a physician, who will generally instill antibiotics to prevent secondary infection, watch for and treat developing scar tissue between lids and globe, and may patch firmly to assist healing of the cornea.

*Foreign Bodies, Including Chemicals.* Foreign bodies of any sort can be extremely irritating to the eye and can cause varying degrees of ocular injury. Foreign objects removed from the eye include cilia (eyelashes), dirt, metal, glass, wood, bee stingers, chunks of lye, and eggshell. These substances may become lodged within the corneal tissue or hidden by the eyelids. Drawing upper and lower lids away from the globe and asking the patient to look in the opposite direction may reveal the offending objects. Everting the upper lid may be of great assistance, but should only be done by one experienced in lid eversion, and only after there is reasonable certainty that the globe has not been ruptured (Figure 14-9).

The cornea is very much more sensitive than the conjunctiva, so if the foreign matter can be moved into the lower cul-de-sac or to one side of the cornea, it can usually be removed without much discomfort to the patient. A good method of doing this is by touching the object lightly, or lifting it, with a sterile cotton-tipped applicator.

If a foreign body is seen to be lodged in the cornea, it will probably require removal by an ophthalmologist or an experienced Emergency Department physician. Keeping the lids lightly closed may increase patient comfort in the meantime.

Foreign substances of greatest potential harm to the eye include acids and alkaline chemicals (bases).

*Acids.* Battery acid and other common acidic substances create immediate damage to the superficial structures of the eye by producing a chemical burn. This kind of injury should be treated by immediate and thorough flushing of the eye with water, or preferably, a balanced salt solution (Figure 14-12). An attempt should be made to flush underneath the lids (see method of elevating lids, above) to counteract pools of acid in these areas. Several liters of fluid should be used. The patient may then be transported for medical attention. The eyes need not be patched, although the patient will probably be more comfortable with the eyes closed.

*Bases.* Alkaline substances are potentially much more damaging to the eye than acidic ones because of their ability to penetrate the coats of the eye and gain access to delicate inner structures. Immediate lavage is called for (as above), but in the case of alkaline chemicals, it should be carried out for twenty to thirty minutes without interruption (Figure 14-12). Only after prolonged rinsing of the eye should the patient be transported. Patching is not necessary, but may be done for comfort.

Medical attention in the case of injury with both acids and bases includes topical antibiotics and patching of the eyes. In the case of

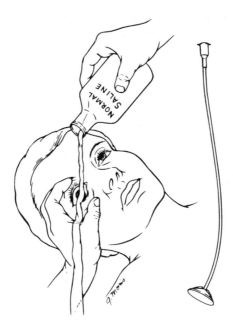

**Figure 14-12.** Caustic burns of the eye are initially treated in the field by copious irrigation with normal saline or Lactated Ringer's solution. The involved eye should be in the dependent position to prevent cross-contamination of the other eye during irrigation. A cup is now available which can be placed directly on the globe and connected to an intravenous line to maintain continuous irrigation.

alkaline injury, it sometimes also includes treatment of damage to the inner eye with anti-inflammatory eye drops and prevention of scar formation between the iris and lens with drops that dilate the pupil. Improper or incomplete attention to alkaline injuries can result in blindness.

## NERVOUS SYSTEM INJURIES (INCLUDING CENTRAL NERVOUS SYSTEM AND HEAD INJURIES)

Because the central nervous system (brain and spinal cord) is protected by the skull and the spine, a significant injury is required to damage it. Closed or nonpenetrating trauma is the most common mechanism of injury to the brain or spinal cord. The brain is a complex structure which receives, stores, interprets, and sends messages. It is this very complexity which makes full functional recovery from injury slow and incomplete. The brain has a high oxygen demand and is very sensitive to hypoxia. It is imperative, therefore, that diagnosis and treatment be completed early to prevent progressive damage. Treatment of head injuries in the field involves maintaining the airway and breathing, supporting the circulation, and protecting the spinal cord.

### Head Injuries

*Scalp Lacerations.* Scalp lacerations are by far the most common injury to the head. The scalp is enormously endowed with blood vessels which can bleed profusely but rarely to the point of producing hemorrhagic shock and death. Minor scalp lacerations may be associated with a major skull fracture or brain injury. On the other hand, complete avulsion of the scalp may be associated with no skull or intracranial injury.

*Treatment*

1. Most scalp lacerations do not require a dressing or further treatment but can be managed at the base station.

2. Large scalp lacerations with bleeding should be managed with a dressing and wrapped for compression.

3. Flaps that have been raised should be returned to their anatomical position and wrapped with a compression dressing.

*Skull Fractures.* Skull fractures can occur with or without scalp lacerations. Many skull fractures are radiologic curiosities and result in no appreciable harm to the patient. A skull fracture, however, does indicate severe trauma to the head. Skull fractures are classified the same as other fractures in the body:

1. Compound (open bone fragments)
2. Comminuted (multiple fragments)
3. Linear
4. Depressed

Compound fractures are potentially more serious since bone is exposed. Depressed fractures may impinge and damage brain tissue.

Another type of skull fracture that may not be visualized by X-ray is the basal skull fracture. These fractures are divided into anterior, middle, and posterior fossa fractures. The posterior fossa basal skull fracture usually produces a hematoma (Battle's sign) behind the ear. A middle fossa brain skull fracture may present with blood-tinged fluid leaking from the ear. This can be confirmed by testing the fluid with a Dextrostix® for glucose (positive in the presence of CSF) or having the fluid drop on a paper towel and watching the clear ring spread from the central portion of blood. This is called the ring test and means cerebrospinal fluid is leaking with the blood. An anterior basal skull fracture may present with clear cerebral spinal fluid or thin bloody fluid leaking from the nose. An anterior fossa basal skull fracture also may present days later with periorbital hematomas and subconjunctival hemorrhages or the so-called "owl's eye" sign. Although these injuries may not produce serious injuries to the brain directly, they are important because bacteria can contaminate the meninges (meningitis) through the cracks in the bone and cause a serious spreading infection to the brain.

*Treatment*

1. Maintain airway and breathing.

2. For open fractures of the skull or exposed brain tissues, sterile, light, compression dressings are in order.

3. If a skull fracture is suspected, the patient must be transported with careful observation of the vital signs and airway.

4. Cerebrospinal fluid leaks are best managed by a sterile dressing over the ear. Avoid insertion of catheters through the nose if an anterior basal skull fracture is suspected.

5. Avoid overadministration of intravenous fluids. If only a head injury is suspected and an intravenous solution is indicated, infuse Lactated Ringer's through a microdrip chamber.

*Intracranial Injury.* By far the most common cause of intracranial injury is that done by the motorcycle or the car. Striking the head on the windshield, top of the car, pavement, or other moving objects applies tremendous force to the head. Other causes of brain injury are gunshot wounds to the head, blows to the head with blunt objects such as baseball bats and baseballs, and stab wounds which enter the eye and pass up to the brain. About 60 percent of all injuries due to traffic accidents involve the head, and in fatal accidents the percentage is 70 percent. In two-thirds of these total cases, the injuries to the head are the cause of death. In head autopsies following head injury, about 30 to 50 percent of patients have an intracranial hemorrhage. If an individual is comatose after an accident, there is an estimated 50 percent chance of intracranial hemorrhage with or without brain damage.

*Types of Injuries.* The types of injury to the brain tissue are classified as follows: (a) concussion, (b) cerebral contusion, and (c) brain laceration.

A concussion is due to a blow on the head. A concussion can be defined as an altered state of consciousness. At present, any head injury without a loss of consciousness and only a brief period of mental confusion is referred to as a mild concussion. The terms "moderate" or "severe" concussion imply a longer period of unconsciousness. In a cerebral concussion, there is little or no demonstrable permanent pathologic damage to the brain.

Structural damage to the brain following injury is called a contusion. Contusions may occur along the base of the frontal lobes or at the tips of the adjacent temporal lobes. There may be injuries to the surface vessels to the brain and/or injuries to the deep structures of the brain.

The brain can be lacerated at any point of substantial force or any point opposite to the point of force (contrecoup). This may produce intracranial bleeding.

*Bleeding After Head Injury.* Following any type of head injury, bleeding can occur between the skull and meninges. This bleeding constitutes an emergency since the patient may deteriorate rapidly because the bleeding is arterial. This bleeding is classified by the layer of the brain in which it occurs. They are: (a) epidural hematoma, (b) subdural hematoma, and (c) subarachnoid hemorrhage.

The middle meningeal artery, which is the major artery to the dura (Chapter 3), enters at the middle portion of the skull in front of the ear and crosses the dura. Fractures of the temporal bone or in the temporal area may transect this artery producing bleeding between the dura and the skull itself. This type of injury can be deceptive because the patient can have an injury followed by a lucid interval and then sudden deterioration of his neurologic signs. This can be particularly deceptive at the roadside and may lull the paramedic into delays in transport. Any laceration or obvious skull fracture anterior and superior to the ear should make one suspicious of an epidural hematoma.

A subdural hematoma is bleeding between the dura and the arachnoid membrane (Figure 14-13). An acute subdural hematoma carries a high death rate. Reduction of mortality can only be achieved by maintenance of the airway and circulation, and rapid transport. A subdural hematoma may not be recognized immediately following injury and slowly progresses. Neurologic changes may not be recognized for two to three days, or even months after the injury.

Subarachnoid hemorrhage is bleeding into the subarachnoid space, which may occur after trauma or after rupture of a cerebral aneurysm. Management of a subarachnoid hemorrhage is no different than the management of other types of brain injuries.

*Signs and Symptoms of Increased Intracranial Pressure.* Intracranial injuries can produce a sequence of neurologic changes which must be understood by the paramedic. The paramedic may encounter the patient any time during the course of his intracranial problem and will

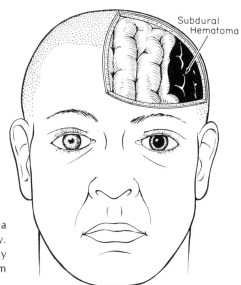

Subdural
Hematoma

**Figure 14-13.** A subdural hematoma occurs following serious head injury. The formation of a blood clot may cause compression of the brainstem and unilateral pupil dilation.

have to assess the direction of neurologic changes. It is for this reason that serial evaluations of the patient are so critical in injuries to the nervous system and evaluation begins in the field.

Following a cranial injury in which intracranial structures have been damaged, intracranial pressure may rise due to bleeding or swelling of the brain itself. The patient may initially complain of headache and dizziness and fainting upon trying to sit up or stand. As intracranial pressure rises in the adult, he may begin vomiting. In a child, vomiting is a nonspecific sign and does not mean that a serious brain injury has occurred. As intracranial pressure increases, a portion of the temporal lobes migrates toward the brainstem. The temporal lobes are then pushed onto the brainstem. This causes partial loss of consciousness. While this is occurring, the patient may experience personality changes as there may be cerebral hypoxia due to restricted blood flow to certain areas of the brain. The patient may also appear to be irrational, overdosed on drugs, or intoxicated. It is incorrect to assume that the latter situation exists since serious intracranial injury will be overlooked. As the patient passes from the irrational stage to the comatose stage, there will be changes in his pupils, breathing pattern, response to pain, and motor function. The progression of the temporal lobe pressure on the brainstem is manifested by a dilatation of one or both pupils. This dilation is caused by compression of the third nerve which supplies the pupil. As pressure increases, both pupils may dilate and become nonreactive to light as the occipital cortex becomes anoxic and unable to respond to a light stimulus. The blood pressure becomes elevated because the swelling has become so severe that arterial perfusion to the brain tissue is compromised. The body responds to this by raising the arterial pressure (Cushing's phenomenon) in an attempt to pump blood into the brain through an obstruction. The slowing of the pulse is a vagal reflex as a result of compression of the brain. These latter vital sign changes are a very late manifestation of increased intracranial pressure and one should not await them to diagnose intracranial problems.

The paramedic must always be looking for changes in neurological signs due to a mass lesion within the skull. Increases in intracranial pressure due to bleeding or destruction of brain tissue can cause brainstem compression and sudden deterioration in the patient's status. The paramedic must be alert for changing neurologic signs which may indicate increasing intracranial pressure.

*Evaluation of Brain Injury.* Field evaluation of the brain injured patient can by no means be complete. It is therefore important to develop an orderly neurologic examination which will give the most information in the briefest period of time. This neurologic examination may be repeated frequently to assess the progress of the neurologic deficit. The four physiologic events to observe are as follows:

Breathing
Response to stimuli
Pupil signs
Motor response

*Breathing.* The type of respiration can be helpful in assessing the depth of coma in a brain injured patient. Normal respirations are commonly noted in a very light stage of coma. Cheyne-Stokes respiration is a form of breathing characterized by shallow inspiration and expiration which gradually increases in rate and depth, then suddenly stops. After a pause this breathing pattern then repeats itself. This respiration is noted in brain injuries involving the upper diencephalon to the upper pons (Chapter 4). Brain injuries to the more caudal portions of the brainstem are more serious and these may be exhibited by evidence of central neurogenic hyperventilation. This form of respiration is characterized by rapid, deep, regular respirations. This is often seen in decerebrate states and implies midbrain or pons dysfunction. Almost any form of respiration can be seen with more severe brainstem injuries including apnea, Cheyne-Stokes breathing, ataxic form of respiration, and apneustic (jerky) respirations; and even occasional normal respiratory states can be seen with very severe brainstem injuries.

*Response to Stimuli.* The patient is evaluated by his response to pain or verbal stimuli. If response to painful stimuli is used the best motor response is recorded. This describes a patient's movement and ability and is graded as follows: (1) follows command, (2) localizes painful stimuli, (3) responds with abnormal flexion to painful stimuli (flexion of one or both upper extremities, formerly decorticate), (4) responds with abnormal extension to pain (formerly decerebrate), and (5) gives no motor response. When a patient is comatose and cannot respond to commands, painful stimuli are used. Painful stimuli can be produced by squeezing the trapezius muscle in the neck, pushing on the sternum by sliding down it with the knuckles, and grabbing the anterior compartment of the calf and squeezing. A familiar in-hospital way of testing painful sensation is squeezing the nipple. This should not be done in the field since people will be observing, especially if the patient is female. If the response to a painful stimulus is to try and wipe away the examiner's hand, this indicates a fairly light state of coma. It also informs the examiner that at the time of examination, the injury was no lower than the rostral diencephalon (Chapter 4).

The deeper state of coma is indicated by a decorticate response to pain. The response is exemplified by flexion of the arms at the elbow and straightening of the legs. The decorticate or flexion response to pain implies a somewhat more serious injury to the brainstem. Usually, this injury is mid-upper brain or lower diencephalon. A more serious form of response to pain is a "decerebrate" response to pain. This pain response involves straightening and hyperpronating the arms as well as extending the legs and possibly the back. It is simpler to remember that the two responses are either (1) flexion or (2) extension. Extension is worse, and it indicates midbrain and upper pons level injury. The most serious response to pain is no response at all and this may be seen in very severe brain injury patients in which the injuries include lower pons and medullary areas. These patients are unlikely to recover.

The best verbal response documents the ability to speak as well as the speech content: (1) answer is appropriate; (2) gives confused answers; (3) makes unintelligible noises; (4) makes no verbal response. In each case, the best response is recorded even if a painful stimulus is required to elicit the response.

Another method to evaluate the level of consciousness is recording eye opening by the required stimulus: (1) spontaneous eye opening, (2) eye opening on command, (3) eye opening to shaking, (4) eye opening to painful stimulus, and (5) no eye opening. The preceding responses give a sensitive and reproducible measure of the patient's neurologic state and supplement the other assessments.

*Pupil Response.* As mentioned previously, as brain swelling occurs, herniation of the temporal lobe at the base of the brain compresses the third nerve which carries the parasympathetic fibers to the pupil. The nerve that is compressed may be on the same or opposite side of the injury. A small degree of pupil inequality is present in many people normally. However, any obvious pupil inequality should be noted. The pupil should also be tested for its response to light stimulation. In broad daylight this can be done by closing the eyelid and rapidly opening one or both eyelids. Normally, pupils react readily and symmetrically by constriction of pupillary dilation in the presence of a bright light. At the other end of the spectrum, when a brainstem is severely injured, the pupils are large and unresponsive to light implying medullary damage and a terminal state (Figure 14-14). Between these two extremes there are intermediate changes that can occur. At the level of the pons, for example, the pupils may be pinpoint in size and unresponsive to light. At the midbrain level, small parts of the reactive pupil may be seen. And, finally, if there is unilateral temporal lobe herniation, a complete third nerve pause of the large unreactive pupil or dilating pupil may be seen (Figure 14-14).

*Motor Response.* The motor response is part of the physical examination since, if the patient is awake, it is necessary to detect weakness in the motor response. This is particularly true in evaluating evolving brain lesions or possible injury to the spinal cord. The motor response is gained by having the patient squeeze the examiner's hands one at a time, and then by dorsiflexing both feet and pushing them down against the examiner's hand. This will assess the strength of

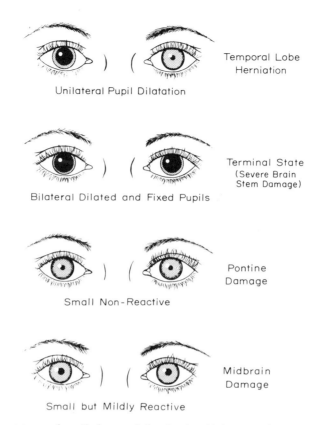

Unilateral Pupil Dilatation — Temporal Lobe Herniation

Bilateral Dilated and Fixed Pupils — Terminal State (Severe Brain Stem Damage)

Small Non-Reactive — Pontine Damage

Small but Mildly Reactive — Midbrain Damage

**Figure 14-14.** The different types of pupil changes following head injury are shown.

movement, whether movement is present, and also aid in subsequent examination to see if the strength is changing.

### Treatment of Central Nervous System Injury

1. Treatment initially need not be involved and complicated. Maintenance of the airway is of primary importance. If the patient is comatose, then an oral airway or an oroesophageal airway is necessary to prevent aspiration of secretions and to promote adequate ventilation. The comatose head-injured patient should be treated with hyperventilation. Reduction in carbon dioxide produces vasoconstriction of cerebral vessels, retarding cerebral edema by altering blood flow. Hyperventilation by itself will also reduce the size of brain tissue.

2. With isolated head injuries, starting intravenous fluids may not be necessary and might be a waste of time in the field. Overhydration and its effect on brain swelling should be avoided. However, if shock is present, it must be treated by infusion of intravenous fluids, application of the MAST suit, and/or rapid transport. Lactated Ringer's is the solution of choice.

3. All head injury patients should be suspected of having a neck fracture also, and the spine should be supported.

4. Significant bleeding from scalp or head wounds should be controlled by direct pressure or compression bandages.

5. A quick but careful neurologic assessment will help the hospital physician determine in which direction the patient's neurologic picture is changing. This information can be radioed ahead or directly transmitted to the physician.

6. Mannitol and corticosteroids have been used for head injury patients to reduce cerebral edema. Their use is controversial. They may mask neurologic changes and present only transient improvement of the patient having definitive therapy. We have used intravenous dexamethasone (Chapter 6) in the field for the past year. Forty milligrams of dexamethasone is given intravenously after establishment of an IV. Although it is controversial whether early administration of dexamethasone is of any benefit, it cannot harm the patient as long as there is no delay in starting an intravenous and giving the medication. Mannitol and steroids are used to control cerebral swelling in the head trauma patient during or following surgical procedures, or during observation in the Intensive Care Unit at the hospital.

7. All other significant injuries should be treated in transport. Fractures should be splinted, hemorrhage controlled, and vital signs monitored.

*Spinal Cord Injury.* Injury to the spinal cord occurs most commonly after automobile accidents, swimming pool or ocean diving accidents, and penetrating injuries to the neck or thoracic spine. Other causes are falls from heights, including telephone lines, horses, buildings, or falls down stairways.

*Mechanisms of Injury.* In general, there are five mechanisms of injury:

1. Flexion injuries—the chin is flexed downward on the chest causing wedging of the body of the vertebrae and fracture dislocation or forward dislocation (Figure 14-15).

2. Rotation with flexion—the head is rotated and flexed at the same time causing a spiraling fracture of the vertebrae.

3. Vertical compression—straight on the vertex with compression fracture and cord compression.

4. Lateral flexion—a wedge fracture of a vertebral body and cord compression.

5. Hyperextension—the result of diving into a swimming pool.

Spinal injuries damage neurostructures by encroaching upon the spinal canal and intervertebral foramen (Figure 14-16). Neurologic involvement ranges from mild and transient to severe and permanent.

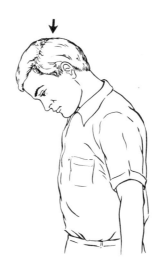

**Figure 14-15.** Direct downward force, such as in a fall on the occiput, will cause fractures at the C-5 and C-6 levels of the spinal column.

*Clinical Findings.* Spinal cord injury may not be apparent upon initial examination by the paramedic, particularly in patients sustaining other more obvious injuries. However, spinal injuries should be considered in the presence of the following findings: (1) all acute injuries to the head and jaw, (2) pain in the occiput spine or limbs, (3) weakness of one or more limbs, (4) spinal deformity, (5) paralysis of accessory muscles of respiration with diaphragmatic breathing, and (6) manifestation of "spinal cord shock" such as priapism (an erected penis), hypo- or hyperthermia, and low blood pressure.

*Physical Examination.* When encountering a patient with a suspected spinal cord injury, the physical examination can be brief yet complete. It should begin with palpation of the cervical spine for a local deformity or tenderness. If the patient's airway is compromised and the head is totally flexed, the head can be straightened with gradual traction, as long as traction is maintained on the head. The airway must be maintained either by an oral airway or insertion of an oroesophageal airway. Mouth-to-mouth resuscitation must be done by the chin lift

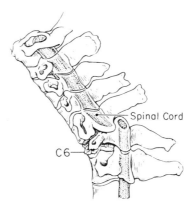

**Figure 14-16.** In cervical fractures, the displacement of the cervical spine of one spine following collapse of another may transect the spinal cord.

technique (Chapter 9). Motor sensation can be appreciated by having the patient grasp the examiner's hands for equality of grip and also by pushing down with his feet against the examiner's hands, first the right and then the left. The area below a spinal cord injury that has lost sympathetic stimulation will be cool and dry to the touch.

*Spinal Cord Injury in Water Accidents.* A common cause of spinal cord injuries is diving into the shallow end of a swimming pool or being tossed by waves onto the sand at the beach. A spinal cord injury in water presents a very special problem and will be discussed in detail here. If the spinal cord injury has been high enough in the cord to cause diaphragm paralysis it is not unusual for the swimmer to drown following the injury. If the accident has been witnessed, the rescuer must support the patient's head out of the water while protecting the spinal cord from further injury. The patient should not be removed from the water until a backboard arrives (Figure 14-17). If a backboard is not available, any wooden or firm structure (surfboard or plank, ironing board, table bench) will suffice. If the patient is floating face down, he should be turned over carefully keeping his head and body aligned.

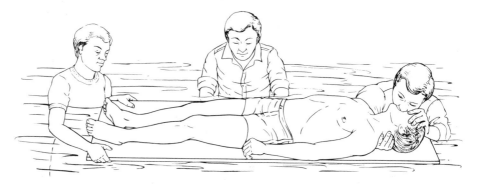

**Figure 14-17.** Swimming pool accidents are common causes of cervical fractures. Protection of the spinal cord as well as cardiopulmonary resuscitation may need to be done simultaneously.

This can be done by maintaining traction on the head, while at the same time locking an arm under one of the armpits and turning the patient. Once he is face up, mouth-to-mouth resuscitation may be necessary if the patient is apneic. The backboard is floated under the patient and the patient is then lifted out of the water. Although this may present an ideal situation, in some circumstances, the damage to the cord is complete and other extenuating circumstances make it imperative that the patient be moved without the use of a backboard (cardiac arrest). With as many persons as are available, an arm stretcher can be formed under the patient and he can then be carried out.

*Treatment:*

1. The treatment of spinal cord injury begins with the high index of suspicion that it may be present. The use of neck collars and backboards are imperative and cannot be overemphasized (Figure 14-18). A suspected spinal cord injury patient should have his body and neck held in one axis and moved as a single unit.

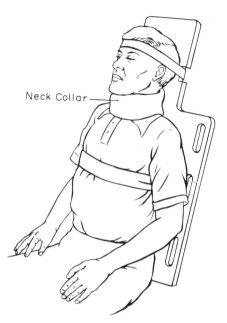

Neck Collar

**Figure 14-18.** The backboard for extrication and movement of a patient following a suspected spinal injury. Chin straps were formerly used to stabilize the jaw, but these may prevent access to the oral airway. A better combination is to use a neck collar with the backboard.

2. If airway obstruction is a problem or if the ventilation is inadequate, the jaw should be opened by displacing it forward. An oro- or nasopharyngeal airway or an esophageal obturator airway may aid mouth-to-mouth or mouth-to-nose resuscitation.

3. Hypotension in these cases may be due to the loss of sympathetic tone from the cord injury and therefore may not require massive fluid resuscitation. Simple elevation of the legs or moderate infusion of a balanced salt solution, such as Lactated Ringer's usually suffices.

4. Remember other life-threatening injuries might make the spinal cord injury of secondary importance. These would include massive hemorrhage from the chest, abdominal or extremity injuries, and upper airway obstruction due to facial or jaw fractures. The choice is always to salvage a life.

5. Remember judicious treatment may save someone from one of the most devastating of all nonfatal injuries, quadriplegia.

Trauma to the chest can occur from either a blunt or penetrating injury. Blunt injuries are often deceiving, since on external examination, the patient may seem to have experienced very little trauma. However, severe damage to the lungs, heart, major vessels, or other intrathoracic structures may have occurred even without rib fracture. Blunt chest trauma is a common occurrence after automobile accidents in which the victim's chest is pinned between the steering wheel or dashboard. Other causes of chest injuries are those due to falls (accidental or attempted suicides) and cardiopulmonary resuscitation.

Penetrating chest wounds are generally caused by knives or bullets. Often the patient with a penetrating chest injury may be quite alert and seemingly in no distress. This should not lull the paramedic into a sense of complacency since a serious injury may have occurred, and sudden deterioration can lead to an irretrievable situation. Much has been written about correlating the entry site of the missile with the probable severity of the underlying trauma. This is certainly true with entry sites in the parasternal or precordial region (Chapter 4). However, lateral chest wounds, depending upon the angle of the missile, may cause just as serious an injury to the heart or major vessels. Each patient must be individually evaluated and appropriately treated. The majority of penetrating chest injuries are managed at the hospital by the insertion of a chest tube and observation. Even massive hemorrhage can be controlled by the evacuation of blood and expansion of the lung. Some patients, however, may have such a serious injury that to salvage them a thoracotomy must be done immediately upon entry to the Emergency Department.

Injuries to the chest can be classified according to the anatomical structures involved. They are classified as follows: (1) ribs and sternum, (2) lung, (3) trachea, (4) diaphragm, (5) heart, and (6) great vessels.

*Ribs and Sternum.* The most frequently injured structures of the chest are the ribs and sternum. The trauma may be well-intentioned, such as the fracture of the costochondral junction which can occur during external cardiac compression for cardiac arrest, or due to a crushing injury to the chest, usually following auto accidents or falls (Figure 14-19). When ribs are fractured, they produce pain directly over the injury site. Costochondral fractures occur along the parasternal region. Examination of the sternum and ribs begins with direct compression of the sternum. This will produce pain if there are rib or costochondral fractures. If the costochondral fracture has been serious, the entire sternum may collapse under the pressure. Palpation along both chest walls should be done feeling for subcutaneous emphysema or rib fractures. Subcutaneous emphysema has a very characteristic feel (like a crinkling sensation under the fingers) and usually means a lung has been lacerated.

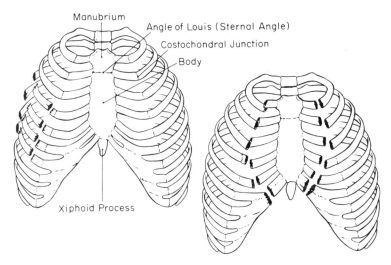

Manubrium
Angle of Louis (Sternal Angle)
Costochondral Junction
Body
Xiphoid Process

**Figure 14-19.** The anatomy of the thorax with common rib fractures. Fractures of the costochondral junction can occur after cardiopulmonary resuscitation with external cardiac massage or steering wheel accidents. The fractures shown will produce a flail chest.

Depending upon the force of injury the rib may snap and bend back into the chest, lacerate the lung, and then return to the anatomic location. Laceration of the lung may lead to bleeding and air leakage into the pleural space (hemopneumothorax).

When there have been extensive rib fractures or fractures of the costochondral arch, there may be obvious paradoxical motion of the chest wall. Paradoxical motion usually occurs if two ribs are broken in two or more places. This is called a flail chest. Sometimes, however, the patient's chest is so thick or muscular that paradoxical motion may not be appreciated. Paradoxical chest wall motion will lead to hypoventilation with carbon dioxide retention and hypoxemia if the fracture is severe enough. The mechanism for these changes in oxygenation and $CO_2$ elimination is based on the paradoxical motion of the chest wall. On inspiration, when negative intrapleural pressure is generated, the flail segment of the rib, instead of moving outward, is sucked in by the negative pressure and compresses the lung underneath it. This expels the gas in that lung to the opposite lung or to areas of the lung on the same side. On expiration, when intrapleural pressure increases, the flail segment balloons out creating a negative pressure area over the lung and it is sucked out with it. This causes gas to rush into the area which is flail, thereby ventilating the portion of the lung with expired gases from other parts of the lung. This type of back-and-forth breathing is called Penduluft breathing. It is important to eliminate this breathing pattern either by splinting the paradoxical area with sandbags or some other device, or in the comatose patient, by insertion of an esophageal obturator airway and positive pressure ventilation.

*Treatment:*

1. Simple rib fractures need no specific treatment. A supporting chest strap may be used.

2. Rib and/or sternal fractures that lead to paradoxical respiration should be treated by sandbag compression or positive pressure ventilation in the comatose patient.

3. Always suspect hemothorax and/or tension pneumothorax with rib fractures.

*Lung.* The lung can be injured either by closed or penetrating trauma. In either case, air leaks from the lung and collects in the pleural space (pneumothorax). Pneumothorax literally means air within the thorax, and in most cases, when not associated with other serious injuries, is well tolerated. A pneumothorax can develop after trauma, but also may spontaneously occur from a ruptured bleb on the lung. If there are no respiratory or significant vital sign changes, a pneumothorax need not be treated in the field and the patient can be transported. On occasion, pneumothorax can be bilateral. This is a surgical emergency since these patients' clinical condition can deteriorate rapidly. Decompression of the pneumothorax can be lifesaving. In the patient with other underlying diseases, such as chronic obstructive pulmonary disease (COPD) and congestive heart failure (CHF), a small pneumothorax is not well tolerated. Early diagnosis and treatment are the best hope for the patient.

Hemothorax occurs when there has been a significant rib fracture with tearing of intercostal blood vessels, or secondary to an injury from a penetrating object to a blood vessel. Hemothorax is easily diagnosed by the decreased breath sounds and the hyporesonance on percussion. Unexplained shock in someone with chest trauma and no other physical findings indicates a significant hemothorax. As much as 3000 ml of blood can collect in the chest over a short period of time, resulting in severe shock. There is no field treatment for hemothorax except to recognize the possibility of this condition. In conjunction with shock, rapid transport to the hospital is in order

*Tension Pneumothorax.* A tension pneumothorax refers to a pneumothorax which compresses the intrathoracic structures. Tension is generated from air that has leaked from the injured lung into the pleural space and cannot escape back through the lung and out the oral airway (Figure 14-20). Air is trapped in the pleural space and, as the patient coughs, strains, or breathes deeply further air is expelled under high pressure into this space and the pressure rises. As the pressure rises, it tends to shift the mediastinum and heart to the opposite side compressing

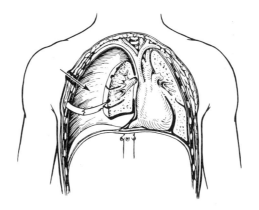

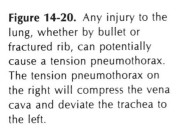

**Figure 14-20.** Any injury to the lung, whether by bullet or fractured rib, can potentially cause a tension pneumothorax. The tension pneumothorax on the right will compress the vena cava and deviate the trachea to the left.

the uninjured lung. At the same time, pressure is placed on the vena cava diminishing venous return to the heart and reducing the cardiac output and blood pressure. The patient with a tension pneumothorax is usually very ill and will have the following signs and symptoms:

1. Dyspnea
2. Chest pain
3. Diaphoresis
4. Cyanosis
5. Deviation of the trachea
6. Hyperresonance on the side of the pneumothorax
7. Wide changes in the blood pressure with respiration
8. Diminished breath sounds on the side of the tension pneumothorax
9. Reduced blood pressure

It is clear from the above description that the diagnosis of a tension pneumothorax can be best made on physical examination since the presenting signs are consistent with many other clinical disorders. Evaluation of these patients should include the recording of blood pressure, pulse, and respiratory rates. Wide variations in blood pressure with deep inspiration and expiration, and marked changes in the quality of the pulse with the same maneuver, indicate the presence of cardiac tamponade or the intrapleural collection of blood or air. Following recording of the vital signs, the trachea is palpated in the suprasternal notch to determine if it is in the midline or has shifted to the right or left (Figure 14-20). In most cases it will shift in the direction opposite the injury. This is a very valuable sign and is usually positive. If the patient has a tension pneumothorax on the left, the trachea will be deviated to the right. In percussing the chest for resonance, the optimum position is with the patient upright so that air can rise to the top of the pleural cavity and the difference in resonant sounds can be appreciated between the two sides of the chest. However, in the field this is impossible, and if the chest is percussed anteriorly, the difference in the two sides can be easily recognized. Hyperresonance indicates a pneumothorax; hyporesonance is consistent with hemothorax.

*Treatment:*

1. If the diagnosis of a tension pneumothorax has been established with certainty it may not necessarily require treatment in the field, but rapid transport to the base station hospital.

2. If the patient's condition is markedly deteriorating, vital signs are poor, ventilation inadequate, and it appears that a life or death situation exists, then a number 12 or 14 large bore cannula can be placed in the mid- or anterior axillary line at the level of the nipple with the patient either lying flat or in a 30° upright position. This maneuver will place the cannula in the fourth or fifth intercostal space. Air will hiss out under pressure like that coming out of a tire and this can be connected to a one-way valve called a Heimlich valve (Figure 14-21).

3. Nasal oxygen.

4. Maintain the airway if the patient is comatose.

5. In any patient who is coughing blood following an injury and if the side of injury can be identified, the patient must be transported in a semiupright position or on his side, with the injured side down. If the patient is placed with the good lung down, bleeding will occur from the injured lung into the good side and will cause aspiration asphyxia and death. The same position should be maintained to the Emergency Department, and subsequently to the operating room if indicated.

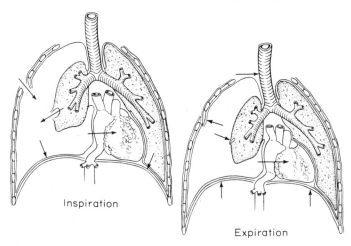

Inspiration

Expiration

**Figure 14-21.** A sucking chest wound allows for ingress of air during inspiration. During expiration a flap of chest wall tissue may close and trap air inside. This type of sucking chest wound will produce a shift in the mediastinum and compression of the heart.

*Sucking Chest Wounds.*    Explosions and other kinds of disrupting trauma may create chest wall defects exposing the lung to the atmosphere. As the patient breathes, air is sucked in and out of the hole. A small sucking chest wound can attract a great deal of attention because of the hissing, sucking, and fluttering noise that is made. There are two types of sucking chest wounds and these produce different physiologic responses. In one type the defect in the chest wall is so great that there is free ingress and egress of air from the thoracic cavity during respirations. Air is sucked in and moves out on expiration. At the same time there may be damage to the lung underneath also contributing to the movement of air in and out through the chest wall. In the second type of injury, the skin may be intact and air is sucked in on inspiration but a flap of chest wall and rib functions as a trap door (Figure 14-22). On expiration this snaps shut and air that has been sucked in through the skin then collects within the pleural space. At the same time there may be injury to the lung underneath and air may be escaping into this pleural space through the lung. This type of injury is a tension pneumothorax. Both types of injury may produce a critically ill patient, but it is more likely that the sucking chest wound in which air cannot escape because of the trap door phenomenon may precipitate deterioration in the patient's clinical status more quickly.

Traditionally, paramedics have been taught to place a tight compression dressing over the sucking chest wound and transport the patient. Although this may be indicated in certain situations, this is not always the correct thing to do. For example, if the lung beneath the chest

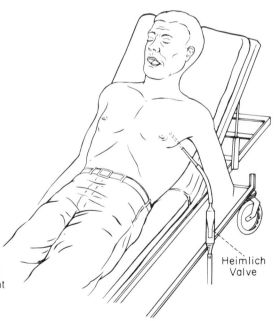

**Figure 14-22.** On rare occasion it is necessary to relieve a tension pneumothorax in the field. This is done by inserting a large Medicut cannula (#10 or #12) and connecting it to a Heimlich valve. The patient is best transported in the semi-upright position.

Heimlich
Valve

wall defect has been damaged, then covering the defect will force the air that is leaking from the damaged lung to collect in the pleural space. This will cause a tension pneumothorax under the dressing, and, unless the patient is monitored very carefully, it may lead to sudden death. The alternative is to leave a light sterile dressing over the chest and be certain that air is moving freely inward and outward. If it appears that air is sucked in from the outside and is being trapped in the pleural space, the best approach would be to use a throat stick, gloved finger, or some other device to keep the pleural space open, or at least keep the skin separated so that air is not trapped in the pleural space. These procedures leave the decision as to the best approach in the field to the paramedic's discretion. As long as air can freely move in and out of the pleural space, there should be no change in the patient's condition over a short period of time (20 minutes).

In our paramedic training program, a laboratory demonstration has repeatedly shown the hazards of tight compression of a sucking chest wound. The experiment consists of anesthetizing a dog and creating a pneumothorax by introducing a needle into the chest cavity and filling the cavity with air. This type of tension pneumothorax will cause a change in the dog's heart rate and respiratory rate as well as the color of his tongue. This is followed by a small thoracotomy in which the pleural space is left open with the animal breathing spontaneously (sucking chest wound). An injury is then made in the lung and the skin is taped over the sucking chest wound and vital signs recorded. Finally, the animal is allowed to breathe spontaneously with the injured lung and the pleural cavity wide open to the atmosphere. As might be expected, the situation in which the animal does the poorest is when the injured lung exists and the skin is taped tightly closed. He shortly develops a tension pneumothorax under the bandage and his vital signs rapidly deteriorate.

*Treatment:*

1. Ideally, the treatment of a sucking chest wound would be to occlude the injured site and insert a chest tube. Clearly this cannot be done in the field and a simple approach to treatment must be used.

2. Place a light, nonocclusive dressing over the wound and rapidly transport the patient. Notify the Base Station Hospital so that they are prepared for chest tube insertion.

*Diaphragm.* Injuries to the diaphragm most commonly occur after blunt injury in automobile accidents. The force on the abdominal viscera is so great that it disrupts the diaphragm, usually on the left side, forcing the bowel contents into the left chest. As time passes, the bowel contents migrate more and more into the chest and as the patient swallows, the bowel and stomach become distended with air. This produces compression of the lung on the side of the injury, as well as a shift in the mediastinum and further compression of the contralateral lung. It is difficult to differentiate this entity from a tension pneumothorax, and only a high index of suspicion will make the diagnosis. If one hears bowel sounds in the left chest, then the diagnosis of a diaphragmatic injury should be strongly suspected. Other physical findings would include diminished breath sounds and hyperresonance. Diaphragmatic injuries rarely occur on the right side because the liver protects the diaphragm from disruption.

*Treatment:*

1. Nasal oxygen.

2. If the diagnosis is suspected and the patient is in shock, only the leg portion of the MAST suit should be inflated (Chapter 15).

3. Transport.

*Hemopericardium.* Penetrating or blunt injury to the chest can cause disruption of one of the major cardiac chambers or vessels with bleeding into the pericardial sac. The blood within the pericardial sac compresses the heart and diminishes the cardiac output. The pulmonary veins, left atrium, and right ventricle are the chambers initially compressed, producing a diminished blood pressure. This phenomenon is called cardiac tamponade and produces three characteristic clinical findings:

*Signs:*

1. Distention of the neck veins

2. Quiet or distant heart sounds

3. Low blood pressure

Pericardial tamponade can also be detected by the use of the blood pressure cuff. By palpation of the pulse at the wrist, and recording serial systolic blood pressures, the pressure will be noted to change remarkably with inspiration and expiration. A 15 mm Hg change in blood pressure with a deep inspiration indicates cardiac tamponade. This change in blood pressure or pulse volume is related to the intrathoracic pressure changes with respiration. During inspiration, negative thoracic pressure forces blood to pool in the left atrium and pulmonary veins. Therefore, as this pooling occurs less blood is emptied from the left ventricle into the aorta. This drops the systemic blood pressure. On expiration, as the intrapleural pressure rises, the pressure in the pulmonary veins and left atrium pushes the blood into the left ventricle and the blood pressure rises. Although this is a normal physiologic response, it is usually not detectable under normal conditions. But in cardiac tamponade, when the ventricular filling is compromised by blood outside the heart, this normal physiologic response is exaggerated and becomes detectable with a blood pressure cuff. This has been incorrectly called pulsus paradoxicus (paradoxical pulse). Cardiac tamponade should be suspected in penetrating or blunt injuries over the precordium. It should be suspected if any of the above physical findings are present. It should always be looked for in any chest injury, regardless of severity.

In major trauma centers in the United States where paramedic teams have been used solely for the source of transport of trauma patients, treatment of heart injuries has improved dramatically. At Houston's Ben Taub Hospital, for example, a large number of cardiac injuries have been treated with excellent results. Paramedics bring the patients immediately to the hospital often without intravenous fluids started, and these patients undergo thoracotomy in the Emergency Department. Many patients have been salvaged.

*Treatment of Hemopericardium:*

1. Nasal oxygen.
2. Maintain airway and breathing.
3. Rapid transport.
4. Time should not be wasted attempting intravenous fluid administration since sudden deterioration can occur, irrespective of fluid replacement.
5. Obviously, the base station should be notified that this diagnosis is considered and that the patient must be transported to a center that can do a thoracotomy in the Emergency Department.

*Blunt Injuries to the Heart.* As mentioned in the previous section, penetrating or blunt injuries to the heart can produce hemopericardium and cardiac tamponade. Blunt injuries can also cause a contusion of the heart muscle. Myocardial injury is nearly identical to an acute myocardial infarction. There may be immediate EKG ST segment changes and/or dysrhythmias. Blunt injuries can also produce disruption of the interventricular septum and tearing of the valve tissues. This can be appreciated on physical examination by the presence of a large murmur.

*Treatment:*

1. Myocardial contusions should be treated as myocardial infarctions.
2. Nasal oxygen.
3. Monitor closely by electrocardiogram.
4. Intravenous fluid administration of Lactated Ringer's.
5. Transport.

*Great Vessel Injury.* Trauma to the great vessels (aorta, innominate and left subclavian arteries) can occur secondary to a penetrating or blunt injury. One of the most serious injuries that can follow deceleration automobile accidents is one to the descending aorta. This type of injury is instantly fatal in approximately 70 percent of the victims who have it. However, 30 percent will survive the injury and can be transported to a proper facility for immediate surgery. This has proved lifesaving and some patients have experienced excellent longterm results. The reason the aorta is injured at this location is that it is weakest at this point and it is surrounded by pleura and intercostal vessels. This anchors it to the posterior mediastinum, whereas the more proximal portion of the aorta is free to twist and move during deceleration. In most cases when this injury occurs, the aorta is disrupted and massive exsanguination into the left hemothorax occurs. In some cases the pleura is strong enough to buttress the disruption, which prevents sudden exsanguination (Figure 14-23). Deceleration injuries to the aorta should always be considered when the blood pressure in the arms is elevated in the absence of a serious head injury. The second finding would be a diminished or absent pulse in the femoral artery when the upper arm artery pulses are full. Blood pressure measurements in the leg can also make this diagnosis. Descending aortic injuries should be suspected when there is an onset of paraplegia without evidence of a spinal injury. The latter can be determined by palpation of the thoracic spines.

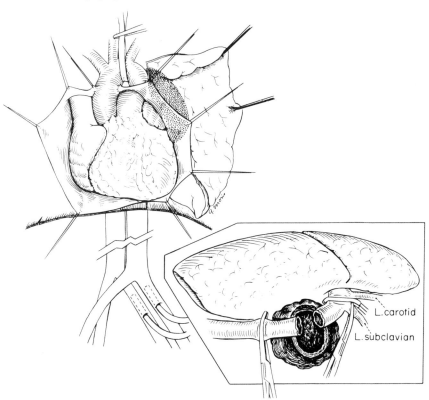

**Figure 14-23.** Disruption of the descending aorta is becoming an increasingly common deceleration injury. Although the aorta is disrupted, it may not burst into the chest since the mediastinal pleura may hold the hematoma. This type of injury can be repaired and patients salvaged.

*Treatment:*

1. Nasal oxygen.

2. Monitor.

3. Intravenous fluid administration of Lactated Ringer's.

4. The MAST suit may be used on the lower extremities if there is hypotension. Although this diagnosis would be difficult to make in the field, an abdominal MAST suit might raise the restriction to flow from the thoracic aorta, causing a potential chance of the disruption of the aorta.

5. Notify the base station of the possibility of a thoracic injury so that the angiography and open heart teams can be alerted.

6. Transport the patient.

ABDOMINAL INJURIES

Abdominal injuries can occur after automobile accidents in which the victim has been thrown against the steering wheel or the dashboard. Usually a seat belt is not attached in such a case. The person who is in the back seat asleep or who has passed out from alcohol is more vulnerable to an injury than the individual in the front seat who is alert and tenses his abdominal musculature just prior to the collision. Penetrating injuries, from either knives or gunshot wounds, may or may not represent injury to the deep structures (ranging from zero to cataclysmic trauma). Often there is no way to tell for certain, in either circumstance, whether a serious injury has occurred.

The major decision in the field regarding abdominal injuries is the determination of a significant blood loss within the peritoneal cavity. Hemoperitoneum is a consequence of any significant abdominal injury, and as much as two or three thousand milliliters of blood can accumulate within a short period of time, with a sudden deterioration in the vital signs. The diagnosis of hemoperitoneum can be made in the field and should be suspected when the following exists:

1. Hypotension with no other visible signs of injury except abdominal injury.

2. Pain or tenderness on palpation of the abdomen, particularly in the right or left upper quadrants.

3. Pain in the shoulder tip without shoulder injury.

4. Obvious abdominal distention.

The above findings, following abdominal injury, would indicate serious bleeding within the peritoneal cavity and immediate transport would be imperative. The following case is an example:

A 15-year-old girl was shot at close range in the left upper quadrant in a motel room. Paramedics responded immediately, and on physical examination the abdomen was found to be markedly distended, the blood pressure was not obtainable, the pulse barely palpable, and the girl was semiconscious. The patient was placed immediately on a stretcher and transported to the base station hospital three minutes away. Notification of these findings had been made and the patient was taken from the Emergency Department directly to the operating room where an abdominal laparotomy was performed. Operative findings revealed that a hole had been blown in the aorta. The time from the accident to surgery was fifteen minutes. The patient made an uneventful recovery.

The preceding case illustrates that an abdominal injury to a major blood vessel will produce massive bleeding within a short period of time. Such an injury will produce abdominal distention and hypotension. Hypotension in the presence of any abdominal injury without other signs of injury is due to blood loss. The best practice in this particular case would have been to quickly place the patient in a MAST suit and transport. At the present time, this would appear to be the best approach, especially if transport may be prolonged more than several minutes. However, the only thing that will salvage a patient of this type is abdominal laparotomy with closure of the hole. This requires no delays in the field. This would also mean that time should not be wasted attempting to start intravenous fluids that would not help significantly. When the patient, within minutes of his injury, has developed virtually no vital signs, rapid transport with surgery offers the only hope ("scoop and run").

The most commonly injured organ producing significant hemoperitoneum is the spleen. As mentioned in the chapter on anatomy, the spleen resides in the left upper quadrant and is a highly vascular organ. It is contained within a thin capsule and can easily be ruptured or torn. The spleen is frequently injured in automobile accidents where the disrupting force is the shearing stress from the sudden rise in intra-abdominal pressure as the steering wheel or dashboard hits the abdomen. The spleen itself is not directly injured, but tears due to the sudden disrupting forces around it. The spleen may also be injured during "horsing around" where one individual hits another in the abdomen, blind-sided. If the person has not tensed his abdominal muscles, the sudden increase in pressure due to the fist blow will cause disrupting forces to the spleen and make it burst. The spleen may rupture due to certain types of infectious disease processes such as infectious mononucleosis in which the speen has become enlarged. In this state, the spleen is very vulnerable to injury, particularly in high school and college students who have a high incidence of infectious mononucleosis. Very innocent trauma, such as a minor injury or jumping, may disrupt an enlarged spleen. The important point to remember is that the spleen can be ruptured by seemingly innocent trauma and present with pain in the left upper quadrant and shoulder tip.

In cases of multiple trauma where the abdomen may not seem to gain primary attention, a ruptured spleen should always be kept in mind. Hemoperitoneum must be suspected, particularly if there has been a sudden deterioration in the vital signs and there are no other obvious signs of bleeding.

The liver is in the right upper quadrant and is often injured in pedestrian accidents in which the individual is run over by a car. If the tire tracks go over the right thorax and abdomen, expect that the liver has been severely fractured. Liver injuries are also frequent in gunshot and stab wounds of the right upper quadrant. Liver injuries can be minor, with sealing off of the injury site without serious bleeding. This may produce only abdominal pain and no change in the vital signs. On the other hand, massive liver disruption can produce a distended abdomen, a moribund patient, and often a fatal outcome within minutes of the injury. Liver injuries present as right upper quadrant and right shoulder tip pain. Accurate diagnosis with immediate transport and use of the MAST suit can salvage these patients.

The aorta traverses the abdominal cavity and divides into two iliac arteries at the level of the lumbar vertebrae. Associated with the aorta are the vena cava and iliac veins. Both the aorta and its major branches as well as the vena cava can be injured either in blunt or penetrating trauma. Usually these injuries will occur after a penetrating trauma, such as stab and gunshot wounds. As described in the preceding case report, the bleeding can be massive within a very short period of time. Vena caval injuries may produce hypotension, but not the sudden deterioration in vital signs caused by arterial injuries. Any abdominal distention after a penetrating or blunt injury in which there is dullness to percussion, or at least no evidence of hyperresonance, the diagnosis of acute blood loss is made. The only treatment for this in the field is application of the MAST suit and transport.

The remaining injuries within the peritoneal cavity of significance include disruption of the pancreas, duodenum, stomach, and small and large bowels. These injuries often do not produce serious bleeding initially, and may even present diagnostic problems for the physician in the Emergency Department. However, there will usually be some guarding or tenderness after any abdominal injury when bowel structures have been disrupted. If the vital signs are stable, these problems can be managed by the administration of intravenous fluids and transport.

Penetrating abdominal injuries which have produced an opening in the abdominal wall will often be the exit point for some portion of the intra-abdominal contents. The most common of these is either the omentum or the small bowel. While these structures may migrate through the hole, it may also be noted on subsequent operation at the hospital that there is no intra-abdominal injury. Although the protrusion of these structures would seem to indicate a serious injury and an urgent situation, they often prove to be of no consequence. The protruding structure is best managed by covering it with a sterile dressing and attending to other problems that may be more pressing.

*Treatment:*

1. Abdominal injuries should be suspected whenever there is pain or distention of the abdomen following trauma.

2. If hemoperitoneum is suspected, application of the MAST suit is indicated.

3. Maintain the airway.

4. Oxygen by face mask.

5. Intravenous fluids are indicated if there does not appear to be massive hemorrhage, in which case rapid transport is in order.

6. Transport.

## INJURIES TO THE MUSCULOSKELETAL SYSTEM

### BONE

Injuries to the bone occur commonly after accidents. Although the bone injury itself is rarely life-threatening, combined with other injuries it may contribute to a fatal outcome. The important concept of bone fractures is to use common sense and remember that healing of a bone takes months and the initial treatment of the fracture begins in the field. It takes a significant injury to fracture a bone. The character of the resulting fracture is dictated by how the force was applied to the bone, the rate of application of the force, and the total amount of imparted force absorbed by the bone during the event. When a fracture occurs, the bone substance itself is disrupted. There will also be varying amounts of disruption of the surrounding soft tissues, including lacerations of muscles and possibly the large vessels and nerves adjacent to the bony structure. The enveloping periosteum and osteum are torn and vessels within the periosteum as well as the intramedullary vessels will be disrupted, resulting in extensive hemorrhage, pain, and often an angulation deformity of the extremity.

Bone is a strong tissue, which, under mechanical compression stress, exhibits superior strength. It is relatively weak in twisting or torsion stress and is weakest in tension stress. Thus, most fractures occur as a result of tension (bending). During bending the fracture always initiates on the convex aspect of the bending bone where tensile stresses are concentrated. The fracture proceeds from the convex to the concave surface. The mechanical configuration of the fracture is often determined by the amount of energy absorbed by the bone during the application of stress. Slow application of energy, particularly associated with twisting stress, may result in long spiral oblique fractures. High energy impacts (as in auto accidents) may, on the other hand, result in multiple fragments of bone referred to as a comminuted fracture. Direct blows may result in relatively transverse fractures without much fragmentation which are referred to as simple fractures.

*Classification of Fractures.* Fractures are classified as (1) simple or closed implying the maintenance of continuity of the overlying skin and as (2) open or compound implying a communication between the outside environment and the fracture site (Figure 14-24). The compounding force may either be from within (a sharp spicule of bone may protrude through the skin from within to the outside environment during the displacement of the limb at the time of fracture) or may be compounded by external objects (e.g., bullets) which penetrate through the soft tissues down to the bone causing it to fracture, and in the process may bring with them pieces of clothing, dirt, glass, and general contamination. The small puncture wound often can be very misleading, as superficial inspection may indicate a rather small wound with ostensibly little problem potential. A bone may protrude an extreme distance from the skin digging into the external environment carrying with it debris and dirt that sets the stage for serious infection. Bone fragments can also be quite sharp and may produce extensive soft tissue injuries, including muscle, nerve, and vessel lacerations.

Fractures can also be classified in relation to the number of fragments that are present. A comminuted fracture exists when multiple fracture fragments are present in the bone (Figure 14-24). This diagnosis is usually made by X-ray.

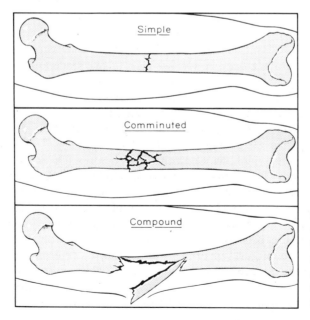

**Figure 14-24.** The various types of fractures. Potentially the most serious is the compound fracture, in which bone is exposed to the environment.

*Diagnosis of Fractures.* In the field, diagnosis of a fracture is usually not difficult to make. The common symptoms of a fracture are pain and inability to move an extremity or joint. The signs of a fracture are localized tenderness, swelling, crepitus with palpation over the injured site, instability, angulation of the extremity or bone, and perhaps bone protruding from the skin. In examining the patient with a fracture, it must be remembered that serious injury may be related to the head, chest, or abdomen. In dealing with fractures in the field, the other systems take priority and the fracture treatment is delayed until it is certain that no other serious disorder is present.

Because of the disruption of the soft tissues and vessels within the surrounding muscle mass, extensive hemorrhage can accompany a major fracture, particularly those of the pelvis and femur. This blood loss may be slow and insidious, so that vital signs must be monitored frequently to recognize the early appearance of shock. The following list demonstrates the amount of blood that can be lost within six hours after a fracture:

1. Pelvis          1300–1500 ml or more
2. Femur           400–800 ml
3. Tibia-Fibula    300–500 ml
4. Humerus         150 ml

It can be seen from the above list that fractures can contribute to a persistent blood loss after multiple injury. If there is more than one fracture, the blood loss becomes greater.

When evaluating fractures it is important to pay attention to the extremity distal to the fracture. This would include the warmth of the skin and presence of pulses and the ability to move parts of the extremity. It would be important to know, for example, that after a fracture of the femur, a pulse was present in the foot. This is especially true if, during the reduction of the fracture, the pulse suddenly disappeared and did not return with change in position of the fracture. This could indicate that the fracture injured or entrapped a vessel, or the vessel was already injured and made worse by straightening out the fracture. The same statement is true for the neurological examination of the distal portion of the extremity to be certain that during reduction or application of traction the nerve was not injured producing a loss of function of the extremity.

## Types of Fractures

*Simple Fractures.* A simple fracture has been defined as a fracture involving injury to the bone without disruption of the skin. These fractures may be obvious on physical examination in the field, or may only be suspected based on physical findings. The main goal in the field treatment of simple fractures is to prevent further soft tissue injury about the fracture site and relieve the patient of pain and discomfort.

The following list defines those simple fractures which occur in the upper and lower extremities based on the bones present and the possible fractures that might occur.

| Upper Limb | Signs and Symptoms | Field Treatment |
|---|---|---|
| **Shoulder and Arm** | | |
| Clavicle | Pain, deformity over clavicle | Sling or figure 8 dressing |
| Humerus | | |
|   Proximal<br>  Midshaft | Unstable arm, pain, deformity. Radial nerve injury, cannot dorsiflex wrist | Sling |
|   Supracondylar<br>  Portion | Pain, distal humerus, deformity. Cool forearm and hand, absent radial pulse | Sling, transport especially in children, this is an orthopedic emergency |
| **Forearm** | | |
| Radius | Pain over proximal midshaft or distal portion. Cannot dorsiflex wrist or pronate forearm | Sling or splint |
| Ulna | Pain over midshaft or distal portion | Sling or splint |
| Carpal Bone (Wrist) (Navicular) | Pain in snuff box space or directly over wrist, pain on dorsiflexion of wrist | Splint |
| **Hand** | | |
| Metacarpals | Pain, deformity | Splint |
| Phalanges | Pain, deformity, loss of flexion | Splint |
| *Pelvis* | | |
| Innominates (2)<br>Ilium<br>Ischium | Pain on compression of pubic bone, pain on barrel hoop compression of pelvis, pain on forced adduction of knees | Child—Splint pelvis with a circumferential splint. Adult—Stabilize fracture with sandbags, MAST suit may be used |
| *Hip and Leg* | | |
| **Femur** | | |
|   Proximal (hip)<br>  Neck | External rotation of foot, short leg, pain on slightest motion of leg, pain directly over trochanter | Traction splint (Hare) Transport |
|   Midshaft | Angulation of thigh, extremely tender to motion, unstable lower limb | Traction splint (Hare) Transport |

| Distal | Pain above knee, deformity, instability, angulation of thigh | Fractures directly above the knee should be splinted with cardboard. |
|---|---|---|
| **Lower Leg** | | |
| Tibia | | |
| Proximal Midshaft | Pain over knee, angulation, instability | Splint (cardboard) |
| Distal | Pain over ankle, pain with motion | Splint (cardboard) |
| Fibula | Pain, usually no instability if the only fracture | Splint (cardboard) |
| Os Calcis | Pain over "heel" line | Pillow splint |
| Foot Fracture | Pain over site | Pillow splint or wrap, crutches |

It can be seen that the preceding fractures are easily treated by splinting. The major fractures that require transport are those of the femur, pelvis, or supracondylar fractures of the upper extremity in children. All of these are considered serious conditions which may lead to major blood loss or a severe loss of function. Supracondylar fractures of the elbow in children, if not treated quickly, can lead to an occlusion of the brachial artery with spasm. The deformity of the fracture causes swelling and the loss of venous return from the forearm. These two factors produce damage to the muscles of the forearm and may leave the patient with a Volkmann's ischemic contracture. This contracture renders the hand virtually useless and is a serious complication.

Pelvic fractures can be suspected in the field by compression of the pubic bones as mentioned. The best way to manage these fractures in the adult is by splinting the pelvis and prevent it from rolling during the motion of transport. This motion is very painful and also aggravates bleeding by causing the fractures to rub against each other, further lacerating tissue. In the child a splint can be wrapped around the entire pelvis to steady the fracture site. Vacuum splints that will encircle the entire pelvis in a child are available and allow for stabilization of the fracture.

Severely angulated simple fractures of the femur and fractures about the knee are best splinted in the position they are found. When traction is placed on these fractures, severe damage to blood vessels can occur. When there is distal loss of pulse in an angulated fracture, gentle reduction may help. However, traction splinting should not be used. The best splint for angulated fractures is a cardboard splint.

*Compound Fractures.* The compound fracture is a special problem and treatment begins in the field. If the extremity is in alignment and the bone has returned into the soft tissue, then a traction splint is indicated. However, if the bone spicule is sticking through the skin and is contaminated with debris, splinting of the bone fragment should be done in the position that the bone is discovered. To relocate the bone fragment may cause additional laceration of soft tissues (nerves and vessels) and also grossly contaminate the deep tissues. All compound injuries should be covered with sterile or clean occlusive dressings to protect the compound fracture site from the external environment. Compound fractures constitute an orthopedic emergency, and undue delay in their treatment should be avoided. The inadequately treated compound fracture can lead to serious infection which may result in osteomylitis and subsequent delayed or nonunion of the fracture site.

## FAT EMBOLISM

Fat embolism is a major catastrophe in the patient with multiple fractures and can in itself be life-threatening, carrying a significant mortality. The reasons for this complication have not been clearly defined. It may represent a general biochemical stress response or a gross embolization of fatty marrow elements aspirated into the disrupted veins within the confines of the fracture. Embolization of fat by whatever mechanism usually manifests itself within 48 hours after the initial injury with probabilities of embolization decreasing with ensuing time. The heralding onset is shortness of breath, increased agitation, and irrational behavior in an otherwise normal patient. In many patients, embolization is inapparent due to the lack of any overt symptoms or signs. There is a definite association of this syndrome in the patient with multiple large bone fractures and repeated handling of fractures from multiple transfers to various hospitals, and repeated manipulations for evaluation and clinical assessment. All persons associated with the management of multiple-injury patients must be cognizant of its potential, minimizing manipulation of fractures, by early and stable splinting, and avoidance of multiple transfers due to poor triage.

## LIGAMENT INJURIES

Ligamentous injuries are called sprains, and can be clinically grouped in three degrees:

> First degree sprain
> Second degree sprain
> Third degree sprain

1. A first degree sprain is a minor stretch of a ligament with associated hemorrhage and increased tissue fluid (edema), which may

result in a minor laxity of the ligament. When stressed, even in the acute and painful stage, the ligament will have integrity and will take additional stress when it is applied manually. Pain is the primary symptom of the first degree sprain and relaxation of the ligament is a minor portion of the disability.

2. A second degree sprain implies further loss of ligamentous integrity due to increased disruption of the substance. Laxity on manual testing becomes more evident and pain continues to be the prominent symptom. Swelling and hemorrhage may also be present. The common second degree ligament sprain is the sprained ankle in which the ligaments from the fibula to the talus are torn.

3. A third degree sprain implies a complete disruption of the substance of the ligament (Figure 14-25). This may be accompanied by some swelling and bleeding, but the pain may be surprisingly minimized due to the fact that the nerve fibers within the substance of the ligament that respond to stretch are no longer stimulated. In the stressing of the third degree ligament injury, increased angulation of the joint in the plane of the ligament without apparent limits is produced, and the stretch of the joint will continue relative to the amount of stress applied.

Ligamentous injuries are important problems because of their role in stabilizing joints. Second degree ligamentous injuries can be treated with splinting and ice packs with transport. A third degree ligament injury may cause instability of the joint. For example, this occurs in third degree ligament injuries to the knee following football injuries. The knee is so unstable that the patient cannot stand or walk. Because ligaments heal by the formation of collagen and scar tissue, it is important that the degree of swelling and injury not be worsened by the type of splinting or by excess manipulation of the joint.

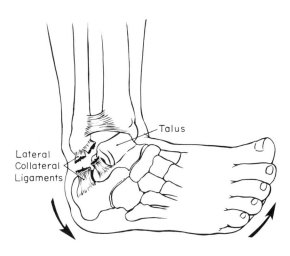

**Figure 14-25.** Injuries to the ankle can be serious even though fracture may not occur. A ligament disruption is a serious ankle injury.

Severe trauma imparted to the skeletal system may also produce dislocations of joints in addition to, or as isolated occurrences from fractures. Symptoms and signs of dislocations are deformity, pain over the joint, and loss of the joint movement. Joints that are commonly involved in dislocations include the shoulder, hip, knee and ankle, but any joint has a potential for a dislocation injury. During dislocation, the capsule and ligamentous investment about the joint is disrupted sufficiently so that gross displacement of the normal relationships of the joint surfaces occurs. These dislocations may be momentary events having a spontaneous relocation of the joint's anatomy or the joint may become displaced and remain dislocated. An example of the latter is posterior dislocation of the hip, which occurs when striking the knee on a dashboard during sudden deceleration. The patient complains of pain in the hip and the foot is turned outward (Figure 14-1). Dislocations should be promptly reduced at a hospital or a comparable facility for several reasons. If prompt reduction is not accomplished, ischemia of bone can occur to produce bone necrosis. This will result in delayed avascular changes in the bone, collapse of the architecture, and subsequent degenerative changes within the joint as a consequence of damage to the articular cartilage. The femoral head, in particular, is susceptible to avascular necrosis associated with a dislocation when it remains dislocated beyond twelve hours from the initial displacement. Assessment of all major joints in trauma should be done to eliminate the presence of an occult dislocation, and this is particularly needed in the comatose or unresponsive patient. Because of the extreme displacement of the joint and stretching of surrounding soft tissues, dislocations can result in nerve and vessel injuries. The following is a list of common joint dislocations and their treatment:

| | *Signs and Symptoms* | *Field Treatment* |
|---|---|---|
| Anterior dislocation of the shoulder | Cannot raise arm, pain over shoulder anteriorly, loss of sensation in the hand and arm and possible brachial plexus injury. | Sling; this dislocation can be reduced by placing the foot in the axilla and pulling on the arm; this can be done in the field, but is not recommended for paramedic personnel. |
| Elbow | Inability to straighten out the elbow, deformity behind the elbow, pain over the elbow joint. | Sling. |
| Wrist and Fingers | Pain, deformity, inability to move joint. | Ice pack. |

| Signs and Symptoms | Field Treatment |
| --- | --- |

| | Signs and Symptoms | Field Treatment |
| --- | --- | --- |
| Hip | Foot outwardly rotated, inability to raise hip, pain and deformity posteriorly over buttock, shortening of the involved leg when compared to the other leg. | Hare traction splint. Transport; this is an orthopedic emergency. |
| Knee | Absent pedal pulses, cool extremity below the knee, marked angulation and deformity of the knee and inability to move it. | Transport, repeated evaluation of pedal pulses. May attempt reduction if transport is delayed and pulses are absent. Otherwise, splint with cardboard in position found. |
| Ankle | Pain, deformity, angulation, swelling. | Ice pack, reduce into the most anatomic position achievable, pillow splint, transport. |

## PRINCIPLES OF SPLINTING

Because any fractured extremity will respond with swelling and an increase in volume, circumferential splinting of an extremity with continued subsequent swelling may result in the delayed onset of increased pressure within muscle compartments leading to a decrease in blood supply. The capillary filling pressure to deep muscle masses is approximately 40 mm Hg. The filling pressure in medium-sized vessels generally is about 90 to 120 mm Hg; thus, the patient may continue to transmit a pulse in larger main arteries, but due to the increased compartmental pressure, cessation of all blood flow may occur to the deep muscle compartments. This may result in extreme ischemia of tissue and loss of muscle mass. It has been estimated that four hours of total ischemia produces a 25 percent loss of muscle; eight hours produces a 50 percent loss; and twelve hours produces complete loss of muscle due to ischemic necrosis. The emergent nature of the problem is evident, and the prompt release of all tight muscle compartments by surgical fasciotomy may be necessary. Any splint that is circumferential and compressive must be applied with this knowledge.

*Types of Splints.* Many types of splints are available either by commercial production or homemade. In general, splints should accomplish splinting of an injury without compression of structures in the extremity.

1. A finger can be splinted with a padded tongue depressor or a padded flexible aluminum strip. The finger is splinted with either of these items and then wrapped with a circular dressing as shown in Figure 14-26.

425

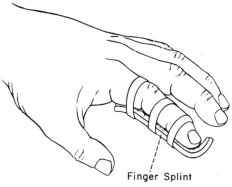

Finger Splint

**Figure 14-26.** A simple finger splint will often relieve the pain of a fractured or dislocated finger.

2. Cardboard splints are ideal for tibial and fibular fractures. They also may be used for upper arm fractures of the forearm or humerus. The reason that cardboard provides a good splint is that it is malleable, sturdy, and inexpensive. These splints are held in place by wrapping with interrupted pieces of cloth or gauze wrapping. The splint is shown in Figure 14-27.

3. The Hare traction splint is ideal for lower extremity fractures or hip dislocations (Figure 14-28). These splints are commercially available and can maintain traction on the foot, but at the same time are not occlusive to the extremity. Velcro straps are utilized to stabilize the leg on the frame anteriorly and posteriorly. Since these straps are

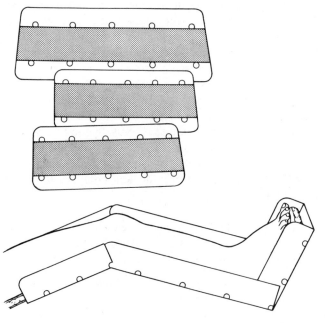

**Figure 14-27.** Cardboard splints are inexpensive and useful.

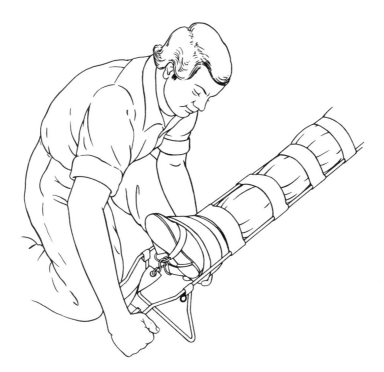

**Figure 14-28.** The Hare traction splint. Injuries around the knee may involve damage to blood vessels and excessive traction could aggravate the damage.

intermittent and their tension can be adjusted, there is no circular occlusion of the extremity. The older ring splints, which had a complete circular ring near the hip, with swelling often caused compression of the vessels in this region. The Hare splint should not be used for severely angulated femur fractures or fractures about the knee. Distal pulses should always be assessed when the Hare splint is used.

4. Homemade splints can be made from any sturdy object. A broom handle, piece of wood, cardboard, or a magazine, etc. have all been used in certain situations in which commercially constructed splints were not readily available (Figure 14-29). The principle of wrapping the

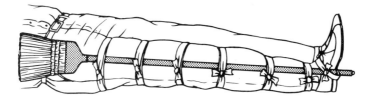

**Figure 14-29.** A makeshift leg splint. Interrupted bandages prevent compression of muscle and blood vessels.

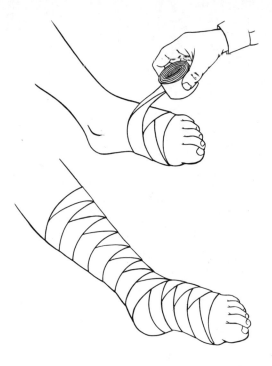

**Figure 14-30.** An ankle injury can be stabilized with an Ace wrap.

extremity to the splint is to use intermittent dressings that are not tightly bound.

5. Ace bandages are elastic bandages that provide some splinting either of the foot, knee, wrist, forearm, or elbow. The Ace wrap is applied with gentle traction starting at the most distal portion to be wrapped and then working proximally. A figure of 8 weave, as shown in Figure 14-30, will give the best stability and prevent motion of the Ace wrap. If the ankle is to be splinted, the wrapping should begin near the toes and carried proximally above the ankle to the midportion of the leg.

6. Pillow splints can either be made out of a pillow or some foam rubber padding. These splints are ideal for ankle dislocations or ankle fractures. A simple pillow splint is shown in Figure 14-31. Cardboard splints are also just as adequate, but do not provide the padding and comfort of a pillow splint for these particular types of injuries.

## GENERAL APPROACH TO MUSCULOSKELETAL TRAUMA

1. Remember that the musculoskeletal injury is of secondary importance when considering the airway, breathing, shock, and bleeding.

2. Splints and splinting techniques vary depending upon preferences of individual paramedic units and base station hospitals. Regardless of

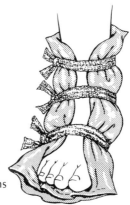

**Figure 14-31.** A pillow splint is a comfortable means of stabilizing an injured ankle.

the type of splint used, the principles of preventing tissue damage as previously outlined are most important.

3. The application of ice to injured parts to help minimize hemorrhage and local tissue reaction is an excellent initial treatment measure. Ice also has a local anesthetic effect and will make the patient more comfortable in transport.

4. Compound fractures in which the bone has been repositioned should be treated by traction splinting. A compound fracture in which the bone fragments are clearly exposed and dirty should not be reduced back into the soft tissue. It is best to splint them in any way possible in the position they were found. All exposed bone or compound sites should be covered with a sterile dressing. All areas of hemorrhage should have an application of bulky dressings.

5. The manipulation of fractures should be minimized and interhospital transport should be eliminated, or at least reduced to as little as possible.

6. Two major orthopedic emergencies are posterior hip dislocation and supracondylar elbow fracture in children. These require immediate attention by specialists who can deal with these problems.

## VASCULAR TRAUMA

Injury to the vascular system can be minor, such as a laceration of a vein in an arm; or it can be major, such as a disruption of the abdominal aorta due to a bullet. Vascular injuries are generally catastrophic events and can either be caused by blunt or penetrating forces. By and large, the most common types of vascular injuries are those due to penetrating injuries such as knives or bullets. The injury may penetrate an artery or vein. When a blood vessel is injured with a penetrating object, it depends on whether the vessel has been severed or only partially severed as to whether hemorrhage will be controlled by vasoconstriction or other forces within the body. A totally transected artery will often go into spasm and bleeding will stop as the blood pressure is reduced from the blood loss. A vessel that has been partially severed so that one portion of the wall is still intact cannot contract to close off its end (Figure 14-32). This type of vessel injury is more serious and bleeding will continue to occur.

The diagnosis of a vascular injury within the chest or abdomen is not always easy. Any penetrating injury of either the chest or abdominal cavity with sudden loss of vital signs indicates a major injury to a vascular structure. Injuries to arteries in the chest that produce a sudden loss in vital signs can only be managed by maintenance of the airway, inflation of the leg portion of the MAST suit, and rapid transport. Injuries to major arteries or veins in the abdomen can be treated by application of the MAST suit (Chapter 15) and rapid transport. Exclusive of these two cavities, injuries to arteries outside of the abdominal and thoracic cavities are directly accessible to management. These would include injuries to the subclavian, carotid, brachial, radial, femoral, popliteal, and pedal arteries. Injuries to veins outside of the abdominal and thoracic cavities are no less important, but are more easily controlled by simple compression or possibly even elevation.

Arterial injuries outside of these two body cavities should be suspected whenever there is a penetrating injury in these areas with sudden swelling. Loss of distal pulses with a cool extremity should always indicate an arterial injury. The five Ps of an arterial injury are:

1. Pain—Due to ischemia.
2. Pallor—Loss of arterial blood.
3. Paralysis—Ischemia to the nerve and muscle.
4. Pulselessness—Loss of distal pulse in any extremity.
5. Paresthesia—Numbness.

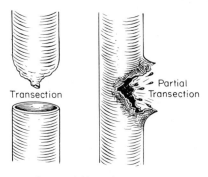

Severed Vessels

**Figure 14-32.** A partially transected vessel cannot retract and may bleed more profusely than the totally transected vessel.

The basic principle of vascular injury when the vessel is accessible to compression is to apply compression and transport. The following is an example:

> A 23-year-old male, while intoxicated, drove his motorcycle through the glass front of a business concern at 2:00 AM in the morning. The police and paramedics were immediately called. Upon arrival, the patient was pale and had several large lacerations with glass protruding from a laceration in the neck over the anterior triangle. Blood was emanating from this particular laceration. The glass shard was removed and direct compression was applied. The patient's blood pressure was not obtainable and he was immediately transported. In the Emergency Department, exploration of the neck revealed a lacerated carotid artery and jugular vein. These were repaired. The patient subsequently died of a neurologic injury.

The important feature of the preceding case is that the diagnosis of vascular injury was made immediately since the patient, shortly after being seen, had no vital signs. Obvious lacerations were present about the head and neck, particularly one in the anterior triangle of the neck suggesting a carotid and jugular vein injury. Removing the impaled object was the correct thing to do since direct pressure could not be placed on the artery with a piece of glass in the incision. Since the artery was bleeding around the glass and the vessel was readily accessible, removal with direct compression with a glove or bare finger was the appropriate choice. In all other situations, however, the impaled object should be left in place since its removal may release bleeding tamponaded by the impaled object. For example, a knife protruding from the epigastrium should not be removed since it may be in the aorta tamponading bleeding. Its removal could cause sudden torrential hemorrhage. In any penetrating injury of the neck, the possibility of an air embolism is present and the patient should be transported in a head-down position (Figure 14-8).

The paramedic should become familiar with all the different points of pulses which have been outlined in the chapter on the history and physical examination. He should be able to find these pulses and practice compression by occluding the pulse proximally and feeling distally. One can practice by occluding the femoral artery and assessing the absence of the dorsalis pedis pulse. The same is true for compression of the axillary artery in the axilla to be sure the radial artery pulse disappears. Since direct finger compression appears to be the most reliable and best method for occlusion, it has gained wide acceptance (Figure 14-33). However, the use of tourniquets should not be abandoned. If it is known that the individual has suffered a serious disrupting injury of the forearm with vessel laceration and major blood loss, the application of a tourniquet is reasonable; especially if the transport is only fifteen minutes and the paramedic placing the tourniquet follows the patient all the way through to the hospital. Application of the tourniquet or blood

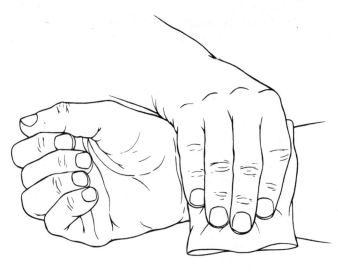

Direct Compression of Artery

**Figure 14-33.** The best method for controlling bleeding from any vessel is by direct compression.

pressure cuff to an extremity to stop bleeding frees the paramedic to treat other victims or to give further attention to his own patient (Figure 14-34). While using a tourniquet, common sense must be maintained and followup by the individual using the tourniquet is mandatory.

It can be seen from these statements that control of bleeding outside of body cavities can be accomplished by direct compression, proximal occlusion of the vessel either with the finger or blood pressure cuff (tourniquet), or by direct compression using the MAST suit. Vascular injuries of the body cavities are more difficult to diagnose and treat. Intraabdominal vascular injuries can be treated with inflation of the leg and abdominal portions of the MAST suit, whereas intrathoracic bleeding is best managed with inflation of the leg portion of the MAST suit and rapid transport.

*Treatment:*

1. Vascular injuries should be suspected whenever there have been penetrating wounds and a sudden loss of vital signs. Abdominal vascular injuries are managed with the MAST suit and transport; thoracic vascular injuries are managed by application of the leg portion of the MAST suit and rapid transport.

2. Vascular injuries that are accessible to compression should be treated by direct digital compression. The use of tourniquets can be helpful and should be used with common sense. The ordinary blood pressure cuff makes an excellent upper arm tourniquet. After the

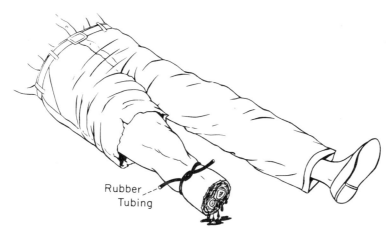

Rubber
Tubing

**Figure 14-34.** In some situations, a tourniquet is indicated and will not jeopardize the limb or the patient's life.

application of a tourniquet, abandoning the patient for other reasons without followup is bad practice. Use of the tourniquet in the field is controversial, but if transport time is rapid and the paramedic will follow the patient, then it can be of extreme value. It is important to inflate the blood pressure cuff above systolic pressure so that the artery, and not just the vein is occluded. The latter may further aggravate tissue swelling and result in further soft tissue injury.

3. When a vascular injury is suspected and the pulses are not palpable, this information should be transmitted to the base station hospital.

## ANALGESICS

The use of analgesics in the field for the treatment of trauma patients is not condoned. Analgesics can suppress respiration, causing hypercapnia and changes in cerebral blood flow. This is particularly detrimental in the patient with head trauma. Analgesics also cloud the sensorium and may alter the patient's response to pain, and may confuse the Emergency Department physician who has to evaluate the patient. Often analgesics are used when the patient seems hysterical, but more often than not, this is related to cerebral hypoxia or low cardiac output. There are very few indications for the field use of analgesics, such as morphine, to manage the trauma patient. The only time it has been used in our experience has been when an individual has impaled an arm or a leg in a machine or structure and cannot be extricated immediately. These patients are often frightened and in extreme pain. Morphine can be used in this situation, but the paramedic must be certain that he has control over the patient's airway, if needed, and should have an IV infusing before the medication is given. Morphine is a venodilator and, if the patient is hypovolemic, the blood will pool in the venous system and cause hypotension and shock.

Summary

The preceding chapter is quite lengthy and complicated in certain areas. However, the appraisal and management of trauma in the field is a very common occurrence for the paramedic. It is necessary to understand basic anatomy and mechanisms of injury before treatment is initiated; that is why we have discussed this area so comprehensively. We hope this type of background will allow the paramedic to operate with a maximum of information and confidence when meeting these situations in the field.

The treatment of trauma begins the same way in every situation. Start with the primary and secondary surveys. Strict attention to the airway, breathing, shock, and blood loss are the initial points of evaluation. Secondary considerations include protection of the spinal cord, stabilization of fractures, and the starting of intravenous fluids.

Movement of the injured victim to the proper facility is of primary importance in the total care of the patient. Sophisticated field care will not compensate for bad Emergency Department or hospital management. The converse is also true. The best way to maintain one's expertise in the management of trauma patients is to practice hypothetical situations in your own mind. What would I do if I saw the following? This mental preparation allows one to be ready when the time comes. The paramedic at the scene is in charge of the injured victim once he has been turned over to him. The victim is no longer a victim, but becomes the patient of the paramedic. Do not make the patient a victim of your treatment.

Important
Points to
Remember

Trauma is the third leading cause of death in the United States (*most* common between 20–40).

The basic tenet in the management of trauma is primarily not to do harm. Skillful extrication, airway management, spinal cord protection, bleeding control, fracture splinting, and rapid transportation are essential.

Primary and secondary surveys of the patient are important in the injured patient. Primary (life-threatening situations):

Airway and breathing

Pulse and circulation

Severe bleeding

Shock

Secondary (various body parts and systems to check for specific injuries).

*Specific helpful things to look for*

1. If spinal injury suspected, stabilize neck and back.
2. Serious bleeding—apply direct pressure.

3. Start examination at scalp and skull and proceed through examination of ears, nose, face, mouth, neck, chest, abdomen, pelvis, back, extremities, and spinal cord.

The history should include mechanism of injury and pattern of injury. The various wounds may be classified as: contusion, abrasion, laceration, avulsion, amputation, and ulcer.

A puncture wound in the skin may be a clue to a deeper injury to structures in the chest or abdomen.

Falls should always include examination for spinal cord injury.

Blows to various body surfaces may be associated with hidden injuries elsewhere.

Fractures of the trachea and larynx due to blunt injury to the neck are often not diagnosed.

Injuries to the eye may be caused by chemical agents, trauma, burns, foreign bodies, and many other substances. Most of the field treatment involves only superficial care, since the majority of problems must be handled in the hospital by an ophthalmologist.

It is imperative that head injuries be suspected and diagnosed quickly to prevent progressive damage. Treatment in the field involves airway maintenance, circulation support, and protection of the spinal cord.

Skull fractures can occur with or without scalp lacerations. Many skull fractures represent no real threat. Compound and especially depressed fractures, however, may cause brain injury.

A hematoma behind the ear may mean a posterior fossa basal fracture. Bloody fluid from the ear may mean a middle fossa fracture. An anterior basal fracture may show a bloody or cerebral spinal fluid leak from the nose.

The most common causes of intracranial injuries are auto or motorcycle accidents.

A concussion is an altered state of consciousness due to a blow on the head.

Intracranial bleeding following head injury may be epidural, subdural, or subarachnoid.

Signs of brain damage, bleeding, or swelling following injury include headache, dizziness, fainting, vomiting, partial to full loss of consciousness, personality changes, pupillary changes, breathing changes, and loss of motor function and response to pain. Elevated blood pressure, slow pulse, and convulsions may also occur.

The four cardinal signs to follow in the field evaluation of a head injury are:

Breathing

Response to stimuli

Pupil signs

Motor response

Treatment of central nervous system injuries includes:

Airway maintenance, support of neck and spine, control of bleeding, careful neurological exam, possible use of steroids (Decadron®).

Spinal cord injuries occur after auto accidents, diving accidents, and penetrating injuries to the neck and thoracic spine.

Thoracic trauma can occur from either blunt or penetrating injuries. Blunt injuries follow automobile accidents and falls. Penetrating wounds are caused by knives or bullets.

The most commonly injured structures of the chest are the ribs and sternum.

Lung lacerations may lead to bleeding and air leakage into the pleural space (hemopneumothorax).

A flail chest is paradoxical motion occurring after extensive rib fractures.

An air leak from the lung into the pleural space is called a pneumothorax. If there are no respiratory or significant vital sign changes, pneumothorax need not be treated in the field.

A tension pneumothorax is one that compresses the intrathoracic structures. Signs include dyspnea, chest pain, sweating, cyanosis, tracheal deviation, unilateral hyperresonance, wide blood pressure changes, and diminished breath sounds on the side of the pneumothorax.

Treatment of a tension pneumothorax need not be undertaken in the field except if the patient is rapidly deteriorating. In this case a 12 or 14 large bore needle is placed in the mid or anterior axillary line and connected to a valve. Oxygen is given and the airway is maintained.

Treatment of sucking chest wounds is best accomplished by placing a light sterile dressing over the chest and being certain that air is freely moving.

Tight compression is no longer indicated for these wounds in all cases. It is important to keep the wound open by whatever means is available.

Blunt trauma may produce hemopericardium, which is recognized by distention of neck veins, distant heart sounds, and low blood pressure. Abdominal injuries can occur after automobile accidents. The major determination in the field is whether there has been significant blood loss within the peritoneal cavity.

The most commonly injured organ in the abdomen is the spleen. Injuries to the aorta and major vessels usually follow penetrating trauma.

Abdominal injuries should be suspected whenever there is pain or distention following trauma. Treatment includes: MAST suit for suspected hemoperitoneum; maintenance of airway, nasal oxygen, and IV fluids when there is not massive hemorrhage; and rapid transport in *case* of hemorrhage.

Bone injuries occur after accidents. They are not usually fatal but combined with other injuries may lead to a fatal outcome.

Fractures are classified as simple (closed), compound (open), or comminuted (multiple fragments).

Signs and symptoms of fractures include pain, inability to move an extremity or joint, tenderness, swelling, crepitus, instability, angulation, and perhaps bone protrusion.

Extensive hemorrhage may follow fractures of the pelvis and femur.

When examining fractures, pay attention to the extremity distal to the fracture.

Field treatment of simple fractures involves mainly prevention of further soft tissue injury and relief of pain and discomfort.

The major fractures that require transport are those of the femur, pelvis, and supracondylar fractures of the upper extremity in children.

Compound fractures may need traction or splinting and always should be covered with a sterile or clean occlusive dressing.

Treatment of injuries to ligaments and joints depends on the involvement and degree of injury.

General facts about musculoskeletal trauma include:

1. Watch for breathing, shock, airway, and bleeding problems.

2. Splinting should be done to protect tissue damage.

3. Ice is useful for anesthesia and minimizing hemorrhage.

4. Manipulation should be minimized.

Vascular trauma may be major or minor. Most are caused by penetrating injuries (knife or bullet). Remember the 5 Ps of arterial injury.

The basic principle of vascular injury when the vessel is accessible is to apply compression and transport.

Tourniquets are occasionally helpful.

Abdominal vascular injuries are managed by the MAST suit and transport; thoracic vascular injuries are managed by rapid transport.

The use of analgesics in the field for the treatment of trauma is not condoned. The one exception may be the use of morphine for a patient who has impaled an extremity in a machine or structure.

*Bibliography*

American Red Cross. *Advanced First Aid and Emergency Care.* New York: Doubleday and Company, Inc., 1973.

Committee on Trauma, American College of Surgeons. *Early Care of the Injured Patient.* Philadelphia, Pa.: W. B. Saunders Company, Inc., 1976.

Dunphy, J. E. and L. W. Way. *Current Surgical Diagnosis and Treatment.* Los Altos, California; Lange Medical Publications, 1977.

Mattox, K. L., A. C. Beall, G. L. Jordan, and M. E. DeBakey. "Cardiography in the Emergency Center." *Journal of Thoracic and Cardiovascular Surgery.* 68:886, 1974.

McCredie, J. A., Ed. *Basic Surgery*. New York: MacMillan Publishing Company, Inc., 1977.

Yeo, M. T., E. J. Domanskis, R. H. Bartlett, and A. B. Gazzaniga. "Penetrating Injuries of the Abdominal Aorta." *Archives of Surgery*. 108:839, 1974.

# Chapter 15

# SHOCK

Descriptions of shock date back to the sixteenth century, but the word first appeared in an eighteenth century treatise on gunshot wounds in its French form, "choc." This was a literal reference to its meaning, impact or collision, not a description of the consequences of collision. Shock has become such a common term in the lay language, as well as in medical and paramedic parlance, that it will not be displaced by any other word in the foreseeable future. It is an indefinite term and has been applied to acute catastrophic organ or whole-body disorders. As it is used in the present context, shock implies a condition of circulatory inadequacy. Most people associate the term shock as synonymous with low blood pressure. However, low blood pressure does not necessarily mean shock, and a complete understanding of the physiologic changes which occur during injury, hemorrhage, acute myocardial infarction, or infection is needed before one can apply methods of treatment. Shock, in the specific sense, means inadequate organ or tissue perfusion, or, in the term more commonly used by physicians, a "low flow state." This means that there is insufficient perfusion (blood flow) to organs to meet their metabolic (oxygen) demands.

## MECHANISMS OF SHOCK

Shock can be produced by essentially three different mechanisms:

Disorders of blood volume
Disorders of the heart
Disorders of the peripheral circulation

### DISORDERS OF BLOOD VOLUME

The most common cause of shock is a disorder of the blood volume. Reduction in blood volume, called *hypovolemia*, can occur after a multitude of different conditions. Blood loss after trauma or a bleeding duodenal ulcer are common examples of conditions that produce hypo-volemia and shock. Hypovolemia may also result from the loss of fluid rather than whole blood. An example of this would be massive diarrhea. In hypovolemia, venous return of blood to the heart is decreased and a fall in blood pressure follows.

## CIRCULATORY DISORDERS

The second category of conditions that can produce shock is related to the heart. This is commonly termed pump failure and may be the result of valve disorders, such as narrowing of the aortic valve (aortic stenosis), or insufficiency (leak) of the mitral valve (Chapter 10). Pump failure may also be related to disorders immediately outside of the heart which are affecting the heart and its function, such as cardiac tamponade (fluid around the heart), hydrothorax (fluid around the lung that com-presses the heart), or even tension pneumothorax. Another more common category of conditions which can produce shock related to the heart is injury to the heart muscle. This occurs (previously described in Chapter 10) with acute myocardial infarction. Dysrhythmias, such as ventricular tachycardia, can cause shock by not allowing the heart enough time to fill and eject blood.

## DISORDERS OF PERIPHERAL BLOOD FLOW

The third disorder, which is the least commonly encountered in the field, applies to disorders of the peripheral blood flow. In this situation there may be normovolemia and the heart may be functioning adequately, but there is not enough blood flow to meet the oxygen demands of the peripheral tissues. The heart cannot keep up with the amount of oxygen demanded and it fails. Such a condition occurs frequently in the hospital during severe infections by gram-negative organisms or during a condition called endotoxic shock. This is shock produced by the release of toxic products from gram-negative organisms into the bloodstream. This could be encountered in the field in patients who have a perforated diverticulitis or appendicitis with peritonitis (Chapter 16).

## PATHOPHYSIOLOGY OF SHOCK

Large numbers of animal experiments have been performed in an effort to learn what changes in normal physiology occur during blood or fluid loss. These studies have led to a better understanding of the consequences of blood and fluid loss in the human. When blood is removed from the body, there is a gradual narrowing of the pulse pressure. The pulse pressure is the difference between the systolic and diastolic blood pressures. For example, the pulse pressure in a patient with a blood

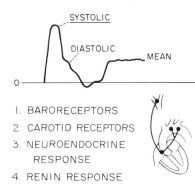

Figure 15-1. Pulse pressure is the difference between the systolic and diastolic pressures. As the pulse pressure narrows (hemorrhagic or cardiogenic shock), this change is sensed by receptors in the carotid artery and aorta, which stimulates a neuroendocrine response.

pressure of 120 mm Hg/80 mm Hg is 40 mm Hg. Narrowing of the pulse pressure is recognized by sensors in the carotid body and in the aortic arch (Figure 15-1). These sensors send signals to the adrenal glands notifying them that the pulse pressure has changed. The adrenal glands respond by secreting epinephrine and norepinephrine. These potent drugs, called catecholamines, produce vasoconstriction raising the peripheral vascular resistance, returning the arterial blood pressure to normal levels (Figure 15-2). Catecholamines also increase the force and rate of the heart action. Arteriolar constriction (vasoconstriction) reduces the blood flow to other organs. The organ having its blood supply reduced first is the skin, followed by the skeletal muscle, kidneys, and the intra-abdominal organs. This restriction of organ flow to raise the blood pressure occurs to protect perfusion of the brain and heart. If blood loss were to stop at this point, the blood pressure would stabilize and the intravascular volume would increase as extracellular and intracellular fluids migrate into the circulation. Then vasoconstriction would gradually subside and normal organ perfusion would be restored. If bleeding

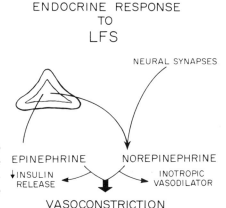

Figure 15-2. The endocrine response to the low flow state (LFS) is based on the release of catecholamines from the adrenal gland. This stimulates the heart rate and constricts peripheral blood vessels.

continues, however, further compensation by vasoconstriction would not be possible and the blood pressure would start to fall. If the hemorrhage progressed, the heart rate would increase dramatically in an attempt to pump more blood to the body until the blood volume was so low that virtual circulatory standstill and cardiac arrest ensued.

During the period of inadequate tissue perfusion, the body cells undergo ischemia. That is, the blood present in the capillaries has normal oxygen tension, but there is not enough of it to deliver oxygen to the cells. This leads to anaerobic metabolism (cellular metabolism in the absence of oxygen). Anaerobic metabolism produces hydrogen ions and leads to metabolic acidosis (Figure 15-3). Although this acidosis begins within the cell and produces intracellular and finally extracellular acidosis, it will eventually produce acidosis in the blood, which will affect the heart and capillaries throughout the body. If the acidosis is severe and the arterial pH drops below 7.25, it will affect the heart function and further aggravate the consequences of shock.

Reduction in the blood volume, or hypovolemia, produces profound direct and indirect effects on the heart. As mentioned previously, the release of catecholamines due to the reduction in pulse pressure increases the heart rate and makes the heart beat more forcibly. At the same time the reduction in blood volume means less blood returns to the heart, which reduces left atrial pressure, left ventricular filling pressure, cardiac output, and blood pressure (Figure 15-4). These changes are compensated for by neural and endocrine responses as well as the reabsorption of fluid back into the vascular space (Table 15-1). The heart rate increase is an attempt to pump more blood and meet the

## "SHOCK"

LOW FLOW STATE – ORGAN AND CELLULAR HYPOXIA

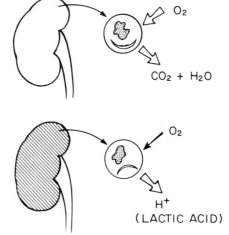

$O_2$

$CO_2 + H_2O$

$O_2$

$H^+$
(LACTIC ACID)

**Figure 15-3.** With inadequate perfusion of organs, cells undergo anaerobic metabolism. This releases hydrogen ion ($H^+$) metabolic acidosis.

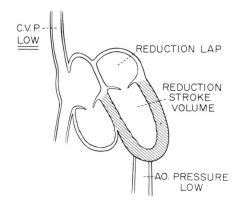

**Figure 15-4.** During hemorrhage, there is a reduction in left atrial pressure and stroke volume.

TABLE 15-1.   INADEQUATE PERFUSION FOR METABOLIC NEEDS

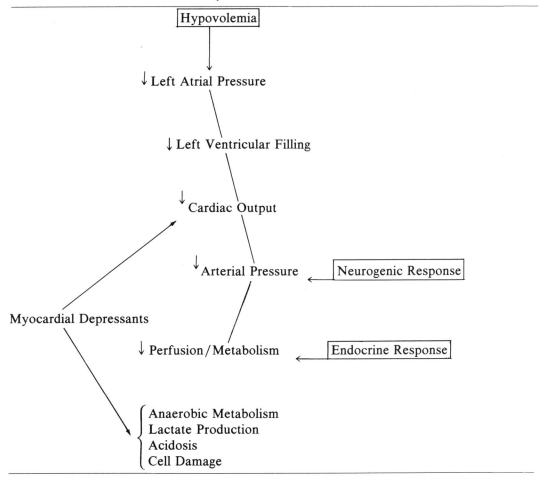

oxygen demands of the peripheral tissues. As shock continues and metabolic acidosis ensues, toxic products are released from anoxic cells, which further depresses the heart function and makes it inefficient in the presence of shock. If left unchecked, the heart will eventually not receive enough perfusion of blood for its own oxygen demands and will fail.

Besides the adrenal catecholamine response to reduction in pulse pressure, endocrine changes occur which attempt to restore homeostasis. One of these is the release of antidiuretic hormone (ADH) from the posterior pituitary gland. This hormone enables the kidney to conserve water which is then returned to the body. Patients in shock will always manifest low to absent urine output. The kidney responds to a fall in mean arterial pressure by secreting a hormone called renin which interacts with the adrenal gland via a plasma protein to release the salt-retaining hormone, aldosterone. Renin also promotes further arteriolar constriction. Renal sodium retention aids in the expansion of blood and extracellular fluid volume. Adrenal corticosteroids are released and they help to conserve sodium as well as to aid in other aspects of metabolism. In shock, the pancreas releases insulin, but its effect is blocked at the cell, and blood glucose levels rise. Epinephrine promotes the mobilization of free fatty acids which become available for energy sources.

## CATEGORIES OF HEMORRHAGE

The most common cause of shock encountered by paramedic personnel is blood loss. Accurate assessment of the patient's blood volume can lead to important decisions regarding priorities. Unless the blood loss is external, it is not always clear that the shock is due to blood loss. An example of this is a ruptured spleen following blunt abdominal trauma. Therefore, it is helpful to keep in mind the different grades or degrees of hemorrhage that can produce changes in appearance and vital signs. It is important to remember that approximately 6 to 8 percent of the body weight of an adult and 10 percent of that of an infant is the predicted blood volume of that individual. For example, a 70 kg female has an approximate blood volume of 4500 ml (6.5% × 70 kg).

Blood loss can be graded into four categories, as follows:

Grade I Hemorrhage
Grade II Hemorrhage
Grade III Hemorrhage
Grade IV Hemorrhage

Grade I hemorrhage approximates 10 percent of the patient's predicted blood volume. Findings would include dizziness on sitting up, modest elevation in the heart rate to 90 to 100 beats per minute, and a slightly cool skin. A 10 percent blood loss in a patient with a blood volume of 5000 ml would be approximately 500 ml. This is equivalent to a single unit donation in a blood bank. One can appreciate this type of blood loss by observing blood donors when they suddenly sit up after venisection. They feel dizzy and usually develop an increase in their heart rate. This type of blood loss may occur after the fracture of a femur, a major scalp laceration, or the puncture of a major vein.

## GRADE II HEMORRHAGE

A Grade II or moderate hemorrhage would be 10 to 20 percent of the predicted circulating blood volume. In a 70 kg female it would be 500 to 1000 ml. This loss would produce cool sweating skin, thirst and anxiety, an increased heart rate to over 100, and elevation in the respiratory rate. There may be a narrowing of the pulse pressure, and hypotension may or may not be present. Usually, the systolic blood pressure is around 100 mm Hg and may fall further when the patient is placed in the upright position. This type of blood loss can occur with a ruptured spleen, a pelvic fracture, or hemorrhage from a duodenal ulcer.

## GRADE III HEMORRHAGE

Grade III or marked hemorrhage refers to a loss of 20 to 40 percent of the predicted blood volume, and would be between 1000 to 2000 ml of blood in a 70 kg female. The signs of blood loss are obvious and include anxiety and fright by the patient, pale to white cold and clammy skin, a heart rate over 120 per minute, and a rapid respiratory rate. The pulse pressure is narrow and the systolic blood pressure is below 100 mm Hg. The longer this type of shock or hypotension is present, the more severe the tissue metabolic acidosis becomes. This type of blood loss may follow a gunshot wound of a major blood vessel, fracture of the liver, or a severe splenic injury.

## GRADE IV HEMORRHAGE

Grade IV or massive blood loss is any blood loss over 40 percent of the predicted blood volume. The patient would appear moribund, cyanotic, semiconscious or unconscious, with a rapid heart rate, obvious respiratory distress, a blood pressure less than 50 mm Hg, and probably unpalpable pulses. This type of massive catastrophic blood loss would be associated with any multiply-injured patient who has simultaneously had a liver, splenic, and pelvic fracture, or has had a rupture of an abdominal aortic aneurysm.

## TREATMENT OF SHOCK

As mentioned previously, the most common cause of shock encountered by paramedic personnel and perhaps by hospital personnel as well is secondary to blood loss. If the patient is hemorrhaging and the blood loss is external, simple measures to stop the bleeding would be an obvious first step. For example, a stab wound of the femoral artery in which the bleeding is in the groin region can be stopped by simple firm digital pressure. On the other hand, bleeding from a ruptured spleen is internal and is not easily dealt with in the field. The first step is to determine that shock is due to blood loss and the second is to attempt some volume replacement either before or while transferring the patient to a hospital facility. The paramedic traveling in his van does not have a blood bank in his back pocket, and therefore cannot give blood as a part of his resuscitative efforts. Even if blood were immediately available to him, the full and complete resuscitation of the patient often requires an immediate operation and cessation of hemorrhage by surgical techniques.

The goal of treating shock in the field is to restore intravascular volume with solutions that are compatible to all types of patients and early and rapid transportation. In most cases, the best treatment of shock due to blood loss following trauma is rapid transport. The use of Lactated Ringer's solution is a common practice and should be the solution of choice in the initial resuscitation of patients in shock. This is true for all types of shock, not just that due to acute blood loss. In most situations, a rapid infusion of one liter of Lactated Ringer's in an adult will often restore blood pressure to a normal level. The use of other types of solutions, such as colloids, would depend upon the situation and the type of injury. Transportation to most facilities is quite rapid. The use of colloid plasma expanders is often not necessary and should not delay transport of the patient. However, this is controversial, and it really matters very little in the initial 1000 to 2000 ml of fluid resuscitation whether the patient is given Lactated Ringer's or an albumin-containing solution, as long as the goal remains to transport the patient to a facility where hemorrhage or shock can be treated in a complete fashion.

If shock has been present for a long period of time and has been profound, the use of sodium bicarbonate may help restore heart function and peripheral circulation. One mEq/kg of sodium bicarbonate (approximately two ampules) in the usual adult patient is a satisfactory initial dose until the patient is transported to a facility and a measurement

of the pH can be done. The use of bicarbonate solutions implies that
the patient is adequately ventilated and, of course, this aspect of the
patient's overall care must not be neglected. Alveolar oxygen concentration should be as great as possible to allow maximal oxygenation of
blood as it passes through the lung. This can be achieved by use of
a face mask with a tight fit and high oxygen flow rates. It may also
be necessary to use the esophageal obturator airway and positive pressure
ventilation when there is full arrest or coma, and no gag reflex.

The recent introduction of the MAST suit (Military Anti-Shock
Trousers) has aided in the treatment of patients with hypovolemia due
to shock (Figure 15-5). This device encases each leg separately as well
as covering the pelvis and abdomen up to the rib cage. The MAST
suit is equivalent to a quick IV of 750 to 1000 ml of blood. It works
by squeezing veins and emptying blood from them to transfuse the patient
as well as compressing veins and arteries that may be injured and bleeding.
This will allow optimal perfusion of the upper half of the body while
the lower half is compressed. It is particularly useful when there is
hypotension due to an abdominal or pelvic injury. The garment is applied
and inflated until there is some return of vital signs. It has become
common practice to place the MAST suit under all serious trauma patients
so it is ready to inflate at any time during transport. The following
are the most simple instructions in setting up the MAST suit for use
in the field:

1. Unfold the MAST suit completely and lay flat.

2. Attach foot pump and open stop cocks.

3. Place the patient on the MAST suit so the top of the garment
will be just below the lowest rib.

4. Wrap the left leg of the garment around the patient's left leg
and secure with velcro strips.

5. Wrap the right leg of the garment around the patient's right
leg and secure with velcro strips.

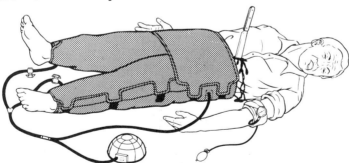

**Figure 15-5.** The MAST suit has allowed for stabilization of many trauma patients
and patients with shock due to blood loss from causes other than trauma. It comes
in three parts. The abdominal portion or each leg portion can be inflated separately.

6. Wrap the abdominal area and secure with velcro strips.
7. Inflate the trousers by using the foot pump until:
   a. the velcro is heard crackling
   b. air exhausts through the relief valve
   c. the patient's systolic blood pressure is maintained at approxi-
      mately 90 to 100 mm Hg
8. Close valves.

The Mast suit is removed at the hospital by a physician, and the sequence is as follows:

1. A physician should be present and in charge of the patient.
2. Fluid should be adequately replaced prior to removal.
3. Anesthesia and surgical teams should be ready to operate immediately.
4. The abdominal section should be removed first.
5. Vital signs should be checked frequently to insure stability of the patient's condition before further sections are removed.

It is common for the patient to arrive in the Emergency Department and the physician will wish to remove the abdominal portion of the suit for a physical examination to look for penetrating injuries. If the patient's condition is unstable and he has been in shock, the patient should be transported to the operating room and the MAST suit removed under anesthesia when early entry into the abdomen can be effected. If the patient arrives in the Emergency Department with stable vital signs and the abdominal portion of the MAST suit is removed, sudden deterioration in vital signs can occur. The MAST suit should immediately be reapplied, and the patient taken to the operating room.

There has been some controversy as to when the MAST suit should not be used. Since it is used for anyone with hypotension and obvious hypovolemia with abdominal injury, such as a gunshot wound or severe blunt injuries, there are a great number of situations in which it can be used. The absolute contraindications for its use are pregnancy and the presence of a diaphragmatic hernia or tension pneumothorax. Even here it can be used by inflating only the leg portion and leaving the abdominal part deflated. There is also some controversy as to whether it should be used in the head-injured patient. However, if the patient is hypovolemic and a blood pressure is not obtainable and there is obvious hemorrhage, its application is mandatory. The theoretical effects it may have on cerebral blood flow and circulation do not outweigh the importance of restoring normal blood pressure. The MAST suit can be used in bleeding not due to trauma (duodenal ulcer), cardiogenic shock, and even during cardiac arrest.

Although bleeding has been emphasized as the most common cause of hypotension, the evaluation of patients in the field should be complete to rule out other causes for low blood pressure. One of the more common mistakes is missing a tension pneumothorax and explaining shock on the basis of blood loss. This occurs after trauma in which the patient looks like he has lost a large amount of blood from his injuries and is shocky, yet his only major problem is a tension pneumothorax. The treatment and diagnosis of this condition is covered in Chapter 14. Some other possibilities include cardiac tamponade, myocardial infarction, and overwhelming infection. The treatment of these conditions varies little from the treatment of hypovolemic shock and the same basic principles are utilized before transporting the patient.

*Summary*

Shock is a condition of inadequate tissue perfusion. It can be caused by many different conditions, but it is basically either due to hypovolemia, disorders of the heart, and/or disorders of the peripheral tissues and circulation. In the field the most common cause of shock is hypovolemia. This can be due to fluid loss, blood loss, or both. The treatment of shock is to control obvious hemorrhage, attempt to restore circulating blood volume in the field or enroute to the hospital, maintain adequate oxygenation, use of the MAST suit and rapid transport. In cases of Grade III or Grade IV shock, there may not be much that can be done in the field except maintaining the airway and rapid transport with advance notification of the situation relayed to the base hospital ("scoop and run").

*Important Points to Remember*

Shock, in the specific sense, means inadequate organ or tissue perfusion or "low flow state." Thus there is insufficient perfusion (blood flow) to organs to meet their metabolic demands.

Mechanisms of shock include:

1. Disorders of blood volume
2. Disorders of the heart
3. Disorders of the peripheral circulation

The most common cause of shock encountered by paramedics is blood loss. Six to 8 percent of an adult's body weight and 10 percent of an infant's weight is blood volume.

Grades of hemorrhage:

Grade I—10% (Dizzy, slight increase in heart rate.)

Grade II—10–20% (Anxiety, thirst, cool skin, increased heart and respiratory rate.)

Grade III—20–40% (cold, clammy, lower BP [under 100], anxiety, fright).

Grade IV—over 40%; Massive (moribund, cyanotic, semiconscious or totally unconscious, respiratory distress, BP less than 50, and unpalpable pulses).

Principles of treatment of shock due to blood loss:

Stop bleeding

Restore intravascular volume (usually 1000 ml of Lactated Ringer's)

Transportation

If of long duration, sodium bicarbonate

Oxygen

MAST suit where indicated

Other causes of shock must be carefully sought out, including pneumothorax, myocardial infarction, and overwhelming infection.

*Bibliography*   Espinosa, M. H., Updegrove, J. H. "Clinical Experience with the G-Suit," *Archives of Surgery*. 101:36, 1970.

Gardner, W. J. "Circumferential Pneumatic Compression," *JAMA*. 196:117, 1966.

McCredie, J. A., Ed. *Basic Surgery*. New York: MacMillan Publishing Company, Inc., 1977.

Nagel, E. L., Hirschman, J. C., Nussenfeld, S. R., et al. "Telemetry—Medical Command in Coronary and Other Mobile Emergency Care Systems," *JAMA*. 214:337, 1970.

Wangensteen, S. L., Ludewig, R. M., Con, J. M. and Lynk, J. N. "The Effect of External Counter-Pressure on Arterial Bleeding," *Surgery*. 64:922, 1968.

# Chapter 16

# EMERGENCY MEDICAL CONDITIONS

The paramedic is most interested in emergency situations where rapid identification and treatment in the field result in saving a life or reducing the degree of illness. The most publicized examples of this type of problem are represented by patients with life-threatening dysrhythmias and those with severe trauma. The field of internal medicine, however, contains numerous other conditions requiring rapid diagnosis and treatment. In fact, many Emergency Department visits are due to conditions not related to trauma. In this chapter we will deal with the most common medical conditions where field recognition is possible, and where initial management significantly affects the future course of the patient's illness. Discussion will center around prominent signs and symptoms and specific disease processes. Medical emergencies will be presented in the following categories:

Neurology
Infectious disease
Gastrointestinal
Endocrine, metabolic, renal
Pulmonary
Psychiatric

## NEUROLOGIC

The sudden onset of brain disorders is frightening to witness or discover. The paramedic is often called because someone cannot be awakened, someone has just had an "attack," or someone has a sudden onset of paralysis and cannot talk. Careful assessment and intervention in these situations may determine how well the patient eventually recovers.

Although there is much about the brain that is unknown, several basic facts should be constantly remembered. These include (1) the brain requires a constant supply of oxygen and glucose, and (2) after ten to twenty seconds without blood flow, a patient becomes unconscious. Irreversible brain damage occurs within five minutes of anoxia. Significant hypoxemia or hypoglycemia (low blood sugar) can also result in coma or seizures, in spite of normal brain blood flow. Once damaged, the brain has almost no capacity for regeneration. Remember, in dealing with patients who have a brain disorder, the first priority is to insure that the patient's brain is receiving adequate blood, oxygen, and glucose.

The brain is enclosed in an unyielding bony box (the cranium) from which there is only one exit, the foramen magnum, which exits to the spinal canal (Chapter 4). The contents within the cranium consist of brain tissue, blood contained within arteries and veins, and the cerebrospinal fluid (CSF). If any of the three components (brain, CSF, or blood) increases significantly in volume, the intracranial pressure rapidly rises. Mild to moderate increases in intracranial pressure cause headache, nausea, vomiting, and double vision. When no additional blood or CSF can be extruded by increased intracranial pressure, the brain is forcibly shifted from one compartment to another or pushed down out of the skull. This process is called "herniation." Herniation may be heralded by lethargy or confusion and sleepiness. Later, the pupil of one eye dilates as the brain presses on the third cranial nerve. This is not always a sure physical finding since 15 percent of normal people have a 0.5 to 1.5 mm asymmetry in pupil size.

Herniation can occur following trauma, hemorrhage into the brain substance, tumor, anoxia, and brain abscess. The changes caused by herniation can occur within seconds or minutes and makes herniation a life-threatening emergency. A further indication of herniation is paralysis or intermittent strange posturing of the limbs on one side of the body, characterized by extension of the leg and flexion or extension of the arm. Respirations may be rapid, irregular, slow, or depressed.

Ventilation plays a key role in the events surrounding increased intracranial pressure. Impaired respiration from any cause, whether brain disease, sedation, or airway obstruction causes retention of carbon dioxide and hypoxia. Hypercarbia dilates intracranial blood vessels, increases intracranial blood volume and pressure, further aggravating the situation. Hypoxia further damages brain cells and they swell, which further increases the intracranial pressure. It follows that clearing the airway, administration of moderate amounts of oxygen, and support of ventilation are absolutely essential in any case of increased intracranial pressure.

## STUPOR AND COMA

Our awareness and ability to react to external stimuli refers to our "state of consciousness." Stupor is defined as partial or nearly complete unconsciousness or reduced responsiveness. Coma, from whatever cause, is a state of unconsciousness from which the patient cannot be aroused,

TABLE 16-1. COMA

| Structural | Metabolic | Drug | Cardiovascular | Respiratory |
|---|---|---|---|---|
| Trauma | Hypoglycemia | Barbiturate | Hypertensive Encephalopathy | Chronic Obstructive Pulmonary Disease |
| Tumor | Diabetic Ketoacidosis | Narcotic | Shock | Inhalation Toxic Gas |
| Epilepsy | Hepatic Failure | Hallucinogen | Anaphylaxis | Pickwickian Syndrome |
| Subarachnoid Hemorrhage | Renal Failure | Depressant | Dysrhythmia | |
| | Thiamine Deficiency | Alcohol | Cardiac Arrest | |
| | | | Stroke | |

even by powerful stimulation. Impaired states of consciousness may take the form of sleepiness, bizarre behavior, delirium, or coma. Coma is the most severe change and may be due to a multitude of disorders as shown in Table 16-1. While the finding of an altered mental status in any patient may herald serious disease that should be brought to medical attention, the comatose patient requires immediate evaluation and intervention.

There are many causes of coma and they are not easily classified. Table 16-1 attempts to classify coma under five broad categories: (1) structural, (2) metabolic, (3) drug, (4) cardiovascular, and (5) respiratory. It is helpful to remember the categories in this fashion since it will give an orderly approach to diagnosis and treatment.

### Causes of Coma

*Structural Causes.*  Structural causes include intracranial bleeding, skull trauma, brain tumors, and any other space-occupying lesion. Even though some causes of coma are due to chronic diseases, such as a brain tumor, the change in consciousness can occur abruptly if bleeding into the tumor has occurred. The mechanism by which structural lesions cause coma is to increase the intracranial pressure or to destroy or compress the brainstem, which is responsible for the state of consciousness (Chapter 14).

*Metabolic Causes.*  The metabolic causes for coma are usually due to undersupply or oversupply of certain substances. Obvious undersupply causes would be lack of oxygen, hypoglycemia, or a thiamine deficiency. Diabetic ketoacidosis will also produce coma. Both liver and kidney failure can produce encephalopathy, which may present as coma. In this situation toxic metabolic products have not been excreted or broken down by these organs.

*Drug Causes.*  Coma in some parts of the country is almost exclusively due to drug overdosage. (Drug abuse is presented in Chapter

17.) Common drugs that produce coma are barbiturates, narcotics (e.g., heroin), hallucinogens, depressants (e.g., Valium₍ᵣ₎), and alcohol. The narcotic addict can be identified by the needle tracks on his arms and the pinpoint pupils. However, the narcotic addict may also drink alcohol and the presence of alcohol on the patient's breath may lead one to think that the coma is secondary to alcohol ingestion. It is best to assume that, although alcohol can produce coma, some other cause is present to explain the coma. It is especially important when it is realized that alcohol can cause hypoglycemia and the patient may benefit from intravenous dextrose rather than detoxification.

*Cardiovascular Causes.*   Cardiovascular conditions that can produce coma are extensive. Hypertensive encephalopathy is a term used to describe a brain disorder in the patient with chronic high blood pressure. The hypertension may be so severe as to make the patient comatose. Any disorder of the cardiovascular system which produces shock, such as hemorrhage, dehydration, and cardiac arrest, can lead to comatose states. The patient who has a fainting episode because of a sinus block or atrioventricular dysrhythmias may present with coma.

Strokes can produce coma and are discussed in a later section.

*Respiratory Causes.*   Respiratory failure is a cause of unconsciousness and coma. This is particularly true in patients with chronic obstructive pulmonary disease who may have become progressively hypercarbic and experience "CO₂ narcosis." Coma is often seen in patients with the "Pickwickian" syndrome in which they are so massively obese that they are unable to breathe properly and thus maintain a chronic hypercarbic state. These patients may present with coma since their carbon dioxide levels go high enough to produce narcosis. Toxic gases can produce coma and cardiovascular changes and should be considered in anyone who has been exposed to them.

*Assessment of the Comatose Patient.*   The paramedic must make an initial assessment of the severity and cause of the brain disorder. At the same time, he must assess the patient's breathing and cardiovascular status. A second paramedic can help by gathering information from relatives, friends, or bystanders. Facts about the patient's past history are extremely important, including whether he is a diabetic, drug user, or alcoholic; and whether he has experienced a fall, or struck his head after a fall. A history of medications used by the patient and information on previous episodes of a similar nature should be obtained also. The paramedic should be assessing the neurologic status of the comatose patient in the same manner as presented for the head trauma patient (Chapter 14).

The evaluation of the patient includes: (1) breathing, (2) responses to stimuli, (3) pupil size and reactivity, and (4) motor response. Further examination of the patient may explain why he/she is comatose. Is

the patient jaundiced? Is he cyanotic (respiratory failure)? Is there
evidence in the room of alcohol or other drugs? Is there an odor to
the breath consistent with alcohol or ketones (fruity smell)? Are there
medications nearby, such as sedatives or insulin? Are there needle tracks
on the forearm or antecubital fossa suggesting a mainline drug user?
When the initial assessment has been completed, treatment is begun.

*Treatment*

1. The initial priority is to make certain the patient has an open
airway and is breathing. If neither are present, steps should be taken
to open the airway, either by holding the jaw forward and pulling the
tongue off the oropharynx, or by inserting an oral airway and beginning
bag and mask ventilation. If the patient is semiconscious, insertion of
an oral airway may induce vomiting and aggravate the situation. If the
patient is exchanging air, but has soft tissue obstruction of the upper
airway, it is best to relieve this without attempting mechanical ventilation.

2. If shock is present, start an intravenous infusion of $D_5W$ and
Lactated Ringer's. Draw a red top tube before the infusion begins. A
serum glucose determination at the hospital will tell if the coma is due
to hypoglycemia.

3. If a dysrhythmia is palpable by pulse or auscultation, monitor
the patient's heart rate.

4. If the cause of the coma is not apparent from the initial
examination, the patient should receive an IV bolus of 50 ml of 50
percent dextrose. This will correct hypoglycemia, which may be the
cause of the coma. This is safe therapy, since, even if the patient is
an uncontrolled diabetic, the hyperglycemia produced by administration
of the glucose will not harm him. On the other hand, if the patient
is hypoglycemic from too much insulin, the administration of glucose
can be lifesaving and the patient will immediately awaken. In the alcoholic
patient who is also hypoglycemic, the glucose may be lifesaving as well.

5. The comatose patient who appears to be an alcoholic by history
or physical examination (bulbous nose with dilated veins, protuberant
eyes, wasting of arm and leg muscles, red skin over the palms, etc)
should also receive 100 mg of thiamine intravenously at the same time
glucose is given. These patients may be suffering from a deficiency
of this vitamin. Failure to give the vitamin may make the condition
worse, while its administration can result in a response almost as dramatic
as that to glucose in the hypoglycemic patient.

6. In the patient who is comatose due to a drug overdose, not
much can be done except to support the patient until arriving at the
hospital. If the overdose is due to heroin, however, an antidote is available
and can be given in the field. This is described in more detail in Chapter
17. Narcan can be given in a dose of 0.4 mg (1 ml should be given
intravenously and repeated in three minutes). Since Narcan ® does not

cause the respiratory depression seen with other narcotic antagonists, repeated doses can be used. However, the duration of its action is shorter than that of the opiate. Therefore, the patient should be monitored closely for relapses. Suspected heroin overdose patients have been given Narcan ® in the field by paramedics, and then transported to the hospital by less skilled personnel. This is a dangerous practice since the Narcan ® can wear off and the patient may relapse into a coma and need the support of paramedic personnel. Narcan ® is an antagonist effective in reversing apnea and coma caused by morphine, heroin, codeine, meperidine, propoxyphene, pentazocane (Talwin ®), and other opium-related drugs.

7. In patients with coma, such drugs as morphine, meperidine, or similar drugs are not indicated and, in fact, are contraindicated. They depress respiration, predispose to vomiting and aspiration, and obscure pupil size and level of consciousness. These important signs will be necessary for the Emergency Department physicians. In the patient with suspected increased intracranial pressure, sedatives or narcotics are contraindicated. When increased intracranial pressure is suspected, intravenous solutions should not be hypotonic, such as $D_5W$ and, if the blood pressure is satisfactory, limited amounts should be given. Hypotonic solutions and overhydration may aggravate increased intracranial pressure.

8. If the patient is comatose but breathing adequately, he is best transported to the hospital in the comatose position (Figure 16-1). Neck support is necessary because it is not known if a coma patient has had trauma. In this position the patient is placed semiprone with one knee drawn up and one arm extended up over the head. The mouth can hang over the side of the stretcher and any vomitus or oral secretions can pour forth from the mouth by gravity. This position prevents aspiration caused by vomiting. Aspiration, whether occurring in the field or in the hospital, is a difficult problem to treat. Many deaths from drug overdose have occurred because of aspiration. The paramedic and

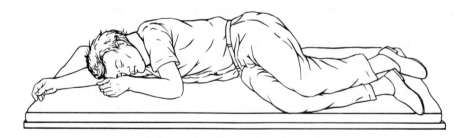

**Figure 16-1.** The coma patient is transported in the semiprone position. The neck collar is used since neck injury may have occurred in the coma patient.

Emergency Department physicians should be on guard to prevent aspiration since it is such a common complication.

## SEIZURES

*Description.* Seizures are often dramatic events that "take" a patient suddenly without warning; it is this abrupt onset that gives rise to the name "seizure." A very important aspect of field treatment is to obtain a detailed description of what happened to the patient. This may come from direct observation by the paramedic, or by asking intelligent questions of people who witnessed the "attack." In order to make proper observations or to ask the appropriate questions, the paramedic must have a clear idea of how seizures are classified.

Seizures are symptoms and may occur in any individual under the right stress, such as hypoxia, sudden elevation in temperature, or very rapid lowering of the blood sugar. Seizures also occur in structural diseases of the brain. The terms epilepsy or epileptic indicate nothing more than the liability to recurrent seizures in circumstances not provoking seizures in most persons. Otherwise, epilepsy has no prognostic or therapeutic meaning.

Those seizures that involve more than transient loss of consciousness are called major seizures. Those seizures with only transient, not very obvious interruption of consciousness are often called minor seizures. Seizures that involve a loss of consciousness from their start are called generalized seizures. Seizures starting in a limited portion of the brain are called focal seizures. Focal seizure discharges may remain confined to a limited portion of the brain or may spread to become generalized.

It is descriptively convenient to refer to certain phases in the sequence of seizures from warning phase to period of recovery.

*Stages*

1. Premonitory or prodromal symptoms are ill-defined warnings, such as irritability, apathy, or withdrawn behavior, which precede single seizures or a flurry of seizures by days to weeks.

2. Before displaying obvious activity, some patients experience an aura. The aura has been misinterpreted as a warning, but is actually part of the seizure. It results from a localized discharge before the loss of consciousness. Since the patient was conscious during the aura, he may recall it. The nature of the aura experienced by a given patient derives its particular character from the area of the brain involved. Some common types of aura include hearing noise or music, seeing floating lights, smelling unpleasant odors, an "odd" feeling in the stomach, or experiencing tingling or twitching of a given body part. The aura may last for only a few seconds.

3. The "onset" is the first portion of the seizure recognizable to an observer and may be focal or generalized.

4. The "seizure proper" is described below.

5. Immediately following a seizure, in the so-called postictal period, there may be nonspecific changes such as loss of corneal reflex (Chapter 8), lethargy, confusion, pounding headache, or sore muscles. Sometimes there is focal postictal deficit (i.e., a deficit suggesting dysfunction of a limited portion of the brain) while consciousness and other functions are retained. One example is hemiplegia. When the postictal deficit persists for as long as one to 24 hours and clears, it is called "Todd's postictal paralysis."

### Types of Seizures

*Generalized Major Motor Seizures ("Grand Mal").* Most people who have seen a seizure are familiar with this variety, which, in full-blown form, can be very striking (Figure 16-2). The patient falls abruptly to the ground. All of the body musculature stiffens (the tonic phase). Diaphragmatic and chest muscular spasm produce a "cry." The eyes turn up or to one side, the jaw tightens, and the patient may bite his tongue. Spasm of the respiratory apparatus prevents breathing and the patient turns blue or red. Shortly, violent jerking movements (clonic

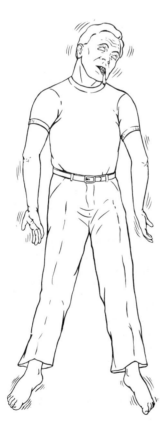

**Figure 16-2.** A grand mal seizure involves the entire body. The eyes are usually drawn upward to the left or right.

phase) of the legs, arms, and head begin, with gasping respiration. Saliva or bloody froth may form on the lips or face, and the patient may lose sphincter control. He is comatose with absent corneal and extensor plantar responses. After a few minutes, he awakens, confused and drowsy. He may have amnesia for the experience, complain of headache or aching muscles, and frequently falls into a deep sleep.

*Focal Seizures.* When there is electrical discharge from a small portion of the brain, only those functions served by that area will have dysfunction. Focal seizures begin as tonic/clonic movements localized in one part of the body. They frequently spread and appear as generalized major motor seizures. For example, a patient may have a seizure begin as twitching on one side of the body and progress to a major convulsion of all limbs with the loss of consciousness. It is very important to document how such seizures begin.

*Psychomotor Seizures.* Psychomotor seizures are often heralded by distinctive auras, including unusual smells, tastes, sounds, or the tendency of objects to look very large and near (macropsia), small and distant (micropsia), or scenes appear familiar (déja vu) or strange (jamais vu). After this the patient begins some unusual behavior. Common examples are staring spells, picking at the clothes, and smacking of the lips. In this "dreamy" state, some automatic activities such as walking or driving an automobile may continue, though the patient does not remember the episode. Many observers, including health personnel, mistakenly interpret the patient's behavior as merely uncooperative or actually psychotic, when in fact it is due to a psychomotor seizure.

*Petit Mal.* Petit mal epilepsy is a rare, idiopathic disorder of early childhood, characterized by brief lapses of consciousness (absences). The absences are, perhaps, two to thirty seconds in duration and may recur up to several hundred times daily. Minimal blinking, nodding, or an upward deviation of the eyes may be associated. Spells are usually so brief that ongoing activities of the child are not disrupted. Petit mal usually begins between 5 and 12 years of age (rarely, if ever, before 2) and almost always ceases by age 20 to 25.

*Myoclonus and Myoclonic Seizures.* Myoclonus is the very abrupt jerk of a portion of a muscle, the whole muscle, or a limb. This may recur at the same site or may skip unpredictably and irregularly from muscle to muscle. Some kinds of myoclonus are normal. Examples are the upward jerking of the arms and legs of an infant who is startled and the abrupt jerks observed in many people who are falling asleep. In general, myoclonus or myoclonic seizures are very difficult to treat and the emergency drug treatment discussed below will not apply.

*Status Epilepticus.* For our purpose, status epilepticus may be defined as a state characterized by recurrent, major, generalized seizures, between which there is no resumption of consciousness. A generalized seizure of fifteen to twenty minutes duration should be considered in the same light. Status epilepticus is a grave emergency and should be contrasted with a single seizure, recurring focal seizures (e.g., twitching of one arm), or minor spells in which the patient is confused. None of these latter forms are life-threatening.

The major problem in status epilepticus is impairment of oxygen delivery relative to brain requirements. This results from spasm of respiratory muscles during the seizure, depression of the nervous system which normally follows a seizure, the increased demand for oxygen caused by a seizure, and the use of CNS depressant drugs to treat seizures.

The most common causes of status epilepticus are withdrawal from (prescribed or nonprescribed) drugs, meningitis, encephalitis, toxemia of pregnancy, hypertensive encephalopathy, brain abscesses, kidney failure, and acute electrolyte disturbances, such as hypernatremia.

*Assessment of Seizures.* It is important to establish the fact that a seizure has occurred. The first health professional on the scene will be in the best position to make this diagnosis by observing the "attack" and by interviewing bystanders who would not be available to hospital personnel after transport. Two groups of clinical problems may be confused with seizures, specifically those that occur episodically, especially if they are of abrupt onset, and those that look something like seizures.

Many things other than seizures occur in episodes. Examples are migraine headaches, cardiac dysrhythmias, low blood sugar after exercise or drug ingestion, and the tendency to faint with a fall in blood pressure upon standing up. This last problem (orthostatic hypotension) most often results from medications used to treat high blood pressure. Two other common examples are breath-holding spells in an angry baby and hyperventilation in a nervous person. Not all causes of hyperventilation (overbreathing) are benign. Heat stroke, diabetic acidosis, and poisoning from drinking wood alcohol also cause hyperventilation.

Another group of problems commonly confused with seizures are those which have an appearance similar to some feature of seizures. Loss of consciousness is most often caused by simple fainting (see below). Stiffness of the limbs can be caused by hyperventilation (patient is still conscious), meningitis or intracranial hemorrhage, certain major tranquilizers, and by decerebrate movements associated with increased pressure inside the head. In case of doubt, the administration of an anticonvulsant medication is more likely to be harmful than helpful.

It is important to be able to distinguish fainting (syncope) from a seizure. Syncope is caused by insufficient blood flow to the brain, resulting from ineffective pumping by the heart; by relaxation of peripheral blood vessels caused by medication, reflex, or disease; or by insufficient blood volume. The most common causes of fainting are either benign vasovagal syncope associated with fatigue, emotion or heart disease. In the field, intraabdominal diseases, heat stroke, severe pain, and blood loss are also important. Because fainting results from poor blood flow to the head, faints almost always start from a standing posture. The patient usually remembers a warning that he knew he was going to faint, and he regains consciousness almost immediately upon hitting the ground. He is briefly pale and motionless, has a slow, feeble pulse and is clammy. This can be compared to seizures, which start in any position without warning and result in jerking movements during unconsciousness. A few people have a brief episode (two to three seconds of jerking) like a seizure at a point in a faint when they fall to the ground. This jerking has no significance.

*Treatment*

1. Seizures provoke anxiety in patients, families, and medical personnel. Do not treat or overtreat your anxiety. Your hand is forced in treating seizures only when the respiration is compromised. In most situations, nasal oxygen and turning the patient on his side to prevent aspiration after vomiting is all that is required. Because the patient may become hypothermic if he is exposed, it is important to keep his body temperature elevated through the use of blankets. If the patient appears hot because of a rapid elevation in his body temperature, heavy outside clothing should be removed. Do not expose the patient to bystanders.

2. In the treatment of status epilepticus, airway management is the most important consideration. Inspect to determine if the patient's jaw is not clamped down, and remove dentures and/or foreign bodies. Turn the patient to one side if there is no fear of a spinal fracture. Manage the tongue and larynx by firm gentle traction on the angle of the mandible. This will lift the jaw forward and raise the tongue off the back of the oropharynx. Hyperextension of the neck is not necessary. If possible, avoid pharyngeal or laryngeal stimulation by oral airways, tubes, and tongue blades, as these may evoke reflex vomiting and aspiration or spasm of the larynx.

3. Low flow nasal oxygen by prongs or catheter (2 to 6 liters/minute) is desirable. An oxygen mask might frighten the patient.

4. If the patient is not breathing on his own, or is breathing with shallow and slow respirations, and has more than brief pauses in respiration with seizures, ventilatory assistance will be required between spasms. During spasms, it will be ineffective. The Ambu bag with mask, as described in Chapter 9, should suffice. If this is not adequate, the esophageal obturator airway may be required to assist ventilation.

5. If the seizure appears to be due to hypoglycemia, drug therapy may be indicated. Start an intravenous infusion of $D_5W$ and Lactated Ringer's with a microdrip chamber at 20 ml/hr. If hypoglycemia is suspected, 50 ml of 50% dextrose should be given.

6. Drug therapy should only be necessary in the field in status epilepticus. Unless the patient has been receiving diazepam (Valium $_®$), this is probably the most useful emergency drug. An adult can usually be given 5 to 10 mg intravenously as a bolus slowly (over one minute), with repetition in five to fifteen minutes. Intravenous Valium $_®$ can cause respiratory arrest when given quickly. The full dose should be repeated only if seizure severity and frequency have not been altered. A total of three or four doses may rarely be necessary enroute to the hospital. Because patients who have received other drugs, such as barbiturates, may stop breathing after intravenous diazepam, the dose should be halved in such cases and resuscitation equipment should be immediately available. The pediatric dose is approximately 2 mg from infancy to age five.

7. If the patient is experiencing any dysrhythmias or blood pressure changes, vital signs should be monitored and the cardiac rate and rhythm monitored with the cardioscope.

8. In the postictal phase, during transport, the patient is best placed in the coma position if the breathing is adequate.

## STROKE

Stroke is the third most common cause of death and, in the middle-aged and older American, is a more frequent cause of disability. A stroke is an illness with a rapid onset and is usually the result of diseased blood vessels. A stroke in medical parlance is termed a cerebrovascular accident (CVA). The patient who has a stroke may die shortly after the onset. However, in many cases the patient survives the initial stroke to be left with a neurologic deficit, or may even recover completely. Most types of strokes are associated with a focal neurologic deficit symptom that is attributable to an involvement of a limited portion of the brain. When there is paralysis, for example, it may be on one side of the body or involve impairment of the language function or speech.

*Causes.* Strokes can be divided into two broad categories. One category of stroke is the result of *infarction*, which occurs when the blood supply to a limited portion of the brain is inadequate and death of nervous tissue follows. Infarction may be caused by embolism or by blood vessel occlusion due to atherosclerosis. Emboli are usually small blood clots arising from diseased blood vessels (carotid) in the neck or from clots or material arising from the heart. Other types of emboli which may cause occlusion of cerebral blood vessels are air, tumor tissue, and fat. An infarction can also occur when there is marked narrowing of the blood vessels in the neck or within the skull due to atherosclerosis. The gradual closure of the vessel produces reduced flow to certain portions of the brain and, if the narrowing becomes severe enough, thrombosis may occur.

The second category is *hemorrhages*, which may occur within the substance of the brain (intracerebral hemorrhage) or into the fluid bathing the surface of the brain in the subarachnoid space (subarachnoid hemorrhage). The development of the hemorrhage is usually sudden and marked by a severe headache and stiff neck. The vast majority of intracerebral hemorrhages occur in hypertensive persons when a small vessel deep within the brain ruptures. Subarachnoid hemorrhages most often result from congenital blood vessel abnormalities or from head trauma. The congenital abnormalities causing hemorrhage are known as aneurysms (weakened, outpouched areas of the blood vessel wall) and arteriovenous malformations (collections of abnormal blood vessels). Aneurysms tend to be on the surface and may bleed into the brain substance or into the subarachnoid space. Arteriovenous malformations may be within the brain substance, and bleeding may be within the brain, subarachnoid space, or both.

Bleeding within the brain substance often tears tissue or separates normal brain tissue, and improvement occurs when the blood clot is slowly reabsorbed. The release of blood into the spinal fluid-containing cavities deep within the brain may paralyze vital centers. If blood in the subarachnoid space impairs the drainage of cerebrospinal fluid, which is constantly formed and reabsorbed, the lack of reabsorption may cause a rise in the intracranial pressure. Herniation or protrusion of brain tissue through a narrow opening in the skull may then occur. Bleeding and recurrence or extension of bleeding is another concern with hemorrhage.

In infarction, the tissue that has died swells. This swelling may cause further damage to nearby tissue that has only a marginal blood supply. If the swelling is serious enough, herniation may result.

*Assessment.* The patient who is suspected of having a stroke requires the same evaluation as described in Chapter 14 for the head trauma patient. The important points of the history are to determine when the patient was last noted to be alert and how his physical condition has altered. Details such as medications used, previous history of strokes, hypertension, cardiac abnormalities, and other underlying medical illnesses, are important. In the neurologic evaluation, the important points to note are the *level of consciousness* upon initial examination and *changes* during the neurologic exam. Unilateral neurologic signs help to localize the lesions.

The patient with a stroke may present with unilateral weakness or paralysis of the arm, leg, and face (drooping of the eyelids and corner of the mouth). For example, a right cerebral hemisphere stroke would produce left facial weakness and left body weakness. This is diagrammed in Figure 16-3, as well as the central nervous system pathways. When the stroke is below the hemisphere in the pontine region near the seventh nerve nucleus, the patient will present with paralysis of the face on

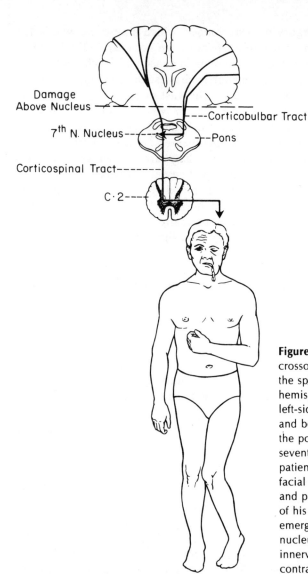

Damage
Above Nucleus

Corticobulbar Tract

7<sup>th</sup> N. Nucleus

Pons

Corticospinal Tract

C·2

**Figure 16-3.** Because there is crossover of motor fibers in the spinal cord, a right hemisphere stroke presents as left-sided paralysis of the face and body. If the damage is in the pons at the level of the seventh nerve nucleus, the patient would present with facial paralysis on one side and paralysis of the other half of his body. The facial nerve emerges in the site of its nucleus, but receives its innervation from the contralateral hemisphere.

the side of the stroke, and paralysis of the rest of his body on the opposite side. This is because the motor fibers pass through this region and then cross over to the opposite side of the body on the lower level of the spinal cord. The seventh nerve, which receives its motor fibers from the cerebral cortex of the opposite hemisphere, emerges on the same side as its nucleus.

Occasionally, patients may have small emboli that produce transient stroke-like symptoms that clear rather rapidly. These patients still require hospitalization to assess the reason for the transient stroke and possible treatment. Transient ischemic attacks (TIAs) are a common manifestation of carotid artery disease, which is due to atherosclerosis and obstruction of the carotid artery in the neck. TIAs can manifest themselves by sudden blindness in one eye (Amaurosis fugax), weakness in one side of the body, loss of speech, and even fainting. This may occur quite rapidly, but the paramedics may already have been summoned. Although not a usual part of the paramedic evaluation, examination of the neck may reveal a murmur over the carotid artery, called a *carotid bruit*. This bruit indicates that there is some narrowing or irregularity at the site of the bifurcation of the carotid artery. It is important for the paramedic personnel to document the exact changes which occurred with the TIA, since this would be of immense help to the hospital physicians. Sometimes the family may insist that the patient is now fully recovered and does not need a physician's care, but a second TIA may follow at any time that may produce irreversible neurologic deficits.

*Treatment*

1. The first goal in treating a patient who has had a stroke is to maintain adequate oxygenation and perfusion to the brain. If there is any suggestion that the condition may not be a stroke, but may be secondary to hypoglycemia, 50 ml of 50 percent dextrose should be given. This treatment may suddenly awaken a patient who has otherwise been diagnosed as having a stroke.

2. If the patient's airway does not appear adequate, the jaw should be lifted forward and the patient turned to the side to allow secretions to flow out as well as helping to keep the jaw forward. With clear evidence of inadequate breathing or ventilation, an oral airway with bag or mask ventilation should be instituted. On occasion, an esophageal obturator airway may be needed. However, it should be emphasized that any patient with a stroke should not be unduly stimulated to produce vomiting. This may cause increased intracranial pressure and further risk from the stroke. If the airway appears to be adequate and air exchange is present, a face mask or nasal prongs with oxygen flow rates of 6 l/min is better than attempting mechanical airway intervention.

3. The vital signs are recorded and if hypotension is present an intravenous infusion of Lactated Ringer's is started. Judicious administration of fluids should be used, since overhydration may aggravate increased intracranial pressure.

4. Because of the impairment of blood flow to the brain, the patient should be kept flat with the head propped up 15° to allow for adequate venous drainage. If there is congestive heart failure, the patient should be maintained in the semiupright position.

5. One should avoid maneuvers that would make straining, coughing, or vomiting possible. Noise, movement, and excitement should be minimized.

6. If increased intracranial pressure appears to be part of the clinical syndrome, then consideration should be given to the administration of corticosteroids or even mannitol in the field. Their use is controversial and will depend upon the preferences of the physicians involved in the management of these patients.

7. Narcotics and sedatives are not indicated and should not be used for these patients. Agitation in these patients most likely represents reduced cerebral blood flow or hypoxia.

## INFECTIOUS DISEASES

The paramedic will frequently encounter patients who have an infectious disease. An infectious disease is an illness caused by an organism, such as a virus, bacteria, or fungus. Common examples of infectious diseases are pneumonia caused by bacteria or viruses; meningitis caused by viruses, bacteria, or fungi; and peritonitis caused by organisms normally found in the intestines.

Some infectious diseases are highly communicable, whereas others are not. For the purposes of this discussion, a communicable disease is a disease process caused by an organism that can be transmitted from one human to another. The common cold caused by a virus is highly communicable, but does not usually produce serious effects. On the other hand, tuberculosis is a communicable disease requiring close exposure for a prolonged period of time for transmission. (The same may be true of leprosy.) However, tuberculosis organisms coughed into one's eye can produce a serious infection based on that one encounter. Therefore, the fundamental questions the paramedic needs to answer in the field include the following:

1. Does the patient have an infectious disease?

2. Has the paramedic protected himself from the infectious disease?

3. Has the paramedic decontaminated his equipment and ambulance?

4. Has he sought advice in terms of the followup on his own behalf based on the knowledge of the final diagnosis of the patient he encountered?

Infectious diseases generally produce systemic symptoms such as fever and tachycardia. When the paramedic suspects an infection, he can confirm this by measuring the patient's temperature and, if it is elevated, he should assume that the patient has an infectious disease. Before initiating treatment, the paramedic should be certain that both he and the patient are wearing a face mask. The patient should be transported to the hospital in this fashion.

If the patient requires ventilatory assistance during transport, then all nondisposable masks and bags should be properly decontaminated by gas sterilization based on hospital protocol. When transporting patients, there should be free circulation of air inside the vehicle in order to reduce the quantity and concentration of the organisms.

The paramedic must protect himself in cases where there has been some type of undue exposure. This would include exposure to a patient with meningococcal meningitis (see next section). Although this is a communicable disease, the chances of its transmission from one person to another are only one in 2000. However, if an individual has been exposed to a patient that was subsequently discovered to have meningococcal meningitis, a prophylactic course of antibiotics may be indicated. The paramedics should consult the physician at the base station hospital for such information. If the paramedic has been struck by a needle or some instrument that has previously been contaminated by a patient with suspected hepatitis, he should also consult the base station physician.

## MENINGITIS

Meningitis may be defined in the broadest terms as an inflammation of the coverings of the spinal cord and brain. It constitutes an emergency because, if left untreated, it can lead to a rapid death; and if treatment is delayed there may be lifelong neurologic sequelae. On the other hand, early treatment of bacterial meningitis usually results in a complete cure.

The inflammation can be due to bacteria, viruses, or fungi. The most common bacteria causing meningitis are *Hemophilus influenzae, Neisseria meningitidis,* and *Streptococcus pneumoniae* (except in the very young and very old).

The infection spreads to the meninges either by direct extension through the skull from the outside, or through the brain itself after being lodged there by the bloodstream (hematogenous spread). Direct invasion can follow trauma or infections of the ear, sinuses, orbit, or scalp. Hematogenous spread occurs in patients with infection of the heart valves, lungs, kidney, or intestines. Therefore, in any patient with meningitis, it is important to search for the originating source of the bacteria.

The hallmarks of meningitis are headache and a stiff neck. Other constitutional symptoms are fever, chills, and weakness. Localizing symptoms vary according to the source of infection. In patients with head trauma and a possible skull fracture, it is very important to ask about drainage from the nose (rhinorrhea) or ear (otorrhea), which may actually be cerebrospinal fluid leaking from around the brain. In patients with overwhelming infections or those left untreated, symptoms of brain injury usually ensue. These include seizures, change in consciousness (delirium, stupor, coma), cranial nerve dysfunctions, and circulatory collapse.

*Assessment.* Physical examination must include detection of neck stiffness by seeing if the patient can touch his chin to his chest or if there is neck stiffness when it is moved forward. Vital signs are important to determine the presence of shock or respiratory compromise. An initial assessment of mental status is also critical. Look for skin eruptions, especially those that appear to be hemorrhagic. This may indicate meningococcal meningitis (especially petechiae, which are tiny purple dots).

There are some pitfalls to the diagnosis. Patients not presenting with classical symptoms include small children, the elderly, the immuno-suppressed, and the alcoholic. In the latter, symptoms of headache, fever, and altered mental status are often attributed to the acute or chronic inebriation, when they may be due to bacterial meningitis. Alcoholics are more susceptible to meningitis than other population groups. Overdiagnosis may occur in patients with arthritis of the cervical spine or those who have sustained an injury to the spine and/or the head.

*Treatment*

1. The paramedic must have a high index of suspicion for the diagnosis of meningitis if he expects to discover it. In any suspected cases, all efforts should be directed towards transporting the patient to the hospital as rapidly as possible.

2. When shock is present, start an IV of $D_5W$ and Lactated Ringer's.

3. Monitor the heart rate.

4. Seizure control with IV diazepam should only be given in status epilepticus, since respiratory depression can occur.

5. Since some bacterial organisms that cause meningitis are highly contagious and may be harbored in the throat (meningococcal organisms), paramedics should take precautions to protect themselves. These include the routine use of a face mask and a bag/mask resuscitator as needed, rather than the use of mouth-to-mouth resuscitation in the case of respiratory arrest.

SEPTIC SHOCK

*Description.* Septic shock is medical slang for a severe systemic reaction to Gram-negative and/or Gram-positive organisms. It usually means that organisms have entered the bloodstream and produce systemic changes. The most common changes are reduction in blood pressure, elevation in heart rate, and alteration in the sensorium. Gram-negative shock is caused by bacterial organisms that usually reside in the gastrointestinal tract and produce profound effects on the patient. An example of Gram-negative shock is that which can occur following a ruptured appendix that has gone untreated. The most common cause of septic shock, however, is in patients with urinary tract infections. Shock can be caused by the organisms themselves or an endotoxin or exotoxin* liberated by the organisms. The patients often present in two general categories. In one situation, the patient's blood pressure is reduced, his temperature is elevated, he has tachycardia, and his skin feels warm. This is called warm septic shock. The patient may also exhibit signs of mental confusion and appear quite ill. In the other situation, septic shock is heralded by hypotension, tachycardia, fever, and cool extremities. In the latter case, the cardiac output may be normal but the peripheral arterioles are constricted, allowing for inadequate tissue perfusion. In either case, septic shock is a serious condition requiring immediate field treatment and transportation to the hospital.

*Treatment*

1. The diagnosis of septic shock can be made by measuring the body temperature, pulse rate, and blood pressure. The patient will often have some other complaint to indicate that septicemia is occurring. However, if the patient is comatose, the diagnosis can only be a guess.

2. Start an IV of $D_5W$ and Lactated Ringer's, and infuse at a rate that will restore vital signs. A blood pressure of 100 mm Hg systolic should be achievable. Most patients in septic shock have an increased fluid requirement. Overhydration with the infusion of 1 liter of Lactated Ringer's in the field would be a rare occurrence.

3. Mask oxygen should be used at a rate of 6 l/ min to provide the maximum alveolar oxygen concentration. Because these patients have metabolic acidosis in the tissues, they will be hyperventilating.

4. The heart rate should be monitored, since these patients are subject to dysrhythmias, especially if coronary artery disease is present and the blood pressure is low.

5. Dopamine has proved very effective in the treatment of Gram-negative shock when volume replacement has not corrected hypotension, and inadequate perfusion persists (cool extremities, clouded sensorium). If hypotension persists and transport is prolonged, consideration should be given to the administration of dopamine in a dose used for cardiogenic shock.

6. Corticosteroids, although recommended for in-hospital treatment of septic shock, probably are not indicated for field use.

---

*A toxin is a poison produced by the organism. Endotoxins are those liberated by the death of an organism which is toxic itself; exotoxins are those released into the bloodstream by an organism which itself is not toxic.

## THE ACUTE ABDOMEN

Abdominal pain may herald a life-threatening illness or be of trivial importance. A detailed explanation of the pain mechanisms and pathways of the abdominal cavity is presented in Chapter 8. The analysis and deductions about the importance of abdominal pain are ultimately made by the physician at the hospital. No area in medicine is more demanding than attempting to determine the cause and severity of abdominal pain.

The acute abdomen is that abdomen with an acute, nontraumatic condition that requires surgical intervention. It is important for the paramedic to assess the severity of the patient's complaints, and to determine if immediate transport is indicated. If the pain does not appear to be serious, the patient can be reassured and transported under less hurried circumstances.

Abdominal pain may originate within the abdominal wall, peritoneal cavity, or within the intraabdominal structures themselves. These intraabdominal structures include the liver, gallbladder, pancreas, spleen, gastrointestinal tract, and the blood vessels serving these various organs Pain can also arise from structures behind the peritoneal cavity such as the urinary tract system or the aorta.

When gastrointestinal contents rupture into the peritoneal cavity, there is immediate irritation, inflammation, and pain. Initial chemical irritation is replaced within six hours by bacterial infection called peritonitis. Gastrointestinal contents can derive from the upper abdomen, as with a perforated duodenal ulcer, or can be from the lower abdomen, as in a perforated diverticulum of the colon. The confusing aspect of abdominal pain is whether the pain is due to peritonitis, rupture of a viscus, or inflammation of the wall of the gastrointestinal tract. The latter is called gastroenteritis and is accompanied by distention of the bowel, often with diarrhea or vomiting. This distention will produce abdominal pain and some tenderness on physical examination.

Swelling or inflammation of the capsule of the liver or spleen may produce vague to severe upper abdominal pain. As mentioned previously, rupture of either the liver or spleen due to trauma will place blood under the diaphragm producing shoulder tip pain secondary to diaphragmatic irritation with referred pain. Acute pancreatitis can be related to severe alcoholism, gallbladder disease, or a duodenal ulcer, and usually produces pain in the upper abdomen in the epigastric region. This type of pain may radiate directly into the back, and the patient can be quite seriously ill. Acute pancreatitis is often hard to differentiate from the rupture of a perforated viscus, such as a duodenal ulcer. Pancreatitis and/or a perforated duodenal ulcer can produce such severe pain that the patient may be writhing and extremely uncomfortable.

Pain outside of the peritoneal cavity can be generated from a kidney stone, which will produce pain in either flank. The pain may migrate and actually present in the lower abdomen on either side. A ruptured abdominal aortic aneurysm can also present with pain in either flank and may be mistaken for a kidney stone.

To add to the difficulties in assessing abdominal pain is the knowledge that pain may arise from other areas of the body and be referred to the abdomen. Such conditions as fracture of the lumbar spine, myocardial infarction, pulmonary embolism, inflamed testicle, and pneumonia may present with abdominal pain as the primary symptom. Abdominal pain is confounding and it often takes skill as well as the back-up of radiologic studies and the laboratory to help in the assessment of the pain. For this reason, the evaluation of pain in the field is limited to detecting the location, probable cause, and severity.

In evaluating the patient with abdominal pain, the history is important in determining the onset of pain, its initial site, and severity. It is important to know what relieves the pain and whether it has occurred before. All of these factors of the history are detailed in Chapter 8. The physical examination includes the complete evaluation of the patient beginning with the recording of vital signs and examination of the neck, chest, and abdomen. A more reliable test to determine if abdominal pain is due to peritoneal irritation or secondary to some distention or swelling of a structure within the abdomen is to have the patient cough. If he can localize the pain upon coughing, this would indicate that the irritation is in the peritoneal cavity and is of greater significance. The most important aspect of the physical examination of the abdomen is palpation. Involuntary and voluntary guarding with gentle palpation indicates peritoneal irritation and usually a serious condition. Tenderness to firm and deep palpation usually means that there is some swelling or inflammation of an organ within the peritoneal cavity and may not be as serious. However, this can be deceptive. The presence of shock with acute abdominal pain or postural hypotension, which is described in the following section on gastrointestinal bleeding, indicates a severe intraabdominal problem. Shock can be due to blood loss or loss of fluid such as is seen in pancreatitis, or to a perforated viscus with peritonitis. Shock with abdominal pain and rapid breathing may indicate the presence of severe metabolic acidosis with a respiratory compensation. The presence of a fever suggests infection. Table 16-2 lists the categories of the more common acute abdominal conditions.

*Treatment*

1. If the patient has stable vital signs, does not have guarding, and shows no other associated illness, he should be reassured and given an explanation of the possible diagnostic considerations. The patient can then be advised to seek help through his own physician or the Emergency Department of the nearest hospital.

TABLE 16-2. CONDITIONS PRODUCING ACUTE ABDOMINAL PAIN

| Condition | Definition |
|---|---|
| 1. Intestinal Obstruction | Intestinal obstruction most often occurs following previous abdominal surgery. Patients will complain of crampy abdominal pain and vomiting, and will have abdominal distention with changes in their bowel sounds. Pain is almost always present and there may or may not be guarding. Intestinal obstruction is an acute emergency only if the fluid loss has been great enough to produce shock. |
| 2. Acute Cholecystitis | Acute cholecystitis is an acute inflammation of the gallbladder. It produces right upper quadrant pain with radiation to the shoulder tip. The sudden onset of pain in the middle of the night may awaken an individual and precipitate a call for help. There is tenderness to palpation in the right upper quadrant. Patients with this condition are frequently obese, female, and in the 30- to 40-year-old age group. |
| 3. Acute Appendicitis | Acute appendicitis has been discussed in Chapter 8. More often than not, the condition begins with epigastric discomfort followed within 6 to 12 hours with right lower quadrant pain. These patients will often have a mild temperature elevation and complain of nausea and an upset stomach. |
| 4. Perforated Duodenal Ulcer | A perforated duodenal ulcer can occur quite suddenly. Sudden soilage of the upper abdominal cavity with gastric secretions produces severe pain. These patients are often in agony and require large doses of morphine to quiet them. The abdomen is rigid like a board, particularly in the upper quadrants. Often a previous history of duodenal ulcer is not present. |

TABLE 16-2. CONTINUED

*473*

*Gastrointestinal*
*Problems*

| Condition | Definition |
|---|---|
| 5. Acute Diverticulitis | Diverticulitis of the sigmoid colon is a common condition in the United States. It is often the result of chronic dietary habits, including lack of bulk in the diet. Patients with acute diverticulitis often have pain in the left lower quadrant. The diverticulitis ruptures into the free peritoneal cavity and there may be severe pain with shock. |
| 6. Abdominal Aortic Aneurysm | An abdominal aortic aneurysm is due to degenerative changes in the abdominal aorta. The aneurysm can often be felt if the patient is thin enough and the aneurysm is large enough. The aneurysm is due to a ballooning out of the artery, producing a large pulsation that can be felt on either side of the umbilicus. Patients with abdominal aortic aneurysms will often have some leakage of blood from the aneurysm and will experience pain directly in the back or in either flank. If the leaking continues, the pain becomes worse and shock will be present. On some occasions the patient may experience sudden pain, then shock, and finally faint. It is very important to know if the patient had a previous history of an aneurysm. |

2. If the patient complains of abdominal pain and has unstable vital signs, or is in shock, the situation is serious. An intravenous infusion of Lactated Ringer's should be started and the patient transported.

3. Mask oxygen at a rate of 6 l/min should be used if respiratory symptoms as well as cyanosis are present.

4. If vomiting is part of the acute abdominal process, the patient should be transported in the right or left lateral decubitis position, so that any vomitus material can be quickly cleansed from the oropharynx or can drain out by gravity.

5. If hypotension is part of the picture, the patient's heart should be monitored and vital signs taken frequently.

6. Under no circumstances should analgesics be given, since pain medication will mask the symptoms and delay the diagnosis at the hospital.

7. When the diagnosis is acute abdominal blood loss with hypotension, the MAST suit is indicated. This is especially true if the diagnosis is a ruptured abdominal aortic aneurysm or other ruptured intraabdominal organ with bleeding.

## ACUTE GASTROINTESTINAL BLEEDING

Bleeding may occur from within the gastrointestinal tract itself. This may manifest itself as the vomiting of blood (hematemesis) or as bloody stools (hematochezia). Nothing is more frightening to the patient than a sudden emesis of bright red blood or diarrhea with bloody stools. This will prompt a call for help more times than not, and in most cases is quite justified.

Bleeding in the gastrointestinal tract is usually from the mucosal surface of the esophagus, stomach, duodenum, small bowel, or colon. The following is a list of common causes of gastrointestinal bleeding (a complete list is so extensive that it would be impractical to present it here). The major categories include (1) inflammatory (peptic ulcer gastritis, inflammatory bowel disease, such as ulcerative colitis), (2) mechanical (a tear of an esophageal blood vessel due to vomiting, diverticulosis, hiatus hernia), (3) vascular (occlusion of a major blood vessel to the intestines, hemorrhoids, esophageal varices, arteriovenous malformation), (4) tumor (any cancers of the gastrointestinal tract), (5) systemic (patients with bleeding problems such as hemophilia and uremia), and (6) drugs (aspirin, steroid compounds, anticoagulants).

*Signs and Symptoms of Bleeding.* Blood in the intestinal tract is an irritant and large amounts will result in vomiting and diarrhea. Hematemesis (the vomiting of bright red or dark blood) localizes bleeding to the upper gastrointestinal tract. If blood remains in the stomach long enough, it is acted upon by hydrochloric acid and changes its chemical composition, which will result in a dark appearance referred to as "coffee ground." Melena (the passage of black or tarry stools), most commonly implies a bleeding site in the upper gastrointestinal tract (stomach, duodenum, small bowel). However, occasionally, bleeding in the lower gastrointestinal tract (right colon) may cause melena. Generally, bleeding from the lower tract results in bright red (hematochezia) or dark blood from the rectum. Occasionally, if transit is rapid, bright red blood may be seen following a massive hemorrhage from the upper tract.

However, black or red vomitus or stools might not represent gastrointestinal bleeding. Color changes in the stool may be due to factors other than bleeding. Iron, bismuth (Peptobismol), and charcoal preparations may cause black stools. However, black stools due to bleeding are black like tar, sticky in appearance, and foul smelling. The ingestion of beets or strawberries may occasionally cause a dull red appearance to the feces.

Not all blood in the gastrointestinal tract *arises* from the gastrointestinal tract. Blood swallowed during bleeding from the nose, mouth, or pharynx may cause melanotic stools. It takes about 60 ml of blood to cause melena. Vaginal bleeding is also sometimes confused with gastrointestinal bleeding.

The rate of blood loss is as important as the total quantity lost in determining the clinical manifestations. The loss of more than one half of the circulating blood volume over a period of several weeks or months may produce only mild pallor and weakness, while the acute loss of 1000 to 1500 ml of blood may result in syncope with many of the clinical findings of hypovolemia (Grade II hemorrhage). Acute massive bleeding may be defined as a 20 to 40 percent reduction of the circulating blood volume, or at least 1000 to 2000 ml over a brief period of up to several hours (Chapter 15). Signs and symptoms of shock or impending shock include dizziness, tachycardia, cold extremities, hypotension, thirst, and apprehension.

When the patient is first encountered, determine immediately if there has been bleeding and, if so, whether the bleeding is still active. The patient's general physical condition should be observed, and evidence of blood noted on the clothing. The examination of any gastric or rectal material that may have been saved by the patient may also yield valuable information. The so-called "tilt test" may be useful for measuring the circulating blood volume and detecting impending shock. This test will give some indication of acute blood loss by measuring the pulse rate and blood pressure in relation to postural changes.

The test is performed by determining the blood pressure and pulse first in the supine position and then in the sitting position. A drop in systolic pressure of 15 mm Hg or more, or an increase of 15 beats per minute or more in the pulse rate indicates a minimum blood loss of 15 percent of the blood volume. It is helpful to remember 15/15/15. In the patient who already has hypotension in the supine position, this test adds little information and may, in fact, be dangerous.

Information may be obtained from relatives or friends on pertinent history which might be related to the present bleeding episode. Such information includes alcohol abuse, the ingestion of aspirin-containing compounds, anticoagulation therapy, or a prior bleeding episode.

*Treatment*

1. If the patient shows no evidence of active bleeding and his vital signs are stable without evidence of shock, he can be transported to the hospital under controlled conditions.

2. If the patient is actively bleeding, which would be manifested by vomiting blood or bloody stools, and signs of impending shock are present, an intravenous infusion should be started. A large bore needle placed in the antecubital space can be used to start an intravenous infusion of Lactated Ringer's. The rate of infusion should be 500 to 1000 ml per hour (or more) in order to reestablish the vital signs.

3. The patient should be kept in a supine position.

4. Mask oxygen should be administered at a rate of 6 l/min.

5. If the patient is hypotensive, the vital signs should be recorded frequently and the patient's heart rate monitored.

6. The patient who is actively bleeding should be rapidly transported to the hospital, saving any vomitus or rectal contents for evaluation at the hospital.

## ENDOCRINE, METABOLIC AND RENAL EMERGENCIES

### THE ENDOCRINE GLANDS

The endocrine glands are anatomically distinct glands that secrete hormones into the blood. These hormones are transported to distant target organs and tissues, and exert specific effects on their anatomy and function. There are medical emergencies related to each endocrine gland, but usually only the pancreas, adrenal, and thyroid glands are involved. (The principal endocrine glands are the pituitary, thyroid, parathyroid, adrenal, and the pancreas.)

*Pituitary Gland.* The pituitary gland weighs approximately 0.5 g and is enclosed in the bony structure at the base of the skull called the sella turcica (Chapter 4). It is composed of the anterior adenohypophysis and posterior neurohypophysis. The anterior portion secretes growth hormone (GH), lactation-stimulating hormone (prolactin), leutenizing and follicle stimulating gonadotropins which regulate gonadal functions, thyroid stimulating hormone (TSH), and adrenocorticotropin (ACTH) which regulates the adrenocortical functions. These hormones are under the control of humoral substances from the hypothalamus. Pituitary disorders as well as injury or disturbance of the hypothalamus can cause endocrine disorders.

The neurohypophysis secretes (1) oxytocin near the end of pregnancy and (2) antidiuretic hormone (ADH). Both of these hormones are actually synthesized in the hypothalamus and transferred by neuronal axons into the posterior pituitary where they are released into the bloodstream. Antidiuretic hormone facilitates the reabsorption of water in the kidneys.

*Thyroid Gland.* The thyroid gland is composed of two lobes connected by an isthmus and is attached to the trachea (Chapter 4). It secretes thyroxine and triiodothyronine, hormones that accelerate oxygen metabolism in the tissues. A lack of these hormones results in hypothyroidism, and an excess leads to hyperthyroidism.

*Parathyroids.*   The parathyroids are four to five small, pea-sized glands attached to the posterior capsule of the thyroid gland. The parathyroid hormone (PTH) stimulates reabsorption of calcium from the bone, kidneys, and possibly the gastrointestinal tract. It also promotes the excretion of phosphate in the urine. The purpose of this hormone is to maintain normal calcium levels for proper function of the nervous system and the heart. Tetany occurs when there is a decreased amount of PTH-producing hypocalcemia. An excess of parathyroid hormone causes elevation of serum calcium and may lead to muscle weakness, loss of appetite, nausea, bone fractures, kidney stones, peptic ulcer disease, and in severe stages, mental confusion and coma. Hypercalcemia can also be caused by other disorders such as metastatic cancer of the breast.

*Adrenal Glands.*   The adrenals are paired glands located in the retroperitoneal fat above the upper pole of the kidneys (Chapter 4). They are composed of the centrally placed adrenal medulla and the superficial adrenal cortex. The medulla is the site of catecholamine secretion, i.e., epinephrine and norepinephrine. These are the so called "stress" hormones, which help to maintain normal blood pressure and blood sugar, support smooth and cardiac muscles, and defend against infections. An excess of these hormones results in hypertension and hyperglycemia. A lack of catecholamines may lead to hypotension and hypoglycemia.
   The adrenal cortex secretes three types of hormones: (1) glucocorticoids (such as cortisol) which regulate the metabolism of protein, carbohydrate and lipids, and prevent excessive inflammation associated with infections and allergic reactions; (2) mineralocorticoids (such as aldosterone) which regulate electrolyte metabolism by increasing the reabsorption of sodium and decreasing the reabsorption of potassium in the kidneys; and (3) androgens which contribute to muscle strength and body hair. Decreased adrenocortical function results in muscle weakness, loss of appetite, nausea, vomiting, hypertension, and chronically increased pigmentation of the skin. This condition is called Addison's disease and may be due to the destruction of the adrenal gland by tuberculosis, surgical removal for high blood pressure or breast cancer, or sudden withdrawal of steroids in a patient who has been on chronic steroid therapy. The sudden withdrawal of steroids from the patient who has been on chronic steroid therapy for renal transplantation or rheumatoid arthritis is an example.

*Pancreas.*   The endocrine function of the pancreas is represented by small (microscopic) islets of specialized tissue that secrete insulin which is necessary for the normal metabolism of carbohydrates, protein, and fat. The pancreas also secretes glucagon, which increases the production of glucose in the liver and also increases the serum glucose level. The absence of insulin or resistance to the action of insulin and an excess of glucagon underlie the clinical condition known as diabetes mellitus. Excessive amounts of insulin cause hypoglycemia.

A medical emergency due to dysfunction of an endocrine organ is characteristically an exaggeration of the symptoms due to a disease of that organ. Therefore, it is clear that the clues to correct the diagnosis are frequently found in the history. The examiner should inquire not only about the symptoms preceding the acute episode, but also about the family history (many endocrine diseases run in families) and the patient's medications. Many endocrine patients wear a bracelet or a necklace that indicates the diagnosis and treatment in case of emergencies (Medi-Alert). Acute symptoms arise when the disease progresses to a critical level, when the hormonal reserve becomes exhausted from injury or infection, or when patients fail to take their replacement medications.

The following endocrine emergencies will be discussed in this chapter, since their early recognition without sophisticated laboratory tests is possible, and since their early treatment is important and relatively simple.

1. Diabetic Ketoacidosis (DKA)
2. Nonketotic Hyperosmolar Coma
3. Hypoglycemic Coma
4. Adrenocortical Insufficiency
5. Thyrotoxic Storm
6. Myxedema Coma
7. Disturbances of Calcium Metabolism

## SPECIFIC ENDOCRINE DISEASES

*Diabetes Mellitus.* Diabetes mellitus is one of the world's most common medical diseases. There are approximately 4.2 million diabetics in the United States. Clinically, there is an insulin deficit resulting in an elevated blood sugar and there may be accelerated atherosclerosis in the vasculature. The atherosclerosis leads to an increased frequency of heart attacks, strokes, blindness, renal failure, and ulceration or gangrene of the extremities. There are approximately 300,000 deaths per year related to diabetes mellitus.

The most common acute life-threatening emergencies in the diabetic result from too little insulin. Insulin regulates the body's supply and use of glucose as a fuel source. When there is just enough insulin, glucose enters the cells at a rate allowing them to function normally, and there is a constant concentration of glucose in the blood. When there is not enough insulin, glucose cannot enter the cell and it accumulates in the blood.

The changes that occur from an acute lack of insulin stem from the accumulation of glucose in the blood and from the body's use of proteins and fats as alternate fuels. When the serum glucose levels rise above a normal concentration in the blood, glucose is filtered into the urine. When glucose molecules are excreted into the urine, water molecules must follow (osmotic diuresis). This results in drastic increases in urine volume and eventual dehydration. Using fat as a fuel permits the body to meet its metabolic needs on a short term basis. However, the breakdown products of fat, called ketone bodies, rapidly accumulate and cause a drastic change in the patient's fluid and electrolyte balance. A severe acidosis (diabetic ketoacidosis) develops which prevents necessary chemical reactions in all of the vital organs, such as the brain and heart. Untreated, the patient will die.

*Clinical Manifestations.* The patient with diabetic ketoacidosis may or may not know he is a diabetic. The life-threatening attack may be the first sign of diabetes. If the patient is still conscious, he will note increased thirst (polydipsia) and frequency of urination (polyuria). He will feel weak, and nausea, vomiting, and abdominal pain will occur in approximately one-third of the patients. Many times ketoacidosis is triggered by an added stress on the patient's metabolism, such as an infection, alcohol excess, pregnancy, or trauma.

The patient's mental status will range from normal to comatose. Vital signs will reveal hyperventilation and, in advanced cases, shock. To compensate for the acidosis, the body reflexly initiates deep, rapid, sustained respirations, called Kussmaul breathing. Another characteristic is the fruity odor of the breath that results from exhaled ketone bodies. Shock intervenes when dehydration is severe, and is accompanied by dry mucous membranes, soft eyeballs, dry skin, and pallor.

*Treatment*

1. In all patients, an intravenous infusion should be started, and for the initial solution normal saline is recommended. Prior to the infusion a red top tube should be drawn and saved for glucose analysis at the hospital. The infusion should be rapid, at a rate of approximately 200 to 300 ml per hour or greater, in order to treat the dehydration and possible hypotension. Vital signs should be monitored and the infusion continued until there is a return of normal vital signs.

2. If the patient is comatose, all the precautions listed in the section dealing with coma or brain disorders should be followed. These may include the administration of concentrated glucose, 50 ml of $D_{50}W$. Although apparently contradictory, the glucose will not hurt the patient and, if the diagnosis is hypoglycemia instead of hyperglycemia, it can be lifesaving. Dipping a Dextrostix® in a sample of blood that has been

drawn may indicate the diagnosis of hypoglycemia. Although the Dextrostix$_®$ is not accurate for determinations on the lower end of the scale, a glucose of 60 mg percent may indicate severe hypoglycemia because this test overestimates the blood glucose. A level of 50 mg percent or below indicates hypoglycemia.

3. The patient's vital signs should be monitored. The heart should be monitored on the cardioscope since hypokalemia can occur with diabetic ketoacidosis, and dysrhythmias may appear.

4. Administer oxygen as needed as shown by clinical evaluation.

5. At the hospital, carefully regulated amounts of insulin can be given according to the results of blood chemistries. The physician will look for underlying causes of the ketoacidosis and will institute medical treatment. The mortality rate from diabetic ketoacidosis is approximately 5 percent when it is appropriately managed.

*Nonketotic Hyperosmolar Coma.*   In diabetics over the age of 60, stupor and coma may also develop with excessive hyperglycemia *without* acidosis. This condition, called hyperosmolar nonketotic coma, occurs typically in diabetes of adult onset where some insulin secretion is preserved. Serum levels of glucose are often above 1000 mg/100 ml (normal, 80 to 120 mg/ml). High concentrations of glucose are also present in the cerebrospinal fluid, and since the entry of glucose into the cells is limited, cerebral cellular dehydration takes place. Osmotic diuresis analogous to diabetic acidosis also is present and this causes severe dehydration.

The diagnosis is dependent upon a history of diabetes or diabetic symptoms with stupor or coma, often provoked by infections, extreme cold, dehydration, or drugs such as cortisone, Dilantin$_®$, or diuretics. Poor skin turgor and dehydration are present, but Kussmaul breathing and acetone on the breath are not. Critical laboratory findings are elevated blood sugar and sugar in the urine *without* ketones.

*Treatment*

1. Treatment in the field consists of rehydration and supporting the airway. Once the airway has been opened and breathing assured, an IV should be started with normal saline or Lactated Ringer's. This can be infused at a rate to restore the vital signs and may be as much as 500 to 1000 ml per hour.

2. Monitor the heart rate since acidosis may contribute to cardiac dysrhythmias.

3. Protect the airway and assure breathing.

4. If hypertonic glucose is given because of suspected hypoglycemic coma, a red top tube should be drawn to save for analysis at the hospital.

5. At the hospital, the patient will be treated with insulin and further hydration. In these patients, small doses of insulin will bring the blood sugar down within the normal range.

## Hypoglycemic Coma

*Background and Chemistry.* Since the brain is almost totally dependent on free glucose, a sudden drop in blood glucose levels results in the immediate loss of normal cerebral function, mimicking a "stroke" with focal neurologic signs, or coma and seizures due to anoxia. Blood glucose is replenished by absorption from the gastrointestinal tract, breakdown of skeletal muscle and liver glycogen into glucose, or the conversion of protein and fat into glucose (gluconeogenesis).

Glycogen is a molecule composed of glucose. Glycogen is stored in the liver and muscles. It is a quick reserve source of glucose for the body, but amounts are limited, and a patient fasting for twelve hours will have largely used up his glycogen stores. Therefore, in the absence of food intake, glucose is not absorbed and the glycogen stores are rapidly depleted, so that gluconeogenesis is practically the only source of blood glucose. This process takes time and may not occur fast enough to supply adequate glucose for metabolism.

Insulin lowers the serum glucose by enhancing the transfer into cells and by stimulating deposition of the glucose as glycogen. In contrast, other hormones, such as glucocorticoids, epinephrine, and glucagon, tend to cause hypoglycemia by stimulating the breakdown of glycogen, or by interfering with the utilization of glucose at the cell level. Hypoglycemia can thus occur with excess insulin or the lack of other hormones which tend to maintain critical levels.

Hypoglycemia can occur after fasting or after food intake. Fasting hypoglycemia can occur in normal individuals, patients with tumors of the pancreas which produces insulin, patients with adrenocortical insufficiency, and those who suffer from chronic alcoholism. Hypoglycemia that occurs after eating may be a manifestation of early diabetes, or may occur in the patient who has had a previous gastric operation. However, the most *common cause of hypoglycemia is probably due to overdose of insulin or other types of hypoglycemic drugs.*

In evaluating the patient who is suspected of having hypoglycemia, the previous diagnosis of diabetes treated with insulin or hypoglycemic agents is a significant piece of information. This is particularly true if the patient took his medication but forgot to eat. Diabetics are very familiar with the symptoms of hypoglycemia and can tell when they have not ingested adequate carbohydrate. In chronic and acute alcoholism, hypoglycemia can occur when the patient does not eat after a "bender." The patient suffering from chronic alcoholism develops changes in the liver that prevent rapid mobilization of glucose. Glycogen stores are also depleted. He can develop hypoglycemia hours later after drinking and then fasting.

*Clinical Picture.* Symptoms of hypoglycemia include weakness, a feeling of hunger, nervousness, restlessness, muscle twitching or spasms, convulsions, depression, sleepiness, blurred vision, loss of concentration, headache, shaking, sweating, palpitations, confusion, aggressive behavior, and irritability. Many of these symptoms are due to the reflex release of epinephrine in a response to attempt mobilization of further glucose from the liver. In other words, patients may experience hypoglycemia and have an epinephrine response from the adrenal gland that may confuse the clinical picture.

Physical findings include sweating and normal or shallow respirations in contrast to the deep Kussmaul breathing of diabetic ketoacidosis. Variable neurologic findings may include pupillary inequality and abnormal reactions, tonic/clonic seizures, sucking and grasping reflexes, and grimacing. The eyeballs are tense in contrast to their softness in diabetic coma. In deep hypoglycemic coma, the corneal reflexes are lost, and the liver may be enlarged. The contrast between hypoglycemia and diabetic ketoacidosis is shown in Table 16-3.

*Treatment*

1. Since the patient in hypoglycemic coma is unconscious, the airway is the first priority. Assure that the patient is breathing and, if not, establish ventilation either by opening the airway or mouth-to-mouth or mouth-to-bag breathing.

2. Start an intravenous with D$_5$W and draw a red top tube before infusion begins. Do a Dextrostix® on the blood.

3. Give 50 ml of 50 percent glucose. (In some areas 25 percent glucose is used.) If the patient awakens suddenly, the diagnosis of hypoglycemia is almost certain. A 10 percent solution of glucose or intermittent injections of 25 or 50 percent glucose may be necessary to keep the patient awake.

4. If an intravenous infusion cannot be started, instant glucose gel (25 g tube) can be given in the mouth on the mucous membranes, and the rapid absorption of glucose will follow.

TABLE 16-3. HYPERGLYCEMIA (KETOACIDOSIS) vs. HYPOGLYCEMIA

| | *Hyperglycemia* | *Hypoglycemia* |
|---|---|---|
| Onset | Hours to days. | Minutes. |
| Inciting Events | Infection, omission of insulin. | Missing meals, heavy exercise, insulin overdose. |
| Symptoms | Thirst, polyuria, headache, nausea, vomiting, abdominal pain. | Hunger, headache, sweating, confusion, stupor. |
| Physical Findings | Kussmaul respirations, fast pulse, soft eyeballs, dehydration, flushed face, appears ill. | Normal or shallow respirations, normal pulse, tense eyeballs, appears well. |

5. If the patient has alcohol on the breath and is unconscious, the diagnosis of hypoglycemia may be accurate. Do not assume because there is alcohol that this is the reason for the coma. In the alcoholic, additional thiamine may be necessary.

6. Any patient with hypoglycemia and coma is subject to cardiac dysrhythmias, and his heart rate should be monitored.

7. If the patient has not responded to glucose, he should be transported in the coma position, and all the other precautions observed.

## Adrenocortical Insufficiency

*Background.* Adrenocortical insufficiency may be caused by the inadequate production of ACTH from the pituitary gland, adrenal suppression due to the chronic use of steroid medications, or previous surgery to remove either the pituitary gland or the adrenal glands. Patients who have adrenocortical disorders are generally familiar with their disease process and can make excellent historians if they are alert. Those on chronic steroid medication are subject to adrenocortical insufficiency because they have not taken their steroids; they have taken them and vomited them; or their steroid dose is inadequate for the stress situation they may be encountering. The stress might be due to an illness or infection. The types of patients who take steroid medications are those who have had arthritis, certain blood disorders, asthma, kidney transplantation, and corticosteroid replacement for previous adrenal or pituitary removal.

*Clinical Picture.* Physical findings for chronic adrenal insufficiency include dark pigmentation of the skin, or even areas of dark and light pigmentation. The patient is generally sweaty and hypotensive. He may appear dehydrated and thirsty. Patients who have developed chronic adrenal insufficiency and who have been on large amounts of steroids will have a "Cushingnoid" habitus. They will have deposition of fat in the face and in the trunk, with thin extremities showing bruises. The skin will be thin and the face will be flushed and may contain excess hair. The individual who is on high doses of steroids may experience adrenal insufficiency if he is not taking the steroid medication, or if he has undergone stress and the steroid dose is inadequate. The types of steroid medications commonly used are Decadron_®, prednisone, Solu-Cortef_®, Solu-Medrol_®, and hydrocortisone.

## Treatment

1. Generally the patient who has been taking steroids for replacement or loss of the adrenal glands is aware of his situation. A Medi-Alert bracelet may indicate that he is a steroid user.

2. The mainstay of treatment is the restoration of intravascular volume and infusion of steroids. The IV should consist of Lactated Ringer's or normal saline. It should be run at a rapid rate to restore

the vital signs. Steroids should be given, and in the field dexamethasone 4 to 10 mg intravenously can be given as an IV push dose.

3. The patient should be transported with monitoring of vital signs and heart rate.

### Thyrotoxic Storm

*Clinical Picture.* Thyroid hormones (thyroxine and triiodothyronine) increase the metabolic rate and oxygen consumption in practically all tissues. Excessive amounts of thyroid hormones lead to acceleration of these processes. In order to satisfy the increased needs for nutrients and oxygen, the heart rate must increase. High levels of thyroid hormones are utimately toxic, and cause cardiac dysrhythmias, congestive heart failure, gastrointestinal hypermotility, loss of weight, muscle weakness, and liver disorders. Thyrotoxic storm is an exaggeration of these symptoms and represents a severe stress that may exhaust the adrenocortical defense function.

Thyroid disease tends to run in families. The crisis is preceded by symptoms such as nervousness, heat intolerance, tremor, palpitations, diarrhea, menstrual disturbances, goiter, and protrusion of the eyes (exophthalmos). The crisis is frequently precipitated by trauma or infection. Young females below the age of 50 years are most frequently affected. The patient is agitated, confused, or stuporous. The skin is thin, moist, hot, and sometimes erythematous or jaundiced. The hair is thin. The systolic blood pressure may be elevated with a wide pulse pressure, but in advanced cases the blood pressure may be low. The pulse is rapid (usually over 150/min). It may be irregular due to atrial fibrillation.

### Treatment

1. Initial treatment is supportive and requires hydration and sedation.

2. Monitor the heart rate and vital signs.

3. Propranolol in 1 to 2 mg IV doses will usually slow down the pulse and alleviate most of the symptoms due to the increased sympathetic activity.

4. Specific treatment at the hospital includes initiation of drugs to suppress thyroid function.

5. As mentioned above, the stress of this condition may exhaust the adrenocortical reserve and large doses of intravenous steroids are indicated.

### Myxedema Coma

*Background and Clinical Picture.* The lack of thyroid hormones may be due to destruction of the gland, impaired biosynthesis of the hormones, or failure of the hypothalamo-pituitary stimulation. The result is a general decrease of metabolic processes and impaired elimination of various metabolic products and water.

Some patients have a history of hyperthyroidism treated by surgery, drugs, or radioiodine. Others are known hypothyroid patients who discontinue their medication for some reason. Typically, the patient is elderly and there is a history of progressive deterioration of his mental, physical, and social functions. Symptoms include cold intolerance, somnolence, loss of memory, constipation, deafness, lethargy, and confusion progressing to coma. An intercurrent disease may be a provocative condition.

The skin is thick, dry, and has a pale yellow color. The tongue is enlarged, and there may be a large goiter or the scar from a previous thyroidectomy in the neck. The pulse is slow and sometimes irregular. The heart is usually enlarged with faint heart sounds due to pericardial effusion. The abdomen is protuberant with hypotonic muscles, and there is a frequently associated umbilical hernia. The comatose state may be associated with circulatory collapse.

### Treatment

1. If coma presents, support the airway and observe the precautions for the coma patient.

2. Monitor vital signs and heart rate.

### Disturbances of Calcium Metabolism

*Background and Clinical Picture.* Calcium is maintained in the serum in a narrow range, between 9 and 10.5 mg/100 ml. Only about 45 percent of this amount is free and biologically active. The rest is bound to serum albumin and is inactive. Free calcium increases with acidosis and decreases with alkalosis. In hypoalbuminemic states the total calcium level is low but the free calcium is usually normal.

Normal levels of calcium are critical for permeability of plasma membranes, excitability of the cells, and generation and transfer of the action potentials. The most obvious consequences of changes in the serum calcium levels are modifications of the neural and neuromuscular activities. In general, a decrease in serum ionized calcium results in an increased neuromuscular excitability, while increased calcium causes depression of the excitatory processes.

A number of mechanisms regulate the serum calcium. The hormones involved are parathyroid hormone (PTH) and vitamin D.

Serum calcium is continuously replenished by resorption from the gastrointestinal tract through vitamin D activity, and conserved by the kidney through PTH and vitamin D activities. Thus, hypercalcemia may be a result of vitamin D or PTH excess, and hypocalcemia may be due to vitamin D or PTH deficiency. Hypercalcemia may also accompany malignancy with osteolytic metastases in the bone, or tumors producing calcium mobilizing substances. The symptoms of hypercalcemia are weakness, anorexia, nausea, vomiting, polyuria, polydipsia, confusion, psychotic behavior, depression, high blood pressure, and peptic ulcer disease. The patient may have bone fractures and renal failure.

Hypocalcemia causes tetany, seizures, muscle cramps, muscle weakness, irritability or apathy, abdominal pain and distention, scaly skin, and increased pigmentation. A tap on the facial nerve in front of the ear may provoke twitching of the upper lip (Chvostek's sign). Inflation of the blood pressure cuff above the systolic pressure for up to three minutes may result in carpopedal spasm (Trousseau's sign). This sign is present when the hand pulls in and the wrist flexes with curling of the fingers.

In hypercalcemia the electrocardiogram reveals shortening of the RST segment of the Q-T interval, while prolongation of this segment occurs with hypocalcemia. The diagnosis of hyper- or hypocalcemia depends upon the measurement of serum calcium at the hospital.

### Treatment

1. Hypocalcemia (tetany) is treated by the intravenous administration of calcium gluconate, 10 to 20 ml of a 10 percent solution.

2. These patients may have electrocardiographic changes; therefore, their heart rates should be monitored.

3. Hypercalcemia is best treated by starting a rapid intravenous infusion of normal saline and the administration of furosemide, 20 mg intravenously. This promotes increased diuresis of sodium as well as calcium.

## METABOLIC DISORDERS

### Acid/Base Balance

*Background.* The disorders of acid/base balance usually occur secondary to an illness or as a response to a drug. Normal metabolism results in the production of organic acids, which must be cleared from the blood by the kidneys and the lungs. In many diseases the final common pathway for sudden deterioration of the patient is the development of severe acidosis or alkalosis. Acid/base abnormalities cannot be diagnosed for certain in the field since blood gas determinations are not possible. However, the paramedic will often encounter a situation where abnormalities of the acid/base mechanism are suspected and immediate treatment is necessary. In preparation for such situations, the paramedic must have a working knowledge of the principles of acid/base balance, the clinical manifestations of these abnormalities, and when an acid/base imbalance constitutes an emergency (Chapter 3).

Acids are chemicals which release hydrogen ions. Bases are chemicals which attract hydrogen ions. In Chapter 4 an ion was described as a charged particle in a solution. In any solution containing ions, there must be equal numbers of positively and negatively charged ions. When the hydrogen ion concentration rises in the blood the condition is called acidemia (Chapter 3). When the hydrogen ion concentration is reduced below physiologic levels, the condition is called alkalemia. In the hospital, measurement of acid/base balance is determined from arterial blood samples, and these concentrations are expressed in terms of pH (Chapter 3). The pH is the inverse of the log of the hydrogen ion concentration and the normal values for human blood are 7.35 to 7.41. A pH of 7.0 represents severe acidosis, and a pH of 7.6 represents severe alkalosis. The four general types of acid/base derangement are: (1) metabolic acidosis, (2) metabolic alkalosis, (3) respiratory acidosis, and (4) respiratory alkalosis.

### Clinical Disturbances

1. *Metabolic Acidosis.* Metabolic acidosis occurs when there is an overproduction of organic acids (diabetic ketoacidosis, lactic acidosis, or salicylate poisoning) and a failure to adequately excrete the hydrogen ion. The accumulation of the hydrogen ion reduces the pH to below 7.35. The body compensates for this by attempting to reduce the hydrogen ion concentration. It does this by combining hydrogen with the bicarbonate ion ($HCO_3^-$), which is then converted to $CO_2$ and water. The $CO_2$ is exhaled by the lung. Consequently, when metabolic acidosis is present, it produces a deep, rapid breathing pattern (Kussmaul breathing) and may also aggravate coma, confusion, fatigue, and shock.

There will also be symptoms of the underlying cause of the metabolic acidosis. For example, the diabetic will have severe thirst, increased urination, and evidence of dehydration. The patient with a metabolic acidosis after an aspirin overdose may have an altered mental status, complain of ringing in his ears, or vomit blood. Lactic acidosis is a metabolic acidosis found in patients who have impaired circulation, such as with cardiac arrest or in shock.

2. *Metabolic Alkalosis.* Metabolic alkalosis usually results from the loss of too many organic acids from the gastrointestinal tract or from the kidney. For example, the patient who has an obstructed duodenal ulcer and has been vomiting for several days, will lose hydrogen ions through the stomach; this will produce a rise in his pH as well as a reduction in his serum potassium and chlorides. Chronically used strong diuretics, such as furosemide (Chapter 6) can produce a metabolic alkalosis. Rarer causes are an increase in hormones by the adrenal gland producing potassium deficiency and alkalosis.

Symptoms of metabolic alkalosis are confusion, muscle weakness, apathy, and even coma. Metabolic alkalosis is usually secondary to some other underlying disorder.

3. *Respiratory Acidosis.* Respiratory acidosis is caused by failure to exhale sufficient amounts of the carbon dioxide produced by the

body. This results in the accumulation of carbonic acid in the blood (hypercarbia). The usual setting where this type of acidosis is seen is in the patient with chronic obstructive pulmonary disease or the patient with acute respiratory failure (Chapter 9). Respiratory acidosis also may occur in patients following cardiac arrest who are being inadequately ventilated. It will occur anytime in anyone who is inadequately ventilated regardless of the underlying cause.

In the field, respiratory acidosis should be suspected in any patient who cannot breathe effectively. These would include those patients with brain injuries and upper airway obstruction, asthmatics, patients with wheezing, and any patient with chronic obstructive pulmonary disease. Respiratory acidosis may or may not be accompanied by hypoxia and the symptoms may include agitation or delirium, confusion, sleepiness, coma, severe "air hunger," and cyanosis in the hypoxic patient.

4. *Respiratory Alkalosis.* Respiratory alkalosis is caused by over-breathing that results in the inappropriate loss of carbon dioxide and, indirectly, hydrogen ions. The loss of carbon dioxide shifts the equation $(H^+ + HCO_3^- \rightarrow CO_2 + H_2O)$ to the right, consuming hydrogen ions. This reduction in carbonic acid may be seen in patients with liver failure or hepatic encephalopathy. It may also occur secondary to metabolic acidosis produced by shock or in diabetic ketoacidosis. (This is the compensation mechanism mentioned earlier for metabolic acidosis.)

Often the patient in hemorrhagic shock presents in the Emergency Department breathing rapidly and with an alkalotic arterial pH. The intracellular pH is reduced because of anaerobic metabolism. The cells stimulate compensation for this through the pulmonary system (hyperventilation). With rapid breathing, carbon dioxide is eliminated, increasing the pH.

More commonly, hyperventilation and respiratory alkalosis are seen in the anxious, but otherwise healthy, person. These patients have the hyperventilation syndrome and may present with tingling of the fingers, spasm of the hand muscles (tetany), lightheadedness, and may also faint.

*Treatment*

1. Treatment of acid/base disorders in the field may be necessary despite the fact that blood gas analysis is not available. In cardiac arrest the patient receives sodium bicarbonate for lactic acidosis. The patient in respiratory arrest must receive assisted ventilation to reduce the accumulation of carbon dioxide in the blood.

2. Patients with acid/base disorders often have other underlying diseases and the acid/base disturbance is only a manifestation of it. An IV of $D_5W$ should be started since life-threatening dysrhythmias may occur.

3. In all patients an attempt should be made to gather data relevant to the diagnosis of the underlying condition so that the wrong drug will not be given.

*Background and Clinical Picture.* The liver is the largest single organ in the body weighing about 1400 grams, and is located in the right upper quadrant of the abdomen. It has a dual blood supply with the portal vein supplying nutrients from the gastrointestinal tract and the hepatic artery providing it with oxygenated arterial blood. The major function of the liver is the regulation of energy and organic metabolism. In addition, it removes substances from the blood which may be toxic to the body. It also stores many carbohydrates and the fat soluble vitamins.

Liver failure may result in a clinical picture that consists of an abnormal mental and neurologic state and is associated with certain characteristic, but nondiagnostic, laboratory and electroencephalographic findings. This clinical state is referred to as hepatic encephalopathy. The mental changes vary from mild clouding of the sensorium, confusion, and inappropriate behavior to lethargy and deep coma. The neurologic changes include tremors, incoordination, muscle twitching, and violent movements. A classic early finding is asterixis, which is a peculiar flapping tremor of the hand. It can be elicited by having the patient outstretch the arms and forearms and bend the hands back at the wrist. The patient will be unable to maintain this position of the hands for more than a few seconds and coarse twitching movements will appear at the wrist. Since asterixis may occur in other diseases it is not exclusively diagnostic of hepatic encephalopathy. However, when it occurs in patients with liver disease, it indicates hepatic encephalopathy.

Hepatic encephalopathy may be divided into four stages based on the mental and neurologic findings. Stage 1: Changes may be minimal and may be missed. There is slowing of the thinking process, mild euphoria, lack of insight, and slight tremor. Stage 2: This represents an accentuation of Stage 1. The patient develops drowziness, inappropriate behavior, and gross tremors of the hands. Stage 3: Sleeps most of the time, but can be aroused and found to be markedly confused. Tremor is usually present if the patient can cooperate. Stage 4: The patient is comatose and cannot be aroused. Tremor is usually absent.

The pathogenesis of hepatic encephalopathy is not clear. Although deranged nitrogen metabolism and the effect of ammonia on brain cells has been implicated, it is by no means established that ammonia is the only substance involved. There is sufficient evidence that other substances are involved.

Hepatic encephalopathy may occur in patients with acute hepatic necrosis or with chronic liver disease. Patients with acute overwhelming viral or toxic hepatitis may present with a fulminant illness characterized by delirium, convulsions, deep coma, and decerebrate rigidity often developing within 24 hours without other obvious precipitating causes. Fulminant hepatic coma (Stage 4) is fatal in about 80 percent of these patients. By contrast, a common pattern in patients with chronic liver disease is a gradual onset of a cloudy sensorium and intellectual impairment. In this group, hepatic encephalopathy is usually precipitated by some specific event, such as gastrointestinal bleeding, diuretics, uremia, infection, excessive protein intake, sedatives, alcohol ingestion, and constipation. Most of these are related to an increased production of ammonia. In this group the encephalopathy may be reversed in about 80 percent of the cases if appropriate therapy is instituted.

### Treatment

1. Patients with acute liver failure may be confused or comatose and unable to give information about their underlying problem. This information might be obtained from persons who may be available and are familiar with the patient. If coma is present, maintain the airway. If breathing is inadequate, ventilate with the bag/mask apparatus. Do not use mouth-to-mouth ventilation since hepatitis due to a virus may be the underlying cause of liver failure.

2. Impaired mental status in an individual who is jaundiced or has signs of chronic liver disease (ascites, telangiectasia of the face and neck, etc.) may not be due to liver failure, but may be due to head trauma with a subsequent subdural hematoma, or to intoxication with alcohol or drugs.

3. A quick evaluation of the patient for the above possibilities should be made, and vital signs quickly obtained. If these are stable and the patient is alert he is taken to the hospital for further evaluation. Intravenous fluids need not be started.

4. If vital signs are unstable and the patient is comatose, one should consider shock as a possible underlying cause and appropriate therapy started. In this case, an IV of Lactated Ringer's is started, and the patient rapidly transported to the hospital with the vital signs and heart rate monitored.

## RENAL PROBLEMS

There are two kidneys located in the retroperitoneal space. They receive about 25 percent of the cardiac output and weigh less than 1 pound each. A single kidney contains approximately one million functional units called nephrons. The nephron is composed of a glomerulus and a tubule (Figure 16-4). The blood enters the glomerulus through a small artery and this same artery continues through the glomerulus and leaves as an arteriole which then circulates around the tubule. The glomerulus acts as a filtration system and approximately 150,000 ml of fluid is filtered through the glomeruli in a normal adult each day. Most of the fluid is reabsorbed so that only about 500 to 2000 ml of urine is formed each day.

The kidney maintains homeostasis (a normal balance) of volume, osmolality, blood pH, and composition of body fluids, despite a wide variation in intake of food, fluids, and chemicals. It also acts to eliminate

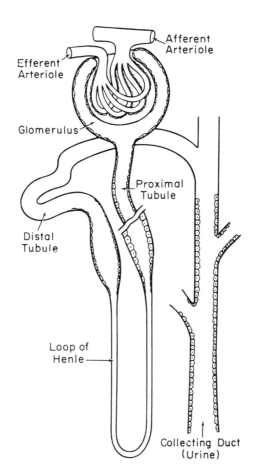

**Figure 16-4.** The microscopic anatomy of a glomerulus and its tubules. There are over a million of these tiny structures in each kidney.

metabolic waste products formed in the body and toxic materials which enter the body through the mouth, skin, or lungs. In renal failure, various metabolic waste products accumulate in body fluids exerting toxic effects on different organs to produce uremic symptoms. The word uremia comes from urea, which is a chemical formed with the breakdown of protein. When urea is not excreted by the kidney it, along with other nitrogen products, builds up in the blood, producing uremia.

Inadequate kidney function can result in fluid retention, hypertension, heart failure, hyperkalemia, and metabolic acidosis. The individual with renal failure is susceptible to a toxic buildup of drugs given in normal doses.

An additional function of the kidney is the manufacture of a hormone which stimulates the synthesis of red blood cells. The kidney also regulates phosphorus and calcium metabolism. A drug called renin is secreted by the kidney and it controls the secretion of a hormone from the adrenal gland called aldosterone. Aldosterone aids in the regulation of sodium metabolism (Chapter 15).

*Renal Failure.*   Depending upon its duration and potential reversibility, renal failure can be classified as acute or chronic.

*Acute Renal Failure.*   Acute renal failure is characterized by rapidly and potentially reversible deterioration of kidney function. It can be caused by conditions which reduce renal blood flow (shock, dehydration), by renal parenchymal injury (trauma, nephrotoxic drugs, infection), or by obstruction to the flow of urine (enlarged prostate, tumor obstruction of the ureters).

*Chronic Renal Failure.*   Chronic renal failure refers to the irreversible component of renal failure and is associated with a loss of the nephron mass subsequent to a variety of insults, such as immunologic, infectious, ischemic, and congenital disorders. A common cause of chronic renal failure is acute glomerular nephritis, which occurs after beta-streptococcal throat infections. There are also many diseases that destroy the arteries in the kidneys and cause chronic renal failure.

When kidney failure occurs, the volume, pH, and composition of body fluids become profoundly abnormal, depending upon the degree of catabolism, exogenous intake of water and solutes, and accumulation of waste products. Consequently, severe renal disease, by producing an abnormal internal environment (body fluids) adversely affects the function of practically all organ systems leading to the clinical picture of the uremic syndrome (Table 16-4). Patients with chronic renal failure will have a specific look about them. Their skin is pasty yellow and they have thin arms and legs. The latter is due to the protein loss which occurs with chronic renal failure and poor nutrition. Urea crystals may form on the skin producing a frostlike appearance to the skin (uremic frost). The patient's face is often puffy and there may be leg and periorbital edema.

Renal failure can produce the following conditions which involve paramedic personnel:

Fluid Overload and Pulmonary Edema
Hyperkalemia
Uremic Pericarditis and Pericardial Tamponade
Uremic Encephalopathy

### Clinical Syndromes of Renal Failure

*Fluid Overload and Pulmonary Edema.*   In patients with severe renal failure and a low urine output, the ability to excrete salt and water is markedly diminished and predisposes the patient to a fluid overload and episodes of noncardiac pulmonary edema. These patients present with severe dyspnea and neck vein distention, and rales are often heard at the lung bases. The basic management is similar to that of cardiogenic pulmonary edema (Chapter 10), but the following points should be kept in mind.

## TABLE 16-4.  CLINICAL ABNORMALITIES ASSOCIATED WITH SEVERE RENAL FAILURE

| Complications | Symptoms | Treatment |
|---|---|---|
| **Fluid and Electrolyte Disorders** | | |
| Dehydration | Hypotension, thirst, rising blood urea nitrogen. | Fluid replacement. |
| Fluid Overload | Dyspnea, hypertension, rales, venous distention. | Salt and water restriction, dialysis. |
| Hyponatremia | Headache, confusion, convulsions. | Water restriction if not dehydrated. |
| Hyperkalemia | EKG changes + weakness or paralysis. | Na bicarbonate, glucose and insulin. Kayexalate$_®$, dialysis, $K^+$ restriction. |
| Metabolic Acidosis | Weakness ± dyspnea. | Na bicarbonate, Ca gluconate, dialysis. |
| Hypermagnesemia | Confusion, weakness, cardiac complications. | Dialysis, avoid Mg in antacids and laxatives. |
| **Cardiovascular** | | |
| Pericarditis | Chest pain ± fever. | Dialysis, pericardiocentesis for tamponade. |
| Cardiac Failure | See Fluid Overload. | See Fluid Overload. |
| Atherosclerosis | Angina, myocardial infarction, cerebrovascular accidents. | Not clearly understood, control risk factors. |
| **Nervous System** | | |
| Uremic Encephalopathy | Insomnia, somnolence, confusion, coma, asterixis. Paresthesia, muscle weakness, and atrophy. | Dialysis or transplantation. |
| Gastrointestinal | Nausea, vomiting, anorexia, diarrhea. | Dialysis. |
| Immunologic | Predisposition to infections. | Dialysis or transplantation. |

*Treatment*

1. When using rotating tourniquets, it is important not to place a tourniquet on an extremity that might have a vascular shunt. (A vascular shunt is discussed in the subsequent section on chronic problems of patients on hemodialysis.) The tourniquet that is placed on an extremity with a shunt may cause it to rupture, thrombose, or, if it is an external shunt, blow apart.

2. Ordinary doses of diuretics may produce no response in the face of kidney failure and much higher doses may be necessary.

3. The usual doses of narcotics may produce profound central nervous system depression and respiratory arrest. If needed, drugs should be given in reduced doses with extreme caution.

4. The most effective means of fluid removal in patients with acute or chronic renal failure is ultrafiltration on a dialysis machine. Notification to the base hospital that the patient has renal failure will allow them sufficient time to prepare for the possibility of dialysis. If a patient is known to be in renal failure and is on a chronic dialysis program, it will be mandatory to transport him to an institution that has dialysis capabilities.

5. *Extremity veins in these patients are to be scrupulously protected.* These vessels are used to construct shunts for vascular access in dialysis. Since their lives may depend upon the integrity of these vessels, extreme caution should be exercised in establishing intravenous lines. Small veins in the dorsum of the feet and hands should be used whenever possible. Avoid using the cephalic vein at the wrist since this vein is often used to construct a fistula for subsequent chronic dialysis.

*Hyperkalemia.* In acute or chronic renal failure, the excretion of potassium, which enters the body through the gastrointestinal tract or from the breakdown of cells, is markedly impaired. The resulting elevation in serum potassium may cause fatal cardiac arrest. When the potassium concentration rises above 6.5 mEq/l, the patient is susceptible to cardiac dysrhythmia and death. The elevation in serum potassium may also cause neuromuscular problems which are initially manifested by hyperexcitability followed by the development of muscle weakness and paralysis.

The diagnosis of hyperkalemia should be suspected in any patient with kidney failure who complains of muscle weakness. The electrocardiographic manifestations of hyperkalemia consist of tall, peaked T waves with decreased amplitude and widening of the QRS complexes, prolongation of the PR interval and disappearance of P waves (Chapter 11). This may progress to an almost S-curve configuration on the electrocardiogram, and subsequently cardiac arrest.

*Treatment*

1. Emergency treatment of severe hyperkalemia is aimed at rapid lowering of the plasma potassium concentration to a safe level. An intravenous infusion of $D_5W$ should be started and 40 to 80 mEq of sodium bicarbonate given. An additional technique is the administration of 25 to 50 ml of 50 percent glucose. As the glucose moves into the body cells, so does potassium. Both maneuvers only temporarily lower the serum potassium concentration by shifting the potassium into the cells.

2. An intravenous infusion of 1 g of calcium chloride can temporarily protect against the toxic effects of hyperkalemia, although it does not lower serum potassium levels. This technique should not be used in patients receiving digitalis and, of course, calcium chloride cannot be given in the same syringe with sodium bicarbonate because precipitation will occur.

3. When the diagnosis of hyperkalemia is made, advanced notification of this information should be relayed to the hsopital and the patient transported to an institution that can institute hemodialysis.

4. In transport, the patient should be given nasal oxygen by nasal prongs at a rate of 6 l/min.

*Uremic Pericarditis and Pericardial Tamponade.* Uremic pericarditis is a complication of acute or chronic renal failure. This is caused by the accumulation of a bloody fluid in the pericardial sac. Patients with uremic pericarditis experience chest pain, fever, and a friction rub may be present. The heart sounds are distant, and the neck vein may be distended with a reduction in blood pressure. A full discussion of cardiac tamponade is presented in Chapter 10. Pericardial tamponade constitutes a medical emergency and, if this is suspected, the information should be relayed to the hospital.

*Treatment*

1. Start an intravenous infusion of normal saline and infuse at a rate of approximately 300 ml over one-half hour. Monitor the vital signs over one-half hour. The rate of fluid administration may be increased or decreased depending upon the patient's response to this fluid challenge.

2. Record vital signs and monitor the cardiac rhythm.

3. Use nasal prongs for oxygen administration at approximately 6 l/min.

4. Avoid administering medications which would reduce venous return. (These would include furosemide and morphine.)

5. Dopamine may be helpful if severe hypotension persists despite a fluid challenge.

*Uremic Encephalopathy.* Mental confusion, somnolence, coma and convulsive seizures may develop in advanced renal failure. As yet, no single substance retained by the failing kidney has been identified as being responsible for these symptoms. Disturbances in intracellular and extracellular sodium and solute concentrations appear to be factors resulting in cerebral edema.

*Treatment*

1. Treat as any patient with a seizure or coma. Maintain the airway.

2. Record vital signs and monitor the heart rhythm.

3. An IV of normal saline should be started and if seizures predominate intravenous Valium₍ᵣ₎ (2.5 mg) is indicated. If the patient is unconscious, this latter treatment may make the coma worse, requiring airway support.

## ACUTE PROBLEMS ASSOCIATED WITH HEMODIALYSIS

Over 40,000 patients in the United States undergo treatment of chronic renal failure through the use of hemodialysis. The dialysis may occur at home, in the hospital, or in dialysis centers outside of the hospital. The basic principle of dialysis is the diffusion of water and solutes across the semipermeable membranes separating two fluid compartments. The factors which govern the migration of fluids and solutes across the membrane include the permeability characteristics of the membrane, the osmotic pressure on each side of the membrane, hydrostatic pressures, chemical concentration gradients, and the size of the molecules in the solution. Since solutes tend to migrate from higher concentrations to lower concentrations when exposed to a normal concentration, solutes will tend to equilibrate over a period of time. This normalization constitutes the basis for dialysis treatment. During dialysis, the patient's blood is brought into contact through a membrane with a physiologic solution called the dialysate. The dialysate contains normal concentrations of electrolytes. Equilibration of the patient's blood with this fluid normalizes the patient's electrolyte composition and eliminates undesirable waste products which the patient's kidney cannot excrete.

By manipulation of the hydrostatic and osmotic pressures, excess fluid can also be removed from the patient. This process is called ultrafiltration and is used to control volume overload in patients with kidney failure. From the above discussion it is apparent that the dialysis process involves three basic elements:

The patient as a source of blood

An artificial kidney with a dialyzing membrane

The dialysis fluid (dialysate)

### VASCULAR ACCESS

In order to be able to dialyze the patient it is necessary to have access to the bloodstream. There are two general types of access. The external arteriovenous shunts, which were the original devices used, are still commonly used (Figure 16-5). The second type is an internal fistula, either made with the patient's own blood vessel or by the use of treated arteries from animals or synthetic arterial conduits. The purpose of an arteriovenous fistula is to allow the artery under high pressure to circulate through a vein with low pressure. This allows for a high flow through

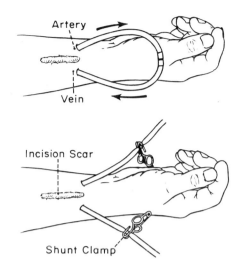

**Figure 16-5.** A Scribner shunt, which is an arteriovenous fistula allowing access to the circulation for hemodialysis.

the shunt and prevents clotting. This also makes the high flow that is necessary for dialysis. External arteriovenous shunts are usually placed in the forearm, groin, or ankle. Between treatments the external shunt is wrapped and protected by a dressing to prevent dislodgment and injury. The internal fistula is in the subcutaneous tissue, usually of the forearm, groin, or, in some cases, in the upper arm. These fistulas can be noted by the bruit related to the flow from the high pressure arterial system to the low pressure venous system. The internal fistula is preferred by most patients because there is not an external device showing, and the patient can bathe or swim and not be concerned about infection, as is the case with the external shunt. Aesthetically, it is also much more pleasing. However, it does require that the patient undergo a needle prick to gain access to the shunt for the purposes of dialysis.

## EMERGENCY COMPLICATIONS ASSOCIATED WITH DIALYSIS

Patients maintained on dialysis are not only susceptible to diseases contracted by the general population, but also to a number of conditions which are more or less peculiar to them. Complications related to dialysis are induced changes in volume and composition of body fluids.

*Hypotension.*   Hypotension is in part due to removal of fluids by ultrafiltration and shunting of blood into the extracorporeal system. It may present as lightheadedness, dizziness, weakness, pallor, cold sweats, reduction in the blood pressure, and syncope. It is treated by reducing the blood flow rate through the dialysis machine, lowering the head, elevating the legs, and infusing intravenous saline.

*Disequilibrium Syndrome.* This is caused by rapid changes of body fluids, sodium concentrations, osmolalities, and perhaps other as yet unidentified alterations. It presents with headache, lethargy, convulsions, and even coma. It usually occurs following the first or second dialysis. This condition can be minimized by giving shorter dialysis when the patient is first starting his dialysis treatments. Valium<sub>®</sub> may be given to treat the convulsions.

## COMPLICATIONS ARISING FROM THE DYSFUNCTION OF THE DIALYSIS APPARATUS AND INAPPROPRIATE DIALYSATE COMPOSITION

*Blood Loss.* This can be caused by rupture of the dialyzer membranes or defects in the tubing system. In this situation, the pump of the dialysis machine should be turned off, and dialysis stopped immediately. If possible, the blood remaining in the system should be returned to the patient and additional intravenous saline given.

*Thrombosis.* Sometimes the blood in the dialyzer and tubing system clots, particularly with inadequate heparinization. When this occurs the blood pump should be turned off and the entire tubing system changed. The blood that is clotting the system is equivalent to blood loss and restoration of fluid volume by intravenous administration of saline may be necessary.

If the dialysate bath is mixed without electrolytes, the patient may become acutely hyponatremic leading to seizures, coma, and possibly death. This is managed by stopping the dialysis and infusing saline into the patient.

*Air Embolism.* Under negative pressure in the venous side of the dialysis tubing, air is sucked in and carried to the right ventricle where, because of its vigorous contraction, the mixture of air and blood turns into massive quantities of foam. The foam is then pumped into the pulmonary artery blocking the passage of blood to the left side of the heart. This will produce severe dyspnea, cyanosis, hypotension, and respiratory distress. When this is recognized, the dialysis machine should be immediately stopped and the patient positioned on the left side, down, with the feet elevated and the head down. Oxygen should be given by nasal catheter.

## COMPLICATIONS RELATED TO THE VASCULAR ACCESS

*Clotting.* Clotting of the shunt or fistula can occur spontaneously or as a result of problems with the shunt itself. A clotted shunt is easy to recognize since the bruit, if it is an internal shunt, will be lost or, in the case of external shunts, clots can be seen in the tubing. For the patient on chronic dialysis, thrombosis of a vascular access represents an emergency and the patient should be informed to return to the hospital for declotting procedures.

*Infection.* Infection can arise in any vascular access from needle punctures or, if the access is external, through the skin tract formed by the external tubing. Patients will manifest a high body temperature, aching, and weakness. These patients are susceptible to infections of heart valves. This complication is treated by antibiotics in the hospital.

*Massive External Bleeding.* Massive external bleeding can occur with separation of arteriovenous fistulas. Rupture of internal fistulas can occur if aneurysms have formed and the shunt ruptures through the skin. For the external shunt, clamps are secured to the dressing covering the shunt and are there to clamp the shunt. If an internal shunt ruptures, the bleeding can be quite frightening and difficult to stop. The best method to stop the bleeding is direct pressure and/or tourniquet and rapid transport.

## HYPERTENSION

### CLINICAL BACKGROUND

Like diabetes mellitus, hypertension is one of the most common chronic diseases in western society. It is defined as a blood pressure greater than 150/90 mm Hg. Blood pressure determinations measure the effective force with which each heartbeat causes a pulse of advancing blood to push against the arterial walls. In a normal individual, the cardiac output, vascular resistance (elasticity), and effective vascular volume are all interrelated so that enough blood is provided to the tissues without stressing the body's vascular tree.

Hypertension results from an unchecked increase in cardiac output, vascular resistance, or blood volume, without any compensating fall in the other two. In 90 percent of patients the precise cause for the hypertension is unknown. Among conditions known to cause hypertension are acute and chronic renal disease, tumors secreting hormones causing increased vascular resistance, narrowing or coarctation of the aorta, and toxemia of pregnancy. Although initially asymptomatic, even mild hypertension can lead to stroke, heart attack, congestive heart failure, and chronic renal failure in ten to twenty years. Because long term treatment can markedly reduce complications of hypertension, it is the responsibility of all health personnel detecting high blood pressure to inform the patient and direct him to appropriate followup. Long term treatment has a definite beneficial effect on survival in this chronic disease.

Life-threatening hypertensive emergencies result when there is an extremely high, sustained elevation of the blood pressure (malignant hypertension), or when there is an extremely rapid (though not necessarily high) rise in blood pressure. This results in spasm of the arteries and rapid organ failure in the brain, heart, and kidneys. Furthermore, there may be specific development of hypertensive encephalopathy with a change in the state of consciousness, intracranial hemorrhage, aortic dissection, or acute left ventricular failure. Diagnosis is based on a history of recent onset of headache, altered mental status or coma, signs of congestive heart failure, specific changes in the arteries of the retina, and proteinuria and hematuria on urinalysis. The blood pressure is usually, but not always, greater than 200/130 mm Hg.

## TREATMENT

With rare exception, the decision to treat a patient with hypertensive crisis should follow some observation. Frequently, an anxious patient will have a blood pressure elevated to high levels for brief periods of time and not need any medicine after calming down. Assess the patient's mental status, look for signs of congestive heart failure, or coronary insufficiency, and measure the blood pressure serially while calming the patient.

Treatment specifics include:

1. If the systolic blood pressure is sustained, give the patient nasal oxygen at 6 l/min.

2. Monitor the heart rate since these patients very often have coronary artery disease and may develop dysrhythmias.

3. Monitor the blood pressure every five minutes with the patient in the supine position.

4. Start an IV with $D_5W$ at a keep open rate only.

5. An intravenous dose of Lasix® (20 to 40 mg) can be used in this situation. It will reduce preload by venous pooling and will also act as a venodilator. Antihypertensive drugs, such as Hyperstat®, are not acceptable for field use because of the profound effect they have on blood pressure. A sudden fall in blood pressure can cause a stroke or myocardial infarction.

6. Transport the patient immediately, notify the receiving center that you are dealing with a patient in hypertensive crisis, and relay the blood pressure findings.

Acute respiratory failure is presented in Chapter 9. This chapter will deal with the specific pulmonary problems created by different clinical disorders. More detail will be given to the pathology and treatment of the specific pulmonary disorders. These disorders include the following:

Spontaneous pneumothorax

Chronic bronchitis and emphysema

Asthma

Hyperventilation syndrome

Pulmonary failure due to massive obesity

## SPONTANEOUS PNEUMOTHORAX

*Clinical Picture.*   Pneumothorax is defined as the accumulation of air within the pleural space (Chapter 14). This space is a potential space and anatomically is located between the lung and the chest wall. Both of the surfaces are lined with pleura. When a pneumothorax occurs without an obvious predisposing incident, such as trauma, the term spontaneous pneumothorax is used. When the collection of intrapleural air progresses and the normally negative intrapleural pressure becomes positive, there is a shift in the mediastinum, known as a spontaneous tension pneumothorax. The pneumothorax without tension is usually not life-threatening, but a tension pneumothorax, as discussed in Chapter 14, can produce sudden death.

As tension rises in the pleural space, the vena cavae are compressed and the venous return to the heart is diminished. At the same time, blood flowing through the lungs is not adequately oxygenated. This contributes to cyanosis and a low blood pressure. Diminished lung volume includes reduced vital capacity and reduced lung compliance. In someone who already has an element of underlying lung disease, such as chronic obstructive pulmonary disease, a small pneumothorax can produce considerable deterioration in the patient's status.

The symptomatic signs and symptoms of a pneumothorax are described in Chapter 14. Patients with spontaneous pneumothorax are often in the age range of 20 to 40. They usually present with a history of reaching or stretching for an object, or coughing, when they suddenly experience chest pain. A short time later they develop shortness of breath. Depending on whether the hole is large and whether the pleural space is free of adhesions, the symptoms may or may not progress. Progression to severe respiratory embarrassment due to tension pneumothorax is a medical emergency. Physical examination in the field will make the diagnosis of a tension pneumothorax. A spontaneous pneumothorax without tension can be suspected by the clinical history and the patient's general condition. Physical examination of the chest is the key in making the diagnosis, and includes palpation of the trachea to ascertain whether or not it is in the midline, percussion for hyperresonance, and auscultation for diminished breath sounds.

*Treatment*

1. Treatment of spontaneous pneumothorax depends upon the severity of the problem. A small pneumothorax of sudden onset often does not even require hospitalization. The patient can be observed in the outpatient clinic or office, and the air will gradually resolve on its own. In some patients the problem is moderately severe and they need to be hospitalized with the insertion of a chest tube and reexpansion of the lung. In another group of patients the symptoms are so severe that rapid transport and mask oxygen may be indicated.

2. If there is hypotension and severe respiratory embarrassment, the tension pneumothorax may need to be relieved in the field. This is not an easy decision but, on the other hand, it is not difficult to accomplish. The proper relief of a tension pneumothorax is described in Chapter 14. The insertion of a large bore needle into the mid- or anterior axillary line in the fourth intercostal space is indicated. A large bore catheter such as a 12 or 14 sheathed needle will suffice. This can be connected to the Heimlich valve (Chapter 14). A sudden hissing of air will relieve the patient's acute symptoms and allow time for transport under controlled circumstances.

3. At the hospital a chest tube will be inserted and the patient observed until the air in the lung seals, at which time the chest tube can then be removed.

4. Patients with spontaneous pneumothorax tend to experience recurrent episodes and they may facilitate the diagnosis in the field by giving a previous history. These patients can always tell when a second pneumothorax has occurred because of the unmistakable sudden tearing sensation in their chests.

## EMPHYSEMA AND CHRONIC BRONCHITIS

In Chapter 9 the patients with chronic obstructive pulmonary disease (COPD) were divided into two general categories; the type A patient (pink puffer) with pulmonary emphysema, and the type B patient (blue bloater) with chronic bronchitis. Chronic bronchitis and pulmonary emphysema are considered to be a part of the spectrum of chronic obstructive pulmonary disease. While COPD is a convenient abbreviation, use of the term confuses the fact that the two components are not identical. Patients suffering from chronic bronchitis have a predominance of airway disease, whereas patients with emphysema have a predominance of lung parenchymal (lung tissue) disease. Both diseases may be associated with a severe obstruction to air flow. In bronchitis this may be due to airway narrowing, while in emphysema this is most likely attributable to loss of elastic recoil of the lung tissue. Frequently, patients suffer from both chronic bronchitis and pulmonary emphysema.

### Chronic Bronchitis

*Clinical Picture.* The pathophysiology of chronic bronchitis may be defined as chronic or excess mucus secretions in the bronchial tree recognized by the presence of a productive cough lasting three months of each year for at least two years. Pathologic studies of the lungs of severe bronchitics have shown (1) an enlargement of mucus glands, (2) increased secretions of mucus and plugging of airway passages, (3) an inflammation of the airway and fibrosis around the bronchial tissue, (4) a decreased number and caliber of airways, (5) abnormalities of the mechanism to move the mucus from the lung, (6) a diminished amount of pulmonary vasculature and (7) cor pulmonale (Chapter 10).

The airway obstruction as described in the preceding pathology of chronic bronchitis is manifested by a reduced rate of inspiratory and expiratory air flow and an increased resistance to this flow. Because of the patchy nature of the abnormality, some areas of the lung are overventilated, while other areas are underventilated. This will lead to a diminished amount of oxygen in the blood and hypercarbia. In addition to this, the arterioles in the lung tissue are chronically constricted giving rise to high blood pressure in the lungs and right ventricular failure.

The patient with chronic bronchitis has a chronic cough with expectoration of mucus, shortness of breath, frequent pulmonary infections, and wheezing. In advanced cases, cyanosis and signs of right ventricular failure (neck vein distention, an enlarged liver and leg edema) may be found (blue bloater). Because of the chronic hypoxemia, the hematocrit rises and the blood becomes more viscous.

### Pulmonary Emphysema

*Clinical Picture.* Pulmonary emphysema is defined as a condition of the lungs characterized by an increase in size of the air spaces accompanied by destruction of the alveolar walls. There are two anatomic types, called centrilobular and panlobular emphysema. In centrilobular emphysema the bronchioles are damaged, and most often this type of emphysema is associated with some element of chronic bronchitis. In panlobular emphysema the alveolar septae are damaged and the lung cannot recoil on its own. Emphysema is a common disorder and has been found in as many as 50 percent of autopsies in the older patient population.

The physiologic abnormalities of emphysema include the reduction in both the rate of air flow and the maximum breathing capacity. This leads to overinflation of the lung, reduction of the diffusing capacity of the lung, and nonuniform ventilation, such as is seen with chronic bronchitis. These symptoms are characteristic of pulmonary emphysema, although pulmonary hypertension and abnormal right ventricular failure can occur late in the disease in advanced panlobular emphysema.

The typical cardinal features of emphysema are shortness of breath and exercise intolerance. A cough is usually minimal or absent and respiratory infections are not that common. The patients often appear thin and asthenic, and sit and breathe with pursed lips in order to raise airway pressure and help maintain inflation of their alveoli (Figure 16-6). These patients often have a normal $Pa\text{CO}_2$ since they must hyperventilate to maintain a normal arterial oxygen tension.

Acute shortness of breath (SOB) is one of the more frequent complaints encountered by paramedics on an emergency call. There are many conditions that give rise to this complaint, but perhaps the greatest difficulty is met in trying to distinguish between an acute exacerbation of chronic obstructive pulmonary disease (COPD), usually due to superimposed infection, and acute left ventricular failure (LVF) in chronic congestive heart failure (CHF). To make matters worse, it is not unusual for one patient to be suffering chronically from both pulmonary and cardiac disorders. The information in Tables 16-5 and

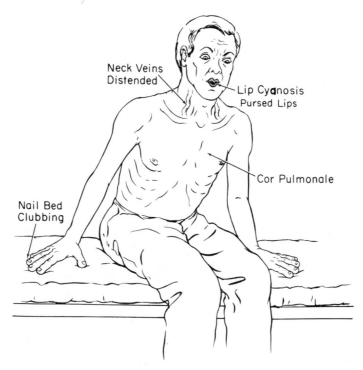

Neck Veins
Distended

Lip Cyanosis
Pursed Lips

Cor Pulmonale

Nail Bed
Clubbing

**Figure 16-6.** In chronic obstructive pulmonary disease there may be cardiac as well as pulmonary problems. The typical patient with COPD has cyanosis with pursed lip breathing and nail bed clubbing.

## TABLE 16-5. CHRONIC OBSTRUCTIVE PULMONARY DISEASE (COPD) VS. CONGESTIVE HEART FAILURE (CHF)

| | COPD With Exacerbation | CHF With LVF |
|---|---|---|
| Past History of Illnesses | "Pneumonia," "asthma," "bronchitis," or "lung surgery" | "Heart attack," "heart surgery," "high blood pressure," or "rheumatic fever" |
| **Past History of Symptoms** | | |
| Cough | Frequent | Occasional |
| Wheeze | Frequent | Occasional |
| Sputum | Often thick or purulent | Infrequent thin, white, mucoid |
| Hemoptysis | Occasional red globs | Occasional, pink froth |
| Paroxysmal Nocturnal Dyspnea (PND) | Usually after asleep for four hours | Typically one-half to one hour after lying down |
| Smoking | Commonly heavy | Less common |
| Ankle edema | Occasional | Common |
| **Present History** | | |
| Onset | Recent upper respiratory infection (URI) with cough | Orthopnea at night |
| Chest pain | Unusual and occurs late May be diaphragmatic soreness or pleuritic Not relieved by Nitroglycerine | Common and occurs at onset Usually precordial and oppressive Relieved by Nitroglycerine |
| **Physical Signs** | | |
| Clubbing | Often | Rare |
| Cyanosis | Often and severe | Unusual and mild |
| Diaphoresis | May be present | May be present |
| "Pursed lips" on Expiration | Often | Rare |
| "Barrel" chest | Common | Rare |
| Distended neck vein | May be present | May be present |
| Florid face | Common | Not common |
| Nicotine stains | Common | Not common |
| BP | Usually normal | Often elevated |
| Previous surgery (scar?) | Lateral thoracotomy | Usually sternotomy |
| Significant murmur | Not common | Often |
| Dysrhythmia | Occasional supraventricular (PACs, PAT, AF) | Occasional ventricular (PVCs) |

TABLE 16-5.  CONTINUED

| | COPD With Exacerbation | CHF With LVF |
|---|---|---|
| Cardiac impulse | May be increased at xiphoid or under sternum | May be increased at apex |
| Rales or rhonchi | Coarse rhonchi, diffuse | Fine rales, basilar |
| Wheeze | More common | Less common |

16-6 may be helpful in the differential diagnosis and in the management of these two conditions.

*Treatment*

1. Patients who have COPD and manifest acute respiratory failure need immediate hospitalization. This is necessary in order to monitor blood gas changes, determine if an underlying disease disorder has not precipitated the pulmonary failure, and if the progress of the disease process can be documented by sophisticated laboratory studies.

2. In the field, the patient with COPD of either general type may need supplemental oxygen. Since blood gas studies are not available, it is important to monitor the patient while giving oxygen. A face mask should not be used; nasal prong oxygen is the method of choice. In Chapter 9 the liter flow rate with nasal oxygen is shown with the probable $FIO_2$ generated. It is best to use only a 2 l/min flow rate of nasal oxygen,

TABLE 16-6. TREATMENT OF CHRONIC OBSTRUCTIVE PULMONARY DISEASE (COPD) VS. CONGESTIVE HEART FAILURE (CHF)

| Treatment | COPD With Exacerbation | CHF With LVF |
|---|---|---|
| $O_2$ | Low concentration, 1–2 l/min (nasal prongs) | High concentration, 6–10 l/min (face mask) |
| Morphine | Contraindicated | Usually indicated |
| Epinephrine (subcutaneous) | May be indicated in bronchial asthma | Contraindicated |
| Furosemide | Not helpful | Usually indicated |
| Orthopnic position | Yes | Yes |
| Transport in van | Chest raised; head to front of van | Chest raised; head to back of van |
| Digitalis | Usually not indicated | May be indicated (atrial fib with very rapid ventricular rate) |
| Rotating tourniquets | Not indicated | Indicated |
| Aminophylline | May be indicated | May be helpful |

which will raise the $FIO_2$ to 28 percent. Further increases in $FIO_2$ may stop respiration by halting the respiratory drive due to hypoxemia.

3. Respiratory failure in these patients is often associated with hypercapnia. If the patient does not appear to be ventilating adequately, it may be necessary to provide positive pressure ventilation with a bag and mask, or even an esophageal obturator airway. The purpose of this treatment is to inflate the lungs and remove $CO_2$, reducing the hypercarbia. Hypercarbia can be suspected in the field by the symptoms outlined in Chapter 9.

4. These patients are subject to cardiac dysrhythmias and may be in either right or left ventricular failure. Their vital signs should be measured and their heart rates continuously monitored.

5. An IV of $D_5W$ with a microdrip chamber should be started at the keep open rate only. Since these patients may be in pulmonary edema, as assessed by rales at the lung bases and neck vein distention, a fluid overload must be avoided. Diuretics in these patients must be used cautiously, since right ventricular failure may be present.

6. The patient with respiratory failure should be allowed to assume the position in which he/she is most comfortable.

7. Because of the hypoxemia and hypercarbia that is often present, the vital signs should be taken frequently and the patient's heart rate monitored.

## ASTHMA

### BACKGROUND

Asthma is a disease process characterized by airway obstruction, usually considered to be reversible. Fixed airway obstruction, however, can develop in chronic cases. Asthmatic symptoms usually have their onset during childhood or adolescence, but they may begin in young adulthood, or occasionally in middle age. The hallmark of asthma is wheezing, although wheezing is generally indicative of airway obstruction and not necessarily specific for asthma. The dictum "all that wheezes is not asthma" should be remembered. Three general types of stimuli seem to precipitate asthmatic attacks: (1) allergy, (2) infection (usually viral), and (3) nonspecific irritants, such as cold air, smog, humidity, pollens, etc. It is important to realize that exposure to the above stimuli does not cause wheezing in nonasthmatic subjects and that many subjects with other proven allergic conditions do not wheeze when exposed to allergens. Hence, it is felt that an underlying hyperreactive airway is present in asthmatic subjects. The underlying abnormality is in the nerve receptors in the bronchial smooth muscle cells.

The airway obstruction in asthmatics can be explained by multiple factors such as spasm of bronchial and bronchiolar smooth muscle, hypersecretion of mucus, bronchial and bronchiolar edema, bronchial and bronchiolar inflammation, and thickening of airway smooth muscle. These conditions produce the following changes in pulmonary function: (1) an increased resistance to air flow, (2) reduced rates of air flow, (3) hyperinflation and air-trapping in the alveoli, (4) reduced vital capacity (Chapter 3), (5) abnormal ventilation, (6) abnormal gas exchange with hypoxemia, and (7) hypoventilation (hypercarbia). If pulmonary mechanics are sufficiently impaired, however, life-threatening hypercapnia and respiratory acidosis may occur.

CLINICAL PICTURE

The clinical feature of the asthmatic is related to airway obstruction. This is manifested by wheezing, usually upon both inspiration and expiration. Prolonged expiratory time and cough are also manifested. The patient invariably appears distressed with tachycardia and tachypnea. Initial auscultation of the chest will reveal breath sounds with high-pitched wheezing on inspiration and expiration. With increasing severity, the breath sounds as well as the wheezing may become quite diminished. This is related to a reduced flow through the bronchial tubes or loss of flow through the tubes. This is an ominous sign. The patient may have intercostal retraction, flaring of the nostrils, and cyanosis. The patient invariably prefers leaning forward in the sitting position and breathing through his mouth with the mouth widely open.

TREATMENT

1. Most asthmatic attacks are relatively mild and easily treated. However, when the asthmatic attack is prolonged, severe, and poorly responsive to treatment, the condition may be termed status asthmaticus. Most deaths from asthma occur during the status asthmaticus attack. Therefore, it follows that death could ordinarily have been prevented by early appropriate therapy.

2. A mild attack of short duration can ordinarily be avoided by inhalation of isoproterenol (Isuprel®) medication. Patients will often already be using such medication.

3. In cases of acute status asthmaticus, an intravenous infusion of $D_5W$ with a microdrip chamber should be started.

4. Oxygen should be given by nasal prongs at 6 l/min flow rates. If chronic obstructive pulmonary disease appears to be part of the clinical process, a 2 l/min flow rate should be used.

5. If the attack is severe and worsening, give 0.3 to 0.5 ml of epinephrine (1:1000) subcutaneously. This can be repeated every fifteen minutes for several doses. In older patients, asthma is less common

and wheezes may be due to congestive heart failure. In that case epinephrine should not be given.

6. If the attack is not controlled with epinephrine, aminophylline should be given. The loading dose is 5 to 6 mg/kg injected intravenously over a ten to fifteen minute period. This is followed by a continuous intravenous infusion at a rate of 0.9 mg/kg/min. (Aminophylline administration in the field is a controversial issue, and its use may vary depending upon local preferences.)

7. In status asthmaticus, aminophylline should be started as described. At the same time, Solu-Medrol$_®$, 80 mg, should be given intravenously. If Solu-Medrol$_®$ is not in the drug protocol, Decadron$_®$, 20 mg, can be given IV. The patient in status asthmaticus should be transported to the hospital.

8. Because of the possibility of hypercarbia and hypoxia, vital signs should be taken frequently and the cardiac rhythm monitored.

## HYPERVENTILATION SYNDROME

### CLINICAL PICTURE

The hyperventilation syndrome is an anxiety state characterized by subjective feelings of fear unrelated to any external stimuli. Acute anxiety attacks usually last from a few minutes to hours, but may go on to a chronic state. This syndrome has been called anxiety neurosis, anxiety state, and anxiety reaction. The acute attack usually begins with a sudden onset of fear accompanied by a restlessness, increased tension, tightness of the chest, breathlessness, palpitations, sweating, flushing, tightness in the throat, and trembling. Hyperventilation may be so marked that a severe respiratory alkalosis from the carbon dioxide elimination will be produced. This may lead to tingling of the fingers, toes, and the periorbital region. The patient often has an impression of impending doom. Following the attack the patient may feel exhausted.

The physical examination may reveal perspiration, elevation in the heart rate, trembling, and possibly even tetany.

### TREATMENT

1. In most cases reassurance of the patient may be of some help. Voluntary control of the hyperventilation can be helpful if the patient is cooperative. This can be augmented by instructing the patient to hold his breath or rebreathing into a paper bag. Mild sedatives such as Valium$_®$ can be tried. In the adult a dose of 0.5 mg given intravenously is often sufficient.

2. Because the hyperventilation syndrome can be mistaken for so

many other more serious conditions, the patients are often transported to the hospital and evaluated in the Emergency Department. Often they will require monitoring of the heart rhythm because they will have chest pain and their syndrome cannot easily be distinguished from a myocardial infarction.

## PULMONARY FAILURE DUE TO MASSIVE OBESITY

### CLINICAL PICTURE

This syndrome has been described for an extremely obese individual. Patients who may weigh 400 lb or more will develop this syndrome. It is characterized by chronic hypoventilation. These patients are so massively obese that they cannot breathe adequately in the supine position because of their great abdominal girth. They seem more comfortable sitting up and allowing gravity to pull their abdomen forward and aid in the motion of the diaphragm. These patients are subject to acute respiratory failure and are frequently subject to pneumonia. The term "Pickwickian syndrome" is used for these patients because of the similarity to Dicken's description of the fat boy in his novel *Pickwick Papers.* Patients with the Pickwickian syndrome often have red cheeks and appear somnolent and sleepy. They may present with cyanosis and altered breathing patterns. If their carbon dioxide retention is severe enough they may be somnolent or even comatose.

### TREATMENT

1. Patients who have respiratory failure due to obesity have hypercarbia and hypoxemia. They need adequate ventilation to remove the carbon dioxide and improve the arterial oxygen saturation.

2. The sudden administration of a large high dose of oxygen in these patients can cause elimination of their hypoxic drive and further aggravate the situation. If the patient is reasonably awake or somewhat alert, nasal oxygen given at 2 l/min flow rates is recommended.

3. If the patient is comatose and ventilation is inadequate, a bag and mask and an oral airway is indicated. Hyperventilation is necessary to eliminate the carbon dioxide. If this is inadequate, an esophageal obturator airway is the next alternative.

4. It will be impossible to start an intravenous infusion in these patients because of their massive obesity. They should be transported, monitoring their heart.

A psychiatric emergency exists when a person loses control of his behavior. These behavioral crises may be related to organic causes, the use of drugs (alcohol, barbiturates), an acute flareup of a previous psychiatric illness, or a reaction to environmental stress. The paramedic may be called to aid in the assessment and control of a psychiatric emergency; therefore, he must know how to deal with these patients. However, the knowledge of psychology and thought processes in the clinical field of psychiatry are not as clear-cut as they are in physical medicine. Psychiatry does not have the objective scientific tools to immediately measure the mental disturbance as the electrocardiogram measures cardiac dysrhymthias. Human behavior is very unpredictable and people can change instantly. For the effective field management of psychiatric emergencies, the paramedic must allow for changes in his own response system.

In this discussion we will attempt to differentiate some of the more common types of psychiatric emergencies. Such insights will help the paramedic to respond in the most useful manner. The psychiatric emergencies to be discussed include the following:

The Family Disturbance Call
The "Jumper"
The "Out of Control" Individual
The Armed Assaulter
The "Panicked" Individual
The Hijacker

## THE FAMILY DISTURBANCE CALL

The family disturbance call is potentially the most dangerous call for the paramedic. The paramedic may be asked to respond in anticipation of physical injury or from harm that has already been inflicted. It is safest to overestimate the danger to yourself and others in the presence of people involved in this type of call. Records indicate that more police officers are injured or killed in family disturbance calls than in any other calls. The disturbed person who has had a feud with someone must be considered a danger to himself, to others, and to you until you have conclusive evidence to the contrary. The difficulty in this circumstance is assessing the risk involved because the degree of danger can only be really determined after a great deal of information is known. This information is generally not available at the time you are forced to make the decision of how to approach the situation.

Sixty-seven percent of the homicides in Los Angeles County last year involved people of kin, i.e., people not necessarily married or blood related, but people with a close ongoing relationship. It is important to understand that the participants involved in the family disturbance call have an ongoing "fat" game between themselves and are periodically going to erupt. Society is forced to intervene when the eruptions of their long-standing game spread to involve children, neighbors, or others who are in their crossfire. This particular group is the largest, the most troublesome to manage, and the one with the least success. These people do not want to make peace or to be reasonable. They are often angry, sometimes destructive, sometimes childish, and if they cannot destroy their partner, they would just as soon take a gun or knife to you—and they will. This kind of game is best illustrated in the movie "Who's Afraid of Virginia Wolf?" where the husband and wife can only have some existence by continuing a relentless chopping at one another, each time involving someone innocent in their struggle.

Remember that these people do not bring out weapons, and generally do not initially threaten the paramedic or police with a weapon. However, just at the time when events seem to have cooled off, the individual will go into another room, pull out a revolver and take a shot at the person who intervened or anyone else around, including themselves. When someone says they want to "chop off your head," an appropriate response would be, "I am leaving and will return when you want to behave reasonably." In contrast, these people continue to feed the game and do not want to stop. This is the real danger to the health professional attempting to stop their destructive interaction. The sensible response of physical separation can be executed by taking one of the warring parties to the nearest psychiatric facility. The physician there can determine if admission, medication, and/or referral to an outside clinic is the most appropriate treatment. Do not underestimate the danger when dealing with these people because it could be a fatal mistake for you or for others.

## JUMPERS

"Jumpers" is a slang word used to describe a group of people whose intention is threatening to jump from high places. It is an oversimplification, and for the purposes of this discussion, jumpers will be divided into two classes.

The first class includes those persons who feel sorry for themselves and desire sympathy and attention. They will exhibit themselves by standing on the ledge of a building, bridge, or high wire, threatening to jump. That individual can be "talked down" most of the time if he is not crowded and you let him control the distance between you. Removing the crowd of observers and isolating him is absolutely essential. The fewer the observers he can appeal to, the better. He should be encouraged to talk about how he was "worked over," mistreated, how unfair life is, how he is going to live without his mate, or whatever else is bothering him. It is important to keep talking to the jumper, building trust, and listening to him as soon as possible. Avoid actions that will make him distrust you, such as sending someone around the back to grab him, because this may force him into jumping.

The paramedic must be able to differentiate the neurotic jumper, as described above, from the psychotic jumper whose motivation for jumping is based on self-made realities; for example, God says he must pay for his sins. The psychotic jumper is more difficult to manage. The attempt to talk down the psychotic jumper may precipitate the destructive action that you want to prevent. It is critical to allow him to control the distance between you. This can be done by asking him, "Can I come up and talk to you?," "Can I give you a megaphone so you can talk to me?" The psychotic, paranoid, delusional jumper will react best to straight, honest, kind, and definitive statements. Do not encourage him to talk about his delusional system because you will have no logical answers for him. This will only agitate him further, cause him to lose control, and force him to jump precipitously. By firmly telling him that you will do everything in your power to prevent his suicide, you are not being hostile, but are showing that you care. Nets, lassoes, and any other equipment necessary to the circumstances should be available and ready for use.

Since there are basically two types of jumpers, it is important to differentiate between them. Obviously, upon arrival at the scene where a man or woman is perched on the ledge of a building, it is impossible to tell immediately whether he or she is neurotic or psychotic. The ability to differentiate comes from the individual's words, and determination can only be made by getting close enough to hear. Remember, let the jumper control the distance between the two of you. Shortly after talking with the jumper, the paramedic should be able to tell which type he is dealing with. In managing both types of patients, it is important to remove the crowd and take away the audience.

## THE "OUT OF CONTROL" INDIVIDUAL

This vague category is purposely used to describe a class of psychiatric emergency because that is the situation as it is. The paramedic will be called to this emergency in anticipation of physical injury. The treatment is prevention of injury, which can best be accomplished by helping the person regain control promptly and safely by exercising as little force as possible.

For example, what do you do with a shouting woman who is waking up everyone in the neighborhood at three o'clock in the morning? What do you do with the man or woman who is running naked down the middle of a street? In either case, this exhibitionistic behavior may be a legitimate expression of their rage, or the individual may be under the influence of hallucinogenic drugs such as PCP or LSD (Chapter 17). An analogous model is that of a four-year-old child who is running amok. The effective treatment for a child is to put him on your lap, hug him tightly with your arms, and tell him that you will not allow him to, for example, run around the edge of a cliff, and that you are going to protect him until he has control of himself.

Unfortunately, the adult who is out of control is much harder to reach with this type of communication. The basic rule is to get control of the situation, make the patient aware of your control, and help him reduce his anxiety with a minimum of force and a maximum of safety precautions. As with so many decisions and actions taken by the paramedic in the field, he must base his response on inadequate data. Therefore, the paramedic's behavior must lean toward excess caution. He must assume that the patient is more dangerous than he really may be, so that both parties are protected. This is best accomplished by exercising caution and making thorough observations until you are forced to execute a response. Obviously, if five or six people are available to grab someone running amok, it is much easier than attempting this action by yourself. Weapons used to threaten this kind of individual allow the potential of supplying him with a weapon for use against you and should probably not be used. Often a significant "other" in the lives of these people, such as a brother, mother, parish priest, or even a psychiatrist, will be of help if there is sufficient time to contact them. It is interesting to note that sometimes the 16-year-old daughter is the strongest and most stable member of the family group and can be very effective in controlling these people.

Individuals who seem out of control or exhibit bizarre behavior can be quite dangerous to both police and paramedic personnel. This is particularly true if the individual has taken the drug PCP. Individuals withdrawing from or under its active influence can be extremely hostile and most dangerous to the people trying to control them. This type of crisis will always arouse great hostility in the families of the victim. It should always be remembered that individuals may be on PCP and they are extremely dangerous and can cause harm to anyone around them.

## THE ARMED ASSAULTER

The individual threatening another person with a weapon should be dealt with according to his choice of weapon, i.e., projectile or nonprojectile. Individuals carrying a nonprojectile weapon can be managed with a sufficient show of force. Four or five people who are intent on taking the weapon away from an individual reduce the risk of his harming himself. Rushing him with a mattress is a very effective defense. The best action for a paramedic may be to stand off and allow the SWAT team to deal with him using such methods as mace, etc.

When dealing with the potential assaulter armed with a lethal projectile weapon, the paramedic's function becomes that of support to law enforcement officers. He must stay out of range of the weapon. Paramedics are trained to help people, not to be killed or mutilated. If you put yourself in a position of danger, you are not going to be able to give medical aid to the police officers, firemen, or assaulter. The situation discussed earlier must be differentiated from the episodic killer who has a lethal weapon. This latter individual cannot be talked out of using his weapon and discussion should be avoided. The psychotic killer will come down and surrender his weapon when he is ready, and verbalizing his fantasies or anxieties will only agitate him. He is so dangerous that usually your own sense of fear will alert you to him.

The armed assaulter may be placed in two categories. The hysteric who is depressed wants attention and plans to kill himself or one specific individual. He may be talked down using a megaphone providing there is sufficient distance for safety. The second category is the psychotic who is a sniper and is intent on killing. He must be dealt with by force. When in doubt about which category the assaulter is in, stay out of range. This sounds like a simple instruction, but it may be the most difficult action to take if you are attempting to administer medical aid to the injured at the scene.

## THE "PANICKED" INDIVIDUAL

The paramedic may be called to see an individual who is in an absolute state of panic. His fear may stem from paranoid ideation or from fact. He may be afraid he is going to die or become injured, and your ability to estimate the reality behind his panic is severely limited. Your best response is to accept his evaluation at face value and allow him to tell you how you can help. For example, if an individual believes he has been poisoned, ask him what poison he thinks he used, and then tell him the antidote (Chapter 17). You can offer to administer it and suggest hospitalization. Based on your physical assessment, you may be skeptical that his fears are well-founded, but if he accepts treatment, it will not hurt him. This reassuring approach may reduce his panic if it is based on a nonreal situation. This treatment will also give him some protection if his panic is based on actual fact.

## THE HIJACKER

Paramedics do not often become involved with hijackers or armed terrorists. However, if the situation should arise, the basic rule is to consider them very serious in their intentions. Do not crowd a hijacker, and buy time by making the assumption that they are hysterical exhibitionists wanting attention. Assume, however, that they are in dead earnest about their intentions. While this does not mean giving in to them, the paramedic should take their threats and demands at face value. Verbal communication will help you to decide if you are dealing with an exhibitionistic person who is making half-hearted gestures, or dedicated individuals. The advantage in these situations is that time is on the side of the law enforcement agency. The demands of the hijacker or terrorist require time and allow for assessment of their behavior, securing of past records, and also time to enlist the help of family members, etc. The most dangerous type of individual is the fanatic who is willing to die for some real or alleged grievance or cause. While the FBI profile for labeling and identifying hijackers is confidential material, by observation he can be identified as an insecure male having extraordinary exhibitionistic qualities who wants to be a hero and, therefore, demands a great deal of attention. Tactics such as limiting the crowd and observers and isolating him are generally helpful. As in all the other situations, it is best to overestimate the risk and protect yourself.

## SUMMARY OF PSYCHIATRIC EMERGENCIES

The risk to the paramedic has been emphasized in this section because of the dangers involved in psychiatric emergencies. If the paramedic is killed or seriously injured, his capacity to help someone is eliminated. Therefore, the paramedic must be constantly aware of the steps to protect himself while administering aid. In most instances in which medical personnel have been injured by disturbed individuals, it has been due to letting their guard down. Never underestimate the risk to yourself. The best principle to remember is, "Do very little, observe a great deal, and intervene only when you are forced to, or until you have adequate data."

*Summary*

This chapter has reviewed some material presented previously and has presented quite a bit of new information. This is in reality a textbook of medical problems which are not day-to-day occurrences, but which may be seen from time to time in the field. It would be well for the paramedic to have an introductory knowledge of this material and to review it occasionally in order to keep the important points in mind.

*Important
Points to
Remember*

The most publicized examples of paramedic intervention are in the areas of trauma and cardiac problems. However, there are numerous other medical conditions that necessitate field recognition and management.

*Neurologic Emergencies.* The brain requires a constant supply of oxygen and glucose. After 10 to 20 seconds without blood flow, a patient becomes unconscious. Five minutes of anoxia causes irreversible brain damage. Significant loss of oxygen (anoxia) or low blood sugar (hypoglycemia) can result in coma and/or seizures. In patients with brain disorders, we must insure adequate blood, glucose, and oxygen.

*Stupor and Coma.* Stupor is partial or nearly complete uncon-sciousness or reduced responsiveness. Coma is a state of unconsciousness from which the patient cannot be aroused.

Causes of coma may include:

1. Structural (trauma, tumor, epilepsy, hemorrhage).
2. Metabolic (hypoglycemia, diabetic acidosis, liver or kidney failure).
3. Drug (barbiturate, narcotic, hallucinogen, alcohol).
4. Cardiovascular (hypertension, shock, anaphylaxis, dysrhythmia, arrest, stroke).
5. Respiratory (chronic obstruction, inhalation of toxic gas).

Evaluation and assessment include:

1. History.
2. Breathing.
3. Response to stimuli.
4. Pupil size and reaction.
5. Motor response.
6. Other physical signs.

Treatment of coma includes:

1. Open airway and breathing.
2. Treat shock (IV infusion).
3. Identify dysrhythmia.
4. If cause not discernible, give bolus of 50% glucose (50 ml).
5. Support vital signs.
6. Administer specific antidote (Narcan₍ᵣ₎ for heroin).
7. Prevent vomiting and aspiration.

Causes of seizures include:

1. Hypoxia.
2. Sudden temperature elevation.
3. Rapid lowering of blood pressure.
4. Structural brain disease.
5. Epilepsy.
6. Trauma.

Types of seizures include:

1. Major motor (grand mal).
2. Focal.
3. Psychomotor.
4. Petit mal.
5. Myoclonic.
6. Status epilepticus.

Treatment of seizures includes:

1. Administer nasal $O_2$ and turn patient to side.
2. Keep temperature normal.
3. Keep airway open.
4. Provide ventilatory assistance if necessary.
5. If due to hypoglycemia, give 50% glucose.
6. In status epilepticus give medication for seizure itself (Valium®
most used here).

*Stroke.* Strokes are cerebral vascular accidents. They are caused by obstruction to cerebral blood vessels by emboli or thrombosis, air or fat, or hemorrhage into the brain.

Assessment for strokes includes:

1. Important history (when last alert).
2. Medical history (medications).
3. Level of consciousness.
4. Changes in neurologic examination.

Treatment of strokes includes:

1. Maintain adequate oxygenation and perfusion to brain.
2. Maintain airway.
3. Watch vital signs.
4. Position patient flat with head up 15°.
5. Avoid noise, movement, excitement, coughing, vomiting.
6. Use NO narcotics or sedatives.

*Infectious Diseases.* Infectious diseases are caused by organisms such as viruses, bacteria, or fungi.

Fundamental field questions include:

1. Does patient have infectious disease?
2. Has paramedic protected himself?
3. Is ambulance and equipment decontaminated?
4. Did paramedic seek medical advice on final diagnosis?

Meningitis is inflammation of coverings of brain and spinal cord. Signs and symptoms include:

1. Headache.
2. Fever.
3. Stiff neck.
4. Chills.
5. Weakness.
6. Convulsions.

Treatment includes:

1. High index of suspicion.

2. Shock treatment.

3. Monitoring of heart.

4. Seizure control.

*Septic shock* is severe systemic reaction to bacteria that have entered the bloodstream. Signs and symptoms include:

1. High or very low body temperature.

2. Low blood pressure.

3. Mental confusion.

4. Severe toxicity.

5. Ill looking.

Treatment includes:

1. IV fluids.

2. Oxygen.

3. Monitoring of heart.

4. Dopamine.

*Gastrointestinal Problems.* The acute abdomen is one with an acute, nontraumatic condition that requires surgical intervention. Some causes of acute abdominal pain are:

1. Intestinal obstruction.

2. Acute cholecystitis.

3. Acute appendicitis.

4. Perforated ulcer.

5. Acute diverticulitis.

6. Abdominal aortic aneurysm.

Treatment of the acute abdomen includes:

1. Reassure.

2. Treat shock (IV).

3. Mask $O_2$.

4. If vomiting, transport in lateral decubitus position.

5. Monitor and treat hypotension.

6. Give NO analgesics.

7. If acute blood loss present, use MAST suit.

*Gastrointestinal bleeding* may present as vomiting blood or bloody stools. Causes include:

1. Ulcer.

2. Inflammation (colitis).

3. Mechanical.

4. Vascular.

5. Tumor.

6. Systemic.

7. Drugs.

Signs and symptoms include:

1. Vomiting.
2. Diarrhea.
3. Vomiting of blood.
4. Bloody stools.
5. Pallor.
6. Weakness.
7. Shock.

Treatment may include:

1. Transport if stable.
2. If active bleeding present, start an IV.
3. Keep patient in supine position.
4. Mask $O_2$.
5. Monitor vital signs.
6. Transport rapidly and save specimen of bloody stool or vomitus.

*Endocrine, Metabolic, and Renal Emergencies.* Endocrine glands secrete hormones into the blood. Usually the glands involved with emergencies are the pancreas, adrenal, and thyroid. Other endocrine glands include the pituitary and parathyroids.

A medical emergency due to dysfunction of an endocrine organ is characteristically an exaggeration of the symptoms due to a disease of that organ.

The more common endocrine emergencies include:

1. Diabetic ketoacidosis.
2. Nonketotic hyperosmolar coma.
3. Hypoglycemic coma.
4. Adrenocortical insufficiency.
5. Thyrotoxic storm.
6. Myxedema coma.
7. Disturbances of calcium metabolism.

Diabetes mellitus is one of the world's most common medical diseases and certainly the most common endocrine disorder causing acute problems. Clinical manifestations of diabetic ketoacidosis (too little insulin) include:

1. Thirst.
2. Polyuria.
3. Weakness.
4. Nausea.
5. Vomiting.
6. Abdominal pain.

7. Eventual coma.

8. Shock.

9. Severe dehydration.

These patients often have deep, rapid respirations (Kussmaul breathing).

Treatment of this disorder involves:

1. IV infusion (saline).
2. Drawing blood for glucose and chemistries.
3. Monitoring vital signs.
4. Treating coma.
5. Treating dysrhythmias.
6. Oxygen.
7. Insulin injection at the hospital.

Hypoglycemia (low blood sugar) may be caused by various endocrine disorders, but the most common cause is an overdose of insulin. Clinical manifestations of hypoglycemia include:

1. Weakness.
2. Hunger.
3. Nervousness.
4. Restlessness.
5. Muscle spasms.
6. Convulsions.
7. Blurred vision.
8. Loss of concentration.
9. Confusion.
10. Sweating.
11. Palpitation.
12. Aggressive behavior.
13. Coma.

Treatment of hypoglycemia involves:

1. Maintaining airway.
2. Ventilating.
3. Injecting IV fluids (50 ml of 50% glucose).
4. Monitoring vital signs.
5. Transporting.

*Metabolic disorders* include the following problems:

1. Acid-base imbalance.
2. Metabolic acidosis.
3. Metabolic alkalosis.
4. Respiratory acidosis.

5. Respiratory alkalosis.

Metabolic acidosis occurs when there is an overproduction of organic acids (diabetes, aspirin poisoning).

Metabolic alkalosis results from the loss of too many organic acids from the gastrointestinal tract or kidney (intestinal obstruction with vomiting).

Respiratory acidosis is caused by failure to exhale sufficient amounts of carbon dioxide (chronic pulmonary disease).

Respiratory alkalosis is caused by overbreathing, which results in the inappropriate loss of carbon dioxide (liver failure, secondary to metabolic acidosis).

Treatment of acid-base disorders depends on the proper history and assessment of the problem.

*Acute liver failure* may result in a picture that consists of an abnormal mental and neurologic state. Signs and symptoms include:

1. Clouding of the sensorium.
2. Confusion.
3. Lethargy.
4. Coma.
5. Tremors.
6. Incoordination.
7. Twitching.

*Flapping tremor of the hand (asterixis)* is known as *hepatic encephalopathy.* This condition may occur in patients with acute hepatic necrosis, chronic liver disease, and hepatitis.

*Renal Emergencies.* Inadequate kidney function can result in fluid retention, hypertension, heart failure, hyperkalemia, and metabolic acidosis. Causes of acute renal failure include:

1. Shock.
2. Dehydration.
3. Trauma.
4. Drugs.
5. Infection.
6. Obstruction to the flow of urine (enlarged prostate or tumor).

Chronic renal failure refers to the irreversible component of renal failure and may be caused by acute glomerulonephritis as well as many other diseases which destroy the renal arteries.

Renal failure can produce the following conditions involving paramedical personnel:

1. Fluid overload and pulmonary edema.
2. Hyperkalemia.

3. Uremic pericarditis and pericardial tamponade.

4. Uremic encephalopathy.

Fluid overload and pulmonary edema will produce a clinical picture of severe dyspnea, neck vein distention, and rales.

Hyperkalemia should be suspected in any patient with kidney failure who has muscle weakness.

Patients with uremic pericarditis experience chest pain, fever, and a friction rub, along with distant heart sounds and neck vein distention.

Uremic encephalopathy presents with somnolence, mental confusion, coma, and convulsive seizures.

Emergency conditions associated with renal dialysis include:

1. Hypotension.

2. Dysequilibrium syndrome.

3. Blood loss.

4. Thrombosis.

5. Air embolism.

6. Clotting.

7. Infection.

8. Massive external bleeding.

*Hypertension* is defined as a blood pressure greater than 150/90 mmHg. Hypertension results from an unchecked increase in cardiac output, vascular resistance, or blood volume without a compensating fall in the other two. Although initially asymptomatic, even mild hypertension can lead to stroke, heart attack, congestive heart failure, and chronic renal failure in ten to twenty years.

Life-threatening hypertensive emergencies result when there is an extremely high, sustained elevation of the blood pressure, or when there is an extremely rapid rise in blood pressure. This may result in organ failure in the brain, heart, and kidneys, or perhaps in the development of hypertensive encephalopathy, intracranial hemorrhage, aortic dissection, or acute left ventricular failure.

Treatment of hypertensive emergencies includes:

1. Administering nasal $O_2$ (6 l).

2. Monitoring heart rate and rhythm.

3. Monitoring BP every 5 minutes.

4. Starting IV with $D_5W$.

5. Lasix₍ᵣ₎ may sometimes be indicated.

6. Transporting and notifying receiving center.

Pulmonary disorders that can present as emergencies include:

1. Spontaneous pneumothorax.

2. Chronic bronchitis and emphysema.

3. Asthma.

4. Hyperventilation syndrome.

5. Pulmonary failure due to massive obesity.

Spontaneous pneumothorax is the accumulation of air within the pleural space. The clinical picture is one of chest pain, shortness of breath, and cough. Treatment depends upon the severity of the problem.

Patients with chronic bronchitis have a predominance of airway disease and those with emphysema have mostly parenchymal disease. Both diseases may be associated with obstruction to air flow. The clinical picture and treatment of emergency conditions may vary greatly. The monitoring of blood gases is essential in the management of these problems.

Asthma is characterized by airway obstruction, and the hallmark is wheezing (but not all wheezing is asthma). The clinical picture of asthma includes:

1. Wheezing (more expiratory usually).

2. Cough.

3. Tachypnea.

4. Tachycardia.

5. There may also be retraction, flaring of the nostrils, and occasionally cyanosis.

Treatment of asthma depends on the severity (from mild to status asthmaticus). This might include:

1. Isoproterenol inhalation.

2. IV fluids.

3. $O_2$.

4. Epinephrine (1:1000).

5. Aminophylline or steroids.

6. Careful monitoring of vital signs, cardiac rhythm, and blood gases.

The hyperventilation syndrome is an anxiety state characterized by subjective feelings of fear not related to external stimuli. The clinical picture includes:

1. Restlessness.

2. Chest tightness.

3. Breathlessness.

4. Palpitations.

5. Sweating.

6. Throat tightness.

7. Trembling.

8. Tingling of the fingers, toes, and periorbital region.

Treatment of hyperventilation involves:

1. Reassuring by paramedic.
2. Holding the breath.
3. Rebreathing into a paper bag.
4. Mild sedatives or tranquilizers.

*Psychiatric emergencies* exist when a person loses control of his behavior. This may be due to the use of drugs or alcohol, an acute flare-up of a previous psychiatric illness, or a reaction to environmental stress. Common psychiatric emergencies include:

1. The family disturbance call.
2. The "jumper."
3. The "out of control" individual.
4. The armed assaulter.
5. The "panicked" individual.
6. The hijacker.

The spectrum of psychiatric emergencies is wide, and the management depends upon many different circumstances. The paramedic would do well to familiarize himself with this type of problem and always remember to protect himself while treating these problems.

*Bibliography*

Daniele, R. P. and R. M. Rogers. "Oxygen and Nonventilatory Therapy of Respiratory Failure in COPD," *Postgraduate Medicine.* 54:145, 1973.

Krupp, M. A. and M. J. Chatton. *Current Diagnosis and Treatment.* Los Altos, California: Lange Medical Publications, 1973.

Sodeman, W. A., Jr., and W. A. Sodeman. *Pathologic Physiology.* Philadelphia, Pa.: W. B. Saunders Company, 1974.

Zschoche, D. A. *Comprehensive Review of Critical Care.* St. Louis, Mo.: The C. V. Mosby Co., 1976.

# Chapter 17

# EMERGENCY TREATMENT
# OF POISONING

COMMON NONABUSE POISONING

A poison or toxin is a substance which when ingested, inhaled, or otherwise presented to body tissues in sufficient amounts has a negative or destructive effect on health.

No event is more frightening than when a parent sees his or her child unconscious with an empty medication bottle nearby (Figure 17-1). The immediate reaction is guilt and this is soon overtaken by the urge to help the child. Accidental poisonings have a marked emotional overlay that will precipitate a call to the paramedics or to some other emergency support service in almost every case.

A consistent and logical approach to the poisoned patient as well as handling grieving and often guilt-ridden relatives are part of the important functions of the paramedic.

MECHANISMS OF EXPOSURE

Poisonous substances abound in our environment. Mechanisms of exposure to toxins include, but are not limited to the following:

1. *INGESTION,* or exposure of the toxin to the gastrointestinal tract. Toxins can result in poisoning either by altering or disrupting the tissues of the mouth, esophagus, stomach or intestines; or by being absorbed systemically through the gastric or intestinal mucosa, possibly affecting other organ systems.

2. *INHALATION,* or exposure of toxic substances to the lung that can result, again, in either local irritation or tissue destruction or systemic absorption.

3. *INJECTION* of toxic substances between or below several layers of skin, or into a blood vessel. This can be the intentional result of

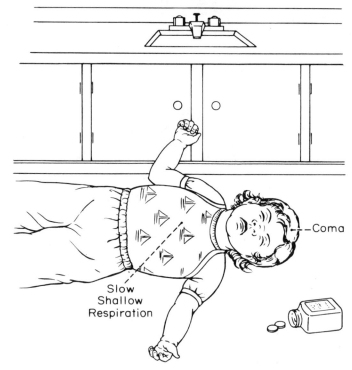

**Figure 17-1.** An unconscious child with a medication bottle nearby is a frightening scene. It is important to know the type of medication and possible amount ingested.

drug abuse, or accidental with respect to venomous stings or bites by insects, marine animals, or snakes.

4. *CONTACT,* or exposure of the surface of the skin to toxic substances. Dermatitis-producing plants such as poison ivy or poison oak fall into this category. Contact of the skin with corrosive and caustic substances such as strong acids and alkalis can result in variable degrees of tissue damage (Chapter 18). In addition, a number of toxic substances can be absorbed through the skin, e.g., pesticides, which may result in systemic effects.

COMMON FACTS ABOUT POISONING

Between three and five million poisonings occur in this country every year, and it is the fifth most frequent cause of accidental death, with only motor vehicle accidents, falls, drownings, and burns more frequent. Over 5000 deaths per year occur due to this problem. Poisonings are responsible for 9 percent of all ambulance transports, 10 percent of all emergency facility visits, and between 5 and 10 percent of medical admissions to hospitals.

Ninety percent of all poisoning cases involve children, with greater than 75 percent under five years of age. The mean age for childhood poisonings is about two years and approximately 50 percent of deaths resulting from poisonings are in this age group.

The UCIMC Poison Control Center in Orange, California, estimates that over 90 percent of poisonings result from ingestion of toxic substances.

## TYPES OF SUBSTANCES INVOLVED

Ingested poisons can be arbitrarily divided into the following classes:

1. *HOUSEHOLD PRODUCTS* (Table 17-1), representing greater than 50 percent of toxic ingestions.

2. *DRUGS* (Table 17-2), about 25 percent of cases.

3. *PETROLEUM PRODUCTS* (Table 17-3), e.g., gasoline, kerosene, paint thinners, and solvents; approximately 10 percent of all cases.

4. *PESTICIDES* (Table 17-4), e.g., insecticides, fungicides, herbicides; about 5 percent.

5. *POISONOUS PLANTS* (Table 17-5) (Table 17-6), between 5 and 10 percent (Figure 17-2).

The incidence of drug-related poisonings has dramatically decreased since 1972, when it became necessary to dispense all prescription and nonprescription drugs containing aspirin in child-resistant containers. Since that time, the known incidence of aspirin ingestions has decreased by about 75 percent.

TABLE 17-1. HOUSEHOLD PRODUCTS IMPLICATED IN POISONINGS

Soaps and detergents
Automatic dishwater detergents (alkali)
Household bleach
Household ammonia
Disinfectants
Adhesives and glues
Drain cleaners (alkali)
Oven cleaners (alkali)
Toilet bowl cleaners (acid)
Metal cleaners and polishes (acids)
Moth balls
Toilet bowl, diaper pail deodorizers
Perfumes and colognes
Cosmetics, lotions, and creams
Furniture polishes
Tile and grout cleaners (acid)

TABLE 17-2.   MEDICATIONS MOST COMMONLY INVOLVED IN CHILDHOOD
(AND ADULT) POISONINGS*

Baby aspirin

Children's multiple vitamins

Iron tablets

Minor tranquilizers

Pediatric antibiotic suspensions and solutions

Nasal sprays

Prescription and nonprescription ointments

Oral contraceptives

Amphetamines, barbiturates, antiepileptic agents

Illicit drugs

*Theoretically, any medication that is kept within sight and reach of small children can be listed. The list above represents those medications for which we have the most statistics.

TABLE 17-3.   PETROLEUM PRODUCTS INVOLVED IN POISONINGS

Gasoline

Kerosene

Paint thinner

Turpentine

Liquid furniture polishes

Motor oil

Transmission fluid

Cleaning solvents

Oil-based paints

Automobile polishes, chrome polish, etc.

TABLE 17-4.   PESTICIDES COMMONLY IMPLICATED IN POISONINGS

Aerosol ant and roach killers

Aerosol-type home fogging agents

Liquid ant killers containing arsenic

Petroleum-based products used in diluted form for spraying vegetables
    and ornamental plants

Warfarin-type rat and mouse killers

Strychnine-based rodenticides

TABLE 17-5.   POISONOUS PLANTS                                                             531
                                                                          *Toxicity Rating*

Gastrointestinal irritants
    Daffodil bulbs
    Philodendron
    Diffenbachia
    Elephant ears
    Caladium
Alkaloidal toxins
    Hemlock
    Night shade
    Castor bean
Glycosides
    Foxglove
    Oleander
    Azalea

TABLE 17-6.   SOME POISONOUS MUSHROOMS

| Species | Common Names | Effects |
|---|---|---|
| *Amanita muscaria* | Fly agaric | Parasympathetic stimulation or depression. |
| *Gyromitra esculenta* | False Morel | Vomiting, diarrhea, convulsions, coma, hemolysis. |

Treatment

| | |
|---|---|
| *Amanita muscaria* | Induce vomiting and catharsis. Save vomitus for analysis. Antidote: Give atropine 2 mg subcutaneously. Repeat at the hospital if no improvement. If atropine symptoms predominate (dry mouth, "mad as a hatter," "red as a beet," etc.), atropine should be discontinued if these symptoms do not abate. |
| Other species | Induce vomiting. Use atropine as above, but discontinue if the atropine effects predominate. |

## TOXICITY RATING

The use of a toxicity rating scale (Table 17-7) to classify the degree of toxicity of a substance has been universal. If the amount of toxin to which a victim has been exposed is known, this scale becomes useful. Unfortunately, in the majority of cases, this amount is not known with

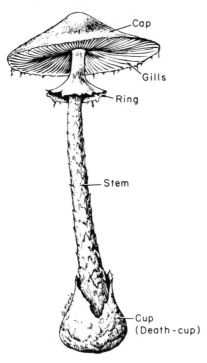

Cap

Gills

Ring

Stem

Cup
(Death-cup)

Destroying Angel
*Amanita Virosa*
(Pure White)

**Figure 17-2.** A poisonous mushroom plant.

any certainty. Moreover, the toxicity rating of a substance is based largely upon animal data that does not directly apply to humans.

A more rational method for assessing toxicity in humans is a TOXICITY RANGE, which combines the lowest dose that has produced toxicity on the one end with the highest dose that has resulted in complete recovery on the other end. A combination of both types of rating systems, if available, would be ideal in assessing the degree to which a patient has been poisoned.

## INITIAL EVALUATION OF THE POISONED PATIENT

When a person has been poisoned, rapid assessment is necessary. It is important to document accurately the circumstances surrounding the exposure, the exact name of the product or substance, the amount of toxin ingested or contacted, and the time since exposure. (Although poisoning by ingestion is the most common, it is important to remember that a person may be poisoned by skin or mucosal contact, and by inhalation.) Consideration of these factors determines further action and the need for professional assistance.

| Toxicity Rating | mg/kg | Probable Lethal Dose for 70 kg man |
|---|---|---|
| (6)  Super Toxic | Less than 5 | A taste (less than 7 drops) |
| (5)  Extremely Toxic | 5–50 | Between 7 drops and 1 tsp |
| (4)  Very Toxic | 50–500 | 1 tsp.–1 oz |
| (3)  Moderately Toxic | 500 mg–5 g | 1 oz.–1 pt |
| (2)  Slightly Toxic | 5 g–15 g | 1 pt.–1 qt |
| (1)  Practically nontoxic | More than 15 g | More than 1 qt |

(Adapted from Gosselin, Hodge, Smith and Gleason, *Clinical Toxicology of Commercial Products*, 4th ed. 1976)

## NAME OF PRODUCT

The name of the product should be documented as accurately as possible. Many products have similar names, so the patient should be encouraged to spell the name of the product, and/or to bring in the container to an emergency facility. The complete name of the product must be given as well as the brand name, since a brand name may be used for a number of products with different ingredients, e.g., Lysol Brand Disinfectant versus Lysol Brand Disinfectant Aerosol Foam Deodorizing Cleaner.

## AMOUNT OF PRODUCT

The amount of a product which is ingested is important so that one can assess the degree of potential toxicity. This information may be unavailable (e.g., with inhalation of toxic fumes, ingestion of petroleum products, or ingestion of liquids from large containers). However, one can usually estimate the largest amount ingested from smaller containers, especially prescription drugs. When the amount of toxic material cannot be determined accurately, it should be assumed that the patient has been exposed to a toxic dose, and treatment instituted accordingly.

## TIME OF EXPOSURE

The time of exposure to a toxic substance is a critical factor in management. For example, with ingestion of a strong base such as lye, immediate administration of large volumes of fluids may prevent esophageal damage. However, the longer the exposure, the more likely it is that significant esophageal impairment will occur. Similarly, ingestion of a toxic quantity of ferrous sulfate (iron) may be managed easily if emesis is induced and charcoal and a cathartic administered immediately. If a delay has occurred, even for two to four hours, generalized supportive care and specific chelation will be required to prevent mortality or serious morbidity.

## QUESTION OF EXPOSURE

Occasionally, circumstances suggest that a poisoning has occurred, but it is not clear whether the patient has actually been poisoned. This conclusion is in evidence when a highly odorous product, such as a petroleum distillate or a perfumed item, is involved, and the product has also been spilled. In this situation, the clothing should be removed and the skin washed. Thereafter, odor of the product on the patient's breath indicates ingestion.

The unknown poison presents problems in diagnosis and treatment. Poisoning should be suspected anytime a patient presents with bizarre symptoms or signs that do not suggest a specific diagnosis. This particularly applies if the patient is a child of a "high-risk" age (one to four years) and/or is unable to relate whether or not poisoning has occurred.

## INITIAL TREATMENT

### REMOVAL

The most important aspect of the initial therapy of poisoning is the removal of the poison. For contact poisons such as poison oak, or topical exposure to caustic/corrosive chemicals, vigorous decontamination of the skin with water and soap, and removal of the clothing is imperative. For inhaled substances such as chlorine gas, ammonia fumes, carbon monoxide, etc., the patient must be removed from the toxic environment. For ingested substances (excluding corrosives), the logical method of treatment is the removal of the toxin from the gastrointestinal tract before systemic absorption. Many times the inactivation of nonremoveable poisons is also indicated.

*Emesis.* The primary method of removing toxic substances from the stomach is emesis. This method is not indicated if the patient is comatose, has no gag reflex, has taken a caustic or corrosive substance, has ingested petroleum products (kerosene or gasoline), or has active gastrointestinal bleeding. It is indicated even several hours after ingestion, and is often possible even if the ingested substance was an antiemetic. In all cases, if the emesis has occurred in the field, the vomitus should be saved for evaluation at the hospital. There are several methods by which to induce emesis:

1. Gagging—Inducing emesis by gagging is the quickest method, and can be accomplished prior to a patient's arrival at an emergency facility. After the patient is given a glass of water or milk, a blunt object, such as a spoon or finger (depending upon the patient's propensity to bite) should be placed well down the throat to elicit gagging and subsequent vomiting. However, not all patients vomit with this method, and when vomiting occurs, it may be incomplete. Care should be taken not to introduce sharp objects, including long fingernails, into the hypopharynx, since puncture wounds can occur. If possible, the patient should be placed on the side, or leaning forward to minimize the possibility of aspiration.

2. Syrup of Ipecac—Syrup of ipecac produces emesis by action on the chemoreceptor trigger zone of the medulla; it may also act secondarily as a direct stomach irritant. It is safe and effective in recommended doses in over 90 percent of the cases. The paramedic can administer this drug after contact and permission with the base hospital. The dose for this substance is as follows:

| | |
|---|---|
| Infants less than 1 year: | 2 teaspoonfuls (10 ml) |
| Children 1 to 12 years: | 1 tablespoonful (15 ml) |
| Over 12 years, and adults: | 2 tablespoonfuls (30 ml, 1 oz) |

Following the administration of the recommended dose, water should be given in as large a quantity as tolerated, both to increase the rate of absorption of the ipecac, and to provide an adequate bolus for emesis. The patient should then be kept active; infants and small children should be kept aroused by physical stimulation if necessary. The time of onset of action for ipecac is about twenty minutes. If emesis does not occur in twenty to thirty minutes, the dose may be repeated. If emesis has still not occurred within forty-five to sixty minutes of the initial dose, the stomach should be emptied with a lavage tube. (The latter is not a field procedure.)

Syrup of ipecac is an appropriate addition to a home drug supply, because of its safety and efficacy; it should also be available in all medical facilities. Physicians should recommend that their patients obtain syrup of ipecac for the home (it can be purchased at pharmacies without prescription in 30 ml quantities), and the phone number of the nearest Poison Control Center should be kept readily accessible for emergency use. This is particularly important if there are preschool children in the household. Parents should be cautioned to treat the ipecac itself as a poison (ipecac, in large doses, can have cardiotoxic effects), and to keep it locked up with the other dangerous drugs in the home. It should be suggested that patients call the Poison Control Center or physician in case of poisoning for instructions. This is safer than giving specific doses of ipecac and having to remember the contraindications to giving this drug, since these are likely to be forgotten or confused in the crisis of a poisoning.

3. Apomorphine—Apomorphine is a prompt-acting (three to five minutes) centrally acting emetic, which must be administered subcutaneously. It is chemically a morphine-related alkaloid, and depresses respiration. It should not be given if the poisoning is due to a respiratory depressant, or if the respirations are slow or labored. The emetic response to this drug may be protracted, and occasionally requires termination with a narcotic antagonist such as naloxone hydrochloride (Narcan®). As with any other emetic procedure, it is important that fluids be administered because emesis does not readily occur, nor is it always effective in poison removal if the stomach is empty.

The usual dose of apomorphine in adults is 6 mg subcutaneously; in children one to two years old, 1 to 2 mg subcutaneously.

4. Other Emetics—The use of warm salt water and/or mustard is dangerous because of the possibility of hypernatremia, and impractical because it is usually difficult or impossible to force children to drink these mixtures. They should *never* be used.

Many packages of commercial products contain inaccurate information regarding treatment of poisoning. Many contain recommendations to use salt water or mustard, or in the case of caustics, to use dangerous treatments. The lay public should be warned to contact a Poison Control Center rather than follow the directions on the package label for treatment of such poisonings.

*Gastric Lavage.* Gastric lavage as a method for poison removal can be useful, but has its limitations. It is recommended when a patient is comatose, has no gag reflex, or when emesis cannot be induced. It is less effective in complete emptying of the stomach than emesis.

When a patient's sensorium is severely depressed, intubation of the trachea with a cuffed endotracheal tube is indicated prior to institution of gastric lavage. In children, because of the small trachea, cuffed tubes are not used. The largest size of lavage tube possible should be used, and copious amounts of the indicated fluid should be used. This is an Emergency Department, not a field, procedure.

The gastric tube can be used as an adjunct to syrup of ipecac in children (or adults) who refuse to drink adequate fluids for absorption of the ipecac and complete emptying of the stomach. In these patients, the tube can be used to introduce liquid into the stomach, while allowing the patient to empty the stomach by vomiting. The tube can also be used to introduce activated charcoal or cathartics. This, however, has not become an accepted field maneuver.

*Activated Charcoal.* Activated charcoal is an effective adsorbent for many toxic substances (Table 17-8). Its action is to adsorb or bind a toxin so that it is not absorbed during its transit through the gastrointestinal tract. It is an innocuous substance, and can be used in all ingestions except cyanide, though it is not effective in all cases. The dosage of

TABLE 17-8. CHEMICAL COMPOUNDS EFFECTIVELY ADSORBED BY
ACTIVATED CHARCOAL

| | | |
|---|---|---|
| Acetaminophen | Hexachlorophene | Phenylpropanolamine |
| Alcohol+ | Iodine* | Phenytoin* |
| Antimony | Ipecac | Phosphorus |
| Antipyrine | Iron | Potassium permanganate |
| Arsenic | Kerosene | Primaquine* |
| Aspirin* | Malathion+ | Probenecid |
| Atropine | Mefenamic acid | Propantheline |
| Barbital | Meprobamate | Propoxyphene* |
| Camphor | Mercuric chloride | Propylthiouracil |
| Cantharides | Methylene blue | Quinacrine |
| Chlordane | Methyl salicylate* | Quinidine |
| Chloroquine | Morphine | Quinine |
| Chlorpheniramine* | Muscarine | Salicylamide |
| Chlorpromazine | Nicotine | Secobarbital |
| Cocaine | Opium | Silver |
| Colchicine* | Oxalates | Sodium salicylate |
| Dextroamphetamine* | Parathion+ | Stramonium |
| Digitalis | Penicillin | Strychnine |
| Digitoxin | Pentobarbital | Sulfonamides |
| Ergotamine | Phenolphthalein | Tin |
| Ethchlorvynol | Phenobarbital | Tricyclic antidepressants |
| Glutethimide | Phenol* | Yohimbine |

*Well adsorbed
+Poorly adsorbed

activated charcoal is 15 to 30 grams (3 to 6 tablespoonfuls taken in a water slurry or given by lavage). The larger the quantity of activated charcoal, the more effective it will be since it functions by adsorbing the toxin to its surface. This can also be administered by the paramedic after contact with and permission from the base hospital.

Charcoal should be used *after* effective emesis to bind residual poisons in the stomach and gastrointestinal tract. This is particularly true when ipecac is used to induce emesis, since the charcoal will adsorb the ipecac itself and render it inactive. If it is necessary to administer activated charcoal prior to emesis, an emetic other than ipecac must be used.

Many people continue to recommend or use the "universal antidote," which is a mixture of activated charcoal, tannic acid, and magnesium oxide. This product is still commercially available, and there are many pharmacy shelves that contain it. This product is not only relatively ineffective, but it can also be dangerous, and its use should be discouraged. Similarly, the use of powdered charcoal for barbecuing or burnt toast as a substitute for activated charcoal is irrational since the charcoal derived from either source has no adsorptive capacity whatsoever.

*Cathartics.* A cathartic used in an acute poisoning acts to increase intestinal peristalsis, promote diarrhea, and thus decrease the amount of toxin absorbed. The ideal cathartic for poisoning promotes activity in both the small and large intestine, and acts rapidly. The following cathartics are recommended for use in acute poisonings:

1. Sodium sulfate, magnesium sulfate (two to six hour time of action)
2. Fleet's Phospho-Soda ® (one to eight hour time of action)
3. Castor oil (two to six hour action, and affects primarily the small intestine).

The use of magnesium salts as cathartics is contraindicated in renal failure or with compromise of renal function. Castor oil is recommended with ingestion of certain oil soluble substances such as phenols, because these preferentially partition into the oil and minimize absorption. Cathartics can be administered concomitantly with activated charcoal if desired.

## SECONDARY SIGNS AND SYMPTOMS

Obviously the paramedic will face many problems secondary to the effects of the poison itself. These may include problems with the respiratory, cardiac, and central nervous systems. Treatment of these conditions may even precede the treatment of the poison. The patient who is comatose with an airway problem needs his airway opened before attempting to determine the type of poisoning. Therefore, evaluation of the poisoned patient would begin similarly to that of the trauma patient with the primary survey to determine the patient's level of consciousness, vital signs, and need for cardiac monitoring. The patient may need oxygen or even positive pressure ventilation with an esophageal obturator airway.

Hypotension and shock should be treated by starting an intravenous infusion of Lactated Ringer's followed by transport. An important consideration to remember in a suspected poisoning is that all available information be brought with the patient to the hospital. The suspected poison, if present, should be brought with the patient.

In some cases a child will be discovered by a neighbor or babysitter to have ingested a poison or medication. The paramedic's first responsibility is to treat the child, but secondarily he should inform local law enforcement agencies so that they can try to contact the parents while the child is being transported to the hospital for treatment.

*Summary*

The effective treatment of poisoning is based upon the prompt recognition of the poisoning and an accurate and thorough initial evaluation of the patient. The basic principle for treatment is the prompt and complete removal of the poison, or the prevention of further absorption, as well as supportive and specific management for the individual toxin. The initial treatment of most noncorrosive/noncaustic toxic ingestions includes emesis or lavage, administration of activated charcoal, and catharsis. If these are completed promptly, the need for additional measures for treating the poisoning will be minimized.

## DRUGS OF ABUSE

### NARCOTICS

The term narcotic in current usage means opium, its derivatives, or synthetic substitutes that produce tolerance and dependence, both psychological and physical. The street names for drugs and the terms commonly used by addicts or drug users is presented in Tables 17-9 and 17-10.

TABLE 17-9. "STREET" NAMES FOR ABUSED DRUGS

Amphetamines—Bennies, Black Beauties (Biphetamine-T), Bombida, Bombita, Browns, Cartwheels, Chicken Powder, Christmas Trees, Co-Pilots, Crank, Crink, Cris, Cristina, Crossroads, Crystal, Dexies, Diet Pills, Eye Openers, Footballs, Hearts, Jelly Babies, Lid Proppers, Meth, Oranges, Peaches, Pep Pills, Purple Hearts, Roses, Speed, Splash, Splivins, Truck Drivers, Uppers, Wake-Ups, Wedges, White Cross, Whites

Chloral Hydrate—Mickey Finn, Peter

Cocaine—Bernice, Bernies Flake, Big Bloke, Big C, Big Rush, Burese, "C", Candy, Carrie, Cecil, Charlie, Cholley, Coke, Corrine, Dama Blanca, Dream, Dust, Flake, Gin, Girl, Gold Dust, Happy Dust, Happy Trails, Heaven Leaf, Her, Jam, Joy Powder, Lady, Leaf, Noise Candy, Nose Candy, Paradise, Pimps, Rich Man's, Rock, She, Smack, Snow, Star Dust, Star-Spangled Powder, The Leaf, White Girl

Codeine—School Boy

Doriden® (Glutethimide)—CB, Cibas, "D", Sleepers

Hashish—Gram, Hash, Keif

Heroin—Big Harry, Bomb, Boy, Caballo, Doojee, Dope, Dujie, Dust, Dynamite, "H", Hairy, Hard Stuff, Harry, Horse, Jack, Joy Powder, Junk, Mexican Horse, Noise, Scag, Scat, Schmack, Skag, Skid, Smack, TNT, White Junk, White Stuff

LSD—Acid, Battery Acid, Berkeley Blood, Big D, Black Sunshine, Blue Acid, Blue Heaven, Blue Microdot, Brown Dots, California Sunshine, Chief, Chocolate Chips, Cupcakes, "D," Domes, Flats, Four-Way, Grape Parfait, Hawaiian Sunshine, Microdots, Orange Barrel, Orange Sunshine, Orange Wedges, Owskey's Acid, Paper Acid, Pearly Gates, Purple Barrels, Purple Flat, Purple Haze, Purple Microdot, Purple Ozoline, Smears, Squirrels, Strawberry Field, Sugar, Sunshine, Twenty-Five, Wedding Bells, Wedges, White Lightning, Window Glass, Window Pane, Yellow Dimples, Zen

Marihuana—Acapulco Gold, Ashes, Baby, Bhang, Block, Bobo Bush, Bomber, Boo, Bush, Butter, Cannibis, Charge, Chiba Chiba, Fu, Gage, Ganja, Giggle Smoke, Gold, Goof Butt, Grass, Grief O, Hay, Hemp, Herb, Indian Bay, Indian Hay, Jay, Jive, Jive Sticks, Joint, Joy Sticks, Kick Sticks, Loco Weed, Log, Love Weed, MJ, Mary Jane, Mary Warner, Mezz, Mohasky, Mootos, Mor A Grif A, Muggles, Mutah, Panama Red, Panatella, Pod, Pot, Reefer, Rope, Sativa, Spliff, Splim, Straw, Sweet Lucy, Tea, Texas Tea, Viper's Weed, Weed

Methadone—Dollies

Morphine—Brown Heroin, Cube Juice, Dreamer, Emsel, Hard Stuff, Hocus, "M", Miss Emma, Morph, Unkie, White Merchandise, White Stuff

Opium—Big O, Black Stuff, Hop, "O", Pin Yen, Skee, Tar

Pentobarbital—Nemmies, Nimbies, Nimby, Nols, Purple Hearts, Sleepers, Yellow Jackets, Yellows

Peyote (Mescaline)—Bad Seed, Big Chief, Cactus, Mesc, Mese, Moon, Pink Wedge, White Light

Phencyclidine—Angel Dust, Angel Mist, Angel Hair, Dusted Parsley, Hawaiian Woodrose, HCP, Hog, Horse Tranq, PCP, Peace Pill, Piperidine, THC

Phenobarbital—Whites

Placidyl—Greenies, pickles

Phenmetrazine HCL (Preludin)—Sweets

Psilocybin—Exotic Mushroom, God's Flesh, Magic Mushroom, Mexican Mushroom

Quaalude®—Sopers, Sopors

TABLE 17-9.   CONTINUED

*541*

*Drugs of Abuse*

Secobarbital—F-40s, Mexican Reds, Pinks, Red Birds, Red Devils,
    Red Lilies, Reds, Seccy, Seggy, Sleepers
STP,DOM— Magic Pumpkin Seeds; Serenity, Tranquility, and Peace
Tuinal®—Double Trouble, Nols, Rainbows, Red & Blues, Sleepers,
    T-Birds, Tooies

TABLE 17-10.   GLOSSARY OF TERMS USED BY DRUG USERS AND ADDICTS

| | |
|---|---|
| Acid | LSD 25 |
| Acid Head | LSD user |
| Bag | A container of drugs |
| Bag Man | Drug supplier |
| Barbs | Barbiturates |
| Bennies | Amphetamines |
| Bindle | A container of drugs |
| Blue Bands | Carbrital (Sodium Pentobarbital—Carbromal) |
| Blue Birds | Amytal® (Sodium Amobarbital) |
| Blue Devils | Amytal® (Sodium Amobarbital) |
| Blue Heaven | Amytal® (Sodium Amobarbital) |
| Blues | Amytal® (Sodium Amobarbital) |
| Bombed | Intoxicated on drugs |
| Bottle Dealer | A person who sells drugs in 1000 tablets or capsule bottles |
| Bread | Money |
| Bummer | A bad trip |
| Burn | To buy phony drugs or to burn the skin when injecting amphetamines |
| Button | Peyote buttons |
| Buy | To purchase drugs |
| Candy | Barbiturates |
| Cap | Capsule containing a drug |
| Carrying | In possession of a drug |
| Cartwheel | Amphetamine tablet (round, white, double-scored) |
| Chicken Powder | Amphetamine powder for injection |
| Christmas Tree | Tuinal® |
| Come Down | To come off from drugs |
| Co-Pilots | Amphetamines |
| Cooker | Bottle cap for heating drug powder with water |
| Crystals | Amphetamine powder for injection |

| | |
|---|---|
| Cube | Sugar cube impregnated with LSD |
| Cut | To dilute a powder with milk, sugar, baking powder, etc. |
| "D" | LSD |
| Dealer | Drug supplier |
| Dexies | Amphetamine tablets |
| Dotting | Placing LSD on a sugar cube |
| Double Cross | Amphetamine tablets (double-scored) |
| Downer | To come off from drugs. Also, means a depressant-type drug such as a barbiturate |
| Fat | Describing someone who has a good supply of drugs |
| Fit | Equipment for injecting drugs |
| Flash | Initial high feeling when injecting amphetamines and other drugs |
| Footballs | Amphetamine tablets (oval-shaped) |
| Freak | A person who injects amphetamines |
| Freak Out | To have a drug party |
| Garbage | Poor quality drugs |
| Goof Balls | Barbiturates |
| Habit | Physically or psychologically dependent on drugs |
| Head | An LSD user |
| Hearts | Dexedrine (orange-colored, heart-shaped tablets) |
| Heat | A police officer |
| High | A drug user who is "up" or under the influence of a drug, usually a stimulant |
| Hit | One dose of a particular drug |
| Hype | A person who takes drugs by injection |
| Hype Outfit | Equipment for injecting drugs |
| Jar Dealer | A person who sells drugs in 1000 tablet or capsule bottles |
| Joy Popping | Irregular drug habit |
| Jug | 1000 tablet or capsule bottle |
| Keg | 25,000 amphetamine capsules or tablets, or more |
| Kick | To stop using drugs |
| "L" | LSD |
| Lab | Equipment used to manufacture drugs illegally |
| Loaded | High on drugs |
| Mainliner | One who injects directly into a vein |
| Man | A drug supplier or a police officer |

TABLE 17-10.  CONTINUED

*543*

*Drugs of Abuse*

| | |
|---|---|
| Mellow Yellows | Pale yellow LSD powder purportedly manufactured by Augustus Owsley Stanley III, or cigarettes made from banana peel scrapings |
| Meth | Amphetamine powder (Methamphetamine Hydrochloride) |
| Micky | Chloral hydrate |
| Mickey Finn | Chloral hydrate |
| Mule | A person who delivers or carries a drug for a dealer |
| Needle | Hypodermic needle |
| Nickel Buy | A $5.00 purchase |
| O.D. | Overdose, death |
| Owsley's Acid | LSD purportedly manufactured by Augustus Owsley Stanley III, also infers that it is good quality LSD |
| Panic | When a drug supply has been cut off |
| Paper | A container of drugs |
| Per | A prescription |
| Pez | Pez candies impregnated with LSD |
| Point | Hypodermic needle |
| Popper | Amyl nitrite in ampule form. Inhaled immediately after taking LSD |
| Powder | Amphetamine powder |
| Rainbows | Tuinal ® (Sodium Amobarbital and Sodium Secobarbital) |
| Reds and Blues | Tuinal ® (Sodium Amobarbital and Sodium Secobarbital) |
| Reds | Seconal (Sodium Secobarbital) |
| Red Birds | Seconal (Sodium Secobarbital) |
| Red Devils | Seconal (Sodium Secobarbital) |
| Righteous | Good quality drugs |
| Roll | A tin foil wrapped roll of tablets |
| Roll Dealer | A person who sells tablets in rolls |
| Run | To take drugs continuously for at least 3 days |
| Score | Make a drug purchase |
| Script | Drug prescription |
| Shooting Gallery | Place where users can purchase drugs and inject them |
| Shoot Up | To inject drugs |
| Skin Popping | Intradermal or subcutaneous injection |
| Sleepers | A depressant-type drug such as barbiturates |

| | |
|---|---|
| Snow | LSD powder, amphetamine powder or cocaine |
| Spatz | Capsules |
| Speed | Amphetamine powder for injection |
| Spike | Hypodermic needle |
| Spoon | A measure for a drug in powder form 16 spoons per ounce |
| Stanley's Stuff | LSD purportedly manufactured by Augustus Owsley Stanley III |
| STP | 4-Methyl 2, 5 Dimethoxy Alpha Methyl Phenethylamine |
| Strung Out | Heavily addicted |
| Stuff | General term for drugs and narcotics |
| Taste | A small quantity of drugs or narcotics, a sample |
| TD Caps | Time disintegrating capsules |
| Travel Agent | A pusher of hallucinogenic drugs |
| Trey | A $3.00 purchase |
| Trigger | To smoke a marihuana cigarette immediately after taking LSD |
| Trip | The hallucinations and/or feelings experienced by a person after taking a drug |
| Turn On | To take a drug |
| Weekend Habit | Irregular drug habit |
| West Coast Turn-arounds | Amphetamine tablets or capsules |
| Whites | Amphetamine tablets |
| Works | Equipment for injecting drugs |
| Yellow Jackets | Nembutal (Sodium Pentobarbital) |
| Yellows | Nembutal (Sodium Pentobarbital) |

*Properties and Effects: Dependence and Addiction.* The relief of physical or psychic suffering through the use of narcotics may result in a short-lived state of euphoria. They also tend to induce drowsiness, apathy, lethargy, decreased physical activity, constipation, pinpoint pupils, and reduced vision. Large doses may induce sleep, but there is an increasing possibility of nausea, vomiting, and respiratory depression.

The initial effects of narcotics are often unpleasant. To the extent that the response is felt to be pleasurable, its intensity may be expected to increase with the amount of the dose administered. Repeated use, however, will result in increasing tolerance; that is, the user must administer progressively larger doses to attain the desired effect, thereby reinforcing the compulsive behavior known as narcotic addiction.

Physical dependence refers to an alteration in the normal functions of the body that necessitates the continued presence of a drug in order to prevent the withdrawal or abstinence syndrome characteristic of each class of addictive drugs. The intensity and character of the physical symptoms experienced during the withdrawal period are directly related to the amount of narcotic used each day.

*Withdrawal.* With the deprivation of morphine or heroin, the first withdrawal signs are usually experienced shortly before the time of the next scheduled dose. Complaints and demands by the addict are prominent, increasing in intensity, and peak from thirty-six to seventy-two hours after the last dose, then gradually subside. Symptoms such as watery eyes, runny nose, yawning, and increased perspiration appear about eight to twelve hours after the last dose. Thereafter, the addict may fall into a restless sleep. As the abstinence syndrome progresses, irritability, loss of appetite, insomnia, goose flesh, tremors, and finally violent yawning and severe sneezing occur. These symptoms reach their peak at forty-eight to seventy-two hours. The patient is weak and depressed with nausea and vomiting. Stomach cramps and diarrhea are common. The heart rate and blood pressure are elevated. Chills alternating with flushing and excessive sweating are also characteristic symptoms. Without treatment, the syndrome eventually runs its course and most of the symptoms will disappear in seven to ten days. However, how long it takes the body to reach full equilibrium is unpredictable.

Infants born to addicted mothers may also be expected to experience withdrawal symptoms, due to the placental transfer of narcotics to the fetus.

Specific drugs (brand names in parentheses) are listed in Table 17-11.

TABLE 17-11.  NARCOTIC DRUGS

| *Drug* | *Comments* |
|---|---|
| Morphine | Most effective for the relief of severe pain and suppression of cough. |
| Codeine | More useful for mild types of pain and as a cough suppressant. Potency about one-half of morphine. Addiction liability much less than morphine. |
| Heroin | Is an effective analgesic; however, high addiction liability makes it undesirable therapeutically. |
| Hydromorphone (Dilaudid) | Shorter duration of action than morphine, but faster onset of action. Approximately ten times stronger than morphine. |
| Hydrocodone (Hycodan) | Most useful as an antitussive. Similar to codeine, but more potent. |

TABLE 17-11. CONTINUED

| Drug | Comments |
| --- | --- |
| Meperidine (Demerol) | Shorter duration of action than morphine, but only one-tenth as potent. Probably most commonly used narcotic. No antitussive properties. |
| Methadone (Dolophine) | Very little addiction liability making it useful for the treatment of narcotic dependence. Duration of action is longer than morphine. |
| Pentazocine (Talwin) | Originally studied as a narcotic antagonist but found to have analgesic properties. Can be addicting and is less active than morphine. |
| Propoxyphene (Darvon) | Propoxyphene is a chemical derivative of opium. Although it is not considered a narcotic by the Dangerous Drug Administration, chronic use of it can produce addiction. Pellets in the Darvon® capsule have been removed and injected intravenously by addicts. It can produce a clinical picture very similar to heroin overdose. |

## DEPRESSANTS

*Properties and Effects.* Depressants have a potential for abuse associated with both physical and psychological dependence.

Therapeutically, they are beneficial in the symptomatic treatment of insomnia, anxiety, irritability, nervousness, etc. In excessive doses they can cause coma, respiratory depression, and possible death. Chronic administration can lead to addiction, especially with barbiturates.

*Abuse.* The pattern of abuse falls into two categories, episodic and habitual. The episodic use is experienced by younger patients who find their source in the illicit market or in their parent's medication cabinet. Their source as well as their use becomes sporadic, and basically the use is aimed for a thrill production. The habitual user shows a tendency toward addiction and has a high incidence of overdosage.

*Tolerance and Overdose.* Tolerance to depressants develops rapidly, narrowing the range between the therapeutic and lethal dose. Depressant drugs in combination with other central nervous system depressants and alcohol multiply the chances for toxicity and overdosage. Moderate depressant overdose closely resembles alcoholic inebriation. The symptoms of severe overdose are coma, weak and rapid pulse, cold and clammy skin, and shallow respirations. If the reduced respiration and low blood pressure are not treated, death usually follows. Thorazine® and Haldol® will produce marked reduction in blood pressure because they are patent vasodilators. Dopamine is used to treat the hypotension if severe.

*Withdrawal.* To abruptly stop the administration of depressants to patients who are addicted will lead to an abstinence syndrome more severe than in an otherwise comparable case of narcotic withdrawal. The symptoms seen with depressant withdrawal are anxiety, agitation, apprehension, anorexia, nausea, vomiting, tachycardia, excessive sweating, insomnia, tremulousness, and muscle spasms. If the addiction is based on large amounts, delirium, psychotic behavior, convulsions, or even death may occur. The withdrawal regimen should consist of the substitution of a long-acting depressant such as phenobarbital for the depressant used, followed by a gradual decreasing of the dose.

Table 17-12 illustrates some of the more commonly used depressants.

TABLE 17-12. DEPRESSANT DRUGS

| Drug | Duration of Action (Hours) |
|---|---|
| Chloral Hydrate | 5 to 8 |
| Pentobarbital (Nembutal) | 4 to 6 |
| Secobarbital (Seconal) | 4 to 6 |
| Phenobarbital | 12 to 16 |
| Tuinal | 6 to 8 |
| Glutethimide (Doriden) | 4 to 8 |
| Diazepam (Valium) | 2 to 4 |
| Chlordiazepoxide (Librium) | 3 to 5 |
| Clorazenate Dipotassium (Tranzene) | 1 to 4 |
| Oxazepam (Serax) | 4 to 6 |
| Meprobamate (Equanil, Miltown) | 2 to 4 |
| Tybamate (Solacen, Tybatran) | 2 to 4 |
| Methaqualone (Quaalude) | 4 to 8 |
| Ethchlorvynl (Placidyl) | 4 to 8 |
| Flurazepam (Dalmane) | 4 to 8 |
| Marihuana, Hashish, and Hashish Oil Phenothiazines | 2 to 4 |
| Chlorpromazine (Thorazine) | 4 to 6 |
| Thioridazine (Mellaril) | 4 to 6 |
| Perphenazine (Trilafon) | 6 to 8 |
| Prochlorperazine (Compazine) | 3 to 4 |
| Fluphenazine (Permitil, Prolixin) | 6 to 8 |
| Trifluoperazine (Stellazine) | 12 |

TABLE 17-12. CONTINUED

| Drug | Duration of Action (Hours) |
|------|:---:|
| Thiothixene (Navane) | 4 to 6 |
| Haloperidol (Haldol) | 2 to 6 |
| Mesoridazine (Serentil) | Undetermined |
| Promazine (Sparine) | 4 to 6 |

## TRICYCLIC ANTIDEPRESSANTS

The tricyclic antidepressants are commonly used in psychotherapy for the treatment of endogenous depression. They are clinically related to the phenothiazine tranquilizers and have similar toxicologic effects. The abuse potential of the tricyclic compounds does not generally lie in their ability to produce a mind-altering state. Rather, because of the nature of the condition for which these drugs are prescribed, patients not uncommonly present with an acute overdose secondary to attempting suicide. Occasionally, tricyclic drugs are a component of mixed drug ingestions.

An overdose of tricyclic antidepressants produces a wide variety of symptoms, the most conspicuous of which is central nervous system depression. Patients may present with symptoms ranging anywhere from lethargy to coma with decreased tendon reflexes. Hallucinations often occur, and convulsions may appear in cases of severe toxicity.

The life-threatening effects of the tricyclics involve the cardiovascular system, including a number of ventricular and supraventricular dysrhythmias, severe hypotension, bradycardia, and shock. The tricyclic compounds also have a number of atropinic or anticholinergic effects, including dry mouth, pupillary dilatation, urinary retention, and decreased gastrointestinal motility.

The biological half-life of these compounds is quite long, averaging three days, and severe overdosage must be monitored continuously. If a patient is suspected of having taken tricyclic antidepressants but presents symptom-free, the use of an emetic, activated charcoal, and a cathartic should be followed by observation for six hours in the event any absorption occurs. Vital signs should be monitored continuously for at least 48 hours if the patient is symptomatic. Hypotension may be managed with appropriate intravenous fluids; pressor agents such as dopamine may be needed.

Physostigmine, a cholinergic agent, may be useful for the treatment of some of the dysrhythmias, hallucinations, and convulsions associated with tricyclic antidepressants, and can be used to diagnose acute anticholinergic poisoning, but should not be administered routinely in comatose patients just to keep the patient awake.

Tricyclic Drugs include:

1. Amitriptyline (Elavil®)
2. Amitriptyline, perphenazine combination (Triavil®, Etrafon®)
3. Desipramine (Pertofrane®)
4. Doxepin (Sinequan®)
5. Imipramine (Tofranil®)
6. Nortriptyline (Aventyl®)

## STIMULANTS

This category of drugs is designed to stimulate the central nervous system, thereby producing a relief from fatigue and increased alertness. Mild CNS stimulants are found in commonly used products such as tobacco (nicotine) and coffee (caffeine). Stronger stimulants have a broad range of activity, and may also produce mood elevation and a heightened sense of well-being. Chronic users tend to rely on stimulants to feel stronger, more confident, decisive, etc. This is often followed by a pattern of taking depressants in the evenings followed by stimulants in the morning.

*Use and Abuse.*   The oral consumption of stimulants may result in a temporary sense of exhilaration, hyperactivity, irritability, anxiety, and apprehension. These effects are intensified when administered by intravenous injection which may produce a sudden sensation known as a "flash" or "rush." A period of depression known as "crashing" occurs after the initial "rush" effect has ended. Heavy users may inject themselves every few hours, a process sometimes continued to the point of delirium psychosis, or physical exhaustion. Tolerance develops rapidly, increasing the probability of overdosage. Very large doses also result in various mental aberrations which include repetitive grinding of the teeth, touching and picking the face and extremities, performing the same tasks over and over, a preoccupation with one's own thought processes, suspiciousness, and paranoia with auditory and visual hallucinations. Dizziness, tremor, agitation, mydriosis (pupil dilatation), hostility, panic, headache, flushed skin, chest pains with palpitations, excessive sweating, vomiting, and abdominal cramps are some of the signs and symptoms of a sublethal overdose. The onset of death may be preceded by high fever, convulsions, and cardiovascular collapse.

*Dependence and Withdrawal.*   The subject of physical dependence with these drugs is debatable. However, there is evidence that chronic high dose users do not easily withdraw or return to normal after the withdrawal. Profound apathy and depression, fatigue, and disturbed sleep up to twenty hours a day characterize the immediate withdrawal syndrome, which may last for several days. Lingering impairment of thought processes may also be present.

Table 17-13 lists some of the stimulant drugs currently in use.

TABLE 17-13.   STIMULANT DRUGS

| Drug | Duration of Action (Hours) |
|------|---------------------------|
| Cocaine | 2 |
| Amphetamines (Dexedrine, Benzedrine) | 2 to 4 |
| Phenmetrazine (Preludin) | 2 to 4 |
| Methylphenidate (Ritalin) | 2 to 4 |

## HALLUCINOGENS

*Effects.*   Hallucinogens can be classified as agents that alter or distort normal behavior, producing changes in the reception of visual and auditory stimuli, and expanding the range of consciousness. They make it difficult to distinguish between reality and fantasy through the production of sensory illusions that result in the apparent perception of unreal sights and sounds. A patient's sense of direction, distance, and time become disoriented. Restlessness and sleeplessness are common until the drug effects diminish. The greatest hazard of the hallucinogens is that their effects are unpredictable each time they are taken.

Phencyclidine (PCP) was first synthesized in 1957. In 1965 human clinical investigation was discontinued because of its obvious hallucinogenic effects. In 1967 it was introduced as a tranquilizing agent and anesthetic for primates. Its first appearance as a street drug was in 1967. On the street it is called Crystal Joint (CJs), Angel Dust, Angel Mist, HCP, Hog, Peace Weed, Rocket Fuel, etc. (see Table 17-9). It can appear as a translucent white rock crystal, coarse white granules, or white powder. It usually comes in 1 g amounts, which is equivalent to four to eight heavy joints, or eighteen to twenty-four street joints. It is usually taken by smoking or snorting. Phencyclidine is available in a liquid or powder form. It can be dissolved in a drink or sprinkled "on mustard" and eaten in a sandwich. Because of it ease of ingestion, PCP has been used as a trick or surprise on unsuspecting people. This is particularly true among high school students, and sudden alterations in consciousness and behavior should alert the examiner to the possibility of PCP ingestion.

The usual amount of PCP is 30 to 90 milligrams for smoking and 5 milligrams for snorting. The effects are listed below:

1. Onset of effects—2 to 5 minutes.

2. Peak or plateau—25 to 30 minutes; user remains loaded for 24 to 48 hours.

3. Return to normal—24 to 48 hours.

PCP may be a stimulant or depressant depending upon the dose. It may be mixed with alcohol or other drugs. In the overdose state, the patient will appear with the following symptoms:

1. Coma with open eyes, pupils reactive to light, miosis.
2. Hypertension.
3. Absence of respiratory depression.
4. Nystagmus.
5. Repetitive motor movements, shivering, muscle rigidity.
6. Vomiting and/or hypersalivation.
7. Incommunicative for 30 to 60 minutes.
8. Manifestation of a low-dose state upon awakening.

The high dose state is characterized by:

1. Normal respirations with occasional apnea.
2. Normal or high blood pressure.
3. Pupillary light reflexes intact, miosis.
4. Opisthotonis posturing.
5. Nystagmus.
6. Vomiting, hypersalivation.
7. Characteristic features include:
    a. Alternating periods of sleeping and waking.
    b. Misperception.
    c. Disorientation.
    d. Hallucinatory phenomena.
    e. Clinical picture of the low-dose state.
    f. Coma for periods of over 12 hours to several days. Subsequent recovery to normal.

Management of these patients is to isolate them and place them in a darkened cushioned room. This is for their own protection. Severely overdosed patients may present in coma and they need the usual management for the coma patient (Chapter 16). When muscle rigidity occurs, IV diazepam (Valium₀) may be necessary to control the subsequent seizures when they occur. PCP is absorbed rapidly and to gavage or induce emesis may be of little benefit.

The important aspect in management of these patients is to realize that they can be sitting staring and appear to be in a state of suspended animation, and then suddenly become quite violent. This change in their physical status must be known by the paramedic or any medical personnel taking care of these patients. They can become incredibly strong and violent, and do harm to themselves and to others. The patient withdrawing from PCP must be watched carefully and there must be ample help available if he becomes violent.

Table 17-14 illustrates some of the commonly abused hallucinogens and relative comments regarding their effects.

TABLE 17-14.   HALLUCINOGEN DRUGS

| *Hallucinogen* | *Comments* |
| --- | --- |
| Peyote (Mescaline) | Mescaline is the active ingredient in peyote cactus. Taken orally, mescaline in a dose of 350–500 mg produces illusions and hallucinations for 5–12 hours. |
| Psilocybin & Psilocyn | Obtained from mushrooms grown in Mexico, taken orally the effects are similar to mescaline except that a smaller dose of 4–8 mg gives an effect for about 6 hours. |
| Lysergic Acid Diethylamide (LSD) | A semisynthetic compound produced from lysergic acid, which is found in a fungus that grows on rye. Frequently sold in the form of tablets, thin squares of gelatin, or paper blotted with the chemical. Oral doses of 100–250 micrograms will normally produce psychedelic "trips." Along with mental changes, physical reactions include dilated pupils, decreased body temperature, nausea, diaphoresis, tachycardia, and elevated blood sugar levels. "Flashbacks" after the pharmacologic effects have worn off are fairly common. |
| DOM (Dimethoxyamphetamine) or STP | Chemically related to mescaline and amphetamines. Sold under the street name of STP (serenity, tranquility, and peace). It is 30–50 times less potent than LSD and 100 times more potent than mescaline. |
| Phencyclidine (PCP) | A veterinary anesthetic (Sernylan₀) that has found popularity for its hallucinogenic effects. It is taken orally, smoked, or sniffed, and has also been sold as LSD, mescaline, or THC (tetrahydrocannabinol). Low dose states produce changes in body image, |

TABLE 17-14. CONTINUED

553

*Management of
Reactions to Drug
Abuse*

| *Hallucinogen* | *Comments* |
| --- | --- |
| | feelings of depersonalization, perceptual distortions, visual and auditory hallucinations, and feelings of apathy and estrangement. A "blank stare" look is seen with low doses. Other effects include drowsiness, difficulty in concentrating, preoccupation with death, and acute psychotic episodes. Common physical signs include flushing and profuse sweating, nystagmus, miosis, ataxia, dizziness, nausea, and vomiting. Use of this drug can cause extreme combativeness and violent behavior. |

## MANAGEMENT OF REACTIONS TO DRUG ABUSE

### RECOGNITION

Although there are laboratory tests to identify levels of barbiturates, opiates, amphetamines, and cocaine, these tests are not always immediately available in the hospital and not at all in the field. Tests for some of the hallucinogens, such as LSD, can only be done in special laboratories; therefore, the diagnosis and treatment of acute drug intoxication or an abstinence syndrome must often be made on the basis of clinical evidence alone. Drugs available on the street are usually adulterated with a variety of other drugs or chemicals, thereby producing a myriad of symptoms.

The route of administration can be an important clue as to the type of drug or chemical abused. For example, sniffing cocaine can lead to inflammation and ulceration of the nasal mucosa; evidence of recent needle tracks or small circular abscesses may suggest opiates or some stimulant such as methamphetamine; a rash may be present around the nose indicating volatile solvent or aerosol use and the breath may smell like gasoline or kerosene in these cases. All of these clues may be useful in helping to determine the agent causing the symptoms.

### TYPE OF SUBSTANCE

#### Narcotics

*Signs.* An overdose of any one of the narcotics produces depressed or absent respirations. The pupils are generally contracted and fixed, although extreme hypoxia or the use of meperidine (Demerol) can be

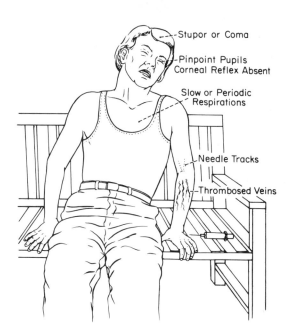

Stupor or Coma
Pinpoint Pupils
Corneal Reflex Absent
Slow or Periodic
Respirations
Needle Tracks
Thrombosed Veins

**Figure 17-3.** An overdosed heroin addict. The needle tracks and thrombosed veins are obvious indications of a chronic drug user.

associated with pupillary dilatation. Shock or pulmonary edema may be present. Look for needle tracks on the flexion surfaces such as the elbow or behind the knee (Figure 17-3). With an overdose of propoxyphene (Darvon), convulsions may be prominent. The illegal narcotics may be adulterated with other drugs such as quinine or lactose, and contaminated with bacteria and fungi. It is often the contaminant that may produce significant clinical problems. Quinine can produce severe reactions and may be more predominant than the heroin itself. Local quinine reactions are characterized by edema, erythema, and blistering of the skin at the injection site. Quinine can also produce laryngeal edema and systemic reactions including headache, fever, shortness of breath, nausea, and diarrhea. Bacteria and fungi, which are present within the narcotic, may infect the patient's heart valves or produce abscesses throughout the body.

*Treatment*

1. Maintain the airway and ventilate the patient if he is not breathing.

2. Record vital signs, and treat shock with an intravenous infusion of Lactated Ringer's. If this does not work, a dopamine drip may be necessary.

3. Monitor the patient's heart since dysrhythmias, including ventricular fibrillation, can occur after heroin overdose.

4. Complete examination of the chest to rule out pulmonary edema. If present, the patient should be treated with intravenous diuretics, such as Lasix₍ᵣ₎.

5. Naloxone (Narcan) is a narcotic antagonist effective in reversing the apnea and coma caused by morphine, heroin, codeine, meperidine, methadone, propoxyphene, pentazocine (Talwin), and other opium-related drugs. It is not effective in barbiturate or other sedative-hypnotic overdoses. However, it can be used as a diagnostic tool; if repeated doses do not improve respirations, opiate overdose is unlikely. A dose of 0.4 mg (1 ml) should be given intravenously and repeated in three minutes. Since naloxone does not cause the respiratory depression seen with other narcotic antagonists, repeated doses can be used. However, the duration of action is shorter than that of the opiate. Therefore, the patient should be monitored closely for relapses.

The abstinence or withdrawal symptoms can be treated with 20 mg of oral methadone and repeated once during the first twenty-four hours of the withdrawal. Some patients may require decreasing doses of oral methadone for one to two weeks or more.

## Depressants

*Signs.* Usually depressants such as sedative-hypnotics and minor tranquilizers in large amounts produce a syndrome resembling acute alcoholic intoxication. Overdosage can lead to coma with depressed respirations and hypotension. The pupils may be unchanged or small, but with glutethimide (Doriden) or in severe poisonings with other depressants, they can be dilated. Drugs such as the benzodiazepines (Valium, Librium, Dalmane) seldom cause serious overdose problems when taken alone. Methaqualone (Quaalude) overdose is associated with hyperirritability, seizures, and hyperactive reflexes (including the gag reflex), which may make airway intubation difficult.

*Treatment*

1. General supportive measures; i.e., maintain the airway or begin assisted ventilation with oxygen.

2. Never administer stimulants in the field.

3. If the patient is conscious and has a gag reflex, an attempt to induce vomiting can be made, or administer ipecac.

4. In the Emergency Department, gavage and activated charcoal are indicated.

5. Monitor vital signs and begin to treat shock with an intravenous infusion of Lactated Ringer's.

6. Unlike withdrawal symptoms seen with narcotics, withdrawal from barbiturates can be life-threatening. This will occur in the hospital and will consist of insomnia, weakness, fever, and restlessness, appearing within twenty-four hours after the last dose. Delirium and convulsions may develop after the second or third day, sometimes resulting in status epilepticus and shock. Withdrawal from nonbarbiturate depressants can

be done by gradual reduction of the dose on which the patient has become dependent.

## Stimulants

*Signs.* Acute intoxication with high doses of amphetamines or cocaine produce the following signs and symptoms: dilated pupils, tachycardia, hyperpyrexia, tremors, paranoia, impulsive-compulsive behavior, psychosis, and convulsions. To a nontolerant person, 100 to 200 mg of dextroamphetamine can be lethal; however, larger doses may have very little effect on tolerant users. To control the psychological disturbances caused by amphetamines, chlorpromazine (Thorazine) can be useful. Cocaine is usually sniffed rather than used intravenously (as are amphetamines). The effects are similar except the duration of the action is brief.

*Treatment.* Gradual detoxification is unnecessary. However, abstinence-like symptoms such as psychological depression, marked fatigue, complaints of body ache, hyperphagia, and hypersomnia may occur. Although true withdrawals have not been seen with cocaine, users suffer a transient depressed state (cocaine blues) when deprived of the drug.

## Hallucinogens

*Signs.* Acute intoxication with hallucinogens such as PCP, LSD, or mescaline will produce a mental state that is highly variable and may include anxiety, panic, and psychosis. The results of these actions may lead to accidental injury or suicidal or homicidal acts.

*Treatment.* Since hallucinogens produce a state of hypersuggestibility, this can be used to try to calm the patient down by speaking to him in a quiet place. To allay the fright and hyperactivity, strong reassurance that the effects will subside is helpful. Focusing on an object helps to reduce the intensity of the experience. When sedation is indicated, Valium® or a barbiturate can be used. Phenothiazines such as chlorpromazine (Thorazine) can also be used; however, care must be taken to avoid the possibility that anticholinergic substances might also have been ingested, since phenothiazine can increase anticholinergic activity.

Even after blood levels of hallucinogens have dropped and the agent has been eliminated from the body, the user may experience a "flashback" phenomenon, which is an acute reoccurrence of the psychedelic-like state. Reassurance that the effect will soon disappear is useful. The use of marihuana or an antihistamine can trigger these reoccurrences. A withdrawal syndrome from the hallucinogens is yet to be described. Prolonged anxiety and psychotic reactions may need to be treated with psychiatric consultation and tranquilizers.

In summary, we have discussed in this chapter the toxic effects *Summary*
of the common and useful drugs and substances, as well as the uncommon
and abused ones. Since the paramedic will often be called upon to be
the first line of medical defense for many patients in these categories,
he would be well advised to gain familiarity with at least the common
problems discussed here. This will enable him to treat this group of
disorders with maximum efficiency.

Mechanisms of exposure include: *Important*
*Points to*
Ingestion *Remember*

Inhalation

Injection

Contact

Ninety percent of all poisoning involves children—mostly under
5 years of age.

Types of substances include:

Household products (50%)

Drugs (25%)—especially aspirin

Petroleum products (10%)—Gasoline, kerosene, paint thinner

Pesticides (5%)

Plants (5%)

*Initial Evaluation:*  Document the circumstances surrounding the
exposure, exact name of substance, amount contacted or ingested, and
time since exposure. Removal is the most important aspect of initial
therapy.

Contact poisons: vigorous skin decontamination with water and
removal of clothes

Inhaled substances: remove person from environment.

Ingestions (except as listed below): removal from gastrointestinal
tract.

Methods of gastrointestinal removal are:

1. Emesis (not if unconscious, or has no gag reflex, or if the
   substance was a petroleum product, or if active bleeding is
   present).
   a. Methods of Emesis:
      Gagging
      Syrup of Ipecac (infants 2 tsp., children 1–12 1 tbsp., over
      12 to adults—2 tbsp.)
2. Lavage (best done at hospital)
3. Cathartics

Secondary signs and symptoms of poisoning must also be looked for and treated in the field. This may include respiratory and circulatory problems.

Drugs of abuse may include:

Narcotics (morphine, codeine, heroin)

Depressants (barbiturates, tranquilizers)

Stimulants [amphetamines, cocaine, methylphenidate (Ritalin)]

Hallucinogens (mescaline, LSD, phencyclidine)

Illegal narcotics may be adulterated with other drugs such as quinine, lactose, or contaminated with bacteria. The contaminant may produce the major problem.

Narcotic overdose is managed by supportive ventilation, oxygen, an airway, and correction of shock with IV fluids. Naloxone (Narcan) is an antagonist which reverses the coma caused by morphine, heroin, codeine, Demerol_®, methadone, Darvon_®, Talwin_®, and other opiates. Dosage is 0.4 mg (1 ml) which can be given IV and repeated in 3 minutes. *Watch for relapses with this drug.*

Treatment of depressant overdose is supportive airway, oxygen, and IV fluids.

Withdrawal symptoms from barbiturates must be treated by hospitalization since this process can be life-threatening.

Treatment of stimulant intoxication may include Thorazine_® for acute states; however, gradual detoxification is unnecessary because of the absence of true addiction or withdrawal.

Acute intoxication with the hallucinogen includes calming down the patient, reassurance, and the occasional use of Valium_® or phenobarbital.

*Bibliography*    Arena, Jay M. *Poisoning* (third ed.) Springfield Ill.: Charles C. Thomas, 1974.

Gosselin, Robert E., Harold C. Hodge, Roger Smith, and Marion N. Gleason. *Clinical Toxicology of Commercial Products: Acute Poisoning* (fourth ed.). Baltimore Md.: Williams and Wilkins Company, 1976.

Dreisbach, Robert H. *Handbook of Poisoning* (eighth ed.). Los Altos, California: Lange Medical Publications, 1974.

Hardin, James W. and Jay M. Arena. *Human Poisoning from Native and Cultivated Plants* (second ed.) Durham, N.C.: Duke University Press, 1974.

Rumack, Barry H., Ed. *Poison Index.* Denver, Colo.: National Center for Poison Information, Rocky Mountain Poison Center, 1977.

# Chapter 18

# THERMAL, ENVIRONMENTAL, AND RECREATIONAL INJURIES

Some of the most devastating accidents can occur without penetration or even severe impact. The most physiologically taxing injury to the human body is that of an extensive thermal injury (burn). Initial field management, Emergency Department management, and finally prolonged hospitalization place strains on the patient and his or her family more than any other single catastrophic illness. In the United States, most major burns are managed in burn centers. Other acute injuries that may be just as devastating include chemical burns, smoke inhalation, cold injury and exposure, heat prostration, electrical injuries including lightning, radiation exposure, hang-gliding accidents, scuba diving injuries, snake and venomous bites, marine animal bites, heat exhaustion, and heat stroke. This chapter will cover all of these acute disorders with emphasis placed on pathophysiology and field management.

## THERMAL INJURY

### THERMAL BURNS

Burns are classified by extent and depth. The extent is an estimate of the body surface area which has been burned. The rule of 9s is an easy way to make this estimate (Figure 18-1). The head and arms are each approximately 9 percent of the body surface, each leg 18 percent, and the front and the back of the torso each 18 percent. For example, a patient with burns involving most of both legs has a 35 percent burn. Burns are caused by house fires, suddenly bursting steam pipes, the opening of an overheated radiator, using gasoline to clean equipment in a garage where a pilot light is burning, attempting to prime a carburetor by pouring gasoline into it, automobile accidents in which gasoline is spilled and flames engulf the car and victim, airplane accidents, etc.

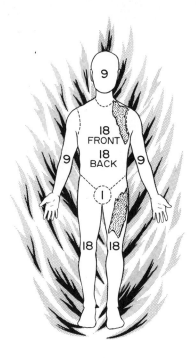

**Figure 18-1.** The rule of 9s for rapid estimation of the percentage of body surface burns. The patient must be examined front and back to make a full assessment.

The depth of the burn is estimated by examining the skin involved (Figure 18-2). Burns are divided into four degrees:

First degree

Second degree

Third degree

Fourth degree

A first degree burn is a mild injury merely causing redness, as in a sunburn. Second degree burns cause severe skin damage, but will heal spontaneously in one to three weeks. Second degree burns are red, covered with blisters or peeling skin, wet with serum, and very

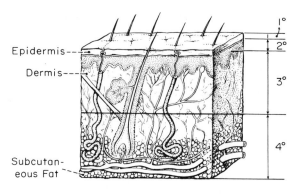

**Figure 18-2.** A cross-section of human skin showing the different layers that describe the degree of the burn.

painful. In third degree burns the skin is completely killed by the injury. This skin will not heal spontaneously and skin grafting must be done after the dead skin comes off. Third degree burns may be white and dead-looking, black and charred, or bright red. External layers of skin may peel off spontaneously, leaving a dry leathery surface. Third degree burns are not painful. Second degree burns are usually caused by scalding or a brief flash of heat; third degree burns are caused by flame. Fourth degree burns are those which extend below the subcutaneous fat into the muscle or bone beneath. The diagnosis of fourth degree burns cannot be made by examining the surface unless the skin has split open.

First degree burns generally do not require medical attention. Second and third degree burns are treated in the same way during the acute phase, and it is often difficult to differentiate between second and third degree burns by examining the surface. Therefore, to say a patient has a 35 percent burn means 35 percent of the body surface is involved with second and/or third degree burns. Since care of the patient will be affected by the size of the burn, it is important to make this estimation as closely as possible at the scene of a burn injury.

*Major burns* are those which carry a high risk of death or disability. Major burns are defined as: (1) those which involve more than 30 percent of the body surface area (ages 2–60) or more than 10 percent of the body surface area at the extremes of age (under 2 or over 60); (2) apparent third degree burns of the hands, face, feet, or genitalia; (3) any burn associated with smoke inhalation; (4) chemical burns (see below); and (5) burns in a patient with major injuries or preexisting illness. *Minor burns* are those which involve a small portion of the body surface and do not require hospitalization. Moderate burns include all those in between. These distinctions are made to facilitate triage of burn patients. Major burns should be cared for in specialized burn care facilities if at all possible, and the patient should be taken there directly. Emergency care units should have a definite plan for major burn patients that is worked out in combination with the nearest burn care facility. Moderate burns can be cared for in burn centers or in general hospitals.

## Treatment

1. At the scene of the accident, all smoldering or burning clothes should be cut and taken off the patient immediately.

2. At the accident scene, other injuries take priority over the burn itself. Respiratory distress, head injuries, and fractures should be managed in the appropriate fashion. If the patient is hypotensive or comatose, the cause is not the burn.

3. When the patient has been evaluated completely, the burns can be treated by a simple covering (i.e., a clean sheet). In some parts of the country prepackaged burn packs are used. Sterile dressings over the burn are not essential.

4. The use of analgesics should be restricted, especially in the presence of a suspected head injury.

5. The depth of the burn injury can be minimized by immediate cooling of the skin, generally by immersion in cold water. This would apply to small burns seen immediately after injury. Surface cooling is important, therefore, in the first few seconds after a burn injury. After that, surface cooling does not do any good, and may do harm. There is never a reason to apply ice packs to a burn surface.

6. Use mask $O_2$, 6 l/min.

7. The pain of second degree burns can be minimized by keeping the surface wet, so if the burn is painful, cover it with towels or sheets moistened with tepid water.

8. Do not apply any creams or ointments: the burn center staff would just have to wash them off.

9. Do not try to remove materials adherent to the burn unless it is a corrosive chemical. Tar, grease, and clothing should be left in place if firmly stuck to the surface. Pour cool solutions over the tar or grease to cool them down. They can be removed by mechanic's soap at the hospital. The simpler the coverage, the better.

10. Transport the patient.

CHEMICAL BURNS

Corrosive chemicals can cause second or third degree burns. These chemical compounds include common alkalis such as sodium or potassium hydroxide (drain cleaners) and lime. Common acids include hydrochloric, nitric, muriatic, and sulphuric. Phenol (carbolic acid) is not soluble in water; therefore, flushing with water helps to wash it off, but alcohol does a better job.

*Treatment*

1. Chemicals should be diluted and washed off with a flood of water, preferably from a hose or faucet (Figure 18-3).

2. Chemical powders (particularly lime) should be brushed off as much as possible first. After washing, neutralize any residual chemical with a weak acid (vinegar in water) or weak base (baking soda in water) if possible.

HOSPITAL MANAGEMENT OF BURNS

For the first few days after the injury, the biggest risk to the major burn patient is hypovolemic shock. This is because capillaries in the damaged skin become very permeable, and plasma leaks out into the

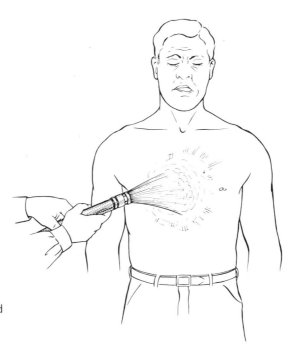

**Figure 18-3.** Corrosive
chemicals should be hosed
off the patient's body with
a flood of water.

interstitial space. In addition to capillary leakage in the area of the
burn, chemicals absorbed from burned tissue (particularly histamine)
cause a generalized increase in capillary permeability, so there is an
extensive plasma "loss," even though the fluid is still inside the body.
The red cells do not leak out of the capillaries, so that the concentration
of red cells (the hematocrit) increases as capillary leakage occurs.
Therefore, following the hematocrit in burn patients is a very accurate
way to determine hypovolemia even though the patient has not lost
any blood. The plasma loss must be replaced by intravenous infusion
of fluids. This is begun soon after the injury, and may require more
than 10 percent of the body weight in fluids in the first two days after
the burn. Because of this, the first priority at the hospital is to establish
one or more intravenous lines and provide for monitoring perfusion
with a urinary catheter, central venous catheter, etc. Because of the
difficulty in finding intravenous sites in the extensively burned patient,
direct IV cutdowns are often required. Even placement of conventional
IVs must be done with great care in burn patients to avoid later infection
at the puncture site. For this reason IVs should not be started in the
field. If the injury occurs a long distance from a treatment facility,
or if several hours have elapsed between the time of the burn and
the time the patient is first seen, then IVs should be started for major
burns, and electrolyte or colloid solutions should be infused at a rate
of 5 ml/kg/hr.

Smoke inhalation syndrome or smoke "poisoning" occurs when partially combustible materials (such as paint, upholstery, wood, etc.) burn in an enclosed space. Smoke inhalation combined with skin burns carries a high mortality. This is the reason burns from house fires (which account for only 5 percent of burn center admissions) cause 50 percent of the the deaths from burns. When smoke inhalation occurs without surface burn, the major risk is to the brain, and the lung damage is minimal. When smoke inhalation occurs with a surface burn, the lung is the target organ. There are three components to smoke inhalation syndrome, any one of which may predominate. These are carbon monoxide poisoning, heat inhalation, and toxic gases.

Carbon monoxide (CO) is a colorless, odorless gas that causes no direct damage but has a very strong affinity for hemoglobin. It attaches to hemoglobin molecules in the lung capillaries forming carboxyhemoglobin, which circulates throughout the body. Carboxyhemoglobin has a bright, cherry red color similar to oxyhemoglobin, so that victims of CO poisoning have a red skin color that simulates the appearance of good oxygenation and perfusion. Carbon monoxide prevents oxygen from binding with hemoglobin, so that the systemic effects are those of severely decreased oxygen delivery. These are confusion; somnolence; stupor; coma; hyperventilation; increased cardiac output, blood pressure, and pulse rate; and progressive severe metabolic acidosis. Emergency treatment of carbon monoxide poisoning, therefore, must be directed at improving peripheral oxygen delivery.

Heat inhalation injury is almost always limited to the upper airway (nose, mouth, pharynx, larynx). Only those victims who inhale live steam sustain actual lung damage from inhalation of heat. The upper airway damage is due to second and third degree burns which present typical findings—blisters, charring, and swelling due to capillary leakage and edema. Like burns on the skin, edema does not occur immediately after injury, and the risk of airway obstruction is greatest twelve to twenty-four hours after the burn. However, it is very difficult to establish an airway after the edema has occurred, so that most patients with heat damage at the level of the pharynx or larynx will be intubated soon after admission to the burn center. This should not be attempted at the scene unless the patient was burned hours before and has severe stridor with each breath. (Most smoke inhalation victims will be hoarse and coughing. This is not stridor.) Airway occlusion is always a potential problem with heat inhalation, however, so that patients with oral or facial burns should be transported to the nearest care center as quickly as possible.

The actual lung damage in smoke inhalation victims is caused by toxic gases. A variety of volatile organic chemicals are released when wood and plastic burn, and some of these compounds cause direct damage to the mucosal lining of the airways, alveoli, and pulmonary capillaries.

Usually the lung will heal well from this kind of insult, unless the problem is compounded by a surface burn with all the resuscitation fluid and potential infection associated with it.

Lung damage from toxic gases occurs progressively during days or weeks, and generally does not cause a problem in the emergent period. Soot particles in smoke do not cause major damage. Every cigarette smoker inhales large quantities of soot (associated with toxic gases) every day. This soot is a convenient marker of the extent of smoke inhalation in patients. This is an important consideration. For example, if a victim has extensive burns in the pharynx and larynx but no soot aspirated from the trachea, the risk of subsequent pulmonary complications is minimal. However, if a patient has a small leg burn from a house fire but coughs up soot for two or three days following the accident, serious, high-mortality risk pulmonary complications can be anticipated.

## TREATMENT

The treatment of smoke inhalation (carbon monoxide poisoning) at the scene is to increase the $FIO_2$ as high as possible by mask or positive pressure oxygen administration. If the patient is alert and able to breathe on his own, then use a tight-fitting mask so that near 100 percent oxygen delivery can be achieved. This will increase the small amount of oxygen dissolved in the plasma and will gradually displace carbon monoxide from hemoglobin.

## ELECTRICAL INJURIES

There are two kinds of injury associated with electrical accidents. The flash from an electrical spark is hot enough to cause burns and ignite clothing. When electrical current passes through tissue, a much more serious type of burn occurs. Third degree burns are seen on the skin where the current entered and exited, but the tissue damage inside is always much worse than the burn on the outside. The electrical current travels along nerves, blood vessels, fascial planes, and through muscle that has the lowest resistance for passage of electrical current. When the current passes through the chest, ventricular fibrillation usually occurs. In many patients, however, the heart rhythm remains regular and serious tissue injury follows. Muscles go into intense spasm. If the contact was made with the hands, this may cause the victim to hold on to the charged object until the current is turned off. The higher the voltage, the more tissue damage.

Extricating a victim from direct electrical contact must be done with care. Direct contact may result in further conducting of electrical current, and sparks with flash exposure may occur when the victim is pulled away from the source. Whenever possible, use dry ropes or nonconductive poles to separate the victim from the source.

TREATMENT

1. As soon as it is safe to touch the victim, institute CPR if necessary.
2. If vital signs are stable, cover the burns and transport the patient to the burn treatment facility.
3. Notify the receiving center prior to transport that the patient has received an electrical burn so the burn unit can be alerted.
4. Monitor EKG during transport since these patients are subject to ventricular dysrhythmias, which may occur at any time.
5. Start an intravenous of Lactated Ringer's.
6. Administer mask $O_2$ at 6 l/min.

# LIGHTNING

Ground-to-air atmosphere electrical discharges occur when water particles in clouds become negatively charged and sufficient positive potential is induced in the earth. Lightning strikes result from broad electrical fields and differ from other electrical injuries in that points of contact are often undefined. High temperatures and electromechanical forces are the primary causes of burn injuries. Injury from lightning may result from (1) direct stroke, (2) side flash in which current discharges from a vertical object through the air to a nearby vertical object, and (3) stride potential where a person standing near the point where lightning strikes develops a potential difference between the legs. In the stride potential, the current enters through one leg and leaves through the other; the heart and brain are spared. Lightning can produce serious injuries and death. It can produce neurological damage without death, including severe brain damage.

Lightning injury prevention must be practiced in areas where there is great risk. Wide-open areas should be avoided during thunderstorms for the risk is thirty times greater in rural areas than in the city. Indoor shelters appear the safest. Contact with metal objects, such as fences, tent poles, golf clubs, and fishing poles, increases the hazard. Taking refuge under a tree increases the risk of a direct strike, side flash, and a ground discharge. A closed car offers good protection. A person caught in the open should curl on the ground on his side with his hands close together to reduce contact points, or squat with his feet together.

TREATMENT

1. Immediate CPR of the lightning victim is the most important aspect of management. Even though resuscitation may be delayed,

successful resuscitation is usually possible as the cardiac standstill often reverts to a sinus rhythm. Myocardial infarctions are frequently reported with lightning strikes, but appear to be a rare cause of death. The heart should be monitored.

2. Extensive skin burns should be covered before transport.

3. Oxygen should be administered by face mask at 6 l/min. Assist ventilation if the patient is not breathing.

4. The patient must be transported to a facility able to handle electrical burns since severe muscle damage may be present.

## FROSTBITE

Local cold injury is called "frostbite." The pathogenesis is very similar to a thermal burn. The outermost layers are most affected and progressive cold exposure causes slowing of blood flow and eventual clotting in capillaries. The metabolism of skin and fat cells is slowed by the cold, so these layers are somewhat protected from the effects of ischemia. The final result after treatment and healing is always much better than would be expected by the initial appearance. Frostbite occurs at the extremes of the circulation where there is little fat for insulation, such as fingers, toes, ear lobes, tip of the nose, etc. Frostbite has the appearance of a third degree burn. The skin is white, cold and dead looking. There is no sensation. Since there is no blood flow and the cells are already damaged, the injury could be made worse by heating the involved parts too rapidly.

### TREATMENT

1. The best emergency treatment is simply to protect the frostbitten area from damage by wrapping in gauze dressings or towels. Separate fingers and toes by placing gauze between them, and allow gradual warming by room temperature and body heat; immersion in tepid water (approximately 100°F) may be used (Figure 18-4).

2. In general, frostbite involving more than tips of fingers and toes should be cared for in a hospital.

## ACCIDENTAL HYPOTHERMIA

Generalized exposure to cold may cause hypothermia (decreased body temperature). Normally, cold exposure causes shivering and increased muscle tone which results in increased metabolism which maintains body temperature. When this increased heat production can no longer keep up with heat lost from the surface (or if shivering is impossible in a

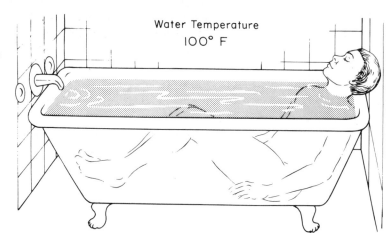

**Figure 18-4.** The hypothermic patient can be warmed in a bathtub. However the water temperature should not be so hot that it scalds the skin.

paralyzed or comatose patient), body temperature falls. As temperature falls, so does the metabolic rate and cardiac output. By this means the body contains mechanisms to preserve the last bit of energy and prevent cell death from low oxygen delivery. Hibernating animals cool down to almost environmental temperature maintaining a very slow heart rate and respiration.

Immersion hypothermia (e.g., falling in a cold lake) is very different from mountain hypothermia. Immersion in cold water leads to rapid loss of body heat, and the victim may lose consciousness and drown within twenty minutes. During immersion, shivering is severe and uncomfortable, and body temperature is well below that believed to be associated with depression of muscular activity. For short periods, shivering may stop and result in an improvement in comfort, which has been described as "basking in the cold." On the other hand, the onset of hypothermia and exhaustion in people exposed to cold air (e.g., skiers) comes on slowly. This may be heralded by changes in mood (usually aggressive behavior). This type of hypothermia is the most treacherous because it is often not suspected until it is too late. This is particularly true in children who are not properly dressed for the mountain climate. There are disturbances in fluid and electrolyte balances and a reduction in blood glucose levels in this group. In immersion hypothermia, fluid shifts are not prominent and glucose levels usually remain high.

There is very little medical data on accidental hypothermia. Through the Paramedic Program, important information can be gathered. This is especially true for dysrhythmias and cardiac monitoring. Via telemetry, heart activity can be recorded and saved for evaluation. In World War

II, the Dachau immersion experiments yielded some information regarding lowering of body temperature (obviously unethical experiments). Ethical body temperature experiments in humans do not go below 34°C (94°F). At this level many of the hypothermic changes have not taken place.

There is no useful way to measure body temperature in the field. Oral temperatures are of no help, and most patients would not tolerate rectal temperature measurements. It is often difficult to judge hypothermia merely by feeling the patient's skin. This is particularly true in mountaineering incidents where exhausted individuals may become confused and lethargic, have cold skin, and still have a normal core temperature. In man, ventricular fibrillation usually occurs at about 27° Centigrade. Ether anesthesia or ingested alcohol smooth out the cooling process and have a protective effect against ventricular fibrillation at lower temperatures. The following is an example of extreme hypothermia with a successful outcome due in large part to the quick action of the paramedics.

A 24-year-old male was in an automobile accident following a heavy drinking episode. The patient drove over a cliff and 300 feet down a ravine. He was thrown from his truck into the snow face down. The patient was discovered eight hours later at 7:00 AM. A Marine helicopter and paramedics were called. In conjunction with the Marines, the paramedics cleared the ravine, placed a monitor on the patient, and inserted an oroesophageal airway. After insertion of the airway, the patient underwent ventricular fibrillation and was transported to the hospital with external cardiac massage. At the hospital (seven minutes later) he was taken immediately to the operating room, where he underwent open chest cardiac massage for one hour. His body temperature in the operating room was 22°C. He was rewarmed to 32°C on cardiopulmonary bypass and then his heart was defibrillated following injection of intracardiac epinephrine. He awoke in the recovery room several hours later and, following a prolonged hospitalization, made a complete and full recovery. There were no neurologic deficits.

The above cases illustrates several points. In the individual with heavy alcohol ingestion, body cooling can occur at a slow enough rate that the body tissues are cooled evenly. If cardiac arrest should result, then the brain is protected from hypoxia by the cold and resuscitation should not be abandoned until all efforts have been made. The patient should not be abandoned even if cardiac arrest occurs after sudden cold immersion. For example, a 19-year-old male who was under ice-cold water for thirty-eight minutes following drowning inside a car made a full recovery following resuscitation.

TREATMENT

1. Emergency management of hypothermic exposure consists of wrapping the patient in blankets and measuring his body temperature and vital signs. Blankets can be warmed by covering them and placing them on the hood of a vehicle, allowing the heat from the running engine to warm them. A useful technique for warming the hypothermic child is to place him in a sleeping bag with an adult. The heat from the adult's body will warm the child.

2. The suspected hypothermic patient should be monitored. They are subject to dysrhythmias, and ventricular fibrillation can occur.

3. Begin CPR if ventricular fibrillation is present and continue during transport to the hospital and operating room. Remember, the hypothermic patient is protected by the hypothermia. CPR should not be abandoned until all efforts have been made to resuscitate the heart.

4. Hypothermic patients are also often hypovolemic. If an IV can be started, give Lactated Ringer's at 250 to 500 ml/hr. However, veins may be constricted and starting an IV may be impossible.

5. Due to the hypothermia, application of the MAST suit is indicated. The MAST suit will squeeze veins and return blood to the heart, improving cardiac output. The suit may also act as insulation and help in the warming process. Notify the hospital of the situation, since cardiopulmonary bypass technique may be necessary in rewarming the patient. The hospital should also be notified in order to have a warming blanket in the Emergency Department to begin the warming process.

6. If the patient is hypothermic but breathing adequately, do not attempt to use an airway since its insertion may stimulate a vagal response and ventricular fibrillation.


HEAT EXHAUSTION AND HEAT STROKE

Heat is generated as a result of body metabolism. The regulation of body temperature occurs in the hypothalamus. Methods by which heat is lost from the body include radiation, conduction, and evaporation. This mechanism is so finely tuned that an individual standing nude in dry air can maintain his body temperature between 98°F and 100°F even though the environmental temperature may range between 60°F and 130°F. The rate of heat loss from the body is increased in two ways. Sweat glands are stimulated to cause increased sweating and when the sweat evaporates it cools the body, and the sympathetic centers in the posterior hypothalamus are inhibited removing the normal vasoconstrictor tone to the skin vessels, thereby allowing vasodilatation and loss of heat from increased blood flow. Prolonged exposure to high environmental temperatures may lead to one of two separate syndromes—heat exhaustion or heat stroke.

## HEAT EXHAUSTION

Heat exhaustion or prostration would be better described as exercise hypovolemia. It usually occurs in otherwise healthy individuals who exercise to the point of exhaustion in a warm environment. Water and sodium chloride are lost through sweating in large amounts (Figure 18-5). This fluid and electrolyte loss combined with generalized vasodilatation leads to low circulating blood volume, venous pooling, reduction in cardiac output, and hypotension. A mild form of this syndrome begins with the development of heat cramps. With the loss of salt and the intake of water, hyponatremia occurs, producing muscle cramps (Chapter 5). This can produce abdominal cramping pain from intestinal peristalsis, as well as skeletal muscle cramps in the arms and legs. As the syndrome progresses, the patient may present with wet, pale skin, tachycardia, thready pulse, and low blood pressure. There may also be vomiting, diarrhea, and fainting. The temperature may be normal or elevated, but not to the inappropriate extremes seen with heat stroke.

### Treatment

1. If the syndrome is minor and just developing, the patient should be placed in the shade and given salt by mouth with water. The muscle cramps can be massaged.

2. If the condition is more extreme, the patient should be treated for hypovolemia and an intravenous infusion started with Lactated Ringer's. The patient should be placed in the supine position in the shade with the legs elevated.

3. Blood pressure and vital signs should be monitored.

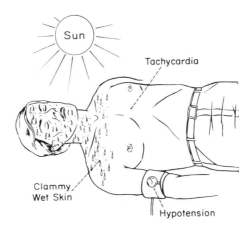

**Figure 18-5.** Heat exhaustion produces hypovolemia and shock by loss of salt and water through sweat.

4. A tube for electrolytes can be drawn and saved for subsequent analysis at the hospital.

5. The patient may require mask $O_2$ and even monitoring.

## HEAT STROKE

Heat stroke is caused by the failure of normal body temperature regulation, specifically the lack of sweating and surface evaporation. Individuals can tolerate an environmental temperature of 200°F if the air is dry. However, if there is high humidity, lower temperatures can produce serious problems since the water will not evaporate from individual body surfaces producing cooling. Heat stroke usually occurs in the elderly, or in individuals exposed to drugs or chemicals which inhibit sweating. This syndrome is characterized by high body temperatures (as high as 44°C, 108°F), dry hot skin, confusion, disorientation, seizures or coma, tachycardia with normal or high blood pressure, and bounding pulses (Figure 18-6).

*Treatment*

1. This is a medical emergency. All efforts should be aimed at reducing the patient's temperature. This can be done by immersion in a cold tub or using cooling blankets.

2. Rectal enemas of cold saline are also effective cooling measures.

3. Start an intravenous of Lactated Ringer's for fluid replacement.

4. Notify the hospital of the situation.

5. Monitor vital signs and start mask $O_2$.

6. Monitor the patient's EKG since cardiac dysrhythmias may occur at any time.

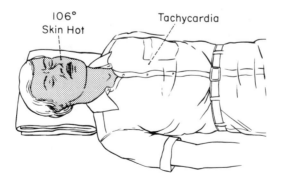

106°
Skin Hot

Tachycardia

**Figure 18-6.** Heat stroke results in a very high body temperature.

If explosions include radioactive material, emergency teams should wait until residual radioactivity has been checked before risking personal exposure. The harmful effects of radiation dissipate rapidly as one moves away from the source, so that it is much safer to be six feet rather than three feet from a radioactive site. Victims exposed to radiation do not themselves become radioactive. However, debris and dust from the explosion may be very radioactive, so that all external clothing should be removed from victims and vigorous washing done at the scene before close contact. Radiation exposure can cause extensive burns and kill internal tissues. However, these effects do not occur for several days, even after massive radiation exposure.

## TREATMENT

1. When handling radiation victims use disposable gloves and coverings.

2. Wrap the patient in blankets.

3. Care for the patient's injuries as in any other trauma case.

4. Transport the patient to the appropriate facility for decontamination.

5. Trained radiation personnel should be notified and the radiation hazards investigated.

6. The paramedic, patient, and all clothing must be monitored and decontaminated as necessary.

## SCUBA DIVING ACCIDENTS

Scuba (Self-Contained Under Water Breathing Apparatus) diving is a very popular recreational sport in southern California as well as on the eastern seacoast. Despite increased legislation and careful monitoring of scuba diving equipment and training, accidents in this sport are very common, especially among inexperienced divers. Scuba diving accidents can occur on the surface, in three feet of water, or at any depth. The more serious accidents occur following the dive. The physiologic principle which explains accidents is that when the temperature of a gas (air) is kept constant, the volume of the gas is inversely proportionate to its pressure. For example, doubling the pressure of a gas mixture will decrease its volume by one-half. The pressure of air at sea level is 14.7 lb/sq in. or 760 mm Hg. This pressure is called one atmosphere absolute or 1 "ata." Two ata equals 33 feet of water, and 3 ata equals 66 feet of water, etc. A scuba diver breathes in air from his tanks and as he goes deeper in the water, the partial pressure of gases in the air (oxygen, nitrogen, carbon dioxide) he breathes increases.

Scuba diving injuries are due to (1) barotrauma (mechanical effect of the pressure differential), (2) cerebral air embolism, (3) compression illness, (4) cold, and (5) panic.

Accidents generally occur at four stages of the dive. These stages include the following: (1) on the surface, (2) during the descent, (3) on the bottom, and (4) during the ascent.

## INJURIES ON THE SURFACE

Injuries on the surface can involve entanglement of lines or entanglement in kelp fields while swimming to the area of the dive. This may lead to panic and drowning. The water may be cold during the swim to the dive area and produce shivering and blackout. Fatigue is always a possibility, especially if entanglement has occurred.

## INJURIES DURING THE DESCENT

During the descent, barotrauma becomes an important consideration. This may produce middle ear pain, if the diver is unable to equilibrate the pressure between his nasopharynx and his middle ear. This will produce pain, ringing in the ears, dizziness, and hearing loss. The trauma may be so severe as to rupture the ear drum. The diver who has an upper respiratory infection and cannot clear his middle ear through his eustachian tube should not dive. A similar lack of equilibration can occur in the sinuses producing severe frontal headaches (squeeze), or pain beneath the eye in the maxillary sinuses.

## INJURIES ON THE BOTTOM

Major accidents involve nitrogen narcosis. This is called the "raptures of the deep" and is due to nitrogen's effect on cerebral function. The diver may appear to become intoxicated and may take risks and forget about his own safety. If the diver becomes entangled or runs out of air, he may panic causing increase in oxygen consumption and further carbon dioxide production. Dives below 40 feet of water require staged ascent to prevent the bends.

## INJURIES DURING THE ASCENT

During the ascent from the dive serious and life-threatening complications can occur. The causes may be related to barotrauma and the diver being unable to equilibrate his inner ear pressure with his nasopharyngeal pressure. This can produce middle ear damage as well as damage to the tympanic membrane. The most serious barotrauma which occurs

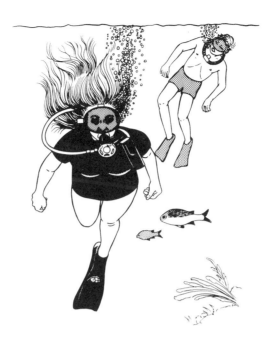

**Figure 18-7.** Since exhalation is not done during ascent, air embolism and pneumothorax can occur.

during the ascent is that to the lung. This type of barotrauma can occur in as little as three feet of water as well as during a deep ocean dive. The barotrauma occurs to the lung while breathholding during the diver's ascent. As he ascends, the air in the lung which has been compressed expands and may rupture the alveoli if the air is not exhaled. This leads to mechanical damage to the lung and air embolism. The lung-injured diver will present with dyspnea, cough, and hemoptysis. There may be mediastinal and subcutaneous emphysema due to diffusion of the gas through the lung into the mediastinum and the neck. The diver may have chest pain, difficulty swallowing, hoarseness, and crepitus in the neck. Also, the blood pressure may be low. Pneumothorax can occur if the alveoli rupture into the pleural cavity (Figure 18-7). Air embolism can occur if the air ruptures into the pulmonary veins and returns to the left atrium and finally into the left ventricle and out the systemic circulation. The most dreaded complication is cerebral air embolism. The diver will present with visual disturbances, confusion, loss of consciousness, and convulsions.

*Treatment*

1. Surface accidents may require cardiopulmonary resuscitation. Vital signs should be checked and the heart rate and rhythm monitored. Body temperature may be reduced because of cold and shivering. It is best to keep the patient warm with blankets.

2. Field management of ruptured ear drums and blood from the ear is best managed by covering the ear with a sterile dressing and transporting the patient.

3. If the patient appears to have sustained a pulmonary barotrauma on ascent with possible cerebral embolism, immediate treatment is necessary if the patient is to be salvaged. This would include immediate decompression in a hyperbaric chamber. Because these chambers are not always accessible and time is necessary to transport the patient, supportive care must be given. This would include administration of oxygen either by mask or esophageal obturator airway, if the patient is unconscious and not breathing, and observation for a pneumothorax and decompression of any tension pneumothorax with an intercostal needle and a Heimlich valve (Chapter 14).

4. Start an IV of Lactated Ringer's if hypotension and signs of shock are present.

5. The patient should be maintained in a head down position with the legs elevated and turned to the left to prevent further accumulation of air. If air transportation to a hyperbaric facility has been arranged, this should be done at the lowest altitude possible to minimize further embolization secondary to reduced atmospheric pressures.

## THE "BENDS"

If the diver has been at a depth greater than 40 feet of water for any prolonged period of time, he must use staged ascent to allow for decompression so nitrogen can be washed from his tissues. If he does not, he may develop the rapid decompression illness called the bends. Abnormally high environmental pressure is usually encountered only in deep water dives. Although the bends is a serious complication, it does not occur that often with scuba divers. The amount of gas (nitrogen, oxygen, and carbon dioxide) which dissolves in blood and body tissues under high ambient pressure is much greater than the dissolved gas at normal (1 atmosphere) pressure. This gas is not deleterious as long as it is dissolved, but if the ambient pressure rapidly drops to atmospheric pressure (as in a rapid ascent from deep water), the gas forms bubbles in the bloodstream, much like the bubbles of carbon dioxide formed when opening a bottle of carbonated beverage. These bubbles form a sort of vapor lock in all capillary beds causing intense pain and muscle cramps (hence, the name the bends) along with multiple organ dysfunction. Carbon dioxide bubbles are very diffusible and rapidly excreted, and oxygen in bubbles is rapidly utilized, so that bubbles of nitrogen, an inert gas, are the major cause of this syndrome. Permanent injury to the brain and other organs can occur if the bubbles are allowed to remain in place for a long period of time.

### Treatment

1. Emergency treatment of the bends consists of giving the patient 100 percent oxygen by mask so that nitrogen gas will be washed out of the body.

2. Start an intravenous of Lactated Ringer's.

3. The patient must be taken as quickly as possible to a hyperbaric chamber. Paramedics working in areas where scuba diving accidents can occur should know the location of the nearest hyperbaric chamber as well as the means of transportation to the chamber. Often the Coast Guard or Marine Corps can assist with helicopter transport. A hyperbaric chamber is a large, reinforced steel room which can be pressurized by filling it with compressed air. As soon as the patient is in the chamber with a physician, the pressure is increased until a level is reached at which nitrogen returns to solution. At that point the symptoms are relieved, and then the pressure is gradually reduced to allow excretion of the dissolved gases at a slow rate. This may require several hours.

## INJURIES DUE TO MARINE ANIMALS

Individuals who swim in the ocean with snorkels or scuba diving equipment are subject to various marine animal injuries. The majority of these injuries are due to contact with jelly fish, sea urchins, and sting rays. Table 18-1 gives a simplified classification proposed by Strauss.*

TABLE 18-1. EMERGENCY TREATMENT FOR INJURIES FROM MARINE ANIMALS

| Class | Mechanism of Injury | Examples | Emergency Treatment |
|---|---|---|---|
| 1 | Traumatic/ Lacerations | Shark | Stop the bleeding |
| 2 | Nematocyst/ Urticarial | Jellyfish Sea Anenomes Hydra Corals | (1) Inactivate with alcohol (2) Coalesce and re-move residual ten-tacles with powder (3) Neutralize with soda or ammonia |
| 3 | Spine/Puncture | Sea Urchin Cone Shells Sting Rays Sculpins | Soak in as hot water as can be tolerated |
| 4 | Fangs/Venom | Sea Snake | Treatment for shock |

*"Injuries to Divers by Marine Animals: A Simplified Approach to Recognition and Management." LCDR Michael B. Strauss, MC, USNR, *Military Medicine,* Vol. 139, p. 129, February, 1974.

## CLASS 1—ANIMALS THAT INFLICT TRAUMATIC INJURIES

A shark can produce serious soft and bony tissue injury. The shark can inflict such an injury as severing an arm or mutilation of the arm or leg. Treatment of this type of injury is to control bleeding and transport the victim. Bleeding often needs to be controlled by tourniquet application. Field management may include the use of intravenous fluids such as Lactated Ringer's and supporting the airway.

## CLASS 2—ANIMALS THAT STING

The animals that sting are listed in Table 18-1. The sting of the animal may produce itching, a prickly sensation, pain, cramps, a sensation of suffocation, and paralysis. In some cases, shock and collapse have occurred immediately after the sting.

### Treatment

1. The area of the sting should be rinsed with an alcohol compound, preferably rubbing alcohol, or even methyl alcohol. The application of a meat tenderizer, for example, Adolph's Meat Tenderizer, is equally effective.

2. Remove the residual tentacles by coalescing them with a drying agent such as flour, baking soda, divers talc, etc. The paste is then scraped away with a blade. Abrasives should not be used since these agents may irritate the nematocysts and cause further release of toxins.

3. Rinse the wound with basic solutions such as baking soda or dilute ammonia hydroxide in order to neutralize the toxins. Antihistamines may be indicated to reduce the inflammatory response.

4. Treat and observe for any respiratory distress or shock.

## CLASS 3—ANIMALS WITH SPINES

A number of animals have venomous attachments on their spines. Regardless of the poison, the spines themselves can produce puncture wounds which are prone to infection. These animals may include the cone shells, sea urchins, and sting rays. The puncture wound tends to be very painful and may produce symptoms similar to the previously described injuries.

### Treatment

1. Soak the involved area with water as hot as can be tolerated. Be careful not to scald the skin.

2. The patient should be transported to an emergency facility since tetanus prophylaxis is indicated.

3. Pain should be controlled by analgesics and antihistamines may be used to reduce the inflammatory response.

4. The spine may be imbedded in the puncture wound and X-rays are often necessary to identify the location of the spine for subsequent removal.

## CLASS 4—ANIMALS WITH POISONOUS BITES

These animals would include the sea snake and the octopus. These bites can produce a delayed response, which includes paralysis and respiratory collapse.

### Treatment

1. The best treatment would include observation of the airway.

2. A loose venous tourniquet should be applied proximal to the bite and loosened every fifteen minutes for ninety seconds. Fluid administration of Lactated Ringer's is indicated to control shock.

3. Cardiopulmonary resuscitation may be necessary if there has been severe shock or respiratory arrest.

## INSECT STINGS AND BITES

Insect bites include those of bees, wasps, spiders, and scorpions. Immediate symptoms produced at the site of the bite include local pain, itching, erythema, and edema. In most cases local treatment may be all that is necessary. However, a certain number of individuals may demonstrate anaphylaxis. Anaphylaxis is a serious condition which may result after many different types of exposures. It may occur after a penicillin injection, or as a consequence of bee, hornet, and wasp stings (Figure 18-8). Anaphylaxis is characterized by flushing, urticaria, angioedema, rapid pulse, hypotension, bronchospasm, laryngeal edema, nausea, vomiting, and abdominal cramps. The onset of anaphylaxis may be immediately after the inciting event or as long as one hour later.

## TREATMENT

1. Treatment of insect bites can include the application of ice to reduce the pain and spreading of the toxins locally. The patient should be kept still and prevented from moving around.

2. Treatment of the anaphylactic syndrome involves the injection of epinephrine 1:1000, 0.3 to 0.5 mg subcutaneously.

3. A light tourniquet should be applied proximal to the bite if it is localized in an extremity.

4. Administer oxygen by face mask at 6 l/min.

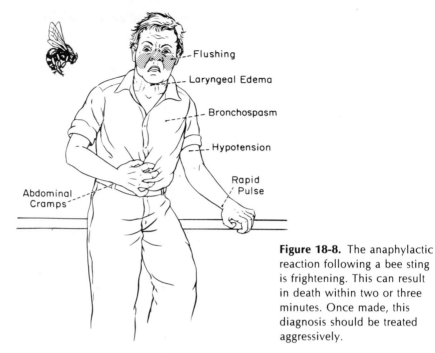

- Flushing
- Laryngeal Edema
- Bronchospasm
- Hypotension
- Rapid Pulse
- Abdominal Cramps

**Figure 18-8.** The anaphylactic reaction following a bee sting is frightening. This can result in death within two or three minutes. Once made, this diagnosis should be treated aggressively.

5. If respiratory symptoms seem to predominate and are becoming worse, 500 mg of Aminophylline® diluted in 250 ml of $D_5W$ can be given slowly over one hour.

6. Begin an IV of Lactated Ringer's solution. Infuse rapidly to restore vital signs if the patient is hypotensive.

7. If the patient is unresponsive to epinephrine or Aminophylline®, give 10 ml of calcium chloride slowly intravenously.

8. Monitor the patient's heart rate and vital signs.

9. Transport.

## SNAKE BITES

In the United States, there are four types of poisonous snakes: (1) rattlesnakes, (2) cottonmouth moccasins, (3) copperheads, and (4) coral snakes. The first three types are called pit vipers. The pit viper has a pit between the eye and the nostril on each side of the head, elliptical pupils, two well-developed fangs, and one roll of plates beneath its tail. The coral snake is a variety of cobra found along the coastlands of the southeastern portions of the United States. It is small and has tubular fangs with teeth behind the fangs and cannot readily attach itself to a large surface, such as a forearm or the calf. It has round eyes and a double row of plates beneath its tail. The coral snake has red, yellow, and black rings around the body and always has a black nose. The pit viper venom and the coral snake venom work on different systems of the body.

Pit viper venom contains hydrolytic enzymes which are enzymes that destroy proteins and other molecules. These enzymes are very stable and can be stored for many years. Phospholipase-A is one of the most widespread of snake venom enzymes. It may produce destruction of red blood cells as well as activate the clotting system within the blood vessels. This will produce infarction and necrosis of tissue, especially at the site of the bite. The venom may cause release of histamine, serotonin, and kinins from within the patient's own tissue. These substances may produce a severe systemic reaction.

The coral snake venom may contain some of the enzymes found in pit viper venom, but it primarily works on neural tissue (neurotoxin). It does not produce the circulatory effects that are present with the pit viper venom.

In the United States during the year 1966, there were approximately 6000 to 7000 snake bites reported. There were fourteen to fifteen deaths as a result of these bites. The incidence of bites was highest in North Carolina, although the fatalities occurred in Arizona, Texas, Georgia, and Florida. The clinical symptomatology of the snake bite varies depending upon the snake, the location of the bite, and the type of toxin injected. The term evenomization means the poisonous effects caused by the bite of an insect or snake.

After a bite from a pit viper, there is free bleeding from the fang punctures and immediate local burning pain. However, in some cases, there may be local numbness and pain may not be a prominent part of the symptomatology. Swelling usually begins around the site of the bite and spreads centrally. This is accompanied by discoloration of the skin and bruising. Blood or serum-filled blebs may appear within a few hours. It must be kept in mind by the paramedic that severe evenomization may occur without these local manifestations. Systemic symptoms include weakness, faintness, sweating, thirst, nausea, vomiting, and diarrhea. Tingling around the face and head are common symptoms with rattlesnake bites. The individual may lose consciousness right after the bite, but then regain it a short time later. In some cases of severe viper evenomization, death from shock may occur within 30 minutes. However, most pit viper bite fatalities in the United States occur within six to thirty hours after injury.

The bite from a coral snake presents differently. There may be no local manifestation, or even any systemic effect for as long as twelve to twenty-four hours after the bite. Early signs are drowsiness, weakness, difficulty in swallowing and speaking, and double vision. There is some degree of mental confusion and euphoria. There may be abdominal pain and vomiting. This may continue on to flaccid paralysis of all the muscle groups, shallow breathing, hypotension, subnormal temperatures, coma, convulsions, and death.

The study of snake bites and the venom of snakes is an extensive field all its own. There are important considerations when dealing with the bite. It has been shown by studies with radioactive-tagged rattlesnake venom that the venom remains within the area of the bite for approximately thirty to sixty minutes. After that time, most of the venom has been absorbed. Therefore, local treatment of the wound one hour after the bite will not appreciably add to the patient's well-being.

## TREATMENT

1. The initial treatment of snake bites is centered around reduction of the absorption of the toxins from the local area of the bite. It is best accomplished by keeping the patient still and as calm as possible. The patient should be supine and not allowed to walk around. The administration of alcohol is to be condemned since it will cause vasodilatation and may aid in the absorption of the toxin.

2. A tourniquet should be applied proximal to the bite on the forearm, finger, or upper arm as the case may be. The tourniquet should only be tight enough to occlude superficial veins and lymphatics. It should not occlude the deep venous system or the arterial system. If it does this, swelling of the arm may occur unrelated to the bite itself. This will confuse the physician taking care of the patient at the hospital. A string tourniquet is more useful here than a rubber tourniquet, which may cause more compression than is needed. The string is inflexible and will only occlude superficial veins and lymphatics if applied properly. One finger should fit snugly under the string (Figure 18-9).

3. Various portions of the United States treat snake bites in different ways. In some areas, the initial hospital treatment is to completely excise the local tissue around the bite area down to the deep tissues and do no further therapy. This is done if the bite victim arrives at the Emergency Department within one hour after the injury. It is important, therefore, that all snake bite victims be transported as quickly as possible—no delays should occur in the field. However, if it appears that the patient, from the time of the bite to the time of hospital treatment, is to be

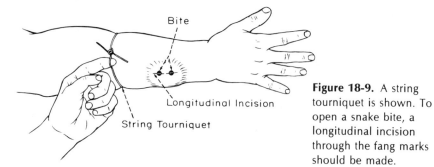

**Figure 18-9.** A string tourniquet is shown. To open a snake bite, a longitudinal incision through the fang marks should be made.

delayed for one reason or another, opening of the snake bite and suction is indicated. Snake bite kits that include a scalpel-like instrument as well as a suction cup are available on a commercial basis. Any clean (or field-sterilized) sharp cutting instrument may be used in circumstances when these kits are not available. The incision should be through the skin only in the long axis of the limb. Do not make the classic cross-cut incision. The incision should be approximately 1 to $1\frac{1}{2}$ cm long over the site of the fang marks (Figure 18-9). If a suction cup is not available, use your mouth to suck the venom out. If the venom is sucked into the mouth, it should be spit out, although swallowing it will not produce any side effects.

4. Do not pack the wound in ice. It may cause further tissue necrosis. A cool, damp cloth may aid in relieving local tenderness.

5. The patient's breathing status should be monitored and any respiratory difficulties treated accordingly.

6. Hypotension and shock should be treated by starting an intravenous infusion of Lactated Ringer's at a rate of 500 ml per hour.

7. Transport the patient to the hospital, giving prior notification that a snake bite victim is enroute, the status of the patient, and attempt to inform them of the type of snake.

8. At the hospital, the patient should receive antitoxin (tetanus), antivenom, and antibiotics.

## HANG GLIDING INJURIES

During the past four years, the sport of hang gliding has developed rapidly in the United States and at the present time there are approximately 60,000 hang gliding enthusiasts. Soaring is a very dangerous sport and should only be done after proper instruction. There were approximately 68 deaths from hang gliding accidents in the United States during the year 1976. Besides death, other injuries usually involving fracture are associated with this sport. Whereas scuba diving injuries often occur to the novice, the most severe hang gliding injuries often occur to the more experienced hang gliders. This is because hang gliding is an exhilarating sport and the hang glider develops a godlike syndrome and with experience feels he is indestructible.

Of the deaths reported, the most common cause appears to be due to cervical fracture with spinal cord injury, and head injuries. Other injuries include forearm and shoulder fractures and leg and sacral fractures. Hang gliders generally land either in the sitting position and can sustain injuries to the sacrum or coccyx, or land flat with the arms extended producing fractures of the forearm or shoulders.

Treatment of these patients does not differ from the patient who has been involved in an automobile accident, or other impact-type injuries.

TREATMENT

1. Do the primary and secondary surveys as outlined in Chapter 14. Remember that most hang gliding accidents are fractures so that the orthopedic examination must be thorough.

2. Remember that the cervical spine is often injured and that the spinal cord must be protected at all times.

3. The victim may be in an inaccessible area and extrication may be delayed. It is therefore necessary to treat shock if present by starting intravenous fluids of Lactated Ringer's. All fractures should be splinted as best as possible and a cervical collar with a back board is indicated.

## DROWNING AND NEAR DROWNING

It is estimated that in the United States, 6000 to 7000 lives per year are lost by drowning, and this number will increase in the future. Next to motor vehicle accidents, drowning is the second leading cause of accidental death in the 1-to-14 year old age group. In Dade County, Florida, for example, drowning accounts for 32 percent of all pediatric accidental deaths. Drownings and near drownings occur in a variety of places and situations, including swimming pools, lakes, bays, bathtubs, jacuzzis, showers, oceans, and reservoirs. The backyard swimming pool is the site for 38 to 60 percent of near drownings in children, whereas for the adult this site accounts for only 11 percent. Drowning and near drowning episodes in the adult occur most often in bays, lakes, and canals.

In the pediatric age group, males are more often involved in both drownings and near drownings, accounting for nearly 85 percent in some series. This is probably the result of cultural influences rather than anatomic or physiologic mechanisms. Little boys are simply more curious and aggressive behavior is expected of them. The average age for little children who drown in pools is approximately three years of age (the range extends up to 5 to 8 years of age). The one-year-old child is curious, but uncoordinated and limited in his mobility; while the four-to five-year-old child is quick, agile, and curious, but possessing some degree of experience. The two- to three-year-old child combines the worst of these traits: he is quick, strong and adventuresome, but lacks experience.

Home pool drownings usually occur on weekends and usually in the late afternoon and evening from about 4:00 P.M. to 6:00 P.M. In one large series, over 97 percent of the pools were fenced and the drowning occurred in the victim's own pool. The setting is this: one or both parents are at home and the child is discovered to be missing. Surprisingly, the pool is one of the last places that is searched, and the child is found floating face down either on the top or the bottom of the pool. Efforts are then made to remove the child from the pool and artificial resuscitation is instituted at the same time the paramedic unit is called.

## PATHOPHYSIOLOGY

It is appropriate at this point to review the sequence of events in drowning or near drowning, as it is important to understand this in the assessment of children and adults who have the sequence interrupted. If the drowning occurs while the victim is conscious, it is usually because he cannot stay afloat for some reason, be it exhaustion, panic, drug or alcohol intoxication, hypothermia, suicide, or a neck injury following a dive. In some instances, drownings occur after the victim has been rendered unconscious. This would include the situation in which an individual is stepping into a bathtub or shower, slips, falls, and strikes his head, rendering him unconscious. He may drown in as little as three inches of water. An individual with a seizure disorder may experience a seizure and be rendered unconscious and drown.

If the victim is conscious during the near drowning, he undergoes a period of complete apnea from one to three minutes. This apnea is probably voluntary in nature as the victim strives to get his head above water. While this is occurring, there is a shunting of blood to the heart and brain (similar to the "diving reflex" which has been shown in seals). When the victim is apneic the $PaCO_2$ in the blood rises to greater than 50 mm Hg and the $PaO_2$ of the blood falls below 50 mm Hg. There are violent inspiratory and swallowing efforts. At this point, copious amounts of water enter the mouth, posterior pharynx, and stomach, stimulating severe laryngospasm and bronchospasm. In approximately 10 percent of drowning victims, and in a much greater percent of near drowning victims, this laryngospasm prevents the influx of water into the lungs and these patients never have problems with aspirated water. This phenomenon has been called a "dry drowning." Regardless, the laryngospasm or airway obstruction due to aspirated water further aggravates the hypoxemia and hypoxia, leading to anoxia. The stimulus from the hypoxia overrides the sedative effects of the hypercarbia, and central nervous system stimulation is a result. This may be seen in many victims as convulsions and/or vomiting. The anoxia results in a deeper coma. Hypotension, bradycardia, and death will supervene in a short period of time. This entire sequence, however, may take up to ten to twenty minutes depending upon many factors, such as hypothermia, the amount of clothing worn, or the presence of additional injuries.

In the lung, the problem of both drowning and near drowning is primarily that of asphyxia from airway obstruction secondary to the aspirated water. If the process does not lead to the death of the patient, then the near drowning episode results in lower airway disease caused by the fluid.

In fresh water near drownings, the large surface area of the alveoli and small airways allows a massive amount of hypotonic water to diffuse across and into the vascular space. This results in a thickening of the alveolar walls with inflammatory cells, hemorrhagic pneumonitis, and destruction of surfactant. Surfactant is a chemical in the alveoli of the lung that is responsible for the stability and patency of the alveoli. When the capillaries of the alveoli are damaged, plasma proteins leak back into the alveoli, resulting in the accumulation of fluid in the small airways. This leads to multiple areas of atelectasis.

In salt water near drownings, however, the hypertonic nature of the fluid draws water from the bloodstream into the alveoli. This results in the failure of oxygenation and produces hypoxemia, since the blood is traveling through the lung tissue without being oxygenated. The damage to the lung may not be readily apparent, but may progress over the next twenty-four hours after the near drowning. Any individual who has experienced near drowning must be hospitalized and observed for at least twenty-four hours to be certain that pulmonary damage has not occurred. The differences between salt and fresh water drownings are presented in Table 18-2.

It should be mentioned that in Denmark, there is a country-wide law that swimming pools must have isotonic saline in them. Drowning in these pools is not associated with the pulmonary complications resulting from fresh water swimming pool drownings in the United States. This is particularly true when it is remembered how many different chemicals, especially chlorine, are placed in fresh water pools. Chlorine itself is damaging to the lung alveoli and aggravates fresh water drownings in the United States.

## AT THE SCENE OF THE DROWNING

When the paramedics arrive at the scene of a drowning, one should assess the patient while the other secures the facts concerning the incident.

> Who?—Name and age of the victim.
>
> When?—What is the best approximation of when the drowning occurred?
>
> How Long?—How long was the victim submerged?
>
> Where?—This may be obvious, but sometimes the victim has been pulled out of the submerged area and it may not be clear. Was the victim submerged in a bathtub and rushed out to the front lawn? Or was he found in the swimming pool and rushed out to the front lawn after he arrested?
>
> State of
> Consciousness—When was the victim last known to have spoken to someone?

| Fresh Water | Salt Water |
|---|---|
| Hypoxia | |
| Alteration in normal surface tension properties of surfactant with a subsequent collapse of alveoli, leading to atelectasis. There is an imbalance between ventilation and perfusion, which tends to aggravate hypoxemia. | Greater degree of hypoxia with fluid in the alveoli, which interferes with ventilation. |
| Blood Volume | |
| Hypotonic water rapidly absorbed into the circulation, producing transient hypervolemia and elevation in central venous pressure. | Hypertonic fluid draws water into the alveolar spaces, producing hypovolemia and shock. |
| Serum Electrolytes | |
| In either case, serum electrolytes are not usually affected. In salt water drownings, sodium is in the fluid and it is difficult to determine from the serum electrolytes exactly what has occurred. | |
| Cardiac Changes | |
| Sufficient water is infrequently aspirated to cause ventricular fibrillation by itself. Ventricular fibrillation is usually the result of hypoxia and hypercarbia. | |
| Hemolysis | |
| Hemolysis can occur after aspiration of at least 11 ml of fluid per kilogram of body weight. | |

How?—Was it an attempted suicide, or exhaustion, or were there drugs or alcohol involved?

What?—What type of fluid was the victim submerged in?

The vast majority of near drowning victims will be in various stages of wakefulness with coughing and varying degrees of depth of respiration. The heart beat can usually be palpated and the peripheral pulses and blood pressure are adequate. In many situations, however, the victim may be apneic, requiring immediate respiratory support. If the victim is apneic and the airway has been opened yet there is no visible breathing, either by watching the chest or by listening at the mouth, then mouth-to-mouth resuscitation should be started. Many of these patients have vomited and have vomitus, rather than just water, in the posterior pharynx. This must be cleared out with the finger, a gauze pad, or a towel. A portable suction apparatus with a tonsil-tip sucker is of extreme value

(Chapter 9). No time should be wasted positioning the patient for drainage of pulmonary fluid or oral secretions, as this will merely delay the establishment of better ventilation.

After the initial attempted mouth-to-mouth breathing, it is often apparent that laryngospasm is present. This can be managed in one of two ways. The abdominal thrust (Heimlich maneuver) can be used. Four upper abdominal thrusts may break the laryngospasm. After these thrusts, mouth-to-mouth ventilation should be attempted again. If this is not successful, the patient can then be physically lifted by the shoulders and dropped down on the knee of the paramedic. This sudden "breaking of the patient" will force air out through the larynx and may break the laryngospasm. After this, mouth-to-mouth breathing should be attempted again.

In approximately 10 to 30 percent of the near drowning victims, the respirations and vital signs will not be adequate. In this situation, cardiopulmonary resuscitation should begin immediately. Following attempts at ventilation and establishment of ventilation, the carotid pulse should be palpated. If it is not present, then external cardiac massage with ventilation should begin. Shortly afterwards, the chest can be smeared with electrode paste and the defibrillator paddles placed on the chest. An immediate reading of the ventricular rhythm can be ascertained. If ventricular fibrillation is present, defibrillation is indicated according to the tables in Chapter 13. Once defibrillation has been attempted, if successful, further ventilatory support should be maintained while vital signs are monitored. If the victim continues to be apneic, then an esophageal obturator airway is inserted and ventilation maintained with 100 percent oxygen. It may be just as prudent to place an oral airway and begin bag/mask breathing with 100 percent oxygen.

In children, the esophageal obturator airway is not used. Mouth-to-mouth resuscitation followed by bag/mask breathing appears to be the only choice at the present time. Resuscitation in an infant or small child is discussed in Chapters 13 and 20.

If a full arrest situation continues, an IV should be started with $D_5W$ and a microdrip chamber. Two ampules of sodium bicarbonate is administered immediately. If there is continued fibrillation, 0.5 to 1.0 ml of 1:10,000 epinephrine should be given intravenously and cardiopulmonary resuscitation continued. The patient may have to be transferred from the pool to the receiving hospital with full CPR underway.

Details of the accident are vital in the complete management of these patients. If the individual had been drinking alcohol, it is important to know if he was found in the shallow end of the pool. This would indicate that a cervical injury is more than likely. If the patient was an epileptic, determine if he had a seizure prior to the drowning incident.

In the management of the child who has drowned, it is best to transport the child as quickly as possible after basic CPR has been undertaken. The reasons for this are that in a very young child it is difficult to start an intravenous. A cut-down at the hospital may be the only way to gain access to the circulation. Adequate ventilation and correct external cardiac compression must be maintained while the child is transported.

In any drowning situation, hypothermia is a potential problem. This is especially true if the near drowning occurred in the winter months in a backyard swimming pool or in the ocean. It is helpful to notify the hospital that you have a near drowning victim who is hypothermic. This will allow the hospital time to have a warming blanket in the Emergency Department where rewarming can begin. During transport, the patient should be warmed by keeping the ambulance warm and placing warm blankets over the patient.

Almost all near drowning victims have a stomach full of water. At the hospital a nasogastric tube can be inserted to remove any additional water present in the stomach to prevent problems of ingested water, which can occur during the in-hospital management of these patients.

## OUTCOME

The vast majority of near drowning victims do extremely well. Greater than 90 percent of near drowning victims of all ages survive without sequelae. All near drowning victims should be admitted to the hospital for twenty-four hours to observe the onset of late coma or other complications. Some of these patients have major problems with pulmonary parenchymal injury, destruction of surfactant, aspiration pneumonitis, or pneumothorax. Hypoxia, hypercarbia, mixed metabolic and respiratory acidosis, and the need for respiratory assistance can plague these victims, often requiring extended hospital stays. The problems of electrolyte disturbances, anemia, and hemoglobinuria complicate the clinical picture only rarely. Treatment of the effects of cerebral hypoxia occasionally continues through and after the hospitalization. Patients who arrive in the Emergency Department with variable neurologic signs, unconscious, and with major respiratory difficulty are the ones who benefit most from the Intensive Care Unit procedures and the modalities of therapy available.

On the other hand, those patients arriving in the Emergency Department pulseless, without cardiac action, and with central nervous system signs of dilated pupils and apnea will usually go on to die. This pessimistic outlook should not limit the activities of the paramedic unit in the field, as it is based on the assessment and monitoring capabilities in the Emergency Department. An often stated fear of successfully resuscitating an individual who may survive but with severe neurologic injury is not justified. An unknown number of these near drowning patients are revived and resuscitated enroute to the hospital. It should be remembered that if the patient survives, the outlook is generally quite good that no temporary or permanent neurologic damage will occur.

The most physiologically taxing injury to the body is that of an extensive burn. Burns are divided into four degrees—first, second, third, and fourth.

First—mild injury causing redness

Second—severe skin damage but will heal in 1–3 weeks (red, blisters, painful)

Third—skin completely killed (skin whitened, black and charred, or red) skin graft necessary. Not painful

Fourth—extend below subcutaneous fat into muscle or bone

Major burns are those which:

1. Involve greater than 30% body surface area (or greater than 10% under 2 years or over 60 years)
2. Are third degree of face, hands, feet, genitals
3. Are associated with smoke inhalation
4. Are chemical
5. Are in a patient with preexisting illness or major injuries.

Principles of burn treatment include:

1. Cut off burning clothes
2. Attend to other major problems (respiratory, circulatory)
3. Cover burn (clean sheet)
4. Cool (cold water)
5. Oxygen mask (6 l/min)
6. Painful second degree burns—wet towels or sheets
7. Do *not:* Use analgesics, remove stuck clothing, or use creams or ointments.

Treatment of chemical burns includes:

Dilute and wash with flood of water

Brush off chemical powders first

Neutralize with weak acid (vinegar) or base (baking soda).

Smoke inhalation syndrome includes:

Carbon monoxide poisoning

Heat inhalation

Toxic gases.

Two kinds of injuries are associated with electrical accidents:

The flash may cause burns and ignite clothing

Tissue damage as the current goes through the body.

Treatment of electrical injuries includes:

As soon as safe to touch patient initiate CPR if necessary.

If vital signs stable, cover burns and transport

Notify Burn Unit

Monitor EKG during transport

Intravenous of Lactated Ringer's

$O_2$ (mask) at 6 l/min.

Treatment of patient struck by lightning:

Immediate CPR

Cover skin burns

$O_2$ (mask) at 6 l/min; assist ventilation when needed

Transport to facility able to handle electrical burns.

Frostbite is a local cold injury; it has the appearance of a third degree burn (skin white, cold, dead-looking).

Treatment of frostbite includes:

Protect area by wrapping in gauze or towels

Separate fingers and toes with gauze

Allow gradual warming by room temperature, body heat, and occasionally tepid (100° F) water

Do not heat too quickly!

Hospital care if more than fingertips involved.

Hypothermia of the body can occur after exposure. Treatment includes:

Wrap patient in blankets

Monitor, including temperature and vital signs

CPR if fibrillation present

Notify hospital of the situation

If hypothermia exists with adequate breathing *do not* insert airway.

Transport.

Heat exhaustion (prostration) occurs in healthy individuals who exercise to exhaustion in a warm environment. Water and salt are lost through sweating. This may produce skeletal cramps, abdominal pain, and subsequently wet pale skin, tachycardia, thready pulse, and low blood pressure, along with vomiting, diarrhea, and fainting. Temperature is normal or slightly elevated.

Treatment of heat exhaustion includes:

If minor, place in shade and give oral salt and water.

If extreme, start IV of $D_5 W$/Lactated Ringer's, place in shade and elevate legs.

Monitor vital signs

Draw blood for electrolytes

Possible mask $O_2$.

Heat stroke is caused by the failure of normal temperature regulation and lack of sweating. Patients have high temperatures (44° C or 108° F at times); dry, hot skin; confusion; seizures; coma; tachycardia; bounding pulses.

Treatment of heat stroke:

A medical emergency!

Reduce body temperature (cold tub or cool blankets)

IV Lactated Ringer's

Notify hospital

Monitor vital signs and mask $O_2$

Monitor EKG.

Scuba diving injuries are due to: Barotrauma (pressure differential), cerebral air embolism, compression, illness, cold, panic. Accidents may occur on the surface, during descent, on the bottom, during ascent.

Management of scuba accidents includes:

1. Surface accidents may need CPR.
2. Monitor vital signs, keep warm.
3. Bleeding ears should be covered with sterile dressing.
4. If pulmonary or cerebral pressure or embolism problems present, use $O_2$, supportive care, airway; watch for pneumothorax, and transport to hyperbaric chamber.
5. IV of Lactated Ringer's.
6. Head down position with legs elevated and turned to left.
7. Bends are treated with 100 percent $O_2$, hyperbaric chamber.

Insect bites may include those of bees, wasps, spiders, and scorpions. Symptoms include pain, itching, redness, and edema. In most cases local treatment suffices.

Patients may develop anaphylaxis due to insect bites or stings. They may have flushing, hives, angioedema, rapid pulse, hypotension, bronchospasm, laryngeal edema, and gastrointestinal symptoms.

Treatment of anapyhylaxis includes:

1. Ice locally
2. Epinephrine 1:1000 (0.3 to 0.5 ml)
3. Tourniquet (proximal part of extremity)
4. $O_2$ (face mask) 6 l/min
5. If respiratory symptoms worsen—Aminophylline₎ 500 mg (250 ml of $D_5W$) in one hour
6. Start IV with Lactated Ringer's
7. If still unresponsive, give 10 ml calcium gluconate IV
8. Monitor and transport.

There are four types of poisonous snakes in the U.S.:

Pit Vipers
{
1. Rattlesnake
2. Cottonmouth moccasin
3. Copperhead
}
4. Coral

Pit viper venom destroys protein and causes hemolysis and severe systemic reactions.

Signs of a pit viper bite may include local signs such as bleeding from site, burning pain, numbness, swelling, discoloration, bruising, blebs, and blood blisters. Systemic signs include weakness, sweating, thirst, nausea, vomiting, diarrhea, tingling around face, unconsciousness, and death may occur from 30 minutes to 30 hours.

Coral snake bites cause few local signs. Systemic signs include drowsiness, weariness, swallowing and speaking difficulty, and double vision. Many other more serious systemic signs and symptoms including coma, convulsions, and death may occur.

Treatment of snake bites is controversial and varies from area to area. General rules include:

1. Keep patient still
2. Proximal tourniquet for superficial veins and lymphatics (string tourniquet)
3. Transport (rapid)
4. If delayed transport—open wound and suction (see text)
5. No ice, use cool damp cloth
6. Monitor vital signs
7. Treat hypotension and shock (Lactated Ringer's)
8. Notify hospital and transfer for specific therapy with antivenom.

Six to seven thousand people in the United States drown each year. Most pool drownings are in the person's own pool.

Drownings may occur while the victim is conscious, because of exhaustion, panic, drug or alcohol intoxication, hypothermia, suicide, or a neck injury following a dive.

Drownings that occur after the patient is unconscious are usually due to his slipping and falling in a tub and striking his head. Patients with seizures may also drown while unconscious. This type of drowning may occur in as little as three inches of water.

The train of events in the drowning of a conscious person include:

1. Apnea of 1–3 minutes.
2. Shunting of blood to brain and heart.
3. Increase in $PaCO_2$ and decrease in $PaO_2$.
4. Violent inspiratory and swallowing efforts.
5. Severe laryngospasm and bronchospasm following water intake.

If the person continues to be immersed in water, there is more hypoxia and hypoxemia and finally anoxia. This leads to central stimulation, convulsions, and vomiting. The final results of this train of events consist of coma, hypotension, bradycardia, and death. The entire sequence may take 10 to 20 minutes.

In the lung, the problem is asphyxia from obstruction of the airway by water. If the process leads only to near drowning, the fluid causes lower airway disease.

There are many differences between drownings in fresh water and those in salt water. These include differences in the amount and type of hypoxia and changes in blood volume due to the production of either hypo- or hyperosmolarity by water or salt.

The paramedic who arrives at the scene of a drowning must rapidly determine:

Who?

When?

How long?

Where?

State of Consciousness?

How?

What?

Findings in a near drowning victim include:

1. Various stages of wakefulness and coughing.

2. Various degrees of depth of respiration.

3. Palpable heart beat, peripheral pulses, and adequate blood pressure.

4. Occasional apnea requiring immediate respiratory support.

If apnea necessitates respiratory support, the following maneuvers are helpful:

1. Mouth-to-mouth breathing.

2. Clearing of upper airway.

3. If laryngospasm is present:

   a. Heimlich maneuver.

   b. Abdominal thrusts.

   c. Lift by shoulder and drop to knee of paramedic.

   d. After above, re-try mouth-to-mouth.

In 10 to 30 percent of near drownings, respiration and vital signs are not adequate; in these cases use cardiopulmonary resuscitation (Chapter 13). In a child who has drowned, transport as quickly as possible after basic CPR is undertaken (because of difficulty of starting an IV). Watch for hypothermia in drowning patients, especially in the winter.

The vast number of near drowning patients do extremely well (over 90 percent survive). All should be hospitalized for at least 24 hours for observation for sequelae. These may include:

1. Late coma.

2. Pulmonary injury.

3. Aspiration pneumonitis or pneumothorax.

4. Hypoxia, hypercarbia.

5. Metabolic and respiratory acidosis.

6. Electrolyte disturbance.

7. Anemia.

8. Various neurologic complications.

A pessimistic outlook should not limit the activities of the paramedic in the field; fear of successfully resuscitating a person who may survive and develop neurologic complications is not justified. If the patient survives, the outlook is generally quite good.

*Bibliography*

Dembert, M. L. "Scuba Diving Accidents," *American Family Physician.* 16:75, 1977.

Minton, S. A. *Venom Diseases.* Charles C. Thomas Publishers, 1974.

Myers, G. J., M. T. Colgan, and D. H. Van Dyke. "Lightning—Strike Disaster Among Children," *JAMA.* 238:1045, 1977.

Rowe, M. I., A. Arango, and G. Allington. "Profile of Pediatric Drowning Victims in a Water-Oriented Society," *Journal of Trauma.* 17:587, 1977.

Snyder, C. C., R. Straight, and J. Glenn. "The Snakebitten Hand," *Plastic and Reconstructive Surgery.* 49:275, 1972.

Sproul, C. W. and P. J. Mullanney. *Emergency Care: Assessment and Intervention.* St. Louis, Mo.: The C. V. Mosby Co., 1974.

# Chapter 19

# CHILDBIRTH

The birth of a child in the field has become so common that the paramedic must be familiar with the complications of pregnancy, techniques for delivering a baby, and aftercare of the mother and infant. It is important to remember that the pregnant woman can develop diseases irrespective of her pregnancy and that most babies can be safely delivered.

## ANATOMY OF THE FEMALE REPRODUCTIVE SYSTEM

Figure 19-1 shows the basic anatomy of the female organs. The ovary and Fallopian tube are situated on either side of the uterus within the

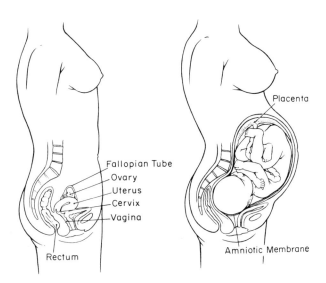

**Figure 19-1.** The female anatomy. On the right, the full-term fetus in position for delivery. The placenta is usually located at the fundus of the uterus.

*597*

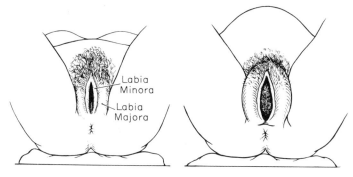

**Figure 19-2.** At left, the normal female perineum. The labia majora and minora are the folds of skin that encircle the vaginal orifice. At right, the baby's head is at the vaginal orifice; hair can be seen.

pelvic cavity. When ovulation occurs, the egg travels from the ovary in the Fallopian tube and insemination occurs somewhere within the Fallopian tube. The fertile ovum then comes to rest within the endometrium (lining) of the uterus. The uterus is a single-cavity organ posterior to the urinary bladder and is composed primarily of smooth muscle. The uterus pares down to an opening called the cervix. In the center of the cervix there is a small hole (os) that dilates during pregnancy. This hole allows for passage of the infant into the vagina. The vaginal opening is located posterior to the urethra. On either side of the vagina are two folds of skin called the labia minorum and the labia majorum (Figure 19-2). Posterior to the vagina is the rectum.

## EMERGENCY SITUATIONS DURING PREGNANCY

Emergencies occurring during pregnancy fall into three general categories:

1. Conditions unrelated to pregnancy.
2. Aggravation of prior disease process by the pregnancy.
3. Conditions related to pregnancy.

An emergency may arise unrelated to the pregnancy. This would include trauma or any other acute medical or surgical problem. A familiar surgical problem is the development of right lower quadrant pain during pregnancy. This is often ascribed to pain in the round ligaments which support the uterus, but it can be due to acute appendicitis.

The second type of emergency is due to a preexisting disease that becomes worse due to the pregnancy. Two of the most serious diseases of this type are diabetes mellitus and essential hypertension. Diabetes becomes notoriously unstable during pregnancy, and unless the insulin requirements and diet are watched carefully, hypo- or hyperglycemic coma can occur (Chapter 16). Essential hypertension is dangerous because eclamptic toxemia may become superimposed on it in late pregnancy.

The added increase in blood pressure can result in cerebral hemorrhage or cardiac or renal failure. In addition, eclamptic seizures may supervene (Chapter 16).

The third type of emergency is that which occurs only during pregnancy; this type will be described in detail. The three most common symptoms that may lead to serious complications are: (1) abdominal pain, (2) uterine hemorrhage, and, (3) generalized convulsions.

## ABDOMINAL PAIN—NORMAL

The most common type of abdominal pains occurring during pregnancy are due to contractions of the uterus. These are called Braxton-Hicks contractions and are felt by the patient as intermittent pains accompanied by hardening of the uterus. When labor commences, the contractions become stronger and increase in frequency from once every twenty to thirty minutes at the commencement of labor to every two minutes shortly before delivery. The pains during labor last from thirty to sixty seconds and the uterus can be felt to harden, or contract, while the pain is present. The uterus relaxes when the pain ceases. The characteristics of labor pains are that they are present during contraction of the uterus and disappear when the uterus relaxes. Between contractions, it should be possible to hear the baby's heartbeat.

## RUPTURED UTERUS

A more serious cause of abdominal pain occurring in late pregnancy or during labor is due to the rupture of the uterus. In late pregnancy, it usually follows previous delivery by a cesarean section, and characteristically the patient complains of a continuous lower abdominal pain becoming progressively worse, as she gradually goes into shock. During labor, rupture occurs if the baby is too large or in an abnormal position, which prevents it from passing through the mother's pelvis. Labor commences normally and progresses with very strong and tumultuous contractions which increase in frequency as the uterus attempts to expel the fetus. Eventually the uterus ruptures and the contractions cease. This is followed by continuous lower abdominal pain, absent fetal heart sounds, and the sudden onset of shock.

Impending rupture should be considered when a pregnant woman is having exceptionally strong and frequent contractions, particularly if she has had a cesarean section or has previously delivered several children. The only alternative diagnosis is that she is about to deliver. The absence of contractions in a patient who has previously had strong labor pains accompanied by lower abdominal pain and the onset of shock is diagnostic of an already-ruptured uterus. Management of these patients consists of starting intravenous fluids to combat shock and transporting the patient to the hospital as quickly as possible. When in the hospital the treatment will be surgical, with either repair or removal of the uterus.

# ABRUPTIO PLACENTA

Usually when the placenta separates from the uterine wall there is external hemorrhage from the vagina. Sometimes hemorrhage occurs behind the placenta, separating it from the uterine wall and later spreading into the uterine muscle without any external evidence of bleeding. This is called abruptio placenta, which produces pain over the uterus and shock due to blood loss. The uterus is tender on abdominal palpation and fetal heart sounds are absent. Abruptio placenta is an emergency that usually results in the death of the baby and, unless treated, progresses to death of the mother from shock. The initial treatment is to start an IV with Lactated Ringer's and transport the mother to the hospital. If fetal heart sounds are present, a cesarean section is occasionally done. Generally, however, this is not the case and labor is induced by rupture of the membranes and the administration of oxytocics in a continuous intravenous drip.

## GYNECOLOGIC CONDITIONS

There are two gynecologic conditions that may produce pain during pregnancy. The first is a degenerating fibroid of the uterus. A fibroid is a benign tumor growing in the uterine muscles. During pregnancy this may degenerate and cause pain localized over the tumor. The condition of the patient is usually good, and the fetus is not affected.

The second gynecologic condition is a torsion of an ovarian cyst. Pain is on one side of the uterus, is constant, and ceases when the cyst untwists. The duration of the torsion is, however, unpredictable and may last a few minutes to several hours. The patient may state that she had the same pains previously and they generally subsided with rest.

A degenerating fibroid will cause pain that abates after several days of bedrest. Torsion of an ovarian cyst requires surgery because of the severity of the pain and the risk of its interference with labor.

Medical and surgical causes of abdominal pain such as pyelonephritis (kidney infection) and appendicitis are managed in the same way as they would be in the nonpregnant woman. In pregnancy, there is the added risk that the disease will cause the onset of premature labor.

## UTERINE HEMORRHAGE

Bleeding from the uterus continues to be the leading cause of maternal death during pregnancy. Bleeding may occur at any time during the pregnancy, but the most common times are early (during the first eight weeks) and late (during the last eight weeks).

The two main causes of hemorrhage in early pregnancy are spontaneous abortion and ectopic pregnancy. Abortion is by far the most common; approximately one in five, or 20 percent, of all pregnancies are aborted, whereas only one in 300, or 0.3 percent, are ectopic pregnancies.

*Abortion.* Typically, an abortion will commence with vaginal hemorrhage due to the separation of the placenta from the uterine wall. Later, cramping pains will occur as the uterus starts to expel the products of conception. The loss of blood may be considerable, producing hypovolemic shock and, if untreated, death of the patient.

*Ectopic Pregnancy.* An ectopic pregnancy is one that occurs outside of the cavity of the uterus. The most common location is in the Fallopian tube. The patient will give a history of missing one or possibly two menstrual periods and will complain of pain in her lower abdomen. The pain is continuous and gradually increases in severity. After onset of pain there is vaginal bleeding. Therefore, unlike an abortion, the pain in ectopic pregnancy precedes the bleeding. The main danger of an ectopic pregnancy is that hemorrhage occurs internally. This takes place when the immature placenta separates from the wall of the tube, or when the tube ruptures. Shock can develop quickly with the loss of 2000 to 3000 ml of blood into the peritoneal cavity. The patient's vital signs will indicate the severity of the bleeding. A rapid pulse and low blood pressure demand immediate intervention. Blood can be seen escaping from the vagina, and the presence of large clots in the bed are evidence of severe hemorrhage. The uterus cannot be palpated since it is still a small organ within the pelvis. In an ectopic pregnancy the lower abdomen may be very tender, with rebound tenderness due to peritoneal irritation.

*Treatment:*

1. Start an IV with a #14 cannula in the arm and infuse Lactated Ringer's at a rate to restore vital signs.

2. Administer oxygen with a face mask at 6 liters/min.

3. If external bleeding due to an abortion appears to be excessive, inject 0.2 mg Methergine® intramuscularly to help the uterus contract.

4. Monitor vital signs and the patient's cardiac rhythm.

5. In severe shock and absence of vital signs, the MAST suit is indicated.

6. Transport the patient to the hospital with advance notice of this diagnosis.

7. At the hospital, abortion is treated with supportive therapy and

a dilatation and currettage to evacuate the uterus. The treatment of ectopic pregnancy is an abdominal operation to remove the involved tube.

## HEMORRHAGE IN LATE PREGNANCY (ABRUPTIO PLACENTA AND PLACENTA PREVIA)

The external bleeding in late pregnancy is due to separation of the placenta from the uterine wall. There are two types, depending on the situation of the placenta. When the placenta is located in its normal position in the fundus of the uterus, the bleeding is called a revealed abruptio placenta (Figure 19-1). When it is attached to the lower one-fifth or lower segment of the uterus, it is called a placenta previa. In both instances the hemorrhage is painless and the onset is spontaneous. Initially the hemorrhage may be slight in amount, the uterus nontender, and the fetal heartbeat present. If the hemorrhage persists, the placenta may separate from the uterine wall, resulting in death of the fetus. As the hemorrhage continues, the patient becomes hypovolemic and will proceed through the state of shock to eventual death. When the placenta separates and the hemorrhage remains behind the placenta, a concealed abruptio placenta is taking place, as previously described.

The history will establish the duration of pregnancy and the presence of pain and external bleeding. On physical examination, the vital signs will provide the most important indication concerning the amount of blood lost. Examination of the abdomen will show whether the patient is in labor and also whether the fetal heart sound is present.

### Treatment

1. Start an IV of Lactated Ringer's and infuse at a rate to restore vital signs.

2. Maintain close evaluation of the patient since further bleeding may occur during the process of moving the patient.

3. Administer oxygen as needed with a face mask at 6 l/min.

4. At the hospital, the patient may be treated with oxytocic drugs to see if the bleeding will stop; if not, a cesarean section may be indicated.

## GENERALIZED CONVULSIONS

The two types of convulsions (seizures) seen during pregnancy are due to epilepsy or eclampsia. They are similar in appearance, having tonic and clonic phases (Chapter 16). Eclamptic seizures are more serious since they are accompanied by hypertension. The latter can cause cerebral hemorrhage and heart or renal failure. It may be possible to distinguish between the two on clinical evaluation. The history from the husband,

Eclamptic seizures generally occur in the latter part of the pregnancy and mainly in the last eight weeks. If the patient has been receiving prenatal care, there may be a history of high blood pressure. High blood pressure may herald the onset of eclampsia.

The epileptic seizure consists of four phases. Initially there is an aura in which the patient senses something unusual, such as flashing lights in front of her eyes. This is followed by a tonic phase in which she becomes rigid, and then the clonic phase in which the actual convulsions take place. It is during this phase that she might injure herself by biting her tongue or striking her arms or head against the wall or floor. Finally, there is a flaccid phase in which she becomes relaxed and may involuntarily lose urine or feces.

The eclamptic seizure is similar to the epileptic seizure except there is no aura. The tonic, clonic, and flaccid phases may be very similar. The severity of the seizures can be judged by the duration of the convulsions and the frequency with which one follows another. On examining the eclamptic patient between convulsions, one should look for evidence of edema as shown by puffiness of the face, hands, and ankles. The blood pressure will be raised, with diastolic levels above 100 mm Hg and systolic levels possibly over 200 mm Hg. Other diagnostic points are protein in the urine and spasm of the retinal blood vessels as seen with an ophthalmoscope. As these latter signs are difficult to elicit, in an emergency situation a presumptive diagnosis of eclampsia should be made if the following are true: (1) there is no history of epilepsy; (2) the patient is in late pregnancy; (3) she is having seizures as described above; and (4) the blood pressure is elevated.

## TREATMENT

1. The initial objective is to prevent the patient from injuring herself by falling or striking an object. It is probably not a good idea to attempt opening the mouth with a tongue depressor during the clonic phase. This may stimulate the patient, causing vomiting and possible aspiration. It is important to observe the patient and make certain the airway does not become obstructed after the seizure when the patient becomes relaxed.

2. Oxygen should be administered to reduce the risk of cerebral hypoxia and possible lack of oxygen to the fetus. Use a face mask with 6 liter flow rates.

3. The eclamptic seizures are very likely to recur and, since they can result in the death of fetus and mother, they must be considered as a serious emergency. If eclamptic seizures are recurring frequently, the use of two drugs should be considered. The first is magnesium

sulfate, which has been used for years in the treatment of eclampsia and which helps to decrease the irritability of nerve endings. An initial dose of 2 ml of a 50 percent solution given intravenously will decrease the frequency of convulsions during transportation. A sedative should also be used. In a situation where seizures are occurring with considerable rapidity, an intravenous dose of 5 to 10 mg of diazepam (Valium) should be given.

4. Transport the patient to the hospital.

5. At the hospital, the treatment will be to control the seizures and reduce the blood pressure by using antihypertensive agents. When the patient is stabilized, labor will be induced. Eclampsia continues to be a cause of maternal mortality and produces a high fetal death rate.

Three emergencies that may be encountered by a paramedic team are presented: abdominal pain, vaginal bleeding, and convulsions. Though each symptom may have a variety of causes, the initial management of a particular symptom in an emergency situation is fairly standard irrespective of the cause. After arrival at a hospital, the cause assumes greater importance and will dictate the further management of the patient. In the management of any patient during an emergency, the basic rules are: (1) keep the patient alive, and (2) transport to a hospital for further treatment.

# NORMAL DELIVERY

## LABOR

*First Stage.* Labor generally starts about 270 days after conception. At this time the uterus has reached its maximum size, is composed of approximately two pounds of muscle, and extends from the pubis to the costal margin. Within the uterus are the fetus, the afterbirth, or placenta, and about one liter of amniotic fluid. At the lower pole of the uterus is the cervix, through which the term fetus will be expelled. It is approximately one centimeter in length and contains a canal leading from the uterine cavity to the vagina, which is less than 1 cm in diameter. In the multigravida, the diameter of the cervical canal may be 2 cm. During the course of labor, the cervix will thin out, or efface, and the cervical canal will dilate to a diameter of 10 cm. This process of effacement and dilatation from 1 or 2 cm to 10 cm is called the first stage of labor. The duration of the first stage depends on a number of factors, one of the most important of which is whether the patient is having her first baby (a primigravida) or has had children before, (a multigravida). The first stage in a primigravida usually lasts about twelve hours and may extend even longer, while in a multigravida the first stage does not generally last more than six hours. The grand multipara, who has had five or more children previously, has a short first stage, which may last less than one hour.

Labor commences with contractions that are felt by the patient as a discomfort or pain starting in the lower back and passing to the front of the abdomen. Initially they are twenty to thirty minutes apart, then gradually increase in frequency, until at the end of the first stage they are occurring every two to three minutes. At first they last thirty to forty seconds, and then as labor progresses they become stronger, lasting forty-five to sixty seconds. At the onset of labor, there may also be a "show," which consists of a small amount of blood mixed with mucus, or a rupture of the membranes, particularly if there is a malpresentation of the fetus.

*Second Stage.* The second stage of labor commences when the cervix is fully dilated (10 cm) and ends with delivery of the baby. In a primigravida, it is usually about one hour's duration; in the multigravida it is much shorter; and it may last only a few minutes in the grand multipara. During this stage, the contractions are strong, lasting forty-five to sixty seconds, and occur every two minutes. The mother has a desire to push, and will generally do so as she feels a uterine contraction, in order to help expel the fetus. As the baby's head is pushed down through the maternal pelvis, signs of imminent delivery will appear. These consist of stretching of the perineum, bulging of the rectal mucosa through the anal orifice, and crowning or appearance of the fetal head at the vulva.

*Third Stage.* The third stage of labor commences with delivery of the baby and terminates with delivery of the placenta. Generally in both primigravidas and multigravidas it is of twenty to thirty minutes duration. When the baby is delivered, the uterus decreases in size and, as this makes the site of placental attachment smaller, the placenta is sheared off the uterine wall. It remains in the uterus, however, until another contraction, when it is pushed into the vagina. The signs of descent of the placenta from the uterus to the vagina are a lengthening of the umbilical cord, a rise and hardening of the uterine fundus, and a small amount of bleeding from the vagina.

## MANAGEMENT

Management of a patient in labor depends on the stage she is in and how much time is available before delivery of the baby. If she is in the first stage of labor, she can generally be moved to the hospital. In the second stage of labor, a primigravida can usually be moved if the signs of imminent delivery are not present. In the case of a multigravida, if she is having strong, frequent contractions and wants to push, it would be safer to prepare for delivery in the patient's home, rather than risk an unprepared delivery during transport.

If the decision is made to deliver the patient, the following steps should be taken.

## STEPS FOR A NORMAL DELIVERY

1. Start an IV drip of $D_5W$ with one-half normal saline. This is a route for administering medication and if extensive blood loss occurs, it will be available to correct the hypovolemia.

2. Lay the patient on her back with her knees flexed. In this position, the paramedic can observe the vulva and handle the baby as it is delivered (Figure 19-2).

3. Encourage the mother to push with her contractions. Between contractions, listen for the fetal heart.

4. If the head crowns, attempt to keep it flexed by gentle pressure on the portion nearest the anus (Figure 19-3). At this point in delivery, the baby's face is towards the anus and the occiput is passing under the pubis (Figure 19-4).

5. As the head delivers, the face will be pointing downwards (Figure 19-4). Mucus must be sucked from the mouth and nose with a rubber suction bulb. This is essential, for if the air passages are not cleared, the infant will inspire the mucus into its lungs.

6. The head will now rotate 45° in one direction or the other, depending on the position of the fetus (Figure 19-5). A further rotation

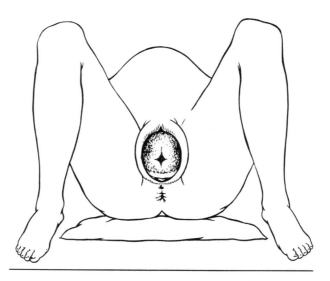

**Figure 19-3.** As the head crowns, the baby's face is usually posterior facing the anus. With further crowning, gentle compression on the occiput and full flexion of the head may prevent further passage of the fetus.

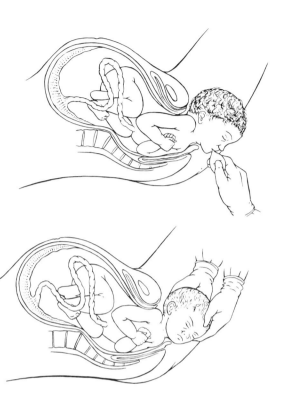

**Figure 19-4.** When the face is delivered, the shoulders reside under the pubis; the mouth and oropharynx should be aspirated.

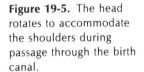

**Figure 19-5.** The head rotates to accommodate the shoulders during passage through the birth canal.

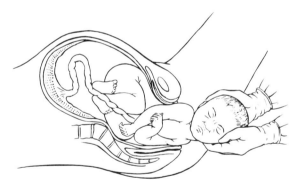

**Figure 19-6.** Following rotation, the shoulders are delivered.

of 45° in the same direction will take place with the next contraction as the shoulders are pushed into the pelvis (Figure 19-6).

    7. The shoulders should deliver with the following contraction. If there appears to be difficulty in expelling the shoulders, the paramedic may help by easing the posterior shoulder out digitally. It is important at this point to ensure that the cord is not around the baby's neck, as it can delay further progress and cause a fetal death. If it is around the neck, the cord should be pushed back over the shoulders. If this is not possible, two clamps should be placed on the cord, which is

then cut in between the clamps with a scissors. The cut ends can then be unwound from the baby's neck and the shoulders delivered.

8. After the shoulders are expelled, the remainder of the baby will be delivered easily (Figure 19-7). The cord should be doubly clamped about four inches from the infant and cut between the two clamps (Figure 19-8). Do not strip the cord to empty blood into the baby. The baby should not be lowered below the vagina, since this will drain placental blood into the infant by gravity. Overtransfusion by either means can cause complications in the neonatal period.

9. The baby is now removed from the bed and laid on its side on a blanket. The air passages are sucked clear of mucus again, at which time the infant generally starts to cry (Figure 19-8). The umbilical cord should be inspected to ensure that the clamp is firmly applied and that no bleeding is taking place. The baby can then be lightly wrapped in a warm blanket and placed on its side in a safe spot. The drawer from a chest of drawers makes an excellent temporary bassinet.

10. The patient is now in the third stage of labor. If her general condition is good and there is no hemorrhage, spontaneous delivery of the placenta can be awaited (Figure 19-9). When the signs of placental descent are observed (lengthening of the cord, rising of the fundus,

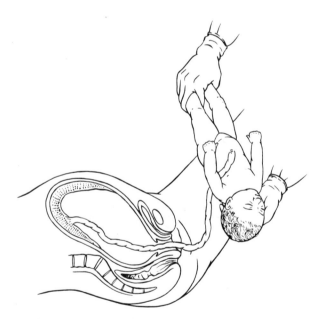

**Figure 19-7.** After delivery of the baby, the head is placed downward to prevent aspiration. The infant can be stimulated by several short slaps on the bottoms of the feet.

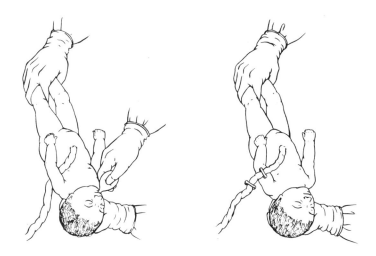

**Figure 19-8.** The oropharynx is aspirated of mucus and other materials. The cord is doubly clamped before division. It is important not to raise the baby higher or lower than the vagina. The former may drain blood from the baby, whereas the latter may overtransfuse the baby through the umbilical vein.

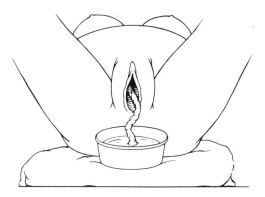

**Figure 19-9.** The amniotic membranes reside in the basin. Yet to be delivered is the placenta and the remainder of the cord.

and slight blood loss), gentle pressure on the fundus accompanied by a push on the part of the mother will expel the placenta.

11. After the placenta has been expelled, the uterus can be stimulated to contract by massaging the uterine fundus and injecting slowly 10 units of Syntocinon® IV.

12. It is very likely that a tear has taken place through the perineum. This generally does not present a problem, and can be repaired after the patient is transported to the hospital. If hemorrhage from a tear should be excessive, pressure should be applied with a sterile pad.

Emergencies during labor are due to abnormalities of the following:

the pelvis

the passenger, or fetus

the powers, or action of the uterine muscle

## PELVIC ABNORMALITIES

The main abnormality of the pelvis consists of its being too small for the fetus to pass through. When this situation is present, the uterine muscle continues to contract and will attempt to force the fetus through. If the disproportion between the fetal head and maternal pelvis is slight, the baby will pass through, but may suffer a skull fracture or damaged brain. When the disproportion is greater, the fetus will not pass through the pelvis. If a cesarean section is not performed, pressure on the fetal skull will produce a cerebral hemorrhage and death of the baby. This will be followed by rupture of the uterus, shock, and possibly maternal death.

Pelvic disproportion should be suspected if a primigravida has had no prenatal care, is having strong frequent contractions, and there are no signs of impending delivery. Absence of the fetal heart sound will add confirmation to this suspicion. Should uterine rupture take place, the signs described in the previous section will be present.

The treatment of cephalopelvic disproportion (CPD) is by cesarean section, which, if performed early enough, will result in a live baby and a live mother. Emergency treatment consists of transporting the patient to the hospital, where a cesarean section can be performed. The patient should be transported after starting an IV of Lactated Ringer's.

## THE PASSENGER (FETUS)

The passenger can produce an emergency situation during labor in two ways. The fetus may be too large to pass through a normal pelvis, or it may be in an abnormal position.

*Size.* Large babies occur when the mother has diabetes mellitus, or with normal genetic development if the husband is a large individual, compared to a relatively small wife. Hydrocephalus causes distention of the fetal head so that it is considerably larger than normal. These abnormalities produce a situation similar to the small or contracted pelvis, resulting in cephalopelvic disproportion.

*Position.* Abnormal positions of the baby can delay the progress of labor or prevent a vaginal delivery.

*Face.* The most common type of malpresentation is an occipitoposterior position of the head. When the baby is delivered in this position, the face looks upwards instead of down when the mother is lying on her back. An occipitoposterior position generally lengthens the duration of labor. In some instances, the head is arrested within the maternal pelvis in the transverse position, necessitating a forceps delivery. In this situation, the baby's scalp may be seen at the vulva, but there is no progress and delivery does not take place. The diagnosis should be suspected if the mother is having strong two to three minute contractions and is pushing, but cannot effect delivery. Management consists of asking the mother to stop pushing, and transferring to the hospital where a forceps delivery can be performed.

A face presentation occurs in one in 300 labors, and consists in presentation of the face rather than the vertex. In this situation, the baby's head is fully extended, rather than fully flexed as it is normally. In the majority of face presentations, the chin lies under the mother's pubic bone and points upwards when she is on her back. Delivery of the head should be effected by flexing the face upwards after the chin has passed under the pubis. The shoulders are delivered as in a normal vertex presentation. When the chin is pointing backwards, or towards the mother's sacrum, spontaneous delivery will not be possible unless the baby is very small. In this situation, the patient should be transported to a hospital, where delivery will be performed by forceps under anesthesia.

*Brow.* If the baby's head is partially flexed, midway between a vertex and face, the presentation is by the brow. When the brow presents, the diameter of the baby's head is too large to enter the pelvis, and so it does not engage and remains above the pelvic brim. This produces a situation identical to cephalopelvic disproportion, and should be managed in the same manner. Delivery will be by cesarean section.

*Transverse.* A particularly dangerous malpresentation occurs when the fetus lies transversely in the uterus instead of longitudinally. The baby cannot enter the pelvis, and vaginal delivery is not possible. If the membranes are not ruptured, a cesarean section will save the baby's life and prevent uterine rupture. Shortly after rupture of the membranes, the fetal heart stops and, if contractions are strong, rupture of the uterus will follow. The position can be diagnosed by observing the width of the uterus and palpating the fetus through the abdomen. Initial treatment is transfer to the hospital after starting an IV of Lactated Ringer's. At the hospital a cesarean section will be performed.

*Compound.* Prolapse of an arm beside the baby's head constitutes a compound presentation, and does not generally cause serious problems. Labor will be slowed but delivery can take place. Management is the same as for a normal delivery.

*Breech.* In a breech presentation, the fetus presents by the buttocks rather than the head. Three percent of babies present in this manner. It is dangerous for the fetus, as the head does not pass gradually through the pelvis, and may be injured by a relatively rapid passage. Delivery should be in a hospital. In a primigravida, there is usually time for transportation, even when the buttocks are beginning to appear at the vulva. In a multipara, or in a primipara when the buttocks are bulging through the vulva, an emergency delivery in the patient's home will be necessary. This should be performed as follows:

1. Lay the mother on her back, transversely across the bed so that her buttocks are at the edge of the bed.

2. Have two paramedics, one sitting on either side of the mother, holding her legs flexed.

3. Allow the mother to push with her contractions, and do not pull on the baby's legs. As she pushes, the baby's buttocks will progress farther out of the vagina, and the legs will eventually flop out.

4. At this point, as the mother's buttocks are at the edge of the bed, the baby's legs will hang down towards the floor. Do not pull on the legs. Further contractions will push the baby down, and the arms will fall out next.

5. Once the arms are out, the baby may be supported gently to prevent injury should the head suddenly be pushed out. Further contractions and the weight of the baby will push the head down until the occiput passes under the pubic arch.

6. Once the head is past the pubis, gentle traction can be exerted until the baby's mouth appears over the perineum. The air passages are then sucked clear of mucus and the head can be delivered.

7. Twins may present abnormalities, but labor is generally slow so that transport to the hospital is possible. If the first twin has to be delivered in an emergency situation, transportation to a hospital should be possible for delivery of the second twin.

POWERS OR ACTION OF THE UTERINE MUSCLE

The third group of problems during labor involve the powers, or action, of the uterine muscle. The type most likely to be seen as an emergency is a precipitate labor. The typical patient is called a grand multipara because she has had five or more children. The contractions are initially weak and irregular, possibly for several hours. Suddenly, without any warning, the contractions become stronger, regular, and more frequent. Their frequency increases and the patient starts to push and rapidly delivers the baby. The total duration from the commencement of strong contractions to delivery of the baby may be fifteen minutes or less. The main danger is to the baby, who may be delivered in unsatisfactory surroundings, and injured. In the management of this abnormality, it is important to know that a woman, particularly if she is a grand multipara, may have weak contractions that can become stronger and effect a rapid delivery. It is a good rule never to turn one's back on a woman in labor, and during transportation always be ready to perform an emergency delivery.

Other abnormalities of uterine action cause delay in labor and can be treated by rest, stimulation, or a cesarean section, depending on the type, in the hospital.

## POSTPARTUM HEMORRHAGE

The third stage of labor, which commences after the baby is delivered, is the most dangerous for the mother because of postpartum hemorrhage. After World War II in London, obstetrical flying squads were started in order to reduce the number of maternal deaths due to postpartum hemorrhage in women who delivered in their homes. Each flying squad consisted of a doctor, nurse, ambulance driver, and assistant. Following a call, the team was transported by ambulance and could be in the patient's home within ten to fifteen minutes. The team was equipped to handle emergency deliveries, start IVs, treat shock, and stop uterine bleeding. The flying squads effectively reduced the number of maternal deaths in the London area, and provided a model for the current paramedic team.

## DESCRIPTION

Postpartum hemorrhage consists of bleeding from the uterus after delivery of the baby. Normally there is little blood loss, but it may become excessive, resulting in hypovolemia, shock, and eventual death. It is difficult to estimate the amount of blood lost when one arrives in a home where a woman has just delivered. The patient's appearance, pulse rate, and blood pressure provide the most valuable clues. If she is showing signs of hypovolemia and is still bleeding, and if the uterus feels soft on abdominal palpation, she will undoubtedly pass into shock. Management consists of stopping the bleeding and treating the hypovolemia with an IV of Lactated Ringer's.

## TREATMENT

With the patient lying on her back, one paramedic should massage the uterus through the abdominal wall. This mechanical stimulation will cause the uterus to contract and will temporarily stop the hemorrhage. Meanwhile, the second paramedic should start an intravenous drip of half normal saline. The speed at which this is infused will depend on the patient's general condition. Ten units of Syntocinon® should be given intravenously rapidly, and a further 10 units placed in the IV solution. The effect of Syntocinon® is to produce a sustained uterine contraction. Until the patient is in the hospital, the uterus must be maintained in contraction by massage and by regulating the rate of the Syntocinon® infusion.

Another drug that will produce a tonic contraction of the uterus is Methergine®. Given intramuscularly in a dose of 0.2 mg, Methergine® produces a uterine contraction in five to ten minutes. It should not be administered intravenously due to the danger of sudden hypertension. Its duration of action by the intramuscular route is about sixty minutes, which is ample time for transport to the hospital.

The above regime can be instituted whether the placenta is in or out of the uterus. After the placenta has been delivered, the uterus generally contracts, but may relax and allow hemorrhage to take place. The basis of treatment is to stimulate the uterus to contract. If the placenta is in the uterus, there is a temptation to attempt its delivery. This is dangerous when the patient has been bleeding, as she can quickly pass into shock due to attempts at delivering the placenta. It is safer to stimulate a tonic uterine contraction, which will control the bleeding. The placenta will be retained in the uterus, but will present no problems and can be removed at a hospital when the uterus relaxes and the patient's general condition has improved.

The fundamentals of treating postpartum hemorrhage whether the placenta is in or out of the uterus consists of: (1) stopping the bleeding by uterine massage, intravenous Syntocinon®, and intramuscular Methergine®; and (2) administering intravenous fluids to compensate for hypovolemia and prevent or treat shock.

## CARE OF THE NEWBORN

Delivery of most babies inside or outside of the hospital is uncomplicated, but sometimes unforeseen problems arise that may severely compromise the newborn. Since there has been a recent increase in the number of home deliveries, more complications are arising from these that require the assistance of trained personnel for intact survival of the infant. The estimated number of home deliveries in Orange County, California, which has a population of approximately 1.3 million, is 500 to 1000 out of 22,000 births annually. With a perinatal mortality rate of 10 per 1000, five to ten infants born at home will die each year, some from preventable causes. Many that survive suffer brain damage. This chapter will cover some of the newborn's physiological changes during the period immediately following birth and the care that should accompany them. A special section covers procedures for the newborn infant in distress.

During intrauterine life all oxygen and nutrition needs of the fetus are provided by the mother via the placenta and the umbilical vessels. The integrity of the placenta is the main factor in normal development, both during this period and also during labor and delivery. The oxygenated blood from the placenta flows through the umbilical vein, vena cava, and then to the right atrium. From there, most of the blood crosses the foramen ovale (hole between the right and left atria) to the left side of the heart. The fetal lungs, which are not expanded, are bypassed and therefore have no role in oxygen exchange before birth. The blood presented to the right ventricle enters the pulmonary artery, and from there flows through the ductus arteriosus to the aorta. It does not flow through the lungs, since the vascular resistance is much higher in the pulmonary bed than through the ductus arteriosus. The vascular resistance in the pulmonary circulation remains high until the infant's first breath, which causes the capillary bed to open in the lungs and allows them to fill with air. This decreases the pulmonary resistance and permits the blood from the pulmonary artery to enter the lung circulation rather than the ductus arteriosus, which then closes off. The pressure also drops lower in the right atrium than in the left atrium, allowing the closure of the foramen ovale. These basic changes permit independent circulation and oxygenation and, therefore, an independent existence.

## GENERAL FACTS ON CARE

*Clamping the Cord.*    The initiation of the first breath is a complex process accomplished by a combination of several interacting conditions in the infant including acidosis, initiation of stretch reflexes, hypoxia, and hypothermia. However, the time of the infant's first breath is not related to the clamping of the cord. The clamping of the cord finalizes the intrauterine existence. The first breath usually occurs within the first few seconds after birth, while at least thirty to forty-five seconds elapse before the cord can be clamped. It is therefore reassuring to know that from 50 to 60 percent of the placental blood volume has automatically passed across to the baby by this time. This is a sufficient volume for the newborn; thus the cord should not be stripped or milked to give the baby more blood.

The infant should be held at the level of the vagina following delivery, as holding it lower will also greatly increase the volume of this placental transfer and may cause an excessive blood transfusion to the infant and severe problems.

During the birth process, fluid is forced out of the infant's lungs into the oropharynx and runs out through the nose and mouth. This fluid drainage is independent of gravity. However, it is recommended that during the stabilization period following birth, the head should be turned to the side and held slightly lower than the rest of the body to facilitate clearing of this fluid.

*Heat Loss in Newborns.* All infants lose heat immediately following birth. The infant's temperature before delivery is approximately 38°C (100.4°F), and an immediate drop of 1°C (2°F) in the core temperature occurs in all newborns. Whether or not further heat is lost is dependent on the care given to the infant. Heat loss may occur by evaporation, convection, conduction, and radiation.

*Evaporation.* The baby is wet when emerging from the birth canal; this water quickly evaporates and changes from a liquid to a gas state. This process draws energy from the infant in the form of heat and results in a decrease of the baby's temperature. The evaporation of water has the same effect as ether when it is applied to the skin. It evaporates and the skin feels cold. Rapid drying will prevent or reduce this heat loss. Evaporation is by far the most extensive form of heat loss immediately after birth.

*Convection.* Heat loss by convection is dependent on the temperature and the velocity of the air in the room. It is therefore advisable to keep the temperature in the room where the baby is delivered at a minimum of 23 to 24°C (74–76°F) and to keep the windows and doors closed to prevent excessive air currents (drafts).

*Conduction.* Conductive heat loss occurs between the infant and colder surfaces in direct contact with him or her. After the baby has been dried, the wet blankets should be removed and new warm dry blankets should be applied.

*Radiation.* Radiant heat loss is a difficult concept to understand, but it helps to remember that the transfer of heat from the sun to the earth is mainly by radiation. The sun's rays pass through absolute zero (i.e., −273°C or −523°F) in the atmosphere, but heat transfer to the earth still occurs. Heat transfer through radiation must therefore be relatively independent of the environmental or room temperature. Radiant heat transfer occurs between two objects in close proximity that have different temperatures. Infants lose heat to colder surfaces or objects in their immediate vicinity. Heat loss by radiation is partially dependent on the environmental temperature, due to the fact that this influences the temperature of the colder objects in the room. The greater the temperature gradient between the "heat source" and the recipient object, the greater the heat transfer. Radiant heat loss may become a severe problem during transport of newborns in ambulances at night, particularly in colder climates. This will be discussed in further detail under transport of newborns.

The importance of thermal control for the newborn cannot be

overemphasized. The smaller the infant, the more crucial thermal control becomes and the smaller the variations that can be tolerated. The paramedic's goal should be to create a neutral thermal environment for each infant. This is defined as the environmental temperature at which the minimum amount of oxygen is used for basic metabolic processes. An increase or decrease in temperature outside of the neutral thermal environment range causes an increase in the infant's oxygen consumption and produces stress. Hypothermia can cause acidosis, resulting in peripheral and pulmonary vasoconstriction, which is a major cause of shock in both preterm and term infants. Generally the vasoconstriction causes anaerobic metabolism with a decrease in pH. This causes further vasoconstriction and predisposes preterm infants to respiratory distress syndrome (hyaline membrane disease) by decreasing the production and release of lung surfactants. Such an increased workload may also cause hypoglycemia, another condition that can lead to shock.

## ROUTINE CARE

When you arrive at a home prior to a birth, make certain everything is ready for the infant as well as the mother. This includes increasing the room temperature to 23 to 24°C (74–76°F) if possible and reducing drafts in the room by closing doors and windows. Warm, clean, and preferably sterile blankets should be ready, as well as a bulb syringe, oxygen, masks, and resuscitation bag.

*Suction.* When the head is delivered, the infant's mouth should be suctioned out with a bulb syringe or DeLee suction unit. Following the delivery, the baby should be covered or placed on a blanket and dried. From thirty to forty-five seconds after the birth, the cord can safely be clamped, leaving a stump of no more than four inches. Following the cord clamping, first dry the infant's face and then the rest of the baby. Further suctioning should be done if required. Intermittent one to two seconds' application of suction pressures of 50 to 60 cm $H_2O$ may be necessary for good clearance. This can be obtained by Venturi effect from oxygen flow or other portable suction units. Once the baby has been dried, the blanket should be changed, and a new warm blanket should be wrapped around the baby.

*Evaluation.* The evaluation of the baby's condition is best done by using the Apgar scoring chart (Table 19-1). This enables you to identify and differentiate between babies who require routine care and those who need further assistance. The scoring should be done both at one and also at five minutes after birth. The scores assigned at these times aid you in: (1) identifying babies who need help; and (2) observing whether or not the help given has had the desired effect. The heart rate is determined by listening to the chest with a stethoscope or by looking

TABLE 19-1.  APGAR SCORING CHART

| Sign | 0 | 1 | 2 |
|------|---|---|---|
| Heart Rate | Absent | Below 100 | Over 100 |
| Respiratory Effort | Absent | Weak cry Hypoventilation | Good, crying |
| Muscle Tone | Limp | Some flexion of extremities | Well flexed |
| Reflex Response to Stimulation | No response | Grimace | Cough or sneeze |
| Color | Blue, pale | Body pink Extremities blue | Completely pink |

at the cord stump where the arterial pulsations frequently can be seen. Respiratory activity is judged by the baby's breathing efforts and rate. The tone is best seen in the extremities in response to stimulation. Reflex activity is best evaluated during suctioning of the naso- and oropharynx or handling of the infant. Most newborns score only 1 for color both at one and five minutes of age, as there is always some degree of peripheral cyanosis (acrocyanosis).

A score of 7 to 10 means an active and vigorous infant who requires only routine care. A score of 4 to 6 indicates a moderately depressed infant who requires stimulation to breathe and the administration of oxygen in addition to routine care. Severely depressed newborns have scores between 0 to 3, and need immediate help with ventilation by bag and oxygen by mask. It is also helpful to use this scoring system during the transport of infants to the hospital. This will enable you to determine if the baby's condition remains stable, improves, or gets worse. After the first five to ten minutes, if the baby is stable and doing well, he or she can certainly be given to the mother for the mutual benefit and enjoyment of both.

DISTRESSED INFANTS

Remember that resuscitation of distressed newborns is primarily concerned with establishing ventilation, oxygenation, and stabilization of the infant and not the use of drugs or cardiac compressions. If these basic procedures can be done correctly in the field, the newborn's chances of survival are high. Intravenous therapy and therefore drug administration in newborn resuscitation are more complicated to achieve away from hospital facilities. Most veins are extremely small and a stable intravenous line is difficult to establish. Proficiency at this requires a level of practice and continued experience on newborns rarely acquired by an individual paramedic.

Peripheral veins are never used for drug therapy during resuscitation in a delivery room. The only method of establishing a stable line rapidly is to pass a catheter equivalent to a central venous catheter into the umbilical vein. This mode of therapy is not recommended for use by paramedics. Therefore, the role of drug therapy in newborn resuscitation will not be covered in this section.

The distressed infant needs prompt and effective action. He or she should first be dried, suctioned, and kept warm before further resuscitation measures are taken. Proceed immediately to the following (do not wait 1 or 2 minutes to see if the infant can do it on his own).

*Stimulation.* Stimulation to breathe and oxygen administration should begin immediately. Respirations may be improved by slapping the soles of the feet (one or two slaps only, not ten or fifteen). The best response is usually achieved by placing your left hand under the baby's back and rubbing your fingers up and down the spine.

*Oxygen.* Simultaneously, oxygen should be administered. This is best done through a plastic line to the baby's face from an oxygen tank at a flow rate of approximately 4 to 5 liters per minute.

There is no way to predict the oxygen concentration given, since the infant is not in a sealed chamber, and the oxygen is directed at the baby's face. The basic principle guiding administration should be to give oxygen if the baby is cyanotic or pale and continue until the baby is pink. A continuing cyanotic color indicates that the oxygen tension must still be too low and thus below levels that are known to cause eye problems (retrolental fibroplasia). There is no safe level of inspired oxygen for newborns. Oxygen therapy must be guided by clinical evaluations. The smaller the infant, the more critical the evaluation becomes; the smaller infant is more prone to eye damage from oxygen than the full-term infant. In the field, however, toxicity from excessive oxygen is unlikely since the duration of administration will be short.

Remember that there is no flow of oxygen through the regular resuscitation bags except when they are compressed. Therefore, use the oxygen line directly to the baby's face. With a new bag that has a reservoir or a tail tube, you can point this end to the baby's face while the oxygen line is still connected to the resuscitation bag.

*Intermittent Positive Pressure Ventilation (IPPV).* If stimulation and oxygen administration do not improve the baby's condition, proceed to the next step, which is assisted ventilation. If a bag and mask device is not available, mouth-to-mouth-and-nose resuscitation is used as described in Chapter 20. Since inflation of the lungs by a bag and mask also causes inflation of the stomach, a nasogastric tube must always be inserted before bagging. In addition, the 15 to 20 ml of fluid in the stomach should be aspirated.

### Airways

1. *Oral.* The oral airway should not be used for resuscitation of newborns: it may be relatively easy to introduce, but it is impossible to keep in place during bagging. It cannot be kept in place by the mask and may be expelled into the mask itself since its position cannot be monitored. You can also waste too much time trying to adjust the oral airway when good ventilation can be achieved with correct positioning of the head and chin.

2. *Masks.* The mask should be made of clear plastic, which allows visualization of the nose and mouth during bagging. This is important for proper position of the mask relative to the nose and mouth and to ensure their patency. A special infant-size mask must be used, as a larger mask will not give an effective seal and inflation cannot be obtained.

3. *Bags.* Only a special infant resuscitation bag should be used to bag the infant. Do not use adult equipment. Thorough knowledge of how these work, including pressures, oxygen concentration, and how to "troubleshoot" them should be mandatory for all users.

A note of warning is appropriate concerning all resuscitation bags. Most bags have pressure limitation valves, but these limits can be exceeded on all bags if the compressions are fast and forceful. Thus, all resuscitation bags are potentially dangerous. The effect of your bagging must be monitored by close observation of the chest expansion.

4. *Bagging Techniques.* The baby's head should be in the neutral sniffing position. You can demonstrate this position on yourself by sniffing and noting that while you extend your neck to a straight position, it is not hyperextended. Apply the mask to cover the infant's nose and mouth, taking care not to compress the nose. It is best to hold the bag in the right hand with the mask in the left. The thumb and index finger of the left hand should apply pressure on the mask to obtain a seal against the face, while the middle finger should be placed under the chin and pulled upwards. Pulling the chin upward allows air to pass behind the tongue.

5. *Pressure.* It is usually necessary to use pressures from 20 to 30 cm $H_2O$ to expand the lungs of normal newborns when a bag and mask are used. Newborns create a negative pressure of 60 to 80 cm $H_2O$ to overcome resistance for their first breath, so pressures higher than 20 to 30 cm $H_2O$ may sometimes be necessary. With bag and mask ventilation, the nasal and oral passages, the stomach, and the lungs will be inflated. In an emergency, there is the tendency to overdo things, and hyperinflation and lung rupture is a frequent complication

from IPPV in the newborn. Practice with bagging on "resuscibabes" is necessary to develop a feel for pressure and compliance. A pressure manometer should be connected in line with the bag. Your best guide during inflation however is to observe closely the baby's chest expansion.

6. *Rate.* If no spontaneous respirations are present, a rate of 30 to 40 breaths per minute should be used. As soon as the baby starts spontaneous respirations, reduce the rate, observe the spontaneous efforts, and administer oxygen to the baby's face. Remember, hyperventilation can remove the $CO_2$ drive to respiration. If this has occurred, the baby may need to be stimulated as described earlier.

*Cardiac Compressions.* During IPPV, the heart rate should be monitored. Observe the umbilical stump for pulsations, or use a stethoscope. If the heart rate is less than 80 beats/minute and falling despite IPPV, initiate cardiac compressions. This should be done by a second person, since the bagging must be continued. The technique that has been found to be most effective is demonstrated in Figure 19-10. Place both thumbs over the lower one-third of the sternum with the palms of the hands placed firmly around the chest. The fingers of both hands should encompass the chest completely. The thumbs should compress the sternum regularly at a rate of 80 to 100 per minute with a three-to-one ratio of compressions to bagging. This should be continued for thirty to forty seconds and then feel for the femoral pulse and listen for spontaneous activity with the stethoscope before resuming compressions. The heart rate can be determined over a monitor if available. It is best to have the person doing the compressing count out loud, "1, 2, 3, bag; 1, 2, 3, bag; etc." This will help improve the coordination of the resuscitative measures. This technique differs from the description of single-person resuscitation of the infant discussed in Chapters 13 and 20.

*Meconium in the Amniotic Fluid.* The presence of meconium in the amniotic fluid means that the infant has had a bowel movement prior

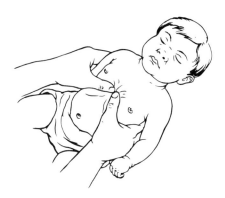

**Figure 19-10.** External cardiac compression in the neonate. The neonate can be ventilated by mouth to mouth-and-nose or bag/mask breathing.

to birth. This occurs as a response to stress, either chronic or acute, and is usually due to placental insufficiency. The meconium itself is sterile, but when it is inhaled, it can cause severe lung inflammation. The thicker or lumpier the meconium, the more severe the lung damage and the more likely it is to be fatal. Therefore, if meconium is found in the baby's mouth, vigorous and frequent suctioning of the oropharynx, nasopharynx, and stomach should be done.

*Transfer of the Infant to a Hospital.* The major problem during transfer of the infant to a hospital is continuous monitoring of the clinical conditions with special reference to: (1) maintenance of body temperature and, (2) continuance of controlled oxygen administration with ventilations if the infant is in distress. The Apgar score may be a useful tool for evaluating the infant's condition and a guide for your therapy throughout the transport.

*Method of Heat Control Before and During Transport*

1. It is essential that you measure the baby's temperature before transfer to obtain a baseline temperature. Rectal temperature should be between 37 and 37.3°C (98.6 to 99°F). The axillary temperature is usually 1°C (2°F) lower. The preventive measures for heat loss have been discussed earlier.

2. Heat the ambulance before the baby is transferred from the house, and maintain the ambulance temperature throughout the transfer.

3. External Heat Sources

In addition to keeping the ambulance warm, you have to use or improvise external heat sources in order to maintain the temperature inside the vehicle.

a. Stable Heat Sources: There are few commercially available heating units that can be used safely for transport of newborns. Radiant heating units can be modified for ambulances, but their justification for use in each paramedic unit is questionable since most interhospital transports are done in specially equipped intensive care ambulances for newborns. The "Porta-warm" mattress is available for use during transports and has been found to be safe, provided the instructions are followed exactly.* After activation, the mattress has a surface temperature of approximately 39° to 40°C (102 to 104°F), which will last for two to three hours. The mattress should not, of course, be applied directly to the infant.

b. Improvised Measures: Hot water bottles can be a useful source of heat, but their temperature should not be allowed to exceed 40°C (104°F). Again, several layers of diapers or blankets

*Marion Scientific Corp., Costa Mesa, California.

(at least four or five) should be placed between the hot water bottle and the infant. Rubber gloves filled with hot water (40°C) can also be used with great success, although they should not be applied directly to the infant either. By wrapping aluminum foil around the baby and these heat sources, further preservation of heat can be obtained. A specially designed commercial aluminum foil wrapper is available for this use. (This type of wrapper should be mandatory equipment in units located in colder climates.)

c. Dangerous Heat Sources: Chemical heat packs should not be used under any circumstances to supply heat to newborn infants. There have been several incidents in which these packs caused third degree burns on newborns despite insulating the heat packs with three or four layers of diapers. Temperatures of these packs can reach 50 to 60°C (122 to 140°F).

One should remember that the babies who are most susceptible to burns from any kind of heating pack are those in shock. With their decreased peripheral circulation, they cannot dissipate the heat away from the area of application. Tissue damage may therefore occur at much lower temperatures in these infants than in stable ones.

Management of sick infants requires practice and repeated exposure to these problems. In any given year, a single paramedic may not see enough problems to maintain his expertise. Therefore, he must constantly update his knowledge by attending in-service and training sessions at the hospital. In managing these patients, the paramedic should also be aware of centers that are able to handle newborn problems. These centers have Newborn Intensive Care Units staffed with doctors and nurses trained in the highly specialized care of the critically ill infant.

In California there are two infant dispatch centers that offer twenty-four hour service in the care of infants in distress and will know where the available beds are at the tertiary care centers. The telephone numbers for these centers are (213) 226-7801 and (415) 497-7342.

# RAPE

Rape is a rapidly spreading form of violence. Law enforcement agencies estimate that only 10 to 20 percent of sexual assault cases are reported annually. Despite reluctance to report this crime, Federal Bureau of Investigation statistics show there were 56,090 known cases of rape in 1975. Sexual child abuse, even less frequently reported, is estimated at 200,000 to 500,000 cases per year. Considering these figures, the likelihood of paramedic involvement in this trauma is high, although partially dependent on geographical location and season of the year.

Rape victim risk rate is highest (73/100,000) in the western United States, followed by the south (50/100,000), north central (47/100,000) and northeast (41/100,000). The crime occurs most frequently in the summer months, peaking in August.

Sex offenders have been classified into three types. One is the rapist with a primary goal of sexual gratification; he rarely inflicts additional harm on his victim. The second type has a deep-seated hatred and aggressive feelings toward women. The third type has a predatory and destructive nature. The latter two groups of assailants impart violent, physical abuse during their assault. It is these attendant injuries of stab wounds, fractures, bites, blunt injuries, etc. that will require immediate assessment and treatment by the paramedic.

Obtaining a history of the sexual assault emergency differs in some ways from the description obtained for the auto accident victim (Chapter 8). DO NOT question the patient about the particulars of the incident. It is not appropriate or beneficial to the patient to describe the assault in detail to the paramedic. She will experience additional emotional stress reporting the crime to the physician, police department, and attorneys. Allow her to talk, but lead the discussion to assessment of injuries, not the act of rape. Avoid the use of "why" questions, i.e., "Why were you alone at this time of night?" The patient's behavior may be hysterical or stoic, but the professional must empathetically reassure her that his immediate concern is for her well-being as a *trauma* patient. This attitude will help to stabilize her emotionally, enabling her to endure further examination more easily. The same approach should be used with parents of a molested child.

It is the police department's responsibility to collect evidence of the crime, but any clothing that must be removed from the patient to facilitate care in-transit should be handled as little as possible and saved as evidence. Do not use plastic containers for blood-stained articles. Plastic enhances continuing bacterial action, which interferes with blood grouping techniques used for determination of suspect identity. Resolution of long-term emotional trauma seen in these patients is partially related to successful capture and prosecution of the assailant and every precaution should be taken to preserve evidence.

TREATMENT

1. Proceed with treatment of injuries as outlined in Chapter 14. Wounds containing debris and other parts of the body should NOT be cleansed. Foreign material on the body, wound debris, fingernail scrapings, and loose pubic hair are all potential samples for analysis.

2. Examination of the genital area must be deferred for the Emergency Department physician unless hemorrhage is present. Genital injuries, although painful, are rarely associated with significant bleeding unless mutilation of the area has been attempted. Examination of female

genitalia in the field, except in childbirth, has serious medical-legal implications. Upon arrival at the hospital in most communities, the physician will follow a rape protocol, which includes written consent for pelvic and rectal examinations.

3. The paramedic's role in this trauma is to treat life-threatening injuries and lessen the immediate emotional trauma by his reassuring, nonjudgmental attitude.

This chapter has reviewed the important aspects of normal labor *Summary* and delivery, care of the newborn, and rape. Abnormalities and complications of pregnancy have also been presented. Most pregnant women will be able to pass through an uncomplicated course of events, and the normal, routine delivery steps will suffice. In the uncommon case of some type of complication, however, it would be best for the paramedic to understand the background of the problem and to know how to approach the management. Care of the neonate need not be complicated, but basic points, such as suction, prevention of body heat loss, and oxygenation, need repeated stressing. The rape victim requires gentle handling and assessment of trauma as for any other trauma patient. Clothing, hair, and other material found at the rape scene must be preserved as evidence.

Emergencies during pregnancy fall into three categories: *Important*
1. Problems irrespective of pregnancy. *Points to*
2. Problems due to preexisting disease. *Remember*
3. Problems occurring only during pregnancy.

The three most common symptoms of a problem unique to the pregnancy are:
1. Abdominal pain.
2. Uterine hemorrhage.
3. Convulsions.

Causes of abdominal pains include:
1. Braxton-Hicks contractions (normal).
2. Normal labor pains.
3. Ruptured uterus (exceptionally strong, continuous contractions with subsequent shock, especially if previous C-section).
4. Abruptio placenta (separation of placenta, hidden bleeding, shock).
5. Gynecologic conditions (torsion of ovarian cyst and degenerating fibroid tumor).

Causes of uterine hemorrhage include:
1. Spontaneous abortion.
2. Ectopic pregnancy (outside of uterus).

Treatment of abortion and ectopic pregnancy include:

1. IV (large bore) with Lactated Ringer's.
2. O$_2$ (mask) at 6 l/min.
3. If bleeding is severe, 0.2 mg Methergine® IM.
4. Monitor vital signs.
5. If in shock, without vital signs, MAST suit.
6. Notify and transport.

The two types of generalized convulsions seen during pregnancy are due to:

1. Epilepsy (preexisting).
2. Eclampsia (accompanied by hypertension and edema).

Treatment of convulsions includes:

1. Prevent injury.
2. O$_2$ (mask) at 6 l/min.
3. Drugs (magnesium sulfate for eclampsia; Valium® for epilepsy).
4. Transport.

The first stage of labor includes dilation and effacement of the cervix. It may last from one to twenty-four hours or more.

The second stage of labor starts when dilation is complete and ends with delivery.

The third stage of labor includes the delivery of the placenta and usually lasts twenty to thirty minutes.

If delivery must be done in the field, the following brief outline is to be followed (see text):

1. IV (dextrose and 0.45% saline).
2. Supine, knees flexed.
3. Push with contractions, monitor fetal heart.
4. Control baby's head.
5. Apply suction.
6. Rotate head.
7. Deliver shoulders.
8. Deliver rest of body.
9. Care for baby (suction, warm, cord).
10. Deliver placenta.
11. Stimulate uterus.
12. Examine for perineal tear.
13. Transport.

Emergencies during labor are due to abnormalities of the:

1. Pelvis (too small for baby or head).
2. Passenger

   a. Size (baby too large or abnormal).

   b. Position (face, brow, transverse, compound, breech).

   c. Twins.

3. Powers or action of uterine muscle

   a. Very rapid delivery.

   b. Very weak contractions.

It is a good rule never to turn one's back on a woman in labor or during transportation. Always be ready to perform an emergency delivery.

Routine Care of Newborn Infants

1. Make certain everything is ready for the infant.

2. Room temperature should be 74–76°F.

3. Close doors and windows.

4. Have warm, clean, sterile blankets ready.

5. When head is delivered, suction mouth with bulb syringe or DeLee unit.

6. Dry baby and cover with blanket.

7. Clamp cord thirty to forty-five seconds after birth.

8. Continue suction, or use suction with pressure if necessary.

9. After drying the baby, use a new warm blanket.

10. Evaluate by Apgar score (see text).

If the infant is distressed, establish ventilation, oxygenate, stabilize; intravenous and drug therapy are not feasible in the field.

Steps that can be taken:

1. Stimulate (1–2 slaps to soles, rub along spine).

2. Oxygen (plastic line to face from tank at 4–5 l/min).

3. If no improvement, use assisted ventilation.

   a. Insert nasogastric tube first.

   b. No oral airway to be used.

   c. Use mask made of clear plastic.

   d. Use only special infant resuscitation bag.

   e. Rates of 30–40/min at pressures of 20–30 cm $H_2O$ are usual.

4. Monitor heart by pulsation of cord or with stethoscope; if below 80/min use cardiac compression.

5. Transfer to hospital; make certain temperature is maintained during transport (see text for particulars on this subject).

The paramedic should be familiar with the stage of regionalization of newborn intensive care in his area and always bring such infants to regional centers with expertise in newborn care.

Only 20 percent of the total number of rape cases are reported, and there were 56,090 known rape cases in the United States during

1975. The paramedic sees the victims of the rapists usually when there has been trauma involved.

Assessment:

1. The history should involve questions about the injury, and not about the sexual assault.

2. DO NOT examine the genitalia region unless bleeding is suspected.

Treatment:

1. Treat injuries as in any trauma case, except do not cleanse wounds or remove materials from the body that can be used as evidence.

2. The paramedic's attitude should be sympathetic, not judgmental.

*Bibliography*    Amlie, R. N. "Neonatal Resuscitation," *Symposia Specialists*. Symposium on Perinatal Medicine, April, 1977.

*Clinical Obstetrics and Gynecology*. 511 Vol. 20, No. 3, September, 1977.

Cohen, M., R. Garofalo, R. Boucher, and T. Seghorn. "The Psychology of Rapists," *Semin. Psychiatry*. 3:307, 1971.

Danforth, David N., Ed. *Obstetrics and Gynecology*. Hagerstown, Md.: Harper and Row, 1977.

George, J. "Rape and the Emergency Department Physician," *Emergency Physician Legal Bulletin*. 1:1, 1975.

Gregory, G. A. "Resuscitation of the Newborn," *Anesthesiology*. 43:225, 1975.

"Manually Operated Resuscitators," *Health Devices*. 3:164, 1974.

Pritchard, Jack A., and MacDonald, Paul C., Ed. *Williams Obstetrics*. New York: Appleton-Century-Crofts, 1976.

*Uniform Crime Reports*. USFBI, 1975 Catalog No. J1147:975, 1976.

Willson, J. Robert, Clayton T. Beecham, and Elsie R. Carrington. *Obstetrics and Gynecology*. St. Louis, Mo: The C. V. Mosby Co., 1975.

# Chapter 20

# CARING FOR
# SPECIAL AGE GROUPS:
# CHILDREN

The infant, child, or adolescent who is critically ill or injured presents special problems to those who care for him. His treatment requires particular attention to both physiologic and psychologic aspects of his condition in order to adequately evaluate, stabilize, and transport him without his suffering additional stress. Although most evaluations and treatment of ill or injured children is identical in principle to adult care, children are different, not only in size, but also in physiologic function, susceptibility to certain disease entities, and frequency of some injuries.

## THE RELATIONSHIP OF GROWTH AND DEVELOPMENT TO ILLNESS AND INJURY

The hallmarks of infancy and childhood are growth and development. The child is normally in a state of flux regarding vital functions, size, and developmental capabilities. His month-to-month changes contribute to the difficulty in assessment and complicate treatment.

Growth refers to an increase in body mass or size. Development refers to a maturation of function, both physiologic and psychologic. Growth and development occur in an interrelated and orderly fashion. Although there are individual variations, predictions based on age can be made about body size, organ function, and motor and reasoning capacity.

When assessing and treating a child who is ill or injured, his age, size, and development level must be considered. Infants and young children are subject to certain diseases that do not ordinarily affect older children and adults. Similarly, the types of injuries for which a small child is at-risk can be predicted from observations of his ability to get himself into certain situations, his curiosity, and the peculiarities

TABLE 20-1.  COMMON SERIOUS ILLNESSES AND INJURIES RELATED TO AGE

| Age of Child | Illnesses | Sources of Injuries |
|---|---|---|
| Newborn, incl. premature | Respiratory distress | Hypothermia |
| 0–2 mo | Septicemia, meningitis, pneumonia | Vehicle accidents, child abuse, hypothermia |
| 2–12 mo | Febrile (6 mo) and other seizures, dehydration, bronchiolitis, meningitis | Vehicle accidents, child abuse |
| 1–6 yr | Croup, asthma, seizures, epiglottitis, meningitis | Vehicle accidents, child abuse, accidental poisoning, burns, drownings, aspiration and ingestion of foreign bodies, car vs. child accidents |
| 6–12 yr | Few (asthma, diabetes) | Vehicle accidents, car vs. child, car vs. bicycle accidents, child abuse, burns, falls, sports injuries, drownings |
| 12–18 yr | Few (asthma, diabetes) | Same as 6–12, plus drug ingestions (abuse) |

of his physical makeup. Some common causes of serious illness and injury according to the age of the child are listed in Table 20-1.


## SPECIAL PROBLEMS IN EVALUATING AND ASSESSING CHILDREN

The ill or injured child is usually frightened, upset, uncomfortable, and fearful of those who are trying to assist him. He is frequently surrounded by adults who are as upset and confused as he is.

### HISTORY

In cases involving children under five years of age, most information about the illness or injury must be obtained from adults, usually the parents. Questioning must be specific and direct, concentrating on the immediate situation, yet considering any prior trauma or illnesses of a similar nature. Assessment should focus on the observed behavior of the child, rather than how he says he feels or how the adult thinks he feels. A child under three who can talk and communicate has a limited vocabulary and experience, compromising his reliability as a historian.

The child over five years of age can be of great help if he is awake and if he is asked questions he understands. Usually the older child can tell what happened or how he feels and is willing to do so. However, the older child who sustains an injury while doing something foolish or forbidden by his parents may be reluctant to disclose details because of the expected consequences.

## APPROACH

The tone of the approach to the ill or injured child is crucial. Unless a child is clearly in need of immediate resuscitation or care for coma, shock, or bleeding, he should be approached slowly and gently to avoid further upset and to encourage cooperation. An initial visual assessment of his position, activity, and behavior can guide subsequent evaluation. When possible, touching or moving a painful or injured body part should be avoided until after the child's confidence has been obtained. All parts of the body should be inspected eventually, but the sequence should be guided by the circumstances. Children with illness or injury change rapidly, and repeated evaluation and appropriate changes in action are necessary. It is common for a child to be overtreated initially and undertreated subsequently, unless repeated assessments are made.

## PHYSICAL EXAMINATION

Following the initial inspection and overview of the child's condition, his vital signs must be measured. Despite difficulties in obtaining accurate values, pulse, respiratory rate, and blood pressure should be measured in all children. Although the "normal" values for these parameters vary widely with age and excitement level, it is possible to establish guidelines for "worry levels" for these measurements. These values and estimates of weights for making emergency calculations are included in Table 20-2. Serial measurements are useful in recognizing changes in the child's condition.

Determination of body temperature is another critical part of the initial evaluation of children. Both fever and hypothermia (low body temperature) can be found in the ill or injured child. The younger the child, the more likely he is to have a temperature above 103°F with even a relatively mild illness. This degree of temperature corresponds in significance to adult temperatures of 101° to 102°F. Conversely, children may have a low body temperature in some illnesses and injuries. This should be noted also, since the complications of hypothermia can be as serious as the underlying disease, particularly in the newborn and small infant. Rectal measurement is fast and reliable, although axillary determination can be used if the thermometer is left in place from three to five minutes. In the alert cooperative child over six years of age, the temperature may be taken orally. *Keep the child warm* if the

TABLE 20-2.  AGE-RELATED SIZE AND VITAL FUNCTIONS FOR FIELD USE

| Age | Weight (Kg)[1] | Pulse[2] | Resp[3] | Blood Pressure[2] |
|-----|----------------|----------|---------|-------------------|
| Birth | 3 | 120–140 | 60 | 60–90/20–60 |
| 3 mo | 5 | 110–140 | 40 | |
| 6 mo | 7.5 | 100–140 | 30 | |
| 1 yr | 10 | 80–140 | 25 | 65–95/25–65 |
| 2 yr | 12.5 | 80–130 | 20 | |
| 3 yr | 15 | 80–120 | 20 | 70–100/30–70 |
| 4 yr | 18 | 70–115 | 20 | |
| 5 yr | 20 | 70–115 | 20 | |
| 6 yr | 25 | 70–115 | 20 | |
| 9 yr | 30–35 | 70–115 | 20 | 90–120/50–80 |
| 12 yr | 40 | 65–115 | 20 | 100–125/55–85 |

[1]Estimates are derived for ease of calculation only; adjustment should be made if child is smaller or larger than usual for age, and accurate weight should be obtained when possible.

[2]Ranges are wide. It is best to compare repeated measurements in the same child for changes.

[3]Estimates are for upper limits of normal, at rest, or with mild excitement.

temperature is low (less than 98°F, 37°C) and *cool him* if body temperature is high (over 103°F, 39.5°C). Axillary temperature is usually lower than both oral and rectal temperature.

A physical feature unique to children under one year of age is useful in evaluation, also. The child of this age has an open anterior fontanelle (''soft spot'') that may indicate the presence or absence of increased intracranial pressure or dehydration. Normally, the fontanelle is level with the surface of the skull, or slightly sunken when the child is sitting and quiet; it may pulsate slightly as well. If the infant is experiencing increased intracranial pressure, the pulsations decrease or disappear, and the fontanelle feels tight and may bulge above the surface of the skull. (It is important that the child remain calm throughout this observation, since tenseness of the fontanelle is normal during crying.) If an infant is dehydrated, the fontanelle dips low below the surface of the skull. Figure 20-1 demonstrates the location of the anterior fontanelle.

The level of consciousness and activity of the ill or injured child may vary widely. Sometimes, the child's behavior and symptoms may be contradictory to the seriousness of the injury or illness. The critically ill child may be lethargic or semiconscious, but when disturbed may become very irritable. The other extreme, the child who is excited and agitated, is also worrisome. However, the extent and nature of such agitation must be viewed in light of the degree of pain and fear the child is experiencing. The infant suffering from increased intracranial

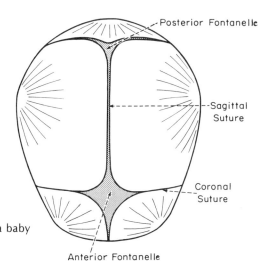

**Figure 20-1.** The skull of a baby showing the anterior and posterior fontanelles.

pressure characteristically has a shrill, high-pitched cry. The infant or child who lies quietly and moans or emits faint expiratory grunting sounds, without apparent respiratory distress, is experiencing severe pain.

Children who are ill or injured may display a wide variety of gastrointestinal disturbances, even when their primary problems seem totally unrelated to the gastrointestinal tract. Most infants and many older children vomit with any problem, including excitement, regardless of its severity. Their parents can be informative as to whether or not this is a characteristic of the individual child. Likewise, the child is subject to ileus (the paralysis of normal intestinal mobility) and also to gastric distention. This causes a painfully distended abdomen which is worsened by the air-swallowing that accompanies crying. Insertion of a nasogastric tube will relieve this distention somewhat and make the child more comfortable. A nasogastric tube should be inserted whenever assisted ventilation is used.

Although stabilizing the patient/victim prior to transport is a major goal of field care, some children may be too difficult to assess or treat in the field. In these cases, assure vital functions (breathing, circulation, and hemorrhage control) and transport, thus avoiding unnecessary time in the field. This is advisable whenever the initial assessment of the problem is either confusing, complicated, or impossible.

## SUDDEN INFANT DEATH SYNDROME (SIDS)

The sudden, unexpected death of a child from Sudden Infant Death Syndrome (SIDS) or "crib death" is a perplexing medical problem for which the cause is unknown. Many tentative theories have been offered to explain these tragic deaths, and some methods for identifying and protecting infants at-risk have been proposed, all to little avail. SIDS presents pressing problems to Mobile Intensive Care and other medical personnel in managing parents who must cope with extreme grief and shock.

The incidence of SIDS is stable and is 2.5 to 3 infants per thousand live births each year. Histories of SIDS victims have revealed some common findings. The usual infant who suffers this sudden, unexpected, and unexplained death is under six months of age, although a few are as old as one year. The peak age for occurrence is four months, and it is more common in boys than in girls. The premature infant, especially one with a history of serious illness related to its prematurity, is at marked risk for SIDS, as are subsequent infants in families where SIDS has occurred.

In the typical case, the infant has been healthy for the days, weeks, and even months prior to death, although a few have had mild "cold" symptoms. Usually, no problem has been suspected until the parent finds the child dead in bed. Occasionally, a parent can recall hearing an unusual noise that prompted a look, or a "feeling" that something was wrong.

Most SIDS deaths occur in the early morning hours before 9 A.M. The infant is found in the crib. There may be some disarray of the bedclothes, suggesting a terminal struggle. There is frequently vomitus in the mouth and sometimes in the trachea. This is thought to be a terminal event, rather than the cause of death. The infant has usually urinated and defecated. Frequently the infant's body is cold and there is postmortem discoloration. Autopsy reveals no specific cause of death.

Occasionally, an infant will be discovered in time to be successfully resuscitated. This is the exception rather than the rule, and many of these resuscitated infants have severe brain damage as a result of the hypoxia. If such an infant is discovered, vigorous and immediate resuscitative efforts should be made. The infant should be transported to a receiving hospital as soon as possible.

In the usual situation, however, it is clear that the infant has been dead for an extended time. Under these circumstances, the parents deserve immediate and sympathetic attention. They should be allowed and encouraged to express their grief. Under no circumstances should accusations be either made or implied as to the parents' role in the death of the infant. The few deaths that appear to be SIDS, but are found later to be the result of another illness or inflicted injury, can be handled later at the time of detection. Parents' normal guilt feelings should be recognized and hopefully diminished at this time. They should be reassured that they, in all likelihood, could not have prevented the death. Field personnel should explain to the parents the need and rationale for notifying the coroner and police and should then make the notification. If the family has a physician, he/she can offer support to the family and should be called immediately.

Laws in many states require postmortem examination, collection of epidemiologic data, and discussion with the parents of SIDS as the presumed cause of death. These procedures are conducted by medical personnel and often include counseling for the parents. Local and national organizations for parents whose children suffered SIDS can be very supportive to grieving parents.

## CHILD ABUSE AND NEGLECT

### PHYSICAL ABUSE

*Background.* Physical abuse should be considered anytime a child has been injured and the cause is not obvious. The types of injuries inflicted upon children are many, and the younger the child, the more likely it is that his injuries are not accidental. It is estimated that up to 10 percent of the injured children under five years seen in Emergency Departments have received those injuries nonaccidentally. If this cause of trauma is not recognized and alleviated, abused children are at continuing risk for further, and usually increasingly severe, damage.

All fifty states have laws which require any professional, who by the nature of his/her work deals with children, to report suspected child abuse. Most of the laws extend protection from civil and criminal liability to reporting professionals and provide punishment for those who fail to comply. Each state has a defined time limit and mechanism for the required reporting.

Child abuse is a problem of the child, the family, and society. For physical abuse to occur in a family, three conditions are necessary: (1) a parent/adult with the potential, (2) a particular child at-risk, and (3) a crisis. There are some recognized characteristics of the family at-risk, although it should be recognized that almost any adult, given the right child and the right circumstances, could physically harm that child. The fact that most are able to control the urge to do harm is fortunate for children.

*The Family.* The abuser is usually a parent (or a parent's boy friend/girl friend) who may come from any geographic, religious, ethnic, occupational, educational, or socioeconomic group. The mother is frequently involved, since she is likely to spend the most time with the child. Most abusers are not insane, but rather injure children in anger or frustration, or after provocation. They frequently have been either abused themselves as children or exposed to much violence at home. They are often lonely, isolated people who feel worthless and who have partners unable to satisfy their needs. They frequently look to the child to fulfill their own needs and are disappointed and disturbed when the child fails. Child abusers feel unable either to ask for help or to use community resources during crises and prefer to attempt solving their own problems without help. Many feel that physical punishment is the only way to teach a child respect for authority. This concept underlies much child abuse found among military families and those with fundamentalist religious beliefs.

The child who is abused is "special." He is somehow different, or seen as different, from his siblings. Perhaps he is more demanding, or handicapped, or in some way does not meet his parents' expectations. The young child (under five years), who tends to be more demanding, more dependent, and less able to communicate without crying than the older child, is at particular risk. Also, the child who was premature, or ill as a newborn, is in danger. Boys are mistreated more often than girls.

The potential abuser and the special child can usually survive together until there is a crisis in the home. The crisis can be either major or just another "little" thing. Common crises are financial stresses, marital reverses, and physical illness in a parent or child.

The abuse incident usually occurs as an "explosion" of behavior, during which the child is injured in either anger or frustration. Usually the abuser feels remorseful immediately. At this point, some parents seek help for even minor injuries, while others ignore major trauma, fearing the potential consequences.

*Types of Injuries.* The types of injuries suffered by abused children are varied and numerous. Some "red flags" for the possible abuse include the presence of any of the following:

1. Any obvious or suspected fracture in a child under 2 years of age,

2. Injuries of various "ages" (different stages of healing),

3. More injuries than usual when compared to children of the same age,

4. Injuries scattered on many parts of the body,

5. Bruises or burns in patterns which suggest purposeful infliction,

6. Obvious or suspected increase of intracranial pressure in an infant, regardless of whether or not there is external evidence of trauma,

7. Suspected intra-abdominal trauma in a young child.

8. Any injury that does not seem to fit the description of its cause.

(All of these "red flags" obviously do not apply in major vehicular trauma or other incidents in locations which indicate the cause of the injury. Most child abuse occurs in the home.) Common signs of abusive injuries are bruises to the buttocks and the backs and sides of the legs, belt or strap marks, and bruises and contusions to the face and head (frequently on both sides). Other indications of abuse are twisting and wrenching injuries to the arms and legs (either with or without fractures), severe shaking injuries to young infants causing increased intracranial pressure and neck damage, and many kinds of burns inflicted for punishment.

Historical clues are useful in assessing trauma that may reflect abuse. Frequently the history does not match the nature or severity of the injury. The account may be vague or change with further questioning. (Most parents know exactly how a child was hurt at home and are very willing to discuss what happened.) The "accident" may be clearly beyond the developmental capabilities of the child, e.g., a two-month-old who fell out of a highchair, or the "accident" may have occurred at an unusual time. ("Accidents" that occur in the middle of the night should raise suspicions.) The injury may be blamed on a third party, or it may be implied that the child willfully injured himself, something children rarely do. There may have been a delay in calling for help, or the child may either be dressed inappropriately or be too clean for the situation. Such statements as "he bruises easily" or "he has soft bones" or "he falls a lot" are common.

*Care of the Abused Child.* The approach to the abused child's injuries differs little from the approach to accidental injuries. Full inspection for all injuries is indicated, as is immediate treatment based on the nature and severity of the trauma. If the child is capable of telling what happened, it is appropriate to ask once. However, most abused children will not answer truthfully in this situation, either because they have been taught not to, or because they are afraid of getting their parents in trouble. Moreover, the children may fear being hurt again or losing their parents' love. They should, therefore, not be pressed to disclose what happened, and it should not be implied that they are lying.

A critical point in the management of nonaccidentally injured children is insuring that these children are transported/accompanied to a receiving hospital. Suspected child abuse victims require complete evaluation, often as inpatients. This hospitalization may further protect the child from additional injuries while an investigation is completed. If parents object, regardless of the severity of the injury, the police should be called to the scene to assure the safety of the child. After the child is delivered to the receiving hospital, the Mobile Intensive Care team should report their suspicions and observations to the hospital staff and/or appropriate agency.

## APPROACH TO THE PARENTS

A sympathetic approach to parents of abused children is warranted, both to maintain cooperation and also to acknowledge the anguish of the parents. Rescue personnel should not make accusations or conduct a detailed "interrogation" under any circumstances. These functions are more properly left to police and social agencies. Expressing the anger normally aroused in medical personnel by the nature and circumstances of the abused child's injuries is always counterproductive. The short-term goal in the field, and later in the hospital setting, should be to treat the injuries and protect the child from further abuse. The long-term goal is to treat the family to reduce the risks for future abuse.

## PHYSICAL NEGLECT

Physical neglect of children is a problem which has its roots in the same type of family setting as physical abuse. Some elements of neglect are seen frequently in abused children, but neglect and its results may be seen in the absence of trauma also. The lesser or more moderate forms of physical neglect are rarely seen alone in the field, but the most severe forms are. Such things as severe malnutrition (with or without dehydration), numerous insect bites on an infant, skin infections of long duration, some forms of severe diaper rash, and extreme lack of cleanliness should arouse suspicion. The approach to this problem should be to recognize and treat the immediate life-threatening problems and transport to a receiving hospital for further evaluation and treatment. In most states, suspected physical neglect must be reported under the child abuse laws.

## CARDIORESPIRATORY ARREST IN CHILDREN

### BACKGROUND

Cardiorespiratory arrest is the lack of effective ventilation and circulation. Tissue damage from hypoxia and acidosis follows within minutes of untreated arrest. Acute airway obstruction, shock, and central nervous system depression are the most common causes of arrest in infants and children.

Poor or absent chest movement and breath sounds, absent pulses, cyanosis or pallor, loss of consciousness, and dilatation of the pupils are the signs of arrest. Resuscitation must be started immediately when these signs are present.

### TREATMENT

The principles of resuscitation are the same in infants and children as in adults:

> Establish an open airway
> Ventilate the patient
> Begin closed-chest massage
> Correct acidosis

Support the circulation
  Administer necessary drugs
  Defibrillate if necessary
  Treat shock

*Establishing an Airway.*   The mouth and throat must be cleared of mucus and debris. Extend the neck slightly to straighten the trachea, taking care not to overextend, or the airway will narrow. (A rolled towel placed under the shoulders is ideal.) Pull the jaw forward to prevent the tongue from obstructing the airway. Insert an oral airway only if convenient.

Tracheal intubation or cricothyrotomy, if permitted, should be done only if ventilation is impossible without one of these procedures. Endotracheal tube sizes for children are listed in Table 20-3.

*Ventilation.*   Ventilation is most easily performed using a bag and tight-fitting mask. Make a seal with the mask, and ventilate deeply enough to cause the chest to rise, and to produce adequate breath sounds. Listen for the breath sounds at the sides of the chest, rather than at the front. If available, use a small bag with a pop-off valve for infants up to two years in order to prevent pneumothorax. Begin ventilating with room air, and add 100 percent oxygen to the bag as soon as possible.

If a bag and mask are not available, begin mouth-to-mouth breathing, after pinching the nose shut. In small infants, breathe into both the mouth and the nose, using small puffs of air (Figure 20-2). Change to the bag and mask as soon as available. If ventilation is not possible, foreign body obstruction may be present. This is treated by inverting the infant on the forearm with back slaps (Figure 20-3). An older child can be placed prone on the thigh and back slaps administered.

In newborns and very young infants, provide sixteen to twenty breaths per minute. The same rate is used in children between one and five years. A rate of ten to twelve is adequate for older children. The ventilations should be synchronized with closed-chest massage.

TABLE 20-3.   ENDOTRACHEAL TUBE SIZES USED AT VARIOUS AGES
IN CHILDREN

| Age of Child | Size (mm) |
|---|---|
| Premature Infant | 2.5 |
| Term Newborn | 3.0 |
| 0–3 mo | 3.0–3.5 |
| 3–18 mo | 3.5–4.0 |
| 18 mo–5 yr | 4.0–5.0 |
| 5–12 yr | 5.0–6.5 |
| 12 yr and up | 6.5–8.0 |

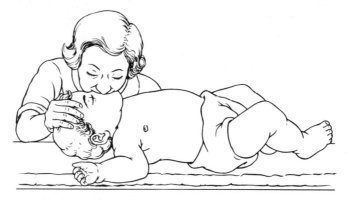

**Figure 20-2.** Infant mouth-to-mouth resuscitation is done by extending the baby's head slightly and breathing into both the nose and mouth. Overextension of the neck will collapse the trachea.

Deliver one ventilation for each five chest compressions. Frequently, the stomach becomes distended with air during assisted ventilation. Insert a nasogastric tube if this occurs. Turning the head slightly during ventilation may prevent this problem.

*Closed-chest Massage.* The child has a much more flexible chest wall than the adult, and his heart is located higher in the chest. Therefore, the technique for closed-chest massage must be modified. In the young infant, massage is most easily accomplished by encircling the chest with both hands, so that the fingers are supporting the back, and the thumbs

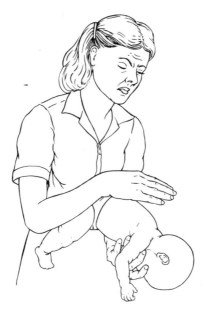

**Figure 20-3.** When a foreign body is suspected in a child, he should be turned prone and tilted head down over the forearm and his back should be slapped with the other hand.

rest over the middle portion of the sternum. The sternum is then compressed by the thumbs, one-half to two-thirds the distance to the spine. As an alternative, one hand can be placed under the infant to support the back, and two fingers of the other hand used to compress the sternum.

In children over one year, first place a firm support such as a backboard under the back. In children from one to five years, use several fingers or the heel of one hand to compress the chest, just below the middle of the sternum. For those over five years, use the heel of both hands to compress the lower third of the sternum (Figure 20-4). Chest compressions must be synchronized with ventilation, providing five compressions for each breath. The rate of massage is eighty to 100 beats per minute for the infant and young child, and eighty beats per minute for older children.

Closed-chest massage should produce a pulse of normal volume, although movement during massage may interfere with palpation. If resuscitation is effective, the patient's pupils should become smaller, and his color should improve.

*Correction of Acidosis.* As soon as assisted ventilation and circulation have begun, an intravenous line should be established. Sodium bicarbonate (1 mEq/kg) should be administered immediately, and repeated every five to ten minutes throughout the resuscitation. Specific therapy is usually ineffective unless acidosis is controlled.

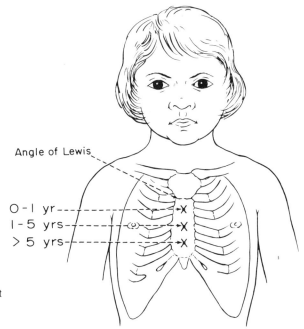

**Figure 20-4.** The sites for extracardiac compression in infants and children. Their bony cages are very flexible and ribs should not be broken during external cardiac massage.

*Further Circulatory Support.* Specific therapy during a cardiorespiratory arrest depends upon the cardiac rhythm, and the effectiveness of any electrical activity of the heart. An electrocardiogram is essential to guide treatment. Drug therapy requires that an intravenous line be available. The intracardiac route of medication administration is hazardous, and should be used only as a last resort. If asystole is present, administer epinephrine (1:10,000) 0.1 ml/kg intravenously. If this is unsuccessful, give further sodium bicarbonate, and repeat the epinephrine dose. Epinephrine may be repeated every three to five minutes, alternating with bicarbonate. If an intravenous line cannot be established, intracardiac epinephrine should be given (Chapter 13).

If there is a sinus rhythm, but ineffective pump action (electromechanical dissociation), calcium gluconate, calcium chloride, or isoproterenol will frequently stimulate the heart (Table 20-4). Calcium gluconate is administered very slowly, through the IV. Isoproterenol is administered by continuous infusion. Atropine may increase the heart rate if the sinus rhythm is very slow (less than 60).

If ventricular fibrillation is present, electrical defibrillation is indicated when acidosis has been controlled. The initial energy dose is approximately 2 to 4 watt-seconds per kilogram (Table 20-5). If initial electrical conversion is unsuccessful, further sodium bicarbonate is indicated before attempting defibrillation. Propranolol (Inderal®) or phenytoin (Dilantin®) may be used to depress electrical irritability of the heart if frequent ventricular fibrillation is a problem. Frequent ventricular ectopic beats may be controlled with lidocaine (Xylocaine®), administered either as an IV bolus or as a continuous infusion (Table 20-4).

Shock must be treated with intravenous fluids if volume loss is a problem. Persistent hypotension can be controlled with infusion of dopamine.

The stress of cardiorespiratory arrest depletes the amount of circulating and stored glucose in the young infant. Concentrated glucose solution, administered intravenously, may improve the infant's response to resuscitation.

## SHOCK

### BACKGROUND

Shock exists when there is not enough blood circulating to provide adequate oxygen to the brain, heart, kidneys, and liver. It may result from the actual loss of blood or fluid such as in hemorrhage, or dehydration from diarrhea and/or vomiting or burns. Septicemia may cause trapping of blood because of relaxation of the blood vessels, or failure of the cardiac pump. Cardiogenic shock is uncommon in children. In infants

TABLE 20-4. DOSAGE GUIDE FOR PEDIATRIC EMERGENCY DRUGS

### Cardiopulmonary Arrest

| | |
|---|---|
| Sodium bicarbonate ($NaHCO_3$) | 1 mEq/kg IV q 5–10 min |
| Epinephrine, 1:10,000 | 0.1 ml/kg IV, max 5 ml |
| Isoproterenol (Isuprel®) | Add 1 mg to 250 ml $D_5W$ = 4 µg/ml<br>Run at 0.1–0.5 µg/kg/min |
| Calcium gluconate, 10% | 0.1 ml/kg, max 5 ml, slowly |
| Calcium chloride, 10% | 1 ml/kg (20 mg/kg) body weight, max 5 ml, slowly |
| Lidocaine | 0.5–1 mg/kg IV push q 5–10 min or add 1 g to 250 ml $D_5W$ = 4 mg/ml. Begin at 1 mg/min |
| Atropine sulfate | 0.01–0.2 mg/kg, max 2 mg |
| Propranolol (Inderal®) | 0.025–0.1 mg/kg/dose q 5 min, Max 3 mg total |
| Dopamine | Add 80 mg to 250 ml $D_5W$ and give 5–10 µg/min/kg |

### Other Emergencies

| | |
|---|---|
| Seizures<br>  Diazepam (Valium®) | 0.25–0.5 mg/kg IV; max 10 mg<br>3–5 mg/kg IM<br>3–10 mg/kg IV push, slowly |
| Asthma, anaphylaxis<br>  Epinephrine, 1:1000 | 0.01 ml/kg SC q 15 min, max 0.3 ml |
| Hypoglycemia<br>  Glucose (Dextrose) | 1 ml/kg of 50% $D_{50}W$, or 2 ml/kg of 25% $D_{25}W$ (the latter is preferable) |
| Other<br>  Naloxone (Narcan®) | 0.01 mg/kg/dose IV (IM, SC) |
| Other<br>  Furosemide (Lasix®) | 1–2 mg/kg IV q 2 hr |

TABLE 20-5. INITIAL ENERGY SETTINGS FOR DEFIBRILLATION IN CHILDREN

| Type of Patient | Weight (kg) | Watt-Seconds* |
|---|---|---|
| Infant | 0–12 | 25–50 |
| Small child | 12–25 | 100 |
| Large child | 25–50 | 100–200 |

*Alternatively, may estimate at 2–4 watt-seconds/kg

and children, body fluid accounts for a larger proportion of weight than it does in adults. The circulating blood volume is proportionately larger also, although the actual volume is much smaller. A relatively small loss of fluid or blood in an adult could be life-threatening to an infant or small child.

## SIGNS

Signs of shock begin to occur when the circulating blood volume is rapidly reduced by 10 to 20 percent. (In the dehydrated child, this occurs when he has lost approximately 15 percent of his body weight.) The heart rate increases, and the systolic blood pressure is reduced. The pulses feel weak and thready. The peripheral veins and capillaries are collapsed. The skin is pale and ashen, and the extremities are cold and sweaty. Initially, the patient is restless and anxious. As shock worsens, he becomes stuporous, and eventually comatose.

## TREATMENT

Rapid administration of intravenous fluids is the treatment for shock in children, since the problem usually is lack of fluid, rather than pump failure. Establish an intravenous route with the largest needle or catheter possible, and administer Lactated Ringer's solution. The initial dose is 10 ml/kg, given over ten to thirty minutes. This dose can be repeated until shock lessens—that is, the pulse becomes stronger and slower; the blood pressure increases; and the patient becomes more alert.

If large volumes of fluid are necessary to correct shock, albumin or plasma should be used for part of the replacement. In children, this is not usually required unless 20 ml/kg of fluid has been given without improvement in the child's condition.

## THE INJURED CHILD

Injuries are the leading cause of death in children and may be accidental or intentionally inflicted. Fortunately, most trauma involves a single organ system, and is relatively uncomplicated. However, the child with multiple injuries presents a challenge in evaluation and management. A careful, systematic initial approach is the key to successful treatment of the multiply-injured child. Avoid the tendency to concentrate on obvious external injury, and anticipate the presence of life-threatening internal injury. This approach differs little from the adult and is presented in more detail in Chapter 14. When first encountering the child, if he is conscious, approach slowly explaining what is happening and reassure him.

Evaluate the respiratory system first. Assure a patent airway by clearing the mouth and throat of foreign material. Administer oxygen if there is cyanosis and a patent airway. Vomiting is common after childhood injury, and aspiration of vomitus (or a dislodged tooth) will complicate the patient's recovery. If there is external chest bruising or abrasion, suspect pneumothorax or hemothorax. Pneumothorax and hemothorax can occur without rib fracture in children. Decreased or absent breath sounds on one side of the chest, tracheal shift, and a shift in the location of the heart sound to the other side in a child with respiratory distress are signs of a tension pneumothorax. Relief of a tension pneumothorax is described in Chapter 14. Multiple rib fractures causing collapse of the chest wall with inspiration (flail chest) may require assisted ventilation and sandbag stabilization of the chest.

Control any obvious external bleeding, since a relatively small volume of blood loss is significant for the small child. Assume shock in a pale child who has a rapid, weak pulse, and administer intravenous fluids. Shock in the absence of serious external bleeding suggests hemorrhage in the abdomen or chest. The restlessness and rapid pulse of the shocky child is often erroneously attributed to fear and pain. If the situation is unclear, infuse 5 ml/kg of Lactated Ringer's over ten to fifteen minutes. If the child improves, the blood volume is low, and more fluid is indicated.

Next, evaluate the central nervous system. Examine the head for swelling, lacerations, and deformity. A severe scalp laceration can bleed enough to cause shock in the infant. Note the level of consciousness, and evaluate the pupils, muscle tone, reflexes, and response to pain. If the fontanelle is open, check for bulging. Loss of consciousness is evidence of a head injury. Head injuries do not cause shock, and shock does not cause coma unless death is imminent.

If the child is conscious, check for neck pain, tenderness, and voluntary movement of the neck and extremities. If the child is comatose, assume a neck as well as a head injury.

Proceed with a more detailed inspection of the entire body, noting bruises, lacerations, and swelling, which offer clues to underlying injuries. If external injuries are concentrated on one side of the body, suspect chest and abdominal injuries on the same side.

Inspect the abdomen for distention. This may be difficult to appreciate in the child under three years, because the abdomen usually protrudes somewhat. When the abdomen is palpated, rigidity or tenderness is consistent with hemoperitoneum. Rigidity of the abdomen in the comatose child signifies injury, unless the child has generalized rigidity.

Most blunt trauma to the abdomen causes a rupture of the spleen or a laceration of the liver, with bleeding. A rupture of the bowel or bladder can also occur. Bulging and tenderness of the flank suggest a kidney injury, with bleeding. Insertion of a nasogastric tube may relieve abdominal distention and increase the child's comfort.

Splint any suspected fractures or dislocations. Do not administer pain medications, since they tend to mask signs of further shock and central nervous system deterioration. Attempt to maintain normal body temperature, especially in an infant. If a neck injury is likely, transport the child on a backboard, with the neck slightly extended and immobilized with a cervical collar. Reassess the child's general condition and measure vital signs frequently during transport.

## THE UNCONSCIOUS CHILD

Coma (unconsciousness from which the patient cannot be aroused) may be caused by central nervous system disorders (injury, infection, seizure, tumor), or by a variety of generalized disorders. Common causes of unconsciousness in children include head trauma, shock, drug intoxication, seizures, and severe infections (meningitis, septicemia).

Initially, assess and support ventilation and circulation. Note the pattern of respiration, as well as its rate. Administer oxygen, and assist ventilation if necessary. If the child is in shock, establish an intravenous route, and administer fluids rapidly. Control any visible bleeding.

Although hypoglycemia is a relatively uncommon cause of coma in children, it can be treated successfully in the field. Administer 25 percent or 50 percent dextrose (glucose) intravenously (Table 20-4). (A Dextrostix® determination can be useful—readings below 45 mg percent are significant.)

After ventilation and circulation are supported, further assessment of the child should be performed. Measure the temperature; then maintain a normal temperature. Assess the pupils for size, equality, and reactivity to light. Check the fontanelle of the young infant for bulging. Inspect for signs of injury, and determine the response to pain. Check the muscle tone (floppy, normal, stiff) and reflexes.

Abnormalities limited to one part of the body, increased muscle tone (stiffness), overactive reflexes, pathologic reflexes, bulging fontanelle, and pupil inequality suggest primary central nervous system disorders, usually with increased pressure. Decreased muscle tone (floppiness), weak or absent reflexes, and lack of localized abnormalities suggest a generalized problem.

As soon as the child is stable, transport to a receiving hospital. If a head injury is possible, assume a neck injury also, and transport the child on a backboard, with the neck in slight extension and immobilized with a cervical collar.

## SEIZURES IN CHILDHOOD

### BACKGROUND AND CAUSES

Seizures or convulsions occur at any age and are among the most common problems for which field assistance is requested. Most convulsions in children are short, generalized, and stop spontaneously without specific treatment; however, a few are prolonged and require therapy.

A seizure is characterized by intense electrical activity in the brain, which causes repetitive jerking movements of the body, and is associated with relative or complete absence of adequate ventilation (Chapter 16). Several causes of seizures, such as fever, are unique to childhood; and others, such as meningitis and shigella infections, are more common in children than in adults. Convulsions are also associated with head trauma, idiopathic epilepsy, and various metabolic disturbances.

Febrile convulsions occur in children between the ages of six months and six years. Approximately half of the children who have had one febrile convulsion are at-risk for further convulsions. Some children with idiopathic epilepsy experience their first seizure in association with fever. The typical febrile seizure is short (less than ten to fifteen minutes) and stops with specific treatment. Fever should be suspected as the cause of seizure in the infant or child whose temperature is over 103°F. A convulsion caused by shigella infection initially may look identical to a febrile seizure, since children with this disease often have a high fever. These children usually have had diarrhea for several hours or days before the seizure, however. Central nervous system infections such as meningitis and encephalitis should be suspected if the child has been feverish and either lethargic or irritable for a time before the seizure, and is found to have a full or bulging fontanelle following the seizure. (The fontanelle will bulge during the convulsion whether or not there is a central nervous system infection.)

## TREATMENT

1. The convulsing child should be assessed quickly to determine whether or not ventilation and cardiac function are adequate. Vomitus or other foreign material in the mouth or throat should be removed. Oxygen should be administered whether or not the child is cyanotic, and the child should be placed on his side with his head slightly lowered to prevent aspiration. If the upper airway appears to be obstructed, an oral airway may be inserted, although this is seldom necessary. Insertion of a tongue blade between the teeth is generally useless and wastes time. History should be obtained on the length of the seizure, prior symptoms and medications, and whether or not there have been prior seizures.

2. The vital signs, including temperature, should be measured and recorded initially and at frequent intervals afterward. If the temperature is above 103°F, cooling measures, including the removal of all clothing and the use of lukewarm wet cloths, should be started. Since hypoglycemia is the most immediately treatable metabolic cause of seizures, a Dextros-tix$_®$ determination of blood sugar should be made. If the reading is less than 45 mg percent, a blood specimen should be drawn when possible for later measurement of true blood sugar, and an intravenous infusion begun. Fifty percent glucose should be administered immediately and

the infusion should be continued with a solution containing 5 percent glucose (Table 20-4).

3. Seizures which persist despite the above measures may be treated with intravenous (not intramuscular) diazepam (Valium®), administered slowly. The use of this or any other anticonvulsant must be accompanied by careful monitoring of the child's cardiorespiratory status, since such drugs depress respiration. If diazepam fails to control or stop the seizure, the patient should be transported to a receiving hospital without delay.

4. Febrile seizures, or other seizures associated with fever, usually stop with control of the fever alone. For seizures that do not respond to cooling within ten to fifteen minutes, some physicians prefer to use intramuscular phenobarbital rather than diazepam. An effect is usually seen in ten to fifteen minutes. Some physicians order phenobarbital as a preventive measure for the child who has had a seizure (even if the seizure has already stopped). When any intramuscular drug is given to control seizures, the possibility of respiratory arrest must be carefully considered. Therefore, some physicians now feel that seizures should be treated by an intravenous anticonvulsant medication rather than intramuscular. Although this point is not entirely agreed upon at the present time, the use of intramuscular anticonvulsant medication in the field is still a quite acceptable procedure.

Immediately following, and up to several hours after a seizure, a child may have unusual and changeable neurologic findings. These changes are part of the expected postictal state, and make evaluation of underlying causes difficult. This usually is more of a problem for the receiving hospital personnel than it is for the paramedic in the field.

## ACUTE RESPIRATORY EMERGENCIES OF CHILDHOOD

Among the most common medical emergencies encountered in a child are those involving the respiratory tract. The most life-threatening of these are characterized by obstruction or blockage of the airway, resulting in failure of adequate air exchange. The clinical picture of the child with respiratory obstruction differs depending on both the level of obstruction and its severity.

### UPPER AIRWAY OBSTRUCTION

Obstruction above, at, or just below the vocal cords causes more difficulty with inspiration than with expiration. The child with this condition usually exhibits stridor (a "crowing" sound with inspiration), a harsh barking cough, dyspnea (labored breathing), flaring of the nostrils, and retraction above the sternum and clavicles and of the chest wall. He is usually agitated. Mild or moderate obstruction can usually be assumed if stridor is loud; the severely obstructed child makes little, if any, noise and appears severely air-hungry and cyanotic. Air exchange to the lungs is either diminished equally from side to side, or absent. Stridorous noises may or may not be audible over the lung fields.

Obtaining accurate historical information is vital in determining the cause of the blockage. Elicit information regarding the time of onset of symptoms, activity of the child immediately prior to the difficulty, presence or absence of fever, and whether or not the child's condition is worsening, stable, or improving. Determine what has been done for the child prior to your assessment.

*Foreign Bodies.* The sudden onset of symptoms and signs of upper airway obstruction in any child over the age of six months who has had no previous problem should immediately suggest the probability of aspiration of a foreign body. The history may be useful in confirming this suspicion, although most children have not been observed directly at the time of aspiration. Correct and prompt performance of back slaps with the infant prone on the forearm and a child prone on the thigh can dislodge a foreign body. If this is not successful, visual and manual exploration of the mouth and throat may be tried. Forceps of any kind should never be used to probe for foreign bodies unless there is direct visualization of the area being explored, since serious damage may result. Failure to remove a suspected foreign body in a deteriorating child necessitates prompt establishment of an airway, with cricothyrotomy if necessary (Chapter 9). Immediately transport once an airway has been established and vital signs are present. Since bradycardia is an indication of hypoxia in the infant or child, the heart rate should be monitored continuously.

*Epiglottitis.* A life-threatening infection that causes upper airway obstruction is epiglottitis, a disease in which the severely inflamed and swollen epiglottis obstructs the larynx. This infection occurs most often in children between two and four years of age, although older children may be affected. Signs of illness appear at least several hours before severe obstruction develops and include fever, sore throat, muffled voice, and reluctance to swallow. As the epiglottis becomes progressively inflamed and swollen, difficulty with breathing occurs. The child has a fever, usually over 102° F, appears very ill and anxious, and prefers to sit up, leaning forward to breathe. His breathing is shallow, and stridor is relatively soft or inaudible, although retractions are moderate or severe. He refuses to swallow liquids and usually drools. This child is at-risk for sudden and complete upper airway obstruction and death. The use of tongue blades and oropharyngeal airways is contraindicated. Manipulation and examination of the mouth and throat should be avoided in order to prevent gagging and resultant airway obstruction by the swollen epiglottis. Emergency care of the child with epiglottitis should include the administration of oxygen by mask or nasal prongs, if tolerated. Transport the child quickly but calmly to a receiving hospital, allowing him to remain in his most comfortable position and without restraint, if possible. Be prepared to assure an airway by a cricothyrotomy at any time, should sudden obstruction occur. Bag-and-mask ventilation is impossible with this condition, and successful orotracheal intubation after complete obstruction is rarely possible. The treatment goal in the field should be to transfer the ill child safely and quickly to a receiving hospital prior to complete obstruction, in order that an appropriate airway (endotracheal tube or tracheostomy) can be placed under controlled conditions, and necessary antibiotic therapy given.

*Croup.* By far, the leading cause of upper airway obstruction in infants and small children is "croup," a term used for several disorders with similar signs and symptoms. The most common of these disorders appears very much like laryngitis in an older person. A respiratory infection, usually viral in origin, causes swelling of the vocal cords and all immediately adjacent structures except the epiglottis. The child with croup is typically between six months and three years of age, and has had symptoms of a "cold" for one to two days. Fever, if present, is minimal, and the child does not seem seriously ill. He awakens at night crying hoarsely, and has a barking cough and loud stridor. Although he makes frightening noises, he exchanges air well and is usually only mildly to moderately obstructed. Although consideration must be given to the possibility of either foreign body aspiration or epiglottitis, the "croup syndrome" is relatively easy to recognize. Most attacks (and the child may have several) respond to the administration of humidified air. Only rarely does a child with croup require endotracheal intubation or tracheostomy. The child with croup should be transported to a receiving hospital for evaluation.

*Injuries.* Injuries to the face and neck can produce upper or lower airway aspiration of blood and tissue, as can direct injury to the laryngeal area. When injury is suspected, it is important to palpate the neck for crepitation due to escaped air and to clear the airway of debris. Treatment of these injuries is the same as in adults (Chapter 14). An anaphylactic reaction may be manifested by laryngospasm and edema, with obstruction. This problem, although unusual in children, can occur with ingestion of foods to which the child is allergic, exposure to drugs, or stings by certain bees or insects. Treatment includes the administration of subcutaneous epinephrine, assurance of an airway, ventilation, and treatment for shock, if present.

*Structural Abnormalities.* A newborn infant may manifest upper airway obstruction because of structural abnormalities. The most serious of these is choanal atresia, a malformation in which the nasal passages are blocked. Because an infant breathes almost exclusively through the nose for the first several months, an affected newborn will show respiratory distress and cyanosis within an hour or so of delivery. This distress is profound when the infant is quiet but disappears when he cries. Insertion of an oropharyngeal airway is lifesaving until definitive treatment can be accomplished. Structural disorders of the oral cavity, larynx, and trachea may also produce obstructive symptoms; although these problems are usually suspected, evaluated, and treated prior to the infant's release from the hospital.

## LOWER AIRWAY OBSTRUCTION

Airway obstruction within the chest cavity, including the lower trachea, results in difficulty with expiration more than with inspiration, because the airways tend to collapse slightly with exhalation. The major features of lower airway block include prolonged exhalation, wheezing, dyspnea, nasal flaring, and retractions of the chest wall. The chest diameter is also increased because of air trapped behind the area of obstruction. Air entry is normal or diminished, and breath sounds may be unequal from side to side if the obstruction is unilateral.

Historical information useful in determining the cause and site of obstruction in a child include the type, severity, and progression of signs and symptoms, suddenness of onset, activity immediately before the onset of symptoms, presence or absence of fever, prior similar episodes, history of asthma, and possibility of injury. Remember a foreign body can lodge in the distal trachea and give the clinical appearance of asthma.

*Asthma.* The most common "wheezing disease" of childhood is allergic asthma, which primarily affects children over the age of two years, but also may occur in younger children. Attacks are usually recurrent and are related to exposure to a substance or environment to which the child is allergic. Symptoms of coughing, wheezing, and respiratory distress may either appear suddenly and progress rapidly or develop over several hours or days. Fever is minimal or absent. The asthmatic child with moderate or severe obstruction is usually uncomfortable and agitated. He is usually relatively dehydrated as well because of decreased water intake and the increased loss of water from the lungs. In addition to audible wheezing, there may be rales, cyanosis, and pallor.

Assessment of the asthmatic child must include a detailed history of medication intake in the twenty-four hours prior to treatment. Specific attention must be given to the type and dosage of any medications used for the wheezing, from over-the-counter drugs to the use of corticosteroids and inhalers. Only after such information is known is it safe to administer drugs.

*Treatment*

1. Administration of oxygen by mask or nasal prongs.

2. The usual initial treatment for the acute attack is aqueous epinephrine 1:1000, administered subcutaneously (see Table 20-4).

3. Rehydration is indicated and fluids may be given either orally or, preferably, intravenously in the child who is severely distressed and/or vomiting.

4. Administration of bronchodilating drugs by inhalation may be useful.

5. Administration of aminophylline in the field is rarely, if ever, indicated in a child.

6. Sedatives should not be given, since they may mask signs of impending respiratory failure.

7. Heart rate must be monitored and blood pressure and respiratory rate measured repeatedly during field observation, treatment, and transport.

*Bronchiolitis.*   Bronchiolitis is a disease which may mimic asthma and occurs in young babies between the ages of two months and two years. It also produces lower airway obstruction, but unlike asthma which causes obstruction because of bronchial spasm, the obstruction here is due to inflammation and mucus collection caused by a virus. The infant with bronchiolitis has usually had nasal congestion and a cough with minimal, if any, fever for several days before signs of obstruction become apparent. He is frequently pale or cyanotic, listless (because he is using all his energy for breathing), and profoundly distressed. He breathes rapidly, with poor air exchange. Rales and wheezes are readily apparent and scattered over the lung fields.

*Treatment*

1. Administer oxygen.

2. Monitor for signs of respiratory failure.

3. Institute assisted ventilation if breathing is labored or stops. In contrast to the asthmatic child, this infant usually does not benefit from the administration of epinephrine or bronchodilating drugs. The disease is usually self-limiting.

Certain infants and children suffer from various forms of chronic obstructive pulmonary disease not unlike adults. These children may have acute and life-threatening difficulty with a respiratory infection. Children with advanced cystic fibrosis, severe asthma, and residual disease and damage from prolonged and severe respiratory diseases of the newborn are included in this group. They require recognition and care must be taken to not overhydrate them or allow carbon dioxide rebreathing with a poorly ventilated face mask. Nasal prongs are preferred.

*Pneumonia.*   Pneumonia (inflammation and infection of the lung tissues) is a common childhood illness. The child with pneumonia usually has had symptoms of a "cold" for a short time, then develops fever, cough, and increasing respiratory difficulty. He breathes rapidly, has nasal flaring and retractions of the chest, and may "grunt" with expiration. He appears ill and may be cyanotic. Breath sounds over the lungs are diminished, and unequal if the inflammation is limited to one area. Crackling or bubbling rales might be present, and the pulse is usually rapid. A young infant sometimes breathes irregularly because he becomes exhausted by the effort to breathe.

### Treatment

1. Administer oxygen if cyanosis is present, or if the child is severely distressed.

2. Assisted ventilation with bag and mask might be required if the cyanosis and distress are not improved with oxygen. Move the child to a receiving hospital for definitive treatment as soon as possible.

*Aspirated Foreign Bodies in the Lower Respiratory Tract.*   The young child who aspirates a small object into a main or smaller bronchus has an episode of coughing or choking at the time of aspiration, but then may be relatively free of symptoms for minutes, hours, or days. Foreign bodies such as peanuts, popcorn seeds, screws, and buttons can pass through the larynx and trachea, and then more often than not lodge in the right main bronchus because of its vertical position. Peanuts and similar organic bodies, if present in the bronchial tree for longer than several hours, cause inflammation of the surrounding tissue. The child with such a foreign body usually has symptoms and signs of localized pneumonia. A history of a prior choking episode is important to obtain and should be passed on to the doctor at the hospital.

An "inert" metal or plastic foreign body causes symptoms of lower respiratory obstruction—cough, respiratory distress, wheezing, and sometimes cyanosis. Breath sounds are decreased or absent over the area of obstruction. Wheezing, if present, may be generalized, or localized to the area of blockage. Rarely, a smooth object will shift its position in the chest; the physical findings will change accordingly.

### Treatment

1. If a child has signs of localized lower respiratory obstruction, try to determine if there was a prior choking episode.

2. Administer oxygen by mask if cyanosis is present or distress is severe.

3. Avoid vigorous assisted ventilation if possible, in order to prevent moving a suspected foreign body further into the bronchus.

*Spontaneous Pneumothorax.* Spontaneous pneumothorax occurs occasionally in older children and adolescents. Its symptoms and signs are similar to those in adults, and fortunately the child is usually old enough to communicate that he experienced sudden chest pain and respiratory difficulty. Evaluation for the presence of air under tension is important (Chapter 14). Transport the patient to a receiving hospital without delay.

## CARDIAC EMERGENCIES

Cardiac emergencies are less common in children than in adults and most children who suffer these conditions have underlying serious congenital heart defects. Congenital heart defects are those present from birth. Infants can acquire heart diseases after birth but most commonly these are due to viral or bacterial infections. Coronary artery disease can occur in children due to viral lymph node disease but these cases are rare in the United States. The following is a simplified classification of heart disease for infants or children:

CONGENITAL

| *Cyanosis* | *Congestive Heart Failure* |
|---|---|
| 1. Tetrology of Fallot | 1. Ventricular Septal Defect |
| 2. Transposition of Great Vessels | 2. Anomalous Left Coronary Artery |
| 3. Pulmonary Atresia | 3. Patent Ductus Arteriosis |
| 4. Tricuspid Atresia | 4. Aortic Stenosis |

ACQUIRED

1. Pericarditis (Tamponade)
2. Myocarditis (Viral)
3. Endocarditis

Congenital defects that produce cyanosis can cause sudden death. Defects that produce congestive heart failure may make the infant or child quite sick, but there is usually time to institute treatment and transport the patient. Cyanosis due to congenital heart disease is due to an anatomic defect and not to a lung problem. Therefore, administration of oxygen may not make much difference in the child's clinical condition but should be used.

Any of the cardiac dysrhythmias can affect a child with heart disease. In this child, an abnormal rhythm may be a response to the defect itself, or to medications, especially digitalis. In the otherwise healthy child, a dysrhythmia should suggest drug ingestion, hypoxia, a metabolic or electrolyte disturbance, or a disturbance in blood volume.

1. Sinus tachycardia occurs in a child with fever, anemia, severe anxiety, or impending shock (low blood volume). Recognition and treatment of its cause is paramount. Sinus bradycardia occurs in normal children, but in the ill or injured child it may be associated with (1) severe shock, (2) increased intracranial pressure or brainstem injury, and (3) severe hypoxia. Again, recognition and vigorous treatment directed at the cause of the problem is critical for survival. In the newborn or very young infant, bradycardia may follow vigorous suction of the mouth, throat, and stomach. Although this rhythm usually is transient, the procedure should be stopped temporarily.

2. Paroxysmal supraventricular tachycardia, especially when seen in normal children, frequently stops without therapy, and is surprisingly well-tolerated. If it continues for over twelve hours, however, congestive heart failure may result. If there is an associated AV block, digitalis overdosage is frequently the cause.

3. Occasional premature ventricular contractions (PVCs) are not uncommon in the child, and do not require treatment. Frequent PVCs, especially in the child with heart disease, may precede a more ominous rhythm—ventricular tachycardia or fibrillation.

*Treatment*

1. Accurate identification of a dysrhythmia must be made by EKG monitoring.

2. Treatment of a supraventricular dysrhythmia should focus on the cause.

3. Ventricular rhythms should be treated promptly if there are changes in vital signs or sensorium. However, because children without underlying heart problems usually tolerate dysrhythmias better than adults do, any treatment should be less risky than the abnormal rhythm itself.

4. Start an intravenous infusion with $D_5W$ and a microdrip. If lidocaine is indicated for premature ventricular tachycardia or ventricular tachycardia, use dose according to Table 20-4.

CONGESTIVE HEART FAILURE

Recognition of congestive heart failure (CHF) can be difficult, especially if the patient is an infant. This condition frequently mimics (and can occur along with) bronchiolitis and pneumonia. The infant or young child has tachypnea, tachycardia, and cyanosis. His heart is enlarged, although this may not be appreciated during the examination. Rales are heard in the lungs if the failure is severe. A heart murmur may be heard over the chest, and gallop rhythm is common. If the abdomen is carefully examined, an enlarged liver will be detected. Edema and distended neck veins are almost impossible to detect in the young infant.

Suspect CHF in the infant or child with respiratory distress and a heart murmur, especially if he has a known heart defect, has had feeding difficulties (tires with eating), and is small for his age.

*Treatment*

1. Administer oxygen by mask, and transport the infant or child in a sitting position if this is more comfortable.

2. If there is pulmonary edema in a child, careful use of rotating tourniquets and intravenous Lasix<sub>®</sub> is indicated. Pulmonary edema is rare in an infant and rotating tourniquets are not used.

## HYPOXIC OR CYANOTIC "SPELLS"

An infant or child with cyanotic congenital heart disease sometimes has episodes of sudden respiratory distress with marked cyanosis. During the "spell," his heart murmur becomes faint, or disappears altogether. Immediate treatment is necessary in order to prevent brain damage or death. The child should be placed in the knee-chest position, and oxygen should be given by mask. Specific treatment includes morphine sulfate and/or propranolol (Table 20-4). Intravenous sodium bicarbonate is indicated for acidosis, and assisted ventilation may be required. Transport the child to a receiving hospital immediately.

## POISONING IN CHILDREN

Children between the ages of eighteen months and three years are especially at-risk for poisoning. Normal curiosity and a relative lack of supervision have major roles in this problem. Older children and teenagers may poison themselves in experimentation with drugs, or in suicide attempts. Most poisoning results from ingestion of toxic substances, although contact may occur through the skin or by inhalation. Drugs, household products, and plants are the most common causes of difficulties.

Poisoning may be suspected in a child with unusual behavior, an altered level of consciousness, vomiting, diarrhea, or a cardiac disturbance. Identify and save any toxic substances, and determine the amount taken, if possible.

1. Any ingested poison should be diluted with water or milk, and removed from the stomach promptly.

2. Vomiting can be induced mechanically, by gagging, or chemically, by administering syrup of ipecac.

3. Emptying the stomach can be effective in removing toxins even if several hours have passed since ingestion, and syrup of ipecac may successfully induce vomiting even if the poison is a drug used to prevent vomiting.

Induction of vomiting is contraindicated in children who are comatose or unusually sleepy, and in those who have ingested acids, caustic substances, and petroleum products (gasoline, kerosene). Vomiting and aspiration of these substances is usually fatal. Removal of poison by lavage is rarely indicated in the field, especially in a comatose child. Children who have swallowed acids, caustics, or petroleum products should be given water or milk to drink and transported immediately. The child should be transported on his side or semiprone.

Very few poisons have specific antidotes. Therefore, the mainstay of treatment is general support. During and after removal of the poison, the patient's status must be monitored closely, and life-threatening complications recognized and treated. (See Chapter 17 for a more complete discussion.)

## MENINGITIS AND SEPTICEMIA

### MENINGITIS

Meningitis is an infection involving the tissues covering the brain and spinal cord. Infants and young children are more at-risk for developing these infections than adults, and the bacteria that cause this illness are usually different from "adult" bacteria. Most organisms that cause childhood meningitis are the kind normally found in the throats of healthy, or reasonably healthy, individuals; therefore, those who have come in contact with the ill children are not particularly at-risk. Viruses may also cause meningitis, although the disease produced is usually more mild than that caused by bacteria.

An infant or child who has meningitis usually has been ill for several days, frequently with an ear or respiratory infection. He suddenly becomes more ill, usually runs a high fever, and is lethargic or irritable. He refuses feedings and seems generally sick. His fontanelle is full or bulging because of brain swelling and he may have a seizure. (The fontanelle is normally closed after twelve to eighteen months of age.)

SEPTICEMIA

Septicemia, or generalized infection of the bloodstream, is another problem more common in children than adults. The child may have been ill for several days, or he may get sick suddenly. His symptoms are similar to those of the child with meningitis, although his fontanelle is usually normal. He may be in shock.

Both septicemia and meningitis are diagnoses that require laboratory confirmation. They can be suspected, however, in a child who is very ill. Field care should include only the recognition that the child is very ill and the administration of necessary cardiorespiratory or circulatory support. Time should not be spent on further evaluation. These children should be transported to a receiving hospital promptly for diagnosis and definitive treatment.

## INTRAVENOUS THERAPY

The intravenous route is the most effective way to administer the medications used in emergencies, and the only way to deliver fluids to a patient who is in shock. In a child, an intravenous line must be established to treat cardiopulmonary arrest, shock, and prolonged seizures. A "keep-open" line is reassuring is almost any field situation.

Although the basic technique of starting an IV is the same regardless of the age of the patient, the procedure can be difficult in infants and very young children. The peripheral veins are small, and tend to be fixed deeply after a tourniquet has been applied, unless the child is in shock. Intravenous lines can be placed in the veins of the hands, feet, arms, scalp, and neck. Search for the largest accessible vein, and insert the largest possible intravenous catheter or scalp vein needle (Figure 20-5).

The veins located along the forehead and temporal areas are useful in infants less than 1 year of age, because they are very superficial, and usually covered by little hair. A rubber band can be stretched around the head just above the eyebrows to distend the veins. Take care that the bore of the needle is pointed toward the face or neck (down), and release the rubber band before running fluid, because the veins are very fragile. Use a 21 or 23 gauge scalp vein needle.

The veins on the tops of the hands and feet are usually large enough to admit a 21 or 23 gauge scalp vein needle. In older children (4 years or older), an adult needle with a plastic sheath (Chapter 7) can be used. Look particularly at the top of the hand between the fourth and fifth metacarpal bones. If the veins of the arms or legs are used, it is critical that the extremity be fixed to an armboard, and the needle be taped securely so that the IV is not dislodged.

If the patient is in shock, attempt to insert a 20 gauge cannula

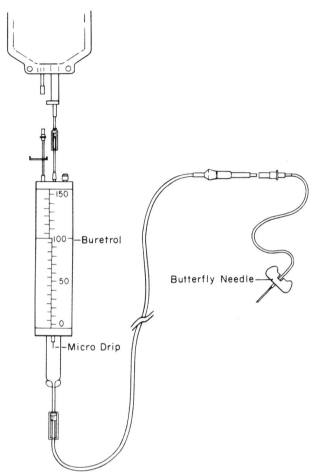

**Figure 20-5.** A typical intravenous set for a child. The butterfly or scalp vein needle is shown. A microdrip chamber is used in infants and small children, but a macrodrip chamber may be used in older children when a large volume of fluid is to be given rapidly.

into the large vein in the antecubital fossa. If this is impossible, and there are no other immediately accessible sites, insert a cannula into the external jugular vein. Use of the jugular veins should be limited to immediately life-threatening situations when no other site can be used.

The choice of fluid to be administered is determined by the child's clinical problem. Except during the first few days of life, when 10 percent dextrose in water is used, IV fluids administered to children should contain saline. "Keep open" IVs can be maintained with $D_5W/0.2$ NS. The dehydrated child should receive $D_5W/0.45$ NS, $D_5W/NS$, or Lactated Ringer's. Administer Lactated Ringer's, $D_5W/NS$, or albumin to the child in shock.

The quantity of fluid given depends upon the size of the child. Control the volume given by inserting a small chamber (Buretrol, Volutrol, Solu-set) between the large bottle and the child, to prevent fluid overload (Figure 20-5). For shock, the correct volume of fluid is "enough." The initial rate in dehydrated or burned children can be as much as 10 ml/kg/hour. For other children, limit the infusion to 5 ml/kg/hour (Chapter 7).

*Summary*

The general approach to the care of the ill or injured child is similar in principle to that of the adult. However, accurate evaluation and adequate treatment in an emergency depends upon an appreciation of the child's difference in size, physiologic function, and susceptibility to various diseases and injuries.

*Important*
*Points to*
*Remember*

Treatment of the infant, child or adolescent presents special problems. Special attention must be paid to both physiologic and psychologic aspects of the condition.

When assessing and treating a child who is ill or injured, the age, size, and developmental level must be considered.

Most information about the child under five is obtained from adults, usually the parents.

Assessment should focus on how the child behaves, rather than how he says he feels.

Unless immediate resuscitation is needed, approach the child gently and slowly.

Children with illness or injury change rapidly—thus repeated observations and evaluations guide subsequent actions.

The soft spot (anterior fontanelle) of a baby under 1 year is useful in evaluation for increased intracranial pressure or dehydration.

Occasionally the child's behavior and symptoms may be contradictory to the seriousness of the illness or injury. Children who are ill or injured may have gastrointestinal disturbances, even when the primary problem lies elsewhere.

Some children may be too difficult to assess or treat in the field; in these cases rapid transport is indicated after assurance of vital functions (breathing, circulation, and hemorrhage control).

The sudden infant death syndrome remains a great problem. These are usually infants under six months (may be a year or older though) who may have been healthy or have had a mild cold and are found dead in their crib.

In sudden infant death cases the parents deserve immediate and sympathetic attention. Guilt feelings must be dealt with in a positive manner. Field personnel should see to the notification of the police and coroner.

Physical abuse should be considered anytime a child has been injured and the cause is not obvious.

All fifty states have laws that require any professional who deals with children to report suspected child abuse.

Child abuse is a problem of the child, family, and society. It usually occurs in a crisis situation where there is an adult with the potential and a child at-risk.

Most child abusers have usually been abused themselves and have many psychological and social problems.

Types of injuries that may lead one to think of abuse include:

1. Fracture (or suspect) in child under two
2. Injuries in different stages of healing
3. More injuries than similar age children
4. Injuries in many parts of body
5. Bruises or burns in patterns suggesting pain infliction
6. Suspected increased intracranial pressure in infant
7. Suspected intra-abdominal trauma in young child
8. Any injury not fitting the description of its cause.

Treatment of the abused child is the same as for other trauma. It is also critical to transport and accompany these children to the hospital. A sympathetic approach to parents of abused children is warranted to maintain cooperation and acknowledge anguish.

Short Term Goal: Treat the injured and protect from further abuse.

Long Term Goal: Treat the family to reduce risks for future abuse.

Cardiorespiratory arrest in children is usually due to acute airway obstruction, shock, and central nervous system depression.

Principles of resuscitation are the same in infants and children as in adults:

Establish open airway

Ventilate patient

Begin closed-chest massage

Correct acidosis

Support circulation

Respiratory rates for resuscitation are:

Infants—16 to 20/min

Children (one to five)—16 to 20/min

Children (over five)—10–12/min.

Closed-chest massage in children differs from adults (see text for details).

Rate of massage is:

Infants: 80–100/min

Young child: 80–100/min

Older child: 80/min

The control of circulation, acidosis and other aspects of CPR are covered elsewhere. See text for comparison in children.

Shock in children usually results from actual loss of blood or fluid and septicemia. Cardiogenic shock is uncommon in children.

Since body fluid accounts for a larger proportion of weight in children, a relatively small loss of fluid or blood is much more dangerous than in adults. Treatment of shock usually involves rapid administration of intravenous fluid. Lactated Ringer's in a dose of 10 ml/kg over 10 to 30 min is given at first and may be repeated.

Most convulsions (seizures) in children are short, generalized, and stop spontaneously. A few are prolonged and require therapy.

Fever is a common cause of seizures in children. They occur from six months to six years of age. Fifty percent of children who have one febrile seizure have subsequent ones.

Other causes of seizures are meningitis, metabolic disorders, shigella infection, head trauma, and epilepsy.

Treatment of convulsions includes:

1. Assessment of ventilation and cardiac function
2. Remove foreign material from mouth
3. Place on side with head lowered
4. Administration of $O_2$
5. Airway insertion if obstructed (tongue blades should not be used)
6. History of prior seizures and medication should be obtained
7. Vital signs measured and monitored
8. Cooling for temperature over 103°F
9. Dextrostix® (if below 45 percent, gives 50 or 25 percent glucose IV)
10. If seizures persist, give IV Valium® (some physicians use IM phenobarbital)
11. Transport if seizures persist

Respiratory emergencies in children are usually characterized by obstruction or blockage of the airway. Obstruction above or just under the vocal cords causes inspiratory difficulty. The child usually exhibits stridor ("crowing" inspiration); a harsh, barking cough; dyspnea; retraction; and flaring of nostrils.

Causes of upper airway obstruction include:

Foreign bodies

Croup

Epiglottitis

Injuries

Structural abnormalities

Obstruction within the chest cavity causes more expiratory difficulty than inspiratory. The child exhibits wheezing, dyspnea, flaring, and retractions.

Causes of lower airway obstruction include:

Asthma

Bronchiolitis

Pneumonia

Foreign body

Spontaneous pneumothorax

Treatment of asthma in children includes:

1. Oxygen by mask or nasal prongs
2. Aqueous epinephrine 1:1000
3. Rehydration
4. Bronchodilating drugs by aerosol
5. Monitor vital signs
6. Transport

Cardiac emergencies are less common in children and most who suffer these conditions have underlying serious congenital heart defects.

Congenital heart disease includes:

Tetrology of Fallot ⎫
Transposition of great vessels ⎬ Cyanotic
Pulmonary atresia ⎪
Tricuspid atresia ⎭

Ventricular septal defect ⎫
Patent ductus arteriosus ⎬ Noncyanotic
Aortic stenosis ⎭

Acquired heart disease:

Pericarditis

Myocarditis (viral)

Endocarditis

Cardiac dysrhythmias commonly seen in children include:

Sinus tachycardia (anemia, fever, anxiety, shock)

Sinus bradycardia (shock, increased intracranial pressure, hypoxia, brainstem injury)

Paroxysmal supraventricular tachycardia (mostly in normal children or secondary to digitalis overdose)

Premature ventricular contractions are not uncommon and except when frequently experienced in children with heart disease do not need treatment.

Meningitis is an infection involving the tissues covering the brain and spinal cord.

Infants and children who have meningitis show the following:

1. Sick several days with upper respiratory infection
2. Become acutely ill
3. High fever, lethargy, or irritability
4. Refusal of feedings
5. Seizure
6. Bulging fontanelle in infant.

Some useful facts on starting intravenous therapy in children:

1. IV lines can be placed in the veins of the hands, feet, arms, scalp, and neck.
2. Insert the largest possible cannula or needle in the largest accessible vein.
3. In infants under 1 year, the veins in the forehead and scalp are useful (use 21 or 23 needle).
4. The veins on the tops of the hands and feet can usually admit a 21 or 23 needle.
5. In older children (4 years or older) an adult cannula is usually used.
6. If shock is present, put a 20 or 22 cannula into the antecubital fossa vein. If impossible, use a catheter in the jugular vein.

Types of IV solutions usually used in children include:

1. "Keep-open"—$D_5W/0.2$ NS
2. Dehydration—$D_5W/0.45$ NS or Lactated Ringer's
3. Shock—Lactated Ringer's, $D_5W/NS$ or albumin.

The quantity of fluid given depends on the size of the child (control by inserting a Buretrol, Volutrol, or Solu-set between large bottle and child.

The initial rate of fluid administration in dehydrated or burned children can be as much as to 10 ml/kg/hr. For other children, limit the rate to 5 ml/kg/hr.

**Bibliography**

Graef, John W. and Thomas E. Cone, Jr. *Manual of Pediatric Therapeutics.* Boston, Mass.: Little, Brown and Company, 1974.

Grosfeld, Jay L., Ed. "Symposium on Childhood Trauma," *Pediatric Clinics of North America.* Vol. 22, May, 1975.

Pasco, Delmer J. and Moses Grossman, Ed. *Quick Reference to Pediatric Emergencies.* Philadelphia, Pa.: J. B. Lippincott Company, 1973.

Smith, Clement A., Ed. *The Critically Ill Child.* Philadelphia, Pa.: W. B. Saunders Company, 1972.

The Surgical Staff, The Hospital for Sick Children, Toronto, Canada. *Care for the Injured Child.* Baltimore, Md.: The Williams and Wilkins Company, 1975.

# RADIO OPERATING PROCEDURES

1. For brevity and reliability, use radio codes (ten-code) and suggested vocabulary. This practice minimizes errors and misunderstandings, and reduces air time. All messages should be as brief as possible, consistent with clarity.

2. Press the transmit switch before you start talking and hold it down until your message is completed. Pronounce words slowly and distinctly. The normal rate of dispatch is approximately forty to sixty words per minute.

3. Emotion tends to distort the voice, making it unintelligible on the radio. Try to keep your voice as emotionless as possible. Keep humor, anger, and impatience off the air. Courtesy is implied and expressions like "thanks" and "you're welcome" are superfluous.

4. Do not guess about questionable messages. Obtain a repeat of any doubtful messages before you acknowledge receipt. This is done by use of 10-9 "entire message," 10-9 "all before," or 10-9 "all after" the part you have received.

5. Always begin instructions with the call sign of the unit for which the instructions are intended; "medic three-one give . . .," "medic five-one push . . ."; DO NOT pronounce call signs as "medic thirty-one," "medic fifty-one."

6. Use accepted, short, clear action verbs to begin transmission of instructions: push, give, prepare and hold. Give orders in standard form: push 1 peds amp bicarb, give intracardiac, 1 amp Epi, piggyback 1 g lidocaine in 2–5–zero $D_5W$.

7. Profane or obscene language is forbidden. Intentionally interfering with another transmission and use of false identifiers are also forbidden.

# RADIO CODES

| | |
|---|---|
| 10-1 | Receiving transmission poorly. |
| 10-2 | Receiving transmission clearly. |
| 10-4 | O.K.; I understand; acknowledge your transmission. |
| 10-5 | Relay information. |
| 10-7 | Not working, subject to call. |
| 10-8 | Unit working, in service. |
| 10-9 | Repeat last transmission. |
| 10-11 | Speak more slowly. |
| 10-19 | Return or returning to base station. |
| 10-20 | What is your location? |
| 10-21 | Call by telephone. |
| 10-22 | Cancel last message. |
| 10-23 | Stand by, do not transmit until I call you back. |
| 10-33 | Stand by for emergency communication. |
| 10-97 | Arrived on the scene. |
| 10-98 | Finished last assignment. |
| 901-K | Ambulance dispatched. |
| 901-N | Ambulance needed. |
| 901-Y | Do you need an ambulance? |
| 902-H | Enroute to the hospital. |
| 914-C | Coroner needed. |
| 914-D | Physician needed, or physician. |
| 914-O | Refuse order. |
| 914-Q | Question medical/nursing orders. |
| 954 | Leaving the radio at the scene. |
| Code 2 | Urgent transport without lights and siren. |
| Code 3 | Emergency transport with lights and siren. |
| URP | Unreliable patient. |
| QDI | Questionable drug ingestion. |

# VOCABULARY

| Use | Do Not Use |
|---|---|
| Advise | Let me know if; can you tell me |
| Affirmative | Yes, uh huh |
| Amp | Ampule, dose, IMS, vial, syringe of |
| Apply | Put on |

| Use | Do Not Use |
| --- | --- |
| Aramine | Metaraminal |
| BP | Blood pressure |
| Bag | Ventilate |
| Begin | Initiate |
| Burn Hydro | Hydrotherapy room |
| Cardiac Care | ICCU |
| Check | Take (VS) |
| Confirm | Is this; did I understand; acknowledge |
| Continue | Keep on with |
| Copy | Receive, interpret, understand |
| CPR | Cardiopulmonary resuscitation |
| Defib | Defibrillate, zap |
| Desire | Want, wish |
| Dextrose | Sugar |
| Digoxin | Dig |
| Epi | Epinephrine |
| ER or ED | Emergency Room or Emergency Department |
| ETA | Estimated time of arrival |
| Fracture | Broken |
| Garbage | Unintelligible EKG tracing; not 60-cycle or motion artifact; may look live V-fib |
| Give | Administer |
| Intensive Care | ICU |
| Intracardiac | IC |
| Isuprel | Isoproterenol |
| IV | Intravenous |
| Maintain | Keep going as is (maintain airway) |
| Monitor | Watch scope |
| Morphine | MS |
| Negative | No, uh uh |
| Neonatal Intensive Care | NICU |
| Normal Saline | NS |
| P (Pappa) Wave | P wave |
| Pearl (PERL) | Pupils equal and reactive to light |
| Pediatric Intensive Care | PICU |
| Piggyback | IVPB |
| Prepare and Hold | Mix this drug but do not administer |

| Use | Do Not Use |
| --- | --- |
| Pulse | Heartbeat, rate |
| Pupils | Eyes |
| Push | IVP |
| Report | Tell me |
| Request | Please |
| Respirations | Breathing |
| Ringer's | Ringer's Lactate |
| Rule Out | See if you can find out if |
| Run | Drip IV |
| Send | Transmit |
| Splint | Immobilize (do not describe splinting) |
| Start | Establish |
| Status | Patient is in |
| Suction | Understood to be done, as needed |
| T (Tango) Wave | T wave |
| Transport | Transfer, take patient to |
| 250 $D_5$ | 250 ml of $D_5W$ |
| 250 $D_5$1/2 Normal Saline | 250 ml $D_5$1/2NS |
| Unable | Can't |
| Understand | Know what you are trying to tell me |
| Valium | Diazepam |
| We | I |

# TABLE OF NORMAL LABORATORY VALUES, WEIGHTS AND MEASUREMENTS

NORMAL VALUES

## HEMATOLOGY

Hematocrit (PCV): Men, 45–52%; women, 37–47%.

Hemoglobin [B]: Men, 14–18 g/100 ml; women, 12–16 g/100 ml.

Red blood count (RBC): Men, 4.5–6.2 million/μ; women, 4–5.5 million/μl.

White blood count (WBC) and differential: 5–10 thousand/μl.

| | |
|---|---|
| Myelocytes | 0% |
| Juvenile neutrophils | 0% |
| Band neutrophils | 0–5% |
| Segmented neutrophils | 40–60% |
| Lymphocytes | 20–40% |
| Eosinophils | 1–3% |
| Basophils | 0–1% |
| Monocytes | 4–8% |

## Chemical Constituents

Amylase: 80–180 units/100 ml (Somogyi*). 0.8–3.2 IU/liter.

Blood Urea Nitrogen (BUN): 20 mg/100 ml.

$CO_2$ Content: 24–29 mEq/liter.

Glucose: 80–120 mg/100 ml.

Lactic Acid: 4–16 mg/100 ml.

*Laboratory method.
Note: Normal laboratory values are subject to variation based on the individual laboratory method.

Osmolality: 285–295 mOsm/kg water.
Oxygen/Arterial PO$_2$ (PaO$_2$): 80–100 mm Hg (sea level).
PaCo$_2$: 35–45 mm Hg.
pH (reaction): 7.35–7.45 (arterial).

*Electrolytes*

Calcium: 4.5–5.3 mEq/liter (varies with protein concentration).
Chloride: 96–106 mEq/liter.
Potassium: 3.5–5 mEq/liter.
Sodium: 136–145 mEq/liter.

## ABBREVIATIONS

### TYPE OF MEDICATION

| | |
|---|---|
| ampule | amp. |
| water | Aq. or H$_2$O |
| capsule | cap. |
| elixir | el. or elix. |
| extract | ext. |
| solution | sol. |
| spirits | sp. or spt. |
| suppository | supp. |
| syrup | syr. |
| tablet | tab. |
| tincture | tr. or tinct. |
| ointment | ung. |

## POUNDS TO KILOGRAMS

| *Lb* | *Kg* | *Lb* | *Kg* | *Lb* | *Kg* | *Lb* | *Kg* | *Lb* | *Kg* |
|---|---|---|---|---|---|---|---|---|---|
| 5 | 2.3 | 50 | 22.7 | 95 | 43.1 | 140 | 63.5 | 185 | 83.9 |
| 10 | 4.5 | 55 | 25.0 | 100 | 45.4 | 145 | 65.8 | 190 | 86.2 |
| 15 | 6.8 | 60 | 27.2 | 105 | 47.6 | 150 | 68.0 | 195 | 88.5 |
| 20 | 9.1 | 65 | 29.5 | 110 | 49.9 | 155 | 70.3 | 200 | 90.7 |
| 25 | 11.3 | 70 | 31.7 | 115 | 52.2 | 160 | 72.6 | 205 | 93.0 |
| 30 | 13.6 | 75 | 34.0 | 120 | 54.4 | 165 | 74.8 | 210 | 95.3 |
| 35 | 15.9 | 80 | 36.3 | 125 | 56.7 | 170 | 77.1 | 215 | 97.5 |
| 40 | 18.1 | 85 | 38.6 | 130 | 58.9 | 175 | 79.4 | 220 | 99.8 |
| 45 | 20.4 | 90 | 40.8 | 135 | 61.2 | 180 | 81.6 | | |

(1 kg = 2.2 lb; 1 lb = 0.45 kg)

In accordance with the decision of several scientific societies to employ a universal system of metric nomenclature, the following prefixes have become standard in many medical texts and journals.

| Symbol | Prefix | Numerical Value |
|--------|--------|-----------------|
| k | kilo- | $10^3$ |
| c | centi- | $10^{-2}$ |
| m | milli- | $10^{-3}$ |
| μ | micro- | $10^{-6}$ |
| n | nano- (formerly millimicro, mμ) | $10^{-9}$ |
| p | pico- (formerly micromicro, μμ) | $10^{-12}$ |
| f | femto- | $10^{-15}$ |
| a | atto- | $10^{-18}$ |

(The prefix nano- is derived from L nanus dwarf; pico- from Sp pico small quantity; femto- from Dan femten fifteen; atto- from Dan atten eighteen.)

## WEIGHTS AND MEASURES

### METRIC MEASURE

| | |
|---|---|
| 1 kilogram | = 1000 grams |
| 1 gram | = 1000 mg |
| 1 milligram | = 0.001 g |
| 1 microgram | = 0.001 mg |
| 1 gamma | = 1 microgram |
| 1 liter | = 1000 ml |
| 1 cc | = 1 ml |

### APOTHECARY WEIGHT

| | |
|---|---|
| 1 scruple | = 20 grains |
| 1 drachm | = 3 scruples |
| | = 60 grains |
| 1 ounce | = 8 drachms |
| | = 24 scruples |
| | = 480 grains |
| 1 pound | = 12 ounces |
| | = 96 drachms |
| | = 288 scruples |
| | = 5760 grains |

### AVOIRDUPOIS WEIGHT

| | |
|---|---|
| 1 drachm | = 27.3 grains |
| 1 ounce | = 16 drachms |
| | = 437.5 grains |
| 1 pound | = 7000 grains |
| | = 16 ounces |

### CONVERSION FACTORS

| | |
|---|---|
| 1 gram | = 15.4 g |
| 1 grain | = 64.8 mg |
| 1 ounce (Av.) | = 28.35 g |
| | = 437.5 g |
| 1 ounce (Ap.) | = 31.1 g |
| | = 480 g |
| 1 pound (Av.) | = 453.6 g |
| 1 kilogram | = 2.68 pounds Ap. |
| | = 2.20 pounds Av. |
| 1 fluidounce | = 29.57 ml |
| 1 fluidrachm | = 3.697 ml |
| 1 minum | = 0.06 ml |

671

| | |
|---|---|
| 1 fluidrachm | = 60 min |
| 1 fluidounce | = 8 fl dr |
| | = 480 min |
| 1 pint | = 16 fl oz |
| | = 7680 min |
| 1 quart | = 2 pt |
| | = 32 fl oz |
| 1 gallon | = 4 qt |
| | = 128 fl oz |

| | |
|---|---|
| 1 teaspoon | = 5 ml |
| | = 1/6 fl oz |
| 1 tablespoon | = 15 ml |
| | = 1/2 fl oz |
| 1 wineglass | = 60 ml |
| | = 2 fl oz |
| 1 teacup | = 120 ml |
| | = 4 fl oz |
| 1 tumbler | = 8 fl oz |
| | = 240 ml |

## CONVERTING °F to °C

For °F to °C, the formula is:

$$5/9 \ (\text{°F minus } 32) = \text{°C}$$

For °C to °F, the formula is:

$$9/5 \ (\text{°C plus } 32) = \text{°F}$$

## DOSE EQUIVALENTS

| Metric Weight | Approximate Apothecary Equivalents | Liquid Measure | |
|---|---|---|---|
| 30 g. | 1 oz. | 1000 ml. | 1 qt |
| 15 g. | 4 dr. | 500 ml. | 1 pt |
| 10 g. | $2\frac{1}{2}$ dr. | 250 ml. | 8 fl oz |
| 6 g. | 90 gr. | 200 ml. | 7 fl oz |
| 5 g. | 75 gr. | 100 ml. | $3\frac{1}{2}$ fl oz |
| 3 g. | 45 gr. | 50 ml. | $1\frac{3}{4}$ fl oz |
| 2 g. | 30 gr. | 30 ml. | 1 fl oz |
| 1 g. | 15 gr. | 15 ml. | 4 fl dr |
| 0.75 g. | 12 gr. | 10 ml. | $2\frac{1}{2}$ fl dr |
| 0.6 g. | 10 gr. | 8 ml. | 2 fl dr |
| 0.5 g. | $7\frac{1}{2}$ gr. | 5 ml. | $1\frac{1}{4}$ fl dr |
| 0.4 g. | 6 gr. | 4 ml. | 1 fl dr |
| 0.3 g. | 5 gr. | 3 ml. | 45 min. |
| 0.2 g. | 3 gr. | 2 ml. | 30 min. |

| Metric Weight | Approximate Apothecary Equivalents | Liquid Measure | |
|---|---|---|---|
| 0.15 g. | $2\frac{1}{2}$ gr. | 1 ml. | 15 min. |
| 0.1  g. | $1\frac{1}{2}$ gr. | 0.75 ml. | 12 min. |
| 60   mg. | 1 gr. | 0.6  ml. | 10 min. |
| 50   mg. | 3/4 gr. | 0.5  ml. | 8 min. |
| 40   mg. | 2/3 gr. | 0.3  ml. | 5 min. |
| 30   mg. | 1/2 gr. | 0.2  ml. | 3 min. |
| 20   mg. | 1/3 gr. | 0.1  ml. | $1\frac{1}{2}$ min. |
| 10   mg. | 1/6 gr. | 0.06 ml. | 1 min. |
| 8    mg. | 1/8 gr. | 0.03 ml. | $\frac{1}{2}$ min. |
| 6    mg. | 1/10 gr. | | |
| 5    mg. | 1/12 gr. | | |
| 4    mg. | 1/15 gr. | | |
| 3    mg. | 1/20 gr. | | |
| 2    mg. | 1/30 gr. | | |
| 1    mg. | 1/60 gr. | | |
| 0.8  mg. | 1/80 gr. | | |
| 0.6  mg. | 1/100 gr. | | |
| 0.5  mg. | 1/120 gr. | | |
| 0.4  mg. | 1/150 gr. | | |
| 0.3  mg. | 1/200 gr. | | |
| 0.2  mg. | 1/300 gr. | | |
| 0.15 mg. | 1/400 gr. | | |
| 0.12 mg. | 1/500 gr. | | |
| 0.1  mg. | 1/600 gr. | | |

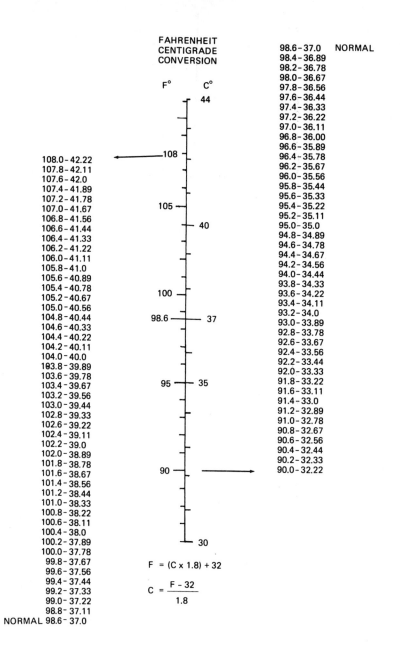

FAHRENHEIT
CENTIGRADE
CONVERSION

F°        C°

| | |
|---|---|
| | 44 |
| 108.0 – 42.22 | ← 108 |
| 107.8 – 42.11 | |
| 107.6 – 42.0 | |
| 107.4 – 41.89 | |
| 107.2 – 41.78 | |
| 107.0 – 41.67 | 105 |
| 106.8 – 41.56 | |
| 106.6 – 41.44 | 40 |
| 106.4 – 41.33 | |
| 106.2 – 41.22 | |
| 106.0 – 41.11 | |
| 105.8 – 41.0 | |
| 105.6 – 40.89 | |
| 105.4 – 40.78 | |
| 105.2 – 40.67 | 100 |
| 105.0 – 40.56 | |
| 104.8 – 40.44 | 98.6 — 37 |
| 104.6 – 40.33 | |
| 104.4 – 40.22 | |
| 104.2 – 40.11 | |
| 104.0 – 40.0 | |
| 103.8 – 39.89 | |
| 103.6 – 39.78 | |
| 103.4 – 39.67 | 95 — 35 |
| 103.2 – 39.56 | |
| 103.0 – 39.44 | |
| 102.8 – 39.33 | |
| 102.6 – 39.22 | |
| 102.4 – 39.11 | |
| 102.2 – 39.0 | |
| 102.0 – 38.89 | |
| 101.8 – 38.78 | |
| 101.6 – 38.67 | 90 → |
| 101.4 – 38.56 | |
| 101.2 – 38.44 | |
| 101.0 – 38.33 | |
| 100.8 – 38.22 | |
| 100.6 – 38.11 | |
| 100.4 – 38.0 | |
| 100.2 – 37.89 | 30 |
| 100.0 – 37.78 | |
| 99.8 – 37.67 | |
| 99.6 – 37.56 | |
| 99.4 – 37.44 | |
| 99.2 – 37.33 | |
| 99.0 – 37.22 | |
| 98.8 – 37.11 | |
| NORMAL 98.6 – 37.0 | |

| | |
|---|---|
| 98.6 – 37.0 | NORMAL |
| 98.4 – 36.89 | |
| 98.2 – 36.78 | |
| 98.0 – 36.67 | |
| 97.8 – 36.56 | |
| 97.6 – 36.44 | |
| 97.4 – 36.33 | |
| 97.2 – 36.22 | |
| 97.0 – 36.11 | |
| 96.8 – 36.00 | |
| 96.6 – 35.89 | |
| 96.4 – 35.78 | |
| 96.2 – 35.67 | |
| 96.0 – 35.56 | |
| 95.8 – 35.44 | |
| 95.6 – 35.33 | |
| 95.4 – 35.22 | |
| 95.2 – 35.11 | |
| 95.0 – 35.0 | |
| 94.8 – 34.89 | |
| 94.6 – 34.78 | |
| 94.4 – 34.67 | |
| 94.2 – 34.56 | |
| 94.0 – 34.44 | |
| 93.8 – 34.33 | |
| 93.6 – 34.22 | |
| 93.4 – 34.11 | |
| 93.2 – 34.0 | |
| 93.0 – 33.89 | |
| 92.8 – 33.78 | |
| 92.6 – 33.67 | |
| 92.4 – 33.56 | |
| 92.2 – 33.44 | |
| 92.0 – 33.33 | |
| 91.8 – 33.22 | |
| 91.6 – 33.11 | |
| 91.4 – 33.0 | |
| 91.2 – 32.89 | |
| 91.0 – 32.78 | |
| 90.8 – 32.67 | |
| 90.6 – 32.56 | |
| 90.4 – 32.44 | |
| 90.2 – 32.33 | |
| 90.0 – 32.22 | |

$$F = (C \times 1.8) + 32$$

$$C = \frac{F - 32}{1.8}$$

674

# CHARTING ABBREVIATIONS

| | | | |
|---|---|---|---|
| a | Before | c/o | Complains of |
| aa | Of each | C-Spine | Cervical |
| abd | Abdominal | c/t | Clot tube |
| ABGs | Arterial blood gases | DC | Discontinue; discharge |
| ac | Before meals | diff | Difficulty |
| a.d. | Right ear | D.M. | Diabetes mellitus |
| ad lib | As desired | DOA | Dead on arrival |
| AMA | Against medical advice | DOE | Dyspnea on exertion |
| amb | Ambulance | dsg | Dressing |
| A.P. | Apical pulse | DTs | Delirium tremens |
| a.s. | Left ear | DU | Duodenal ulcer |
| ASAP | As soon as possible | Dx | Diagnosis |
| a.u. | Each ear | EBL | Estimated blood loss |
| ax | Axillary | EDC | Expected date of confinement |
| bid | Twice a day | | |
| bilat | Bilateral | EEG | Electroencephalogram |
| BP | Blood pressure | EKG (ECG) | Electrocardiogram |
| BS | Bowel sounds | E&R | Equal and reactive |
| BSP | Bowel sounds present | est | Estimated |
| c̃ | With | ETA | Estimated time of arrival |
| cap | Capsule | ETOH | Ethyl alcohol |
| CC | Chief Complaint | F.B. | Foreign body |
| cl | Clear | FHTs | Fetal heart tones |
| CNS | Central nervous system | Flds | Fluids |
| Comp | Compound | FUO | Fever of unknown origin |

NOTE: For cardiac terminology and abbreviations, refer to Table 12-1.

| | | | |
|---|---|---|---|
| Fx | Fracture | MBL | Minimal blood loss |
| G | Gravida | MCA | Motorcycle accident |
| GB | Gallbladder | med(s) | Medication(s) |
| GE | Gastroenteritis | menst | Menstrual |
| GI | Gastrointestinal | ML | Midline |
| GSW | Gunshot wound | mod | Moderate |
| gtt(s) | Drop(s) | MR | Mental retardation |
| GU | Genitourinary | MS | Mitral stenosis; multiple |
| h | Hour | | sclerosis; morphine sulfate |
| h/a | Headache | mult | Multiple |
| HBD | Had been drinking | NAD | No acute distress |
| Hct | Hematocrit | nb | Newborn |
| Hgb | Hemoglobin | NC | Nasal cannula |
| Hosp | Hospital | neg | Negative |
| Ht. | Height | NES | Not elsewhere specified |
| HTN | Hypertension | N/G | Nasogastric |
| HS | At bedtime | NIAL | Not in active labor |
| Hx | History | noc | Night |
| IC | Intracardiac | NOS | Not otherwise specified |
| ID | Intradermal | NPO | Nothing by mouth |
| IM | Intramuscular | NRC | Nearest receiving center |
| IV | Intravenous | NROM | Normal range of motion |
| IVP | IV push | NS | Normal saline |
| IVPB | IV piggyback | NSVD | Normal spontaneous |
| jt | Joint | | vaginal delivery |
| KUB | Kidney, ureter, bladder | N&V | Nausea and vomiting |
| l | liter | -0- | None |
| L | Left | occ | Occasional |
| lac | Laceration | OD | Overdose |
| lg | Large | o.d. | Right eye |
| liq | Liquid | o.s. | Left eye |
| LLE | Left lower extremity | o.u. | Each eye |
| LLQ | Left lower quadrant | P | Pulse |
| LMP | Last menstrual period | p̄ | After |
| LOC | Loss of consciousness | PB | Piggyback |
| L-Spine | Lumbar | p.c. | After meals |
| LUE | Left upper extremity | PD | Police department |
| LUQ | Left upper quadrant | PE | Pulmonary edema |
| m | Murmur | ped | Pedestrian |

| | | | |
|---|---|---|---|
| PEEP | Positive end expiratory pressure | SAH | Subarachnoid hemorrhage |
| PERLA | Pupils equal reaction to light and accommodation | SBO | Small bowel obstruction |
| | | SL | Sublingual |
| | | sl | Slight |
| PMD | Private medical doctor | sm | Small |
| PND | Paroxysmal nocturnal dyspnea | SOB | Shortness of breath |
| | | Sol | Solution |
| P.O. | Postoperative | SQ | Subcutaneous |
| po | By mouth | $\overline{s}$ | Without |
| poss | Possible | S-Spine | Sacral |
| POV | Privately owned vehicle | $\overline{ss}$ | Half |
| PP | Postpartum | SST | Skeletal, stabilization and transport |
| PR | Per rectum | | |
| prn | When necessary, as needed | STAT | Immediately |
| | | Supp | Suppository |
| prox | Proximal | SW | Stab wound |
| pt | Patient | Sx/Sx | Signs and symptoms |
| PTA | Prior to arrival (admission) | Syr | Syrup |
| | | T | Temperature |
| q | Each, every | Tab | Tablet |
| qid | Four times a day | TB | Tuberculosis |
| qod | Every other day | TC | Traffic collision |
| qs | Sufficient quantity | TIA | Transient ischemic attack |
| R | Right; rectal; respiration | tid | Three times a day |
| RBCs | Red blood cells | TIE | Transient ischemic episode |
| RC | Receiving center | | |
| RDS | Respiratory disease syndrome | TLC | Tender loving care |
| | | TPR | Temperature, pulse, respiration |
| re | Regarding | | |
| req | Request | tr | Tincture |
| RLE | Right lower extremity | T-Spine | Thoracic |
| RLQ | Right lower quadrant | Tx | Transport |
| R/O | Rule out | U/A | Urinalysis |
| ROJM | Range of joint motion | u.d. | As directed |
| ROM | Range of motion | UGI | Upper gastrointestinal |
| RSR | Regular sinus rhythm | Unc | Unconscious |
| Rt | Routine | URI | Upper respiratory infection |
| RUE | Right upper extremity | | |
| RUQ | Right upper quadrant | URP | Unreliable patient |
| Rx | Treatment | UTI | Urinary tract infection |

| VD | Venereal disease | WD/WN | Well developed/well |
| WB | Whole blood | | nourished |
| WBCs | White blood cells | WNL | Within normal limits |
| W/C | Wheelchair | wt | Weight |
| | | y/o | years old |

## CHARTING SYMBOLS

| ↑ | Increasing; elevate; up; above | p̄ | After |
| ↓ | Decreasing; down; lower; below | c̄ | With |
| > | Greater than | s̄ | Without |
| < | Less than | = | Equal |
| Ⓛ | Left | − | Negative |
| ® | Right | + | Positive |
| × | Times | | |

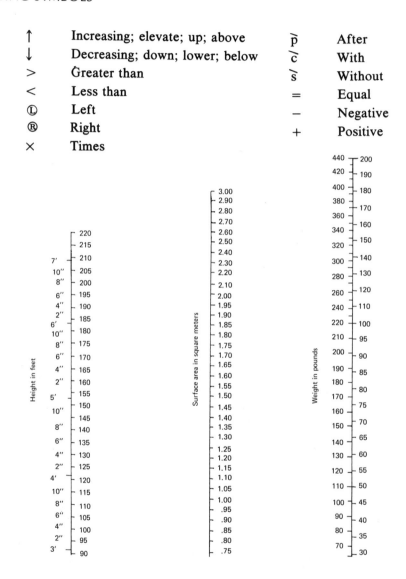

Nomogram for the determination of body surface area of children and adults. (Reproduced with permission from Boothby & Sandiford: Boston MSJ 185:337, 1921.)

American Diabetes Association
New York City, New York
212/697-7760

American Lung Association
New York City, New York
212/245-8000

American Association of Zoological Parks and Aquariums
Antivenin Index Center
Oklahoma City, Oklahoma
405/271-5454
24 hour, 7 day/week information regarding the availability of antivenom
for venomous snake bites from native and exotic species.

Center for Disease Control
Atlanta, Georgia
404/633-3311 (Day)
404/633-2176 (Night)

Epilepsy Foundation of America
Washington, D.C.
202/293-2930

Intermountain Regional Poison Control Center
Salt Lake City, Utah
801/581-2151
Information concerning poisonous plant ingestions

National Center for Prevention of Child Abuse
Denver, Colorado
303/321-3963

National Institute of Drug Abuse
Rockville, Maryland
301/443-2954

National Sudden Infant Death Syndrome Foundation
Chicago, Illinois
312/663-0650

The Soap and Detergent Association
New York City, New York
212/725-1262

U.S. Navy Experimental Diving Unit
Panama City, Florida
904/234-4351 (24 hour emergency hotline)
The Unit will supply the name and telephone number of the nearest
hyperbaric unit.

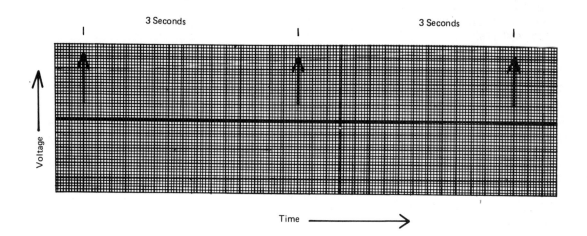

1 small square = 1 mm
1 large square = 5 mm
2 large squares = 10 mm = 1 mv
1 mv = standardization

25 mm/sec = running speed
 1 mm = 1 small square = 0.04 sec
 5 mm = 5 small squares = 1 large square = 0.2 sec
25 mm = 25 sm sq = 5 large square = 1.0 sec

*To Calculate Rate:*

1.  If rhythm is irregular, count the number of complexes in 6 seconds or 15 cm (150 mm) and multiply by 10.

    150 mm = 150 sm sq = 15 lrg sq = 6 sec
    150 mm = 15 cm = 6 in

2.  If rhythm is regular:

    A.  Count the number of small squares between two complexes and divide this number into 1500.

    B.  Count the number of large squares between two complexes and divide this into 300.

    C.  Rapid estimate can be made by counting the number of large squares between two complexes. One large square = 300; 2 large squares = 150; 3 large squares = 100.

# GLOSSARY

**Abduction.** Movement away from the midline.

**Abortion.** Birth of an embryo or fetus prior to the stage of viability (approximately 20 weeks gestation). Note: Infants born after this 20-week period are known as premature.

**Abrasion.** A scraping away of the epidermis of the skin or mucous membrane.

**Abruptio placenta.** Premature detachment of a normally situated placenta.

**Abscess.** A circumscribed cavity containing a collection of pus.

**Abscissa.** One of two coordinates used as a frame of reference. The abscissa (X axis) is the horizontal point coordinate in a plane at right angles to the Y or vertical axis (ordinate). When suitable values have been assigned to each axis, the corresponding data can be plotted.

**Acid.** A compound of an electronegative element or radical with hydrogen; yields hydrogen ion in a polar solvent.

**Acidosis.** A state characterized by actual or relative decrease of alkali in body fluids in proportion to the content of acid.

**Acute.** Of short or sharp force; not chronic.

**Adduction.** Movement of a limb toward the central axis of the body.

**Adipose.** Fatty or relating to fat.

**Aerobic.** Living in air.

**Afferent.** Going toward a center, or bringing to or into a center; denoting certain arteries, veins, lymphatics or nerves.

**Affinity.** Attraction.

**Agonist.** A drug capable of combining with receptors to initiate drug action.

**Albumin.** A type of water-soluble protein with a molecular weight of 68,000. It is located in the vascular space and is a primary component of human blood.

**Alkali.** A strongly basic substance; alkaline in reaction.

**Alkalosis.** Alkaline intoxication; abnormally high alkaline reserves of the blood and other body fluids with a tendency for an increase in the pH of the blood, although it may remain normal.

**Alveolus.** An air cell; one of the terminal sac-like dilatations of the alveolar ducts in the lung.

**Amaurosis fugax.**  A transient episode of monocular blindness lasting 10 minutes or less, usually due to embolization of diseased carotid arteries in the neck.

**Amino acid.**  An organic acid in which one of the hydrogen atoms ($H^+$) has been replaced by ammonia ($NH_3$).

**Ammonia.**  A colorless alkaline gas ($NH_3$) soluble in water which forms $NH_4^+$ when combined with hydrogen ($H^+$).

**Amnesia.**  Loss or impairment of memory; inability to recall past experiences.

**Amniotic fluid.**  The fluid that surrounds the fetus within the amniotic sac. The amount at term varies between 500 and 2000 ml.

**Amputation.**  The cutting off of a limb or part of a limb, the breast, or some other projecting part.

**Anaerobic.**  Living without oxygen.

**Analgesia.**  State of freedom from pain.

**Anaphylaxis.**  Increased sensitivity or hypersensitivity to a toxin or drug.

**Anastomosis.**  An operative union of two hollow or tubulous structures, such as blood vessels.

**Anemia.**  Any condition in which the number of red blood cells or the amount of hemoglobin in blood are less than normal.

**Aneurysm.**  A circumscribed dilation of an artery.

**Angina pectoris.**  Severe constricting pain in the chest, often radiating from the precordium to the left shoulder and down the arm due to ischemia of the heart muscle; usually caused by coronary disease.

**Angioneurotic.**  Denoting spasm or paralysis of the vascular system. Angioneurotic edema is usually the result of swelling due to a vascular disorder.

**Anion.**  An ion that carries a negative charge, going therefore to a positively-charged anode.

**Ano-.**  Relating to the anus.

**Anorexia.**  Diminished appetite or aversion to food.

**Anoxia.**  A decreased amount of oxygen in the organs and tissues.

**Antagonist.**  Something opposing or resisting the action of another.

**Antibiotic.**  A soluble substance derived from mold or bacteria that inhibits the growth of other microorganisms.

**Antibody.**  A body or substance evoked in man or other animals by an antigen in some demonstrable way.

**Anticoagulant.**  A substance that prevents blood from clotting. Two common anticoagulants are Heparin and Coumarin drugs.

**Anticholinergic.**  Antagonist to the action of parasympathetic or other cholinergic nerve fibers.

**Anticonvulsive.**  An agent that tends to prevent or arrest convulsions.

**Antigen.**  Any of various sorts of materials (examples include microorganisms, toxoids, exotoxins, foreign proteins) that, as a result of coming into contact with appropriate tissues of an animal body, after a latent period, induce a state of sensitivity and/or resistance to infection or toxic substances, and will react in a demonstrable way with serum from the sensitized subject.

**Antihistamine.**  A drug whose action is antagonistic to that of histamine. Usually used in treatment of allergic symptoms.

**Aphasia.**  Weakening or loss of the facility of transmission of ideas by language in any of its forms (reading, writing or speaking); or failure in the appreciation of the written, printed or spoken word. This is usually independent of disease of the vocal cords, but due to abnormalities of the appropriate sensory neural apparatus in the brain.

**Apnea.** Absence of respiration.

**Arrest.** Stoppage or interference with, or checking of the regular course of a disease or symptom or the performance of a function. Commonly used to mean a loss of effective cardiac function.

**Arrhythmia.** Any variation from the normal rhythm of the heart beat.

**Arteriole.** A minute artery with a muscular wall; a terminal artery continuous with the capillary network.

**Artery.** A blood vessel conveying blood in a direction away from the heart.

**Ascites.** Accumulation of serous fluid in the peritoneal cavity.

**Asepsis.** The absence of living pathogenic organisms.

**Asphyxia.** Suffocation. Lack of oxygen in the inspired air, resulting in apparent or actual cessation of life.

**Aspiration.** 1. Removal by suction of air or fluid from a body cavity where an unusual collection has accumulated. 2. The inspiratory sucking into the airways of fluid or a foreign body, as in the aspiration of vomitus.

**Atresia.** Term describing structures of the body that have not developed.

**Atrial.** Relating to the atrium of the heart.

**Atrium.** The upper chamber of each half of the heart, which receives the blood from the vena cava and the coronary sinus on the right side, and from the pulmonary veins on the left, and transmits it to the ventricle on the same side.

**Auscultation.** Listening to the sounds made by the thoracic or abdominal viscera, or to sounds in any of the other internal parts of the body.

**Avulsion.** The act of or tearing away.

**Bifurcation.** A forking or division into two branches.

**Bile.** A substance secreted by the liver to aid in digestion. Bile is stored in the gallbladder.

**Biliary system.** The drainage ducts of the liver which carry bile to the duodenum. This system includes the hepatic ducts, gallbladder and common ducts.

**Biotransformation.** The alteration of an ingested drug in the body by enzymes.

**Blackout.** A temporary loss of consciousness due to decreased blood flow to the brain.

**Blood pressure.** The pressure of the blood on the walls of the arteries; dependent on the energy of the heart action, the elasticity of the walls of the arteries, the resistance of the capillaries, and the volume and viscosity of the blood.

**Bolus.** A fairly large amount of a substance, usually a drug, to be taken all at once.

**Brady-.** Prefix meaning slow.

**Bradycardia.** Abnormal slowness of the heart beat as evidenced by slowing of the pulse rate to 60 or less.

**Bronchiole.** One of the finer subdivisions of the bronchial tubes, less than 1 mm in diameter.

**Bronchospasm.** Spasmotic narrowing of the lumen of a bronchus.

**Bronchus.** One of the subdivisions of the trachea serving to convey air to and from the lungs.

**Bruit.** An auscultatory sound or murmur, especially an abnormal one.

**Buccal.**   Pertaining to, or adjacent to the cheek within the mouth.

**Buffer system.**   The ability of the blood to compensate for acid-alkali fluctuations without disturbing the pH.

**Cachectic.**   Term referring to general lack of nutrition and wasting that occurs in the course of a chronic disease or emotional disturbance.

**Cannula.**   A tube that is inserted into a cavity by means of a trochar filling its lumen. After insertion, the trochar is withdrawn, leaving the cannula as a channel for escape of fluid from the cavity.

**Capillary.**   A type of very tiny blood vessel, usually connecting an arteriole to a venule.

**Cardiac.**   Pertaining to the heart.

**Cardiac output.**   The effective volume of blood expelled by either ventricle of the heart per unit of time; equal to the stroke output multiplied by the number of beats per unit of time.

**Cardiogenic.**   Originating in the heart; caused by a condition affecting the heart.

**Carina.**   The point at which the trachea divides into the right and left bronchus.

**Catheter.**   A hollow cylinder or tube designed to be passed through any canal or opening of the body.

**Cation.**   An ion carrying a charge of positive electricity, and therefore going to a negatively-charged cathode.

**Cell.**   The living active basis of all plant and animal organization, composed of protoplasm enclosed in a delicate membrane and containing a nucleus.

**Cerebral.**   Relating to the cerebrum or brain.

**Cervical.**   Relating to the neck.

**Chills.**   A sensation or feeling of cold with shivering and pallor often accompanied by an elevation of temperature in the interior of the body. This is usually a prodromal symptom of an infectious disease due to invasion of the blood by toxins.

**Chronic.**   Of long duration; denoting a disease of slow progress.

**Chronotropic.**   Affecting the rate or time of contraction, especially of cardiac muscle fibers. For example, digitalis is a drug that has a chronotropic effect on the heart.

**Circumduction.**   Movement of a part of the body, such as the eye or an extremity, in a circular direction.

**Clubbing.**   A broadening and thickening of the ends of the fingers, often seen in chronic pulmonary disease.

**Coagulation.**   The process by which a blood clot or thrombus is formed. Generally divided into three stages: (1) the formation of thromboplastin; (2) the formation of thrombin; and (3) the formation of fibrin.

**Colic.**   Spasmotic pains in the abdomen.

**Colloid.**   Aggregates of atoms or molecules in a finely divided state dispersed usually in a liquid medium and resisting sedimentation, diffusion, and filtration (thus differing from precipitates).

**Coma.**   A state of profound unconsciousness from which one cannot be aroused.

**Communicable.**   Capable of being communicated or transmitted; usually pertaining to diseases.

**Compliance.**   The quality of yielding to pressure or force without disruption. When a lung becomes stiffer due to fibrosis, its compliance decreases.

**Concave.**   Having a depressed or hollow surface.

**Condyle.**   A rounded articular surface at the extremity of a bone.

**Conscious.** Aware; having present knowledge or perception of oneself, one's acts and the surroundings.

**Constriction.** Binding or contraction of a part.

**Contraindication.** A drug or therapeutic modality that is not only inappropriate in specific situations, but may also produce harm.

**Contralateral.** Relating to the opposite side.

**Contusion.** A bruise.

**Convex.** A surface that is evenly curved or bulging outward.

**Convulsion.** A violent spasm; often used to describe a seizure.

**Countershock.** Electrical stimulation of the heart to change a rhythm.

**Coronary.** Relating to the vessels supplying the heart muscle.

**Coronary bypass.** Use of artery substitutes to bypass diseased coronary arteries. One to five vessels in the heart can be bypassed to restore normal blood flow to the heart.

**Cricothyrotomy.** The opening of the cricothyroid membrane to gain access to the airway.

**Crystalloid.** A soluble substance, usually a salt, dissolved in a liquid. A common crystalloid solution is Lactated Ringer's.

**Cutdown.** Dissection of a vein for insertion of a cannula or needle for the administration of intravenous fluids or medication.

**Cyanosis.** A dark bluish or purplish coloration of the skin and mucous membranes due to deficient oxygenation of the blood.

**Cystic.** 1. Relating to the urinary bladder or gallbladder. 2. Relating to a cyst. 3. Containing cysts.

**Defecation.** The discharge of excrement from the rectum.

**Defibrillation.** The arrest of fibrillation of the cardiac muscle with restoration of the normal rhythm (accomplished by use of electrical energy).

**Dehydration.** Deprivation of water or reduction of water content.

**Delirium.** A condition of extreme mental and usually motor excitement marked by rapid succession of confused and unconnected ideas, often with illusions and hallucinations.

**Dementia.** General mental deterioration due to organic or psychological factors.

**Depressant.** An agent that lowers nervous or functional activity; a sedative.

**Depression.** 1. A hollow or sunken area, a sinking below the surrounding level. 2. Dejection, a sinking of spirits.

**Derm-.** Prefix signifying skin, or having to do with the skin.

**Dextrose.** A white crystalline powder obtained by the hydrolysis of starch. It is used to make sugar solutions for intravenous therapy.

**Diagnosis.** The determination of the nature of a disease.

**Diaphoresis.** Sweating, especially profuse sweating.

**Diarrhea.** Any abnormally frequent discharge of more or less fluid fecal material from the bowel.

**Diastole.** The dilatation of the heart cavities during which they fill with blood. Alternates rhythmically with systole, or contraction of the heart muscle.

**Diffusion.** The random movement of free molecules, ions or small particles in solution toward a uniform distribution throughout the available volume.

**Digitalis.** A drug originally derived from a plant. This medication improves myocardial contractility and may slow the conduction system of the heart.

**Dilation.** Enlargement of a cavity, canal, blood vessel or opening occurring physiologically, pathologically or artificially.

**Diplopia.** Double vision.

**Discharge.** That which is emitted or evacuated as an excretion or secretion.

**Distal.** Farthest from the center or the median line; farthest from the trunk when referring to the segments of the extremities; opposite of proximal.

**Distend.** Stretch.

**Diuresis.** Excretion of urine; commonly denotes production of unusually large volumes of urine.

**Diuretic.** A substance or agent that increases the amount of urine produced.

**Diverticulitis.** Inflammation of an outpouching of the colon. It is commonly seen in inflammation of the sigmoid colon.

**Dorsiflexion.** Turning the foot or toes upward.

**Dys-.** Prefix meaning bad or difficult.

**Dyspnea.** Subjective difficulty or distress in breathing. Frequently denotes rapid breathing, usually associated with serious disease of the heart or lung.

**Dysrhythmia.** A defective rhythm usually relating to the heart.

**Eclampsia.** Convulsions and coma occurring in a pregnant woman, usually associated with hypertension, edema and/or proteinuria.

**Edema.** An accumulation of excessive amounts of fluid in the cells, tissues or serous cavities.

**Efferent.** Conducting fluid or a nerve impulse outward or centrifugally. Impulses from the brain to skeletal muscles are efferent impulses.

**EKG (ECG).** Abbreviation for electrocardiogram. A graphic tracing of the electric current produced by the contraction of the heart muscle. The normal electrocardiogram shows upward and downward deflections, the result of atrial and ventricular activity. The first upward deflection, P, is due to contraction of the atria and is known as the *atrial complex.* The other deflections, Q, R, S, T, are all due to the action of the ventricles, and are known as the *ventricular complexes.*

**Electrolyte.** Any ionizable substance in solution, such as sodium, potassium, chloride or bicarbonate.

**Embolism.** The obstruction or occlusion of a vessel by a transported clot or vegetation, massive bacteria or other foreign material.

**Emesis.** Vomiting, or having to do with vomiting.

**Emphysema.** An abnormal collection of air in tissues or organs. Pulmonary e. refers to an overinflation of lung tissue with trapping of air in that tissue.

**Encephalopathy.** Neurologic changes that may lead to depression of brain function and even coma. It can be due to high blood pressure or liver failure.

**Endocardium.** The inner lining of the heart.

**Endocrine.** Denoting or relating to a gland that furnishes internal secretions, usually hormones.

**Endotracheal tube.** A plastic tube inserted into the trachea to allow for positive pressure ventilation or the aspiration of secretions.

**Enterocolitis.** An infection or toxic inflammation of the small and/or large bowel.

**Epicardium.** The outside lining of the heart.

**Epidemic.** A disease attacking many people in a community simultaneously, usually coming from outside that community.

**Epistaxis.** Nosebleed.

**Erythema.** Redness of the skin or inflammation due to congestion of the capillaries.

**Ethanol.** Alcohol.

**Eversion.** A turning outward.

**Exacerbation.** An increase in the severity of a disease or any of its signs or symptoms.

**Excretion.** The waste material of a tissue or organ that is to be passed out of the body.

**Exophthalmos.** Protrusion of the eyeballs.

**Exostosis.** A bony tumor or protrusion springing from the surface of a bone.

**Expiration.** 1. The act of exhaling or breathing out. 2. Termination or death.

**Exsanguination.** Blood deprivation; the forcible expulsion of blood from a part.

**Extension.** The act of bringing the distal portion of a joint in continuity with the long axis of the proximal portion, i.e., the straightening out of a joint.

**Extrasystole.** A premature or ectopic beat or contraction of the heart.

**Extravasation.** The act of escaping from a vessel into the tissues of blood, lymph or serum.

**Extremity.** A limb or member; one of the arms or legs.

**Feces.** Excrement; the matter discharged from the bowel during defecation.

**Fever.** A bodily temperature above the normal of 98.6°F.

**Fibrillation.** Exceedingly rapid contractions or twitching of individual muscle fibers, commonly occurring in the atria or ventricles of the heart.

**Fissure.** A furrow, cleft or slit.

**Fistula.** A pathologic or abnormal passage leading from an abscessed cavity or a hollow organ to the surface, or from one abscessed cavity organ to the other.

**Flaccid.** Relaxed, flabby, without tone.

**Flatulence.** The presence of an excessive amount of gas in the stomach and intestines.

**Flexion.** The bending of a joint so as to proximate the parts that it connects.

**Fontanelle.** A soft spot, such as one of the membrane-covered spaces remaining in the incompletely ossified skull.

**Fracture.** A break, especially of a bone or cartilage.

**Fungus.** 1. Any one of a class of vegetable organisms of a low order of development, including mushrooms, toadstools, molds, etc. 2. A growth on the body resembling a fungus, a spongy mass of morbid granulation tissue.

**Gait.** Manner of walking.

**Gangrene.** Necrosis due to obstruction of blood supply.

**Gastric, Gastro-.** Relating to or denoting the stomach.

**Gastrointestinal.** Relating to both the stomach and intestines.

**Genitourinary.** Relating to reproduction and urination; denoting the organs involved in these functions.

**Globulin.** A large protein molecule located in human blood which has many functions, including that of an antibody.

**Glomerulus.** A single unit of the kidney. It is responsible for the filtration of plasma to make urine. There are approximately 1 million glomeruli in each kidney.

**Glycogen.** A sugar form manufactured and stored primarily in the liver. When it is broken down into simpler forms, it provides sugar (energy) for the metabolic functions of tissues.

**Glycolysis.** The breakdown of glycogen into simpler compounds.

**Goiter.** Chronic enlargement of the thyroid gland.

**Gonad.** Testis or ovary.

**Hallucination.** Subjective perception of something that does not exist, or is not there.

**Hallucinogen.** A chemical, drug or agent that produces hallucinations.

**Hematemesis.** Vomiting of blood.

**Hematocrit.** The volume percentage of erythrocytes in whole blood.

**Hematoma.** A localized mass (tumor) of extravasated blood, usually partly clotted.

**Hematuria.** Any condition in which the urine contains blood or red blood cells.

**Hemiparesis.** Slight paralysis affecting only one side of the body.

**Hemiplegia.** Paralysis of one side of the body.

**Hemodialysis.** The removal of certain elements from the blood by virtue of the difference in the rates of their diffusion through a semipermeable membrane.

**Hemoglobin.** The oxygen-carrying pigment of the erythrocytes, formed by the developing erythrocyte in bone marrow. Inactive h. is hemoglobin that does not combine with oxygen. Oxygenated h. is the hemoglobin of arterial blood, combined with oxygen. Reduced h. is the hemoglobin of venous blood, blood that has given up its oxygen in the tissues.

**Hemoptysis.** Pulmonary hemorrhage; the spitting of blood derived from lungs or bronchial tubes.

**Hemorrhage.** Bleeding, especially if it is very profuse.

**Hemostasis.** 1. The arrest of bleeding. 2. The stagnation of blood.

**Hepatic.** Relating to the liver.

**Hepatitis.** Inflammation of the liver, which may be caused by a virus, bacteria or drugs. Hepatitis may produce chronic scarring of the liver and liver failure. Infectious h. is a subacute disease of worldwide distribution; it is caused by a virus and tends to occur in children and young adults. The liver is diffusely enlarged and the symptoms include fever, gastrointestinal distress, headache, anorexia and jaundice. The incubation period varies from one to six weeks. Serum h. is indistinguishable clinically from infectious hepatitis, but is caused by an immunologically distinct virus which is transmitted by inadequately sterilized syringes and needles; by procedures like tatooing; and by administration of infectious blood, plasma or blood products. The incubation period is 8 to 22 weeks.

**Hernia.** The protrusion of an organ or part of an organ or other structure through the wall of a cavity that normally contains it.

**Hives.** *See* urticaria.

**Histamine.** A molecule located in many cells of the body whose functions include: (1) dilation of capillaries; (2) increase of capillary permeability;

and (3) constriction of bronchial smooth muscle. Histamine is released in anaphylactic reactions.

**Homeostasis.**   The tendency to stability in the normal body states. It is achieved by a system of control mechanisms through positive and negative feedbacks.

**Hormone.**   A chemical substance formed in one organ or part of the body and carried to the blood, and thus to another organ or part of the body. Hormones can alter the functional activity and sometimes the structure of just one organ or various numbers of them.

**Hyper-.**   Prefix denoting excessive or above normal.

**Hyperalimentation.**   The ingestion or administration of a greater than optimal amount of nutrients.

**Hypercapnea.**   Excess carbon dioxide in the blood.

**Hyperglycemia.**   Abnormally increased level of sugar in the blood.

**Hyperkalemia.**   Abnormally high level of potassium in the blood.

**Hypernatremia.**   Excess sodium in the blood.

**Hyperpnea.**   Abnormal increase in the depth and rate of the respiratory movements.

**Hypersensitivity.**   1. Abnormally increased sensitivity. 2. The specific or general ability to react with characteristic symptoms to the application or contact with certain substances (allergens) in amounts innocuous to normal individuals.

**Hypertension.**   Abnormally high tension, especially high blood pressure. Benign h. is essential hypertension, which exists for years without producing symptoms. Essential h. is high blood pressure occurring without discoverable organic cause. Malignant h. is essential hypertension with an acute stormy onset, the development of neuroretinitis, a progressive course and a poor prognosis.

**Hyperthermia.**   Abnormally high body temperature; fever.

**Hypertonic.**   1. Pertaining to or characterized by an abnormally increased tonicity or tension. 2. Having an osmotic pressure greater than that of the solution with which it is compared.

**Hypertrophy.**   The morbid enlargement or overgrowth of an organ or part due to an increase in the size of its constituent cells.

**Hyperventilation.**   1. Entrance of an increased amount of air into the pulmonary alveoli, resulting in reduction of the carbon dioxide tension. 2. Abnormally prolonged, rapid and deep breathing, frequently used as a test procedure in epilepsy and tetany.

**Hypervolemia.**   Abnormal increase in the volume of circulating fluid (plasma) in the body.

**Hypo-.**   Prefix denoting a diminution or deficiency of, or a lower than normal level.

**Hypoalimentation.**   Insufficient nourishment.

**Hypocapnea.**   Deficiency of carbon dioxide in the blood (acapnia).

**Hypochondriasis.**   Morbid anxiety about one's health, often associated with a simulated disease and more or less pronounced melancholia.

**Hypoglycemia.**   An abnormally diminished level of glucose in the blood.

**Hypokalemia.**   Abnormally low level of potassium in the blood.

**Hyponatremia.**   Deficiency of sodium in the blood; salt depletion.

**Hypopnea.**   Abnormal decrease in the depth and rate of the respiratory movements.

**Hyposensitive.** 1. Exhibiting abnormally decreased sensitivity. 2. Having the specific or general ability to react to a specific allergen, alleviated by repeated and gradually increasing doses of the offending substance.

**Hypotension.** Diminished tension; lowered blood pressure. Orthostatic h. is lowered blood pressure when changing from a supine to an erect position.

**Hypothermia.** Low temperature; especially a state of low body temperature induced as a means of decreasing metabolism of tissues and thereby the need for oxygen, as used in various surgical procedures, especially on the heart. Endogenous h. is abnormally reduced temperature resulting from physiologic causes, due to dysfunction of the central nervous system or of the endocrine system.

**Hypotonic.** 1. Having an abnormally reduced tonicity or tension. 2. Having an osmotic pressure lower than that of the solution with which compared.

**Hypoventilation.** A reduced amount of air entering the pulmonary alveoli, resulting in elevation of the carbon dioxide tension.

**Hypovolemia.** Abnormally decreased volume of circulating fluid (plasma) in the body.

**Hypoxemia.** Deficient oxygenation of the blood.

**Hypoxia.** Low oxygen content or tension; deficiency of oxygen in the inspired air.

**Icteric.** Relating to or marked by jaundice.

**Incontinence.** The inability to prevent the discharge of any of the excretions, especially of urine or feces.

**Infarction.** The necrotic changes resulting from obstruction of an end artery.

**Inflammation.** The body's response to the presence of foreign agents, such as bacteria or chemicals. Inflammation usually produces invasion of white blood cells, swelling and pain.

**Infusion.** The introduction of fluid other than blood, for example saline solution, into a vein.

**Innervation.** Nerve stimulation to a part.

**Inotropic.** Referring to drugs that improve the contraction of the heart.

**Insertion.** 1. The act of implanting. 2. The place of attachment of a muscle to the bone that it moves.

**Inspiration.** Inhalation; the act of breathing in.

**Insufflate.** To blow into; to fill the lungs of an asphyxiated person with air, either by means of an apparatus or from the lungs of an operator.

**Intoxication.** Poisoning, especially by a toxic product of bacteria or poisonous animals.

**Intravenous.** Referring to drugs or solutions given through a vein. A common nickname is IV.

**Intravenous piggyback.** The hanging of a second solution to an initial IV line. One solution is piggybacked onto another.

**Intrinsic.** Inherent; belonging entirely to a part.

**Intubation.** The passage of an oral or nasotracheal tube for anesthesia or control of pulmonary ventilation.

**Inversion.** A turning inward or upside down.

**Ion.** An atom or group of atoms carrying an electrical charge.

**Ischemia.** Local anemia due to mechanical obstruction of the blood supply, usually caused by arterial narrowing.

**Isosorbide.** A drug used to dilate the coronary arteries.

**Isotonic.** Denoting solutions possessing the same osmotic pressure.

**-itis.** Suffix indicating inflammation.

**Jaundice.** A yellowish staining of the integument, sclera and deeper tissues, and the excretion of bile pigments.

**Juxta-.** Prefix signifying near or close by.

**Kailuresis.** The excretion of potassium in the urine, most often seen with diuretics such as Lasix₍ᵣ₎.

**Kalemia.** The presence of potassium in the blood. (*See* hyper-, hypokalemia)

**Kerato-conjunctivitis.** Inflammation of the cornea and conjunctiva.

**Kernicterus.** A condition caused by prolonged and severe elevation of bilirubin in the blood; it usually occurs in newborns who are jaundiced and it may produce irreversible brain damage.

**Ketoacidosis.** Acidosis caused by elevation of ketones in the blood and body tissues; usually seen in diabetic acidosis.

**Ketone bodies.** Formed after the oxygenation of fat.

**Kilogram.** A unit of weight in the metric system equivalent to 2.2 lb avoirdupois.

**Kimmelstiel-Wilson Syndrome.** The degeneration of kidney glomeruli which occurs in diabetics.

**Laceration.** A tear or torn wound.

**Lateral.** On the side or outer side, as distinguished from medial.

**Laparotomy.** Incision through any part of the abdominal wall.

**Laryngospasm.** Spasm of the vocal cords within the larynx, producing severe airway obstruction. It can be caused by stimulation, aspiration or anaphylactic reaction.

**Lavage.** The washing out of a hollow organ, such as the stomach or lower bowel.

**Lesion.** A wound or injury; generally any pathologic change in the tissues.

**Lumbar.** Relating to the part of the back and sides between the ribs and the pelvis.

**Lumen.** The space in the interior of a tubulous structure, such as an artery or intestine.

**Malinger.** To feign an illness, usually in order to escape work, excite sympathy or gain compensation.

**Malnutrition.** Faulty nutrition resulting from malassimilation, poor diet or overeating.

**Mania.** An emotional disorder characterized by great activity, excitement, a rapid passing of ideas, exultation and unstable attention.

**MAST Suit.** Military Anti-Shock Trousers. Useful in hypovolemic or cardiogenic shock, the trousers are applied to the legs and abdomen and then inflated, compressing the veins and increasing venous return to the heart.

**Medial.** Relating to the middle or center.

**Miosis.** Constriction of the pupil.

**Melena.** The passage of dark colored tarry stools due to the presence of blood altered by intestinal juices.

**Meningitis.** Inflammation of the meninges, which are the cover linings of the brain. This infection can be due to a virus, bacteria or tuberculosis.

**Menstruation.** The periodic discharge of bloody fluid from the uterus.

**Metabolism.** The sum of the chemical changes whereby the function of nutrition is affected.

**Metastasis.** The transfer of disease from one organ or part to another not directly connected with it. The term is commonly used to refer to diseases caused by cancer: when the cancer spreads, it metastasizes from one point to another.

**Morbidity.** The ratio of sick to well in a given population.

**Mortality.** Statistically, the death rate; the ratio of the number of deaths to a given population.

**Mucosa.** Any mucous membrane (i.e., the surface of the stomach, oral cavity, trachea, etc.).

**Mute.** A person who does not have the faculty of speech.

**Mydriasis.** Dilation of the pupil.

**Myocardiopathy.** Heart failure due to damage of the heart muscle or myocardium.

**Narcotic.** A drug which, used in moderate doses, produces stupor, insensibility or sound sleep.

**Nausea.** An inclination to vomit; sick to the stomach.

**Necropsy.** The study of dead tissues. This word may be used in a similar fashion as autopsy.

**Necrosis.** The pathologic death of one or more cells, or of a portion of a tissue or organ, resulting from irreversible damage.

**Necrotizing.** A spread of infection that causes death of tissue.

**Necrotizing enterocolitis.** Death of tissues in the small and large bowel due to infection within the bowel wall.

**Neonate.** A newborn baby.

**Neurosis.** A peculiar state of tension or irritability of the nervous system; any form of nervousness.

**Noxious.** Injurious.

**Nystagmus.** Rhythmical oscillation of the eyeballs, either horizontal, rotary or vertical.

**Obese.** Extremely fat.

**Occlude.** To close or bring together.

**Occlusion.** 1. The act of closing or the state of being closed. 2. The contact between the surfaces of the upper and lower teeth.

**Ocular.** Relating to the eye.

**Olfactory.** Relating to the sense of smell.

**Opiate.** Any preparation derived from opium.

**Opisthotonis.** A form of tetanic spasm following neurologic damage to the brain in which the head and the heels are bent backward and the body bowed forward.

**Oral.** Relating to the mouth.

**Ordinate.** One of the lines used as a base of reference in graphs, it is the vertical line which crosses the abscissa at right angles.

**Orthopnea.** Discomfort on breathing in any but the erect sitting or standing position.

**Orthostatic.** Relating to or caused by erect posture.

**Osmolality.** The osmotic concentration of solute per kilogram of solvent.

**Osmolarity.** The osmotic concentration of a solution expressed as osmoles of solute per liter of solution.

**Osmosis.** The passage of certain fluids and solutions through a membrane.

**Pacemaker.** Any rhythmic center controlling the heart's activity; normally the sinus node.

**Pallor.** Paleness of the skin.

**Palpable.** That which can be felt with the fingers or hand.

**Palpation.** Examination by means of the hands; the sense of touch.

**Palpitation.** Forceful pulsation of the heart perceptible to the patient; usually results in an increase in frequency with or without irregularity in rhythm.

**Palsy.** Paralysis; often used to connote partial paralysis or paresis.

**Pancreatitis.** Inflammation of the pancreas due to trauma, alcohol abuse or gallstones. It is a serious condition attended by pain and tenderness of the abdomen, tympanites and vomiting.

**Papilledema.** Edema of the optic disc; may be due to raised intracranial pressure or part of a diffuse retinal edema, as in malignant hypertension.

**Paralysis.** Loss of power of voluntary movement in a muscle through injury or disease of its nerve supply.

**Paraplegia.** Paralysis of both lower extremities and the lower trunk in general.

**Parasympathetic.** A division of the autonomic nervous system.

**Parenteral.** Entrance by other means than through the intestinal canal; referring particularly to the introduction of material into veins and subcutaneous tissues.

**Paresthesia.** An abnormal spontaneous sensation, such as of burning, pricking, numbness, etc.

**Patent.** Open; unobstructed.

**Pathognomonic.** Signs or symptoms that are specific for a certain disease process.

**Pathology.** The study of abnormal changes in tissues or blood.

**Pelvic.** Relating to the pelvis.

**Penetrate.** To pierce; to pass into the deeper tissues or into a cavity.

**Peptic.** Gastric secretions containing enzymes and acids, called peptic juices.

**Percussion.** A diagnostic procedure designed to determine the density of a part by means of tapping the surface with the finger(s) or a hammer.

**Perfusion.** Artificial passage of fluid through blood vessels.

**Pericardium.** A membranous sac covering the heart.

**Peripheral.** Relating to or situated at the periphery, or the outer edge.

**Peritoneum.** The lining of the abdominal cavity. The peritoneum is divided into visceral, that peritoneum lining the bowel; and parietal, that peritoneum lining the abdominal wall.

**Peritonitis.** Inflammation of the peritoneum, usually due to bacterial organisms. It is attended by abdominal pain and tenderness, constipation, vomiting and moderate fever.

**Petechiae.** Purplish-red, nonraised spots of pinpoint to pinhead size in the skin caused by intradermal or submucus hemorrhage; the spots later turn blue or yellow.

**pH.** An indication of the acidity or alkalinity of a solution; specifically a symbol for the logarithm of the reciprocal of the hydrogen ion concentration.

**-phagia.** Suffix meaning eating or swallowing.

**-phonia.** Suffix signifying relation to sound or to the voice.

**Pigment.** Any organic coloring matter, such as that of the red blood cells, of the hair, of the iris, etc.

**Placebo.** An indifferent or inert substance in the form of a medicine given for the suggestive effect alone.

**Placenta.** The organ formed within the mother's uterus as the result of insemmination of the egg by the sperm. This organ secretes hormones as well as providing the blood vessel union between mother and infant. Gas exchange between the mother's and baby's blood occurs through the placental blood vessels. At term, the placenta weighs about 500 grams, the proportion to weight of child being about 1 to 6.

**Plantar.** Relating to the sole of the foot.

**Plasma.** The fluid portion of the circulating blood.

**Pleural.** Relating to the pleura, or the serous membrane enveloping the lungs and lining the walls of the thoracic cavity.

**-pnea.** Suffix indicating relation to breathing or respiration.

**Pneumo-.** Prefix indicating the presence of air or gas, or the relation to breathing.

**Pre-.** Prefix signifying that which goes before.

**Preeclampsia.** Symptoms that occur prior to the onset of eclampsia. These symptoms may be elevation in weight, blood pressure and edema. Condition is usually seen during the third trimester of pregnancy.

**Pronation.** The act of assuming or being placed in the prone or face-down position.

**Prophylactic.** Related to the prevention of disease.

**Proteinuria.** Protein in the urine.

**Protoplasm.** The essential ingredient of the internal environment of animal cells. It is composed of proteins, fats, carbohydrates, inorganic salts and nucleic acids.

**Proximal.** Nearest the trunk or point of origin.

**Pruritus.** Itching.

**Psychogenic.** Of mental origin or causation.

**Psychosis.** A severe emotional illness.

**Pulmonary.** Relating to the lungs.

**Pulse.** The rhythmic dilatation of an artery produced by the increased volume of blood thrown into the vessel by the contraction of the heart.

**Quadrant.** One quarter of a circle. The abdomen is often divided into quadrants.

**Quadriplegia.** Paralysis of all four limbs.

**Quadruplet.** One of four offspring produced during one gestation.

**Radiation.** 1. The act or condition of diverging in all directions from a center, e.g., radiating pain. 2. Radiating energy of any kind, such as light, short radio waves, ultraviolet or X-rays.

**Rale.** A sound of varied character heard on auscultation of the chest, in many cases in disease of the lungs or bronchi.

**Rash.** Any skin eruption; may be localized or generalized.

**Receptor.** A site usually in the autonomic nervous system that receives stimulation from drugs, chemicals or nervous impulses. A receptor may also be a specific location on a cell or a point of attachment for an antibody. An adrenergic receptor is one that responds to norepinephrine, whereas a beta adrenergic receptor responds to epinephrine.

**Rectal.** Relating to the rectum.

**Reflex.** An involuntary movement in response to a stimulus applied to the periphery and transmitted to the nervous centers in the brain or spinal cord, e.g., knee jerk.

**Rehydration.** The return of water to a system after its loss.

**Renal.** Relating to the kidney.

**Respiration.** Breathing, or the sound of air moving into the bronchi and lungs heard on auscultation.

**Rhabdomyolysis.** Disintegration or dissolution of muscle, associated with excretion of myoglobin (contributes to the color of muscle and acts as a store of oxygen) in the urine.

**Rhin-.** Prefix denoting or pertaining to the nose.

**Rhonchus.** A loud rale, especially a whistling or sonorous rale produced in the larger bronchi or the trachea.

**Rigid.** Stiff.

**Rotation.** Turning or movement of a body around its axis.

**Sacral.** Relating to or in the neighborhood of the sacrum, which comprises the lowest part of the vertebral column.

**Secretion.** The product of cellular or glandular activity; a secretion is stored up in or utilized by the animal. It thereby differs from an excretion, which is intended to be expelled from the body.

**Sedative.** An agent that quiets nervous excitement.

**Senile.** Relating to or characteristic of old age.

**Sepsis.** The presence of various pus-forming and other pathogenic organisms or their toxins.

**Sequestration.** A net increase in the quantity of blood inside and outside of vascular channels; the loss of fluid into the lung from capillaries.

**Serum.** The fluid portion of blood obtained after removal of the fibrin clot and blood cells.

**Shock.** A state of profound physical and mental depression consequent upon severe physical injury or emotional disturbance.

**Sign.** Any abnormality indicative of disease, discoverable by the physician upon his examination of the patient.

**Sinus.** 1. A hollow in bone or other tissue. 2. A fistula or tract leading to a separating cavity.

**Slough.** The shedding of dead tissue from the body. For example, after the skin has been burned, it will begin to slough off within 10 to 14 days.

**Somatic.** Relating to the body.

**Spasm.** An involuntary muscular contraction. If painful, it is usually referred to as a cramp; if violent, it is referred to as a convulsion.

**Sprain.** An injury to a joint with possible rupture of some of the ligaments or tendons, but without discoloration or fracture.

**Sputum.** Expectorated material, especially mucus or mucopurulent material spit up during diseases of the air passages.

**Stenosis.** A narrowing of any canal; a stricture, especially of one of the cardiac valves.

**Sterile.** Aseptic; free from all living microorganisms and their spores.

**Stridor.** A harsh, high-pitched respiratory sound that may be heard during inspiration and expiration. It is most commonly audible during upper airway obstruction in the larynx.

**Stimulation.** Arousal of the body, or any of its parts or organs, to increase functional activity.

**Stroke.** A blow or a sudden attack, such as sunstroke or paralytic stroke.

**Stroke volume.** The quantity of blood pumped from each ventricle during a single heart beat.

**Stupor.** Lethargy or unconsciousness.

**Subcutaneous.** Beneath the skin (SQ).

**Sublingual.** Beneath the tongue.

**Supinate.** To turn the forearm and hand palmar side upward.

**Suppuration.** The formation of pus.

**Sympathetic.** A division of the autonomic nervous system.

**Symptom.** Any morbid phenomenon or departure from the normal in function, appearance or sensation experienced by the patient and indicative of a disease.

**Syncope.** Fainting; a sudden fall in blood pressure or failure of the cardiac systole, resulting in cerebral anemia and more or less complete loss of consciousness.

**Synergism.** Working together; cooperative action.

**Systemic.** Relating to any system, specifically the somatic system.

**Systole.** The rhythmical contraction of the heart, especially the ventricles, by which the blood is driven through the system.

**Tachy-.** Prefix meaning rapid.

**Tachycardia.** Excessive rapidity in the action of the heart. The term is usually applied to a pulse rate above 100 per minute.

**Tachypnea.** Excessive rapidity of respiration; a respiratory neurosis marked by quick, shallow breathing.

**Tamponade.** Compression of the heart resulting from accumulation of fluid in the pericardial sac.

**Tetany.** A disorder marked by intermittent tonic muscular contractions accompanied by tremors, paresthesias and muscular pains. The hands are usually first affected; the spasm occurs later in the face, trunk and sometimes the laryngeal muscles.

**Thoracic.** Relating to the thorax.

**Thrombosis.** The formation of a thrombus.

**Thrombus.** A plug or clot in a blood vessel or in one of the cavities of the heart, formed by coagulation of the blood and remaining at the point of its formation.

**Torsion.** Twisting or rotation of a part upon its axis.

**Toxemia.** Clinical manifestations observed during certain infectious diseases assumed to be caused by toxins.

**Toxin.** A noxious or poisonous substance.

**Trauma.** Wound; an injury inflicted usually more or less suddenly by some physical agent.

**Tremor.** Trembling or shaking.

**Turgor.** Fullness. T. vitalis is the normal fullness of the blood vessels and capillaries. When the surrounding tissues lose their normal resistance, this turgor increases and swelling results.

**Ulcer.** A lesion on the surface of the skin or mucous surface caused by superficial loss of tissue, usually accompanied by inflammation.

**Unconscious.** Not conscious; insensible.

**Urticaria.** Hives; an eruption of itching weals, usually of systemic origin. It may be due to a state of hypersensitivity to food or drugs, a focus of infection or psychic stimuli.

**Vaccine.** Any microbial preparation used for active prophylaxis.

**Vagolysis.** The operation of tearing off the esophageal branches of the vagus from the esophagus for the relief of cardiospasm.

**Vagus nerve.** The tenth cranial nerve.

**Varix.** An enlarged and tortuous vein, artery or lymphatic vessel (pl. *varices*).

**Vaso-.** Prefix meaning relating to a blood vessel.

**Vasodilator.** An agent (motor nerve or chemical compound) that causes dilation of the blood vessels.

**Vasopressor.** Stimulation of contraction of the muscular tissues of the capillaries and arteries, resulting in a rise in blood pressure.

**Venipuncture.** The puncture of a vein for any purpose (phlebotomy).

**Ventilation.** The cyclic process of exchange of air; breathing.

**Vertigo.** Dizziness, giddiness; a sensation of irregular or whirling motion, either of oneself or of external objects.

**Viscera.** Generally, any organ or organs of the body.

**Vitamin.** One of a group of organic substances present in minute amounts in natural foodstuffs which are essential to normal metabolism, and the lack of which in the diet causes deficiency diseases.

**Volkmann's Contracture.** A contraction of the fingers and sometimes of the wrist, accompanied by loss of power, which develops rapidly after a severe injury in the region of the elbow joint or improper use of a tourniquet.

# INDEX

Drugs *(Contd.)*
  in pregnancy, 160
  response, 157
  tolerance, 161, 163–64
  toxic effects, 164–66, 529, 530
Duodenal ulcer, perforated, 472
Dyspnea, 238, 287, 289, 680
Dysrhythmia, 206, 278, 307, 308, 318–38, 680

Ear, 96, 222, 226
Eclampsia, 602–4, 680
Ectopic pregnancy, 601, 626
Edema, 74, 151, 281
  pulmonary, 492
Efferent fibers. *See* Motor fibers
Efferent neurons, 103
Electrical injuries, 565–66
Electrocardiogram (EKG), 3, 47, 49, 71, 72, 284, 307–15, 328–30, 338
Electrolytes, 143, 144, 147–50, 155
  abnormalities and disturbances, 205, 206, 209, 313–14, 493
  concentration, 150
  loss, 207, 208, 571
Embolism, 462, 575, 680
  air, 498
  fat, 422, 576
Emergency Medical Care (EMC), 2, 7, 8
Emergency Medical Services System (EMSS), 41, 42, 44, 46
Emergency Medical Services System (EMSS) Act of 1973, 3–5, 19
Emergency Medical Technicians (EMT), 2, 44
Emesis, 534–36
Emphysema, 244, 502, 503–7, 680
EMT. *See* Emergency Medical Technicians and Paramedics
Endocardial pacer, 337
Endocarditis, 279
Endocrine system, 83, 476–78, 720
Endotoxin, 469
Endotracheal intubation, 249, 256
Enzymes, 68, 75, 77
Epicardial electrode, 337
Epididymis, 135
Epigastrium, 116
Epiglottitis, in children, 649–50
Epilepsy, 602, 603
Epinephrine. *See also* Adrenalin. 73, 83, 179, 180–81, 183, 192, 240, 300, 348–49, 350, 642
Esophageal obturator airway, 40, 249, 254, 256, 257
Esophagus, 92, 114
Eustachian tube, 96
Evaporation, and heat loss, 616
Eversion, of eyelid, 391
Excision, of skin around snake bite, 582
Excretion, of drugs, 161, 162, 193
Exotoxin, 469
Exposure
  to elements, 591
  to infectious diseases, 467
  to toxins, 527–28
Extension, 129–31
Extracellular fluid, 74–75, 83, 146, 147, 205
Extraocular muscle, 95
Extremity, distal to fracture, 419
Extrication, 25, 26, 54, 56, 565–66
Eye, 94–95, 222, 226, 386–92

Fainting. *See* Syncope
Fascicles, 306
Fat. *See also* Obesity
  in body, 154
  and sex, 143
Fatty acids, 68, 75
Federal Communication Commission, 41, 43, 45–46, 52

Femoral nerve, 108
Femur, 124, 125, 129, 133, 421
Fever, 147, 148
Fibrillation, 681
  atrial, 294, 319, 325–26, 338
  ventricular, 285, 327, 569
Fibrin thrombus formation, 282
Fibrinogen, 77
Fibrinolysin, 77
Filling pressure, of heart, 70
Finger probe technique, 261
Fire Department, role in emergency situations, 21, 60, 61
Flap avulsion, 377, 378
Flexions, 127–31
Fluid
  abnormalities and disorders, 209, 493
  balance, in body, 490
  drainage, from newborn's lungs, 615–16
  losses, 440, 571
    in children, 644
    external, 152–53, 206–8
    internal, 151, 208–9
    overload, 492
  regulatory mechanisms, 253
  volume, maintenance of, 153
Focal seizures, 459
Fontanelle, 632, 645, 647
Food
  effects on drug absorption, 158, 162
  obstructing airway, 343–44
Forceps delivery, 611
Forearm, muscles of, 131
Forehead, injuries to, 384–85
Foreign bodies
  in airway, 259–62
  aspiration, 258–59, 253–54
  in children, 640, 649
  in eye, 391
Fowler's position, 287
Fractures, 232, 233, 276, 417
  of cervical, 374, 401
  of chest, 373
  classification, 418
  compound, 421–22, 429
  diagnosis, 419
  of facial skeleton, 380, 389–90
  of jaw, 384
  open. *See* Fractures, compound
  of pelvis, 373, 421
  of skull, 393
  simple, 418–21
  of trachea, 386
Frontal plane, of body, 88
Frostbite, 567
Functional residual capacity (FRC), 81
Furosemide, 181, 288, 290, 300

Gallbladder, 118
Gas
  dissolved in blood and tissues, 576
  exchange, and death, 245
  toxic, 564–65
Gastric lavage, 536
Gastroenteritis, 470
Gastrointestinal system, 222, 470–76, 519, 633
Genitourinary system, 133–36
Glossopharyngeal nerve, 105
Glucola, 182
Glucose, 176–77, 205–6
  and brain, 452
  and heart metabolism, 275
  level in blood, 478–81
  solution, 182
Glucose gel, 182
Glucotal, 182
Glycogen, 481
Gram-negative shock, 468–69
Grand mal, 458–59
Great vessel injury, 412

Gun wounds, 380, 386

Haldol, 546–47
Half-life, of a drug, 161, 163
Hallucinogens, 550–52, 556
Hang gliding, injuries from, 583–84
Hartmann's solution. *See* Lactated Ringer's solution
Head, 89–99, 222, 226, 392–95
Hearing, and airway problem diagnosis, 247
Heart, 114–16. *See also* Cardiac
  block, 318, 330–36
  blunt injuries to, 412
  diagnosis, 305–15
  disorders, 276–95
  drugs for, 295–302
  electrophysiology of, 305–15
  failure
    congestive, 206, 504–6, 655–56
    prevention of, 287–88
  rate, 273–74, 319
    in newborns, 617–18, 621
  system, 69–71, 273–75
  valve, disorders of, 277–79
Heart attack. *See* Myocardial infarction
Heart control
  of ill or injured children, 631–32
  for infants, 616–17, 622–23
Heat exhaustion, 570, 591
Heat inhalation, 564
Heat stroke, 570, 572, 591–92
Heimlich maneuver, 261
Hematemesis, 474
Hematochezia, 474
Hematrocrit, 75, 76, 147
Hematologic system, 74–77
Hematoma, 682
Hemoglobin, 75, 78–79, 238, 682
Hemopericardium, 411
Hemoperitoneum, 414, 416
Hemorrhage, 233, 444–46
  of the brain, 463
  in eye, 379–80
  and fluid loss, 154
  with fracture, 419
  intraperitoneal, 373
  postpartum, 613–14
  and strokes, 463
  of the uterus, in pregnancy, 601–2
Hemostasis, 371
Hemothorax, 406
Hepatic encephalopathy, 489–90, 522
Hepatitis, 682
Heroin, 192, 540
Hijacker, 515–16
Hip, 119, 124, 129, 132, 429
Histamine, 682–83
History, of patients, 211–23, 375, 586–87, 630–31. *See also* Assessment
Homeostasis, 683
Homicide, 511
Hormones
  adrenocortical, 83
  and arterioles, 71
  and blood volume regulation, 153
  and cellular chemical reactions, 68
Humerus, 118
Hydrocephalus, 610
Hydrocodone, 545
Hydrocortisone, 83
Hydrogen ions, 79
Hydromorphone, 545
Hydrostatic pressure, 74
Hyperbaric chamber, 577
Hypercalcemia, 314, 485–86
Hypercapnea, 238, 432
Hypercarbia, 238, 240, 488
Hyperglycemia. *See* Ketoacidosis
Hyperkalemia, 313, 315, 494–95
Hyperkinesis, and chest pain, 285

SA node. *See* Sinoatrial node
Sagittal plane, 88
Salt. *See* Sodium chloride
Salt solutions, 196–97, 198, 208
Saphenous vein system, 139
Sciatic nerve, 108
Sedatives. *See also* Barbiturates, Drugs
  and respiratory failure, 242
  and strokes, 466
Seizures, 206, 457–62, 517–18
  assessment of, 460–61
  children, 646–48, 662
  petit mal, 459
  in pregnancy, 602–3
  treatment of, 461–62, 647–48
Seminal vesicles, 136
Semi-permeable membranes, 74, 150
Sensory fibers, 106–8
Sepsis, 689
Septic shock, 468–69, 519
Septicemia, in children, 658
Shivering, 567–68
Shock, 69, 83, 165, 172, 208, 233, 371,
  439–50, 538, 554
  with abdominal pain, 471
  in children, 642, 644, 662
  defined, 439
  fluid losses, 154
  hypovolemic, 562
  treatment, 446–49
Shortness of breath (SOB), 504
Shoulder, 127, 131
Sick sinus syndrome, 318, 322, 331–32
Sight, and airway problem, 247
Sinoatrial (SA) node, 286, 305, 321
Sinus, 330–31
  bradycardia, 286, 319, 331, 655
  in children, 655
  dysrhythmia, 286
  sick sinus syndrome, 331–32
  tachycardia, 319, 655
Sinuses, 97
Skeletal muscle, 130–31
Skeletal system, 120–26
Skull, fracture of, 393
Smoke inhalation, 564–65, 590
Snake bite, 580–83, 592–93
Sodium bicarbonate, 147, 176, 179, 192–93,
  202, 446–47, 642
Sodium chloride, 147, 148–49, 155, 571
Sodium losses, 153
Sodium sulphate, 538
Somatic nervous system, 106, 107
Sphygmomanometer, 72
Spinal board, 53, 55
Spinal cord, 100, 102–5, 106
  functions, 103
  injury to, 107, 374, 400
    and respiratory failure, 243
    in trauma, 372
    treatment of, 402
  protection of, 392, 435
Spleen, 117, 415
Splinting, 46, 421, 425–28
Sprains, 422–23
Stabbing, injuries from, 379–80
Stabilization, of neck and back, 8, 372
Staphylococcus aureus, 278
Starling, Frank, 70, 274
Sterile techniques, of drug administration,
  171, 172, 173
Sternum, 109–11, 113, 648
  injury of, 404
Steroid medication, 176, 483
Stethoscope, 224, 225
Stimulants, 549–50, 556
Stimuli, use in evaluating brain injuries,
  397–98
Stings, 579–80
Stokes-Adams attacks, 329

Stomach pains. *See* Abdominal pain
*Streptococcus viridans*, 278
Stress, 83
Stridor, 247, 648, 689
  defined, 239
Stroke, 230, 242, 462–66, 518
Stroke volume, 70, 71, 273–74
Stupor, 452, 517
Subcutaneous administration, of drugs,
  158–59, 171
Sublingual administration, of drugs, 173
Sucking chest wounds, 408–10
Suction equipment, battery powered, 40
Sudden Infant Death Syndrome (SIDS),
  632–35, 660
Sugar solution, 197, 198
Suicide, 512–13
Supracondylar fractures, 421
Supraventricular trachycardia (SVT), 322–
  23, 337–38
Surface evaporation, 572
Survey, of multiply injured patients, 370–
  71
Sweating, 153, 570, 572
Swelling, 425
Sympathetic receptors, 73
Syncope, 460, 461, 475
Synergism, 166
Syntocinon, 190, 614
Systemic arterial pressure, 274
Systemic vascular resistance, 70
Systems approach, to emergency medical
  care, 3
Systems, review of, 222–23
Systolic pressure, 72–73, 274

T wave, 307
Tachycardia, 239, 690
  defined, 320
  in infectious disease, 466
  junctional, 321
  paroxysmal atrial (PAT), 298, 321–24
  and premature ventricular contraction,
  286
  supraventricular, 337–38
  ventricular, 329–30
Tachydysrhythmias, 294, 296, 298
Tachypnea, 82, 238
Talus, 126
Talwin, 188, 546
Tamponade, 279–80, 292, 411, 440, 495,
  690
Telemetry, 40, 44, 46, 47, 49
Temperature, body, 567–68
Tendons, 130, 231
Tension pneumothorax, 406–8, 410, 501
Testes, 135
Tetany, 690
Theophylline, 174
Third space losses, 151, 208
Thoracic vertebrae, 103, 111, 112
Thorax, 109–16, 405
  examination of, 227–29
  internal structures, 113–16
  thoracotomy, 404, 412
  topographical anatomy, 109–13
Thorazin, 546, 556
Throat, 222, 226
Thrombosis, 77, 232, 498
Thrombus, 77, 690
Thyroid gland, 476–77, 484–85
Thyrotoxic storm, 484
Tidal volume (TV), 81–82
Tilt test, 475
Tongue, relaxation, 249
Topographic anatomy, 89–92, 109–20
Total body water, 146, 155
Total lung capacity (TLC), 81, 82
Tourniquet, 290, 293, 431–33
Toxemia, 690

Toxic effects, of drugs, 164–66
Toxicity rating, 531–33
Trachea, 91–92, 98, 386
Tracheostomy, 251, 258
  water loss, 153
Transcapillary refilling, 154
Transection, 430
Transport, of patients, 19, 21, 22, 41, 56–58,
  409, 412
  by air, 59
  with cardiac arrest, 354–55, 366
  comatose, 456–57
  with fractures, 421
  immobilization, 57
  newborns, 622–23
  safety in MIC unit, 8
  in shock, 446
  snake bite victims, 582–83
Transverse position, of fetus, 611
Trauma, 20, 51, 208, 369–438
  abdominal, 217–18
  blunt, 389–90, 410–11
  in children, 644–46
  to eyes, 388–90
  head, 101
  multiple, 370, 416
  penetrating, 388–89
  to spinal cord, 104–5, 107
Treatment, 63
  of myocardial ischemia or infarction,
  284–87
  priorities, 248, 249, 262, 294
Triage, 61–65
Tricuspid valve, 71
Trifascicular block (TFB), 318
Triphasic QRS, 319
Trophic volume, 83
Tubing, 33–34, 199–200
Twins, delivery of, 612

Ulcer, 378, 690
  perforated duodenal, 472
Umbilical cord, 607–8, 615
Upper airway obstruction, 648–51
Uremia, 491, 495–96
Ureter, 135
Urinary bladder, function of, 104–5
Urinary tract infection, 469
Uterus
  in difficulties of childbirth, 612–13
  hemorrhage of, 600–602, 625
  rupture of, 600

Vagus nerve, 105–6
Valium, 177, 323, 462, 551, 556
Valves, heart, 71
Vascular system, 71–74, 136–40
  examination of, 232–33
  injury to, 429–42
  resistance, 70
Vas deferens, 136
Vasoconstriction, 73, 441–42
  and control of hemorrhage, 430
Vasodilation, 73, 274, 691
Vasopressor, 691
Venipuncture, 203–5
Venom, 581–82
Venous system, 70, 74, 101–2, 138–40,
  202–3
Ventilation
  in children, 639–40
  and death, 245
  of infectious patients, 466–67
  IPPV, 619–21
  techniques, 81
Ventricles, 69, 70, 306–7
  aneurysm, 277
  contraction phases, 72
  fibrillation, 285, 296, 317, 327, 341–42,
  364, 569, 570, 642

T5-BYL-085

# THE ESSENTIAL
# Vygotsky

# THE ESSENTIAL
# Vygotsky

Edited by

## Robert W. Rieber
*City University of New York*
*New York, New York*

and

## David K. Robinson
*Truman State University*
*Kirksville, Missouri*

In collaboration with

<table>
<tr><td>

### Jerome Bruner
*New York University*
*New York, New York*

</td><td>

### Michael Cole
*University of California-San Diego*
*La Jolla, California*

</td></tr>
<tr><td>

### Joseph Glick
*City University of New York*
*New York, New York*

</td><td>

### Carl Ratner
*Institute for Cultural Research and Education*
*Trinidad, California*

</td></tr>
</table>

### Anna Stetsenko
*City University of New York*
*New York, New York*

## Kluwer Academic/Plenum Publishers
*New York, Boston, Dordrecht, London, Moscow*

Library of Congress Cataloging-in-Publication Data

Vygotskii, L. S. (Lev Semenovich), 1896–1934.
  [Collected works of L. S. Vygotsky. English Selections]
  The essential Vygotsky / edited by Robert W. Rieber, David K. Robinson ; in collaboration with Jerome Bruner . . .
[et al.].
    p. cm.
  Includes bibliographical references and index.
  ISBN 0-306-48552-4 (hardcover)—ISBN 0-306-48553-2 (e-book)
    1. Psychology. I. Rieber, R. W. (Robert W.) II. Robinson, David Kent. III. Bruner, Jerome S. (Jerome Seymour) IV.
Title.
BF121.V94213   2004
150—dc22                                                                                                  2004047336

ISBN 0-306-48552-4

© 2004 by Kluwer Academic/Plenum Publishers, New York
233 Spring Street, New York, New York 10013
http://www.kluweronline.com

10 9 8 7 6 5 4 3 2 1

A C.I.P. record for this book is available from the Library of Congress.

Permissions for books published in Europe: permissions@wkap.nl
Permissions for books published in the United States of America: permissions@wkap.com

Printed in the United States of America

*Dedicated to the memory of Alexander Luria
and with gratitude to the Vygotsky family,
especially G. L. Vygodskaya*

# Prologue: Reading Vygotsky

MICHAEL COLE, *Laboratory of Comparative Human Cognition,*
*University of California, San Diego*

Writing a prologue for a collection like this is truly astonishing to me for many reasons. It is now more than forty years since I first encountered the name of Lev Semenovich Vygotsky, a Russian scholar born just before the start of the twentieth century. By virtue of my education in the middle of the twentieth century as an experimental psychologist who specialized in learning, I was reasonably well trained in that form of positivist behavioral sciences that took it as a simple truth that the errors of the originators of the discipline of psychology were a thing of the past. To my generation of experimental psychologists, the history of psychology was the uplifting story of that long trail of errors that had been overcome by recent scientific advances. Such history served primarily as a cautionary tale about not succumbing to the temptations of subjective, unscientific speculation but instead mastering the quantitative methods that had been pioneered during recent years, leading psychology out of its dark past into a genuinely scientific future that will benefit humankind.

A corollary of this scientific worldview was a strong claim for the continuity of species, such that general laws of human behavior could be studied at least as effectively by studying the behavior of rats as by studying the behavior of college sophomores; the choice of "subject" was merely a matter of convenience. Rats had the advantage that one could control their histories with moral impunity, while at least some consideration had to be given to avoiding harming undergraduates. On the other hand, rats had to be taken care of over the weekend, while undergraduates were the responsibility of university officials who enforced the procedures of *in loco parentis.*

Needless to say, the same notions of continuity applied to age differences. The study of children was a relatively small, and relatively low-status, enterprise. The major mechanism of developmental change favored by psychologists was learning from the environment, using procedures which were often directly modeled on procedures initially developed to study rats, dogs, and cats.

Yet another widely held belief, which admitted of a few exceptions, was that, by and large, scientific psychology could be adequately mastered by knowing how to read only English and, moreover, by restricting one's reading primarily to research conducted in the United States. The few exceptions to this rule do not, so far as I can tell, form any pattern. Frederick Bartlett's experiments on remembering were well known, but his book on thinking was not. Pavlov was of course required reading because American behaviorists of the 1920s and 1930s adopted conditioned reflexes as a major mechanism of learning, but his physiological theories were largely ignored.

This situation was, of course, about to change. In retrospect the signs of change were pervasive. Some were geopolitical. When the Soviet Union put a satellite into space, the term "sputnik" entered the English language, and suddenly a psychology of learning that could transform American education became a compelling national need. Outstanding physicists, biologists, and mathematicians began joint research projects with psychologists. Perhaps not accidentally, the psychologists began to consider the possibility that rats did not, after all, offer an adequate model of learning in college students. I take it as more than accidental that the "cognitive revolution" began in Cambridge, Massachusetts, where somehow professors from a few departments at Harvard and MIT discovered different disciplines and even the other end of Massachusetts Avenue (which connects those revered institutions).

## Why Is Vygotsky Relevant Today?

So, one of the first things we might want to think about is why you are reading the prologue to a selection of essays by a Soviet, Jewish, Belorussian psychologist who died seven decades ago after a brief career. Little of his work was published during his lifetime, even in Russian, and the number of copies of those publications was very small. Some of his work was known to a few specialists in human development and abnormal psychology during his lifetime, thanks in large part to the efforts of Alexander Luria, a contributing editor to the *Journal of Genetic Psychology*, and in part to Eugenia Hanfmann (1953), who replicated Vygotksy's research on concept formation and published in English. Nevertheless, Vygotsky was not well known within his own country and had nothing of the international stature of his great contemporary, Piaget, nor of Werner, Kohler, Gesell, and other "father figures" of the study of human development. It is only in the past two decades that Vygotsky's work has become influential in Russia and on the international scene, where some of his work has been translated into many languages. It has been influential not only among developmental psychologists, but has become increasingly important to other disciplines, such as anthropology and sociology, and in the application of psychology in such areas as education, human–computer interface design, and the organization of work. What can account for this "Vygotsky boom" of recent years?

## The Publication of *Thought and Language*

Prior to 1962, when MIT Press published a translation of Vygotsky's *Thought and Language,* he was best known in the United States for a block-sorting task that resembled classification methods used by American psychologists. This translation was blessed by two circumstances. First, the lead translator, Eugenia Hanfmann, was the daughter of a Russian émigré who had studied in Germany with Kurt Lewin, and for whom Vygotsky was more than a myth of the past. Second, Jerome Bruner, a leader in organizing the cognitive revolution in the United States, wrote the book's preface. (He has also contributed an introduction to the present volume.)

Bruner's education had included time with William McDougall, an Englishman who became one of the giants of early American psychology. At that time the Department of Social Relations at Harvard retained a historically oriented, interdisciplinary faculty who respected the intellectual contributions of past psychologists from many countries, as well as the potential contributions of other social sciences to psychology. Consequently, Bruner was able to draw connections between Vygotsky's ideas and those of other, previously influential scholars in a way that created an "intergenerational bridge" to the 1960s. Moreover, Bruner was himself turning to the study of the role of culture in child development with a special focus on education, and hence he could appreciate the importance of Vygotsky's formulation of cultural–historical psychology and convey that importance in a clearly understandable manner.

Despite these auspicious advantages, the publication of *Thought and Language* did not evoke massive interest in Vygotsky, although his work did gradually begin to attract more attention. There are several potential reasons for its modest impact. First, the threat of conflict between the United States and the USSR reached its zenith that year in the Cuban missile crisis. To display enthusiasm for a Soviet psychologist who declared himself to be a Marxist was, at the very least, to court suspicions of one's allegiances. The translators, in fact, excised a significant portion of the book on grounds that it was either repetitive or polemical. Nonetheless, Marx, Engels, and Plekhanov all remain in the text, even if their appearance was abbreviated. Second, the book still required reasonable familiarity with a wide range of early-twentieth-century psychologists and presumed an interest in developmental psychology, features which were unlikely to find a broad audience at the time. Nor, with the exception of the block-sorting experiment, did it offer a simple experimental paradigm that could be expanded to encompass a major part of the field of cognitive development. Perhaps also significant at the time was the American fascination with Piaget, who did offer easy-to-repeat cognitive tasks and who directly challenged the dominant American notion that learning is the major force in cognitive development, thus generating an entire industry of research designed to prove him wrong.

As fate would have it, I had only minimal familiarity with Vygotsky's work when I went to the USSR in the fall of 1962 as a postdoctoral fellow working under the direction of Alexander Luria. I did not choose to work with Luria because he was a colleague of Vygotsky. I did not know he had been, and I would have made little of the fact even if I had known. I was attracted, instead, by research that Luria had published using Pavlovian conditioning methods to study the acquisition of word meaning, what was termed "semantic conditioning." I divided my year in Moscow between research on the retention or loss of semantic conditioning in patients with lesions in different parts of their brains, the study of avoidance conditioning in dogs at a laboratory in the Institute of Higher Nervous Activity, and research with E. N. Sokolov and his students on orienting reflexes and psychophysics.

Although Luria occasionally encouraged me to read Vygotsky (indeed, *Thought and Language* was published in 1962 owing to his initiative), I actually spent very little time trying to understand Vygotsky's work. The only version of his writings to which I had access was in Russian (mail traveled slowly between Cambridge and Moscow at that time). And as far as I could tell, there was little difference between Vygotsky, with his idea that words begin to mediate thought when children acquire language, and the American neobehaviorists who, starting with Margaret Kuenne in the late 1940s, had made pretty much the same argument (Kendler &

Kendler, 1962; Kuenne, 1946). I was not particularly interested in child development at the time, and I did not see the general significance of such claims.


## Discovering Vygotsky

I have written elsewhere of the long, slow, process through which I came to appreciate and eventually greatly admire the work of Vygotsky and his students (Cole, 1979). And, of course, Luria was responsible for a good deal of this process, just as he played a central role in bringing Vygotsky to the attention of world psychology.

One critical event was totally serendipitous. I was sent to Africa to worry about development and education, and in a state of total ignorance about the appropriate literature to consult on this topic, I contacted Luria to ask about his work in Central Asia, work he had planned with Vygotsky. In part I wanted to get a better specification of the tasks that he had used, since they could possibly provide a useful point of departure for my own work, whatever that might turn out to be. But I also wanted to understand what the *theoretical* relevance of their cross-cultural work was, with respect to issues such as semantic conditioning and recovery from brain injury. And why was there such an emphasis on development?

The second crucial event was a simple extension of Luria's unflagging efforts to get more of Vygotsky's work published in English. Appreciative of the efforts he had extended on my behalf while I was a postdoctoral fellow in Moscow, I agreed to help in two intertwined projects. One was the translation and publication of two of Vygotsky's books; *The History of the Development of Higher Psychological Functions* and *Tool and Symbol in Child Development*, the latter perhaps co-authored with Luria, although I did not suspect that at the time. (See Vygotsky, 1987–99, vols. 4 and 6, respectively, for the fullest translations of these works.) The other project was the editing and publication of Luria's autobiography (Luria, 1979), a brief version of which I had translated earlier for the series on the history of psychology in autobiography (Luria, 1974).

Both projects turned out to be extraordinarily difficult. I enlisted the help of my colleagues, Vera John-Steiner and Sylvia Scribner with the translation of the Vygotsky works, and I spent a lot of time becoming familiar with the sources of Luria's ideas by working through the citations in his autobiography. It soon became clear that the two projects were related, because a great number of the "old-fashioned" citations I encountered while reading Vygotsky were the same citations I found in Luria. Combined with my research in Africa, which carried me inevitably into the topics of culture, cognitive development, and education, the conditions were created which allowed me to make some sense of both Luria and Vygotsky.


## The "Vygotsky Boom"

I received the Vygotsky manuscripts from Luria in the early 1970s. But even with the expert help of able colleagues and a good translation to work from, I could not convince the publisher, with whom Luria had made arrangements, that the manuscripts were worth publishing. All of the problems that I had experienced earlier remained in place. The work seemed dated, the polemics either opaque or outdated, and the overall product was certain to produce fiscal disaster, not to say personal embarrassment.

Faced with this seemingly insurmountable barrier and with help from Luria, whom I visited every year or two and with whom I corresponded regularly, we were able to produce a reasonable selection of readings from the two manuscripts he had given me. To these we added several essays of an applied nature so that readers could see how the abstract theoretical arguments played out in practice. The result, entitled *Mind in Society,* was published in 1978. I heaved a great sigh of relief: I had finally discharged my obligation to Luria and the publisher, thanks in good measure to the hard work of my colleagues.

What happened next was totally unexpected. For reasons I have never learned, the philosopher Stephen Toulmin (1978) was assigned the book to review for the *New York Review of Books.* He entitled his article "The Mozart of Psychology." This review argued, as Sylvia Scribner and I had in our introduction, that Vygotsky's work was of great *contemporary* relevance, despite the fact that it had first been published forty years earlier. In effect, and in brief, the shortcomings of psychology against which Vygotsky struggled in the 1920s—in particular, the failure to recognize the centrality of culture and history to human psychological functioning—had not been overcome by his scientific successors. Instead, his dissatisfactions with psychologists of the early twentieth century applied with at least as great justification at the century's end.

Our group had become convinced that Vygotsky and his colleagues had, indeed, formulated a metapsychology that encompassed the phylogeny, cultural history, ontogeny, and moment-to-moment dynamics of human psychological functioning as a life-long process of becoming. Toulmin, to our great surprise, agreed and strongly conveyed his judgment to a very wide readership.

It is now twenty-five years since the publication of *Mind in Society.* Recently, within a very few years, Vygotsky has become a fad, and, as with all fads, the greater notoriety brought with it both genuine evolution and dimestore knockoffs. Within the former USSR, Vygotsky, who was virtually a forgotten man in 1978, except for a few of his aging followers and a handful of younger scholars, has become a cottage industry generating not only books and articles but entire departments and institutes.

Within the United States there have now been two additional translations of *Thought and Language* (Vygotsky, 1986; "Thinking and Speech," in Vygotsky, 1987–99, vol. 1, pp. 37–285), and there are dozens of books devoted to his ideas, their origins, their virtues, their shortcomings, etc. This book provides the reader with carefully chosen selections from a wide range of his writings. The largest collection of Vygotksy's writings, but not all of them, can be found in *The Collected Works,* now available in English due to the long labors of the general editor, Robert Rieber (Vygotsky, 1987–99).

With introductory essays by various scholars who have made careful studies of Vygotsky, the reader will find here a fine sampling of Vygotsky's work from the main domains that he investigated. The reading will not be easy. It requires patience and reflection. Speaking from my own life experience, the time and effort required will more than recompense the reader and will open new vistas in thought about human nature, any one of which could provide the material for a life's work.

# References

Cole, M. (1979). Epilogue. In *The making of mind: A personal account of Soviet psychology* by A. R. Luria (pp. 189–225). Cambridge: Harvard University Press.

Kendler, H. H. & Kendler, T. S. (1962). Vertical and horizontal processes in problem solving. *Psychological Review, 69,* 1–16.

Kuenne, M. (1946). Experimental investigation of the relation of language to transposition behavior in young children. *Journal of Experimental Psychology, 36,* 471–490.

Luria, A. R. (1974). A. R. Luria (M. Cole, Trans.). In *A history of psychology in autobiography* (Vol. 6, G. Lindzey, Ed.; pp. 251–292). Englewood Cliffs, NJ: Prentice Hall.

Luria, A. R. (1979). *The making of mind: A personal account of Soviet psychology* (S. Cole & M. Cole, Eds.). Cambridge: Harvard University Press.

Toulmin, S. (1978, September 28). The Mozart of psychology. *The New York Review of Books,* 51ff.

Vygotsky, L. S. (1962). *Thought and Language* (E. Hanfmann & G. Vakar, Eds. and Trans.). Cambridge: MIT Press.

Vygotsky, L. S. (1978). *Mind in society: The development of higher psychological processes* (M. Cole, V. John-Steiner, S. Scribner & E. Souberman, Eds). Cambridge: Harvard University Press.

Vygotsky, L. S. (1986). *Thought and Language* (A. Kozulin, Ed. and Rev.). Cambridge: MIT Press.

Vygotsky, L. S. (1987–99). *The collected works of L. S. Vygotsky* (6 Vols.) (R.W. Rieber, Ed.). New York: Kluwer Academic/Plenum.

# Preface

ROBERT W. RIEBER, *City University of New York* and
DAVID K. ROBINSON, *Truman State University*

*The Essential Vygotsky* is a selection of the writings of Lev Semenovich Vygotsky (1896–1934), taken from the six volumes of *The Collected Works of L. S. Vygotsky* that have appeared both in Russian (1982–84) and in English translation (1987–99). The editors have endeavored to choose the most important and most interesting contributions from all types of Vygotsky's writings, and thus from all six volumes, so as to reflect the overall purpose of the program that Vygotsky was developing at the time of his early death.

The introductory essays for each section to follow will explore various aspects of Vygotsky's biography in order to explain certain parts of his work and his writing, but the essentials of his life can be noted briefly here. Lev Semenovich Vogodsky was born to a well-educated Jewish family in the Russian empire, in Orsha, Belarus, on November 5, 1896. Soon the family moved to the larger city of the region, Gomel, where the father worked in a bank. (How the psychologist came to change the spelling of his name, replacing *d* with *t*, remains mysterious.) There were eight children, and Lev was the second. Lev was tutored at home, and in 1911 he entered a private classical school. Receiving the gold medal upon graduation (first place in his class), Vygotsky enrolled in Moscow Imperial University in 1913 and studied in the Faculty of Law. Simultaneous with legal studies, he took courses in the Faculty of History and Philology in Shanyavsky University, a coeducational and otherwise avant-garde institution in prerevolutionary Moscow. It seems likely that Vygotsky made many contacts in both schools, and he gained the reputation of a brilliant, busy student. We know, for example, that he took courses with P. P. Blonsky, G. G. Shpet, and G. I. Chelpanov in the recently opened Institute of Psychology in Moscow.

As Russia suffered terrible defeats in the Great War, Vygotsky finished his university courses. For Shanyavsky University he wrote a thesis in 1916, "Tragedy of Hamlet Prince of Denmark," his first important writing (some of which is included in Vygotsky, 1971). Because of the wars and the revolution, the events of the next period of Vygotsky's life are unclear, but they were undoubtedly very difficult. He returned to his family in Gomel, where he worked as a schoolteacher and/or instructor in a teacher-training school, and he remained there during German occupation, the Bolshevik Revolution, and the Civil War, a time of starvation for the people in that region. In 1920, Vygotsky suffered his first, acute attack of tuberculosis, the disease that repeatedly interrupted his life and would eventually kill him.

Vygotsky's return to the center of Russian intellectual life was marked by his participation in the Second All-Russian Psychoneurological Congress in Petrograd (soon to be renamed Leningrad) held in January 1924. He gave a lecture that was later published as "Consciousness as a problem in the psychology of behavior." By the end of that year, notable for Lenin's death, Vygotsky had married and accepted a position in the Moscow Institute of Psychology, whose directorship had recently passed from G. I. Chelpanov to K. N. Kornilov. His early work there concentrated on what the Russians called (and still call) "defectology," a combination of abnormal psychology and special education. Vygotsky worked directly with children who had been orphaned and damaged by the ravages of the recent wars and revolutionary upheavals. In summer 1925 he even traveled to Western Europe to present some of this work. The next year, however, Vygotsky suffered a second life-threatening attack of his disease, so he spent time in bed reading and rethinking his theoretical approaches. By this time he had clearly emerged as a leading thinker in the Institute, and even psychologists who had arrived there before him, such as A. N. Leontiev and A. R. Luria, were clearly under his influence.

In 1929 Vygotsky and a study group visited Tashkent. Luria remained there to carry out extensive ethnopsychological studies until 1931, his mentor being too sickly to stay on. As Vygotsky continued his writing and research in Moscow, Stalinist repression began to take a toll on his students and colleagues. P. P. Blonsky and A. B. Zalkind, leaders in the wider educational movement called "pedology," lost their lives. Others were scattered by internal exile, and an important group, including Luria and Leontiev, sought refuge in Kharkov, the Ukrainian capital at the time. Vygotsky made some trips there and to Leningrad as his failing health allowed, but on June 11, 1934, following a month of serious hemorrhages, he died in a Moscow sanatorium and was buried in Novodevichy Cemetery. Stalinist ideology eventually settled on Pavlovian "reflexology" as the appropriate Soviet approach to human psychology, and Vygotsky's students and admirers were unable even to refer to their teacher's name in their publications until well after Stalin's death.

There has been a gradual increase of appreciation of Vygotsky's work, long overdue. He appeared on the horizon of professional psychology briefly, after World War I; then his work was lost in the waves of Stalinist repression and the Cold War. Although a few writings of Vygotsky began to appear in Russian a bit earlier, the first breakout may actually have been in the United States, rather than in the Soviet Union: the MIT Press publication of an English translation of *Thought and Language* (Vygotsky, 1962). Certainly, Vygotsky had been continuously revered, at least in private, by a select number of people, an avant-garde in Russia and elsewhere, during a period when behaviorism was the dominant paradigm for the mainstream of psychology. After working in Moscow with Luria and others who were inspired by Vygotsky, Michael Cole joined forces with a few other Westerners (including Jerome Bruner) and, in the late 1960s, started to bring Russian work in psychology, including that of Vygotsky, to a Western audience.

This interest gradually increased through the 1980s in the United States (and, interestingly, in the Soviet Union as well); the greater attention corresponded with increased interest in qualitative research in psychology. Cole (1996), for example, has even related this trend back to Wilhelm Wundt's original project, the marriage of the experimental and the natural–historical approaches to psychology. During the 1980s, social constructionists (for example, Gergen, 1994, and Gergen & Davis, 1985) enhanced interest in Vygotsky, as did the rising interest in theoretical psychology in Europe. At the same time, in many venues, there was a growing interest in neuropsychology, which drew attention to the contributions of Luria, one of Vygotsky's most important associates.

The European Theoretical Psychology Activity Theory Group started in the 1980s, their name derived from a concept promoted by Leontiev. Since 1986, the International Society for Cultural and Activity Research (ISCAR) has been meeting annually, under changing titles and acronyms. Although few of the members would identify themselves as Vygotsky disciples, they clearly find inspiration in the cultural–historical approach, Vygotsky's hallmark. Interest in Vygotsky grew during the climax of the Cold War in the 1980s and during the optimistic time of its ending; the interest continues today, as people are concerned about disappointing, potentially tragic developments in the post-Soviet countries. We could call these groups neo-Vygotskian; they often invoke his name, analyze his works in light of present concerns, and otherwise are influenced by Vygotsky's thought.

The editors decided to follow the structure of the English version of the *Collected Works,* which has a different order than that chosen by the Soviet editors. It could easily be argued that the Soviet ordering would be better, or perhaps a chronological or some other order would be ideal. However, our chosen arrangement has the convenience that the serious reader can use *The Essential Vygotsky* as an introductory textbook and then easily turn to the six volumes of the English language *Collected Works* for more extensive reading. To give the reader a taste of the resources in the six volumes, we have included the references and notes (by Russian and by English editors) for Section I only. Any citations in the other sections refer to materials in the corresponding volumes of *Collected Works.*

The following list shows the order of volumes in the English edition of *Collected Works* (1987–99), the direct source of *The Essential Vygotsky,* with corresponding volume numbers and titles of the Russian edition (1982–84):

| | |
|---|---|
| Vol. 1. Problems of General Psychology | 2. *Problemy obshchei psikhologii* |
| Vol. 2. Fundamentals of Defectology | 5. *Osnovy defektologii* |
| Vol. 3. Problems of the Theory and History of Psychology | 1. *Voprosy teorii i istorii psikhologii* |
| Vol. 4. History of the Development of Higher Mental Functions | 3. *Problemy razvitiia psykhiki* |
| Vol. 5. Child Psychology | 4. *Detskaia psikhologiia* |
| Vol. 6. Scientific Legacy | 6. *Nauchnoe nasledstvo* |

Actually, a note of caution about text is in order. Even using the Russian "original text," *Sobranie sochineni* (1982–84), we cannot be assured of the purity of Vygotsky's text. The Russian editors, inspired by Luria, and ably chaired by A. V. Zaporozhets, surely did their best, and psychologists and intellectual historians will ever be in their debt for their monumental work. All the same, close work with the manuscript materials, most of them still held by Vygotsky's family, remains to be done (see Vygodskaya & Lifanova, 1996). The Russian editors themselves admit that the "collected works" are not the "complete works"; they particularly draw attention to many reviews and early essays that could not be included.

Doubts about the text involve even some of the most important ones. One example is discussed in the introduction to Section III of this volume. Elkhonon Goldberg told one of the editors (RWR) the story of another textual problem. When Luria began the project for the collected works, he was of course interested in finding the complete text of "Tool and sign," which had become an important Vygotskian concept in the intervening years. (see Section VI) However, looking in Vygotsky's papers, they could only locate an *English* version of this famous work. Luria assigned Goldberg the task to produce the Russian version by translating the English one! The Russian original had apparently been lost.

This brings up an interesting line of questions. Why was there an English text, which to that time had never appeared in print? Was there ever a Russian original? As Goldberg recounts, Luria and Vygotsky had both planned to attend a conference at Yale University in 1929. Luria actually did attend and presented his paper, "The new method of expressive motor reactions in studying affective traces" (1930). Vygotsky had apparently planned to attend also, to present "Tool and sign," but probably illness (or perhaps politics or some pressing personal matter) had prevented him from making the trip to the New World. It is interesting, now, to think that Vygotsky was planning to come to Yale, now that so many classes in psychology in the United States, particularly courses in child development, regularly invoke the name of Vygotsky. This is only one extreme example of the efforts the Russian editors had to make in order to collect the work of this seminal thinker in psychology. Critical studies of the source materials and manuscripts remain to be done. Maybe people who are becoming acquainted with this interesting writer by reading this book will do them someday.

In his review of *Mind in Society*, an important article that marked the rediscovery of Vygotsky for a wider Western readership, Stephen Toulmin (1978) called Vygotsky the "Mozart of psychology." Likely he chose this term because, like the great composer, Vygotsky was a very influential Wunderkind who died at an early age. Toulmin might just as well have called him the "Leonardo of psychology," since Vygotsky explored the psychology of art as well as the fundamentals of science; also, he left lots of unpublished work and had a hidden or delayed influence on his followers. The dedicated reader of *The Essential Vygotsky* can join in the process by which this important thinker will surely be raised to the highest ranks in the history of psychology.

## References

Cole, M. (1996). *Cultural psychology: A once and future discipline.* Cambridge, MA: Harvard University Press.

Gergen. K. J. (1994). *Reality and relationships: Soundings in social construction.* Cambridge, MA: Harvard University Press.

Gergen, K. J., & Davis, K. E. (Eds.). (1985). *The social construction of the person.* New York: Springer-Verlag.

Luria, A. R. (1930). The new method of expressive motor reactions in studying affective traces. In *Ninth International Congress of Psychology, held at Yale University, New Haven, Connecticut, September 1st–7th, 1929, Proceedings and Papers* (J. M. Cattell, Ed.). New York: Psychological Review.

Toulmin, S. (1978, September 28). The Mozart of psychology [Review of the book, *Mind in society*]. *New York Review of Books,* 51–57.

Vygodskaya, G. L., & Lifanova, T. M. (1996). *Lev Semenovich Vygotskii: Zhizn,' deyatel'noct,' shtrikhi k portretu* [Lev Semenovich Vygotsky: Life, activity, and sketches for a portrait]. Moscow: Smysl.

Vygotsky, L. S. (1962). *Thought and Language* (E. Hanfmann & G. Vakar, Eds. and Trans.; J. S. Bruner, Intro.). Cambridge, MA: MIT Press.
Vygotsky, L. S. (1971). *The psychology of art.* Cambridge, MA: MIT Press.
Vygotsky, L. S. (1978). *Mind in society* (M. Cole, S. Scribner, V. John-Steiner & E. Souderman, Eds. and Trans.). Cambridge, MA: Harvard University Press.
Vygotsky, L. S. (1982–84). *Sobranie sochinenii* (6 vols., A. V. Zaporozhets, Ed.). Moscow: Pedagogika.
Vygotsky, L. S. (1987–99). *Collected works* (6 vols., R. W. Rieber, Ed.). New York: Kluwer Academic/Plenum.

## Acknowledgments

The production of a book such as this one requires the efforts of a collective, as Vygotsky would have had it. The editors wish to thank all the contributors, whose introductory essays not only provoke thought but also reflect patience and cooperation. Mariclaire Cloutier, Sharon Panulla, Herman Makler, and Joseph Zito at Kluwer/Plenum have our undying gratitude for their talent and professionalism. The junior editor (DKR) also thanks his student assistants—Ryan Buck, Greg Mueller, and Thomas Stuart—without whom he simply could not have finished his part of the work.

# Contents

There is a kind of hypocritical complaint always paid to an originality, with this inconsistent purpose: that mankind are eager to receive what is new provided it is told in the old way.

—JAMES RUSH, The Philosophy of the Human Voice, 1893[1]

# A Dialogue with Vygotsky[2]

ROBERT W. RIEBER, City University of New York

> *This dialogue and book is for you, and you paid the price.*
> *Therefore, make its meaning come through by reading it twice.*

*Interrogator: What is a theory and what is it for?*
*Vygotsky:* It's a plan or a set of guiding principles that provide an explanation about human intentions.

*I: I see, but where does the theory come from?*
*V:* Oh, you mean what causes you to theorize? That's a rather complicated issue, but let's make one thing clear from the start. You're not born with a theory, and it didn't come out of the head of Zeus.

*I: You created it yourself, is that it?*
*V:* Not exactly. Let me put it to you this way; you build on ideas that are already out there, and you construct them so that they will facilitate your ability to discover the answers to the questions that you are interested in.

*I: A plan of action, like a battle plan, is that it?*
*V:* Exactly.

*I: Does it come from your brain, your mind, or something outside of you?*
*V:* You have to be careful, or you may fall into a trap when you pose a question like that. It doesn't come from any one place—from your brain, from your mind, or from here or there or from Red Square.

---

1. "James Rush and the theory of voice and mind," in *Psychology of Language and Thought: Essays on the Theory and History of Psycholinguistics*, eds. Peter Ostwald and R. W. Rieber (New York: Plenum, 1980), pp. 105–119.
2. This is a metalogue, i.e., an imaginary dialogue, with Vygotsky sometime during the last years of his life. The view he expresses is based on ideas discussed in this book (see parenthetical notes for their location). Nevertheless, the statements of his ideas in this metalogue are my interpretations of what I believe that Vygotsky probably meant. Interpretations are unavoidable when attempting to understand the writings of great thinkers. It is my hope that my interpretations will stimulate and facilitate your interpretations in such a way that they may emerge even more accurate than mine.

*I:* *How do you avoid the trap then?*

*V:* By assuming that your plan and your objective—that is, your answers to your questions—are not "things in themselves" but processes that have multiple levels of abstraction and determination. For example, they are historical, social, and personal, but not any single level in isolation.

*I:* *How do you determine one from another?*

*V:* What you must keep in mind is that you should not look for entities. Your objective is to pay attention to the interaction processes.

*I:* *But surely, one aspect may turn out to be more important than another.*

*V:* Maybe, but the question should be reconstructed to ask: important for what?

*I:* *Oh, I never thought of that.*

*V:* Good, now you can start thinking about it.

*I:* *Hmm, what do you mean by thinking?*

*V:* You might consider this concept of thinking to be something like the contemplation of an action, but it comes out of interaction processes within me, by which I was stimulating an activity in you. Consider for a moment the possibility that, in the communicative act, I'm really not sure exactly what I think until I've heard myself say it. In other words, my thinking or my interactive dialogue with myself, which is not yet expression-ripe, obtains meaning from the feedback I get as I'm listening to myself. (See the introductions by Bruner and Rieber to Section I on thinking and speech.)

*I:* *You mean, my thinking is not just in my head alone? Is that what you mean by inner speech?*

*V:* That's right. It can't be all in you alone because you are a social and political animal, as Aristotle pointed out many years ago. What we are talking about emerges not only from your internal monologue, but also from your history and the history of our history.

*I:* *That is very complex. What is the history of our history? Can you simplify it a bit?*

*V:* Oh sure, you can simplify almost anything. But I don't want to misdirect your thinking. The history of our history is a metaphor for the relationships between your own personal development and society's development and the development of the species in general. (See introduction to Section IV, on higher mental functions.) Your personal history of your life cannot be entirely separated from other peoples' lives in general. In other words, I'm talking about the relationship between ontogeny and phylogeny as applied to society at large.

*I:* *You seem to be implying that everything is connected in some way.*

*V:* Yes, I am. The reason that I emphasize this is that there is a great danger if you break the patterns of these connections. In fact, when you realize that they are broken, you must mend them. If you don't, you are bound to create a dangerous epistemological trap. It is true that you may have to extract certain abstractions or elements of the whole process to discover or test something that you are interested in. But your major purpose must always be kept in mind, and this purpose is to see how it all fits into the total pattern of things. In other words, if you break the pattern that connects the learning from the cognitive, emotional, and connotative aspects of mind, you create the danger of interfering in your ability to understand the natural view of human nature.

*I:*  *I see, so when you obtain your evidence as you suggested, how do you know if it's worth anything?*

*V:*  There are many ways. Surely you must put that evidence to the test to see how it works in real life.

*I:*  *It sounds like you are traveling on the "royal road to pragmatism."*

*V:*  If you like, yes. Our purpose is to obtain as much practical information as possible from our theoretical inferences to see whether they make a difference and positively affect our way of life.

*I:*  *How can you tell whether that information makes a difference?*

*V:*  You can tell by observations, and consensual validations of the observations, as to whether or not you have changed things in the direction that matched your inferences. For example, a change in A may result in a change in B. If it does, you produced a difference.

*I:*  *Okay, suppose the difference doesn't make a difference. Then what?*

*V:*  You're right, all differences are not equal, and some are more equal than others. But any new information you discover will make a difference. You then have to explore the qualities and quantities of the differences you have obtained and make a value judgment about them.

*I:*  *Okay, that sounds fine, but I think I am a bit confused about the difference between what is called theory and what is called method.*

*V:*  I'm not surprised. Too many people tend to bifurcate theory from method, and that seems to me to be unnatural. There are reciprocal relationships between the two. (Several section introductions discuss the relationship between theory and method; for example, Section IV, on higher mental functions.)

*I:*  *So it looks like indirect reciprocities are responsible for differences you find in trying to answer your questions.*

*V:*  In a sense, yes. However, one must be careful with regard to the questions that you ask. They may help you with your solutions or distract you from them. Nevertheless, impertinent questions can give rise to pertinent answers. Remember, in the eighteenth century Joseph Priestley actually discovered oxygen by asking some impertinent questions.[3]

*I:*  *How can you tell which way things will go in this endeavor; that is, which is theory and which is method?*

*V:*  Now, don't you see how your questions have been misleading you? Why does it have to be one or another when they are both part of an interaction process? Consider the possibility that your theory is going to help you recognize the most important or the most useful method.

*I:*  *How does that happen?*

*V:*  It happens if the methods produce a useful result.

---

3. Joseph Priestley, *Priestley's Writing on Philosophy, Science, and Politics*, ed. J. A. Passmore (New York: Collier's, 1965), pp. 139–150.

*I:* *Is this discussion related to your Zone of Proximal Development?*

*V:* Yes, exactly. My theory opened the door to the notion of the Zone of Proximal Development because the theory led to the idea of mental abilities, not just as entities alone inside the organism. You see mental abilities can emerge during childhood from many different sources. These sources are processes that are both internal and external to the organism. When it comes to measuring mental abilities, namely intelligence tests, psychology, particularly American psychology, metaphorically speaking, is attempting to measure the "size of the child's mind" by the shadow it casts. Conversely, I wish to measure the child's mind by the assisted light that it emits. (See Bruner's introduction to Section I, and the introduction to Section IV, for more on the ZPD.)

*I:* *Hmm. That's a different idea. It must have taken you a lot of time and effort to achieve all this.*

*V:* Of course, any positive result takes a lot of work, time, and effort.

*I:* *They say you are a driven person and that you produce too much too quickly.*

*V:* They are probably right, but you've got to realize that I am responding to the conditions of the times. We want to start a new way of helping psychology do its work for society and the people that live within it. Don't forget that the Romanov regime was an abomination for the Russian people.

*I:* *Of course, I understand that, but why is going back in time so important for your theory?*

*V:* Don't misunderstand, it's not just going back in time that is important, although it is important to understand your historical roots. You also must know how to capitalize on history's interest for the present as well as for the future. In order to not make the same mistakes, one must know how the past influences the present.

*I:* *My God, you sound like William James—even like a capitalist.*

*V:* Well, I do like William James, but I am not a capitalist. You must not misinterpret words that are meant to represent concepts figuratively.

*I:* *You're right, and I am sorry. This is a bad habit that many people have.*

*V:* I understand. Let's get on with this interview. Time is running out, and I do have a meeting shortly.

*I:* *Before you became a psychologist, you studied literature at the university, didn't you?*

*V:* Yes, formally speaking, but you must remember that literature is not divorced from psychology either. Shakespeare, Dostoevsky, and many other great literary figures were in many ways psychologists in spite of themselves. Take *Hamlet* for example. It's full of psychological insights.

*I:* *You wrote about* Hamlet *and Shakespeare early in your career, didn't you?*[4]

*V:* Yes, I did, and I am sure it had something to do with my becoming a psychologist.

*I:* *More and more, I think you sound like William James.*

---

4. See L. S. Vygotsky, *The Psychology of Art* (Cambridge: MIT Press, 1971).

*V:* Well, I told you that I am very fond of his work, but I am not William James. I like his work because we have been able to see further because of his insights. I acknowledge that old Newtonian idea that we see further if we stand on the shoulders of giants, but I also acknowledge the importance of avoiding the problems that come from a tendency to stand on the shoulders of midgets who think they are giants. We should not divide the importance of the past from its effect upon the present, and it is very important to turn our visions into useful activity for the benefit of society at large.

*I:* *You were critical of Pavlov, Bekhterev, and others, but didn't they also try to do what you just said?*
*V:* Maybe, but their theories limited them and their methods followed suit. It is important to recognize that there is now a clear and present crisis in the profession of psychology and in the culture at large.

*I:* *I suppose that's why you wrote the book you called The crisis in psychology.*
*V:* Yes, I hoped that it would wake us all up out of our deep sleep. In order to change something we first have to recognize what the problem is, and we must make our changes now before it's too late. We have to keep in mind that the word "crisis" implies opportunity as well as danger. Therefore, we must take advantage of the crisis situation before it takes advantage of us. (See Section III, on the "crisis.")

*I:* *Seems reasonable enough. Nevertheless, some psychologists think that you are too polemical and pessimistic about the current state of affairs. You have a tendency to put most other theories down.*
*V:* I am well aware of what you are saying; nevertheless, to repair anything you must have a clear vision of the problems before you can make any changes. It's the only way to stop a misdirected runaway system. Perhaps I am sometimes a bit too critical, but we have been wading in the backwash of old theories and methods too long.

*I:* *I suppose you're right, but you nevertheless do have a tendency to alienate other psychologists with in-your-face criticisms and with your pessimism.*
*V:* If you mean by pessimism that I seem to see the world the way it really is rather than the way I would like it to be, then I plead guilty to pessimism.

*I:* *Now that sounds sarcastic and maybe just a bit like semantic quibbling.*
*V:* Maybe. Have it as you will, but to make a difference is to change things now. We cannot afford to pussyfoot around; we've got to take a strong stance.

*I:* *John Dewey came to Russia in the early 1920s, and he seemed to like the new Russian plan for their educational system. If I am not mistaken, he even thought it was better than what they had in America, and he agreed to make recommendations for improvements to the Russian authorities. Why do you think they did not accept his recommendations?*
*V:* You must understand that I admire Dewey's work very much, and I have praised him in my writings. But this is a long and complicated story. In short, I can tell you that many of Dewey's educational reforms were already in our pedagogical plan. That's why we were so interested in his ideas. Nevertheless, Dewey thought that there was a danger in our system that would interfere with individual freedoms, or "individualism," as he called it—

whatever he meant by that.[5] Having said that, the authorities decided to see how our ideas would work, and we experimented with them ourselves.

*I:   Do you think there was a danger of undermining the individual by stressing the social too much?*
V:   Maybe, but we had to go with what we had, one step at a time. We liked many of Dewey's ideas, but Dewey was not Russian; he did not understand the Russian soul.

*I:   I'd like you to clarify for me the role of the individual in your theory. I understand that the individual is not the main focus but a part of an interactive system. But after I read your material (Section IV, on higher mental functions, and Section V, on child psychology), it is as if the individual is insignificant. Is that the way you mean it?*
V:   I'm not sure I understand what you mean by "insignificant." Certainly, we do not deny that there are individuals, but what we are trying to guard against is the "individualism" which most psychology has been advocating up until now. Having said that, what you must understand is that whatever the role of the individual may be, one cannot answer the question in the abstract; that is, it can only be answered meaningfully in reference to the particular situation related to the question you're asking. I'm sure you remember the saying of John Dunne that "no man is an island unto himself."

*I:   What role does intentionality play in your theory?*
V:   The notion of intentionality has been a matter of controversy for a very long time. Brentano raised it in his classic work: Psychology from an empirical standpoint. My approach is to claim that surely intentionality plays an important role in human nature; nevertheless, intentionality is not a separate thing from mind. Rather, I would suggest that people have many intentions. The nature of these largely depends on what happens to you at a particular point in your life. The time of your life span, the circumstances that surround you, and so forth, are all major factors that produce different kinds of intentions. For example, some intentions aren't intentions until some condition is satisfied. In other words, intentions are contingent intentions. They are the "springs of action" or the motivating forces of life. Life is contingent upon many circumstances. (The introduction to Section VI, on tool and sign explains that "mental processes are more than simply mental.")

*I:   Is that similar to being ready for activity?*
V:   Exactly. And when they are a part of the activity, the intentions are realized. You see this question of intention is one of the murkiest and most difficult concepts to clarify in any interactive process, particularly when you are dealing with an interactive process that deals with mind and society. This is all quite crucial when it comes to dealing with antisocial behavior, that is, whether a person is or is not to be held responsible for his or her actions.

*I:   I gather that you leave room for intentions to be something like secrets of the individual. Is that correct?*
V:   There is no question that people often conceal their intentions, deliberately or unconsciously.

---

5.  See, for example, J. Dewey, *Experience in Nature* (New York: W. W. Norton, 1929), p. 167.

*I:* *In other words, you can have unconscious intentions like unconscious motivations. Is that what you mean?*

*V:* Yes. Certainly people can be motivated by things they aren't aware of. Sometimes, however, it is better to be aware, and sometimes it is not. It depends on the circumstances. If you were aware of every stimulation that was coming from inside or outside of you, you wouldn't be able to process anything at all and would probably become inactivated.

*I:* *How does your theory differ from Freud's theory regarding unconscious intention?*

*V:* Freud's work was very important in the history of psychology. Luria and myself were both interested in Freud's work when it first came out in Russia.[6] But we soon discovered that Freud's theory originated from the individual and that he only gradually realized the importance of the social part of psychology. Yes, he had a diachronic perspective of sorts, but even when he got to the social part of his theory, he brought it all back to his misguided foundations that they were all a part of: "instinctual drives, libido and aggression." This is all too dualistic and reductionistic for my taste. (Section III criticizes psychoanalysis. For discussions of interactionism as opposed to reductionism, see the introductions to Sections IV and VI.)

*I:* *What about Adler?*

*V:* Now, of course, he broke off from Freud for reasons I just mentioned, and he was a good socialist in his politics, but he didn't seem to care much about Marxist philosophical ideas. But to make things worse, he called his psychology individual psychology and he was also a dualist of sorts in the sense that social factors didn't seem to play a role in the causation of mental problems. Of course he had this idea of social interest, but the way he described it, it seems all to be an individual affair.

*I:* *You seem to have similar opinions about Henri Bergson.*

*V:* Yes, Bergson also appears to be dualistic and comes too close to becoming materialistic, and I was concerned, since he was so popular, that nowadays many would be misdirected if they embraced his theory. But don't misunderstand me, he is a great philosophical thinker, but his psychology is not something we would want to promote.

*I:* *Let me pose a question to you that may seem to be impertinent, but I assume you will provide a pertinent answer. What makes the world go 'round? What I mean is, who and what runs the world?*

*V:* I assume you mean, what is my worldview? What makes things happen in world culture? Social institutions are first and foremost in determining what makes the world the way it is.

*I:* *Can you be more specific?*

*V:* Well, for example, you might first mention these three institutions together: government, corporations, and organized crime because, in most of the Western World, they are so much related it is hard to tell which is which at any point in time. But then you also have the institution of education and the institution of science. Remember that all these institutions are interrelated to one another; each has an affect on the other. Events are in the saddle driving

---

6. On the suppression of Freudian psychology in the Soviet Union, by the time of Vygotsky's death in 1934, see Martin A. Miller, *Freud and the Bolsheviks: Psychoanalysis in Imperial Russia and the Soviet Union* (New Haven : Yale University Press, 1998).

individuals and institutions toward the better or the worse. Individuals are part of the process, but if you don't make the institutions work, the individuals are lost. Psychology's job is to discover the best way to help both the process and the individuals that are part of it.[7]

*I:*  *What did you mean by the epitaph at the beginning of your book on the crisis in psychology (Section III in this volume), which reads, "the stone which the builders rejected has become the cornerstone?"*

*V:*  It signifies that they left out the time, place, and people that built it. We placed the cornerstone where it really belonged—they didn't.

*I:*  *If you could start your career all over again, would you do it any differently?*

*V:*  Let me oversimplify, because I see I am late for my conference. I'd probably do it pretty much the same way. But the experiment has really never been carried out, and we can't know whether it will be successful unless we try.

*I:*  *Fascinating, I never thought of it that way, and I can't argue with you.*

*V:*  Good, let me go to my meeting. And so, as Shakespeare liked to say, "Be of good cheer."

*I:*  *Most honored and grateful.*

*V:*  Not at all.

* * *

With an active, Spinozaesque cognitive style, Vygotsky turned life inside out—driving semiotic cultural evolution into personal history—scaffolding brain levels into developmental stages as he fused the external into the internal world. With all of that a new theory was born. In short, Vygotsky was a revolutionary intellectual. All that we have mentioned surely places him outside the mainstream of psychological thought. If he were in any 'mainstream,' it might be such a mainstream as defined by the seminal thought of the great London clinician, Hughlings Jackson, who also discussed inner speech, biological development, evolution, and dissolution (a concept that was influenced by Spencer and then influenced him in turn). Nevertheless, even Jackson did not emphasize a historically diachronic perspective on psychological development, which must stand as Vygotsky's most important contribution to psychological thought.

---

7.  Compare the revealing anecdote that opens a book by another social psychologist of the time: Floyd Henry Allport^, *Institutional Behavior: Essays Toward a Re-interpretation of Contemporary Social Organization* (Chapel Hill: University of North Carolina Press, 1933), p. 3.

    At a meeting of the faculty of a certain large university a proposal for a new administrative policy was being discussed. The debate was long and intense before a final vote of adoption was taken. As the professors filed out of the room an instructor continued with one of the older deans.

    "Well," observed the latter official, "it may be a little hard on some people; but I feel that, in the long run, the new plan will be for the best interests of the institution."

    "Do you mean that it will be for the good of the students?" inquired the younger man.

    "No," the dean replied, "I mean it will be for the good of the whole institution."

    "Oh, you mean that it will benefit the faculty as well as the students."

    "No," said the dean, a little annoyed, "I don't mean *that;* I mean it will be a good thing for the institution itself."

    "Perhaps you mean the trustees then—or the Chancellor?"

    "No, I mean the institution, the *institution!* Young man, don't you know what an institution is?"

# I

## Introduction to *Thinking and Speech*[1]

JEROME BRUNER, *New York University*

Twenty-five years ago, I was privileged to write an introduction to the first translation of Vygotsky's classic, *Thought and Language* (1962). In the opening paragraph of that introduction, I remarked:

> Lev Semenovich Vygotsky . . . in his student days at the University of Moscow . . . read widely and avidly in the fields of linguistics, social science, psychology, philosophy, and the arts. His systematic work in psychology did not begin until 1924. Ten years later he died of tuberculosis at the age of 38 [actually 37—eds.]. In that period, with the collaboration of such able students and co-workers as Luria, Leontiev, and Sakharov, he launched a series of investigations in developmental psychology, education, and psychopathology, many of which were interrupted by his untimely death. The present volume, published posthumously in 1934, ties together one major phase of Vygotsky's work, and though its principal theme is the relation of *Thought and Language*, it is more deeply a presentation of a highly original and thoughtful theory of intellectual development. Vygotsky's conception of development is at the same time a theory of education.

Before the translation of that book in 1962, there were no extended writings of Vygotsky available in English, and only a few shorter articles. Since then, many important works have reported or commented upon his work—the volume of Michael Cole and his collaborators (Vygotsky, 1978); the rich volumes of Alexander Romanovich Luria (1961, 1976, 1979), presenting and expanding many of Vygotsky's ideas; and James Wertsch's useful synoptic volume (1985) on Vygotsky's thought. All of them have suggested that *Thought and Language* is, as it were, only the tip of an iceberg, that Vygotsky's depth was far greater than the book suggested. The six volumes of the *Collected Works* (1987–99) confirm that point dramatically. And so we open *The Essential Vygotsky* with chapters from this work, retranslated and republished in 1987 as *Thinking and Speech*.

Vygotsky was not only a psychologist, he was also a cultural theorist, a scholar deeply committed to understanding not simply man, conceived as a solo "organism," but Man as an

---

1. This is a very slightly altered version of "Prologue to the English Edition" in *The Collected Works of L. S. Vygotsky, Volume 1: Problems of General Psychology (Including the volume* Thinking and Speech) (Robert W. Rieber and Aaron S. Carton, Eds.; Norris N. Minick, Trans.) (pp. 1–16). New York: Plenum Press, 1987.

9

expression of human culture. When I remarked a quarter-century ago that Vygotsky's view of development was also a theory of education, I did not realize the half of it. In fact, his educational theory is a theory of cultural transmission as well as a theory of development. For "education" implies for Vygotsky not only the improvement of the *individual's* potential but the historical expression and growth of the human culture from which Man springs. It is in the service of both a psychological and a cultural theory that Vygotsky places such enormous emphasis upon the role of language in man's mental life and upon its cultivation during growth. For Vygotsky, language is both a result of historical forces that have given it shape and a tool of thought that shapes thought itself. In the end, as we shall see, it is also a liberator: the means whereby man achieves some degree of freedom from both his history and his biological heritage. In mastering language in all its forms—in scientific, artistic, and spontaneous dialogue—the individual reflects history. But Vygotsky did *not* subscribe to the Soviet Marxist dogma that then viewed man as a mere "product" of history and circumstance. For him, the heart of the matter is the interaction between man and his tools, particularly the symbolic tool of language. In the end, Vygotsky flirts with the idea that the use of language creates consciousness and even free will.

Never for a moment overlook Vygotsky's objective. Like Karl Marx, he was in search of a theory of development that would embrace a scientific, historical determinism and a principle of spontaneity as well. Spontaneity is not so much "overcoming" history as it is turning it to new uses, converting it, so to speak, from a fate into a tool. And, of course, one of the chief boons of human history is language and its ways of use. He was forever intrigued with the inventive powers that language bestowed on mind—in ordinary speech, in the novels of Tolstoy, the plays of Chekov, the *Diary* of Dostoevsky, in the stage directions of Stanislavsky, in the play of children.

Vygotsky's Marxism is closer to Althusser (1978), Habermas (1971), and the Frankfurt School than to the Soviet Marxism of his times or of late. It is not surprising, then, that his work was suppressed in the early 1930s. It was appealing enough, however, to circulate underground from hand to hand, and by the testimony of Luria it affected an entire generation of psychologists. The official reason given for the suppression was that his monograph on the Kazakhistan and Kurdistan peasants flouted the interdiction against attributing faulty mental processes to peasants, particularly at a time when Russia's peasantry were undergoing collectivization. My own surmise is, rather, that Vygotsky's vigorous espousal of the place of consciousness in mental life made him suspect to the increasingly rigid Stalinist ideologues who overlooked matters psychological. After the suppression was lifted, the "battle of consciousness" moved officially to center stage in Soviet psychology, with Vygotsky's followers arrayed against such orthodox Pavlovians as Ivanov-Smolensky. In time, with the acceptance of Pavlov's theory of "Second Signal System," the atmosphere improved. Vygotskian theory could be restated in the language of the Second Signal System in a way that captured the distinction between stimuli acting directly on the nervous system (the First Signal System) and those that were mediated by language and concepts (the Second).

It is quite evident once again that instrumental action is at the core of Vygotsky's thinking—action that uses both physical and symbolic tools to achieve its ends. He gives an account of how, in the end, man uses nature and the toolkit of culture to gain control of the world and of himself. But there is something new in his treatment of this theme, or perhaps it is my new recognition of something that was there before. For now there is a new emphasis on the manner in which, through using tools, man changes himself and his culture. Vygotsky's reading of Darwin is strikingly close to that of modern primatology (e.g. Washburn & Howell, 1960), which also rests on the argument that human evolution is altered by man-made tools whose use then creates a technical-social way of life. Once that change occurs, "natural" selection becomes dominated by cultural criteria and favors those able to adapt to the tool-using, culture-using way of life. By Vygotsky's argument, tools, whether practical or symbolic, are initially "external," used outwardly on nature or in communicating with others. But tools affect their users: language, used first as a communicative tool, finally shapes the minds of those who adapt to its use. His chosen epigraph from Francis Bacon, used in *Thinking and Speech*, could not be more apposite: neither hand nor mind alone suffices; the tools and devices they employ finally shape them.

Vygotsky was an engaged intellectual and a child of his revolutionary times. He did not treat psychological issues in isolation from the issues that then preoccupied Russian intellectual life. He was closely in touch with linguistic thinking as represented by Jakobson, Trubetskoy, and the so-called Leningrad Formalists. Indeed, his studies of linguistics preceded his formal work in psychology. Emphasis upon meaning, for example, was central in that linguistic tradition. It was Jakobson (1978), after all, following in the footsteps of his teacher Baudouin de Courtenay, who first enunciated the principle that even the sound system of language was not to be understood through analysis based on the muscle groups implicated in sound production, but through an understanding of how sound changes affected meaning—the famous concept of the phoneme.

And in those days, Vladimir Propp (1968) was formulating a theory of the structure of the folktale that conceived of the characters and the elements of plot as functions or constituents of the plot structure as a whole. The spirit of the work of that time was decidedly "top-down": higher functions controlled lower functions, whether it was lexemes dominating phonemes or plots dominating character and episode. Indeed, Roman Jakobson was fond of asserting years later that Vygotsky's approach to psychology as well as to language was far more in the "high Russian intellectual tradition" than was the bottom-up approach of the Pavlovian reflexologists.

The same can be said of Vygotsky's treatment of the role of consciousness, which I shall discuss more fully later. Russian literary theory (particularly poetics)—and Vygotsky was well versed in its debates—placed great emphasis on poetic language as an instrument for arousing consciousness. The critic Viktor Shklovsky (1965), for example, had introduced the concept of *otstranenie*, the "making strange of the ordinary," and proposed that it was the means that the poet used for creating consciousness in the reader. And poets like Mayakovsky, Mandelshtam, and Akhmatova thought of themselves as engaged in a struggle for new consciousness. So when Vygotsky argued that "climbing to higher ground" conceptually with the aid of language also increased consciousness, he was not making his proposal in a cultural vacuum. For all that, let it be said that he vociferously opposed any Bergsonian view of autonomous consciousness. Such "bourgeois idealism" was not for him. Rather, consciousness emerges out of the interaction of higher mental processes with the tool of language. But for all his appeals to dialectical materialism, he never quite escaped the suspicion of the official ideologists. If his being Jewish did not arouse their distrust, his cosmopolitanism did, for his writings are full of references to the work of German, French, Swiss, and American investigators.

Later I shall also want to say more about the Russian roots of Vygotsky's ideas about the role of dialogue in language and consciousness. Here he was influenced by the ideas of the stage director Stanislavsky (whom he cites) and possibly indirectly by those of the linguist Bakhtin (1981). He rejected the notion that human development could be viewed as a solo achievement. It starts initially as a conversational, dialogical process, and then moves inward and becomes the "inner speech" of thought. Let me turn directly to that issue now.

\* \* \*

The "moving inward" of speech is nowhere better illustrated than in Vygotsky's now famous idea about the Zone of Proximal Development (ZPD). It is a stunning concept on its own, but it also serves to give connectedness to a wide range of Vygotsky's thought. It refers to the brute fact, perhaps first celebrated by Plato in the *Meno*, where he discusses the young slave's apparent "knowledge" of geometry while being questioned appropriately by Socrates, that ignorant learners can do far better in understanding a matter when prompted or "scaffolded" by an expert than they can on their own. The idea of the ZPD focuses attention on the role of dialogue as a precursor to inner speech, in this case the dialogue between a more expert teacher and a less expert learner. Once a concept is explicated in dialogue, the learner is enabled to reflect on the dialogue, to use its distinctions and connections to reformulate his own thought. Thought, then, is both an individual achievement and a social one.

There is another outcome that results from such "assisted" learning, and that bears upon consciousness and volition. For when one climbs to higher conceptual ground—as in going from arithmetic to algebra with the aid of a teacher—one achieves conscious control of the knowledge, what Piaget in another context calls a *prise de conscience,* a taking into consciousness. Vygotsky (like Plato, Piaget, and others who have confronted this riddle) was obviously never fully able to explain how consciousness takes over. "Inner speech" was plainly implicated, but *how* language serves as an instrument of consciousness escaped Vygotsky as it has escaped us all. His student Luria (1976), studying the role of language in the actions of very young children, made a start toward untying this riddle with an experiment showing that one role of language in thought is to help inhibit action, the inhibition being in the form of a command to oneself. The implication (and we shall return to it later) is that consciousness and direct action stand in an inverse relation to each other. But inhibition of action was only one function of inner speech.

Far more important for both Vygotsky and Luria was a general "organizational" function of inner speech whereby a complicated world of stimuli was consciously rendered into a meaningful and syntactically well-formed structure. An example was pro- vided years later in a study of conditional learning in young children carried out again by Luria (1976). They were to discriminate between the silhouette of an airplane when it was displayed against a yellow background and when it appeared against a gray background. At first they could not make the discrimination. But when the children consciously and deliberately learned the formula "planes can only fly in sunny weather, but not in cloudy weather," they mastered the task. Without the intermediation of this verbal formula, they failed.

But this was not enough either (though it would have pleased Vygotsky). Rather, he was interested as much in how it was that language and thought managed to fit together so well, so well indeed that there was scarcely a situation in which one would not find words to fit the experience. Recall that he believed that there were two independent "streams," one of thought and the other of language, and that they "flowed" together with the effect that language gave shape and conscious direction to thought. How do we get over the seemingly "uncrossable Rubicon that separates thinking from speech?" His proposed solution is strikingly different from the one proposed by Benjamin Lee Whorf (1956), who saw the fit between language and thought in the form of a correspondence between lexicon and grammar on the one side and concepts on the other. Vygotsky rejects such correspondence notions. To explicate his point (in the concluding chapter of *Thinking and Speech*), he turns to the literary arts and makes the following remark:

> The theater faced this problem of the thought that lies behind the word earlier than psychology. In Stanislavsky's system in particular, we find an attempt to recreate the subtext of each line in a drama, to reveal the thought and desire that lies behind each expression. Consider the following example: Chatskii says to Sophia: "Blessed is the one who believes, for believing warms the heart." Stanislavsky reveals the subtext of this phrase as the thought: "Let's stop this conversation." We would be equally justified, however, in viewing this phrase as an expression of a different thought, specifically: "I do not believe you. You speak comforting words to calm me." It might express still another thought: "You cannot fail to see how you torture me. I want to believe you. For me, that would be bliss." The living phrase, spoken by the living person, always has its subtext. There is always a thought hidden behind it.
>
> In the examples given above where we tried to show the lack of correspondence between the psychological and grammatical subject and predicate [an earlier reference to the fact that *topic* did not always correspond to subject, nor *comment* to predicate, a central point made by Jakobson and the Prague Circle], we broke off our analysis at midpoint. We can now complete it. Just as a single phrase can serve to express a variety of thoughts, one thought can be expressed in a variety of phrases. The lack of correspondence between the psychological and grammatical structure of the sentence is itself determined by the way the thought is expressed in it. By answering the question, "Why has the clock stopped?" with "The clock fell," we can express the thought: "It is not my fault that the clock is broken; it fell!" However, this thought can be expressed through other words as well: "I am not in the habit of touching other's things; I was just dusting here." Thus, phrases that differ radically in meaning can express the same thought.
>
> This leads us to the conclusion that thought does not immediately coincide with verbal expression. Thought does not consist of individual words like speech. . . . Thought is always something whole, something with significantly greater extent and volume than the individual word. . . . It does not arise step by step through separate units in the way that . . . speech develops. *What is contained simultaneously in thought unfolds sequentially in speech.* . . .
>
> Therefore, the transition from thought to speech is an extremely complex process which involves the partitioning of the thought and its re-creation in words. That is why thought does not correspond with the word, why it does not even correspond with the word meanings in which it is expressed. The path from thought to word lies through meaning. There is always a background thought, a hidden subtext in our speech. The direct transition from thought to word is impossible. The construction of a complex path is always required. This is what underlies the . . . lamentation that the thought is inexpressible . . . (pp. 105–106).

And this leads him to the final step in this astonishingly modern argument, one that gets him very close to Austin's (1962) and Searle's (1969) Speech Act Theory and to Grice's (1968) distinction between utterer's meaning and timeless meaning.

> We must now take the final step in the analysis of the internal planes of verbal thinking. Thought is not the last of these planes. It is not born of other thoughts. Thought has its origins in the motivating sphere of consciousness, a sphere that includes our inclinations and needs, our interests and impulses, and our affect and emotion. The affective and volitional tendency stands behind thought. Only here do we find the answer to the final "why" in the analysis of thinking. . . . A true and complex understanding of another's thought becomes possible only when we discover its real, affective-volitional basis. The motives that lead to the emergence of thought and direct its flow can be illustrated through the example we used earlier, that of discovering the subtext through the specific interpretation of a given role. Stanislavsky teaches that behind each of a character's lines there stands a desire that is directed toward the realization of a definite volitional task. That which is re-created here through the method of specific interpretation is the initial moment in any act of verbal thinking in living speech. . . . A volitional task stands behind every expression (p. 107).

What is especially interesting about Vygotsky's conception is that not only is each act of speech guided by illocutionary intention, as in Austin or in Searle, but that illocutionary intentions are, so to speak, multiple. That is to say, an utterance is driven by such conventional and manifest communicative intentions as requesting, indicating, promising, and so forth, but it is also guided by a more latent subtext of intended meaning that is idiosyncratic in nature and related entirely to the interaction of the characters involved in the exchange. This is where the Stanislavsky method serves him as his model. And you will find at the conclusion of the final chapter of *Thinking and Speech* a detailed *explication du texte* of an exchange between three characters in a play illustrating this multileveled interpretation that must be carried on between interlocutors if they are to grasp meaning fully. Then he concludes with the following characterization of "the living drama of verbal thinking":

> Understanding the words of others also requires understanding their thoughts. And even this is incomplete without understanding their motives or why they expressed their thoughts. In precisely this sense, we complete the psychological analysis of any expression only when we reveal the most secret internal plane of verbal thinking—its motivation. With this, our analysis is finished.

And so we see Vygotsky revealed. We see him as an interpretivist who, in Geertz's (1973) sense, urges that "thick interpretation" is indispensable for the extraction of meaning, interpretation that takes into account not only grammar and lexicon and the conventions of the social setting but also the underlying intentions and desires of the actor in the situation. In any act of speech, then, cultural and historical, as well as personal and idiosyncratic, demands are expressed by the speaker and must then be interpreted by the listener. Learning to *speak*, acquiring the *use* of language, must then be viewed not simply as the mastering of words or of grammar or of illocutionary conventions, but of how to textualize one's intent and to situate a locution appropriately in a personal context involving another person with whom one shares a history, however brief. That is what Vygotsky is seeking to illustrate in his citation of Stanislavsky's stage directions.

I mentioned earlier the involvement of Vygotsky in the literary–linguistics debates of the postrevolutionary Russia of his formative years. Let me say a word further about other ideas that may have grown out of that involvement. For the Russian Formalists, for example, the essence of literature was the relation between a *fabula* and its *syuzhet*—between a timeless "theme" or thought that lay behind a story and its sequential linearization in both plot and language. Vygotsky too saw the relation of *Thinking and Speech* in this way. Thought was, as it were, simultaneous; language was successive. The problem for the speaker was to convert his all-present thought into the linear form of speech in a particular situation. It was no happenstance that Vygotsky found his inspiration in Stanislavsky. This was more of the "high Russianness" of Vygotsky.

Let me add one further word to this discussion about the place of "consciousness." I have already mentioned its centrality in Russian literary debates—particularly in the debates of the Symbolists, Acmeists, and Futurists that swirled first in the coffeehouses of Leningrad and then spread throughout literary Russia in the 1920s and 1930s. As noted earlier, the critic Shklovsky (1965) typically proclaimed the consciousness-raising function of poetry and invoked *otstranenie* ("making the familiar strange") as its principal linguistic tool. Others were concerned in different ways with the question of what shapes imagination. One such voice was Bakhtin's (1978), whose discussion of the "dialogic imagination" also touched on the arousal and shaping of consciousness and meaning. His interest was in the idea of "voices" that enter into the construction of fiction, and the manner in which voice in this sense was an element in imagination and thought. It is hard to know how well Bakhtin and Vygotsky were acquainted with each other. But obviously the idea of dialogic imagination was very current in postrevolutionary Russia, and even the avidly modernist and eccentric Anatoly Lunacharsky, Lenin's eccentric Commissar of Public Education, appreciated its significance for a Marxist theory of mind and culture and gave it his public blessing (e.g., Hughes, 1981). Unfortunately, Lunacharsky did not last long in office; his blessings were never turned into official action. Bakhtin, opposed by what had already become the Old Guard, was exiled to far Kazakhstan, and Vygotsky's work was banned. But, ironically, the discussion of the role of dialogue in the shaping of thought and imagination has today an even higher place on the agenda of contemporary debate in literary theory and psychology than it did when first introduced. Bakhtin and Vygotsky have become posthumous world figures: what was once a Russian issue in danger of cultural extinction has become a topic of worldwide discussion.

The renowned Russian linguistic theorist V. I. Ivanov (1982), eulogizing Roman Jakobson, characterized him as a "visitor from the future." I believe that describes as well the whole postrevolutionary generation of literary–linguistic–philosophical thinkers of which Vygotsky was so incandescent a part. They were indeed "visitors from the future," as will be evident to the reader perusing the pages of this volume.

* * *

Vygotsky's six lectures on human development reveal the true derivational depth and detail of his thinking. (Lectures 1 and 4 are reproduced in the present publication as chapters 4 and 5; all six are in Volume 1 of *Collected Works*.) Though written half a century ago, and though based on the research findings of that distant time, they have an uncanny ring of modernity. They deal successively and cumulatively with the classic problems of psychology:

perception, memory, thought, emotion, imagination, and will, all treated from the perspective of development. They are timeless masterpieces: elegantly and powerfully argued, full of surprises, swift. The philosopher Stephen Toulmin (1978) once referred to Vygotsky as "the Mozart of psychology." Reading these lectures is like listening to the Hafner or the Jupiter. You understand why Vygotsky's reputation shone so brightly for those sophisticated Moscow students a half-century ago and why his banned writing circulated so widely among them.

I propose to set forth the argument of each lecture in turn so that the reader not familiar at first hand with the form in which the issues are raised will be helped to understand the scope and daring of Vygotsky's approach. At the end, I shall try to put them together in a broader perspective.

In the opening lecture on the development of perception (Lecture 1, included in the present volume), Vygotsky begins with a riddle. If we accept the work of the Gestalt psychologists, as we must, how can we account for the fact that adult perception differs so strikingly from perception in the young child? How can early perception be both organized and immature? Vygotsky, like the Gestaltists, rejects the associationist approach to perception on grounds that a theory of memory (which is what a theory of association necessarily is) cannot explain perception. How can the past, organized by memory, explain a present perception? How did memory, in the first place, take its current form unless it had been shaped as well by the nature of perception? No present mental function can be "explained" by association without begging this question. There must also be principles that operate within perception and that precede any influence that memory may have upon it, associative or otherwise.

To make his point, he explores several classic phenomena in perception: the *constancies* (why white looks white even in shadow, or a dinner plate circular even at an angle, why people, for example, do not seem to change size as drastically as the size of their retinal images in our eye when they walk away from us, etc.); the compellingness of *meaning* in perception (how difficult it is for anything to seem totally meaningless); and how we perceive in a two-dimensional picture what it represents in a three-dimensional world. He laments that Gestalt psychology does no better at accounting for the development of any of these phenomena than the associationists whose errors they deplore.

I will not recapitulate his argument in full here lest I steal the reader's pleasure, for the lectures are full of suspense. But let me whet the reader's appetite with an example. The constancies develop over time during development: that much is known. Akin to the constancies is the size–weight illusion: of two lifted objects of equal physical weight, the smaller will almost invariably be judged heavier. Vygotsky sees it as a form of "density conservation." If the illusion does not develop with age, it is usually symptomatic of severe mental subnormality. This strongly suggests that some other mental function is "fusing" with perception in the course of growth that permits the taking in of more related stimulus information (both the size *and* weight of an object).

We also know that some subnormal children are not as likely to "perceive meaning" in events. Consider the emergence of various phenomena in the development of picture perception as children grow older. The youngest children, faced with pictures to interpret, first report isolated objects. Then, as they grow older, they report the objects in action. Still older, they report features or properties of the objects. And finally they reach an age when they can report the overall scene. How can one reconcile this finding with a common one, reported by Gestalt psychologists in studies of nonpictorial, real-world perception, that children first perceive the global properties of the visual world and only gradually are able to isolate its parts?

Vygotsky notes that there is something different about perceiving the world and interpreting a picture that the latter involves more than perceptual processing. Some other process is involved. He comments (almost with glee!) that the order of emergence of the child's "stages" of picture perception corresponds precisely to the order of acquisition of parts of speech: first he learns nouns for objects, then verbs for actions, then adjectives for features or properties, and finally sentences for the overall scene. He offers a hypothesis: does not the developing organization of the percept of a picture depend on the fusing of language-dependent thought with the process of perception? Is it not better thought of as perception entering the sway of higher-order processes that can then use lower-order processes instrumentally? Obviously the *potential* to deal with the whole scene is there from the start, but it is not yet organized analytically, as would be required for the interpretation of pictures. He says, half tongue in cheek, "It would be extraordinarily difficult if the child actually achieved the *potential* of perceiving the whole meaningful situation only between the ages of ten and twelve!" (p. 298; emphasis added). What the child can report in an artificialized task (like picture interpretation) depends on how his perceptual capacities interact with other mental functions.

He then reports a study of his own that turns the whole question on its head. Let another function interact with perception, this time imaginative play with other children. Now the child who in a strict picture-viewing experiment could name only isolated objects will describe the *full* scene to his companions with considerable imagination: "at each stage in the child's development we observe changes in interfunctional connections and relationships" (p. 299). The interacting functions bring into being new powers and create new functional systems. One cannot consider perception in isolation, but must always take into account other mental functions with which it interacts. Perceptual development is the development of new functional connections between perception and other functions.

The lecture on memory (Lecture 2, not included in this work) centers immediately on the problem of representation. After rejecting "bourgeois idealist" efforts to cope with the relation of mind and brain, to see memory as the "bridge between consciousness and matter," he takes as his starting point the well-known experiments of Gottschaldt and of Zeigarnik. The former showed that no matter how much one practiced remembering certain abstract geometric forms, practice had no effect whatever on how well one was able to recognize those same figures when they were embedded and masked in more complex figures. This demonstrated for Vygotsky that memory depends on structural laws governing mental activity, in this case laws of figural integrity. So too Zeigarnik's finding. In her still well-known experiment, subjects were better able to recall uncompleted tasks than ones that they had completed. This immediately implicates the role of *intention* in memory. For Vygotsky, both studies show that memory is not autonomous, that it takes multiple forms, and that it cannot be explained by a single generalization such as the laws of association. For what have such laws to do with such matters as intention?

Finally, we know that memory depends on the meaningful organization that we can impose upon the material to be remembered. Where initially meaningless material can be represented in a meaningful way, remembering is guaranteed by a single encounter.

When we turn to children's memory, the first thing we note is how astonishingly good their raw memory is, language learning being the prime example. So what develops? One must distinguish between *direct* and *mediated* memory, the latter made possible by all manner of memory aids, from strings on the fingers to note taking and precis making. The principal tool of mediated memory is, of course, the verbal formulation or reformulation of what has been encountered and needs to be remembered. By means of such formulation and reformulation, memory is converted from an involuntary, automatic activity into a conscious, intentional, instrumental function. The progress from direct to indirect memory, moreover, characterizes not only the development of the child but the emergence of man into modern culture. So at the start of life, the child's thinking depends on memory. With time and development, memory comes increasingly to depend on thinking, on acts of formulation and reformulation.

And so to the lecture on thinking, a polished gem of Russian intellectual argumentation (Lecture 3, not included in this volume). It begins with an attack on association, his favorite opening target in all the lectures. The associationists, he charges, have such an abstract and undifferentiated conception of thought that they are forced forever to bring in special mechanisms to account for newly observed events. So, for example, they need special processes to deal with such commonsense matters as the fact that thought is generally goal-directed and that it very often exhibits a quite logical, orderly pattern. To account for these ordinary matters, they invoke the idea of perseveration. Perseveration counterbalances association: the flow of thought is thereby slowed from "a gallop or whirlwind of ideas" (the flow of association) and yet, thanks to the balance of the two processes, is kept from being mired in static obsession (perseveration). Imbalances between the two tendencies are invoked by the associationists to account for various mental diseases. The development of thought in the child is also accounted for in these terms. The terminus of growth is the balancing of the two tendencies.

But for Vygotsky all the balance in the world cannot account for why, in the first place, thought tends toward a logical form and serves in the fulfillment of human intentions. Vygotsky sees the shortcomings of associationism as having provoked three corrective efforts. The first, behaviorism, restated the old position in "objective" terms, but to no avail. Frequency and reinforcement, related to overt behavior, do no better than the old mentalistic laws of association in accounting for the intentionality and orderly logic of thought. The second corrective was the idea of a "determining tendency" that propels thought toward goals. However it might account for intentionality, it still left the internal logic of thought unexplained. The third corrective effort was Act Psychology which argued (and tried to demonstrate) that thought was nonsensory or "imageless" and therefore not governed by association. "Rationality" is then stipulated as a feature of this nonsensory process, just as associativeness is stipulated as a property of image processes. Vygotsky dismisses this as rank dualism and charges the Act Psychologists with dragging vitalism into the explanation of mind. Vygotsky dismisses all three views—behaviorism, determining tendencies, and Act Psychology—as grossly insufficient for dealing with questions of human development.

He then turns to Piaget appreciatively, but with a critical edge. His critique will be familiar territory to the modern reader and needs little further comment. In effect, he applauds Piaget's description of the process of growth, but complains about the total lack of a mechanism in his system to account for how or why growth takes place at all—a not unfamiliar complaint a half-century later.

Vygotsky proposes to approach the problem in a new way. For him, of course, the key issue is the relationship between thought and speech during development. He rejects both the Wurzburg proposal that "the word is nothing but the external clothing of thought" and the behaviorist's formula that thought is speech, but going on subvocally. A paradox serves Vygotsky as his point of departure. It is this: in the child's mastery of uttered or vocal speech, he progresses from single words to two-word phrases to simple sentences, and so on. Yet at the semiotic or "meaningful" level, the meanings that are inherent in the child's utterance begin as though expressing full sentences (the so-called holophrase) and only gradually differentiate to express meanings that correspond to phrases or single words. In short, external speech grows from part to whole; meaning from whole to part. We would express this idea today by saying that early language is highly context dependent or intentionally imbedded, and that, as Grace de Laguna argued, it cannot be comprehended without knowing the context and state in which it is uttered. Only gradually does the child's meaning come to be more or less directly mappable onto his actual utterance. Vygotsky argues that it is for this reason that the child, though only able to *utter* single words, is nonetheless able to *act out in play* the full meaning contained in "one-word utterance." For acting out in play entails different processes than talking out in speech.

The next step in his argument is an important one and is already familiar to the reader. In speech, generally, syntactical or grammatical forms do *not* map uniquely on only one meaning. Lexically and grammatically, *polysemy* prevails. Meaning is never fully determined by, and does not correspond directly to, utterance. The last chapter of *Thinking and Speech* includes a quotation from Dostoevsky's, *The Diary of a Writer.* Five drunken workmen carry out a complicated dialogue for five minutes, though the only word any of them utters is a forbidden noun not used in mixed company. Intonation and circumstances determine its meaning in context. Vygotsky concludes that if language operates in this way, then "the child's work on a word is not finished when its meaning is learned" (p. 322). He cannot be said to have mastered the language when, at five or six, he has mastered its lexicon and grammar. He must also understand when, under what conditions, and how to combine language with his intentions and how, then, to do so with appropriate subtlety. What is at issue, as we would say today, is mastering the pragmatics of a language—the forms and functions of its use.

With the development of higher mental functions, the child is finally able to reflect, to turn around on his own language and thought, and to differentiate and integrate them still further. To readers of later Piaget, of course, this attainment will be recognized as akin to "formal operations" where the object of thought is no longer the world as such but propositions about the world. But for Vygotsky, unlike Piaget, there is no "stage" but only a progressive unfolding of the meaning inherent in language through the interaction of speech and thought. And as always with Vygotsky, it is a progression from outside in, with dialogue being an important part of the process.

Vygotsky then moves on to emotion. (Lecture 4 is included in this volume as Chapter 5.) He begins this time with a trenchant critique of post-Darwinian thought. Since Darwin's publication of *The Expression of the Emotions in Man and Animals* (1872/1965), emotions have always been interpreted "retrospectively": as remnants of the expression of animal instinct. Emotions are rudiments, "the gypsies of our mind." "Fear is inhibited flight; anger—inhibited fight . . . remnants that have been infinitely weakened in their external expression and their inner dynamics" (p. 326).

The result of childhood was a tale of suppression and weakening. He mocks Ribot as absurd for celebrating "the glorious history of dying out of this entire domain of mental life."

While the James–Lange theory had the effect of freeing emotion from its phylogenetic roots, the formula "we are sad because we cry" still keeps emotion tied to its old status as an accompaniment of more or less primitive instinctive action. It endows emotion with a "materialistic nature." In time, indeed, James modified his view and proposed that the original theory held only for the lower emotions inherited from lower animals, but not for the higher, subtler ones like religious feeling, aesthetic pleasure, and the rest. These were, he felt, *sui generis*. Vygotsky finds James's retreat even worse than the original formulation. For him, the James–Lange theory was a step backwards from Darwin. It introduced a misleading psychophysical dualism in psychology and, once James excepted the tender emotions as arising *sui generis*, ended in a metaphysical muddle in which there were now purely "mental" emotions whose historical derivation was left unexplained.

It is not surprising then, says Vygotsky, that the James–Lange theory soon came under attack, led by W. B. Cannon. Cannon's classic book on pain, hunger, fear, and rage (1929) had been translated into Russian, and we know from record that he had lectured in Russia and visited Pavlov's laboratory. I do not know whether Vygotsky heard his lectures, but Lecture 4 reveals a close knowledge of Cannon's work. For while Cannon paid lip service to James, his research conclusions left James's theory in shreds and provided Vygotsky with just the key he needed. "James argued that we grieve because we cry. Cannon suggested that this formulation needs to be modified to read that we grieve, feel tenderness, feel moved, and generally experience the most varied emotions, because we cry. . . . Cannon rejected the concept that there is any simple connection between an emotion and its physical expression. He demonstrated that the physical expression is nonspecific to the emotion" (p. 329). Then later Cannon showed that even when animals were sympathectomized, their viscera entirely desensitized, emotional reactions could still be elicited by appropriate situations. And still later, it was discovered that injection of adrenaline in human subjects did not necessarily produce emotional reactions, but that more often than not, the result was "cold emotion" in which one felt aroused but did not know what one was aroused about. These were the openings that Vygotsky needed.

He concludes from Cannon's research that the original function of emotion must have been the facilitation or priming of appropriate instinctive action. What recedes in man is not emotion, but its original links to instinctive actions. In man, with his attenuated instinctual system, emotion takes on new functions. Emotion moves from the periphery to the center, as it were; to the cerebral cortex where it has an equivalent status to other cerebral, central processes. It now can interact with those other processes. As with other processes, then, the development of the emotions cannot be understood separately from their connections with other mental processes. And it is from that vantage point that Vygotsky begins his inquiry.

Freud is the pioneer in rejecting the organic primacy of emotions. It was he who gave them a role in mental life proper. But Vygotsky dismisses Freud's substantive claims as "false," though commenting, "there is a great deal of truth in what he says if we limit ourselves to the formal conclusions based on his studies" (p. 333)—for example, Freud's finding that conflict is a source of anxiety. He also applauds Freud for recognizing that the emotions of the child and adult are different.

But his most approving words are for Karl Bühler and his now all-but-forgotten distinction between *Endlust, Funktionslust,* and *Vorlust:* pleasure derived respectively from the *consummation* of an act, from the actual *performance* of the act, and from the *anticipation* of it. Instinctive activity is characterized by *Endlust.* But the development of skills in an action, even an initially instinctive one, depends on the growth of pleasure in the performance itself, *Funktionslust.* Finally, planfulness and the weighing of alternatives becomes possible only with *Vorlust.* This progression Vygotsky sees as providing a model for the development of emotion.

He couples these distinctions with two other sets, one attributed to Claparede, the other to Kurt Lewin. Claparede distinguishes between emotion and feeling: the former is affect accompanied by action, the latter affect without action. Lewin's distinction is between direct and displaced affect—part of his notion of substitution whereby affect aroused by one mental process can be displaced onto other mental processes that have substitute value for the first.

Bühler, Claparede, and Lewin, by Vygotsky's reckoning, demonstrate ways in which emotion is converted from an *external* to an *internal* role in mental life—the "movement to the center" of human emotion, a process in which emotion becomes increasingly dominated by central processes rather than being peripherally excited as in the James–Lange theory. Once one recognizes this centripetal developmental trend in emotion, it becomes possible to understand more clearly such matters as the deranged mental activity of the schizophrenic. In that illness, emotional "autistic" processes come to dominate mental life and to use rational problem-solving processes as their instrument, rather than *vice versa,* as in normal imagination. This idea leads Vygotsky directly to his penultimate lecture.

It is on the development of imagination (Lecture 5, not included in this volume). "The very foundation of imagination is the introduction of something new . . . the transformation . . . such that something new . . . emerges" (1987–99, Vol. 1, p. 339). Imagination, of course, contains representations of the past; but to these it brings something that is productive as well, something that goes beyond memory. But even the flight of fantasy, however transformed it may be, is lawful and determined. "Thus, a given [fantasy] representation can remind the individual of its opposite, but not of something entirely unrelated," for imagination "is deeply rooted in memory" (1987–99, Vol. 1, p. 341).

Where does the productive, transformative activity of imagination come from? Vygotsky first considers Piaget's idea of egocentrism, which he takes to be an extension of Freud's idea of primary process: that the young child's thinking is at first wishfully pleasure seeking, unrelated to such reality constraints as means–ends compatibility. It is also unconscious and uncommunicable. But Vygotsky finds this view unconvincing from a phylogenetic perspective. It is impossible to imagine that thinking first arose in a primitive form with the function simply and solely of yielding pleasure without regard to reality. Moreover, observations of children do *not* reveal that children get satisfaction from imagined rewards but rather from the real thing, from the satisfaction of *real* needs. They are notably inconsolable by imaginary pleasures.

Finally, one has to question the "nonverbal" nature of early imagination in view of the striking lack of playful imagination in children who, through deafness, autism, or other defects, are retarded in the development of speech. If playful imagination were nonverbal, this deficit should not be present. Moreover, aphasics who lose their capacity for speech also show a marked decline in playfulness and imagination and even lose the capacity to pretend. "Speech gives the child the power to free himself from the force of immediate impressions and to go beyond their limits" (1987–99, Vol. 1, p. 346). From this one must conclude that the growth of imagination is linked not only to the development of language but also to its developing concurrent mental processes. On this line of reasoning, there must be something deeply flawed, Vygotsky concludes, in both Freud's and Piaget's giving primacy to either primary process or egocentrism in the growth of imagination.

Thus, he rejects the view that imagination is a process driven by passions or emotions, even initially. He even questions whether unrealistic imagination or fantasy are always more emotional than reality-oriented thought. How "cool" are we when, for example, we plot something complicated whose outcome is crucial to our well being? We would do far better, in Vygotsky's view, to look more closely at the different forms that imagination takes—whether realistic or fantastic—and inquire what they entail by way of the interaction of different mental processes in producing their effects.

A first conclusion from such an examination is that we must stop drawing a contrastive distinction between "autistic" or "daydreaming" imagination, on the one hand, and "realistic," productively inventive imagination and thought, on the other. Both entail the use of language. Both may be conscious or not. Both may be affectively charged or not. The difference between them is relative not absolute. It would seem that the starting point of each is related to the appearance of speech, and imagination and speech seem to develop as a unity. Moreover, when we examine effective, "reality oriented" thinking, it becomes plain that there are many aspects of it that are quite fantastic. "No accurate cognition of reality is possible without a certain element of imagination, a certain flight from the immediate, concrete, solitary impressions in which this reality is presented in the elementary acts of consciousness" (1987–99, Vol. 1, p. 349).

Yet, it would be in error *not* to distinguish in some way between realistic thinking and imagination. Though both, to be sure, free one from the here and now, they do so by different means and with different purposes. And it is to this matter, the issues of purpose and intention, that Vygotsky's last lecture is devoted (Lecture 6, not included in this volume). How by an act of will does one "free" oneself by leaps of imagination or of thought?

He begins by rejecting theories that reduce volition to nonvolitional processes. With a first lance, he disposes of his *bete noir,* associationism. However elaborate a chain of associations one supposes to exist, he argues, its elaboration cannot yield volition—unless one covertly posits some step of "volition" entering along the way. Even Ebbinghaus's associationist trick—claiming that when an act leads to a result, the association between them becomes reversible and thereby lets the person anticipate each from the other—fails, for one has to bring in "anticipation" as a *deus ex machina.*

He also rejects theories that introduce volitional, vitalistic processes operating *ab initio.* As for Herbartian and other theories that introduce an extraneous will, they fail to specify how this extraneous force arises and how it comes then to interact with other processes. But what is revealing about Herbart's and other theories of autonomous volition is that they always insert the operation of will into the processes of problem solving in order to account for rational action being kept on track, for that seems to be where a directive process is needed.

How does one steer between the Scylla of a futile determinism about the will and the Charybdis of a vapid teleology? How does one maintain a scientific approach while still honoring what is most essential about voluntary action—its freedom. Vygotsky was greatly impressed by the approach of Kurt Lewin to this dilemma. Lewin, to simplify the argument, demonstrated a difference between adults and children in terms of the latter's capacity to initiate and to sustain an "arbitrary" intention, one not naturally related to the situation in which the person finds himself. Not only can adults pursue arbitrary intentions, but they can even transform the situation in which an arbitrary act occurs into one that seems more "rational" to them. If, for example, we have to wait for something to happen whose time of occurrence is randomly scheduled (unbeknownst to us, of course), we find ways of "making sense" of the arbitrariness—what Lewin called "changing the psychological field." All of which suggests to Vygotsky that "will" involves an ability to talk oneself into an action, no matter how arbitrary, and to transform or rationalize the situation in which one must act into a form that makes some sense. He even goes so far as to cite a neurological observation of Kurt Goldstein's suggesting that this form of "self-instruction" may involve a unique neurological structure. He ends with a characteristic Vygotskian query: might it be that the route to the learning of self-instruction is through learning to repeat internally to ourselves the commands that others have given us from outside, until, finally endowed with the fullness of language, we can make up our own novel and even arbitrary commands and use them at will?

Vygotsky's argument on the nature and the growth of "will" is not, alas, an overwhelmingly convincing one. Like philosophers and psychologists before him (and after), he is thrown off his usual thumping stride by this intractable set of issues. But, for all that, he makes his points and manages at least to do so in a fashion consistent with the previous lectures. He strikes materialists and idealists hip and thigh. He points to the importance of the integration of functions. Finally, he manages to make an interesting, if not a convincing, case for the centrality of language and inner speech in mediating "willed" action.

Volition is a topic that rarely comes up for discussion in contemporary psychology. It is usually concealed in theories of motivation or attention or in discussions of Self—in all of which contexts its philosophical dilemmas can be handily disguised behind a mass of data. I think that Vygotsky *had* to confront the issue of will, not so much because he was a child of his times but because he was so dedicated to the concept of self-regulation, a concept that demands one take a stand on the issue of will. It is not surprising that the reflexive use of language is given so prominent a place in the "attainment" of will. For language is the linch-pin in his system of cultural–psychological theory. Man, who lives by his history, learns that history through language. In the end, man frees himself from that history by the very tool that history placed in his hands—language. It is a Promethean thread that Vygotsky weaves.

\* \* \*

Now let me sum up what appears to be, at least for this reader, the forming themes of Vygotsky's thought, both in *Thinking and Speech* and in the six lectures. Perhaps I can do best in the style of linguistics, setting forth a list of critical contrasts that structure his thinking. At a minimum, the list should contain the following:

Inner (central) versus Outer (peripheral)
Interdependent versus Autonomous
Ordered versus Chained
Symbolic versus Biological
Depth versus Surface
Historical versus Ahistorical

For Vygotsky, becoming human implies the "centralizing" or cerebralization of mental processes, whether in development, in cultural history, or in phylogenesis. Emotion moves inward and escapes peripheral control. Speech starts externally and ends as inner speech. Imagination is play gone inward.

Processes go inward, and they are thereby made amenable to interaction with other processes. Interactiveness, "interfunctionality," becomes the rule of maturity. The existence of autonomous processes is a sign of immaturity, of pathology, of phylogenetic primitiveness. Perception operating on its own, for example, yields the symptomatology of mental subnormality.

Through interaction, human mental processes become ordered, systemic, logical, and goal-oriented. By the achievement of generative order in interaction, we become free of the immediacy of sensation, free of the chaining of associations, capable of applying logic to practical action. Kurt Goldstein once said in a seminar that wherever you find associative mental activity, you are sure to find pathology. Vygotsky would have applauded.

The chief instrument of integration and order in human mental life is language, language used in the service of other higher mental functions. Language for Vygotsky, however, is not to be taken in Saussure's (1955) sense as a system of signs, but as a powerful system of tools for use—for use initially in talk, but increasingly and once inwardness is achieved, in perception, in memory, in thought and imagination, even in the exercise of will. In contrast, there is the biological system, operating by what would later be called the First Signal System. For Vygotsky there appears to be a Rubicon that is crossed, going from biological to cultural evolution, some point at which Prometheus steals the fire of the gods.

Because of the mediation of the language system in mental life, and because natural language is necessarily polysemic, the conduct of mental life requires interpretation. This implies that all human action, because it is mediated by language, is subject to multiple interpretations. There will always be a "surface" manifestation that constitutes the superficial interpretation of what seems to be going on in human behavior. Yet, there is also an alternative interpretation of what something "means," and it is this existence of "subtexts" in human behavior that gives depth to human behavior and to its interpretation, in life as in art.

Finally, insofar as language is not only a tool of mind but a product of man's history, man's mental functioning is a product of history. But, paradoxically, it is the systemic productivity of man's language use that makes it possible for him to rise above history and even alter its course: to reach higher ground never before populated by a member even of our language-using species.

Vygotsky was one of the great theory makers of the first half of this century, along with Freud, McDougall, Piaget, and a very few others. Like them, his ideas are situated in his times, but like the best of them those ideas still point the way to the future of our discipline.

# References

Althusser, L. (1978). *Politics and history: Montesquieu, Rousseau, Hegel, Marx.* New York: Schocken.

Austin, J. (1962). *How to do things with words.* Oxford: Oxford University Press.

Bakhtin, M. M. (1981). *The dialogic imagination* (M. Holquist, Ed.). Austin: University of Texas Press.

Cannon, W. B. (1929). *Bodily changes in pain, hunger, fear, and rage.* Cambridge, MA: Harvard University Press.

Darwin, C. (1872/1965). *The expression of the emotions in man and animals.* Chicago: University of Chicago Press. Originally published in 1872.

Geertz, C. (1973). *The interpretation of cultures.* New York: Basic Books.

Grice, H. P. (1969). Utterer's meaning, sentence meaning, and word meaning. *Foundations of Language 4,* 1–18.

Habermas, J. (1971). *Knowledge and human interests.* Boston: Beacon Press.

Hughes, R. (1981). *The shock of the new.* New York: Knopf.

Ivanov, V. (1982). *In eulogies to Roman Jakobson.* The Hague: de Ritter.

Jakobson, R. (1978). *Six lectures on sound and meaning.* Cambridge, MA: MIT Press.

Luria, A. R. (1961). *The role of speech in the regulation of normal and abnormal behavior.* New York: Liveright.

Luria, A. R. (1976). *Cognitive development, its cultural and social foundations* (M. Lopez-Morillas & L. Solotaroff, Trans.; M. Cole, Ed.). Cambridge, MA: Harvard University Press.

Luria, A. R. (1979). *Higher cortical functions in man.* New York: Basic Books.

Propp, V. (1968). *The morphology of the folktale.* Austin: University of Texas Press.

de Saussure, F. (1955). *Course in general linguistics.* New York: Philosophical Library.

Searle, J. (1969). *Speech acts.* Cambridge: Cambridge University Press.

Shklovsky, V. (1965). Art as technique. In *Russian formalist criticism: Four essays* (L. T. Lemon & M. Reis, Eds. and Trans.). Lincoln: University of Nebraska Press.

Toulmin, S. (1978, September 28). The Mozart of psychology [Review of the book *Mind in society*]. *New York Review of Books,* 51–57.

Vygotsky, L. S. (1962). *Thought and Language.* Cambridge, MA: MIT Press.

Vygotsky, L. S. (1978). *Mind in society* (M. Cole, S. Scribner, V. John-Steiner & E. Souderman, Eds. and Trans.). Cambridge, MA: Harvard University Press.

Vygotksy, L. S. (1987–99). *The collected works of L. S. Vygotsky* (6 Vols., R. W. Rieber, Ed.). New York: Kluwer Academic/Plenum.

Washburn, S. L., & Howell, F. C. (1960). Human evolution and culture. In *The evolution of man* (S. Tax, Ed.). Chicago: University of Chicago Press.

Wertsch, J. V. (Ed.). (1985). *Culture, communication, and cognition: Vygotskian perspectives.* Cambridge: Cambridge University Press.

Whorf, B. L. (1956). *Language, thought, and reality: Collected writings* (J. B. Carroll, Ed.) New York: Wiley.

# Problems of General Psychology
## *Thinking and Speech*

ROBERT W. RIEBER, *City University of New York*

This section includes three chapters from Vygotsky's book *Thinking and Speech* (Russian original, 1934), as well as two related lectures on psychology. The Russian editors of Vygotsky's collected works recognized this book as the best known of his works. "It is a summary of the findings of his scientific efforts and an attempt to identify possible directions for further research" (1987, p. 375). *Thinking and Speech* was published in the year of the psychologist's death, gathering some articles that had been published since 1929 and culminating in Chapter 7, "Thought and Word," written especially for the completed book. This was the first book by Vygotsky to be published in English: an abridged translation entitled *Thought and Language* (1962), with a foreword by Jerome Bruner and an afterword by Jean Piaget. When Kluwer Academic/Plenum published the *Collected Works* in English translation, the editors chose to bring out first the volume containing this book, whereas the Russian edition had made it Volume 2, with *Problems of Theory and History of Psychology* (see Section III below) as the first volume. Obviously, the people who initiated the growing interest in Vygotsky in the West agree with the Russian editors and consider *Thinking and Speech* to be the best introduction to Vygotsky's thought, mature as it was at the time of his early death. Bruner wrote a new foreword to the first volume of *Collected Works*, which is reproduced in this volume. Because Bruner discusses every chapter of *Thinking and Speech* and all the related lectures, this introduction will add only brief comments.

It is important to remember that *Thinking and Speech* addresses not only psycholinguistics and psychology of speech; in many ways it represents Vygotsky's approach to general psychology. More than this, Vygotsky's psychological thought characterizes his approach to cultural theory. Vygotsky exercised his full intellectual powers during the exciting (but ultimately tragic) early period of the Soviet Union (1924–1934), so his writings represent an optimistic striving, an energy that can still inspire.

From that broadest context of Vygotsky's work, let us turn to the essentials of his theories on thinking and speech, in particular their development in the child. Indeed, *Thinking and Speech* appeared after nearly a decade of Vygotsky's work with children in special education (see Section II on defectology). As regards the relationship between language and cognition, Vygotsky envisions the development of language out of internalized developmental processes within the child. Cognition and language emerge from a preverbal internalized process in which meaning takes place during cognitive development, before the child is even able to engage in interpersonal relationships using words. Understanding this internalized thinking-and-speaking integrative process, sometimes referred to as "inner speech," is crucial to understanding the later developments in the child's life experience. Consciousness grows out of this early process of diffusion of thought and word during the preverbal period. Thinking and speech are not independent; rather both develop out of the same "mind stuff." Vygotsky recognizes the importance of symbolic signs and their meaning: they are essential to building upon different levels of achievement, as tools for building the scaffolding of knowledge.

Vygotsky sees language as the tool of tools in the development of mental processes. Changes that occur in the development of the child's construction of the real world cannot take place without a solid basis for inner language events, as well as for socialization and interpersonal communication. Psychological reality, for Vygotsky, comprises the experiential emerging and unfolding of the child's connections between cognitive and affective experiences; thus, this reality is empirically determined by the building-block events experienced in life. The history of the child's culture is intertwined with the child's personal history, as that culture forms the foundation for a child's development of a shared ability to communicate with others via the symbolic tool of speech. The genetic capacity for language is not deterministic in any sense, in terms of producing the final by-product of language behavior; rather it is seen as a capacity with which, all things being equal, all children are born.

The cognitive and linguistic activities of the developing child are not primarily understood in terms of egocentric events but as socially influenced processes that evolve the self, always in relationship to significant others and external events in the child's life. These processes are indistinguishable from egocentric wishes and desires by themselves. During the course of development, the qualitative and quantitative aspects of cognition and language do not develop in parallel but emerge from an interactive whole; cognition and language progress sometimes more in concordance with one another and sometimes less. Thinking and speaking may have entirely different roots in their genetic development. Cognition and speech can emerge along different modalities, which may be more or less dependent or independent of one another. Furthermore, this relationship between cognition and language is not necessarily constant over the course of the child's development. The pre–language phase in the development of the cognitive and communicative aspects of the child's behavior is very important, and emotional experiences in the first five years of life are important social events that may affect future developments in the child's life.

On the problems of thinking and speech, it is useful to compare Vygotsky's approach and theories with other well-known ones, particularly the theory of cognitive development of Jean Piaget (whose early works Vygotsky read and criticized) and the psychological approach to structural linguistics of Noam Chomsky (whose career began well after Vygotsky's death). All three deal with similar problems (Rieber, 1983). For Piaget (and similar to Vygotsky), all cognitive abilities, including language, result from a process of construction, from basic biological processes to the highest scientific thought. For Chomsky, much of language and cognition is innate or at least preprogrammed, and it is the structure of this programming that deserves highest attention: Chomsky's characterization of this structure involves his transformational-generative grammar and "deep structures."

In a small pamphlet inserted in some copies of the 1962 publication of *Thought and Language* (Vygotsky, 1962), Piaget highlighted his differences with Vygotsky (Piaget, 1962). Piaget insists that he does not embrace individualism of the type that precedes relations with other people, as Vygotsky charges. However, Piaget believed that Vygotsky is correct in pointing out that he (Piaget) has oversimplified the resemblances between egocentrism and autism, without pointing out the differences sufficiently. Piaget uses examples such as children's play and dreams, and he relates the observed phenomena to Bleuler's notions of nondirected and autistic thought. Piaget describes this in his own terminology as the predominance of assimilation over accommodation in the early play of children. He then goes on to agree that Vygotsky is correct again in his objection that the "pleasure principle" genetically emerges before the "reality principle," as Freud stated. Piaget admits that he oversimplified this sequence without being critical of it. Piaget nevertheless objects to Vygotsky's criticism that he meant to separate thought from behavior, or that he (Piaget) emphasized linguistic aspects more than he should have.

Piaget notes that he could probably have avoided some of Vygotsky's criticism had he written *The Moral Judgment of the Child* (1932) before he wrote, *The Language and Thought of the Child* (1923/26). However, the order of those publications cannot be changed in retrospect. For his source on Piaget, it turns out that Vygotsky actually used a Russian translation (1932) that included two of Piaget's works, *The Language and Thought of the Child* and *Judgment and Reasoning in the Child* (French original, 1924), but not the 1932 work on moral judgment (See editor's footnote, Vygotsky, 1993, p. 332).

Piaget agrees with Vygotsky that linguistic forms are equally socialized and differ only in function. He nevertheless claims that Vygotsky's concept of socialization is ambiguous and prefers to clarify it in the following way: egocentric speech is confusing because it can have two meanings, which should be differentiated into (1) speech that cannot be rationally shared with others and (2) speech that is not meant to be shared with others. Piaget insists that Vygotsky does not make this differentiation and thus introduces confusion on the role of socialization in egocentric speech.

Chomsky recognizes the importance of environment in the growth and structure of language; however, he seeks to tease out the distinct contributions of biology and environment. For Piaget, as for Vygotsky, there is no question of such a separation: verbal and nonverbal systems are interrelated; language does not constitute the framework of logic but is molded by a logic that is generated by learning within a culture. Whereas Piaget emphasized the child's cognitive development within the world of things (and his stages of development have become hypostatized in the literature of developmental psychology), Vygotsky was primarily concerned with the child's development in society, in the world of minds, and saw the process more as a continuous, incremental give-and-take rather than according to distinct stages.

In his "Afterword to the Russian edition," Alexander Luria (1982/87) describes the chapters of *Thinking and Speech* and the four lectures of psychology. Chapter 1, "Problem and Method of Investigation," notes that studies of the relationship between thinking and speech are nothing new, having been prominent in traditional association psychology, but that the problem is largely unexplored in modern scientific psychology. The Wurzburg School of thought psychology had struck out in a promising direction, but the American behaviorists and the Soviet reflexologists had simply avoided the issue. Vygotsky briefly outlines his own approach to the problem in the first chapter. Chapter 2, "The Problem of Speech and Thinking in Piaget's Theory," and Chapter 3, "Stern's Theory of Speech Development," are omitted in the present volume. These chapters review and criticize the work of prominent child psychologists before Vygotsky proceeds to his own approach.

In Chapter 4, "Genetic Roots of Thinking and Speech," Vygotsky attacks the common assumptions that the word is always the carrier of the concept and that the concept provides the foundation for thinking. He proposes instead that human thinking developed from two independent roots: from *practical actions* of animals and from *animal use of speech* for social interaction. He proves this distinction by referring to Wolfgang Köhler's studies with apes, which carried out complex tasks without related speech. The present volume omits the next two chapters. Chapter 5, "An Experimental Study of Concept Development," features the Vygotsky–Sakharov experiments on concept formation in normal and pathological children and adults. Chapter 6, "The Development of Scientific Concepts in Childhood," analyzes the narrower issue of the development of the *scientific concept*, as Vygotsky called the nonspontaneous concept.

Chapter 7, "Thought and Word," deals with the *inner mechanism* of the formation of word meaning. Thought begins as an intention or general tendency of the subject, not already embodied in the word but completed and formed in it. Thought develops from the whole, whereas word develops from the part. Thought is turned into the developed expression through *inner speech*, which preserves all the functions of social interaction, the site of the transition of egocentric speech into inner speech. Such a dynamic hints at the relationships between other forms of speech, e.g., written and oral. The rest of the chapter explores the *sense* and *subtext* of word and expression, using examples from Russian literature. Vygotsky emphasizes that the final link in understanding word meaning, the expression's goal and motive, is laden with emotion and personality.

In the spring of 1932, Vygotsky delivered a course of six lectures at the Leningrad Pedagogical Institute, and the present volume reproduces two of them. Lecture 1 "Perception and Its Development in Childhood," reviews important experimental work on perception, with particular appreciation of the Gestalt School in Germany, which emphasized an integral approach to mental phenomena, as Vygotsky himself did. Lecture 4, "Emotions and Their Development in Childhood," criticizes narrow biological approaches to understanding emotions, including the James–Lange theory, as well as one proposed by Walter Cannon. Vygotsky indicates that emotions are better understood by analyzing the relationships created between emotions and the structure of activity, i.e., a systems approach. The present volume omits the lectures on memory, thinking, imagination, and the problem of the will (Chapters 2, 3, 5, and 6, respectively), all of which are oriented toward child development.

## References

Luria, A. R. (1982/87). Afterword to the Russian edition. In *The Collected works of L. S. Vygotsky, volume 1: Problems of general psychology, including the volume* Thinking and Speech (R. W. Rieber & A. S. Carton, Eds.; pp. 359–373). New York: Kluwer Academic/Plenum. (Russian original 1982)

Piaget, Jean (1923/26). *The language and thought of the child* (M. Warden, Trans.). New York: Harcourt Brace. (French original 1923)

Piaget, Jean (1932). *The moral judgment of the child* (M. Warden, Trans.). New York: Harcourt Brace.

Piaget, Jean (1962). *Comments on Vygotsky's critical remarks concerning The Language and Thought of the Child, and Judgment and Reasoning in the Child.* Cambridge: MIT Press. (Pamphlet included with Vygotsky, 1962)

Rieber, R. W. (Ed.) (1983). *Dialogues on the psychology of language and thought: Conversations with Noam Chomsky, Charles Osgood, Jean Piaget, Ulric Neisser, and Marcel Kinsbourne.* New York: Kluwer Academic/Plenum.

Vygotsky, L. S. (1962). *Thought and Language* (E. Hanfmann & G. Vakar, Eds. & Trans.; J. S. Bruner, Intro.). Cambridge, MA: MIT Press.

Vygotsky, L. S. (1987). *Collected works, Volume 1: Problems of general psychology, including the volume* Thinking and Speech (R. W. Rieber & A. S. Carton, Eds.). New York: Kluwer Academic/Plenum.

Vygotsky, L. S. (1993). *Collected works, Volume 2: The fundamentals of defectology (abnormal psychology and learning disabilities)* (R. W. Rieber & A. S. Carton, Eds.). New York: Kluwer Academic/Plenum.

Vygotsky, L. S. (1997). *Collected works, Volume 3: Problems of theory and history of psychology, including the chapter on the crisis in psychology* (R. W. Rieber & J. Wollock, Eds.). New York: Kluwer Academic/Plenum.

# 1

## The Problem and the Method of Investigation

The first issue that must be faced in the analysis of thinking and speech concerns the relationship among the various mental functions, the relationship among the various forms of the activity of consciousness. This issue is fundamental to many problems in psychology. In the analysis of thinking and speech, the central problem is that of *the relationship of thought to word*. All other issues are secondary and logically subordinate; they cannot even be stated properly until this more basic issue has been resolved. Remarkably, the issue of the relationships among the various mental functions has remained almost entirely unexplored. In effect, it is a new problem for contemporary psychology.

In contrast, the problem of thinking and speech is as old as psychology itself. However, the issue of the relationship of thought to word remains the most confused and least developed aspect of the problem. The atomistic and functional forms of analysis that dominated psychology during past decade led to the analysis of the mental functions in isolation from one another. Psychological methods and research strategies have developed and matured in accordance with this tendency to study separate, isolated, abstracted processes. The problem of the connections among the various mental functions—the problem of their organization in the integrated structure of consciousness—has not been included within the scope of the research.

There is, of course, nothing novel in the notion that consciousness is a unified whole, that the separate functions are linked with one another in activity. Traditionally, however, the unified nature of consciousness—the connections among the mental functions—have simply been accepted as given. They have not been the object of empirical research. The reason for this becomes apparent only when we become aware of an important tacit assumption, an assumption that has become part of the foundation of psychological research. This assumption (one that was never clearly formulated and is entirely false) is that the links or connections among the mental functions are constant and unvarying, that the relationships between perception and attention, memory and perception, and thought and memory are unchanging. This assumption implies that the relationships among functions can be treated as constants and that these constants do not have to be considered in studies that focus on the functions themselves. As we mentioned earlier, the result has been that the problem of interfunctional relationships has remained largely unexplored in modern psychology.

Originally appeared in English translation as Chapter 1 in *The Collected Works of L.S. Vygotsky, Volume 1: Problems of General Psychology* (Robert W. Rieber and Aaron S. Carton, Eds.; Norris Minich, Trans.) (pp. 43–51). New York: Plenum Press, 1987.

Inevitably, this had a serious impact on the approach to the problem of thinking and speech. Any review of the history of this problem in psychology makes it immediately apparent that the central issue, the issue of the relationship of thought to word, has been consistently overlooked.

Attempts to resolve the problem of thinking and speech have always oscillated between two extreme poles, between an *identification* or complete *fusion* of *thought and word* and an equally metaphysical, absolute, and complete *separation* of the two, a *severing* of their relationship. Theories of thinking and speech have always remained trapped in one and the same enchanted circle. These theories have either expressed a pure form of one of these extreme views or attempted to unify them by occupying some intermediate point, by moving constantly back and forth between them.

If we begin with the claim made in antiquity that thought is "speech minus sound," we can trace the development of the first tendency—the tendency to identify thinking and speech—through to the contemporary American psychologist or the reflexologist. These psychologists view thought as a reflex in which the motor component has been inhibited. Not only the resolution of the problem of the relationship of thought to word but the very statement of the issue itself is impossible within these perspectives. If thought and word coincide, if they are one and the same thing, there can be no investigation of the relationship between them. One cannot study the relationship of a thing to itself. From the outset, then, the problem is irresolvable. The basic issue is simply avoided.

Perspectives that represent the other extreme, perspectives that begin with the concept that thinking and speech are independent of one another, are obviously in a better position to resolve the problem. Representatives of the Wurzburg school,[1] for example, attempt to free thought from all sensory factors, including the word. The link between thought and word is seen as a purely external relationship. Speech is represented as the external expression of thought, as its vestment. Within this framework, it is indeed possible to pose the question of the relationship between thought and word and to attempt a resolution. However, this approach, an approach that is shared by several disparate traditions in psychology, consistently results in a failure to resolve the problem. Indeed, it ultimately fails to produce a proper statement of the problem. While these traditions do not ignore the problem, they do attempt to cut the knot rather than unravel it. Verbal thinking is partitioned into its elements; it is partitioned into the elements of thought and word and these are then represented as entities that are foreign to one another. Having studied the characteristics of thinking as such (i.e., thinking independent of speech) and then of speech isolated from thinking, an attempt is made to reconstruct a connection between the two, to reconstruct an external, mechanical interaction between two different processes.

For example, a recent study of the relationship between these functions resulted in the conclusion that the motor processes associated with speech play an important role in facilitating the thinking process [3], in particular, in improving the subject's understanding of difficult verbal material. The conclusion of this study was that inner speech facilitates the consolidation of the material and creates an impression of what must be understood. When inner speech was included in the processes involved in understanding, it helped the subject to sense, grasp, and isolate the important from the unimportant in the movement of thought. It was also found that inner speech plays a role as a facilitating factor in the transition from thought to overt speech.

As this example illustrates, once the researcher has decomposed the unified psychological formation of verbal thinking into its component elements, he is forced to establish a purely external form of interaction between these elements. It is as if he were dealing with two entirely heterogeneous forms of activity, with forms of activity that have no internal connections. Those who represent this second tradition have an advantage over those who represent the first in that they are at least able to pose the question of the relationship of thinking to speech. The weakness of this approach is that its statement of the problem is false and precludes any potential for its correct resolution. This failure to state the problem correctly is a direct function of the method of decomposing the whole into its elements, a method that precludes studying the internal relationship of thought to word. The critical issue, then, is method. If we are to deal with the problem successfully, we must begin by clarifying the issue of what methods are to be used in studying it.

The investigation of any mental formation presupposes analysis, but this analysis can take either of two fundamentally different forms. All the failures that researchers have experienced in their attempts to resolve the problem of thinking and speech can be attributed to their reliance on the first of these two forms of analysis. In our view, the second represents the only means available for moving toward a true resolution of this problem.

The first of these forms of analysis begins with the decomposition of the complex mental whole into its elements. This mode of analysis can be compared with a chemical analysis of water in which water is decomposed into hydrogen and oxygen. The essential feature of this form of analysis is that its products are of a different nature than the whole from which they were derived. The elements lack the characteristics inherent in the whole and they possess properties that it did not possess. When one approaches the problem of thinking and speech by decomposing it into its elements, one adopts the strategy of the man who resorts to the decomposition of water into hydrogen and oxygen in his search for a scientific explanation of the characteristics of water, its capacity to extinguish fire or its conformity to Archimedes law for example. This man will discover, to his chagrin, that hydrogen burns and oxygen sustains combustion. He will never succeed in explaining the characteristics of the whole by analyzing the characteristics of its elements. Similarly, a psychology that decomposes verbal thinking into its elements in an attempt to explain its characteristics will search in vain for the unity that is characteristic of the whole. These characteristics are inherent in the phenomenon only as a unified whole. When the whole is analyzed into its elements, these characteristics evaporate. In his attempt to reconstruct these characteristics, the investigator is left with no alternative but to search for external, mechanical forms of interaction between the elements.

Since it results in products that have lost the characteristics of the whole, this process is not a form of analysis in the true sense of that word. At any rate, it is not "analysis" *vis à vis* the problem to which it was meant to be applied. In fact, with some justification, it can be considered the antithesis of true analysis. The chemical formula for water has a consistent relationship to all the characteristics of water. It applies to water in all its forms. It helps us to understand the characteristics of water as manifested in the great oceans or as manifested in a drop of rain. The decomposition of water into its elements cannot lead to an explanation of these characteristics. This approach is better understood as a means of moving to a more general level than as a means of analysis as such, as a means of partitioning in the true sense of the word. This approach is incapable of shedding light on the details and concrete diversity of the relationship between thought and word that we encounter in our daily lives; it is incapable of following the phenomenon from its initial development in childhood through its subsequent diversification.

The contradictory nature of this form of analysis is clearly manifested in its applications in psychological research. Rather than providing an explanation of the concrete characteristics of the whole that we are interested in, it subordinates this whole to the dictates of more general phenomena. That is, the integral whole is subordinated to the dictates of laws which would allow us to explain that which is common to all speech phenomena or all manifestations of thinking, to speech and thinking as abstract generalities. Because it causes the researcher to ignore the unified and integral nature of the process being studied, this form of analysis leads to profound delusion. The internal relationships of the unified whole are replaced with external mechanical relationships between two heterogeneous processes.

Nowhere are the negative results of this form of analysis more apparent than in the investigation of thinking and speech. The word is comparable to the living cell in that it is a unit of sound and meaning that contains—in simple form—all the basic characteristics of the integral phenomenon of verbal thinking. The form of analysis that breaks the whole into its elements effectively smashes the word into two parts. The researcher concerned with the phenomenon of verbal thinking is then faced with the task of establishing some external mechanical associative connection between these two parts of the integral whole.

According to one of the most important spokesmen of contemporary linguistics, sound and meaning lie unconnected in the word. They are united in the sign, but coexist in complete isolation from one another. It is no surprise that this perspective has produced only the most pathetic results in the investigation of sound and meaning in language. Divorced from thought, sound loses all the unique features that are characteristic of it as the sound of human speech, the characteristics that distinguish it from the other types of sound that exist in nature. As a result of the application of this form of analysis to the domain of verbal thinking, only the physical and mental characteristics of this meaningless sound have been studied, only that which is common to all sounds in nature. That which is specific to this particular form of sound has remained unexplored. As a consequence, this research has not been able to explain why sound possessing certain physical and mental characteristics is present in human speech or how it functions as a component of speech. In a similar manner, the study of meaning has been defined as the study of the concept, of the concept existing and developing in complete isolation from its material carrier. To a large extent, the failure of classic semantics and phonetics has been a direct result of this tendency to divorce meaning from sound, of this decomposition of the word into its separate elements.

This decomposition of speech into sound and meaning has also provided the basis for the study of the development of the child's speech. However, even the most complete analysis of the history of phonetics in childhood is powerless to unite these phenomena. Similarly, the study of the development of word meaning in childhood led researchers to an autonomous and independent history of the child's thought, a history of the child's thought that had no connection with the phonetic development of the child's language.

In our view, an entirely different form of analysis is fundamental to further development of theories of thinking and speech. This form of analysis relies on the partitioning of the complex whole into *units*. In contrast to the term "element," the term "unit" designates a product of analysis that possesses *all the basic characteristics of the whole*. The unit is a vital and irreducible part of the whole. The key to the explanation of the characteristics of water lies not in the investigation of its chemical formula but in the investigation of its molecule and its molecular movements. In precisely the same sense, the living cell is the real unit of biological analysis because it preserves the basic characteristics of life that are inherent in the living organism.

A psychology concerned with the study of the complex whole must comprehend this. It must replace the method of decomposing the whole into its elements with that of partitioning the whole into its units.[2] Psychology must identify those units in which the characteristics of the whole are present, even though they may be manifested in altered form. Using this mode of analysis, it must attempt to resolve the concrete problems that face us.

What then is a unit that possesses the characteristics inherent to the integral phenomenon of verbal thinking and that cannot be further decomposed? In our view, such a unit can be found in the inner aspect of the word, in its meaning.

There has been very little research on this aspect of the word. In most research, word meaning has been merged with a set of phenomena that includes all conscious representations or acts of thought. There is a very close parallel between this process and the process through which sound, divorced from meaning, was merged with the set of phenomena containing all sounds existing in nature. Therefore, just as contemporary psychology has nothing to say about the characteristics of sound that are unique to the sounds of human speech, it has nothing to say about verbal meaning except that which is applicable to all forms of thought and representation.

This is as true of modern structural psychology as it was of associative psychology.[3] We have known only the external aspect of the word, the aspect of the word that immediately faces us. Its inner aspect, its meaning, remains as unexplored and unknown as the other side of the moon. However, it is in this inner aspect of the word that we find the potential for resolving the problem of the relationship of thinking to speech. The knot that represents the phenomenon that we call *verbal thinking* is tied in word meaning.

A brief theoretical discussion of the psychological nature of word meaning is necessary for clarifying this point. Neither associative nor structural psychology provides a satisfactory perspective on the nature of word meaning. As our own experimental studies and theoretical analyses will show, the essence of word meaning—the inner nature that defines it—does not lie where it has traditionally been sought.

The word does not relate to a single object, but to an *entire group or class of objects*. Therefore, every word is a concealed *generalization*. From a psychological perspective, word meaning is first and foremost a generalization. It is not difficult to see that generalization is a *verbal act of thought;* its reflection of reality differs radically from that of immediate sensation or perception.

It has been said that the dialectical leap [4] is not only a transition from matter that is incapable of sensation to matter that is capable of sensation, but a transition from sensation to thought. This implies that reality is reflected in consciousness in a qualitatively different way in thinking than it is in immediate sensation. This qualitative difference is primarily a function of a *generalized reflection of reality*. Therefore, generalization in word meaning is an act of thinking in the true sense of the word. At the same time, however, meaning is an inseparable part of the word; it belongs not only to the domain of thought but to the domain of speech. A word without meaning is not a word, but an empty sound. A word without meaning no longer belongs to the domain of speech. One cannot say of word meaning what we said earlier of the elements of the word taken separately. Is word meaning speech or is it thought? It is both at one and the same time; it is a *unit of verbal thinking*. It is obvious, then, that our method must be that of semantic analysis. Our method must rely on the analysis of the meaningful aspect of speech; it must be a *method for studying verbal meaning*.

We can reasonably anticipate that this method will produce answers to our questions concerning the relationship between thinking and speech because this relationship is already contained in the unit of analysis. In studying the function, structure, and development of this unit, we will come to understand a great deal that is of direct relevance to the problem of the relationship of thinking to speech and to the nature of verbal thinking.

The methods we intend to apply in our investigation of the relationship between thinking and speech permit a synthetic analysis of the complex whole. The significance of this approach is illustrated by yet another aspect of the problem, one that has remained in the background in previous research. Specifically, the initial and the primary function of speech is communicative. Speech is *a means of social interaction*, a means of expression and understanding. The mode of analysis that decomposes the whole into its elements divorces the communicative function of speech from its intellectual function. Of course, it is generally accepted that speech combines the function of social interaction and the function of thinking, but these functions have been conceptualized as existing in isolation from one another, they have been conceptualized as operating in parallel with no mutual interdependence. It has always been understood that both functions are somehow combined in speech. But traditional psychology left entirely unexplored issues such as the relationship between these functions, the reason that both are present in speech, the nature of their development, and the nature of their structural relationship. This is largely true of contemporary psychology as well.

However, in the same sense that word meaning is a *unit of thinking*, it is also a unit of both these speech functions. The idea that some form of mediation is necessary for social interaction can be considered an axiom of modern psychology. Moreover, social interaction mediated by anything other than speech or another sign system—social interaction of the kind that occurs frequently in non-human animals for example—is extremely primitive and limited. Indeed, strictly speaking, social interaction through the kinds of expressive movements utilized by non-human animals should not be called social interaction. It would be more accurate to refer to it as *contamination*. The frightened goose, sighting danger and rousing the flock with its cry, does not so much communicate to the flock what it has seen as contaminate the flock with its fear.

Social interaction based on rational understanding, on the intentional transmission of experience and thought, requires some *system of means*. *Human speech*, a system that emerged with the need to interact socially in the labor process, has always been and will always be the prototype of this kind of means. Until very recently, however, this issue has been seriously oversimplified. In particular, it has been assumed that sign, word, and sound are the means of social interaction. As one might expect, this mistaken conception is a direct result of the inappropriate application of the mode of analysis that begins with the decomposition of the whole into its elements. It is the product of the application of this mode of analysis to the entire range of problems related to the nature of speech.

It has been assumed that the word, as it is manifested in social interaction, is only the external aspect of speech. This implied that sound itself can become associated with any experience, with any content of mental life, and consequently, that it can be used to transmit or impart this experience or content to another human being.

A more sophisticated analysis of this problem and of related issues concerning the processes of understanding and their development in childhood has led to an entirely different understanding of the situation. It turns out that just as social interaction is impossible without signs, it is also impossible without meaning. To communicate an experience or some other content of consciousness to another person, it must be related to a class or group of phenomena. As we have pointed out, this requires *generalization. Social interaction presupposes generalization and the development of verbal meaning;* generalization becomes possible only with the development of social interaction. The higher forms of mental social interaction that are such an important characteristic of man are possible only because—by thinking—man reflects reality in a generalized way.

Virtually any example would demonstrate this link between these two basic functions of speech, between social interaction and generalization. For example, I want to communicate to someone the fact that I am cold. I can, of course, communicate this through expressive movements. However, true understanding and communication occur only when I am able to generalize and name what I am experiencing, only when I am able to relate my experience to a specific class of experiences that are known to my partner.

Children who do not possess the appropriate generalization are often unable to communicate their experience. The problem is not the lack of the appropriate words or sounds, but the absence of the appropriate concept or generalization. Without the latter, understanding is impossible. As Tolstoy points out, it is generally not the word itself that the child fails to understand but the concept that the word expresses (1903, p.143). The word is almost always ready when the concept is. Therefore, it may be appropriate to view word meaning not only as *a unity of thinking and speech* but as a *unity of generalization and social interaction, a unity of thinking and communication.*

This statement of the problem has tremendous significance for all issues related to the genesis of thinking and speech. First, it reveals the true potential for *a causal genetic analysis of thinking and speech.* Only when we learn to see the unity of generalization and social interaction do we begin to understand the actual connection that exists between the child's cognitive and social development. Our research is concerned with resolving both these fundamental problems, the problem of the relationship of thought to word and the problem of the relationship of generalization to social interaction.

However, in order to broaden our perspective on these problems, we would like to mention several issues that we were not able to address directly in our research, issues that became apparent to us only as we were carrying it out. In a very real sense, our recognition of the significance of these issues is the most important result of our work.

First, we would like to raise the issue of *the relationship between sound and meaning in the word.* We have not dealt with this issue extensively in our own research. Nonetheless, recent progress on this issue in linguistics seems to relate directly to the problem of analytic methods that we discussed earlier.

As we have suggested, traditional linguistics conceptualized sound as independent of meaning in speech; it conceptualized speech as a combination of these two isolated elements. The result was that the individual sound was considered to be the basic unit of analysis in the study of sound in speech. We have seen, however, that when sound is divorced from human thought it loses the characteristics that makes it unique as a sound of human speech; it is placed within the ranks of all other sounds existing in nature. This is why traditional phonetics has been primarily concerned not with the psychology of language but with the acoustics and physiology of language. This, in turn, is why the psychology of language has been so helpless in its attempts to understand the relationship between sound and meaning in the word.

What is it, then, that is the most essential characteristic of the sounds of human speech?

The work of the contemporary phonological tradition in linguistics[4]—a tradition that has been well received in psychology—makes it apparent that the basic characteristic of sound in human speech is that it functions as a sign that is linked with *meaning*. Sound as such, sound without meaning, is not the unit in which the various aspects of speech are connected. It is not the individual sound but the *phoneme* that is the basic unit of speech. Phonemes are units that cannot be further decomposed and that preserve the characteristics of the whole, the characteristics of the signifying function of sound in speech. When sound is not meaningful sound, when it is divorced from the meaningful aspect of speech, it loses these characteristics of human speech. In linguistics, as in psychology, the only productive approach to the study of sound in speech is one that relies on the partitioning of the whole into its units, units that preserve the characteristics of both sound and meaning in speech.

This is not an appropriate place for a detailed discussion of the achievements that have been attained through the application of this mode of analysis in linguistics and psychology. In our view, however, these achievements are the most effective demonstration of its value. We have used this method in our own work.

The value of this method could be illustrated by applying it to a wide variety of issues related to the problem of thinking and speech. At this point, however, we can only mention a few of these issues. This will allow us to indicate the potential for future research utilizing this method and to clarify the significance of the method for this whole system of problems.

As we suggested earlier, the problem of the relationships and connections among the various mental functions was inaccessible to traditional psychology. It is our contention that it is accessible to an investigator who is willing to apply the method of units.

The first issue that emerges when we consider the relationship of thinking and speech to the other aspects of the life of consciousness concerns the connection between *intellect and affect*. Among the most basic defects of traditional approaches to the study of psychology has been the isolation of the intellectual from the volitional and affective aspects of consciousness. The inevitable consequence of the isolation of these functions has been the transformation of thinking into an autonomous stream. Thinking itself became the thinker of thoughts. Thinking was divorced from the full vitality of life, from the motives, interests, and inclinations of the thinking individual. Thinking was transformed either into a useless epiphenomenon, a process that can change nothing in the individual's life and behavior, or into an independent and autonomous primeval force that influences the life of consciousness and the life of the personality through its intervention.

By isolating thinking from affect at the outset, we effectively cut ourselves off from any potential for a causal explanation of thinking. A deterministic analysis of thinking presupposes that we identify its motive force, that we identify the needs, interests, incentives and tendencies that direct the movement of thought in one direction or another. In much the same way, when thinking is isolated from affect, investigating its influences on the affective or purposive aspects of mental life is effectively precluded. A deterministic analysis of mental life cannot begin by ascribing to thought a magical power to determine human behavior, a power to determine behavior through one of the individual's own inner systems. Equally incompatible with a deterministic analysis, is the transformation of thought into a superfluous appendage of behavior, into its feeble and useless shadow.

The direction we must move in our attempt to resolve this vital problem is indicated by the method that relies on the analysis of the complex whole into its units. There exists a dynamic meaningful system that constitutes *a unity of affective and intellectual processes.* Every idea contains some remnant of the individual's affective relationship to that aspect of reality which it represents. In this way, analysis into units makes it possible to see the relationship between the individual's needs or inclinations and his thinking. It also allows us to see the opposite relationship, the relationship that links his thought to the dynamics of behavior, to the concrete activity of the personality.

We will postpone the discussion of several related problems. These problems have not been the direct object of our research in the present volume. We will discuss them briefly in the concluding chapter of this work as part of our discussion of the prospects that lie before us. At this point, we will simply restate the claim that the method that we are applying in this work not only permits us to see the internal unity of thinking and speech, but allows us to do more effective research on the relationship of verbal thinking to the whole of the life of consciousness.

As our final task in this first chapter, we will outline the book's general organization. As we have said, our goal has been to develop an integrated approach to an extremely complex problem. The book itself is composed of several studies that focus on distinct though interrelated issues. Several experimental studies are included, as are others of a critical or theoretical nature. We begin with a critical analysis of a theory of speech and thinking that represents the best thought on the problem in contemporary psychology. It is, nonetheless, the polar opposite of our own perspective. In this analysis, we touch on all issues basic to the general question of the relationship between thinking and speech and attempt to analyze these issues in the context of our current empirical knowledge. In contemporary psychology, the study of a problem such as the relationship of thinking to speech demands that we engage in a conceptual struggle with general theoretical perspectives and specific ideas that conflict with our own.

The second portion of our study is a theoretical analysis of data related to the development (both phylogenetic and ontogenetic) of thinking and speech. From the outset, we attempt to identify the genetic roots of thinking and speech. Failure in this task has been the underlying cause of all false perspectives on the problem. An experimental study of the development of concepts in childhood, a study that is composed of two parts, provides the focus for this second part of the investigation. In the first part of this study, we consider the development of what we call "artificial concepts," concepts that are formed under experimental conditions. In the second, we attempt to study the development of the child's real concepts.

In the concluding portion of our work, we attempt to analyze the function and structure of the general process of verbal thinking. Theory and empirical data are both included in this discussion.

What unifies all these investigations is *the idea of development,* an idea that we attempt to apply in our analysis of word meaning as the unity of speech and thinking.

# 2

# The Genetic Roots of Thinking and Speech

## 1

The basic fact we encounter in a genetic analysis of the *relationship* between thinking and speech is that this relationship is not constant. The quantitative and qualitative significance of this relationship changes in the course of the development of thinking and speech [9]. These functions do not develop in parallel, nor is their relationship constant. The curves that represent their development converge, diverge, and cross one another. At one point in the process, these curves may move smoothly along a parallel course, even merging with one another. At another, they may branch away from each other once again. This is true of the development of speech and thinking in both phylogenesis and ontogenesis.

Later, we will attempt to demonstrate that the *relationship* between thinking and speech is not the same in all instances of disturbance, delay, reverse development, or pathological change. Rather, this relationship assumes a specific form characteristic of particular pathological processes. With respect to the issue of development, we must say first that thinking and speech have entirely different genetic roots, a fact firmly established by a whole series of studies in animal psychology. Moreover, these processes develop along different lines in virtually all animals.

Recent studies of speech and intellect in the higher apes conducted by Kohler (1921a), Yerkes[5] (Yerkes & Learned, 1925), and others have been decisive in establishing this basic fact.

Kohler's experiments demonstrate clearly that the rudiments of intellect or thinking appear in animals independent of the development of speech and are absolutely unconnected with the level of speech development. The "inventions" of the higher apes, their preparation and use of tools, and their use of indirect paths in the solution of problems, clearly constitute an initial *pre-speech* phase in the development of thinking.

In Kohler's view, the basic implication of his research is that the chimpanzee displays rudiments of intellectual behavior of the type characteristic of man (Kohler, 1921a, p. 191). The absence of speech and the limited nature of stimulus traces (i.e., representations) are the basic causes of the large differences between the anthropoid apes and the most primitive man. Kohler writes that:

> The absence of this infinitely valuable technical auxiliary means (i.e., language) and the limitations in the most important intellectual material (i.e., representations) are why even the most rudimentary forms of cultural development are beyond the capacity of the chimpanzee (ibid., p, 192).

Originally appeared in English translation as Chapter 4 in *The Collected Works of L.S. Vygotsky, Volume 1: Problems of General Psychology* (Robert W. Rieber and Aaron S. Carton, Eds.; Norris Minich, Trans.) (pp. 101–120). New York: Plenum Press, 1987.

*The presence of a human-like intellect combined with the absence of human-like speech—and
the independence of intellectual operations from speech*—are the basic findings of Kohler's research
on the anthropoid apes that are relevant to the problem in which we are interested.

Kohler's research has been widely criticized. The number of these critical works and the
variety of theoretical perspectives they represent have grown considerably. Psychologists of various traditions and schools do not agree on the theoretical explanation of Kohler's empirical data.

Kohler himself carefully limited the problem he attempted to address. He made no attempt
to develop a theory of intellectual behavior (ibid., p. 134). He limited himself to the analysis
of empirical observations. He dealt with theoretical explanation only to the extent that this was
necessary to demonstrate how intellectual reactions differ from reactions that develop
through trial-and-error processes, through the selection of successful reactions and the mechanical combination of movements.

By rejecting the theory that the development of the chimpanzee's intellectual reactions
can be explained in terms of chance, Kohler limited himself to *a purely negative* theoretical position. His rejection of the idealistic biological conceptions underlying Hartman's theory of the
unconscious, of Bergson's[6] conception of a "vital impulse" *(elan vital),* and of the neovitalist and
psychovitalist assumption of a "purposeful force" in all living matter was equally decisive and
equally negative. In Kohler's view, these theories lie beyond the legitimate boundaries of science
because either overtly or covertly they revert to supersensual agents or simple miracles in their
explanations (ibid., pp. 152–153). Kohler writes: "I must emphasize emphatically that the alternatives of chance and supersensual agents simply do not exist *(Agenten jenseits der Erfahrung)*"
(ibid., p. 153)

Thus, neither in established psychological traditions nor in Kohler's own writings do
we find a complete or scientifically convincing theory of intellect. On the contrary, both biological (Thorndike,[7] Wagner,[8] and Borovskii[9]) and subjectivist psychologists (Buhler, Lind-
vorskii, and Jaensch) contest Kohler's basic position. Biological psychologists dispute his position that intellect cannot be reduced to trial and error. Subjectivists criticize his position that
the intellect of the human and the chimpanzee are similar, that the anthropoids have thinking
that is comparable to that of humans.

In their mutual acceptance of Kohler's empirical observations, those who see nothing
more in the chimpanzee's actions than the mechanisms of instinct and trial and error learning, "nothing more than the familiar processes of habit formation" (Borovskii, 1927, p. 179),
are in accord with those who fear lowering the roots of intellect even to the level of the more
advanced forms of ape behavior. That both groups recognize the accuracy of Kohler's observations and the independence of the chimpanzee's actions from its speech makes the situation yet
more interesting.

Buhler is fully justified in writing that "the chimpanzee's action is *completely independent
of speech.* Even the most advanced forms of human technical and instrumental thinking *(Werkreug-
denken)* are less closely linked with speech and concepts than are other forms of thinking" (1930,
p. 48). We will return to this idea later. At this point, we will say only that what we know of
this issue from experimental research and clinical observation indicates that the relationship
between intellect and speech in the adult is in fact neither constant nor identical for the various forms of intellectual and speech activity.

Disputing Hobhouse,[10] who ascribed "practical judgement" to animals, and Yerkes, who found processes of "ideation" among the higher apes, Borovskii posed the following question: "Do animals have anything like the speech habits of man? . . . Given our current knowledge, it seems to me that we must answer that there is no basis on which to ascribe speech habits to the apes or any animal other than man" (1927, p. 189). The matter would be easily resolved if we did not find rudiments of speech in the apes. However, recent studies have shown that developed forms of "speech" are present in the chimpanzee, In several respects, particularly in its phonetic characteristics, the chimpanzee's speech resembles that of man. Of particular interest in the present context, however, is the fact that the chimpanzee's speech and intellect function independently on one another.

Based on years of observation at the research station on Tenerife, Kohler writes that "without exception, these phonetic manifestations express the frustrations and subjective states of the chimpanzee. They are always emotional expressions, never signs representing something objective" (Kohler, 1921a, p. 27).

The large number of sound elements in chimpanzee phonetics (comparable to that of human phonetics) makes it possible to state with conviction that the absence of "human-like" language in the chimpanzee cannot be explained in terms of these kinds of peripheral factors. In full agreement with Kohler's conclusions concerning the language of the chimpanzee, Delacroix is justified in suggesting that the gestures and mimicry of the ape show not the slightest traces of expressing or signifying something objective, that is, of *fulfilling the function of a sign* (Delacroix, 1924, p. 77). In this context, of course, the issue of peripheral causes does not arise.

Chimpanzees are highly social animals and their behavior can be understood only when they are observed in interaction. Kohler described a wide range of "verbal social interaction" in the chimpanzee. Emotional-expressive movements are the most common form. These movements are rich and clear in the chimpanzee (e.g., mimicry, gestures, and sound reactions). Kohler also observed movements that expressed social emotions, gestures of recognition and contact for example. However, Kohler writes that these social gestures and expressive sounds do not signify or describe anything objective.

The chimpanzee understands mimicry and gesture exceedingly well. Using gestures, they express not only their own emotional states but their wishes and impulses, wishes and impulses that may be directed toward other apes or toward objects. The most common mode of communication in this situation is for the chimpanzee to *begin* that movement or action that it wants to carry out or that it wants to prompt another animal to carry out. For example, the chimpanzee may nudge another animal or make initial walking movements when it wants the other animal to accompany it; it may make grasping movements when it wants a banana. Each of these gestures is directly connected with the action itself.

These observations seem to support Wundt's concept that while the indicative gesture (the most primitive stage in the development of human language) is not found in most animals, it is found among the apes in a *transitional stage* that stands between the grasping movement and the indicative movement. In any case, this transitional gesture is an extremely important step in the genetic transition from purely emotional speech to objective speech.

Elsewhere, Kohler has shown that gestures of this kind are used to achieve primitive forms of explanation, that they function as a substitute for verbal instructions. This type of gesture stands closer to human speech than the ape's fulfillment of orders given by Spanish guards. The latter phenomenon is not essentially different from similar phenomena observed in the behavior of domestic animals such as the dog in responding to calls.

The chimpanzees Kohler observed used colored clay to "paint" during play. Initially they used their lips and tongue, but later they used paintbrushes (Kohler, 1921a, p. 70). Nonetheless, while these animals generally transferred modes of behavior between contexts of play and more serious activity, Kohler never observed the creation of signs through painting. Buhler wrote that "as far as we know, there is no reason to believe that a chimpanzee ever saw a graphic sign in a mark" (1930, p. 320). He argued elsewhere that this fact is critical for the proper evaluation of the chimpanzee's "human-like" behavior.

There are facts that would caution against the over valuation of the chimpanzee's behavior. No traveler has ever mistaken a gorilla or chimpanzee for a person. None has found traditional tools and techniques varying from one group to the next that indicate the transmission of discoveries from generation to generation. We do not find marks on sandstone or clay that could be taken for a picture *illustrating* something nor, even in play, do we find etched patterns. There is no depictive *language*, no sounds or names of equivalence. There must be some internal basis for all this (ibid., pp. 42–43).

Yerkes seems to be the only contemporary researcher studying the higher apes who believes that the absence of human-like language in the chimpanzee is a function of something other than "internal factors." His research on the intellect of the orangutan produced results very similar to those of Kohler. His interpretation of these results, however, differs significantly from Kohler's. In his view, one finds "higher ideation" in the orangutan, though at a level of development not exceeding that of the three year old child (Yerkes, 1916, p. 132).

However, a critical analysis of Yerkes's theory uncovers a basic flaw in his thinking. Simply stated, there is no objective proof that the orangutan solves problems using processes of "higher ideation," using representations or stimulus traces. Ultimately, it is the external similarity of the behavior of man and that of the orangutan that underlies Yerkes's claim that there is "ideation" in the latter.

Obviously, this is not a convincing basis for a scientific argument. We would not want to suggest that using an analogy of this kind is unacceptable in any research on the behavior of the higher animals. Kohler has clearly demonstrated that such analogies can be used within the limits of scientific objectivity. Later, we will have occasion to use this kind of analogy in our own discussion. However, it is not scientifically acceptable to base a conclusion solely on an analogy of this kind.

Kohler relied on exacting experimental analysis to show that the actual optical situation is decisive for the chimpanzee's behavior. In the early stages of experimentation, in particular, the task of using a stick (as a tool) to obtain a piece of fruit (the goal) was made more difficult or even impossible for the chimpanzee by moving the stick slightly to the side of the fruit so that the two did not lie in the same optical field.

Similarly, when two sticks used to make a lengthened tool by inserting one into an aperture in the other crossed and assumed an "X" form in the hands of one chimpanzee, the operation of lengthening the tool (one that had been frequently repeated before) became impossible.

We could cite scores of other experimental findings relevant to this issue. It is sufficient, however, to note the following:

1. In Kohler's view, the actual optical situation (or the primitive situation) is the general, basic, and consistent methodological condition required for any research on the chimpanzee's intellect. One cannot force the intellect of the chimpanzee to function in isolation from this situation.

2. In Kohler's view, the most basic and general feature of the chimpanzee's intellectual behavior is precisely the limited nature of its representations (i.e., its "ideation").

These two positions are sufficient to cast doubt on the validity of Yerkes's basic conclusion. We would add that Kohler's positions are not merely general convictions developed in some unspecified manner. They are the only logical conclusions that can be drawn from his experiments.

Yerkes's most recent studies on the chimpanzee's language and intellect are linked with this assumption of "ideational behavior" in the higher apes. These studies do not extend, deepen, or delimit earlier findings on the intellect. They simply provide additional support for the findings established in previous research by Yerkes and others. However, his experiments and observations do provide new empirical material on speech, including a bold attempt to explain the absence of human-like speech in the chimpanzee.

Yerkes writes that "vocal reactions are both frequent and varied in the young chimpanzee, but speech in the human sense of the term is absent" (Yerkes & Learned, 1925, p. 53). He argues that the development and function of the chimp's vocal apparatus is comparable to man's, but the tendency to imitate sounds is absent. Imitation is limited almost exclusively to the field of visual stimuli, to actions rather than sounds. The young chimpanzee is not able to do what the parrot does. "If the imitative tendency of the parrot were found in the chimpanzee, the latter would undoubtedly possess speech. The chimpanzee has a vocal mechanism comparable to that of man and an intellect that would be entirely adequate for the use of sounds for speech' (ibid.).

Yerkes used four experimental methods in his attempt to teach the chimpanzee the human use of sounds. In each case, the results were negative. Of course, in and of themselves, negative results can never have decisive significance for a fundamental issue of this kind. Kohler has demonstrated, for example, that the negative results obtained by previous experimenters on the question of whether the chimpanzee possesses intellect were a function of the improper organization of their experiments, a function of their misunderstanding of the "zone of difficulty" within which the chimpanzee's intellect can be manifested. Thus, these failures reflected the experimenters' ignorance of the basic characteristics of the chimpanzee's intellect, of its close link to the actual optical situation. Thus, a negative finding is frequently a function not of the phenomenon being studied, but of the researcher's understanding of it. That an animal fails to solve a given task under a specific set of conditions does not imply that it lacks the capacity to solve any such task under any conditions. Kohler correctly states that "research on mental endowment inherently tests not only the subject but the experimenter himself' (1921a, p. 191).

However, while we would not want to rely solely on the results of Yerkes's experiments as the foundation for our perspectives on language in apes, there is good reason to use his findings in combination with other information we have on this issue. In this context, Yerkes's experiments indicate once again that not even the rudiments of human-like speech exist in the chimpanzee. It would seem reasonable to assume that they could not exist in the chimpanzee, (Of course, it is important to distinguish the actual absence of speech from the possibility that speech could be imparted artificially under experimental conditions.)

Experiments by Yerkes's colleague, Learned, indicate that factors such as the underdevelopment of the vocal apparatus or phonetic limitations are insufficient to explain the absence of human-like speech in the chimpanzee. In Yerkes's view, the explanation is to be found in the absence or weakness of the chimpanzee's imitation of sounds. Of course, Yerkes is justified in suggesting that the absence of vocal imitation was the proximal cause of the failure of his own experiments. He is hardly justified, however, in arguing that this is the underlying reason for the absence of speech in apes. None of what we know of the chimpanzee's intellect supports this proposal, a proposal that Yerkes nonetheless advances categorically as an objectively established fact.

What objective basis does Yerkes have for his assertion that the chimpanzee's intellect is characterized by the type and degree of development necessary for the creation of human-like speech? Yerkes had an excellent experimental means available to him for verifying this thesis. Unfortunately, he failed to make use of it. If the necessary materials were available, we would be eager to use them in the experimental resolution of this question.

The exclusion of the factor of vocal imitation would be fundamental to our approach. Speech is not only encountered in vocal forms, The deaf and mute have created and use a visual form of speech. Deaf and mute children are taught to understand our speech by reading lip movement. As Levy-Bruhl has shown (1922), gestural speech exists alongside vocal speech and plays an important role in the language of primitive peoples. It should also be remembered that speech is not necessarily linked to a specific material carrier. Consider written speech for example. As Yerkes himself points out, it might be possible to teach the chimpanzee to use its fingers in communication in a manner similar to the use of sign language by the deaf and mute.

If the chimpanzee's intellect is indeed capable of acquiring human speech, if the difficulty is merely that it lacks the parrot's tendency for vocal imitation, it should be able to master a conditioned gesture, one that would correspond functionally with a conditioned sound. Rather than sounds such as those used by Yerkes (i.e., "va-va" or "pa-pa"), the chimpanzee's speech reactions would consist of certain hand movements, movements such as those used in the representation of the alphabet by the deaf and mute. The critical issue is not the use of sounds, but the *functional use of signs* in a manner appropriate to human speech.

Since experiments of this kind have not been carried out, we cannot predict with any certainty what the results would be. However, nothing that we know of chimpanzee behavior, including the empirical evidence from Yerkes's experiments, gives us any basis to anticipate that the chimpanzee will actually achieve the functional mastery of speech, We know of no evidence of sign use by chimpanzees. The objective data we have on the chimpanzee's intellect do not indicate the presence of "ideation." They merely indicate that under certain conditions the chimpanzee has the capacity for the preparation and use of the simplest tools and for the use of indirect means of obtaining some end.

We do mean to imply that the presence of "ideation" is a necessary condition for the appearance of speech. This question requires further empirical research. Nonetheless, in Yerkes's thinking, there is a direct link between the assumption of "ideation" as basic to the intellectual activity of the anthropoids and the claim that they are capable of human speech. This link is so obvious and so important that it may be worthwhile to critically examine Yerkes's thesis concerning "ideation" and develop an alternate theory of the chimpanzee's intellectual behavior, since his belief in the chimpanzee's capacity to acquire human-like speech will fall at the same time.

If "ideation" forms the foundation of the chimpanzee's intellectual activity, why can we not assume that, like the human being, the chimpanzee can solve problems presented verbally or through some other type of sign, just as it solves problems with the use of tools? (This would, of course, be nothing more than an assumption, not an established fact.) At this point, we need not evaluate the viability of the analogy between the use of tools and the meaningful use of speech. We will have occasion to address this issue in our discussion of speech development in ontogenesis. It is sufficient to remember what we have said of "ideation" to see the precarious nature of Yerkes's theory of chimpanzee speech and the total absence of any empirical foundation for it.

It is precisely the absence of "ideation," the absence of the capacity to operate on the basis of non-actual or absent stimuli, that is most characteristic of the chimpanzee's intellect, The presence of an actual, optical, and easily visible situation is a condition that is necessary for the ape to attain true tool use. Are there conditions in this type of situation where the chimpanzee would discover the functional use of the sign, that is, the use of speech? (We will intentionally speak only *of one condition,* and that a *purely psychological one,* since we constantly have Yerkes's experimental situation in mind.)

No special analysis is necessary to answer this question in the negative. Moreover, under no situation could the use of speech become a function on the basis of the optical structure of the perceptual field. Speech requires another type of intellectual operation, *not one of the type or degree* that is present in the chimpanzee. Nothing that we know of the chimpanzee's behavior indicates the presence of this type of operation. On the contrary, as we have shown above, the majority of investigators see the absence of this operation as the essential feature distinguishing the intellect of the chimpanzee from that of man.

In any event, two theses can be considered beyond dispute. First, the rational use of speech is an intellectual function that cannot under any condition be determined by the immediate optical structure. Second, in tasks defined by a structure other than the actual optical one (e.g., tasks defined by mechanical structure), the chimpanzee abandons intellectual forms of behavior for trial and error. What for the human is a simple operation such as placing one box on another to balance it or removing a ring from a hook is consequently almost beyond the capacity of the chimpanzee's "naive statics" and mechanics (Kohler, 1921a, pp. 106 and 177). This is true of all non-optical structures. The logical implication of these two theses is that the chimpanzee's potential for mastering human speech is, from a psychological perspective, very limited.

It is interesting that Kohler used the term *Einsicht* (insight) (i.e., "reason" in the common meaning of the word) to designate the chimpanzee's intellectual operations, Kafka correctly points out that Kohler's use of the word in this context implies a purely optical perception in the literal sense (Kafka, 1922, p, 130), and only then the more general perception of relationships which is often contrasted with a blind mode of action. Kohler provided neither a definition nor a theory of "perception." As a result, the term acquired a dual meaning in his descriptions of empirical data. On the one hand, he used the term to designate the characteristics of the operations that the chimpanzee carried out, to designate the structure of the chimpanzee's actions. On the other, he used it to designate the internal psychophysiological processes involved in preparation for these actions. Here, the chimpanzee's actions were portrayed as nothing more than the fulfillment of an internal plan of operation. Buhler, in particular, insists on the internal character of this process (1930, p. 33). In much the same way, Borovskii suggests that if the ape "does not carry out an observable probe or trial (i.e., if it does not extend its arm), it still "tests the action" in its muscles " (1927, p. 184).

We will not address this inherently important issue in the present context, A detailed discussion of the problem would not be appropriate at this point, since empirical data sufficient for its resolution simply do not exist. What one says on this issue inevitably depends more on general theoretical considerations and on analogies between higher and lower forms of behavior (i.e., between thinking in man and the trial and error behavior of animals) than on empirical data.

Kohler's experimental data do not permit a definitive answer to this question. The nature of the mechanism of intellectual reactions cannot be answered even hypothetically on the basis of his experiments. Nonetheless, regardless of how we conceptualize this mechanism (whether we localize it psychophysiologically in the brain or in muscular innervation) the proposition as to the actual determination as opposed to the trace-determination remains in force. In the present context, the critical point is that the intellect of the chimpanzee does not function outside the actual optical situation.

On this issue, Kohler writes that "the best tool easily loses all its significance for the given situation if it cannot be perceived simultaneously, or quasi-simultaneously, in the same visual field as the goal of the action" (Kohler, 1921a, p. 39). By quasi-simultaneous perception, Kohler is referring to those cases where the separate elements of the situation are not perceived by the eye directly and simultaneously with the goal, but have nonetheless been perceived in immediate temporal sequence with it or been frequently associated with the situation in previous experience. Such elements are "simultaneous" in psychological function. In contrast to Yerkes, this somewhat extended analysis brings us time and time again to the conclusion that even if the chimpanzee had the parrot's vocal imitative tendencies and capacities, it would not master speech. Moreover, while the chimpanzee has a rich and in many respects human-like speech, this speech has little direct relationship with its highly developed intellect. This is the most important aspect of the entire problem.

Learned compiled a vocabulary of chimpanzee language based on 32 "words" or elements of "speech." Phonetically, these elements are highly reminiscent of human speech. Moreover, they have definite meanings in the sense that they are characteristic of specific situations. For example, various elements are characteristic of situations or objects that elicit desires or pleasures, dissatisfaction or spite, and attempts to escape danger or an object of fear (Yerkes and Learned, 1925, p. 54). These "words" were collected and recorded while the animals were waiting for food, while they were eating, while they were in the presence of people, and while the animals moved as a group.

This vocabulary is composed of emotional meanings. These are more or less differentiated vocal-emotional reactions that generally appear in conditioned reflex connection with stimuli associated with feeding. In essence, this vocabulary affirms what Kohler said of the chimpanzee's speech; it is emotional speech. Three factors associated with this characteristic of the chimpanzee's speech are of interest in the present context, First, this link between speech and expressive emotional movements (which become particularly marked at times of strong affective arousal) is not unique to the higher apes, This phenomenon is common to many animals with a vocal apparatus and probably underlies the origin and development of human speech. Second, emotional and affective states are an extremely unfavorable behavioral domain for the functioning of intellectual reactions. Kohler noted that emotional, and especially affective reactions, completely destroy the chimpanzee's capacity for intellectual operations.

Third, as is the case with other animals, the chimpanzee's speech is not limited to this emotional function, Chimpanzee speech constitutes not only an expressive-emotional reaction, but a means of psychological contact with other members of the species. There is, of course, a genetic link between this function of animal speech and the corresponding functions of human speech.* Kohler's apes and Yerkes's chimpanzees clearly manifested this speech function. This function, however, had no link with the animal's intellectual reactions, its thinking. These were emotional reactions constituting a clear and indisputable part of the emotional symptom-complex. There is no similarity between this reaction and intentional, meaningful communication. It is an instinctive reaction, or something very similar to it.

This speech function is a biologically ancient form of behavior. In animal societies, it is linked genetically with the group leader's optical and audio signals. Recently, in his studies of the *language of bees*, Von Frisch[11] has described extremely interesting and theoretically important forms of behavior that promote connection or contact (Von Frisch, 1928). In spite of the unique character of these forms of communication and their clearly instinctive origin, one cannot help recognizing the common heritage between this behavior and the speech of the chimpanzee (cf. Kohler, 1921a, p. 44). Correspondingly, one can hardly doubt the total independence of the chimpanzee's speech from its intellect.

We are can now summarize several key points. Our concern has been the relationship between thinking and speech in their phylogenetic development. To address this issue, we have analyzed experimental studies and observations of the intellect and language of the higher apes. We can summarize our basic conclusions, and the problems that demand further analysis, in the following way:

1. Thinking and speech have different genetic roots.
2. The development of thinking and speech move along different channels, independently of one another.
3. The relationship between thinking and speech is not constant over the course of phylogenetic development.
4. The anthropoids manifest an intellect similar to that of humans in their rudimentary tool use. Their speech is also similar to human speech, but here the similarity is linked with different aspects of the psychological function. It is linked with the

---

* In animals, Hempelmann recognizes only the expressive function of language, though he does not reject the notion that vocal signals of warning or alarm have an objective communicative function (1926, p. 530).

phonetics of speech, the emotional function of speech, and the existence of the rudiments of social speech.

5.   The anthropoids do not manifest the close link between thinking and speech that is
     characteristic of man. In the chimpanzee, the two are not connected in any way.

6.   In the phylogenesis of thinking and speech, we can almost certainly identify a pre-
     speech phase in the development of intellect and a pre-intellectual phase in the devel-
     opment of speech.


# 2


The lines of development representing thinking and speech in ontogenesis are significantly more obscure and intricate than in phylogenesis. Nonetheless, without claiming that
there is a parallel between ontogenesis and phylogenesis in this context, we can identify different genetic roots and different lines of development for thinking and speech in ontogenesis
as well. Recent objective experimental evidence has demonstrated that the development of the
child's thinking passes through a pre-speech stage. Kohler's experiments on chimpanzee intellect, with appropriate modifications, were carried out with children who had not yet acquired
speech (Kohler had frequently noted the importance of this type of comparative experimentation with children). Buhler has conducted a systematic study of the child along these lines.
He writes that the child's actions are:

> Nearly identical to the actions of the chimpanzee. Therefore, it is not unreasonable to call
> this phase of the child's life the chimpanzoid age. For this child, the period extended from
> the 10th to the 12th month. . . . During this period, the child makes his first inventions,
> extremely primitive ones to be sure, but ones that mark an extremely important point in his
> mental development (1930, p. 97).

As was true of Kohler's experiments with the chimpanzee, the primary theoretical significance of Buhler's experiments is that they demonstrate that rudimentary intellectual reactions occur independently of speech. Buhler makes this point himself:

> It has been said that speech stands at the initial formation of man *(Menschwerden* [human-
> ization]). While this may be true, we must not forget the existence of instrumental think-
> ing *(Werkzeugdenken* [tool thinking]), the understanding of mechanical connections and the
> invention of mechanical means for mechanical ends. Action is subjectively intelligent and
> consciously purposeful before the appearance of speech (ibid., p. 48).

In contrast to this pre-speech phase in the development of intellect, the pre-intellectual
roots of speech in the child's development have been recognized for some time. Crying and babbling are clearly demarcated phases of speech development. These, as well as the child's first
words, are pre-intellectual. They have nothing in common with the development of thinking.

It is generally accepted that the child's speech is primarily an emotional form of behavior in the first year of life. The most recent research—that of C. Buhler[12] and others on the
child's first forms of social behavior and his reactions in the first year of life, and the research
of C. Buhler's colleagues (i.e., Gettser and Tuder-Gart) on the child's early reactions to the

human voice—has shown that the social function of speech develops extensively during this pre-intellectual stage.

The child's rich and complex social contact leads to an early development of means of social connection. It has been clearly demonstrated that simple though unique reactions to the human voice are present in the third week of life (i.e., the presocial reactions) and that the first social reactions appear by the second month (Buhler, 1927, p. 124). Laughter, babbling, pointing, and gesture emerge as means of social contact in the first months of the child's life. During the first year, then, we find in the human child both of the speech functions that we encountered in our discussion of speech in phylogenesis.

However, the most important event in the development of the child's thinking and speech occurs at approximately two years of age. It is at this point that the. lines representing the development of thinking and speech, lines that up to this point have moved in isolation from one another, cross and begin to coincide. This provides the foundation for an entirely new form of behavior, one that is an essential characteristic of man.

Stern provided the first and best description of this extraordinarily important event in the child's mental life. He demonstrated that a vague consciousness of the significance of language and the will to master it is awakened in the child. The child makes what is the most significant discovery of his life, the discovery that "each thing has its name" (1922, p. 92). This critical moment, the moment when speech becomes intellectual and thinking verbal, is marked by two clear and objective symptoms. These signs provide a foundation for reliable judgments concerning whether this turning point in. speech development has occurred. In cases of abnormal or arrested development, they make it possible to determine the extent to which development has been delayed since these two symptoms are closely linked. First, the child who has attained this level of development begins to *actively expand his vocabulary* by asking the name of each new thing he encounters. Second, these efforts result in an extremely rapid increase in the child's vocabulary.

As is well known, animals can master the words of human speech and use them in appropriate situations. Before the child reaches this critical point in development, he also masters individual words that are for him nothing more than conditioned stimuli or substitutes for objects, people, actions, states, or desires. At this point in his development, however, the child knows words only to the extent that they are given to him by the people around him.

A new situation emerges with the new stage in the child's development mentioned above. On seeing a new object, the child asks what it is called. He finds himself in need of a word and actively strives to master the sign belonging to the object, the sign that permits naming and communication. As Meumann has shown, the first stage in the development of the child's speech is an affective-volitional stage. At this critical point in the child's life, speech begins the intellectual phase of its development. The child "discovers" the symbolic function of speech.

Stern writes:

> Only the process described here can confidently be defined as thinking activity in the true sense of the word. The understanding of the relationship between sign and meaning manifested in the child at this stage is something fundamentally different than the simple use of representations and their associations. The requirement that each object, whatever its nature, has its name, can perhaps be considered the child's first general concept (ibid., p. 93).

It is here, in the intersection of thinking and speech in ontogenesis, that the knot that is called the problem of thinking and speech is first tied. However, we must ask whether Stern correctly interprets this critical moment, this "greatest discovery" in the child's life."

Buhler compares this discovery with the inventions of the chimpanzee: "However this circumstance is viewed or interpreted, the decisive point will always be the psychological parallel with the chimpanzee's inventions" (Buhler, 1923, p. 55). Koffka develops the same idea:

> The naming function *(Namengebung)* is a discovery or invention by the child that fully parallels the chimpanzee's inventions. We have seen that the latter is a structured action. Consequently, we can see that naming is a structured action. We would say that the word enters into the structure of the thing just as the stick enters into the structure of the situation, into the desire to obtain the fruit (Koffka, 1925, p. 243).

It is not clear to what extent this analogy between the child's discovery of the signifying function of the word and the chimpanzee's discovery of the functional significance of the tool is correct. There are clearly important differences between these operations. We will address this issue in our discussion of the functional and structural relationship between thinking and speech. What should be emphasized at this point is that this "greatest discovery in the child's life" becomes possible only at a rather advanced stage in the development of thinking and speech. To "discover" speech, the child must think.

Our conclusions can be briefly summarized in the following way:

1. As we found in our analysis of the phylogenetic development of thinking and speech, we find that these two processes have different roots in ontogenesis.
2. Just as we can identify a "pre-speech" stage in the development of the child's thinking, we can identify a "pre-intellectual stage" in the development of his speech.
3. Up to a certain point, speech and thinking develop along different lines and independently of one another.
4. At a certain point, the two lines cross: thinking becomes verbal and speech intellectual.

### 3

However one resolves the complex and still disputed theoretical issue of the relationship between thinking and speech, the significance of the processes of inner speech for the development of thinking must be recognized. Inner speech is so important for all our thinking that many psychologists have identified these two processes with one another, representing thinking as an arrested or soundless form of speech. Nonetheless, the manner in which the transformation from external to inner speech occurs has not yet been clarified. Psychology has not identified the approximate age at which this important transition occurs, how it occurs, what elicits it, or what its general genetic characteristics are.

Watson, who identifies thinking with inner speech, has correctly stated that we do not know "at what point in the organization of the child's speech the transition from overt speech

to the whisper, and then to covert speech, is completed." This question has 'received only incidental investigation'" (1926, p. 293). However, given our own experiments and observations
and what we know generally of the child's development, it seems to us that Watson has stated
the problem incorrectly.

There is no good basis for the assumption that the development of inner speech is a purely
mechanical process, that is, a process that consists of a gradual reduction in speech volume.
To state the problem more directly, there is no evidence that the transition from external overt
speech to inner covert speech moves through the whisper. It is simply not the case that the child
gradually begins to speak more and more softly, ultimately achieving soundless speech. Thus,
we reject the notion that the development of the child's inner speech is based on the genetic
sequence: audible speech whisper inner speech.

A second thesis advanced by Watson cannot salvage his position on this issue. Watson
suggests that "perhaps all three forms of speech develop together from the outset" (ibid.). No
objective data support this contention. There are profound functional and structural differences
between overt speech and inner speech. This single fact, of which everyone including Watson
is aware, contradicts Watson's basic assumptions.

Watson writes that young children "truly think out loud." With good reason, he sees the
cause of this phenomenon in the fact that "their environment does not demand a rapid transformation of external speech into covert form" (ibid.). Developing this thought further, he
writes that:

> Even if we were able to open up all the covert processes involved and record them, these
> processes would be so abbreviated and economical that they would be incomprehensible.
> This would be true, at least, if we failed to trace the formation of these processes from the
> outset, where they are completely social in character, through to the final stage where they
> serve as a form of individual rather than social adaptation (ibid., p. 294).

Functionally, external speech serves social adaptation and inner speech serves individual
adaptation. Structurally, through processes of abbreviation and economization, inner speech
comes to differ so radically from external speech that it is nearly incomprehensible. What reason do we have to assume that processes so different from each other in functional and structural terms develop in parallel with one another? What reason do we have to think that they
move either simultaneously or in some connection with one another through a third transitional process, that is, the whisper? The whisper occupies a position between external and inner
speech only in a purely mechanical, formal, and externally quantitative sense (i.e., phenotypically). It is not transitional *vis-à-vis* external and inner speech in either functional or structural terms (i.e., genotypically).

We were able to evaluate this thesis experimentally in a study of the whispered speech of
young children. Our research demonstrated that: (1) in structural terms, there are no significant
differences between whispered and normal speech and, more importantly, that whispered speech
manifests none of the characteristics of inner speech; (2) in functional terms, whispered speech
is again profoundly different from inner speech, manifesting not the slightest tendency of convergence with it and, finally; (3) in genetic terms, whispered speech can be elicited very early, but
there is no evidence of development or change in its nature from this point through school age.

The sole support for Watson's thesis is the fact that under social pressure even the three year old child (with difficulty but in a very short time) develops speech with a reduced volume.

Watson's perspectives are widely known and typical of this general approach to the problem of thinking and speech. In addition, by focusing on Watson's views, we have been able to present a clear contrast between phenotypal and genotypal approaches to this issue. However, these factors were not our primary motivation for focusing on Watson's views in this context. Our primary consideration was of a more positive nature. Specifically, we feel the basis for a correct methodological resolution of the whole problem can be found in Watson's approach.

The methodological resolution of this problem requires that we find a middle link that unites the processes of external and inner speech, a link that is transitional between these two processes. As we have attempted to demonstrate, Watson's belief that this middle link is to be found in the whisper has no objective support. All that we know of the child's whisper contradicts the notion that it is the middle link in the transition between external and inner speech. However, the attempt to find this middle link—an attempt which is absent from most psychological investigations of this problem—is correct.

In our view, the transition between external and inner speech is to be found in the child's egocentric speech, a phenomenon that has been described by the Swiss psychologist [Jean] Piaget. Observations of the inner speech of school age children by Lemaitre and others support this thesis. These observations have demonstrated that the school child's inner speech is still comparatively labile, that it is not yet fully established. This indicates, of course, that at this age we are dealing with what is still a genetically new process, one that is not yet sufficiently formed or defined.

Alongside the purely expressive function of egocentric speech, its tendency to simply accompany the child's activity, this process *becomes thinking in the true sense of the term*. It assumes the function of a planning operation or the function of resolving a problem that arises in behavior. If this proposition is supported by further research, we will be able to draw a conclusion of extraordinary theoretical significance. Specifically, we will have evidence that speech becomes inner psychologically before it becomes inner physiologically. Egocentric speech is speech that is inner in function. It is speech for oneself, speech on the threshold of becoming inner. It is already half incomprehensible to others. At the same time, however, it is still external in a physiological sense. There is no evidence which would indicate that it is being transformed into a whisper or any other kind of semi-soundless speech.

This leads us to an answer to another fundamental theoretical question, the question of *why* speech becomes inner. The answer would be that speech becomes inner because its function changes. The sequence underlying the development of speech would then be something different from that suggested by Watson. Rather than the stages of overt speech, the whisper, and soundless speech, we would have the stages of external speech, egocentric speech, and inner speech. At the same time, we would have gained something even more important in methodological terms. We would have gained a mode of studying inner speech, a means of studying its structural and functional characteristics in their living form and in the process of their formation. All the characteristics of inner speech would be observable in a form of external speech, a form of speech which we could experiment on and subject to measurement. Our research will demonstrate that the development of this form of speech is subordinated to the same laws as is the development of all mental operations depending on the use of signs, including mnemonic memory and the processes of calculation.

By studying several operations of this kind experimentally, we have established that this development passes through four basic stages. In the first stage, what can be called the primitive or natural stage, we find the operation in the form in which it has developed on primitive stages of behavior. This stage of development corresponds with the pre-intellectual speech and pre-verbal thinking that we discussed earlier.

The next stage is what we will call the stage of "naive psychology" in analogy with the phenomenon that researchers in the field of practical intellect call "naive physics." The phrase "naive physics" is used to refer to the naive experience of the animal or child with the physical characteristics of its own body and the objects and tools that surround it. It concerns the naive experience that defines the child's basic use of tools and the first operations of his practical mind. The child's naive experience of the characteristics of his more important mental operations is, in a similar manner, formed in his behavior. However, as in the development of practical actions, this naive experience usually turns out to be inadequate, imperfect, and naive in the true sense of the word. It leads, therefore, to inadequate use of the mind's characteristics, including the use of stimuli and reactions. In the domain of speech development, this stage is clearly expressed in the fact that the mastery of grammatical structures and forms precedes the mastery of the corresponding logical structures and operations. The child masters the subordinate clause (forms of speech such as "because," "since,.... if,.... when," or "but") long before he masters the corresponding causal, temporal, and conditional relationships. The child masters the syntax of speech earlier than he masters the syntax of thought. Piaget's research has demonstrated beyond doubt that grammatical development in the child leads to logical development, that the child masters the logical operations corresponding to grammatical structures relatively late.

With the gradual accumulation of naive mental experience, the child reaches the stage of the external sign and external operation. Here, the child solves the internal mental task on the basis of the external sign. This is the familiar stage where the child counts on his fingers in the development of arithmetic skills and where external mnemonic signs are used in remembering. In the development of speech, this stage corresponds with the appearance of egocentric speech in the child.

This stage is followed by a fourth that we will call the stage of "rooting" because it is characterized by the movement of the external operation to the internal plane, by the transformation of the external operation into an internal operation. Of course, in the process, the operation undergoes profound change. In this stage, we find operations such as counting in the mind or mute arithmetic. This is the stage of what is called logical memory, a form of memory that utilizes internal relationships in the form of internal signs. In the domain of speech, this stage corresponds with inner or soundless speech. In this context, the most significant characteristic of this stage is that there is a constant interaction between external and internal operations, that is, operations constantly move from one form to the other. We see this most clearly with inner speech. As Delacroix has demonstrated, the more closely inner speech is connected with external speech in behavior, the more similar they become. For example, inner speech may take a form identical with external speech when it occurs in the preparation of an upcoming speech or lecture. In this sense, there is no sharp metaphysical boundary between the external and the internal in behavior. One can easily be transformed into the other and each develops under the other's influence.

Moving now from the issue of the genesis of inner speech to the issue of how it functions in the adult, the first question we encounter is one that we have addressed earlier in connection with issues of phylogenesis and ontogenesis: Are thinking and speech necessarily connected in the adult's behavior? That is, can the two processes be identified with one another? All that we know that is relevant to this issue forces us to answer this question in the negative. The relationship of thinking and speech in this context can be schematically represented by two intersecting circles. Only a limited portion of the processes of speech and thinking coincide in what is commonly called verbal thinking. Verbal thinking does not exhaust all the forms of thought nor does it exhaust all the forms of speech. There is a large range of thinking that has no direct relationship to verbal thinking. In this category, we could include the instrumental and technical thinking that has been described by Buhler and what is commonly called practical intellect.

As is well known, the Wurzburg school has established that thinking can occur without any participation of speech images or movements. The most recent experimental work has also shown that activation and inner speech do not stand in any direct objective connection with movements of the tongue or larynx. In the same sense, there is no psychological basis for relating all forms of speech to thinking. For example, when I reproduce a poem that I have learned by heart in inner speech or repeat a phrase assigned in an experimental context, there is no evidence that would relate these operations to the domain of thought. Watson, who makes the mistake of identifying thinking and speech, is forced to consider all speech processes as intellectual. As a result, he associates with thinking even the processes involved in the simple reproduction of a verbal text in memory. We should also note that speech that is emotional expressive in function or speech with a lyrical coloring can hardly be associated with intellectual activity in the true sense of the word.

In the adult, the fusion of thinking and speech is a limited phenomenon that is of significance only in the domain of verbal thinking. The domains of non-verbal thinking and non-intellectual speech are only indirectly influenced by this fusion. They are not linked with it in a direct causal manner.

## 4

Based on data made available to us by comparative psychology, we have attempted to trace the genetic roots of thinking and speech. We have seen that with the contemporary state of knowledge in this field no complete analysis of the genesis of pre-human thinking and speech is possible. One of the most basic issues, the issue of whether the higher apes possess an intellect of the type found in man, remains in dispute. Kohler answers this question positively but others answer it negatively. Nonetheless, however this dispute is ultimately resolved, one thing is clear even at this point. The *paths* that lead to the emergence of human intellect and human speech do not coincide. The genetic roots of thinking and speech are different.

Even those who are inclined to reject the notion that intellect is present in Kohler's chimpanzees do not and cannot reject the fact that we are dealing here with an important element in the development of human intellect, that we are dealing with the roots of intellect, with a more highly developed form of habit. Even Thorndike found ape behavior to be more advanced than the behavior of other animals (1901).* Others, Borovskii for example, reject the very concept of a higher stage of behavior, a stage of behavior constructed on a foundation of habits but deserving the special name of intellect. These scholars deny the presence of this type of behavior not only in animals but in humans. Of course, in discussions with this group, the very question of a human-like intellect in the apes must be framed somewhat differently.

In our view, whatever one's perspective on the higher behavior of the chimpanzee, this behavior is clearly the root of human behavior in that it is characterized by the use of tools. Kohler's discovery is no surprise for Marxism. Marx wrote that "the use and creation of the means of labor, though found in embryonic form in several animal species, is the characteristic feature of the human labor process" (Marx & Engels, *Collected Works*, v. 23, pp. 190–191). Along the same lines, Plekhanov[13] wrote that "whatever the nature of the underlying process, zoology gave to history a man who already possessed the capacity to invent and use primitive tools" (1956, v. 2, p. 153).

Thus, the most recent developments in zoological psychology are not entirely new *theoretical* developments for Marxism. It is interesting to note that Plekhanov clearly wrote not about instinctive behavior (e.g., the constructions of the beaver) but about the capacity to invent and use tools, about intellectual operations.†

For Marxism, the notion that the roots of human intellect are to be found in the animal world is not novel. In clarifying the meaning of Hegel's distinction between reason and intelligence, Engels wrote that:

> We share with animals all forms of intelligent activity: *induction, deduction* (and, consequently, even *abstraction*) (Didot's species concepts: four-legged and two-legged), *analysis* of unfamiliar objects (breaking a nut is already a form of analysis), *synthesis* (in the sly tricks of animals), and, as the unification of both, the *experiment* (where new barriers or difficult positions are encountered). According to their type, all these methods, all the recognized logical means of scientific investigation, are identical in man and animals. It is only as a matter of degree (in accordance with the level of their development) that they differ (Marx and Engels, *Collected Works*, v. 20, p. 537).‡

---

* In experiments with lower apes (i.e., marmosets), Thorndike observed a *sudden* acquisition of new movements that brought the animal closer to attaining a goal as well as a rapid and often instantaneous cessation of useless movements. He wrote that the speed of this process compared favorably with similar phenomena in man. What Thorndike observed here differed from problem resolution in the cat, dog, or chicken, which are characterized by a gradual elimination of movements that do not contribute to the achievement of the goal.

† In the chimpanzee, of course, we find not the instinctive use of tools, but the rudiments of their rational use. Plekhanov continues: "It is as clear as day that however undeveloped the use of tools, their use presupposes a comparatively advanced development of the mental capacities (1956, v. 2, p. 138).

‡ Elsewhere Engels writes: "We would not, however, presume to reject the notion that animals possess the capacity for planned, intentional actions" (i.e., actions of the type that Kohler finds in the chimpanzee). And further: "An image of the action exists in embryonic form wherever protoplasm, living protein, exists and reacts." This capacity "has attained an advanced level in the mammals (Marx and Engels, *Collected Works*, v. 20, p. 495).

Engels expressed himself with equal decisiveness on the issue of the roots of speech in animals: "Within the limits of its own range of representations, it can learn and understand what it says." Engels provides *objective* criteria for this "understanding":

> If you teach a parrot a swear word so that it attains a representation of its meaning (a common diversion of sailors returning from tropical countries) and tease him, you will quickly discover that it can apply its swear word just as well as any merchant in Berlin. The situation does not change when he begs for a tidbit (ibid., p. 490).*

We would not want to ascribe to Engels the idea that we find human, or even human-like, speech and thinking among animals. We would certainly not want to defend this thesis ourselves. We will attempt to clarify the *proper limits* and true meaning of Engels's assertions on this issue later. At this point, we would simply emphasize that there is no basis for rejecting the presence of the genetic roots of thinking and speech in the animal world. Moreover, the paths along which these forms of behavior develop are distinct.

An advanced capacity for learning speech like that we find in the parrot, is not directly associated with highly developed forms of thinking. Correspondingly, advanced development of the rudiments of thought is not necessarily linked with advanced forms of speech. Each of these processes has its own developmental course. Each develops along separate lines.†

Regardless of one's views on the relationship between ontogenesis and phylogenesis, recent experimental studies have shown that the genetic roots of intellect and speech and the processes involved in their development differ in ontogenesis. That is, up to a certain stage, we can trace the pre-intellectual growth of the child's speech and the pre-verbal growth of his intellect. It is only later that, in Stern's words, *the two lines of development intersect.* Speech *becomes* intellectual and thinking verbal. Stern sees this as the *child's greatest discovery.*

Stern's perspectives on the convergence of speech and intellect are rejected by Delacroix and others who question the universal significance of the distinction between the first age of childhood questions and the second (i.e., the four year old's repeated question: Why?). In any event, these scholars reject the significance that Stern ascribed to this first stage of childhood questions. They reject his argument that it is a symptom of the child's discovery that "everything has its name (Delacroix, 1924, p. 286). Wallon suggests that for a certain period of time the "name" is more an attribute of the object than a substitute for it.

When the one-and-a-half year old asks the name of an object, he observes a connection that he has discovered. However, there is nothing to indicate that he sees in one anything other than a simple attribute of the other. Only a systematic generalization of questions would indicate that what we are seeing here is not an accidental and passive connection, but a tendency of an existing function to seek out the symbolic sign for all real things (Delacroix, 1924, p. 287).

---

* Elsewhere, Engels writes that: The little that the latter, even the most developed, have to communicate to one another can be communicated even without the use of differentiated speech" (ibid., p. 489). In Engels view, domesticated animals may experience the *need* for speech. "Unfortunately, their vocal organs are so specialized that their experienced need is of no use. Where, however, the animal has an organ that approaches that required for speech, the incapacity for speech can disappear to a certain extent" (ibid.). The parrot is a good example.

† Smidt notes that the level of speech development is not a direct indicator of the level of development of mind or behavior in the animal world. Both the elephant and horse fall behind the pig and chicken in their level of speech development (1923, p. 46).

As we have seen, Koffka takes a position that lies somewhere between these two perspectives. On the one hand, following Buhler, he emphasizes the analogy between the invention or discovery of the nominative function of language in the child and the invention of tools in the chimpanzee. On the other, he limits this analogy by saying that the word enters into the structure of the thing but not necessarily into the functional meaning of the sign. The word enters into the structure of the thing as a part of it, alongside it. For a time, it becomes for the child a characteristic of the thing alongside its other characteristics.

However, this particular characteristic of the thing, its name, is separable from it *(verschiedbar)*. Things can be seen when their names are not heard in much the same way that the eyes are a stable but separable aspect of the mother that are not seen when the mother averts her face. "The situation is precisely the same even for us. The blue dress remains blue even when in the dark we cannot see its color. The name is a characteristic of all objects and the child supplements the structure of all objects in accordance with this rule" (Koffka, 1925, p. 244). Buhler points out that any new object presents the child with a situation or task that he resolves in accordance with this general structural scheme, by naming it with the word. Where he does not have a word adequate for designating a new object, he demands it from adults (Buhler, 1923, p. 54).

In our view, the perspective that most closely approximates the truth and effectively eliminates many of these difficulties emerges in the argument between Stern and Delacroix. Data from ethnic and child psychology (see Piaget, 1923) indicate that for the child the word is for some time *more a characteristic of the thing than a symbol for it*. As we have seen, the child masters the *external structure earlier* than the *internal structure*. He first masters the *external* structure-word-thing. Only later does this *become* a symbolic structure.

We are once again faced with an issue that has not been empirically resolved. We are faced with several hypotheses and can only select the one that is the more probable. Our own tendency would be to reject out of hand the attribution of the discovery of the symbolic function of speech to the one-and-a-half year old child. First, such a discovery is a conscious and very complex intellectual operation which does not seem to correspond with the general level of the child's mental development at this age. Second, the experimental data indicate that the functional use of the sign, even of sign forms that are less complex than the word, appears at a later stage of the child's development. It is completely inaccessible to the child at this stage. Third, data on the child's speech indicate that it does not attain conscious awareness of the symbolic significance of speech for a long time and uses the word as one of the characteristics of the thing. Fourth, observations of abnormal children (Helen Keller[14] in particular), observations that are cited by Stern himself, indicate that if one traces how this critical moment emerges in the speech of deaf children one finds no "discovery" that can be identified with temporal precision. On the contrary, there is a whole series of "molecular" changes (Buhler, 1923).

All this evidence indicates that Stern's position was improperly based on an external interpretation of the child's questions, that is, on a *phenotypal* interpretation of these questions. However, our basic conclusion that thinking and speech move along different genetic paths in ontogenesis, that their developmental courses intersect only at a given point, does not fall along with Stern's perspective on this issue. Whether Stern's position or any another stands or falls, this basic conclusion remains. All agree that the child's initial intellectual reactions, reactions established experimentally by Kohler and others, are as independent of speech as are the chimpanzee's actions (Delacroix, 1924, p. 283). Moreover, all agree that the initial stages in the development of the child's speech are pre-intellectual.

With respect to the infant's babbling, the thesis that the initial stages of the child's speech are pre-intellectual is obvious and undisputed. In addition, however, this thesis has recently been affirmed with respect to the child's first words. It is true that several authors have recently disputed Meumann's position that the child's first words are affective-volitional in nature and that objective meaning is foreign to them, his position that they represent "wishes or feelings" (Meumann, p. 1928). Stern has argued that the elements of the object have not yet been differentiated in the initial words (Stern, p. 1928), and Delacroix sees a direct link between the initial words and the objective situation (Delacroix, p. 1924). However, both authors agree that the word has no constant or stable objective meaning at this point and that it is similar in this respect to the parrot's swear word. The word is linked with the objective situation only to the extent that wishes, feelings, and emotional reactions are linked with it. This does not constitute a rejection of Meumann's basic position (ibid., p. 280).

We can now summarize our analysis of the development of speech and thinking in ontogenesis. As was the case in phylogenesis, the genetic roots and the course of development of thinking and speech are different up to a *given point*. What is unique to human ontogenesis is the *intersecting of these paths of development*. That this intersection occurs is not disputed. Whether it occurs at a single point or many times, whether it occurs suddenly and catastrophically or develops slowly and gradually, whether it is the result of a discovery or of a simple structural action and an extended functional transformation, whether it occurs near the age of two or nearer school age, the basic fact remains unquestioned. These two lines of development intersect.

We must also summarize our analysis of inner speech. Once again, we find several hypotheses. However, whether inner speech passes through the whisper or through egocentric speech, whether it develops simultaneously with external speech or arises at a comparatively late stage of development, whether inner speech and the thinking associated with it are considered a distinct stage in the development of cultural forms of behavior, the basic facts remain. Inner speech develops through a long cumulative series of functional and structural changes. It branches off from the child's external speech with the differentiation of the social and the egocentric functions of speech. Finally, the structure of speech that the child masters becomes the basic structure of his thinking.

A basic, indisputable, and decisive fact emerges here: thinking depends on speech, on the *means of thinking*, and on the child's socio-cultural experience. The development of inner speech is defined from the outside. As Piaget's research has shown, the development of the child's logic is a direct function of his socialized speech. This position can be formulated in the following way: the development of the child's thinking depends on his mastery of the social means of thinking, that is, on his mastery of speech.

Here, we approach the formulation of the fundamental thesis of our work, a thesis of great methodological significance for the correct statement of the problem of thinking and speech. This thesis stems from our *comparison* of the development of inner speech and verbal thinking in man with the development of speech and intellect as it occurs in the animal world and the earliest stages of childhood. This comparison demonstrates that the former does not represent a simple continuation of the latter. The very type of development changes. It changes from a biological form of development to a socio-historical form of development.

As the preceding section clearly demonstrated, verbal thinking is not a natural but a socio-historical form of behavior. It is therefore characterized by a whole series of *features and laws* that do not apply to natural forms of thinking and speech. The most important point, however, is that this recognition of the historical nature of verbal thinking requires that in analyzing it we apply the same methodological theses that historical materialism applies to the other historical phenomena of human society. We can anticipate that the basic features of the historical development of behavior in this domain will be directly dependent on the general laws that govern the historical development of human society.

In this way, the problem of thinking and speech grows beyond the boundaries of natural science. It is transformed into the central problem of the historical psychology of man. It becomes the central problem of social psychology. The methodological statement of this problem is also transformed. While we did not deal with this issue in its entirety, we attempted to address the *central points*. In methodological terms, these points are extremely difficult, but they are central to any analysis of human behavior. We have attempted to address them on the foundations provided by dialectical and historical materialism.

This second problem of thinking and speech, as well as many other aspects of the functional and structural analysis of the relationship between these processes, must be left for future studies.

# 3

# Thought and Word

*I forgot the word that I wanted to say,*
*And thought, unembodied, returns to the hall of shadows.*
O.E. MANDELSHTAM, *The Swallow*

## 1

Our investigation began with an attempt to clarify the internal relationships between thought and word at the most extreme stages of phylogenetic and ontogenetic development. In the prehistoric development of thinking and speech, we found no clearly defined relationships or dependencies between the genetic roots of thought and word. Thus, the internal relationships between thought and word with which we are concerned are not primal. They are not something given from the outset as a precondition for further development. On the contrary, these relationships emerge and are formed only with the historical development of human consciousness. They are not the precondition of man's formation but its product.

With the anthropoids—the ultimate development of the animal world—we find forms of speech and intellect that are phenotypically similar to their counterparts in man. However, they are not connected with one another in any way. In the initial stages of child development, we can clearly identify a preintellectual stage in the formation of speech and a pre-speech stage in the development of thinking. Once again, the connection between thought and word is neither inherent or primal. This connection emerges, changes, and grows with the development of thought and word.

As we tried to show at the outset, however, it would be incorrect to represent thinking and speech as processes that are externally related to one another, as two independent forces moving and acting in parallel with one another or intersecting at specific points and interacting mechanically. The absence of a primal connection between thought and word does not imply that this connection can arise only as an external connection between two fundamentally heterogeneous forms of the activity of consciousness. On the contrary, the basic methodological defect of nearly all studies of thinking and speech—that which underlies the fruitlessness of this

Originally appeared in English translation as Chapter 7 in *The Collected Works of L.S. Vygotsky, Volume 1: Problems of General Psychology* (Robert W. Rieber and Aaron S. Carton, Eds.; Norris Minich, Trans.) (pp. 243–285). New York: Plenum Press, 1987.

work—is the tendency to view thought and word as two independent and isolated elements whose external unification leads to the characteristic features of verbal thinking.

We have attempted to demonstrate that those who begin with this mode of analysis are doomed to failure from the outset. To explain the characteristics of verbal thinking, they decompose the whole into the elements that form it. They decompose verbal thinking into speech and thinking, elements that do not contain the characteristics inherent to the whole. This closes the door to any real explanation of these characteristics. We have compared the researcher who takes this approach to one who decomposes water into hydrogen and oxygen in the attempt to explain why water extinguishes fire. As we noted, this researcher would find to his surprise that oxygen sustains combustion while hydrogen is itself combustible. We also argued that decomposition into elements is not analysis in the true sense of the word but *a process* of *raising the phenomenon to a more general level.* It is not a process that involves the internal partitioning of the phenomenon which is the object of explanation. It is not a method of analysis but a method of generalization. To say that water consists of hydrogen and oxygen is to say nothing that relates to water generally or to all its characteristics. It is to say nothing that relates to the great oceans and to a drop of rain, to water's capacity to extinguish fire and to Archimedes's law. In the same way, to say that verbal thinking contains intellectual processes and speech functions is to say nothing that relates to the whole of verbal thinking and to all its characteristics equally. It is to say nothing of relevance to the concrete problems confronting those involved in the study of verbal thinking.

From the outset, then, we have tried to frame the entire problem in a new way and apply a new method of analysis. We attempted to replace the method based on decomposition into elements with a method of analysis that involves partitioning the complex unity of verbal thinking into units. In contrast to elements, units are products of analysis that form the initial aspects not of the whole but of its concrete aspects and characteristics. Unlike elements, units do not lose the characteristics inherent to the whole. The unit contains, in a simple, primitive form, the characteristics of the whole that is the object of analysis.

We found the unit that reflects the unity of thinking and speech in the *meaning* of the word. As we have tried to show, word meaning is a unity of both processes that cannot be further decomposed. That is, we cannot say that word meaning is a phenomenon of either speech or thinking. The word without meaning is not a word but an empty sound. Meaning is a necessary, constituting feature of the word itself. It is the word viewed from the inside, This justifies the view that word meaning is a phenomenon of speech, In psychological terms, however, word meaning is nothing other than a generalization, that is, a concept. In essence, generalization and word meaning are synonyms. Any generalization—any formation of a concept—is unquestionably a specific and true act of thought. Thus, word meaning is also a phenomenon of thinking.

Word meaning, then, is a phenomenon of both speech and intellect. This does not, however, represent a simultaneous and external membership in two different domains of mental life. Word meaning is a phenomenon of thinking only to the extent that thought is connected with the word and embodied in it. It is a phenomenon of speech only to the extent that speech is connected with thought and illuminated by it. Word meaning is a phenomenon of verbal thought or of the meaningful word. It is a unity of word and thought.

No further evidence is needed to support this basic thesis. Our experimental studies have consistently supported and justified it. They have shown that by taking word meaning as a unit of verbal thinking we create the potential for investigating its development and explaining its most important characteristics at the various developmental stages. The primary result of this work, however, is not this thesis itself but a subsequent conclusion that constitutes the conceptual center of our investigation, that is, the finding that word meaning *develops*. The discovery that word meaning changes and develops is our new and fundamental contribution to the theory of thinking and speech. It is our major discovery, a discovery that has allowed us to overcome the postulate of constancy and unchangableness of word meaning which has provided the foundation for previous theories of thinking and speech.

From the perspective of traditional psychology, the connection between word and meaning is associative; it is a connection established as a result of a repeated coincidence in perceptual consciousness of the word and the thing the word designates. The word reminds an individual of its meaning in the same way that a person's coat reminds him of the person. From this perspective, word meaning cannot develop or change once it has been established. Associations that connect word and meaning can be reinforced or weakened. It can be enriched through connections with other objects of the same type, extended in accordance with similarity or contiguity to a wider circle of objects, or contracted as this circle of objects narrows or becomes more restricted. In other words, the association may undergo a series of quantitative and external changes, It cannot, however, change its internal psychological nature. This would require that it cease to be what it is, that it cease to be an association. From this perspective, the development of the meaningful aspect of speech—the development of word meaning—becomes inexplicable and impossible.

This is expressed in linguistics and in the psychological study of both child and adult speech. Having assimilated the associative conception of the word, the field of linguistics that is concerned with the study of the meaningful aspect of speech (i.e., semantics) has continued to view the word as an association between the word's sound-form and its object content. Word meanings—from the most concrete to the most abstract—are assumed to have a single common structure. Since the associative connection that unites the word and its meaning constitutes the foundation not only for meaningful speech but for processes such as being reminded of a person because we have seen his coat there is nothing unique to speech as such. The word forces us to remember its meaning in the same way that one thing reminds us of another. Because there is nothing unique in the connection of the word with its meaning, semantics cannot pose the question of the development of the meaningful aspect of speech, the question of the development of word meaning. The entire process of development is reduced to changes in the associative connections between words and objects. The word may initially designate one object and then become connected with another through the processes of association. The coat, being transferred from one owner to another, may initially remind us of one person and subsequently of another. The development of the meaningful aspect of speech is reduced to the changes that occur in the object content of words. The notion that the semantic structure of word meaning might change through the historical development of language is completely foreign to linguistics. Linguistics cannot perceive the possibility that the psychological nature of meaning changes, that linguistic thought moves from primitive forms of generalization to higher and more complex forms, that the very nature of the reflection and generalization of reality in the word changes with the emergence of abstract concepts in the process of the historical development of language.

This associative perspective on word meaning also leads to the view that the development of the meaningful aspect of speech in ontogenesis is impossible and inexplicable. The development of word meaning in the child is reduced to purely external and quantitative changes in the associative connections that unite word and meaning, to the enrichment or reinforcement of these connections. The notion that the structure and nature of the connections between word and meaning might change during the development of the child's speech—the fact that they do change during ontogenesis—is inexplicable from the associative perspective.

Finally, this perspective leads to the notion that there is nothing in the verbal thinking of the adult other than an unbroken, lineal, associative movement from the word to its meaning and from the meaning to the word. The understanding of speech is conceptualized as a chain of associations that arise in the mind under the influence of familiar word forms. The expression of thought in the word is conceptualized as the reverse movement along this same associative path, beginning this time with the representation of objects in thought and moving to their verbal designation. These kinds of mutual connections between two representations are always insured by associations. At one point, the coat may remind us of the person who wears it, while at another the form of the person may remind us of his coat. Thus, there is nothing in the understanding of speech nor in the expression of speech in thought that is new or unique when compared to other acts of remembering or associative connection.

The inadequacy of associative theory was recognized and demonstrated (both experimentally and theoretically) some time ago. This has not, however, influenced the associative understanding of the word and its meaning. The Wurzburg school considered its main task to be that of demonstrating that thinking cannot be reduced to an associative flow of representations, that the movement, cohesion, and recall of thoughts cannot be explained in associative terms. It assumed the task of demonstrating that the flow of thought is directed by several unique laws. However, the Wurzburg school not only failed to reanalyze the associative perspective on the relationship between word and meaning but failed to see why this kind of reanalysis was necessary. Instead, it separated speech and thinking, granting to God what is God's and to Caesar what is Caesar's. It liberated thought from all images and from everything sensual. It liberated thought from the power of associative laws, transforming it into a purely mental act. In the process, it returned to ideas that have their roots in the prescientific spiritualistic conceptions of Augustine and Descartes.[15] The final product was an extreme subjective idealism that surpassed even that of Descartes. In Kulpe's words: "We not only say: 'I think therefore I am.' We argue that 'the world exists only as we establish it and define it'" (1914, p. 81). Since thinking belonged to God it was granted to God. As Kulpe himself recognized, this opened the door for the psychology of thinking to move toward the ideas of Plato.

Having liberated thought from any sensual component and returned it to a pure, unembodied, mental act, these psychologists simultaneously tore thinking from speech and assigned the latter entirely to the domain of associative laws. Thus, the connection between the word and its meaning continued to be viewed as a simple association. The word was seen as the external expression of thought, as its clothing. The word had no place in the inner life of thought. Never have thinking and speech been as isolated from one another in psychological theory as they were in the Wurzburg epoch. The process of overcoming associationism in the domain of thinking led to its reinforcement in the domain of speech. As Caesar's, speech was granted to Caesar.

Psychologists who have extended this line of thought within the tradition of the Wurzburg school have not only failed to transform it but have continued to deepen and develop it. Having demonstrated the complete inadequacy of the constellational theory of productive thinking (ultimately, the inadequacy of the associative theory of productive thinking), Seltz replaced it with a new theory that deepened and strengthened the gap between thought and word that was inherent in the works of this tradition from the outset. Seltz continued to analyze thinking in and of itself, estranged from speech. He concluded that man's productive thinking is identical in its fundamentals to the intellectual operations of the chimpanzee. To the extent that the word introduced nothing new to the nature of thought, thinking remained independent of speech.

Even Ach, who made special studies of word meaning and who first made the move toward overcoming associationism in concept theory, was unable to go beyond a recognition that determining tendencies were present alongside associative tendencies in the process of concept formation. He did not escape from the earlier understanding of word meaning. He identified the concept with word meaning, excluding any potential for change and development in concepts. Ach assumed that once meaning emerged, it remained unchanged and constant. He assumed that the development of word meaning is finished at the moment of its formation. The psychologists Ach criticized assumed the same thing. Thus, though Ach and his opponents differed in their representations of the initial moment in the formation of word meaning, both assumed that the initial moment and end point in the process of concept development coincide.

We find the same thesis concerning the theory of thinking and speech in contemporary structural psychology. This tradition has made a more profound and consistent attempt to overcome associative psychology. Therefore, it has not been limited to the indecisive resolutions of the question characteristic of its predecessors. It has attempted to remove not only thinking but speech from the domain of associative laws, to subordinate both to the laws of structural formations. However, this tradition not only failed to advance in its theory of thinking and speech but took a profound step backward in comparison to its predecessors.

First, this new theory preserved a fundamental break between thinking and speech. The relationship between thought and word was represented as a simple analogy, as a reduction of both to a common structural denominator. Within this tradition, researchers conceptualized the origin of true meaningful words in the child as analogous to the intellectual operations of the chimpanzee in Kohler's experiments. They argued that the word enters the structure of things and acquires a certain functional significance in the same way that the stick entered into the structure of the situation of attaining fruit for the chimpanzee and acquired the functional significance of a tool. The connection between the word and meaning is no longer thought of as an associative connection. It is represented as a structural connection. Of course, this is a step forward. However, if we carefully consider the foundations of this new perspective, we quickly find that this step forward is an illusion, that we remain in the rut laid down by associative psychology.

The word and the thing that it designates form a single unified structure. However, this structure is analogous to any structural connection between two things. There is nothing that is unique to the word. Any two things, whether they are a stick and some fruit or a word and the object it designates, merge into a unified structure in accordance with the same laws. Once again, the word turns out to be just one thing among other things. It is a thing which is united with other things in accordance with the general structural laws that unite all things. What distinguishes the word from other things? What distinguishes the structure of the word from other structures? How does the word represents the thing in consciousness? What makes the word a word? All these questions remain outside the researcher's field of view. The rejection of the unique character of the word and its relationship to meaning, the dissolving of these particular connections into the sea of all structural connections, is no less characteristic of the new psychology than it was of the old.

To clarify the concept of the word's nature in structural psychology, we can once again use the example of the man and his coat. That is, we can use the same example we used in clarifying the concept of the connection between word and meaning in associative psychology. The word reminds us of its meaning in the same way that the coat reminds us of the man on which we are accustomed to seeing it: this thesis preserves its force for structural psychology. Here, the coat and the man that wears it form a unified structure, a structure which is entirely analogous to the word and the thing it designates. The fact that the coat may remind us of its owner and that the man's form may remind us of his coat are once again explained in this new psychology through a single set of structural laws. The principle of association is replaced with the principle of structure.

*Like the principle of association, this new principle is extended* to *all relationships, extended universally and without differentiation.* Representatives of the old psychology argue that the connection between the word and its meaning is formed in the same way as the connection between the stick and the banana. Is this not the same connection that we have discussed in our example? In the new psychology, as in the old, any possibility of explaining the unique relationships between word and meaning is excluded. There is no fundamental distinction between these relationships and other object relationships. In the twilight of universal structural relations, all cats are gray. As had earlier been the case in the twilight of universal associative connections, it is impossible to distinguish them.

Ach attempted to overcome the concept of associations by using the concept of the determining tendency. Gestalt psychology made the same attempt, relying on structural principles. In both cases, however, two basic features of the old theory were preserved. First, Ach and the Gestalt psychologists preserved the concept that the connections between word and meaning are fundamentally identical to the connections between other things. Second, they preserved the notion that the word—by its nature—does not develop. The concept that the development of word meaning is completed at the moment the word emerges is as basic to Gestalt psychology as it was for traditional psychology. This is why the succession of research traditions in psychology—while producing sharp advances in areas such as perception and memory—appear to be ceaselessly marking time or revolving in a circle in their treatment of the issue of thinking and speech. One principle is replaced by another and the new is in radical opposition to what has preceded it. In their understanding of the relationship between thinking and speech, however, the old and new are like identical twins. In the words of the French proverb, the more things change the more they stay the same.

In its theory of speech, the new psychology retains the thesis of the old; it preserves the concept that thought is independent of word. In its theory of thinking, however, it actually takes a significant step backward. First, Gestalt psychology tends to reject the notion that there are laws that are specific to thinking as such; it tends to merge the laws of thinking with general structural laws. The Wurzburg school raised thought to the rank of a purely mental act, leaving the word in the domain of unchanging sensory associations. As we said, this was its basic flaw. Nonetheless, the Wurzburg school was able to differentiate the laws that govern the coupling, movement, and flow of thoughts from the more elementary laws that govern representations and perceptions. This psychology was more advanced than Gestalt psychology in this respect. Reducing the domestic chicken's perception, the chimpanzee's intellectual operations, and the child's first meaningful word to a common structural denominator, Gestalt psychology has not only erased any boundary between the structure of the meaningful word and the structure of the stick and banana—it has erased the boundary between the highest forms of thinking and the most elementary perception.

If we summarize this modest critical outline of the basic contemporary theories of thinking and speech, we find two basic theses inherent to them. First, none of these theories has grasped what is most basic and central to the psychological nature of the word; none has grasped what makes the word a word and without which it would no longer be one. All have overlooked the generalization that is inherent in the word, this unique mode of reflecting reality in consciousness. Second, these theories consistently analyze the word and its meaning in isolation from development. These two points are internally linked. Only an adequate conception of the word's mental nature can lead us to an understanding of the possibilities that exist for the development of the word and its meaning. These features are preserved at each stage in this sequence of research traditions, To this extent, they merely repeat one another. Thus, the conflicts among the various research traditions in the contemporary psychology of thinking and speech are reminiscent of Heine's humorous poem where he tells of the reign of the old and venerable Template (Schablon) who was killed by a dagger raised against him:

> *When they had finished with the coronation,*
> *The new heir to kingdom and throne*
> *Seemed to those who called him New Template*
> *Like the Old Template they'd already known.*

## 2

The discovery of the changeable nature of word meanings and their development is the key to liberating the theory of thinking and speech from the dead end where it currently finds itself, Word meaning is inconstant. It changes during the child's development and with different modes of the functioning of thought. It is not a static but a dynamic formation. To establish the changeable nature of meaning, we must begin by defining it correctly. The nature of meaning is revealed in generalization. The basic and central feature of any word is generalization. All words generalize.

It is important to emphasize, however, that the fact that the internal nature of word meaning changes implies that the relationship of thought to word changes as well. To understand the changeable and dynamic relationship of thought to word, we need to take a cross-section of the genetic scheme of changes in meaning that we developed in our basic research. We need to clarify *the functional role of verbal meaning in the act of thinking.*

We have not yet had the opportunity to consider the process of verbal thinking as a whole. However, we have brought together all the information necessary to outline the basic features of this process. At this point, we will attempt to outline the complex structure of the actual process of thinking, the complex movement from the first vague emergence of a thought to its completion in a verbal formulation. For this purpose, we must move from a genetic to a functional plane of analysis. That is, we must now analyze not the development of meanings and their structure, but the process through which *meanings function in the living process* of *verbal thinking.* If we succeed in this, we will have shown that with each stage in development there exists not only a specific structure of verbal meaning, but a special relationship between thinking and speech that defines this structure. Functional problems are resolved most easily when we are studying the higher, developed forms of some activity, where the whole complexity of the functional structure appears in a well articulated, mature form. Therefore, we will consider issues of development only briefly, turning then to the study of the relationships of thought to word in the development of consciousness.

When we attempt to realize this goal, a grand and extraordinarily complex picture emerges before us, a picture that surpasses in subtlety the architectonics of researchers' richest expressions. In the words of Tolstoy, "the relationship of word to thought and the formation of new concepts is the most complex, mysterious, and delicate process of the spirit" (1903, p. 143).

Before moving on to a schematic description of this process, we will state our leading concept. This central idea—a concept we will develop and clarify in the following discussion—can be expressed in the following general formula: The relationship of thought to word is not a thing but a process, a movement from thought to word and from word to thought. Psychological analysis indicates that this relationship is a developing process which changes as it passes through a series of stages. Of course, this is not an age related development but a functional development. The movement of thinking from thought to word is a developmental process. Thought is not expressed but completed in the word. We can, therefore, speak of the establishment (i.e., the unity of being and nonbeing) of thought in the word. Any thought strives to unify, to establish a relationship between one thing and another. Any thought has movement. It unfolds. It fulfills some function or resolves some task. This flow of thought is realized as an internal movement through several planes, as a transition from thought to word and from word to thought. Thus, the first task in an analysis of the relationship of thought and word as a movement from thought to word is to analyze the phases that compose this movement, to differentiate the planes through which thought passes as it becomes embodied in the word. To paraphrase Shakespeare, much opens up before us here of which "even wise men have not dreamed."

Our analysis leads first to the differentiation of two planes of speech, Though they form a unity, the inner, meaningful, semantic aspect of speech is associated with different laws of movement than its external, auditory aspect. The unity of speech is complex, not homogeneous. This differentiation in the movement of the semantic and sound aspects of speech is reflected in several factors related to the ontogenesis of speech development. In the present context, we will note only two major factors.

First, we know that the development of the external aspect of speech in the child begins with the initial single word utterance and moves to the coupling of two or three words, then to the simple phrase and the coupling of phrases, and still later to the complex sentence and connected speech composed of a series of complex sentences. Thus, in mastering the external aspect of speech, the child moves from the part to the whole. In its meaning, however, we know that the child's first word is not a one word sentence but a whole phrase. Thus, in the development of the semantic aspect of speech, the child begins with the whole—with the sentence—and only later moves to the mastery of particular units of meaning, to the mastery of the meanings of separate words. The child begins with the whole and only subsequently partitions its fused thought which is expressed in the one word sentence into a series of separate though interconnected verbal meanings. Thus, the development of the semantic and external aspects of speech move in opposite directions. The semantic aspect of speech develops from the whole to the part or from the sentence to the word. The external aspect of speech moves from the part to the whole or from the word to the sentence.

This alone is sufficient to demonstrate the necessity of distinguishing the development of the meaningful and the external aspects of speech. Movement along these two planes does not coincide; it does not merge into a single line. As this example indicates, it can follow lines that move in opposite directions. Of course, this does not imply a rupture in the relationship between these two planes of speech. It does not imply that they are autonomous to one another. On the contrary, the differentiation of these two planes is a first and a necessary step in establishing their internal unity. This unity presupposes that each of these two aspects of speech has its own movement and that the relationships between these movements are complex. We can analyze the relationships underlying the unity of speech only after we have differentiated the aspects of speech among which these complex relationships exist. If both these aspects of speech appeared as one— if they coincided with one another and merged in a single line—we could not speak of their relationship, since it is impossible to have a relationship between a thing and itself. The internal unity of these two aspects of speech emerges no less clearly than their lack of correspondence. The child's thought emerges first in a fused, unpartitioned whole. It is for precisely this reason that it must be expressed in speech as a single word. It is as though the child selects the verbal garment to fit his thought. To the extent that the child's thought is partitioned and comes to be constructed of separate parts, his speech moves from parts to a partitioned whole. Correspondingly, to the extent that the child moves in his speech from parts to the partitioned whole of the sentence, he can move in his thought from an unpartitioned whole to parts.

Even at the outset, then, thought and word are not cut from a single mold. In a certain sense, one can say that we find more opposition than agreement between them. The structure of speech is not a simple mirror image of the structure of thought. It cannot, therefore, be placed on thought like clothes off a rack. Speech does not merely serve as the expression of developed thought. Thought is restructured as it is transformed into speech. It is not expressed but completed in the word. Therefore, precisely because of their contrasting directions of movement, the development of the internal and external aspects of speech form a true unity.

A second fact of no less importance characterizes a later phase of development. As we noted earlier, Piaget established that the child masters the complex structure of the subordinate clause (composed of conjunctions such as "because," "despite," "since," and "although") earlier than he masters the semantic structures that correspond with these syntactic forms. In other words, the child's grammar develops before his logic. Over the entire extent of the school age, the child uses conjunctions correctly and adequately in spontaneous speech in expressing causal, temporal, adversative, conditional, and other dependencies. He is not, however, consciously aware of the semantic aspect of these conjunctions nor is he able to use them voluntarily. Once again, then, the movements of the semantic and external aspects of the word in the mastery of complex syntactic structures do not coincide. Analysis of the word indicates, however, that this lack of correspondence does not exclude the unity of grammar and logic in the development of the child's speech. In fact, this lack of correspondence is fundamental to the internal unity of meaning and word that is expressed in complex logical relations.

This lack of correspondence between the semantic and external aspects of speech emerges less directly but even more clearly in the functioning of developed thought. To see this, we must shift our analysis from the genetic to the functional plane. First, however, it is important to note that the facts which have emerged in our discussion of the genesis of speech allow us to draw several important conclusions concerning the nature of functional relationships. We have seen that the development of the meaningful and external aspects of speech move in opposing directions during the entirety of the early childhood period. It is, therefore, no surprise that we would never find complete correspondence between them at any point in the developmental process.

A more striking set of facts can be taken directly from the functional analysis of speech, facts that are well known to psychologically oriented contemporary linguistics. Of many relevant facts, the most significant are those which indicate a lack of correspondence between the grammatical and the psychological subject and predicate.

Fasler argues that it is wrong to use a grammatical framework in interpreting the meaning of linguistic phenomena, since the psychological and grammatical articulation of speech do not always correspond. Uland[16] begins the prologue to "Herzog Ernst Shvabskii" with the words: "A severe spectacle opens up before you." Grammatically, "severe spectacle" is the subject of this sentence and "opens up" is the predicate. If we consider the psychological structure of the phrase, however, "opens up" is the subject and "severe spectacle" the predicate. The poet is trying to say here that what is going to occur before us is a tragedy. In the listener's consciousness, what is represented first is that he is going to observe a spectacle. This is what the phrase speaks about. It is the psychological subject of the phrase. What is new—what is said about this subject—is that the spectacle will be a tragedy. This, then, is the psychological predicate.

The following example clarifies this lack of correspondence between the grammatical and psychological subject and predicate still more clearly. Consider the phrase, "The clock fell." Here, the "clock" is the grammatical subject and "fell" the predicate. This phrase can be used in different situations and can express different thoughts while retaining this form.

Consider two situations. In the first, I notice that the clock has stopped and I ask why. I am told: "The clock fell." Here, the clock is in my consciousness initially. It is the psychological subject that is spoken about. The representation that it fell arises second. Here, "fell" is the psychological predicate. It is "fell" that says something about the subject. Here, there is

3. Thought and Word

correspondence between the grammatical and psychological partitioning of the phrase. However, this kind of correspondence is not inevitable.

Consider the following situation: I am working at my desk. I hear a noise from a falling object and ask what it was that fell. The same phrase is used to answer my question, but here it is the falling that is initially represented in consciousness. "Fell" is what is spoken about in this phrase; it is the psychological subject. The clock is what is said of this subject, what arises in consciousness second; it is the psychological predicate. This thought might better be expressed as follows: "What fell is the clock." In the first situation, the psychological and grammatical predicate correspond. In the second, they do not.

Any part of a complex phrase can become the psychological predicate and will carry the logical emphasis. The semantic function of this logical emphasis is the isolation of the psychological predicate. According to Paul[17], the grammatical category is to some extent a fossil of the psychological category. It therefore needs to be revived by a logical emphasis that clarifies its semantic structure. Paul demonstrates that a wide variety of meanings can reside in a single grammatical structure. Thus, correspondence between the grammatical and psychological structure of speech may be encountered less frequently than we generally assume. Indeed, it may merely be postulated and rarely if ever realized in fact. In phonetics, morphology, vocabulary, and semantics—even in rhythm, metrics, and music—the psychological category lies hidden behind the grammatical or formal category. If the two appear to correspond with one another in one situation, they diverge again in others. We can speak not only of the psychological elements of form and meaning, not only of the psychological subject and predicate, but of psychological number, gender, case, pronouns, superlatives, and tenses. Thus, what is a mistake from the perspective of language may have artistic value if it has an original source. Consider Pushkin's poem:

> Like rosy lips without a smile, I would not love Russian speech,
> Without grammatical errors.

This has a more profound meaning than is generally assumed. Only in mathematics do we find a complete elimination of incongruities in the use of common and unquestionably correct expressions. It appears that it was Descartes who first saw in mathematics a form of thinking that has it origins in language but has nonetheless surpassed it. We can say only one thing: In its oscillation and in the incongruity of the grammatical and the psychological our normal conversational language is in a state of dynamic equilibrium between the ideals of mathematics and the harmony of imagination. It is in the state of continuous movement that we call evolution.

These examples demonstrate the lack of correspondence between the external and the semantic aspects of speech. At the same time, however, they show that this does not exclude their unity. On the contrary, it presupposes such a unity. This lack of correspondence does not interfere with the realization of thought in the word. Indeed, it is necessary for the movement from thought to word.

To clarify this internal dependency between the two planes of speech, we will give two examples of how changes in the formal and grammatical structure of speech lead to profound changes in its sense. Krylov, in the fable, "The Dragonfly and the Ant," substituted the dragonfly for La Fontaine's grasshopper while retaining the inapplicable epithet "the jumper." In

French, the word grasshopper is feminine. It is, therefore, well suited to embody the image of a carefree attitude and feminine lightheadedness. In Russian—because the grammatical gender of "grasshopper" is masculine—this nuance of meaning critical to the illustration of frivolity would have disappeared had the fable been translated literally. Therefore, Krylov took grammatical gender over actual meaning—substituting the dragonfly for the grasshopper—while preserving characteristics of the grasshopper such as jumping and singing that are clearly not characteristic of the dragonfly. Thus, to adequately translate the sense of the tale, the feminine grammatical gender had to be preserved.

We find something similar in the Russian translation of Heine's poem, "The Fir and the Palm." In German, "fir" is masculine in gender. Thus, in German, the poem symbolizes love for women. To preserve the sense of the German text, Tiutchev substituted a cedar for the fir, since in Russian "cedar" is masculine. In contrast, by translating the poem literally, Lermontov lost this sense. As a consequence, his translation gives the poem a fundamentally different sense, one that is more abstract and generalized. Thus, a change in a single, seemingly insignificant, grammatical detail can lead to a change in the whole meaningful aspect of speech.

We can summarize what we have learned from this analysis of the two planes of speech in the following way. First, these two planes do not correspond. There is a second, inner, plane of speech standing beyond words. The independence of this grammar of thought, of this syntax of verbal meanings, forces us to see—even in the simplest of verbal expressions—a relationship between the meaningful and the external aspects of speech that is not given once and forever, a relationship that is not constant or static. What we do see is movement. We see a continuous transition from the syntax of meanings to the grammar of words, a transformation of sense structure as it is embodied in words.

Obviously, if the external and the semantic aspects of speech do not correspond, the verbal expression cannot emerge directly in its fully developed form. As we have seen, the semantic and the verbal syntax arise neither simultaneously nor together. Transition and movement from one to the other is inherent in the process. Moreover, this complex process involved in the transition from meanings to sounds itself develops. This development constitutes an important aspect of the development of verbal thinking. The partitioning of speech into semantics and phonology is not given at the outset. It arises in the course of development. The child must differentiate these two aspects of speech. He must become consciously aware of the different nature of each to permit the gradual descension that is presupposed in the living process of meaningful speech. In the child, we initially find a lack of conscious awareness of verbal forms and verbal meanings. The two are not differentiated. The word and its sound structure are perceived as a part or characteristic of the thing. They are not differentiated from its other characteristics. This phenomenon appears to be inherent in any primitive linguistic consciousness.

Humboldt[18] relates an anecdote about a peasant who was listening to student astronomers as they were discussing the stars. At one point, the peasant turned to the students and said: "I understand that people have measured the distance from the Earth to the most distant stars with these instruments, that they have identified their distribution and movement. What I want to know is how they learned their names." Here, the peasant has assumed that the names of the stars can only be learned from the stars themselves. Simple experiments with children have shown that children explain the names of objects by referring to their characteristics even in the preschool age: "A cow is called 'cow' because it has horns, a calf 'calf' because his horns are still small, a horse 'horse' because it has no horns, a dog 'dog' because it has no horns and is small, and an automobile 'automobile' because it is not alive at all." When asked if one could substitute the name of one object for another (e.g., calling a cow "ink" and ink 'cow') children answer that this is impossible because you write with ink and a cow gives milk. The characteristics of the thing are so closely connected with its name that to transfer the name means to transfer the characteristics.

The difficulty the child has in transferring the name of one thing to another becomes apparent in experiments where the child is asked to establish temporary names for objects. In one experiment, the names of "cow and dog" and those of "window and ink" were interchanged. The child was asked: "If the dog has horns, does the dog give milk?" The child answered: "It'll give." The child was then asked: "Does a cow have horns?" The child answered: "It has." The experimenter responded: "Cow—that is a dog. Does a dog really have horns?" The child answered: "Of course. Here the dog is a cow. If it is called a cow there must be horns. With the kind of dog that is called a cow there must be little horns." Here, we can see how difficult it is for the child to distinguish the name of the thing from its characteristics. We can see how its characteristics follow the name in the way that property follows its owner. Similar results emerged with questions about the characteristics of ink and window when their names were exchanged. Though with great difficulty, correct answers were initially given to questions. However, we received a negative answer to the question of whether ink is transparent. The experimenter responded: "But 'ink' is 'window' and 'window' is 'ink.'" The child countered: "It doesn't matter. Ink is ink and non-transparent."

This example illustrates the thesis that the *auditory aspect of the word is an immediate unity* for the child, that it is undifferentiated and lacking in conscious awareness. One extremely important line of speech development in the child is the *differentiation of this unity and emergence of conscious awareness of it*. Thus, in early development we have a merging of the two planes of speech. With age, there is gradual differentiation. The distance between the two planes increases. To each stage in the development of verbal meaning and the emergence of conscious awareness of these two planes, there corresponds a specific relationship of the semantic and external aspects of speech and a specific path from meaning to sound. The inadequate differentiation of these planes of speech in the earlier ages is linked with a limited potential for expressing and comprehending thought.

If we consider what we said at the outset about the communicative function of meanings, it becomes clear that the child's social interaction through speech is immediately linked with his differentiation and conscious awareness of verbal meanings. To clarify this thought, we must consider an extremely important characteristic of word meanings that we discussed in the analysis of our experimental findings. In our analysis of the word's semantic structure, we distinguished between its object relatedness and its meaning. We tried to show that the two do not coincide. In functional terms, this caused us to differentiate the word's indicative and nominative function from its signifying function. If we compare these structural and functional relationships in the initial, middle, and end points of development, the following genetic sequence becomes apparent. Initially, we have only object relatedness in the structure of the word. The word's function is exclusively indicative and nominative. Meaning independent of object relatedness, signification independent of the indication and naming of the object, arises later, developing along the path that we attempted to outline earlier.

This makes it apparent that from the moment these structural and functional characteristics of the word emerge in the child they diverge from the characteristics of the word in both its opposing aspects. On the one hand, the word's object relatedness is expressed more clearly and more strongly in the child than in the adult. For the child, the word is part of the thing. It is one of the characteristics of the thing. Thus, the child's word is much more closely connected with the object than the adult's. This underlies the much greater relative weight of object relatedness in the word of the child. On the other hand, precisely because the word is connected more closely with the object for the child—precisely because it is a part of the thing— it can more easily be isolated from the object than can the adult's word. It can more easily take an independent place in thought, more easily live an independent life. In this way, the insufficient differentiation of object relatedness and word meaning in the child leads to a situation where the child's word is simultaneously closer to reality and further from it than the adult's. The child does not initially differentiate between word meaning and the object nor between the meaning and the sound form of the word. In development, this differentiation occurs in accordance with the development of generalization. It is only with the completion of the developmental process—at the point where we find true concepts—that the complex relationships between the partitioned planes of speech first arise.

This ontogenetic differentiation of the two speech planes is accompanied by the development of the path that thought follows in the transformation of the syntax of meanings into the syntax of words. Thought imprints a logical emphasis on one word in a phrase, isolating the psychological predicate. Without this, no phrase would be comprehensible. Speaking requires a transition from the internal to the external plane. Understanding presupposes movement in the reverse direction, from the external plane of speech to the internal.

## 3

We must take an additional step to penetrate the internal aspect of speech more deeply. The semantic plane is only the first of the internal planes of speech. Beyond it lies the plane of inner speech. Without a correct understanding of the psychological nature of inner speech, we cannot clarify the actual complex relationships between thought and word.

There has been more confusion in attempts to address this problem than with any of the other issues associated with the theory of thinking and speech. Much of this confusion has its source in a lack of terminological clarity. The term "inner speech" or "endophasia" is used in the literature to refer to a wide variety of phenomena. This has led to a great deal of misunderstanding, with researchers often arguing about very different things that are designated by a single term. Until some terminological clarity *is introduced,* it will be impossible to systematize our knowledge of the nature of inner speech. It is because this work has not yet been done that there currently exists no systematic presentation of even the simplest empirical data on this problem.

Initially, it appears that the term "inner speech" referred to verbal memory. I can learn a poem by heart and reproduce it only in memory. Like any object, the word can be replaced by a mental representation or image in memory. Within this framework, inner speech differs from external speech in the same way that a representation of an object differs from the object itself. It is in precisely this sense that inner speech was understood by French scholars in their studies of the memory images through which this reproduction of the word is realized (i.e., autistic, optical, motoric, or synthetic images). Of course, memory is one feature that defines the nature of inner speech. However, memory alone does not exhaust the content of this concept. It does not even correspond with it directly. The older scholars consistently equate the reproduction of the word through memory with inner speech. However, these are two different processes that must be carefully distinguished.

The second meaning commonly attributed to the term "inner speech" implies an abbreviation of the normal speech act. Here, inner speech is called unpronounced, silent, or mute speech. In accordance with Miller's well known definition, it is speech minus sound. According to Watson, inner speech is precisely the same as external speech with the exception that it is not completed. Bekhterev[19] similarly defined inner speech as a speech reflex where the motor component is not manifested. Sechenov[20] defined it as a reflex that is cut off when two thirds of its course is completed. Recently, Shilling has proposed the term "speaking" [govorenie], using this term to designate the concept of inner speech that is shared by the authors we have just mentioned. This concept differs from inner speech qualitatively in that it incorporates only the active, not the passive, processes of speech activity. It differs qualitatively from inner speech in that it refers to the initial motor activity of the speech function. From this perspective, inner speaking is only part of the function of inner speech. It is a speech motor act of an initial character, an impulse that is not completely expressed in articulatory movements or one that is manifested in movements that are silently and unclearly expressed but nonetheless accompany, reinforce, or hinder the thinking function. These ideas identify a feature basic to a scientific concept of inner speech. Once again, however, this conception does not exhaust the concept inner speech nor even correspond with it entirely.

The third and most diffuse of all conceptions of inner speech reflects an extremely broad interpretation of the concept. For example, Kurt Goldstein[21] uses the phrase to refer to all that precedes the motor act of speaking, the entire internal aspect of speech itself. He breaks this down into two components. The first is the linguist's inner speech form or Wundt's speech motive. The second is an experience specific to speech. It is an experience that is neither sensory nor motor in nature and is well known to all—though it defies precise characterization. Thus, uniting the entire internal aspect of speech activity in the concept of inner speech—fusing the French scholars' conception of inner speech with the German word-concept—Goldstein places inner speech at the center the whole speech process. This conception of inner speech correctly addresses the negative aspect of the phenomenon's definition. Sensory and motor processes do indeed have a subordinate significance in inner speech. However, the positive aspect of Goldstein's definition of inner speech is extremely confused and, consequently, false. The center of the entire speech process cannot be identified with an experience consecrated only in intuition, an experience that is not submitted to any objective analysis—whether functional or structural. It is equally wrong to identify this experience with inner speech. The identification of inner speech with this experience dissolves the structural planes that have been distinguished through psychological analysis. In fact, precisely because this speech experience is common to all forms of speech activity it is useless as a means of isolating inner speech as a unique speech function. If we take Goldstein's perspective to its conclusion, we find that inner speech is not speech but thought and affective-volitional activity. It includes speech motives as well as the thought that is expressed in the word. What this concept actually refers to are all the internal processes that occur before the act of speaking, that is, the entire internal aspect of external speech.

If we are to understand this phenomenon, we must begin with the thesis that *inner speech is a psychological formation that has its own unique nature,* the thesis that inner speech is a unique form of speech activity that has unique characteristics and stands in complex relationships to other speech forms. To study the relationships of inner speech to thought and to the word, we must identify what distinguishes inner speech from thought and word. We must clarify its unique function.

In our view, it is important in this connection that in one case I am speaking to myself and in the other to another. Inner speech is speech for oneself. External speech is speech for others. This is a fundamental functional difference in the two types of speech that will have inevitable structural consequences. In our view, then, it is incorrect to view the difference between inner and external speech as one of degree rather than of kind (as Jackson and Head, among others, have done). The presence or absence of vocalization is not a cause that explains the nature of inner speech. It is the consequence of its nature.

Inner speech is not merely what precedes or reproduces external speech. Indeed, in a sense, it is the opposite of external speech. External speech is a process of transforming thought into word; it is the materialization and objectivization of thought. Inner speech moves in the reverse direction, from without to within. It is a process that involves the evaporation of speech in thought.* This is the source of the structure of inner speech, the source of all that structurally differentiates it from external speech. Inner speech is among the most difficult domains of psychological research. As a consequence, most theories of inner speech are arbitrary and speculative constructions based on little empirical data. The experiment has been used primarily as a demonstration or illustration. Research has centered on attempts to identify subtle shifts in articulation and respiration, factors that are at best three stages removed from the phenomenon of inner speech. This problem has remained almost inaccessible to the experiment because genetic methods have not be utilized. Development is the key to understanding this extremely complex internal function of human consciousness. By identifying an adequate method for investigating inner speech, we can move the entire problem from its current stalemate. The first issue we must address, then, is that of method.

Piaget was apparently the first to recognize the special function of egocentric speech in the child and to understand its theoretical significance. Egocentric speech is a common phenomenon in the child, one familiar to all who deal with children. Piaget did not overlook its significance. He attempted to study it and interpret it theoretically. However, he remained entirely blind to the most important characteristics of egocentric speech, that is, to its genetic origins and its connections with

---

* It is apparent from the context that in using the expression "the evaporation of speech in thought," Vygotsky is referring to a qualitative change in the speech process with the act of thought, not to the disappearance of the word. Editors' note.

inner speech. As a consequence, his interpretation of its nature was false in functional, structural, and genetic terms.

Using Piaget as a point of departure, our research has focused on the relationship between egocentric and inner speech. As a consequence, we have identified a means for studying inner speech experimentally.

Earlier, we outlined the basic considerations that caused us to conclude that *egocentric speech passes through a several stages that precede the development of inner speech.* These considerations can be classed in three groups. First, in functional terms, we found that egocentric speech fulfills an intellectual function similar to that of inner speech. Second, we found that the structure of egocentric speech is similar to that of inner speech. Third, in our genetic analysis, we combined Piaget's observation that egocentric speech atrophies in the school-age child with several facts that forced us to associate this event with the initial development of inner speech. This led to the conclusion that as egocentric speech atrophies it is transformed into inner speech. This new working hypothesis concerning the structure, function, and ontogenetic fate of egocentric speech facilitated a radical restructuring of our entire theory of the phenomenon. More importantly, however, this new hypothesis provided an access route to the problem of the nature of inner speech. If our proposal that egocentric speech is an early form of inner speech is verified, the problem of finding a method of studying inner speech is resolved.

This implies that egocentric speech is the key to the study of inner speech. Egocentric speech is still vocal and audible. Though internal in function and structure, egocentric speech is external in manifestation. In any investigation of a complex internal process, we must externalize that process to allow experimentation; we must connect it to some form of external activity. This permits an objective functional analysis based on observable external aspects of the internal process. With egocentric speech, we have what might be called a natural experiment. *Egocentric speech—a process internal in nature but external in manifestation—is accessible to direct observation and experimentation.* Thus, the study of egocentric speech is the method of choice for the study of inner speech.

The second advantage of this method is that it allows us to study egocentric speech dynamically in *the process of its development.* It allows us to study the gradual disappearance of certain characteristics and the gradual development of others. This provides us with the potential for understanding the trends characteristic of the development of inner speech. By analyzing what drops out in the developmental process, we can identify what is inessential to inner speech. Correspondingly, by analyzing what tends to be strengthened, what emerges more and more clearly in the developmental process, we can identify what is essential to it. Relying on methods of interpolation, we can follow the development from egocentric to inner speech and draw conclusions concerning the nature of inner speech itself.

Before we discuss the results we have obtained by using this method, we must first clarify its theoretical foundation by outlining our general conception of egocentric speech. We will begin by contrasting Piaget's theory of egocentric speech with our own.

According to Piaget, the child's egocentric speech is a direct expression of the egocentrism of his thought. In turn, the child's egocentrism is a compromise between the initial autism of the child's thinking and its gradual socialization. This compromise differs with each stage in the child's development. It is a dynamic compromise. As the child develops, the elements of autism decrease while those of socialized thought increase. The result is that egocentrism in both thinking and speech is gradually reduced to nothing.

Piaget's view of the structure, function, and fate of egocentric speech flows directly from this understanding of its nature. In egocentric speech, the child need not accommodate himself to adult thought. As a consequence, his thought remains maximally egocentric. This is reflected in the incomprehensible nature of egocentric speech, in its abbreviation, and in several other structural characteristics. Functionally, egocentric speech does nothing more than accompany the basic melody of the child's activity, changing nothing in the melody itself. It has no independent functional significance. Because it is simply the expression of the child's egocentrism—a phenomenon that is doomed to atrophy in the course of the child's development—the genetic fate of egocentric speech is to disappear along with the egocentrism of the child's thought. Thus, the development of egocentric speech follows a falling curve. The apex of this curve lies at the beginning of the developmental process and drops to nothing at the threshold of the school age.

Thus, we can say of egocentric speech what Liszt said of the child prodigy: Its whole future lies in its past. Egocentric speech has no future. It does not arise and develop with the child; it simply atrophies. With egocentric speech, change is not an evolutionary but an involutionary process. At any stage of the child's development, this speech reflects the insufficient socialization of speech, the insufficient socialization of a speech that is initially individual in nature. Egocentric speech is the direct expression of the inadequate and incomplete socialization of speech.

In contrast, our own theory suggests that the child's egocentric speech is one aspect of the general transition from inter-mental functions to intra-mental functions, one aspect of the transition from the child's social, collective activity to his individual mental functions. As we have shown in one of our earlier works,* this transition constitutes the general law of the development of all higher mental functions. Initially, these functions arise as forms of cooperative activity. Only later are they transformed by the child into the sphere of his own mental activity. Speech for oneself has its source in a differentiation of an initially social speech function, a *differentiation* of speech for others. Thus, the central tendency of the child's development is not a gradual socialization introduced from the outside, but a gradual individualization that emerges on the foundation of the child's internal socialization.

This changes our perspective on the structure, function, and fate of egocentric speech. Having received a new assignment, speech is naturally reconstructed and takes on a new structure that corresponds with its new functions. We will consider the structural characteristics of inner speech in more detail later. At this point, we would only emphasize that these characteristics do not atrophy. They are not smoothed away and reduced to nothing. They are strengthened and grow. They evolve and develop in correspondence with the child's age. Like egocentric speech as a whole, they follow a rising not a falling curve.

Our experiments make it clear that the function of egocentric speech is closely related to the function of inner speech. It is not an accompaniment of the child's activity. It is an

---

*    Here, Vygotsky is referring to "The Development of the Higher Mental Functions." See Section IV. Editors' note.

independent melody or function that facilitates intellectual orientation, conscious awareness, the overcoming of difficulties and impediments, and imagination and thinking. It is speech for oneself, a speech function that intimately serves the child's thinking. The genetic fate of egocentric speech is much different from that depicted by Piaget. Egocentric speech develops along not a falling but a rising curve. Its development is not an involution but a true evolution. It has no relationship to the processes of involution so well known to biology or pediatrics, to processes such as the healing and shedding of the umbilical cord or the obliteration of Botallov's channel and the umbilical veins in the newborn. It is more comparable to processes of the child's development that are directed forward, processes that are by nature constructive and creative and have an entirely positive significance for development. Our hypothesis suggests that egocentric speech is speech that is internal in its mental function and external in its structure. It is fated to develop into inner speech.

This hypothesis has several advantages over Piaget's. It allows a more adequate explanation of the structure, function, and fate of egocentric speech. It is in closer agreement with the experimental data we obtained which indicate that the coefficient of egocentric speech increases with the introduction of difficulties that require conscious awareness and reflection. These facts are not explained by Piaget.

The decisive advantage of our hypothesis, however, is that it explains an important and pervasive characteristic of the development of egocentric speech that is paradoxical and inexplicable from Piaget's perspective. According to Piaget's theory, egocentric speech atrophies as the child gets older. Its quantitative significance decreases in accordance with the level of the child's development. This perspective would cause us to anticipate that the unique structural characteristics of egocentric speech would become less and less prominent as egocentric speech disappears. It is difficult to imagine that the process through which egocentric speech gradually atrophies would be reflected in the quantity of egocentric speech but not in its internal structure. If the structural characteristics of egocentric speech are rooted in the child's egocentrism, one would expect that they would fade into the background as the child's egocentrism atrophies. That is, one would expect that the structural characteristics of egocentric speech—characteristics expressed primarily in its incomprehensibility for others—would gradually disappear entirely along with egocentric speech itself. The internal structure of egocentric speech should become increasingly similar to that of socialized speech. It should become increasingly comprehensible.

What do we find when we look at the empirical data? Is the three year old's egocentric speech in fact less comprehensible than that of the seven year old? Among the most important and decisive empirical findings of our research is that the structural characteristics of egocentric speech that differentiate it from social speech—the characteristics that make it incomprehensible to others—increase rather than decrease with age. At three years of age, the differences between egocentric and social speech are minimal. They reach their peak at seven years of age. Thus, these characteristics do not atrophy but evolve, reversing the pattern that characterizes the coefficient of egocentric speech. While the latter steadily decreases, dropping to nothing at the threshold of the school age, the structural characteristics of egocentric speech continue to develop in the opposite direction. That which is unique to egocentric speech increases from almost nothing at three years of age to nearly one hundred percent.

Piaget's theory cannot explain how this atrophy of childhood egocentrism and egocentric speech can be associated with the rapid development of the characteristics that distinguish egocentric speech from social speech. Our own hypothesis allows us to reconcile these facts. Moreover, it helps us understand why the coefficient of egocentric speech decreases as the child develops, that is, it helps explain the phenomenon that provided the foundation on which Piaget constructed his entire theory of egocentric speech.

What is the fundamental significance of the finding that the coefficient of egocentric speech decreases as the age of the child increases? As we have seen, the structural characteristics of inner speech and its functional differentiation from external speech increase with age. Only one characteristic of egocentric speech fades away—its vocalization. Does this fading of vocalization indicate that the whole of egocentric speech atrophies? Such an assumption leaves the development of the structural and functional characteristics of egocentric speech entirely unexplained. The reduction of the coefficient of egocentric speech becomes fully comprehensible and meaningful, however, if we consider it in the context of the development of the other characteristics of egocentric speech. In fact, the contradiction between the rapid disappearance of one symptom of egocentric speech (i.e., its vocalization) and the equally rapid strengthening of its other symptoms (i.e., its structural and functional differentiation) is only apparent.

Our data indicate that the structural and functional characteristics of egocentric speech develop along with the development of the child. At three years of age, there is little difference between egocentric and communicative speech. By seven years of age, nearly all the functional and structural characteristics of egocentric speech differ from those of social speech. In our view, this finding indicates the progressive differentiation of the two speech functions, *the isolation of speech for oneself and speech for others from a general, undifferentiated speech function* that fulfills both these tasks in early childhood, There is no question about this. It is a fact, and it is widely known that it is difficult to argue with facts.

Once this is understood, related issues are immediately clarified. The structural and functional characteristics of egocentric speech—its internal structure and its mode of activity—develop and differentiate it from external speech. To the extent that these specific characteristics of egocentric speech develop, *its external, acoustic aspect will inevitably atrophy.* Its vocalization and external expression will become less prominent and, in the end, disappear. This in fact occurs, and is expressed in the drop in the coefficient of egocentric speech that has been observed between the ages of three and seven years. To the extent that the function of egocentric speech is differentiated from that of social speech, its vocalization becomes functionally superfluous and meaningless. We know our own phrase before we pronounce it. Moreover, to the extent that the structural characteristics of egocentric speech develop, vocalization becomes impossible. Speech for oneself is very different in its structure from speech for others. It simply cannot be expressed in the foreign structure of external speech. This structurally unique form of speech *must have a special form of expression;* its structure and organization has ceased to correspond with that of external speech. The development of the functional characteristics of egocentric speech, its isolation as an independent speech function, and the gradual formation of its independent internal nature, inevitably lead to a situation where its external manifestations become impoverished, It is at this point that its vocal aspect is lost. At a certain moment in development, when speech for oneself is finally differentiated from speech for others, it must cease to be vocal speech. This creates the illusion that it disappears or atrophies entirely.

However, this is precisely an illusion. It is as much an error to view the drop in the coefficient of egocentric speech as a symptom of its disappearance as it would be to assume that the moment when the child stops using his fingers to count—the moment when he moves from counting aloud to counting in his mind—indicates that counting itself has disappeared. In both cases a systematic disappearance, a negative symptom of involution, masks an entirely positive content. As we have shown, the drop in the coefficient of egocentric speech—the fading of its vocalization—is closely linked with the internal development and differentiation of this new speech form. What appear to be negative, involutionary symptoms are in fact evolutionary symptoms indicating that development is moving forward. They are symptomatic *not of a process of atrophy but of the emergence of a new form of speech.*

Thus, the fading external manifestations of egocentric speech reflect its developing abstraction from the vocal aspect of speech, that is, from a feature that is fundamental to external speech. It is, then, simply one aspect of the broader progressive differentiation of egocentric from communicative speech. It is a sign of the child's developing capacities to think or represent words while not pronouncing them, to operate not with the word itself but with its image. The drop in the coefficient of egocentric speech has a clearly defined significance. It is part of the process where the development of the functional and structural characteristics of egocentric speech is realized. It is part of the development of egocentric speech toward inner speech. The fundamental difference between inner and external speech is the absence of vocalization in the former.

Inner speech is mute, silent speech. This is its basic distinction. It is precisely in this direction, in the gradual emergence of this distinction, that the evolution of egocentric speech occurs. Its vocalization fades. It becomes mute speech. This is inevitable, however, if egocentric speech is an early stage in the genesis of inner speech. That the disappearance of vocalization is a gradual process, that egocentric speech is differentiated from social speech in its function and structure before it is differentiated in its vocalization, is an extremely important fact. It indicates that the development of inner speech does not have its roots in the external weakening of the vocal aspect of speech; it does not move from speech to whisper and from whisper to mute speech. It indicates that the development of inner speech begins with its functional and structural differentiation from external speech, that it moves from external to egocentric speech, and then from egocentric to inner speech. This concept is the foundation of our hypothesis concerning the development of inner speech.

The contradiction is only apparent. The drop in the coefficient of egocentric speech is a symptom of the development of a basic characteristic of inner speech, its abstraction from the vocal aspect of speech. It is a symptom of the final differentiation of inner and external speech. Thus functional, structural, and genetic analysis—indeed all the data we have on the development of egocentric speech (including that of Piaget)—provide consistent support for a single idea, the idea that *egocentric speech develops in the direction of inner speech.* The development of egocentric speech can be understood only as a gradual and progressive growth of the basic distinguishing characteristics of inner speech.

In this, we see irrefutable support for the hypothesis that we have developed concerning the nature and origin of egocentric speech. Moreover, in our view, this proves that the study of egocentric speech provides the foundation for understanding inner speech. However, for our hypothetical proposal to be transformed into a theoretical certainty, we must find a critical experiment, an experiment that will resolve which of these two conceptions of egocentric speech and its development corresponds with reality. We will turn to this critical experiment.

Consider the theoretical problem this experiment must resolve. In Piaget's view, egocentric speech arises from the inadequate socialization of what is initially an individual form of speech. In our view, it arises from the inadequate individualization of an initially social speech, from the inadequate isolation and differentiation of egocentric from social speech. In the first case, egocentric speech is a point on a falling curve that culminates in its disappearance. Here, egocentric speech has nothing but a past. In the second case, egocentric speech is a point on a rising curve, the culmination of which lies in the future in inner speech. Here, egocentric speech has a future. In the first case, speech for oneself—inner speech—is introduced from the outside in the socialization process in accordance with the principle mentioned earlier through which the red water is forced out by the white. In the second case, speech for oneself arises from egocentric speech; it develops from within.

To decide which of these views is correct, we had to demonstrate experimentally the direction of the effects of two types of changes in the situation in which egocentric speech occurs, specifically, changes that weaken the social aspects of the situation and changes that reinforce them. The data we have introduced in support of our conception of egocentric speech up to this point—though of tremendous significance in our view—provide only indirect support for our conception. Their significance depends on one's general framework of interpretation. In contrast, this experiment can provide a direct answer to our central question. It is an *experimentum crucis.*

If the child's egocentric speech stems from the egocentrism and inadequate socialization of his thinking, then any weakening of the social aspects of the situation, any seclusion or liberation of the child from his links with the collective, any increase in his psychological isolation, any loss of psychological contact with other people—anything that liberates the child from the necessity of adapting to the thought of others and using socialized speech—should lead to a sharp increase in the coefficient of egocentric over socialized speech, This would create the most favorable conditions possible for the liberation and full manifestation of the child's inadequately socialized thought and speech. If, on the other hand, egocentric speech stems from the inadequate differentiation of speech for oneself from speech for others, if it flows from an inadequate individualization of what is initially a social form of speech, these changes in the situation will be reflected in a sharp reduction in egocentric speech.

This is the question that motivated our experiment. As a point of departure for the construction of this experiment, we selected features of egocentric speech identified by Piaget himself, As a consequence, there can be no question of their empirical relationship to the circle of phenomena we are studying.

Though Piaget did not attribute any theoretical significance to them—describing them merely as external features of egocentric speech—three characteristics of egocentric speech struck us from the outset:

1. The fact that egocentric speech is a collective monologue, that it accompanies the child's activity in the collective (i.e., in the presence of other children) but not when the child is by himself.
2. The fact (noted by Piaget) that this collective monologue is accompanied by an illusion of understanding. The child believes and assumes that the egocentric expressions that he addresses to no one are understood by those around him.
3. The fact that speech for oneself has the character of external speech, that it is similar to socialized speech. It is not pronounced in a whisper for oneself.

These three essential characteristics of egocentric speech cannot be accidental. Egocentric speech has not yet been adequately differentiated from social speech. This is true subjectively, from the child's perspective. The result is the illusion of understanding. It is also true objectively, in terms of the situation. The result is that egocentric speech has the characteristic of collective monologue. Finally, this is true with respect to form. The result is that egocentric speech is vocalized. This alone causes us to question the validity of the notion that the source of egocentric speech lies in inadequate socialization. On the contrary, these characteristics of egocentric speech indicate that socialization is too extensive, that there is an inadequate differentiation of speech for oneself from speech for others. Egocentric speech, speech for oneself, seems to emerge in the objective and subjective conditions characteristic of social speech, of speech for others.

Our evaluation of these three features of egocentric speech is not the product of our own assumptions. In fact, Grunbaum reached a similar conclusion on the basis of Piaget's data. Grunbaum argues that superficial observation will frequently indicate that the child is entirely immersed in himself. This false impression is a function of our expectation that the three year old will relate logically to those around him. Because a logical relationship to reality is in fact not typical of the child, we falsely assume that he lives immersed in his own thought and fantasy, that he has an egocentric set. When they are engaged in joint play, children between three and five years of age are frequently occupied only with themselves. Each speaks only to himself. If this talk is printed, it looks like conversation. Analysis indicates that it is a collective monologue where the participants do not listen or respond to one another. In reality, however, this prototype of the child's egocentric set demonstrates the social connectedness of the child's mind. The collective monologue does not represent an intentional isolation from the collective, an autism as that is defined by modern psychiatry, Indeed, it is symptomatic of the opposite mental structure. Even Piaget, who takes the child's egocentrism as the cornerstone of his whole theory of the child's mental characteristics, recognizes that children believe that they are speaking and listening to one another in the collective monologue. It is true, of course, that they do not attend to one another. This, however, reflects a shared assumption that the thoughts of each are the common property of all, even if these thoughts are expressed inadequately or remain entirely unexpressed.

Grunbaum argues that this demonstrates the inadequate differentiation of the child's individual mind from the social whole. However, the final resolution of this question cannot be found in a particular interpretation of these facts. A critical experiment is required. Our experiment involved the variation of the three characteristics of egocentric speech mentioned earlier:

its vocalization, the illusion of understanding, and the fact that it is collective monologue. To clarify the nature and origin of egocentric speech, we systematically strengthened and weakened each of these characteristics through variations introduced into the experimental setting.

*In the initial series* of experiments, we attempted to destroy the illusion that egocentric speech is understood by other children by placing our subjects either among children who were either deaf or spoke a different language. In other respects, the experimental situations were no different from those where the coefficient of egocentric speech had been measured earlier with the same subjects, situations similar to those in Piaget's experiments. The sole variable in the experiment was the illusion of understanding. In the original experimental situation this illusion had emerged naturally. In these new experiments it was carefully excluded. We found that when the illusion of understanding was excluded the coefficient of egocentric speech fell sharply. In the majority of cases it fell to nothing. In the remaining cases, it was reduced on the average by a factor of eight.

Thus, the illusion of understanding is not accidental. It is not a by-product, an appendage or an epiphenomenon of egocentric speech but is functionally connected with it. These results are paradoxical for Piaget's theory. The less psychological contact between the child and the children around him, the weaker the child's connection with the collective, the less the situation presents the child with demands for socialized speech and for adapting his thought to the thought of others, the more freely egocentrism should be manifested in the child's thinking and, consequently, in his speech. If the child's egocentric speech is actually a function of the inadequate socialization of his thought and speech, no other conclusion is possible. From this perspective, when we exclude the illusion of understanding we should find not an increase but a decrease in the coefficient of egocentric speech. Our hypothesis suggests the true source of egocentric speech is the inadequate individualization of speech for oneself, the failure to differentiate it from speech for others. These data indicate that egocentric speech cannot live and function in isolation from social speech. When we exclude the illusion of understanding—a critical psychological feature of social speech—egocentric speech atrophies.

*The second* series of critical experiments differed from the basic series on the variable of collective monologue. As in the first series of critical experiments, we initially measured the coefficient of egocentric speech in the basic situation where it appeared as collective monologue. We then transferred the child's activity to a situation where the potential for collective monologue was excluded. Specifically, we either placed the child with unfamiliar children (children with whom he did not enter conversation before, during, or after the experiment), placed him behind a table in the corner of a room in isolation from other children, or placed him in complete isolation. In each of these situations, the experimenter left midway through the experiment leaving the child alone. In general, the results of these experiments correspond with those of the first series. Excluding the collective monologue led to a sharp drop in the coefficient of egocentric speech, though the drop was generally less dramatic than in the first experiments. The mean relation of the coefficient of egocentric speech in the basic and second experiments was six to one. The various methods of excluding the collective monologue were associated with different levels of egocentric speech. However, the basic tendency toward a reduction was clearly manifested.

The argument we developed in our discussion of the first series of experiments can be repeated here. Obviously, collective monologue is not an accidental characteristic of egocentric speech. It is not a mere epiphenomenon. It has functional connections with egocentric speech. From the perspective of Piaget's hypothesis, this again presents a paradox. By excluding the collective, we should give full play to the manifestation of egocentric speech. If the source of egocentric speech for oneself actually lies in the inadequate socialization of the child's thinking and speech, the exclusion of the collective should lead to a rapid increase in the coefficient. If, on the other hand, the foundation of egocentric speech lies in the inadequate differentiation of speech for oneself from speech for others, the exclusion of the collective monologue should lead to a reduction in the coefficient.

*In the third and final series* of experiments, we focused on the vocalization of egocentric speech. After measuring the coefficient of egocentric speech in the basic situation, the child was transferred to a situation where the possibility for vocalization was restricted or excluded. Three arrangements were used. In the first, the child was seated in a large hall far from other children. In the second, an orchestra or some other loud noise was used to drown out the child's own voice as well as the voices of others. In the third, the child was forbidden to speak loudly. He was instructed to carry on conversation only quietly or in a soundless whisper. In each of these critical situations, we observed a drop in the coefficient of egocentric speech. The reduction in the coefficient was expressed in a somewhat more complex form that it had been in the second series of experiments. The relationship of the coefficient in the basic and critical experiments was five-and-four-tenths to one. The differences associated with the various modes of excluding or interfering with vocalization were even greater than in the second series. However, the basic pattern once again emerged clearly. When vocalization was excluded, there was a reduction in the coefficient of egocentric speech. Again, these data present a paradox for Piaget's hypothesis while providing direct support for our own.

These three series of experiments had a single goal. They focused on three phenomena that are associated with almost any expression of the child's egocentric speech; they focused on the illusion of understanding, the collective monologue, and vocalization. These three characteristics are shared by egocentric and social speech. In our experiments, we compared situations where these phenomenon were present and absent. We found that where these features were excluded, where we excluded the features of speech common to speech for oneself and speech for others, there was inevitably a reduction in egocentric speech.

This provides a basis for our claim that the child's egocentric speech is a special form of speech. It provides a foundation for our claim that egocentric speech is a form of speech that is being differentiated functionally and structurally from social speech, but has not yet been fully differentiated from it. Egocentric speech has not become fully differentiated from social speech, the womb where it steadily develops and matures.

Consider the following situation: I sit at a desk and converse with a person who is behind me, a person whom I do not see. Unnoticed, this person leaves the room. However, I continue to speak guided by the illusion that I am heard and understood, Here, my speech is externally reminiscent of egocentric speech (i.e., speech in private and for oneself). Psychologically, however, it is social speech.

Compare this to the child's egocentric speech. Piaget assumes that the psychological nature of the child's egocentric speech is the opposite of that in our illustration. From the perspective of the child (i.e., psychologically and subjectively) his speech is egocentric; it is speech for himself. Only in its external manifestation is it social speech. Thus, its social character is an illusion, just as in the illustration the egocentric character of my speech is an illusion.

Our hypothesis suggests that the situation is much more complex. Functionally and structurally, the child's speech is egocentric. It is a special and independent form of speech. The special and independent nature of this form of speech has not, however, developed fully. It has not attained conscious awareness as inner speech either subjectively or psychologically. The child has not yet isolated it from speech for others. Objectively, this speech function has been differentiated from social speech. However, this process has not been completed. Thus, this speech continues to function only in situations where social speech is possible. If we consider both subjective and objective criteria, then, egocentric speech is a mixed speech form, a speech form that emerges in the transition from speech for others to speech for oneself. This constitutes the basic law of the development of inner speech. Speech for oneself (i.e., inner speech) becomes more internal in its function and structure—in its psychological nature—than in the external forms through which it is manifested.

This provides the empirical foundation required for the thesis we have advanced. The key to the investigation of the psychological nature of inner speech lies in the investigation of egocentric speech, in the analysis of the development of the characteristics fundamental to its function and structure. We can turn, then, to the basic results of our investigation, to a brief characterization of the third plane in the movement from thought to word, to the plane of inner speech.

4

Studying the development of inner speech in the child's egocentric speech has convinced us that the former is not speech minus sound but a speech function that is unique in its structure and function. Correspondingly, it has an entirely different organization than external speech. It has its own syntax. One characteristic of egocentric speech that manifests a clear developmental tendency is its fragmentation and abbreviation.

This observation is not new. All who have carefully studied inner speech have recognized that this fragmentation and abbreviation is its central feature. Even those such as Watson who have studied it from a behaviorist perspective have recognized this fact. Inner speech has been seen as a mirror image of external speech only by those who reduce it to the reproduction of external speech in memory. As far as we know, however, no one has gone beyond the descriptive study of this characteristic. Indeed, a systematic descriptive analysis has not been completed. There are many phenomena associated with inner speech that find their expression in its fragmentary and abbreviated nature, Previous analyses have left these phenomena tangled in a single confused knot.

Through genetic analysis, we have attempted to partition the separate phenomena that characterize inner speech from this confused tangle and clarify their respective causes and explanations. Watson argued that this characteristic of silent speaking or thinking had its roots in the phenomenon of short circuiting common to habit development generally, He argued that even if we could record these hidden internal processes, their abbreviations, short circuits, and economies would make them unrecognizable unless we followed their genetic development from beginning to end, that is, from the point where they are complete and social in character to the point where they serve not social but individual adaptation.

Differing only in that it develops before our eyes, an analogous phenomenon can be observed in the development of the child's egocentric speech, a developmental process that culminates on the threshold of the school age as egocentric speech begins to approximate inner speech. As Piaget noted, if you do not know the situation where it arises, egocentric speech is abbreviated and incomprehensible. Studies on the dynamics of this development leave no doubt that if it were extended further it would lead to the complete incomprehensibility and abbreviation characteristic of inner speech. Thus, by studying the development of egocentric speech we can trace the gradual development of these features of inner speech, creating the possibility of isolating them from one another and explaining them.

If we take abbreviation as the first independent phenomenon, a genetic analysis shows us directly how and why it arises. As egocentric speech develops, it does not manifest a simple tendency toward abbreviation or the omission of words, a simple transition toward a telegraphic style. On the contrary, it manifests a tendency toward a form of abbreviation where the predicate and related words are preserved while the subject is omitted. This tendency toward a predicative syntax in inner speech was manifested in all our experiments. With almost no exceptions, its development is extremely regular. Interpolating, we can assume that the syntactic form of inner speech is that of pure and absolute predicativity.

To help us understand how and why this feature of the syntax of inner speech develops, we will consider the kinds of situations where it is manifested in external speech. A purely predicative syntax is manifested in external speech in two basic situations, either where a question is being answered or where the subject of the discussion is known to both the interlocutors. First, no one would answer the question, "Do you want a glass of tea?" with the fully expanded phrase: "No, I do not want a glass of tea." Again, no one would answer the question, "Has your brother read this book?" by saying: "Yes, my brother read that book." In both cases, the answer would be purely predicative. In the first case the answer might be "No"; in the second "Yes" or "He read it." This type of predicative sentence is possible only because its subject—what the sentence speaks about—is implied by the interlocutors.

An analogous situation occurs where the subject of an expression is known to the interlocutors. Imagine that several people are waiting at a stop for the "B" tram. Having sighted the approaching tram, none of these people would say: "The 'B' tram, which we are waiting for to go somewhere, is coming." The expression will always be abbreviated to a single predicate: "It's coming" or "B." Here, we find the predicative sentence in external speech because the subject and associated words are known directly from the situation where the interlocutors find themselves.

In both cases, pure predication arises where the subject of the expression is present in the interlocutors' thoughts. If their thoughts coincide, if both have the same thing in mind, complete understanding can be realized through a single predicate. If the predicate is related to different subjects, however, inevitable and often humorous misunderstandings arise.

We find many examples of the abbreviation of external speech—of the reduction of external speech to a single predicate—in the works of Tolstoy (an author who dealt regularly with issues related to the psychology of understanding). Consider, for example: "No one heard what he [i.e., the dying Nikolai Levin L.V.] had said; only Kitty understood. She understood because she constantly followed his thought so that she might know what he needed" (1893, v. 10, p. 311). Because Kitty followed the thought of the dying man, her thoughts contained the subject to which the word that no one had understood was related. The most striking example of the phenomenon of abbreviation in Tolstoy's works is found in the interchange between Kitty and Levin in which they communicated using nothing more than the initial letters of words:

"I have long wanted to ask you one thing."

"Please, ask."

"Here," he said and wrote the initial letters: W, Y, A, M, I, C, B, D, T, M, N, O, T." These letters meant: "When you answered me, 'It cannot be,' did that mean never or then?" It seemed impossible that she would understand this complex phrase.

Blushing, she said, "I understand."

"What is this word?," he asked, indicating the "N' that represented the word "never."

"That word means "never," she said. "But that is not right." He quickly erased what was written, gave here the chalk, and waited.

She wrote: "I, C, N, A, O, T."

He quickly brightened; he understood. It meant: "I could not answer otherwise then."

She wrote the initial letters: "C, Y, F, A, F, W, H, H." This meant: "Can you forget and forgive what has happened?"

He took the chalk, breaking it with his tense and trembling lingers, and then wrote the initial letters of the following: "I have nothing to forget and forgive. I never stopped loving you."

"I understand," she said in a whisper.

He sat and wrote a long phrase. She understood all. Taking the chalk she answered immediately. For a long time he was not able to understand what she had written. He glanced frequently into her eyes. His mind was blank with happiness. He could not fill in the words that she had in mind, but in her lovely, radiant eyes he understood all that he had to know. He wrote three letters. He had not finished writing when she had read beyond his hand and finished herself, writing the answer, "Da." In their conversation everything had been said: that she loved him; that she would tell her father and mother; that tomorrow he would arrive in the morning (Anna Karenina, Chap. 13, Part 4).

This example is of extraordinary psychological significance, because it was borrowed from Tolstoy's own biography, as indeed was the entire love affair between Levin and Kitty. This was precisely the way that Tolstoy declared his love for his future wife, C.A. Bers.

Like that which preceded it, this example is closely related to the problem of abbreviation in inner speech. When the thoughts and consciousness of the interlocutors are one, the role of speech in the achievement of flawless understanding is reduced to a minimum. Tolstoy turned to our attention the fact that understanding through abbreviated speech is more the rule than the exception for people who live in close psychological contact.

> Levin had grown used to being able to speak his thought without clothing it in precise words. He knew that, in intimate moments such as this, his wife would understand what he wanted to say on the basis of nothing more than a hint or allusion; and she did (1893, v. 11, p. 13).

Studying this kind of abbreviation in dialogic speech, Yakubinskii[22] concluded that where there is common knowledge of the matter at hand, where we find this understanding through allusion and conjecture, the commonality of the interlocutors' apperceptive mass plays a tremendous role in the speech exchange. The understanding of speech requires a knowledge of the matter at hand. In Polivanov's[23] view, everything we say requires a listener who understands the nature of the matter at hand. If we had to include everything we wanted to say in formal word meanings, we would have to use many more words to express each thought than we do. We speak through hints and allusions. Yakubinskii was right in claiming that where we find these abbreviations we have a unique speech syntax with tremendous objective simplicity compared with that of more discursive speech. The simplification of syntax, the minimization of syntactic differentiation, the expression of thought in condensed form and the reduction in the quantity of words all characterize this tendency toward predicativity that external speech manifests under certain conditions.

The comic misunderstandings that we referred to earlier are the polar opposite of this understanding based on abbreviated syntax. A useful illustration is found in this well known parody, where the thoughts of the interlocutors are completely unconnected:

Before the deaf judge two deaf men bow.

The first cries: "Judge! He stole my cow."

"Beg pardon," says the second, in reply,

That meadow was my father's in days gone by."

The judge: "To fight among each other is a shame.

Neither one nor the other but the girl's to blame."

These two extremes are the poles between which the abbreviation of external speech moves. Where the thoughts of the interlocutors focus on a common subject, full understanding can be realized with maximal speech abbreviation and an extremely simplified syntax. Where they do not, understanding cannot be achieved even through expanded speech. Thus, two people who attribute different content to the same word or who have fundamentally different perspectives often fail to achieve understanding. As Tolstoy says, people who think in original ways and in isolation find it difficult to understand the thought of others. They also tend to be particularly attached to their own thought. In contrast, people who are in close contact can understand mere hints which Tolstoy called "laconic and clear." They can communicate and understand the most complex thoughts almost without using words.

5

Having discussed these examples of abbreviation in external speech, we return enriched to the analysis of this phenomenon in inner speech. As we have said, abbreviation is not something that is manifested in inner speech only in special situations. It is a consistent feature of inner speech. The significance of abbreviation becomes apparent when we compare external speech to written and inner speech.

Polivanov has noted that if we included all that we wanted to say in the formal meanings of the words we use, we would need to use many more words to express each of our thoughts than we do. This is precisely the situation we find in written speech. To a much greater extent than in oral speech, thought is expressed in formal word meanings. Written speech is speech without the interlocutor. It is, therefore, maximally expanded and syntactically differentiated. Because of the separateness of the interlocutors, understanding through hints and predicative expressions is rarely possible in written speech. The differing situations in which the interlocutors find themselves in written speech preclude the presence of a common subject in their thought. Thus, compared with oral speech, written speech is maximally expanded as well as syntactically complex. As Thompson has pointed out, we commonly use words, expressions, and constructions in written expositions that would seem artificial in oral speech, Griboedov's phrase, "and you speak as you write," refers to the comic transfer of the word-rich and syntactically complex language of written speech to oral speech.

In linguistics, this problem of the *variation in speech functions* has recently attracted a good deal of attention. It turns out that even from the linguist's perspective, language is not a single form of speech activity but a collection of varied speech functions. Researchers have begun to focus on the functional analysis of language, an analysis of language that focuses on the conditions and goals of the speech expression. As early as Humboldt, linguists addressed the issue of the functional variety of speech in their distinction between the language that is used in poetry and that which is used in prose. Poetry and prose differ from one another in their intention as well as their means. They can never merge because poetry is inseparable from music while prose belongs exclusively to language. In Humboldt's view, prose is distinguished by the fact that language enjoys its own advantages here, though they are subordinated to the governing goal. By subordinating and collecting sentences in prose, there develops a logical eurhythmy that corresponds to the development of thought, a logical eurhythmy in which prose constructs its own goal. Each of these forms of speech is characterized by its unique modes of selecting expressions, using grammatical forms, and incorporating words syntactically into speech.

According to Humboldt, then, speech forms that differ in their function have their own unique lexicon, grammar, and syntax. This is an extremely important concept. Neither Humboldt nor Potebnia—who adopted and developed Humboldt's ideas—understood the full significance of this thesis. Neither went significantly beyond the initial differentiation between poetry and prose, though there was an additional differentiation within prose between forms of conversation that are filled with thoughts and forms of mundane conversation or chatter that serve only for the communication of daily matters. For a period of time, linguists largely forgot this basic concept. As Yakubinskii notes, the very statement of this problem is foreign to linguistics. It is an issue that has generally not been mentioned in collections on general linguistics. However, this concept has tremendous significance for the psychology of language and linguistics and is currently enjoying a rebirth.

Though following its own path, the psychology of speech has also become involved in this task of differentiating the functional varieties of speech, For the psychology of speech and for linguistics the differentiation of dialogic and monologic forms of speech has become particularly important. Written speech and inner speech are *monologic* speech forms. Oral speech is generally *dialogic*.

Dialogue always assumes the interlocutors' knowledge of the crux of the matter. As we have seen, this knowledge allows abbreviations in oral speech. In certain situations, it produces purely predicative statements. Dialogue presupposes visual perception of the interlocutor (of his mimics and gestures) as well as an acoustic perception of speech intonation. This allows the understanding of thought through hints and allusions. Only in oral speech do we find the kind of conversation where (as Tardeés[24] has stated it) speech is only a supplement to the glances between the interlocutors.

Because we discussed the tendency of oral speech toward abbreviation earlier, we will limit ourselves here to a discussion of its acoustic aspects. Dostoevskii's[25] writing provides us with an excellent example of the extent to which intonation facilitates subtle differentiations in the comprehension of word meaning.

Dostoevskii describes the language of several drunks which consisted of a single unprintable noun:

> Once on Sunday, near evening, we happened to walk alongside a crowd of six drunken workers for fifteen paces. I suddenly became convinced that it is possible to express all thoughts and sensations—even a whole chain of reasoning—through a single short noun. One member of the group sharply and energetically pronounced a word, expressing his own scornful rejection of something they had been talking about. In response, another repeated this same noun using an entirely different tone and sense, expressing serious doubt about the validity of the first speaker's rejection. A third, suddenly becoming indignant with the first, sharply and heatedly entered into the conversation. He shouted the same noun at the first but with a sense that was abusive and reproachful. Here the second reentered, indignant with the third (i.e,, the offender); he cautioned him: "Why did you fly in like that? We were talking calmly and in you come swearing." He expressed this thought using the same venerable word, the name of a single object. His speech differed from the others only in that he raised his hand and took the third speaker by the shoulder. Suddenly a fourth speaker—the youngest who previously had been silent—discovered a solution to the difficulty that had initially given rise to the argument. He raised his hand in delight and shouted. . . . "Eureka," . . . "I found it, I found it!" No, not, "Eureka," nor, "I found it": he merely repeated that same noun, only the one word. But he said it with delight, a visage of ecstasy. This seemed too strong. The sixth, a sullen individual and the oldest in the group, did not like it. He quickly snubbed the naive delight of the younger. He turned to him and sullenly repeated that same noun—a noun forbidden to women—with a nasal base tone. His meaning was clear and precise: "What are you screaming about?" Not saying another word, then, they repeated their pet word six times in sequence and understood each other completely. I was a witness (1929, pp. 111–112).[26]

Here we see another of the sources that underlie the tendency for abbreviation in oral speech. Dostoevskii writes that it is possible to express all thoughts, all sensations—even a whole chain of argument—through a single word. Here, this becomes possible when we use intonation to transfer the internal psychological context, that is, the context within which the word's sense can be understood. In this conversation, this context consists in sharp rejection, doubt, or indignation. When the internal content of thought can be expressed through intonation, speech will tend to become abbreviated.

Thus, we have identified two features that facilitate abbreviation, that is, the interlocutors' shared knowledge of the subject and the direct transfer of thought through intonation. Written speech precludes both. This is why we have to use more words to express a thought in written than in oral speech. As a consequence, *written speech has more words, is more precise, and is more expanded than any other form of speech*. In written speech, we must use words to transmit what is transmitted in oral speech through intonation and the immediate perception of the situation,

Shcherba[27] notes that dialogue is the most natural form of oral speech. He argues that monologue is to a large extent an artificial language form, that language reflects its true nature only in dialogue. This is true. In psychological terms, the initial form of speech is dialogic. Yakubinskii expresses this idea in his argument that dialogue—though clearly a cultural phenomenon—is still much more a natural phenomenon than monologue. Monologue is a higher, more complex speech form. It developed later than dialogue. In this context, however, we are interested only in the tendency of these two speech forms toward abbreviation, in their tendencies to be reduced to purely predicative utterances.

The rapid tempo of oral speech is not conducive to the development of speech activity as a complex volitional action, that is, as an action characterized by reflection, the conflict of motives, and selection. The rapid tempo of oral speech presupposes a simple volitional action, one with significant elements of habit. This is simply an observation. In contrast to monologue, and written speech in particular, dialogic social interaction implies immediate expression. Dialogue is speech that consists of rejoinders. It is a chain of reactions. In contrast, written speech is connected with consciousness and intentionality from the outset. Therefore, the potential for incomplete expression in inherent in dialogue. There is no need to mobilize the words that must be mobilized for expressing the same complex of thought in monologic speech. In contrast to dialogue's compositional simplicity, monologue is characterized by a compositional complexity that introduces speech facts into the field of consciousness. It is much easier to focus attention on speech facts in monologue than in dialogue. In monologue, the speech relationships become the determinants or sources of the experiences that appear in consciousness.

It is no surprise that written speech is the polar opposite of oral speech. The situation that is clear to the interlocutors in oral speech, and the potential for expressive intonation, mimic, and gesture, is absent in written speech. The potential for abbreviation is excluded from the outset. Understanding must be produced through words and their proper combination. Written speech facilitates speech as a complex activity. This underlies the use of the rough draft. The path from the rough to the final draft is a complex activity. However, even without the rough draft, the process of reflecting on one's work in written speech is extremely powerful. Frequently, we say what we will write to ourselves before we write. What we have here is a rough draft in thought. As we have tried to show in the preceding chapter, this rough draft that is constructed in thought as part of written speech is inner speech. Inner speech acts as an internal rough draft in oral as well as in written speech. We must, therefore, compare the tendency for abbreviation in inner speech with that of oral and written speech.

We have seen that the tendency for abbreviation and pure predicativity of expression arises in two circumstances in oral speech—where the situation being referred to is clear to the interlocutors and where the speaker expresses the psychological context of his expression through intonation. We have also seen that both circumstances are excluded in written speech. Again, this is why written speech does not manifest the tendency for predicativity characteristic of oral speech. This is why it is the most expanded speech form.

What do we find if we analyze inner speech from this perspective? Our detailed discussion of predicativity in oral speech permits the clear expression of one of the most subtle and complex theses to which our research on inner speech has led us, the thesis that inner speech is predicative. This thesis is fundamental to the resolution of all related issues. In oral speech, the tendency for predicativity arises frequently and regularly in particular types of situations. In written speech, it never arises. In inner speech, it is always present. It is the basic and indeed the only form assumed by inner speech. Inner speech consists entirely of psychological predicates. We do not find a predominance of predicate over subject. We find absolute predicativity. As a rule, written speech consists of expanded subjects and predicates. In inner speech, however, the subject is always dropped. Only the predicate is preserved.

Why do we find this complete, absolute, and consistent predicativity in inner speech? The predicative nature of inner speech can be demonstrated experimentally. Our task here, however, is to explain and interpret this fact. This task can be approached in two ways. We can follow the ontogenetic development of pure predicativity or we can conduct a theoretical analysis of the tendencies of written and oral speech for abbreviation and compare these with the same tendency in inner speech.

We will begin with the second approach, with a comparison of inner speech with oral and written speech. In fact, we have nearly completed this task, having prepared the foundation for our final clarifying thought. Simply stated, the circumstances that sometimes create the potential for purely predicative expressions in oral speech, circumstances that are absent entirely in written speech, are a consistent characteristic of inner speech. They are inseparable from it. As a consequence, this same tendency for predicativity is a consistent characteristic of inner speech. It is expressed here in its pure and absolute form. Thus, written and oral speech are polar opposites because the former is maximally expanded, because it is characterized by a complete absence of the circumstances that result in dropping the subject. Correspondingly, inner, and oral speech are also polar opposites, but in the reverse sense, with absolute and constant predicativity governing inner speech, Oral speech occupies a middle position between written, and inner speech in this respect.

Let us analyze the circumstances that facilitate abbreviation in inner speech in more detail. Remember, with oral speech, elision and abbreviation arise where the subject of the expression is known to the interlocutors. In inner speech, we always know what our speech is about; we always know our internal situation, the theme of our inner dialogue. Piaget once noted that we easily believe our own word, that the need for proof and the ability to provide evidence for our thought emerges only in the encounter between our own ideas and the foreign ideas of others. In the same way, it is particularly easy to understand ourselves through hints and allusions. In inner speech, we are always in the kind of situation that arises from time to time in oral dialogue, the kind of situation that we have illustrated in our examples. Inner speech always occurs in a situation comparable to that where the speaker expressed an entire thought at the tram stop through the single predicate "B." We always know our own expectations and intentions. We never need to resort to the expanded formula: "The B tram that we are waiting for to go somewhere is coming." In inner speech, the predicate is always sufficient. The subject always remains in the mind, just as the remainders beyond ten remain in the student's mind when he is doing multiplication or addition.

Moreover, we always have the capacity to express our thought in inner speech without clothing it in precise words. This was what happened in the conversation between Levin and his wife. As we indicated above, the mental intimacy of the interlocutors creates a shared apperception[28] that is critical for attaining comprehension through allusions, critical for the abbreviation of speech. This shared apperception is complete and absolute in the social interaction with oneself that takes place in inner speech. Therefore, the nearly wordless yet laconic and clear communication of complex thoughts is a consistent characteristic of inner speech, where in external speech it is possible only where there is a profound internal intimacy between the speakers. In inner speech, we never need to name the subject. We limit ourselves to what needs to be said of this subject, to the predicate. This is the source of the dominance of predicativity in inner speech.

Thus, analyzing the tendency for predicativity in oral speech has allowed us to conclude that this tendency arises where the subject is known to the interlocutors, where it is present in the speakers' shared apperception. The fact that these characteristics are found in their extreme and absolute form in inner speech helps us to understand the absolute dominance of pure predicativity that we find here. We have also seen that in oral speech these conditions lead to the reduction of syntactic complexity and differentiation, that is, to a unique syntactic structure. However, what we find expressed weakly in oral speech is manifested in its absolute form in inner speech. In inner speech, we find the ultimate syntactic simplification, the absolute condensation of thought, and an entirely new syntactic structure. We find the complete abolition of the syntax of oral speech in a purely predicative sentence structure.

Our analysis of oral speech also indicated that it is the functional change in speech that leads to structural changes. Once again, the structural changes we found in oral speech are found in absolute form in inner speech. Our genetic and experimental studies demonstrated that what is initially only a functional differentiation of egocentric and social speech leads directly and systematically to structural changes as well. With the development of functional differentiation, we find structural changes in egocentric speech that gradually approach the complete abolition of the syntax of oral speech.

We can trace the developing predicativity of inner speech. Initially, the structural characteristics of egocentric speech are identical to those of social speech. As egocentric speech develops and becomes functionally isolated from social speech, as it becomes an independent and autonomous speech form, we find increasing manifestations of the tendency for abbreviation, continual reduction in the levels of syntactic differentiation, and increasing tendencies for condensation. Before it atrophies, before it is transformed into inner speech, the syntax of egocentric speech is almost purely predicative.

Experimental observations illustrate the nature of the process through which this new syntax of inner speech develops as well as the source of that development. The child talks about what he is occupied with at the moment. He speaks of what he is doing, of what is before his eyes. As a consequence, he increasingly drops, abbreviates, and condenses the subject. Increasingly, speech is reduced to a single predicate. The remarkable law that these experiments establish can be stated in the following way: *As the functional character of egocentric speech is increasingly expressed, we begin to see the emergence of its syntactic characteristics. We begin to see its simplicity and its predicativity.* We see this clearly if we compare that egocentric speech which assumes the role of inner speech and acts as a means of interpreting problems and difficulties with that egocentric speech which is manifested in isolation from these intellectual functions. The stronger the specifically intellectual function of inner speech, the more clearly its unique syntactic structure emerges.

The predicativity of inner speech is not the only phenomenon that lies hidden behind its obvious abbreviation. When we analyze the abbreviation of inner speech, we find an entire series of structural characteristics reflected in it. In the present context, we will mention only a few of the most important.

First, the abbreviation of inner speech includes a reduction in its phonetic aspect. We have seen several examples of this already in the abbreviation of oral speech. The conversation between Kitty and Levin based on only the initial letters of words indicates that the role of verbal stimuli is reduced to a minimum where there is a shared orientation in consciousness. Once again, this reduction in the role of verbal stimuli is taken to its extreme in inner speech. Here, the shared orientation of consciousness is complete.

This situation—a rarity in oral speech—is a consistent aspect of inner speech. In inner speech, we are always in a situation comparable to that in which the conversation between Kitty and Levin took place. In inner speech, we are always guessing the meaning of the complex phrase through nothing more than the initial letters of the words. In Lemetre's studies of inner speech, we find striking analogies to the conversation between Kitty and Levin. In one of his studies, twelve year olds thought the phrase, "Les montagnes de la Suisse sont belles," as a series of letters (l, m, n, d, l, s, s, b) behind which there was a vague outline of a row of hills (Lemetre, 1905, p. 5). In the initial stages of the formation of inner speech, we find an analogous mode of speech abbreviation. The phonetic aspect of the word is reduced to its initial letters. We ever have the need to pronounce the word fully in inner speech. In our intention, we already understand the word we will pronounce.

This comparison is not meant to imply that the word is always replaced by its initial letters in inner speech. Nor do we mean to imply that speech unfolds through identical mechanisms in inner and external speech. Our point is much more general. Simply stated, the role of verbal stimuli is reduced to a minimum in oral speech where there is a shared orientation of consciousness. In inner speech, this reduction in the phonetic aspect of speech is pervasive and consistent. Inner speech is speech carried out almost without words. This is why we find such a profound similarity in these examples of inner and external speech. The fact that we find a reduction of words to their initial letters in certain cases in both oral and inner speech and that the same mechanism seems to be operating in both cases further convinces us of the close relationship between the phenomena of oral and inner speech that have been compared here.

The abbreviated nature of inner speech masks a second feature of substantial significance for understanding the psychological nature of this phenomenon. So far, we have named two sources of the abbreviated nature of inner speech, that is, its predicativity and its reduced phonetic aspect. Both indicate that in inner speech we find an entirely different relationship between the semantic and phonetic aspects of speech than we find in oral speech. In inner speech, the syntactic and phonetic aspects of speech are reduced to a minimum. They are maximally simplified and condensed. Word meaning advances to the forefront. Thus, in inner speech, the relative independence of word meaning and sound is graphically illustrated.

To explain this, we must analyze a third source of abbreviation in inner speech, that is, its unique semantic structure. The syntax of meanings—indeed the whole structure of the meaningful aspect of inner speech—is no less unique than its syntax or sound structure. In our studies, we were able to establish three basic characteristics of the semantics of inner speech. These characteristics are interconnected and together constitute its unique semantics.

First, in inner speech, we find a predominance of the word's sense over its meaning. Paulhan[29] significantly advanced the psychological analysis of speech by introducing the distinction between a word's sense and meaning. A word's sense is the aggregate of all the psychological facts that arise in our consciousness as a result of the word. Sense is a dynamic, fluid, and complex formation which has several zones that vary in their stability. Meaning is only one of these zones of the sense that the word acquires in the context of speech. It is the most stable, unified, and precise of these zones. In different contexts, a word's sense changes. In contrast, meaning is a comparatively fixed and stable point, one that remains constant with all the changes of the word's sense that are associated with its use in various contexts. Change in the word's sense is a basic factor in the semantic analysis of speech. The actual meaning of the word is inconstant. In one operation, the word emerges with one meaning; in another, another is acquired. The dynamic nature of meaning leads us to Paulhan's problem, to the problem of the relationship between meaning and sense. Isolated in the lexicon, the word has only one meaning. However, this meaning is nothing more than a potential that can only be realized in living speech, and in living speech meaning is only a cornerstone in the edifice of sense.

The fable, "The Dragon-fly and the Ant," as translated by Krylov, can be used to illustrate the difference between the word's meaning and its sense. The word "dance" with which the fable ends has a definite and constant meaning. This meaning is identical in all contexts. In the context of this fable, however, it acquires a much broader intellectual and affective sense. It simultaneously means "be merry" and "die." This enrichment of the word through the sense it acquires in context is a basic law of the dynamics of meaning. The word absorbs intellectual and affective content from the entire context in which it is intertwined. It begins to mean both more and less than it does when we view it in isolation. It means more because the scope of its meaning is expanded; it acquires several zones that supplement this new content. It means less because the abstract meaning of the word is restricted and narrowed to what the word designates in this single context.

Paulhan states that the word's sense is complex, fluid, and constantly changing. To some extent, it is unique for each consciousness and for a single consciousness in varied circumstances. In this respect, the word's sense is inexhaustible. The word acquires its sense in the phrase. The phrase itself, however, acquires its sense only in the context of the paragraph, the paragraph in the context of the book, and the book in the context of the author's collected works. Ultimately, the word's real sense is determined by everything in consciousness which is related to what the word expresses. According to Paulhan, the sense of the Earth is the solar system, the sense of the solar system the Milky Way, and the sense of the Milky Way. . . . We never know the complete sense of anything, including that of a given word. The word is an inexhaustible source of new problems. Its sense is never complete. Ultimately, the sense of a word depends on one's understanding of the world as a whole and on the internal structure of personality.

Paulhan's most important contribution, however, lies in his analysis of the relationship between word and sense. Paulhan demonstrated that the relationship between a word and its sense is not characterized by the same direct dependency as the relationship between a word and its meaning. Words can be disassociated from the sense that is expressed in them. It has long been known that words can change their sense. More recently, it has been noted that we must also study how senses change their words or, more precisely, how concepts change their names. Paulhan provides several examples illustrating how the word can remain after sense has evaporated. He analyzed stereotyped phrases such as, "How are you doing?" as well as other situations that illustrate the independence of word from sense. Paulhan also shows how sense can be isolated from the word that expresses it, how it can become fixed in another word. He argues that in the same way that the word's sense is connected not with each of its sounds but with the word as a whole, sense is connected not with each of the words that constitute the phrase but with the phrase as a whole. This creates the potential for one word to take the place of another, for sense to be isolated from the word yet still preserved. However, the word cannot exist without sense nor can sense exist without the word.

Once again, we will use Paulhan's analysis to identify a phenomenon in oral speech that has a kinship with a characteristic of inner speech. In oral speech, we generally move from the more stable and constant element of sense—from the word's meaning—to its more fluid zones, that is, to its sense as a whole. In inner speech, on the contrary, the predominance of sense over meaning that we find in oral speech in unusual situations approaches its mathematical limit. It is manifested in absolute form, The prevalence of sense over meaning, of the phrase over the word, and of the whole context over the phrase is the rule rather than the exception in inner speech.

This characteristic of the semantic aspect of inner speech is the source of two of its other characteristics, both of which are associated with the process of word unification. The first is comparable with agglutination, a means of unifying words basic to some languages though comparatively rare in others. In German, the single noun is frequently formed from several words or an entire phrase that carry the functional meaning of a single word, In other languages, this type of agglutination is pervasive. Wundt argues that these complex words are not accidental word aggregates, that they are formed according to definite laws. These languages take words that designate simple concepts and unite them into words that express complex concepts, concepts that nonetheless continue to designate each of the particular representations they contain. In this mechanical connection or agglutination of linguistic elements, the greatest accent is given to the main root or main concept, facilitating ease of comprehension. Thus, in the Delaware language, there is a complex word formed from the three words "to obtain," "boat," and "us." The literal meaning of the word is "to obtain something for us on the boat" or "to ferry something to us on the boat." The word is most commonly used, however, as a challenge to an enemy to cross a river. This word is conjugated in all the many moods and tenses of other Delaware verbs. Two aspects of this situation should be noted. First, the words that constitute the complex word often undergo phonetic abbreviation as they are incorporated in it. Second, the complex word has the function and structure of a unified word. It does not act as a unification of independent words. Wundt notes that the complex word is viewed in precisely the same way as the simple word in the American Indian languages—that it is declined and conjugated in the same way.

Something analogous can be observed in the child's egocentric speech. As egocentric speech begins to approximate inner speech, agglutination emerges with increasing frequency and clarity as a means of forming unified complex words that are used to express complex concepts. The increasing manifestations of this tendency for an asyntactic fusing of words in the child's egocentric expressions parallels the drop in the coefficient of egocentric speech.

The third and final semantic characteristic of inner speech can once again be illustrated by analyzing a phenomenon found in oral speech. Word sense—broader and more dynamic than word meaning—is characterized by different laws of unification and fusion. We have referred to the unique mode of word unification that we observed in egocentric speech as the *influence* of sense, understanding the word "influence" here both in its literal sense (i.e., that of infusion) and in its broader commonly accepted meaning. Senses infuse or influence one another such that one is contained in or modifies the other.

With external speech, similar phenomena can be observed most frequently in literary speech. Passing through a work of literature, the word acquires all the varied units of sense included within it. Its sense becomes equivalent to that of the work as a whole. The title of a literary work clearly illustrates this. The title has a different relationship to the work in literature than it does in poetry or music. It expresses and crowns the entire sense content of the work much more than it does in painting. Words such as "Don Quixote," "Hamlet," "Eugene Onegin," or "Anna Karenina" express this law of sense influence in its pure form. The sense content of the entire work can be contained in a single word.

Gogol's work, "Dead Souls," provides a remarkable example of this law of sense influence. Initially, these words designate dead serfs who have not been removed from official lists, dead serfs that can therefore be bought and sold like the living. These words are used in this sense throughout the poems, poems that focus on the trafficking in these dead souls. As they pass through the poems, however, these two words acquire an entirely new and an immeasurably richer sense. As a sponge absorbs the ocean mist, these words absorb the profound sense of the various chapters, Only toward the end do they become completely saturated with sense. By this time, however, these words designate something entirely different than they did initially. "Dead souls" refers not only to the dead, yet still counted, serfs but to all the poems' central characters, characters who live but who are spiritually dead.

There is an analogous phenomenon in inner speech, though it is again taken to the extreme. Here, the word assumes the sense of preceding and subsequent words, extending the boundaries of its meaning almost without limit. In inner speech, the word is much more heavily laden with sense than it is in external speech. Like the title of Gogol's poems, it is a concentrated clot of sense, To translate this meaning into the language of external speech, it must be expanded into a whole panorama of words. This is why the full revelation of the sense of the title of Gogol's poems requires the entire text of "Dead Souls" for its development. However, just as the entire sense of the poems can be included in these two words, tremendous sense content can be fit into a single word in inner speech.

These characteristics of the meaningful aspect of inner speech result in the incomprehensible nature of egocentric and inner speech that has been noted by all who have observed them. It is impossible to understand the child's egocentric expression if you do not know what is referred to by the predicates that constitute it, if you do not see what the child is doing and seeing. Watson suggested that inner speech would remain completely incomprehensible even if one were to succeed in recording it. Though noted by all observers, the incomprehensible nature of inner speech—like its abbreviated nature—has not been subjected to analysis. What analysis indicates is that, like the abbreviation of inner speech, its incomprehensible nature is a product of many factors. It is the summary expression of a wide variety of phenomena.

A sufficient explanation and clarification of the psychological nature of the incomprehensibility of inner speech has been provided by our discussion of its characteristics, that is, its unique syntax, its phonetic reduction, and its special semantic structure. Nonetheless, we will consider two additional factors that lead to the incomprehensible nature of inner speech. The first is the integral consequence of all the characteristics of inner speech listed above. It stems from the unique function of inner speech. Inner speech is not meant for communication. It is speech for oneself. It occurs under entirely different internal conditions than external speech and it fulfills an entirely different function. Thus, we should not be surprised by the fact that inner speech is incomprehensible but by the fact that we expect it to be comprehensible

The second is associated with the unique nature of the sense structure of inner speech. We will again clarify our thought through an illustration from external speech. In *Childhood, Adolescence,* and *Youth,* Tolstoy notes that among people who live the same life a special dialect or jargon often emerges that is comprehensible only to those who have participated in its development. The brothers Irten'ev had their own dialect, as do street children, Under certain conditions, the usual sense and meaning of a word changes and it acquires a specific meaning from the conditions that have led to this change. It should be no surprise that this kind of inner dialect also arises in inner speech, In its internal use, each word gradually acquires different colorations, different sense nuances, that are transformed into a new word meaning as they become established, Our experiments show that word meanings are always *idiomatic* in inner speech, that they are always untranslatable into the language of external speech. The meaning of the word in inner speech is an individual meaning, a meaning understandable only in the plane of inner speech. It is as idiomatic as an elision or password.

The infusion of varied sense content into a single word constitutes the formation of an individual, untranslated meaning—an idiom. What occurs here is similar to what we found in the conversation among the six drunken workmen that was described by Dostoevskii. However, once again, what is the exception for external speech is the rule for inner speech, In inner speech, we can always express all thoughts and sensations—even a whole chain of reasoning—through a single word. Of course, the meaning of this word cannot be translated into the language of external speech. It is incommensurate with the word's common meaning. It is because of this idiomatic nature of the semantics of inner speech that it is so difficult to comprehend and translate inner speech into normal language.

With this we can end our outline of the characteristics of inner speech. It is important to emphasize that we first identified these characteristics in our experimental investigation of egocentric speech. We have analyzed analogous or closely related phenomena in external speech in order to more fully understand their nature. This comparison was important because it provided a means of generalizing the data we found in our experiments. Even more significantly, however, this comparison demonstrated that the potential for the formation of these characteristics is already present in external speech.* This provides additional support for the hypothesis that egocentric and external speech constitute the source of inner speech. Given the proper circumstances, all these characteristics of inner speech (i.e,, the tendency for predication, the reduction in the phonetic aspect, the predominance of sense over meaning, the agglutination of semantic units, the influence of word sense, and idiomatic speech) can be found in external speech. This is an extremely important fact, since it demonstrates that the word's nature permits the emergence of these phenomena. In our view, this provides the best support for the hypothesis that inner speech has its origins in the differentiation and circumscription of the child's egocentric and social speech.

This outline of the characteristics of inner speech leaves no doubt concerning the validity of our basic thesis, the thesis that *inner speech is an entirely unique, independent, and distinctive speech function,* that it is completely different from external speech. This justifies the view that inner speech is an internal plane of verbal thinking which mediates the dynamic relationship between thought and word. After all that we have said about the nature of inner speech, about its structure and its function, there is no question that the movement from inner to external speech is incomparable to the direct translation of one language to another. The movement from inner to external speech is not a simple unification of silent speech with sound, a simple vocalization of inner speech. This movement requires a complete *restructuring* of speech. It requires a transformation from one distinctive and unique syntax to another, a transformation of the sense and sound structure of inner speech into the structural forms of external speech. External speech is not inner speech plus sound any more than inner speech is external speech minus sound. The transition from inner to external speech is complex and dynamic. It is the transformation of a predicative, idiomatic speech into the syntax of a differentiated speech which is comprehensible to others.

We can now return to the definition of inner speech and the contrast of inner and external speech which served as the point of departure for our analysis. We said then that inner speech is a unique function that can be considered the polar opposite of external speech. We rejected the view that inner speech is what precedes external speech, that it is the latter's internal aspect. External speech is a process that involves the transformation of thought into word, that involves the materialization and objectivization of thought. Inner speech involves the reverse process, a process that moves from without to within. Inner speech involves the evaporation of speech into thought. How-

---

* The present Russian text reads "inner" where I have translated "external." Earlier versions read "external," which is clearly indicated by the context. N.M.

ever, speech does not disappear in its internal form. Consciousness does not evaporate and dissolve into pure spirit. Inner speech is speech. It is thought that is connected with the word. However, where external speech involves the embodiment of thought in the word, in inner speech the word dies away and gives birth to thought. To a significant extent, inner speech is thinking in pure meanings, though as the poet says "we quickly tire of it." Inner speech is a dynamic, unstable, fluid phenomenon that appears momentarily between the more clearly formed and stable poles of verbal thinking, that is, between word and thought. Consequently, its true role and significance can be clarified only if we take an additional analytic step inward, only if we establish some general representations about the next stable plane of verbal thinking.

This plane is thought itself. The first task of our analysis is to isolate this plane, to partition it from the unity where we always encounter it. We have said that any thought strives to unite something with something else. Thought is characterized by a movement, an unfolding. It establishes a relationship between one thing and another. In a word, thought fulfills some function. It resolves some task. Thought's flow and movement does not correspond directly with the unfolding of speech. The units of thought and speech do not coincide, The two processes manifest a unity but not an identity. They are connected with one another by complex transitions and transformations. They cannot, however, be superimposed on one another.

This can best be seen where the work of thought is unsuccessful, where—in Dostoevskii's words—thought does not move into word. Once again, consider an example from literature, an observation made by one of Uspenskii's[30] characters. In the relevant scene, the unfortunate character has failed to find the words to express a thought that possesses him. He tortures himself helplessly as he wanders in silence, hoping that God will provide the concept and relieve his unspeakable burden. There is no essential difference between what this poor dispirited mind is experiencing and the similar tormented words of the poet or thinker. He speaks with almost the same words:

> " . . . My friend, our sort does not have language . . . .What I say seems to shape up as thoughts,
> . . . but not in language. That's our sorrow and stupidity. At times the fog clears . . . and, like a
> poet, we think that at any moment the mystery will assume a familiar image" (1949, p. 184).

Here, the boundary that separates thought from word, the uncrossable Rubicon that separates thinking from speech for the speaker, becomes apparent. If thought coincided directly in its structure and tendency with speech, this situation described by Uspenskii would be impossible. Thought has its own special structure and course. The transition from this to speech can be extremely difficult.

The theater faced this problem of the thought that lies behind the word earlier than psychology. In Stanislavskii's system in particular, we find an attempt to recreate the subtext of each line in a drama, to reveal the thought and desire that lies behind each expression. Consider the following example: Chatskii says to Sophia: "Blessed is the one who believes, for believing warms the heart." Stanislavskii reveals the subtext of this phrase as the thought: "Let's stop this conversation." We would be equally justified, however, in viewing this phrase as an expression of a different thought, specifically: "I do not believe you. You speak comforting words to calm me." It might express still another thought: "You cannot fail to see how you torture me. I want to believe you. For me, that would be bliss." The living phrase, spoken by the living person, always has its subtext. There is always a thought hidden behind it.

In the examples given above where we tried to show the lack of correspondence between the psychological and grammatical subject and predicate, we broke off our analysis at midpoint. We can now complete it. Just as a single phrase can serve to express a variety of thoughts, one thought can be expressed in a variety of phrases. The lack of correspondence between the psychological and grammatical structure of the sentence is itself determined by the way the thought is expressed in it. By answering the question, "Why has the clock stopped?," with, "The clock fell.," we can express the thought: "It is not my fault that the clock is broken; it fell!" However, this thought can be expressed through other words as well: "I am not in the habit of touching other's things. I was just dusting here." Thus, phrases that differ radically in meaning can express the same thought.

This leads us to the conclusion that thought does not immediately coincide with verbal expression. Thought does not consist of individual words like speech. I may want to express the thought that I saw a barefoot boy in a blue shirt running down the street today. I do not, however, see separately the boy, the shirt, the fact that the shirt was blue, the fact that the boy ran, and the fact that the boy was without shoes. I see all this together in a unified act of thought. In speech, however, the thought is partitioned into separate words. Thought is always something whole, something with significantly greater extent and volume than the individual word. Over the course of several minutes, an orator frequently develops the same thought. This thought is contained in his mind as a whole. It does not arise step by step through separate units in the way that his speech develops. *What is contained simultaneously in thought unfolds sequentially in speech.* Thought can be compared to a hovering cloud which gushes a shower of words.

Therefore, the transition from thought to speech is an extremely complex process which involves the partitioning of the thought and its recreation in words. This is why thought does not correspond with the word, why it doesn't even correspond with the word meanings in which it is expressed. The path from thought to word lies through meaning. There is always a background thought, a hidden subtext in our speech. The direct transition from thought to word is impossible. The construction of a complex path is always required. This is what underlies the complaint of the word's incompletion, the lamentation that the thought is inexpressible:

How can the heart express itself,

How can the other understand . . .[31]

or:

If only it were possible to express the spirit without words![32]

To overcome this, attempts arise to fuse words, to create new paths from thought to word through new word meanings. Khlebnikov[33] compared this kind of work with the construction of a road from one valley to another. He spoke of it as the direct path from Moscow to Kiev rather than one that goes via New York (he called himself a language traveler).

We said earlier that experiments have shown that thought is not expressed but completed in the word. However, as with Uspenskii's character, sometimes thought remains uncompleted. Did Uspenskii's character know what he wanted to think? He knew in the way that those who want to remember something—but fail to remember—know. Had he begun to think? He had begun as they have begun to remember, But had his thought succeeded as a process? To this question we must give a negative answer. Thought is not only mediated externally by signs. It is mediated internally by meanings. The crux of the matter is that the immediate communication of consciousness is impossible not only physically but psychologically. The communication of consciousness can be accomplished only indirectly, through a mediated path. This path consists in the internal mediation of thought first by meanings and then by words. Therefore, thought is never the direct equivalent of word meanings. Meaning mediates thought in its path to verbal expression. The path from thought to word is indirect and internally mediated.

We must now take the final step in the analysis of the internal planes of verbal thinking. Thought is not the last of these planes. It is not born of other thoughts. Thought has its origins in the motivating sphere of consciousness, a sphere that includes our inclinations and needs, our interests and impulses, and our affect and emotion. The affective and volitional tendency stands behind thought. Only here do we find the answer to the final "why" in the analysis of thinking. We have compared thought to a hovering cloud that gushes a shower of words. To extend this analogy, we must compare the motivation of thought to the wind that puts the cloud in motion. A true and complex understanding of another's thought becomes possible only when we discover its real, affective-volitional basis. The motives that lead to the emergence of thought and direct its flow can be illustrated through the example we used earlier, that of discovering the subtext through the specific interpretation of a given role. Stanislavskii teaches that behind each of a character's lines 'there stands a desire that is directed toward the realization of a definite volitional task. What is recreated here through the method of specific interpretation is the initial moment in any act of verbal thinking in living speech.

Because a volitional task stands behind every expression, Stanislavskii notes the desire that underlies the character's thought and speech in each line of a play. As an example, we will present the text and subtext in an interpretation that is similar to that of Stanislavskii's.

| *Text of the play* | *Parallel desires* |
| --- | --- |
| SOPHIA: Oh Chatskii, I am glad to see you. | Wants to hide her confusion. |
| CHATSKII: You're glad, that's good. Though, can one who becomes glad in this way be sincere? It seems to me that in the end, People and horses are shivering, And I have pleased only myself. | Wants to appeal to her conscience through mockery. Aren't you ashamed! Wants to elicit openness. |
| LIZA: But, sir, had you been behind the door, Not five minutes ago, You'd have heard us speak of you, Miss, tell him yourself! | Wants to calm Chatskii and to help Sophia in a difficult situation. |
| SOPHIA: It is always so—not only now. You cannot reproach me so. | Wants to calm Chatskii. I am guilty of nothing! |
| CHATSKII: Let's assume it is so. | Let us cease this conversation. |

Blessed is the one who believes,
And warm his life.

Understanding the words of others also requires understanding their thoughts. And even this is incomplete without understanding their motives or why they expressed their thoughts, In precisely this sense we complete the psychological analysis of any expression only when we reveal the most secret internal plane of verbal thinking—its motivation.

With this, our analysis is finished. We will now briefly consider the results to which it has led. In our analysis, verbal thinking has emerged as a complex dynamic whole where the relationship between thought and word is manifested as a movement through several internal planes, as a transition from one plane to another. We carried our analysis from the most external to the most internal plane. In the living drama of verbal thinking, movement takes the reverse path. It moves from the motive that gives birth to thought, to the formation of thought itself, to its mediation in the internal word, to the meanings of external words, and finally, to words themselves. However, it would be a mistake to imagine that this single path from thought to word is always realized. On the contrary, the current state of our knowledge indicates that extremely varied direct and reverse movements and transitions from one plane to another are possible. We also know in general terms that it is possible for movement to be broken off at any point in this complex path in the movement from the motive through the thought to inner speech, in the movement from inner speech to thought, or in the movement from inner to external speech. However, our task was not to study the varied movements that are actually realized along the trajectory from thought to word. Our goal was merely to show that the relationship between thought and word is a dynamic process. It is a path from thought to word, a completion and embodiment of the thought in the word.

We followed several unusual paths in this investigation. We attempted to study the internal aspect of the problem of thinking and speech, what is hidden from immediate observation. We attempted to analyze word meaning, a phenomenon that has always been as foreign to psychologists as the other side of the moon, a phenomenon that has always remained unstudied and unknown. The sense aspect of speech, indeed the entire internal aspect of speech that is oriented toward the personality, has until recently been unfamiliar territory for psychology. Psychology has primarily studied the external aspects of speech, those that are oriented toward us. The result has been that the relationships between thought and word have been understood as constant, eternal relationships between things, not as internal, dynamic, and mobile relationships between processes. The basic conclusion of our investigation can therefore be expressed in the thesis that these processes—which have previously been thought of as connected permanently and uniformly—in fact have changing and dynamic connections. What has previously been considered a simple construction has turned out to be a complex structure. Our desire to differentiate the external and sense aspects of speech, word, and thought has concluded with the attempt to illustrate the complex form and subtle connections of the unity that is verbal thinking. The complex structure of this unity, the complex fluid connections and transitions among the separate planes of verbal thinking, arise only in process of development. The isolation of meaning from sound, the isolation of word from thing, and the isolation of thought from word are all necessary stages in the history of the development of concepts,

Our goal has never been to provide an exhaustive account of the complex structure and dynamics of verbal thinking. Our goal was to illustrate the tremendous complexity of this dynamic structure. Our only remaining task at this point is that of summarizing the general understanding of the relationships between thought and word that has emerged in this investigation.

Associative psychology represented the relationship between thought and word as an external relationship that is formed through repetitive connections between two phenomena. In principle, this relationship was thought to be analogous with the associative connections that arise between two meaningless words. Structural psychology replaced this representation with one based on a structural connection between thought and word. However, it left unchanged the underlying postulate that this connection is non-specific. It placed this connection alongside all other structural connections that can arise between two objects such as the stick and the banana in the chimpanzee experiments.

All theories that have attempted to resolve this question have remained polarized around two opposing positions. At one pole is the behaviorist[34] conception of thinking and speech, expressed in the formula that thought is speech minus sound. At the other is extreme idealism, a view developed by the Wurzburg school and Bergson in their conception of the complete independence of thought from word and in their view that the word distorts thought. Tiutchev's line, "Thought verbalized is a lie" expresses the essence of this view. This is the source of the attempts of psychologists to isolate consciousness from reality. In Bergson's words, it is the attempt to grasp our concepts in their natural state, in the form in which they are perceived by consciousness, by destroying the parameters of language.

These perspectives share a common point that is inherent to nearly all theories of thinking and speech, They share a profound and fundamental antihistorical perspective. All these theories oscillate between the poles of pure naturalism and pure spiritualism, They view thinking and speech in isolation from their history. However, only an historical psychology, only *an historical theory of inner speech, has the capacity to lead us to a correct understanding of this complex and extraordinary problem*. This is the path that we have attempted to follow in our research.

The basic finding of our research can be expressed in a few words: The relationship of thought to word is a vital process that involves the birth of thought in the word. Deprived of thought, the word is dead. As the poet writes:

> And as the bees which have sunk into their silent Yule season,
> So do dead words sink.[35]

However, in the words of another poet, thought that is not embodied in the word remains a Stygian shadow, it remains in the "mist, bells, and radiance." In Hegel's view, the word is existing, vitalized thought. This kind of existence is absolutely necessary for our thoughts.

The connection between thought and word is not an primal connection that is given once and forever. It arises in development and itself develops. "In the beginning was the word."[36] Goethe answered this Biblical phrase through Faust: "In the beginning was the deed."[37] Through this statement, Goethe wished to counteract the word's overvaluation. Gutsman has noted, however, that we can agree with Goethe that the word as such should not be overvalued and can concur in his transformation of the Biblical line to, "In the beginning was the *deed*." Nonetheless, if we consider the history of development, we can still read this line with a different emphasis: "In the *beginning* was the deed." Gutsman's argument is that the word is a higher stage in man's development than the highest manifestation of action. He is right. The word did not exist in the beginning. In the beginning was the deed. The formation of the word occurs nearer the end than the beginning of development. The word is the end that crowns the deed.

* * *

In concluding, we should say a few words about the prospects that lie beyond the present study, Our investigation has brought us to the threshold of a problem that is broader, more profound, and still more extraordinary than the problem of thinking. It has brought us to the threshold of the problem of consciousness. In our investigation, we have tried to consistently keep in view that aspect of the word which has been unfamiliar ground for experimental psychology. We have tried to study the word's relationship to the object, its relationship to reality. We have tried to study the dialectical transition from sensation to thinking and show that reality is reflected in thinking differently than it is reflected in sensation. We have tried to show that the word's distinguishing feature is a generalized reflection of reality. In the process, however, we have touched on an aspect of the word's nature whose significance exceeds the limits of thinking as such, an aspect of the word that can be studied only within the framework of a more general problem, the problem of the relationship between the word and consciousness.

The consciousness of sensation and thinking are characterized by different modes of reflecting reality, They are different types of consciousness. Therefore, *thinking and speech are the key to understanding the nature of human consciousness.* If language is as ancient as consciousness itself, if language is consciousness that exists in practice for other people and therefore for myself, then it is not only the development of thought but the development of consciousness as a whole that is connected with the development of the word. Studies consistently demonstrate that the word plays a central role not in the isolated functions but the whole of consciousness. In consciousness, the word is what—in Feuerbach's[38] words—is absolutely impossible for one person but possible for two. The word is the most direct manifestation of the historical nature of human consciousness.

Consciousness is reflected in the word like the sun is reflected in a droplet of water. The word is a microcosm of consciousness, related to consciousness like a living cell is related to an organism, like an atom is related to the cosmos. The meaningful word is a microcosm of consciousness.

# 4

# Perception and Its Development
# in Childhood

The theme of our lecture today[1] is the problem of perception in child psychology. You know, of course, that no chapter of contemporary psychology has been as fundamentally rewritten in the past 15–20 years as that concerned with the problem of perception. You know that the skirmish between the representatives of the old and the new psychology has been more intense here than in any other domain of research. Nowhere has the structural tradition placed its new conceptions and experimental research methods in such sharp opposition to the old, associative tradition. If we consider concrete experimental material, the chapter on perception has clearly been more extensively rewritten than any other chapter of experimental psychology.

Though you are probably aware of the essence of this revision, I will outline it briefly.

Taking the law of association as a point of departure, associative psychology represented memory as the basic and general law of connection of the separate elements of mental life. Memory served as the model for the construction and interpretation of all other functions. Thus, perception was understood as a product of the association of a whole complex of sensations, as the sum of separate sensations constructed through their mutual association. This process was assumed to occur in accordance with the same law that leads to the association of separate representations or memories in the creation of a unified picture in memory. These associations were thought to explain the connectedness of perception.

How is it that we perceive not separate, disparate, and dispersed points but a whole figure reflecting the outline of a body's surface? How is it that we perceive the meaning of this body? This is how the associative school stated the question. They answered that connectedness in perception appears in the same way that it does in memory. The separate elements are connected, chained, or associated with one another, producing a unified, connected, integral perception. This theory assumes that the physiological correlate of connected, integral visual perception is a similar picture that is summarized in equivalent disparate points on the retina. It is assumed that each of the separate points of the object excite the corresponding stimulation in the disparate points of the retina. All these stimuli, summarized in the central nervous system, are thought to create a complex excitation, the object's correlate.

The inadequacy of this theory of perception served as the point of departure for the rejection of associationism. The initial attack on associative psychology was not waged on its fortress—

Originally appeared in English translation as Lecture 1 in *The Collected Works of L.S. Vygotsky, Volume 1: Problems of General Psychology* (Robert W. Rieber and Aaron S. Carton, Eds.; Norris Minich, Trans.) (pp. 289–300). New York: Plenum Press, 1987.

on its theory of memory. In fact, the "structural" attack on associative psychology continues to be weakest on this point. Structural psychology's[2] attack began with the demonstration of the structural and integral origins of man's mental life in the domain of perception.

The structural perspective began with the notion that the perception of the whole precedes the perception of the separate parts. Structural psychologists argued that the connected whole of objects, things, and processes is not the product of a summary of separate, disparate, and dispersed sensations. They argued that the physiological substratum of perception is not a group of separate excitations that come to be associated. In several brilliant experimental demonstrations, structural psychologists have collected data representing different stages of development that can only be adequately understood on the basis of the new structural theory. The foundation of this theory is the concept that mental life is not constructed from separate sensations or representations and their mutual association, but from separate integral formations, structures, and images that are called Gestalten. This basic principle has been extended to other domains of mental life. In each domain, structural psychologists have tried to show that the integral formations of mental life arise as integral formations. All this has been demonstrated clearly in several experimental studies.

Consider Kohler's experiment with domestic chickens. This experiment showed that the chicken does not perceive a pair of colors as a simple associative union but as the relationship between these colors. The perception of the field precedes and indeed defines the perception of its separate parts. The colors constituting the colored field can be changed while the general law governing the perception of the field remains the same. These experiments were transferred from the lower animals to the humanoid apes and, with certain modifications, were also carried out with children. They demonstrated that perception is an integral process. The general character of perception is preserved though the separate parts have changed. The structure that forms the integral perception may change, but this change produces a different integral perception.

Folkelt's experiment with spiders demonstrated this in still more integral form, though with less experimental elegance. Folkelt demonstrated that a spider that reacts correctly and adequately when a fly has fallen into its web, that is, when the whole situation is preserved, loses this capacity when the fly is torn from the web and placed in the spider's nest.

Similarly, in one of Gottshaldt's late experiments, he presented the separate parts of a complex figure to his subjects several hundred times until they had learned them thoroughly. He found, however, that if these figures were presented in a different aggregation, and if this whole was unfamiliar to the subject, the old figure remained unrecognized in the new structural perception.

I will not summarize additional experiments. I will say only that they have been extensively developed in zoopsychology and in child psychology. Analogous experiments conducted with adults have also supported this notion that our perception is not atomistic but integral in nature. This thesis is sufficiently well known that there is no need to dwell on it. It is another aspect of the dispute between these traditions that is of particular interest to us here. Specifically, what framework does each provide for understanding child development? How is the question of the development of the child's perception stated by the new structural theory?

Within the associative framework, the theory of the development of the child's perception was entirely analogous to the general theory of mental development. In accordance with this perspective, the key factor of mental life is given at the outset, soon after birth. This factor is the capacity for association, that is, the connecting of elements that are experienced either simultaneously or in close sequence. In the child, however, the material that is pasted or soldered together through these associative connections is extremely limited. The child's mental development consists of the constant accumulation of this material, resulting in new, more extended, and richer associative connections among separate objects. The child's perception is constructed and grows with this development of associative connections. The child moves from the perception of separate sensations to the perception of interconnected groups of sensations, from the perception of interconnected groups of sensations to the perception of interconnected groups of objects, and, finally, to the perception of the whole situation. The infant's initial perception is thought to be chaotic, as Buhler expressed it, a wild dance of uncoordinated sensations.

When I was a university student, the infant's perception was viewed in precisely this way. The infant was thought to be capable of perceiving taste (i.e., bitter or sour) or temperature (i.e., warm and cold). In addition, it was thought that soon after birth he is capable of perceiving sound and color. However, these were thought to be uncoordinated sensations. It was thought that because the groups Of sensations belonging to a single object were repeated frequently in a given combination, they began to be perceived complexively by the child, that is, through a simultaneous grasping. This was thought to be the foundation of perception in the true sense of the word.

Though they agreed that separate sensations are present from the outset, researchers differed in their view of which month in the first year of life is associated with the development or emergence of these complex perceptions. Some argued that the infant's perception is a connected integral process by the fourth month of life. Others argued that this type of perception emerges only in the seventh or eighth month.

Like the idea of deriving the complex mental whole from the sum of its separate isolated elements, this representation of the development of the child's perception is inadequate from the perspective of structural psychology. Structural psychology valued data obtained in the lower stages of development that indicated that our perception is integral in nature from the outset. In his work, Human Perception, Kohler attempted to show that the same basic laws are manifested in human and animal perception. For Kohler, human perception is a perfection of animal perception. It is where these laws find their most subtle, precise, and developed expression.

Structural psychology fell into a dangerous trap in its treatment of the child's perception. In Folkelt's experiments, structural psychology indicated that the structural character of perception can be demonstrated in the earliest stages of the child's development, indeed, in the first month of the infant's life. The structural character of perception is primal; it emerges at the outset. It is not the product of an extended development. If one accepts these arguments, what constitutes the development of the child's perception? Where are we to find development if the most essential feature of perception (i.e., its structural integral nature) is present both at the beginning of the developmental process and at its culmination in the adult?

This is among the weakest empirical and theoretical aspects of structural psychology. Nowhere does structural psychology manifest its inadequacy more clearly than in its theory of perception. Several attempts to construct a theory of the child's mental development based on the structural perspective are well known. Though it may seem strange, the weakest aspect of these attempts to develop a theoretical analysis of the psychology of the child's development from the perspective of structural theory has been in the treatment of the child's perception. The refusal, in principle, to view the child's perception in the context of its development is connected with the basic methodological assumptions of this theory. These assumptions attribute a metaphysical character to the concept of structure.

As a product of these assumptions, we have two works that have appeared following that of Gottshald. The first, Koffka's study of the phylogenetic problem, rejected the very possibility that the nature of this difference could be clarified. In the second, Folkelt relied on an experimental study of very young children to conclude that we are dealing here with features of perception that characterize a primitive integral structure at various stages of development. Utilizing Goethe's catchword, Folkelt attributed these the characteristics of the eternal, unchanging child to the category of that which is preserved throughout man's development.

To illustrate the path taken by researchers striving to avoid this dead end, or by those who return to this problem again and again in the hope of avoiding it, I must consider what is commonly called the orthoscopic nature of the child's perception. This is an old problem. Several psychophisiologists first stated the problem and made the initial attempts to resolve it. It had a particularly important place in the research of Helmholtz. [4] Following these early efforts, the problem was largely abandoned. In the past two decades, however, it has emerged once again.

The essence of the problem is that the perception of contemporary adults is distinguished by several mental characteristics that seem to be unexplained or incomprehensible. Which characteristics of our perception are the most important? What characteristics of perception, when lost, lead to the pathology of perception? Before all else, our perception is characterized by the fact that we see a more or less constant, ordered, connected picture wherever we direct our eyes.

As we partition this problem into its separate aspects, they must be named in a specific order corresponding to the order of their emergence in experimental psychology.

First, we will consider constancy in the perception of magnitude. If I hold two objects of identical length before an infant's eyes, two identical pencils for example, there will be two representations of identical length on the retina. If I hold one pencil that is five times greater in length than the other, the corresponding representations will be found on the retina. It would appear, then, that my perception of one pencil as longer than the other is a direct function of retinal representation. I continue the experiment, however, and hold the larger pencil at a distance five times greater than the other. The size of its representation on the retina decreases by a factor of five. Thus, the two representations on the retina will be identical in size. How do we explain the psychological fact that the pencil that is removed to five times the distance does not seem to be reduced in size by a factor of five? Why, when it is removed at a distance, do I continue to see it as the same size? With the similarity of the two representations on the retina, what allows me to see the larger pencil as larger but located at a distance.

How can we explain that the object preserves its size despite the increase in its distance from the eye? Even more remarkable, how do we explain that this occurs even though objects actually have a tendency to seem smaller at a greater distance (i.e., at a great distance a large ship seems like a small point)? The experiment is well known in which one holds an object close to the eye and then quickly moves it away. The object dances in the eyes and becomes smaller. How do we explain the finding that objects seem smaller in accordance with their distance from the eye but nevertheless retain a relative tendency for the preservation of size? This question becomes still more interesting when we remember its tremendous biological significance. On the one hand, perception would not fulfill its biological function if it did not have this orthoscopic character, that is, if the size of the object changed with its distance from the subject. To the animal that fears the beast of prey, the latter at one hundred steps must not seem one hundred times smaller. On the other hand, if perception did not have this tendency, the impression of an object's proximity or distance would not arise. Clearly, the biological mechanism that allows the object to preserve size constancy with distance from the eye—and at the same time to lose it—must be extremely complex.

We should also consider constancy in the perception of color. Hering[5] demonstrated that a piece of chalk reflects ten times more white light at midday than at dusk. Still, at dusk, chalk is white and coal is black. Though the quantity of rays falling on the object and the color of this illumination may change the quality of the immediate stimulus, other colors are also characterized by a relative constancy. Of course, there is also constancy in the perception of form. Though I look on it from above, the briefcase lying before me appears to me as a briefcase, an object with a definite form. As Helmholtz notes, a painting instructor goes to a good deal of effort to show his pupil that he does not see the entirety of the chair, but only a portion of it.

We could supplement the analysis of constancy in the perception of size, form, and color with a discussion of constancy in the perception of several other features. This is the general phenomenon called orthoscopic perception. Orthoscopic (on analogy with orttzographic) means that we see objects correctly. Despite the varying conditions of perception, we see an object of a certain size, form and color. The orthoscopic nature of perception makes it possible to perceive stable features of objects that are independent of accidental conditions such as the angle of view or of the subject's own movements. In other words, it allows a comparatively eternal, stable picture which is independent of subjective and accidental aspects of the observation.

Interest in this problem has grown because we have found that analogous perceptual phenomena have different characteristics. In particular, you probably are aware that after-images manifest characteristics of orthoscopic perception that are the opposite of those manifested by real perception. If we fix a red square on a grey background and then remove it from this background, we see the square illuminated by its complementary color. This experiment demonstrates what our perception would be like if it was not orthoscopic. If I move the screen away, the size of this square increases. If I move the screen closer by a factor of two, the square is reduced in size by a factor of two. The perception of the square's size, position, and movement is a function of movement, the angle of vision, and all the other factors that our actual perception is independent of. In my view, the emergence of an ordered, constant perception raises several important questions. It indicates the developmental path of the child's perception in a place where associative and structural schools have closed the door for the researcher.

How can we explain these facts? In his attempt, Helmholtz himself suggested that orthoscopic perception is not primal, that it arises in the developmental process. He considered some precarious yet interesting data. In particular, he discussed memories of distant childhood. For example, when passing a bell tower, the child may think that the people there are tiny. Describing similar observations by other children, Helmholtz concludes that orthoscopic perception does not exist from the outset. One of Helmholtz's pupils argued that it is only this gradually acquired perception of a constant picture that can reflect constant object characteristics. He suggested that the acquisition of this constant picture constitutes a major feature of the development of the child's perception.

Helmholtz's explanation of orthoscopic perception relied on the concept of unconscious inference. He assumed that the pencil that is removed from the eye at 10 times the distance of another is actually perceived as a pencil reduced in size by a factor of ten. At this point, however, he felt that perception adds several unconscious judgments. The subject knows from previous experience that this is an object that he has seen up close and that it is now some distance from the eye. Thus, a correction is made on the initial portion of the perception, introducing the unconscious inference.

Numerous experimenters have scoffed at this kind of explanation and immediate experience does indicate the naivete of the way that Helmholtz states the question. In real perception I do not perceive a pencil that has decreased in size, while consciously knowing that it has been removed to a distance. The simplest data of immediate experience indicate that Helmholtz's explanation is inadequate. However, several experiments have shown that he was moving in the right direction. Helmholtz was right when he said that the orthoscopic character of perception should not be taken as something given from the outset, when he said that we should understand it as a product of development. This is the first point. The second point is that we need to understand that constancy of perception does not arise from changes in the internal constitution and characteristics of perception itself. The emergence of this feature of perception has its roots in the fact that perception begins to act within a system that involves other functions.

Helmholtz's reference to unconscious inference is an unscientific hypothesis that has hindered the search for a solution to this problem for years. However, contemporary research shows that the orthoscopic nature of perception, visual perception in particular, arises from truly complex available stimuli and from stimuli that are fused with them, stimuli that act simultaneously with them. I said that in Helmholtz's view the pencil that is removed 5 times further from the eye must appear to be reduced in size by a factor of five. Suppose, on the other hand, that we have before us not a pencil but its representation as an after-image. If the object itself is taken away and the screen is removed to a distance 5 times further from the eye, the law of Emert indicates that the pencil will increase in size by a factor of five. However, if the screen was moved away from the eyes the size of the object must not change. Consequently, I must perceive the object and its retinal image as mutually compensating for one another. The image increases by a factor of five in accordance with the distance of the screen, while the object decreases in size by a factor of 5. Thus, if the object is fused with the after-image, the available stimulus would remain unchanged.

The initial experimental studies moved in this direction. Can this fusion of the available perception with the after-image be created in such a way that the alter-image would be given simultaneously with the perception? Experimenters quickly resolved this task. The subject was asked to fixate on a red square on the screen, but the square was actually an illustration in red light, not an actual square constructed of paper. This red square was then taken away. The subject saw the green complementary image. Unnoticed by the subject, a real red square was then substituted. The experimenter then moved the screen away from the subject, producing a violation of Emert's law.

At the same time, experimenters made a bold and brilliant attempt to produce constancy in the image. They tried to find conditions under which the size of the image would increase nonproportionally with distance, diverging in this respect from Emert's law. If this hypothesis were correct, it would become impossible to explain why an object at a greater distance seems smaller. For this to occur the object must be quickly (i.e., instantaneously) removed from the eye, so that I would not notice its decrease in size.

This type of complete constancy in perception would be as bad in biological terms as complete changeability of perception. If we lived in a world of constantly changing objects, absolute stability of perception would mean that we could not perceive the distance that separates the object from us. Experiments carried out by the Marburg school indicate that the explanation for this characteristic of perception must take as its point of departure not the after-image but the eidetic image. An entirely independent line of research has shown that the eidetic image that we see on the screen after an object has been removed is not susceptible to Emert's law. As it is removed to a greater distance, the increase in the size of the eidetic image is much slower than it would be if it were proportional.

Research carried out in accordance with the method described, that is, research that elicits a fusion of the real light illustration with the eidetic image, has shown that this fusion produces an experimental effect much more similar to that of real perception. The size of the theoretically calculated error here turns out to be $1/10$ while the error that is found experimentally differs by only $1/5$.

Before I attempt to summarize this discussion and draw theoretical conclusions, it would be useful to consider two additional closely related problems. This should allow us to draw several theoretical conclusions more easily and on better empirical foundations.

The first of these two problems is that of the meaningful nature of perception. Taking the developed perception of the cultured adult as our point of departure, we face a problem that is analogous to that I have just developed for you. The orthoscopic nature of adult perception is one of its prominent characteristics. Another is the meaningful nature of our perception. It has been shown experimentally that we cannot create conditions that will functionally separate our perception from meaningful interpretation of the perceived object. I now hold a notebook in front of myself. I do not perceive something white with four corners and then associate this perception with my knowledge of the object and its designation, that is, with my understanding that this is a notebook. The understanding of the thing, the name of the object, is given together with its perception. Studies have in fact shown that the perception of the object's distinct objective characteristics depends on the meaning or sense that accompanies the perception.

You are probably aware that several experimenters have continued the experiments begun by Rorshach. Recently, these studies have been presented systematically and definitively by the young Bleuler. These studies have shown that the problem of the perception of meaningless ink spots posed by Binet[7] is a truly profound one, one that leads us to the problem of the meaningful interpretation of our perception. Why is it that I don't see a certain form, weight, or size? Why do I know simultaneously that what I have before me is a chair or table? Binet proposed the following experiment. Have the subject look at a simple inkblot on a piece of paper that has been folded in two such that the spot is symmetric, meaningless, and entirely accidental. Binet notes that, remarkably, in every case the resultant inkblot seems to be similar to something. The children with whom he carried out his initial experiments were almost never able to perceive this meaningless inkspot as a spot. They always perceived it as a dog, a cloud, or a cow.

Rorshach created a systematic series of these meaningless colored symmetrical figures and used them in his experiments. His experiments have shown that only in a state of dementia, particularly in an epileptic state, can the spot be perceived as entirely meaningless. It is only in this situation that subjects say that this is nothing more than a spot. The normal subject sees a lamp, a lake, or a cloud. The nature of the meaningful interpretation changes, but the tendency to see the spot meaningfully is consistent.

Buhler used this tendency toward the meaningful interpretation of any perception as a means for analyzing the meaningful nature of our developed perception. He showed that to the extent that developed forms of perception are stable and constant, they are also meaningful or categorical. I do not see a series of separate external forms of an object. I see the object. I immediately perceive the object as such, with all its meaning and sense. I see a lamp, a table, a person, or a door. In Buhler's words, my perception is an inseparable part of my concrete thinking. Simultaneously with that which is seen, I am given the categorically ordered nature of the visual situation that is the object of my perception.

Related research has indicated that this kind of complex meaningful interpretation arises in immediate perception and occasionally leads to illusion. Consider, for example, Sharpant's illusion. If the subject is asked to determine (either simultaneously or successively) the heaviness of two cylinders that are identical in weight and form but differ in size, it will always seem that the smaller of the two is the heavier. Even if we see the two cylinders weighed and are convinced that they are of equal weight, when we take them in our hands we cannot escape the sensation that the smaller is the heavier.

Many explanations have been offered for Sharpant's illusion. However, several studies concerning the problems we have just discussed have demonstrated that this mistake arises because this apparently mistaken perception is actually, in a certain sense, a correct perception. Those who have studied this illusion have noted that when we judge the small object to be the heavier our evaluation is correct with respect to the object's relative weight or density, that is, with respect to the relationship of the object's weight to its volume. In this sense, the smaller object actually is "heavier." The immediate perception of heaviness is subordinated to the meaningful perception of heaviness in relation to volume. This results in the distortion of the immediate perception. If we close our eyes, we perceive these objects as equally heavy. Nonetheless, those who have been blind from birth experience Sharpant's illusion. Though they do not see the cylinders, the cylinder that they perceive through their developed tactile sensation as the smaller is perceived as heavier. It is in the meaningful perception that the immediate sensation of heaviness is compared with the object's volume. Experiments have shown that, though they can see, deaf and mute children are not susceptible to Sharpant's illusion.

Research has also shown that this illusion has an important diagnostic significance. The absence of Sharpant's illusion among profoundly retarded children is referred to as Demor's symptom. The perception of these children remains nonmeaningful. The smaller cylinder does not seem heavier. When there is a need to differentiate diagnostically between profound retardation and a lesser degree of retardation in a child of between 9–10 years, the presence or absence of Demor's symptom is an extremely important criterion. Extending this line of reasoning, Claparede suggested that Sharpant's illusion could be used as a criterion in the analysis of the development of the child's perception. Studies have demonstrated that before five years of age normal children are not susceptible to Sharpant's illusion.

It is clear, then, that the phenomenon observed by Sharpant emerges in development. It does not occur in profoundly retarded children or in the majority of deaf and mute children. It does appear in the blind and it can serve as a reliable diagnostic criterion in the differentiation of profound retardation from lesser degrees of retardation.

Thus, experimentation in this domain has led to findings similar to those that have resulted from the study of orthoscopic perception. On the one hand, experiments have shown that the meaningful character of the adult's perception is not inherent in the perception of the child. This characteristic of perception emerges at a certain stage. It is not given at the outset, but is the product of development. On the other hand, experiments have shown that much as the stability and constancy of our perception is a function of the fusion of perception with the eidetic image, what we have in meaningful perception is an immediate fusion of the processes of concrete thinking and perception such that the two functions are inseparable. One function works within the other as its constituent. The two form a cooperative unit that can only be partitioned through experimental means. It is only in the psychological experiment that we can achieve meaningless perception, that we can partition immediate from meaningful perception.

The third problem of perception that we will consider here, the problem of true categorical perception, is closely related to this problem of meaningful perception. A typical example of studies in this domain are the experiments with the perception of pictures, experiments that have a long history. Early researchers believed that this experiment was the key to the study of the general development of the child's meaningful perception. In their view, a picture represents some portion of reality. They felt that by selecting pictures, showing them to children of various ages, and studying the development of changes in the perception of these pictures, statistical methods could be used to summarize the thousands of facts accumulated. Through this process, they hoped to identify the stages through which the developing child passes in his perception of reality.

These stages have been defined and described in a variety of ways. Stern, for example, classified these stages differently at various points in his career. However, the majority of authors agree that there are four basic stages in the child's perception of pictures. Initially, in the object stage, the child perceives separate objects. Then, in the action stage, the child begins to name objects and indicate the actions that are being carried out with them. In the next stage, the stage of qualities or features, the child begins to indicate the features of the perceived object. Finally, the child begins to describe the picture as a whole, beginning with it as an aggregation of parts. On the basis of these experiments, investigators (in particular, Stern in Germany and Blonskii here) have suggested that we can identify basic stages in the development of the child's meaningful perception. Blonskii argues that in the beginning the child perceives the picture, that is, the world, as a collection of objects. Later he begins to perceive it as a collection of acting and moving objects and then begins to enrich this collection of action objects with qualities or characteristics. Finally, the child attains the perception of an integral picture. This is the analogue of the real, meaningful, integral situation, the perception of an integral reality. The strength of these arguments is that they are actually supported consistently in experiments. That is, Blonskii's experiments, conducted here, have produced the same basic results as the experiments of Stern, Neuman, Rollof, Mukhov, and many other researchers internationally.

Only 15 years ago, this was considered a basic law of the development of the child's perception. However, in the past 15 years experimental psychology has undertaken critical work that has left this concept with little credibility.

Given what we do know of perception, it is difficult to imagine that the child moves from the perception of separate objects to the unification of objects with actions, then to the unification of the object with its features, and finally to the perception of the whole. Experimental data have shown that the structural and integral nature of perception are inherent to the earliest stages of development. The perception of the whole precedes the perception of its parts. The data from these experiments stand in glaring contradiction to what we know of the structural character of perception.

Associative atomistic psychology naturally presupposes that the child moves from the part to the whole, that he supplements the parts with actions and qualities, perceiving the whole situation only as a final achievement. From the perspective of structural psychology, on the other hand, the notion that the child moves fromthe perception of separate parts and then, by summarizing them, to the perception of the whole, is nonsense. We know the development of perception follows the opposite path. Structural psychology has shown that the small child does not perceive separate objects. Daily observation supports this perspective. Whether the situation is that of play or feeding, the child perceives the whole situation. The infant's perception, not to mention that of the older child, is consistently determined by the integral situation. It would be extraordinarily difficult if the child actually achieved the potential of perceiving the whole meaningful situation only between the ages of ten and twelve! It is difficult to imagine the actual implications this would have for the child's mental development. (We will not even consider, in this context, the experiments that have shown that the perception of movements and actions is often found much earlier than the perception of objects.)

These considerations concerning the experimental verification of this law make it necessary to resolve two questions. First, if this law is a false representation of the sequence of stages in the development of the child's perception, how should this sequence actually be represented? Second, if this law incorrectly represents the sequence of stages, why is there such massive support for the notion that younger children describe the picture by isolating objects while in subsequent ages children isolate actions and features?

Attempts to resolve this problem have begun in a variety of countries and have taken different paths. The most interesting research has been carried out by Piaget and Eliasberg. Eliasberg has shown that the younger child's perception is not the perception of separate objects. Indeed, it is composed of completely undifferentiated connections. Similarly, Piaget's research has demonstrated that the younger child's perception is syncretic. That is, it is associated with groups of objects that are not isolated, objects that are globally interconnected and perceived as a unified whole. These studies indicate that Stern's point of departure was false. In general terms, current research has shown that this proposed sequence of stages cannot withstand criticism.

This brings us to the two questions mentioned above. It would be inadequate to merely refute Stern's perspective. We need to show why the child's description of pictures follows a developmental path that is the opposite of his actual perceptual development. Stated crudely, the question is that of how we are to explain the finding that the child moves in perception from the whole to its parts, while in the perception of pictures he moves from the parts to the whole? Stern attempted to explain this by saying that the structural development of perception from the whole to its parts is characteristic of immediate perception, while the sequence described earlier is characteristic of meaningful perception, perception that is fused with concrete thinking. This Ehasberg experiment, however, initially dealt with nonmeaningful material. This material was then replaced with meaningful material. There was no difference in Eliasberg's findings related to the type of material used. Eliasberg demonstrated that meaningful material contradicts the findings that would be anticipated on the basis of Stern's data.

At the International Psychotechnics Congress in Moscow, we had the opportunity to hear Eliasberg's report on his new studies as well as his discussion with Stern. Stern's argument was clearly unsuccessful. Studies have demonstrated that this question is resolved both more simply and more complexly than Stern has imagined. Simple observation indicates that while this sequence of stages (i.e., the stages of objects, actions, qualities, and relationships) is not a useful description of the development of the child's perception, it does coincide with the development of his speech. The child always begins with the pronunciation of separate words. Initially, these words are substantive nouns. Later substantive nouns are supplied with verbs, giving rise to the two word sentence. Adjectives appear in the third period. Finally, with the acquisition of a certain supply of phrases, we find extended accounts in the description of pictures. Thus, this sequence of stages is related not to the development of perception, but to the development of speech.

This fact becomes particularly interesting when we analyze it experimentally. For the sake of simplicity, I will allow myself a slight immodesty and cite our own published experiments in which we attempted to resolve this problem. If we ask the child to tell us what is depicted in a picture, we indeed do find evidence for the set of stages identified by previous researchers. However, if a young child is asked to represent the picture in play, he never merely plays with the separate objects (assuming, of course, that the conditions depicted in the picture are accessible to his understanding). For example, if the picture depicts a man with a bear on a chain that he is showing to a group of children, the child will not first take the role of the bear and then that of the children. The child does not reproduce several separate details in his play. He consistently represents the picture as a whole. When the child is asked to represent the picture in this way, the developmental sequence looks much different.

I do not have the time to discuss many other important problems. This would leave us with no time for theoretical conclusions, without which even the best material would lose its sense. To make my conclusions more complete, however, I will however permit myself a brief comment on several new studies concerned with the development of man's primitive perceptions.

Experimental psychology has recently begun to address problems associated with the senses of smell and taste. These experiments, though still in their infancy, have led researchers to surprising genetic conclusions. It seems that the immediate connection of perception and concrete thinking is absent in primitive perceptions. With smells, for example, we cannot produce generalizations either in everyday practice or in scientific theory. In the early stages of development, the child does not have a general concept of the color red. He knows only the concrete manifestations of red. In much the same way, we lack the ability to generalize smells.

We designate them much like primitive peoples designate colors. It seems that categorical perception is not found in several biologically rudimentary phenomena, phenomena that have lost their adaptive significance, that no longer play an essential role in man's cultural development. The perception of smells is one such phenomenon. In this context, I would cite Henning's work. This work has opened up an entire epoch in the theory of the primitive forms of perception, forms of perception that have clearly regressed in man if we compare him to many of the higher mammals.

Permit me a few minutes to outline some conclusions. Whether we consider orthoscopic perception, meaningful perception, or the connections between perception and speech, we find a single fact of extraordinary theoretical importance. Specifically, at each stage in the child's development we observe changes in interfunctional connections and relationships. In the child's development a connection arises between the function of perception and the functions of eidetic memory. As a consequence, a new unified whole arises, a whole within which perception acts as an internal constituent. There is a fusion of concrete thinking and perception. We can no longer separate categorical from immediate perception. We can no longer separate the perception of the object as such from its meaning or sense. Experiments indicate that it is here that the connection between perception and speech, the connection between perception and the word, arises. They indicate that the typical course of the child's development changes if we view this perception through the prism of speech, if the child not only perceives but tells about what is perceived.

We find these interfunctional connections everywhere. It is because of the emergence of these new connections, these new unities that include perception and other functions, that we find the extremely important developmental changes that lead to the emergence of the distinctive characteristics of developed adult perception. If we view the evolution of perception in isolation, if we fail to recognize that it is part of the complex development of consciousness as a whole, these changes and these characteristics will remain unexplained and inexplicable. Of course, this is precisely what associative and structural psychologies have done.

If we remember that the characteristic features of perception are the same in the earlier and later stages of development, it becomes clear that theories that have viewed, and continue to view, perception outside its connections with other functions, will be powerless to explain the distinctive characteristics of perception that arise in the developmental process. These new complex formations of mental functions are not separate functions. What we are speaking of here is a new unity. For lack of a better term, I will call these formations psychological systems. Throughout the child's development, then, new systems constantly emerge within which perception acts. Within these systems, and only within these systems, perception acquires new characteristics that are not inherent to it outside that developmental system.

It is also important to understand that with the formation of new interfunctional connections in development, perception is freed or emancipated from connections characteristic of it in earlier stages. In the early stages of its development, perception is immediately connected with the motor system. It is a feature of an integral sensorimotor process. Only gradually, over the years, does perception begin to acquire a significant degree of independence, to renounce this particular connection with the motor system. Lewin, who has worked most extensively on this problem, argues that only with the passage of years is the child's perception expressed dynamically in the internal processes. In particular, Lewin has shown that it is only with the liberation or differentiation of perception from this form of integral psychomotor process that its connection with concrete thinking becomes possible.

Folkelt, Knaeger, and other researchers of the Leipzig school have shown that, in the early stages of perception's development, it is equally inseparable from emotional reactions. Krueger has suggested that in these early stages perception should be called "sensual" or "emotional" perception. His studies have shown that only with the passage of time is perception gradually liberated from its connections with the child's immediate affect or emotion.

We are indebted to the Leipzig school, because it established the extremely important fact that in the beginning of the developmental process we generally cannot identify fully differentiated mental functions. What we find at this stage are much more complex undifferentiatedunities that give rise to the separate functions during development. Perception is one of these separate functions. However, further research cannot follow the path established by the Leipzig school. The development of perception will become comprehensible only if research is carried out on the basis of entirely different methodological foundations.

# 5

# Emotions and Their Development in Childhood

The theory of emotions and its development are unique among the various domains of psychological research. Until recently, this domain was completely dominated by a pure naturalism of a kind profoundly foreign to other domains of psychological investigation. These other domains have shifted to purely naturalistic theories only with the emergence of behaviorism and similar behavioristic research traditions. Methodologically, the entire future of behaviorism is contained in the old theory of emotions, since both have developed as a reaction to the forms of spiritualistic introspective psychology that preceded them. Developing primarily on a naturalistic plane, research on the emotions stood out like a white raven from other domains of psychological research contemporary to it.

There are many reasons for the uniqueness of the theory of emotions. In this context, however, we need only note the proximal cause, a cause connected with the name of Charles Darwin. Bringing to completion an old and extensive tradition in biology, Darwin's "The Origin of the Expressive Movements in Man" linked man's emotions with the corresponding affective and instinctive reactions that can be observed in the animal world. In sketching the evolution and origin of human expressive movements, Darwin was pursuing his basic evolutionary concept. As he noted in a letter that has recently been published in Russian, it was important to him to show that man's feelings, considered until then the inner "sanctum" of the human soul, have the same animal origins as does man as a whole. Of course, the connection between man's emotional expressions and the emotional expressions of animals similar to man on the evolutionary scale is so obvious that it has rarely been disputed.

As a contemporary historian has noted, the English psychology of this period was temporarily dominated by scholastic thought and by the associated religious traditions rooted in the middle ages. The response of these psychologists to Darwin's arguments on the human emotions was shrewd. They accepted the Darwinian position as developed by Darwin's students with a great deal of sympathy. From their perspective, Darwin had shown that man's earthly passions, those concrete inclinations and emotions connected with his physical concerns, actually do have animal origins. This provided an immediate impetus for two directions in psychological thought. On the one hand, extending the positive tradition of the Darwinian concept, psychologists began to develop the idea that human emotions al origins in the affective and

Originally appeared in English translation as Lecture 4 in *The Collected Works of L.S. Vygotsky, Volume 1: Problems of General Psychology* (Robert W. Rieber and Aaron S. Carton, Eds.; Norris Minich, Trans.) (pp. 325–337). New York: Plenum Press, 1987.

instinctive reacti ns of animals (e.g., Spencer[9] and his students, the French positivists such as Ribot[10] and his school, and the biol riented German psychologists). This led to the development of the theory of cmotions that is included in nearly all psychological textbooks, a theory commonly called the rudimentary theory of emotions.

This theory holds that the expressive movements that accompany human fear are rudimentary remnants of the animal reactions of flight and defense, that the expressive movements that accompany human anger are the remnants of movements that once accompanied the reaction of attack in our animal predecessors. According to one formula, fear is inhibited flight; anger—inhibited fight. In other words, all expressive movements came to be viewed retrospectively. Ribot noted that the emotions, like "a state within a state," are the sole domain of the human mind that can only be understood retrospectively. The emotions are "a dying tribe." They are "the gypsies of our mind." From this perspective, the only possible conclusion for psychological theory is that man's affective reactions are remnants of his animal existence, remnants that have been infinitely weakened in their external expression and their inner dynamics.

The general impression created is that the curve representing the development of the emotions moves downward. Recently, a student of Spencer has argued that if we compare animals with man, the child with the adult, or the primitive with the cultured man, we see that the emotions fall back to a less prominent plane as the developmental process moves forward. This gives rise to the concept that the man of the future will be without emotion, that the process will be taken to its logical end and man will lose the final remaining links to the emotional reactions whose significance is found in an ancient epoch of his existence.

From this perspective, the only chapter of the psychology of emotions that can be adequately developed is that concerned with the emotional reactions of animals and with the development of emotions in the animal world. It is indeed this chapter that has been most extensively and most thoroughly developed by contemporary psychology. Any potential for an adequate investigation of the specific characteristics of human emotions was excluded by the way these psychologists stated the issue. Rather than facilitating the investigation of the enrichment of the emotions in childhood, this statement of the issue led to the assumption that the emotional order characteristic of early childhood is suppressed and weakened. With respect to the issue of change in the strength of emotions from primal man to the present, we find the assumption of a direct continuation of an evolutionary process based on the premise that a step forward in the development of the human mind implies a step backward in the development of the emotions. According to Ribot, this is the glorious history of the dying out of this entire domain of mental life.

While a biological analysis of the emotions would seem to indicate that this whole sphere of mental life dies out, our immediate psychological experience and our experimental research demonstrate the absurdity this position.

Independently of one another, Lange[11] and James[1] assumed the task of locating the source of the vitality of the emotions in the human organism itself. In this way, they liberated themselves from the dominant retrospective approach to human emotions. Each followed his own path, James consciously as a psychologist and Lange as a physiologist. Both found the source of the vitality of the emotions in the organic reactions that accompany emotional processes, This theory is widely known, so there is no reason to discuss it in detail. I will remind you only that the key to this theory was the introduction of a change in the traditional view of the sequential relationship between the various components of the emotional reaction.

Before James and Lange, psychologists represented the emotional process in the following way. The first component is the external or internal event. The perception of this event elicits the emotion (an encounter with danger for example). This is followed by the experience of the emotion (ie,, the feeling of fear). Finally, we observe physical and organic expressions of the emotion (ie,, palpation, turning pale, shivering, and a dry throat). Rejecting this sequence of "perception—feeling—expression," James and Lange argued that the immediate perception of an event gives rise to reflexively elicited organic change (for Lange this was primarily vasiomotor change; for James, While a biological analysis of the emotions would seem to indicate that this whole visceral change, change in the internal organs). These reflexive changes accompanying fear and other emotions can be perceived. Indeed, James and Lange argued that this perception of our own organic reactions provides the foundation for the emotions.

In their attempts to demonstrate their opposition to this theory, others have misinterpreted it in a variety of ways. James' classic formula, however, can be statzd in the following manner: While we usually assume that we cry because we feel grief or that we shiver because we are frightened, we in fact feel grief because we cry and are frightened because we shiver.

According to James, one need only suppress the external manifestation of the emotion and it will disappear; one need only elicit an emotion's expression and the emotion itself will ensue.

This theoretically refined and comparatively developed theory has two strengths. First, it actually provides what seems to be a natural-scientific, biological basis for the emotional reactions. Second, in contrast to many other theories, it actually provides an explanation for the continued existence of the emotions, an explanation for why these remnants of our animal existence seem to remain so close to the nucleus of the personality (everyone knows that the experience that is most emotional is that which is inner and personal).

The James-Lange theory (the two theories were quickly united into a single general theory) initially met with substantial criticism because of its "materialistic nature." Critics argued that James and Lange wanted to reduce human feelings to the reflection of organic processes in consciousness. However, James' perspective was hardly materialistic. In his textbook on psychology, he replied to these initial reproaches with the following statement : "My theory cannot be called materialistic." Indeed, his theory was not materialistic, though there was some foundation for the perception that it was in its use of materialistic methods. However, James' theory led to results that were in direct opposition to materialism. Nowhere, for example, were the higher and the elementary functions separated so clearly as in James' theory of emotions. The further development of his theory was consistently based on this initial separation of the higher and lower emotions.

In answer to his critics, James took the path identified in Darwin's time in response to the criticism of the English scholastic psychologists. That is, he attempted to grant to God what is God's and to Caesar what is Caesar's. He argued that it is only the lower emotions such as fear, anger, despair, and rage, emotions inherited by man from his animal predecessors, that have an organic origin. What James called the "subtle" emotions, emotions such as religious feeling, the love of a man for a woman, or the esthetic experience, do not. Thus, James sharply differentiated the lower and the higher emotions, particularly in the intellectual domain (a domain of emotional experience that had not generally been noticed prior to James but has recently become the focus of experimental research). He isolated the emotional experiences that are directly intertwined with our thinking processes, those that constitute an inseparable part of the integral process of judgment, from organic foundations. He viewed these emotional experiences as processes sui generis, processes with a unique nature.

As a pragmatist, James had little interest in the nature of the phenomena that he studied. As far as society's practical interests are concerned, he argued that it is sufficient to be aware of the difference between the higher and lower emotions as it is The James-Lange theory (the two theories were quickly united into a single genmanifested in empirical research. From a pragmatic perspective, what was important was that the higher emotions were saved from a materialistic or quasimaterialistic interpretation.

This theory led to a dualism similar to that characteristic of intuitive and descriptive psychology. Bergson himself, an extreme idealist whose psychological and philosophical perspectives coincided in several respects with those of James, adopted James' theory of emotions, appending his own theoretical and empirical considerations. With the dualism inherent in this distinction between the higher and the lower emotions, this theory cannot be called materialistic, as James himself correctly noted. It contains not a grain more materialism than does the assertion that we hear because our auditory nerve is stimulated by our oscillating eardrum. Not even the most deliberate spiritualist or idealist has rejected the simple fact that our sensations and perceptions are connected with the material processes that stimulate our sense organs, James' assertion that the emotions emerge as the consequence of an internal perception of organic changes is no closer to materialism than is the claim of parallelism that the light wave that elicits the stimulation of the visual nerve leads to the movement of a neural process which occurs in parallel with the mental experience of color, form, or size.

Finally, our third and most important point is that these theories provided the foundation for a variety of metaphysical theories of the emotions. In this respect, when compared with the works of Darwin and the Darwinian research tradition, the theories of James and Lange constitute a step backward. It was perhaps necessary to save the emotions, to show that they are not a dying tribe. In his attempt to accomplish this, however, James attached the emotions to organs associated with the most primitive levels of mankind's historical development. According to James, the internal organs provide the foundation for the emotions; the emotions are constructed from the perception of the subtlest reactions of the intestines and heart, of the internal cavity and the internal organs, and of vasomotor reactions and similar vegetative, visceral, or humoral changes. This theory stripped the emotions from consciousness, completing a task that had been started much earlier.

I have mentioned that Ribot and others represent the emotions as a state within a state in the human mind. They conceptualize the emotions in isolation. The emotions are torn from the unified whole, from the rest of man's mental life. The James-Lange theory provided the anatomical and physiological foundation for this notion. James himself emphasized this point, arguing that the organ of human thought is the brain, while the emotions are associated with the vegetative internal organs. Thus, the substratum of the emotions was transferred from the center to the periphery, Moreover, the theories of James and Lange made it even more difficult to pose the question of the development of emotional life. With a retrospective approach to the emotions, the human emotions were represented as phenomena that emerged at a certain point in the developmental process. James' theory excluded any potential for imagining the genesis of human emotions, despite of the emergence of new emotions in man's historical life.

Completing the circle, then, James and his followers returned to an idealistic conception of the emotions. James himself argued that it is in the historical period of man's development that higher human feelings of a kind unknown to animals have been developed and perfected. What man received from the animal has remained unchanged, since it is a simple function of organic activity. Thus, Darwin's theory, initially advanced to demonstrate the animal origin of the emotions, ended with the proof that there is no connection between what man received from the animal and what emerged in the historical period of man's development. What was God's was granted to God; what was Caesar's -to Caesar. The attempt was made to demonstrate the purely spiritualistic nature of the higher emotions and the purely organic or physiological nature of the lower. The experimental attack on this theory came from both physiological and psychological laboratories.

The former played the role of traitor to the theories of James and Lange. Physiologists had initially been inspired by these theories. Year after year, they introduced new data in support of them. These theories obviously contained some truth. There are extremely rich and varied organic changes that are specific to emotional reactions. If we compare what James had said in this connection with what we know now, it is obvious that James and Lange opened up a fruitful area for empirical studies. Their contribution was enormous.

Cannon's well known book[12] now translated into Russian, assumed the treasonous role for the physiological laboratories. A duality which permeated this book was not immediately noted, partly because it was associated with an early stage in the development of this area of physiological research and partly because Zavadovskii's[13] introduction to the Russian translation recommended Cannon's book as concrete proof for the James-Lange theory. Still, a careful analysis of Cannon's experiments indicates that they lead to a rejection of the theory.

Two concepts were fundamental to the James-Lange theory. First, in biological terms, emotions are the reflection of physiological states in consciousness. Second, these physiological states are specific to each of the emotions.

You have probably read several books concerning the most recent work of Cannon and his school. Using extremely complex research methods that included extirpation, psychopharmacological agents, and complex biochemical analysis Cannon's experiments on cats, dogs, and other mammals have demonstrated that the states of rage, anger, and fear are associated with profound humoral changes, changes that are linked to reactions of the endocrine glands (especially the adrenal gland). These changes are also associated with profound changes in the entire visceral system to which all the internal organs react. As a consequence, each emotion is connected with significant changes in the state of the organism.

Even in his earliest work, however, Cannon encountered an extremely important fact. Specifically, the organic expressions of different emotions such as rage, fear, fright, and anger are identical. Thus, even in the book that Zavadovskii cited in support of the James-Lange theory, Cannon introduced a correction to the formula that had been advanced by James. James argued that we grieve because we cry. Cannon suggested that this formulation needs to be modified to read that we grieve, feel tenderness, feel moved, and generally experience the most varied emotions because we cry. On the basis of his experimental data, Cannon rejected the concept that there is any simple connection between an emotion and its physical expression. He demonstrated that the physical expression is nonspecific to the emotion. Data associated with a cardiogram, with humoral and visceral changes, with chemical analysis, or with the analysis of the blood, cannot help us distinguish whether an animal is experiencing fear or rage. We find identical physical changes associated with what are, psychologically, very different emotions.

However, while he rejected the notion that there is a simple connection between a given type of emotion and the particular organization of its physical expression, Cannon did 330 Lectures on Psychology not question James' basic thesis, the thesis that the emotions are the reflection in consciousness of organic changes. On the contrary, Cannon produced experimental data which indicated that organic changes are varied. This provided support for the James-Lange theory.

In his subsequent studies, however, Cannon was forced to conclude that the nonspecific nature of the physical expression of emotion required the rejection of the James-Lange theory. Though he repeatedly varied the situations used to elicit intense emotions in animals, Cannon found an unvarying physical expression of these emotions. It became clear that the clarity of these physical expressions was a function not of the quality of the emotion but of its strength.

Subsequently, Cannon conducted several complex experiments in which a significant part of the animal's sympathetic nervous system was removed. This eliminated any organic reaction. Two cats were compared, In the first, the sympathetic nervous system had been eliminated. Fear and rage did not stimulate the flow of adrenalin or other humoral changes. The second was a control in which these reactions were elicited by fear and rage. These cats behaved identically in analogous situations. The same emotions were observed in the cat whose sympathetic nervous system had been eliminated as in the control; she reacted in the same way when a dog approached her or her kittens, when food was taken away, or when she looked at food through a narrow aperture.

This experiment refuted a basic element of James' theory, his position concerning the subtraction of emotional symptoms. According to James, if we mentally subtract shivering, the bending of the knees, and the stopping of the heartbeat from the emotion of fear, we will find that nothing remains of the emotions. Cannon attempted this subtraction experimentally and found that the emotions remain. This research demonstrated that emotional states are present in animals that lack the corresponding vegetative reactions.

In another series of experiments, Cannon injected first animals and then humans to elicit artificial organic changes analogous to those observed in association with intense emotions. In animals, these organic changes were elicited with no manifestation of emotion. The changes in blood sugar and blood circulation characteristic of the emotional state were observed, but the emotions themselves did not appear.

In this way, James' second assertion met the same fate as his first. When we elicit the external expression that accompanies the emotion, the emotion itself does not appear.

The results of Cannon's experiments on human subjects were more complex. With most of his subjects, no emotions appeared. In a few, however, the injection did elicit an emotion. However, this occurred rarely and only when the subjects were to a certain extent ready to explode with emotion, only when they were prepared for an emotive discharge. In the subjects' explanations that followed the experiment, it became apparent that all the subjects who experience emotion had an external cause for grief or gladness. The injection acted as a source of excitation that reproduced these emotions. Moreover, introspective accounts indicated that none of the subjects actually felt fear, anger, or shyness, The subjects explained their state in the following way: I felt as if I were afraid, as if I were experiencing anger. Thus, the attempt to create an internal experience for the subject, the attempt to elicit the conscious perception of internal organic change, led to a state reminiscent of emotion. Emotion in the true psychological sense, however, was absent.

These experiments based on introspective analysis introduced an important correction to Cannon's data. They demonstrated that the organic expression of the emotions is not as insignificant as Cannon had suggested on the basis of his experiments with animals.

The general implications of Cannon's research, and of other studies in this domain, can be stated in the following two basic propositions. First, these studies have led Cannon, and all other physiologists and psychophysiologists working in this domain, to reject the James-Lange theory. The James-Lange theory did not stand up to experimental evaluation. It was not verified by the facts. One of Cannon's works is entitled "An Alternative to the James-Lange Theory."

Second, as a biologist, Cannon had to explain the paradox that emerged from his experiments. If the profound organic changes that occur with intense emotional reactions in animals are completely inessential for the emotions, if the emotions are preserved despite the elimination of all these organic changes, why are these changes necessary from a biological perspective? In his earliest work, Cannon demonstrated the biological significance of the changes that occur in association with the emotions. Now Cannon was faced with the question of why the cat that had been deprived of its sympathetic nervous system, and thus the humoral and visceral reactions that accompany the affect of fear, still reacted to a threat to its kittens in the same way as the cat in which these reactions have been preserved. From a biological perspective, if these reactions do not play an essential role in the biological changes that occur in association with the emotions, they become incomprehensible and unnatural.

Cannon explained the contradiction in the following way: An intense emotional reaction in an animal is not the end but the beginning of an action. A reaction of this kind arises in a situation of critical life significance for the animal. Thus, the logical conclusion of an intense emotional reaction in an animal is a heightened level of activity. The logical conclusion of fear is flight. The logical conclusion of rage or anger is struggle or attack. The organic reactions associated with emotions exist not for the emotion as such but for what logically follows the emotion. All these changes, the increase in blood sugar and the mobilization of the organism's strength for struggle and flight, are important because an increase in the intensity of muscular activity will follow an intense emotional reaction. Whether this activity is flight, struggle, or attack is not significant. The preparation of the organism must occur. Cannon argued that under laboratory conditions the cat that lacked the physiological symptoms of emotion behaved in the same way as the one in which these symptoms were present. However, this is true only under experimental laboratory conditions. Under natural conditions, the cat in which these symptoms are absent will die sooner. The animal with unorganized visceral processes, processes that fail to prepare the organism, will die sooner than a normal animal.

Other experiments carried out by Cannon provide the most significant experimental foundation for this hypothesis. First in experiments Cannon conducted with animals, and subsequently in experiments carried out by his students with people, intense muscular activity was elicited. In one experiment, for example, Cannon forced a cat into a channel in which there was a steadily flowing current (Durov[14] has conducted similar experiments here). This forced the animal run at maximum speed to save himself. It was found that this simple muscular work, these intense movements, resulted in the same organic changes as intense emotions. This indicated that the vegetative symptoms are merely the companions of the emotions; they are the expressions not of the emotions as such but of intense muscular activity.

Cannon's critics argued that these animals may have been frightened by the situations that were created in these experiments. In response to these arguments, Cannon conducted a further set of experiments that did not include elements that might frighten the animal. Here as well, Cannon found that an increase in muscular activity elicited the changes that have generally been viewed as the companions of the emotions, changes that Cannon himself had earlier seen an essential feature of the emotions. Thus, these symptoms are not so much the companions of the emotions as supplements to certain emotional factors that are associated with instincts.

Cannon notes that Darwin's theory receives unexpected support from this perspective. There is no question that the expressive movements associated with several human emotions can actualLy be viewed as rudimentary in comparison with the expressive movements associated with these emotions in animals. The weakness of Darwin's theory is that he was unable to explain the progressive development of the emotions. He was only able to see their attenuation. What Cannon demonstrated was that it is not the emotions themselves that die away, but only their instinctive component. The role of the emotions in the human mind is different. They are isolated from the instinctive domain and transferred to an entirely new plane.

Thus, if we consider the theory of emotions within the general framework of its historical development, it quickly becomes apparent that while it originates from several different directions it has moved in a single direction. The basic conclusion of the work I have reviewed so far concerns the displacement of emotional life from the periphery to the center. This research has shown that the actual substratum of the emotional processes is not the biologically ancient internal organs, not the extracerebral mechanisms that led to the concept that the emotions are a separate state, but a cerebral mechanism. The basic result of this research has been that of connecting the mechanism of the emotions with the brain. This displacement of the center of emotional life from the organs of the periphery to the brain brings the emotional reactions within the same general anatomical-physiological context as the rest of the psychological functions. It creates an intimate connection between the emotional reactions and the rest of the human mind.

The result of this psychophysiological research becomes particularly significant when considered in the context of the work done by researchers concerned with the psychological aspect of the problem. This psychological research has demonstrated the intimate connection and dependency that exists between the development of the emotions and the development of other aspects of mental life.

This work has done for psychology something analogous to what Cannon and his students have accomplished in the domain of psychophysiology: It has shifted the emotions from the periphery to the center. In psychophysiological research, investigators began to recognize that the mechanism of the emotions is cerebral rather than extracerebral. This research demonstrated that the emotions are dependent on the same organ that controls all other reactions associated with the human mind. In psychological research, we again find the demise of the theory that man's emotional life constitutes "a state within a state." Experiments have identified a whole series of connections and dependencies that make it clear that the separation of the emotions into higher and lower forms (a separation that resulted from the James-Lange theory) into two classes that have nothing in common with one another, led to an impossible situation.

Chronologically, Freud is the first psychologist we must discuss in this connection. Freud, whose work was not experimental but clinical, was among the first to move in a direction of theory development compatible with later research in this domain. In his analysis of the psychopathology of emotional life, Freud rejected the primacy of analysis of the organic components that accompany the emotions. He suggested that there is nothing of less importance for the definition of the psychological nature of fear than knowledge of the organic changes that accompany it. Freud rejected the one-sided organic psychology of James and Lange, arguing that they had studied the husk and left the psychological kernel unexplored. In its investigation of the activity of the organs that express the emotions, Freud felt that this psychology had contributed nothing to the study of the emotions as such. Freud provided extensive documentation of the extraordinary dynamics of emotional life.

Though the basic claims Freud makes in this connection are false, there is a great deal of truth in what he says if we limit ourselves to formal conclusions based on his studies. Freud's explanation of fear is based on the argument that a series of neurotic processes transform the sexual inclination into fear. Within this conceptual framework, fear becomes a neurotic state. It is the equivalent of inadequately suppressed or displaced desires. Freud successfully demonstrates how ambivalent this emotion can be in the early stages of development. His explanation of this ambivalence in the emotion is false. He is right, however, in his claim that the emotion of fear does not exist at the outset, that there is a differentiation of a kernel that contains opposing feelings.

Freud's major contribution in this domain is his demonstration that the emotions were not always as they are in adult life. The emotions characteristic of the young child are different from those of the adult. The emotions are not "a state within a state." They cannot be understood outside the dynamic of human life. It is within this context that the emotional processes acquire their meaning and sense. Of course, Freud was as much a naturalist as James. He interpreted the human mind as a purely natural process, approaching the dynamic changes of the emotions only within specific naturalistic limits. That, however, is a separate issue.

A comparable achievement in the development of the theory of emotions was made by Adler[15] his school. Through observational methods, they demonstrated that in man the unctional significance of the emotions is not linked exclusively to the instincts as it is in animals. The emotions are one of the features which constitute the character of an individual's general view of life. The structure of the individual's character is reflected in his emotional life and his character is defined by these emotional experiences.

This conception of character and emotion led to a situation where the theory of emotions became an inseparable and central aspect of the theory of human character. This provides a striking contrast to earlier perspectives, where the emotions had been perceived as a unique phenomenon, a dying tribe. Here the emotions are conceptualized in connection with character, in connection with the processes involved in the formation of the basic psychological structure of the personality.

Buhler's theory reflected an extremely interesting shift in how the emotions were treated in psychology, a shift associated with the relationship of the emotions to other mental processes. Buhler's experimental findings (his experiments are the best aspect of his work) can be stated crudely and schematically in the following way. First, Buhler takes the critique of the Freudian perspective on emotional life as his point of departure. He emphasizes that the early stages in the development of the child's mental life and activity are not exclusively defined by the pleasure principle. More significantly, however, he argues that pleasure itself—as what impels an act or deed—migrates, wanders, and shifts its position within the system of mental functions. Linking this concept to his division of the development of behavior into three stages (ie,, instinct, training, and intellect), Buhler attempts to show that the point when pleasure occurs in an activity shifts in accordance with the degree of the child's development, changing its relationship to other mental processes with which it is connected.

The first stage in this developmental sequence is referred to by Buhler as *Endlust*. Here, pleasure comes at the end of the action. In Buhler's view, this stage is characteristic of instinctive processes. It is connected primarily with hunger and thirst, experiences that themselves have an unpleasant character. The initial moments of satiation are accompanied by a clear expression of pleasure. Thus, when the instinctive act is completed, *Endlust* appears. The emotional experience lies at the end of instinctive activity. The primitive and primal form of human sexual tendencies is of this nature. The central pleasurable moment is at the end. The end is the decisive moment for the instinctive act. In Buhler's view, the emotions generally, and the emotion of pleasure in particular, have this kind of ending or completing role in instinctive life. The emotions are the feature of mental life that insure the completion of the instinctive act.

According to Buhler, the second stage in this sequence is that of functional satisfaction *(Funktionslust)*. This stage is manifested in the early forms of the child's play, when the child receives satisfaction not so much from the result of the activity as from the process itself. Here, pleasure is transferred from the end of the process to its content, its functioning. Buhler notes, for example, that this is a common characteristic of the child's eating. In late infancy, the child begins to express pleasure not only with satiation or the quenching of thirst but with the process of eating itself. The process itself acquires the potential for pleasure. The fact that the child can become a glutton reflects the emergence of *Funktionslust*.

Finally, Buhler distinguishes a third stage connected with the anticipation of pleasure. Here, the emotional coloring of experience emerges with the onset of the process itself. Neither the result of the action nor the actual process of carrying it out is the focal point of the child's integral experience, The focal point shifts to the beginning of the action (Vorlust). This is characteristic of the processes involved in creative play, finding the answer to a riddle, or solving a problem. Here, the child finds the solution and then realizes what he has found. What he receives as a consequence of the action has no essential significance for him.

If we consider the significance of these stages, it becomes apparent that they correspond with the three stages in the development of behavior outlined by Buhler. First, with instinctive activity, the dominant organization of emotional life is that connected with the final moment

(Endlust). Second, pleasure received from the process of an activity is a necessary biological feature for the development of a skill or habit. Here, not the result of the activity but the activity itself must become the sustaining stimulus. Finally, the essence of early intellectual activity is what Buhler refers to as the reaction of "searching for the answer" (ie. the "aha-reaction"). Here the dominant organization of emotional life is the child's experience of emotion at the beginning of the activity. Pleasure itself leads to a situation where the child's activity develops differently than it does in the two planes referred to earlier.

Another general conclusion of Buhler's research is that the emotional processes are not settled but nomadic, They do not have a secure, firmly established position. My own data convince me that the shift of pleasure from the result of the action to its anticipation is but a pale expression of the diverse range of potential shifts in emotional life, shifts that constitute the actual content of the development of the child's emotional life.

In concluding the empirical aspect of today's lecture, I will briefly mention several recent works, those of Claparede in particular. The unique value of Claparede's work lies in that he has combined research on normal and abnormal children with experimental studies of adults. In addition, I would like to discuss the works of the German structural psychologist, Lewin, who has studied the psychology of affective and volitional life, I will briefly note the central findings of these and several other works and then move directly to my conclusion.

Claparede's work is significant primarily because of his experimental success in differentiating the concepts and manifestations of emotion and feeling. In Claparede's view, though emotions and feelings are frequently encountered in similar situations, they are fundamentally different. In this lecture, however, we must focus not on the classification of the emotions but on their nature. We will therefore have to ignore Claparede's theory concerning emotions and feeling and focus on the close connections he has identified between the emotions and the other processes of spiritual life and on his view of the diversity of the emotions themselves.

Freud was the first to question the traditional theory of the biological utility of the emotions. In his observations of the neurotic state in children and adults, Freud saw something that no psychologist could ignore. Specifically, the neurotic child or adult clearly illustrates how spiritual life can be disordered and deranged as a consequence of an emotional disturbance. Traditional perspectives assumed that the emotions are a biologically useful adaptation. Within this framework, it is difficult to understand why the emotions cause such profound and extended behavioral disorders, to understand why we cannot think consistently when we are ill, cannot act with consistency or according to plan when our feelings are disordered, cannot be responsible for our own behavior and control our actions in an intense affective state. In other words, why does an abrupt change in the emotional processes result in a change in the whole of consciousness, a change that displaces the normal dynamics of the functions that ensure the normal life of consciousness? Primitive biological and naturalistic interpretations of the human emotions make it impossible to understand why biological adaptations that are as ancient as man himself and as necessary as the need for food and water lead to such complex disturbances of human consciousness.

Claparede posed the second half of this question. Specifically, if the primary functional significance of the emotions is their biological utility, how do we explain the fact that human emotions become more varied with every step mankind takes on the path of historical

development. This development and differentiation of the emotions leads not only to the kind
of disorders of mental life that have been explored by Freud, but to the entire vast and diverse
content of mankind's mental life including domains such as art. Why does every step in human
development elicit these "biological" emotions? Why are the individual's intellectual experiences
associated with such intense emotion? Why is every critical moment in the fate of the adult or
child so clearly colored by emotion?

In his attempt to answer these questions, Claparede discusses the frightened rabbit which
is afraid and runs, but fails to save himself precisely because he is afraid, because his running
is disturbed. Taking this as his point of departure, Claparede attempts to demonstrate that alongside biological useful emotions there exist processes that can be called feelings. These feelings
have catastrophic effects on behavior and arise where a biologically adequate reaction to a situation is impossible. When an animal becomes frightened and runs, this is an emotion.
When an animal becomes frightened to the extent that it cannot run, we are dealing with a
qualitatively different process.

The same is true of man. Despite the apparent similarity between feelings and emotions,
these processes have different roles in mental life. Compare the man who is aware of a danger
and arms himself in advance with the man who is not aware and is attacked, or compare the
man who can run with the man who discovers the danger by surprise. In other words, compare
the man who can find an adequate exit from the situation to the man who cannot. The psychological nature of the processes that are involved in the two situations are very different. In his
experiments, Claparede studied reactions with different outcomes, leading to the differentiation of affective life into emotions and feelings. This distinction has tremendous significance
because the old psychology mechanically confused these aspects of emotions and feelings, ascribing both to processes that do not exist.

Finally, we must note Lewin's work, where he demonstrated that the complex dynamics
of the emotional reactions are part of the general system of mental processes. Lewin conducted
the first experimental investigation of processes identified by the phrase "depth psychology,"
processes that in the hands of Freud and Adler were considered inaccessible to experimental
investigation. Lewin demonstrated how one emotional state is transformed into another, how
one emotional experience is substituted for another, and how an unresolved and uncompleted
emotion may continue to exist in covert form. He also demonstrated how an affect enters
into any structure with which it is connected.

Lewin's basic concept was that affective or emotional reactions cannot be found in isolation as a special element of mental life, an element of mental life that is subsequently united
with others. The emotional reaction is the unique result of a particular structure of mental
processes. Lewin demonstrated that the primary emotional reactions can emerge in sporting
activity based on external movements or in activity such as chess that is carried out in the mind.
Different contents arise in correspondence with different reactions, but the structural position
of the emotional processes in the whole remains the same.

In conclusion, we can say that both the major research traditions that I have discussed
in this lecture have moved the emotions from the periphery to the center, Anatomical and
physiological research has shifted the center of emotional life from extracerebral mechanisms
to the brain itself. Psychological research has moved the emotions from the hinterlands to the

forefront of the human mind, no longer treating them as an isolated "state within a state," but including them within the same structure as the other mental processes. As is always the case in the study of mental life, these two lines meet in psychopathology.

Developing in complete independence from researchers such as Cannon and Claparede, we find a splendid analogue in psychopathology that has provided clinicians with the foundation for formulating both sides of the thesis that results from the unification of the two sides of this single general theoretical perspective.

On the one hand, with nervous disorders and illnesses resulting from brain disease (particularly those associated with a disorder of the visual tuberal in the subcortical area), clinicians frequently observe cases where there is a forced laugh or smile that occurs every few minutes. Characteristically, this state is not associated with an emotion of gladness, but is experienced as torment. The imposed grimace sharply contrasts with the individual's actual state. I had the opportunity to study and describe a case characterized by this kind of imposed movement, a case that resulted from encephalitis. This woman experienced profound torment associated with the terrible contrast between what her face expressed and what she actually experienced. In the novel *The Man Who Laughed,* Victor Hugo used his imagination to produce something comparable to this pathological condition.

On the other hand, several clinicians have observed the reverse phenomenon (among these are Jackson and Head, to whom psychology owes such a great debt). With a onesided disorder of the visual tuberal, there can be an extremely intense transformation in emotional life. For example, a man who experiences a normal emotional reaction to a stimulus coming from the right side of his body, may experience a disturbed reaction to a stimulus coming from the left. I have had the opportunity to observe several similar cases. If you apply a poltice the right side of the body of this kind of individual, he may experience the usual pleasant sensation. If you apply it to the left, he may experience an immeasurable delight, with the feeling of pleasure increasing to pathological proportions. The same thing may occur when he touches something smooth or something cold. Kretschmer described a patient who had very different experiences depending on the ear with which he heard music,

These studies provide psychological data that support Cannon's position and demonstrate that the anatomical substratum of emotional reactions is apparently a cerebral mechanism located in the subcortical area (more precisely, in the area of the visual tuberal, an area connected by many pathways with the cortical lobes). As a consequence, the cortical-subcortical localization of the emotions has been defined as closely as the localization of the motor speech centers in Broca's[16] sensory speech centers in Wernicke's[17] area.

These studies are also of relevance to psychopathology in the narrow sense of the term, to the pathology of schizophrenia in particular. Bleuler has shown that changes in emotional life are often observed in cases of pathology. In his view, the basic emotions are preserved, but the normal position of these emotions in the individual's spiritual life shifts and changes. The individual is able to react emotionally, but there is a disturbance of consciousness which reflects the fact that the emotions have lost their former structural position in spiritual life, The result is the emergence of a unique system of relationships between thinking and the emotions.

The autistic thinking that Bleuler has studied, and whose existence has been verified by K. Schneider, provides the clearest example of this kind of new psychological system. Autistic thinking has an analogue in normal consciousness, but is itself an expression of a psychopathological state. In autistic thinking, thought is directed not by the tasks the individual faces but by emotional tendencies. As a consequence, autistic thinking is subordinated to the logic of feelings. The way autistic thinking was initially conceptualized was inadequate. Our own thinking, which can be validly contrasted with autistic thinking, is not without its emotional components. Realistic thinking often elicits more significant and intensive emotions than autistic thinking. The investigator working with interest and inspiration on a problem is linked to emotional experiences no less and no more than the schizophrenic immersed in autistic thought. There is a certain synthesis of intellectual and emotional processes in both autistic and realistic thinking, In realistic thinking, however, the emotional process plays a supporting and subordinate role rather than a leading role. In autistic thinking, the emotional process takes the leading role. The intellectual process assumes the supporting role.

In short, contemporary research on autistic thinking has shown that it is a unique psychological system. What is disordered in this system is not the intellectual or emotional processes themselves, but their relationship. Autistic thinking must be compared to the imagination of the adult and child. This will be the topic of our next lecture, where I hope to discuss an extremely important concept. We will see that in the development of emotional life there is a systematic migration or change in the position of the mental function within the system and that this is what determines the significance of the mental function over the entire course of the development of emotional life.

In this way, we will be able to follow a consistent thread from today's lecture to our next. In discussing the theme of imagination, we will be concerned with another concrete psychological system of the kind that we have identified in our analyses of thinking and the emotions. With this I will conclude, postponing theoretical conclusions for the next lecture.

## REFERENCES TO SECTION I

Marx, Karl and Frederick Engels. Sochenenie [Works].
Lenin, V. I. Polnoe sobranoe sochenenie [Complete Collected Works], v. 29.

\* \* \*

Bleuler, E. Autisticheskoe myshlenie [Autistic Thinking], Odessa, 1927.
Borovskii, V.M. Vvedenie v sravnitel'nuiu psikhologiiu [Introduction to Comparative Psychology], Moscow, 1927.
Buehler, K. Dukhovnoe razvitie rebenka [The Spiritual Development of the Child], Kiev, 1916.
Gezell, G.A. Pedologiia rannego vozrasta [Pedology of the Early Ages], MoscowLeningrad, 1932.
Groos, K. Dushevnaia zhizn' rebenka [The Mental Life of the Child], Kiev, 1916.
Dostoevskii, F.M. Dnevnik pisatelia [Diary of a Writer], Leningrad, 1929.
Krechmer, E. "Meditsinskaia psikhologiia myshleniia" [The Contemporary Psychology of Thinking], in: *Novye idei v filosofii* [New Ideas in Philosophy], 1914, No. 16.
Levy-Bruhl, L. Pervobytnoe myshlenie [Primitive Thinking], Moscow, 1930.
Plekhanov, G.V. Izbrannye filosofskie proizvedeniia v 5-ti tom [Selected Philosophical Works in Five Volumes], Moscow, 1956, Volume 1.

Sakharov, L.S. "O medotakh issledovaniia poniatii" [On Methods of Studying Concepts], *Psikltlogiia*, 1930, Volume III.

Tolstoi, L.N. Pedagogicheskie stat'i [Pedagogical Articles], Moscow, 1903.

Tolstoi, L.N. Sobrannie sochinenie v 11-ti t. [Collected Works in 11 Volumes], Moscow, 1983, Volumes 10 and 11.

Uznadze, D.N. Psikhologicheskie issledovaniia [Psychological Investigations], Moscow 1966.

Uspenskii, (G.1. Izbrannye proizvedeniia [Selected Works], Moscow, 1949.

Watson, J. Psikhlogiia kak nauka o povedenii (Psychology as the Science of Behavior], Moscow, 1926.

Folkelt G. Eksperiniental'naia pskhologiia doshol'nika [Experimental Psychology of the Preschooler], Moscow, 1930.

Shif, Zh.I. Razvitie zhiteiskikh i nauchnykh poniatii [The Development of Everyday and Scientific Concepts], Dissertation, Moscow, 1933.

Shif, Zh.1. Razvitie zhiteiskikh i nauchnykh poniatii [The Development of Everyday and Scientific Concepts], Moscow 1935.

Stern, William. Psikhologiia rannego detstva do shestiletnego vozrasts [The Psychology of Early Childhood Prior to the Age of Six], 1922.

Buehler, C. Soziologische und psychologische Studien uber das erste Lebenjahr. Leipzig. 1927.

Buehler K. Abriss der geistigen Entwicklung des Kindes. Leipzig, 1923.

Delacroix H.S. Le langage et la pensée. Paris, 1924.

Frisch K. Die Sprache der Bienen. Wein, 1928.

Hempelmann F. Tierpsychologie vom Standpunktedes biologen, 1926.

Kafka G. Handbuch der vergleichenden Psychologie. Munchen, 1922.

Koffka K. Grundlagen der psychischen Entwicklung. Berlin, 1925. Kohler W. Aus Psychologie des Schimpanzen. Psuch. Forschung, 1921, No. 1.

Kohler W. Intelligenzprufungen und Menschenaffen. Berlin, 1921.

Leamer W.S. A School System as a Educational Library. Cambridge, Mass., 1914.

Lemaitre A. Observations sur le langage interieur des enfants. Archives de Psychologie, 1905, N. 4.

Levy-Bruhl L. Les fonctions mentales dans les societés primatives. Paris 1922.

Meumann E. Die Entstehung der ersten Wortbedeutung beim Kinde. Philosophische Studien, 1928, v. XX.

Piaget, Jean. Le Langage et la pensee chez l'enfant. Paris, 1923.

Piaget, Jean. La causalite physique chez l' enfant. Paris, 1926.

*Piaget, Jean. Judgement and Reasoning in the Child, New York Harcourt, Brace, & Company, 1928.

*Piaget, Jean. The Language and Thought of the Child, London, Routledge & Kegan Paul, 1932a.

Piaget, Jean. Rech' i Myshlenie Rebenka [The Speech and Thinking of the Child], Moscow-Leningrad, 1932b.

Piaget, Jean. Psychologie de l'enseignement de l'histoire. Bulletin trimestriel de la Conference Internationale pour l'enseignement de l'histoire, 1933, N.2.

*Piaget, Jean. The Construction of Reality in the Child, New York, Basic Books, 1927.

*Piaget, Jean. The Child's Conception of Physical Causality, Totowa, New Jersey, Littlefield, Adams & Co., 1966.

Rimat F. Intelligen zu Untersuchungen anschliessend und die Ach'sche Suchmethode, Leipzig, 1925.

Smidt B. Die Sprache und andere Ausdruchformen der Tiere. Berlin, 1923.

Stern W. Person und Sache, I Band. Leipzig, 1905.

Stern C., Stem W. Die Kindersprache. Berlin, 1928.

Thorndike E.R. The Mental Life of Monkeys. N.Y., 1901.

Yerkes R.M. The mental life of monkeys and apes. Behavior Monographs, 1916, III-I.

Yerkes R.M., Learned E.W. Chimpanzee Intelligence and Its Vocal Expression. Baltimore, 1925.

*The bulk of Vygotsky's discussions of Piaget are based on a Russian translation that combined The Language and Thought of the Child and Judgement and Reasoning in the Child into a single volume (e.g., Piaget, Jean. Rech' i Myshlenie Rebenka [The Speech and Thinking of the Child], Moscow-Leningrad 1932). As a consequence, when reading Vygotsky, it is often difficult to know which of these two books by Piaget he is discussing or citing. To facilitate attempts by readers to analyze Vygotsky's discussion of Piaget, we have used the English rather than the Russian translations of Piaget's works for quotations and citations in this volume. The few significant discrepancies between the English and Russian translations are discussed in footnotes.

## Notes (from the Russian Edition) to pp. 33–110

*Thinking and Speech,* from which Chapters 1, 4, and 7 are taken, was published in 1934 and is the best known of Vygotsky's works. It is a summary of the findings of his scientific efforts and an attempt to identify possible directions for further research.

By the end of 1933 and the beginning of 1934, Vygotsky and his colleagues (A.N. Leont'ev, A.R. Luria, A.V. Zaporozhets, L.S. Sakharov, Zh.I. Shif, L.I. Bozhovich, N.G. Morozova, L.S. Slavina, I.M. Solov'ev, L.V. Zankov, E.I. Pashkovskaia, and others) had completed their initial research within the framework of cultural-historical theory. The hypothesis that provided the foundation for this theory, that the higher mental functions are mediated by "psychological tools," had been verified on the basis of material relevant to most of the mental functions (for example, on memory see: A.N. Leont'ev, *Razvitie Pamiati* [The Development of Memory], Moscow, 1931; on attention see: L.S. Vygotsky, "The Problem of the Child's Cultural Development," *Pedalogiia* [pedagogy], 1928, No.1; on thinking see L.S. Sakharov, "Methods for the Study of Concepts," *Psikhologiia* [Psychology], 1930, vol. 3, no. 1; Zh. I. Shif, *Razvitie Nauchnykh Poniatii u Shkol'nika* [The Development of Scientific Concepts in the Schoolchild], Moscow, 1935. All these studies were carried out under Vygotsky's supervision in 1932.). This produced the need to summarize these works and identify prospects for further research.

However, there were also important external circumstances motivating this work. What had formerly been a unified "Vygotskian school" had divided. Leont'ev, Zaporozhets, Bozhovich, and several others had moved to the Ukrainian Psychoneurological Academy in Khar'kov where they had begun to develop their own theoretical program. Because of this, and because of the sharp criticism that was being directed on the basic positions of cultural-historical theory, Vygotsky felt the necessity of explicating his perspectives. This was the purpose of his 1931–1932 manuscript *Istoriia Razviliia Vysshikh Psikhicheskikh Funktsii* [The History of the Development of the Higher Mental Functions] (Part I of this manuscript was published in 1960 in L.S. Vygotsky, *Razvitie Vysshikh Psikhicheskikh Funktsii: Iz Neopublikovannykh Trudov* [The Development of the Higher Mental Functions: from the Unpublished Works]; Part II is published for the first time in the third volume of this collected works), of the conference that had been planned for 1933–1934 to address basic issues in Vygotsky's theory (see: L.S. Vygotsky, "From the Unpublished Materials," in: *Psikhologiia Grammatiki* [The Psychology of Grammar], Moscow, 1968), and of his work *Thinking and Speech.*

*Thinking and Speech* is a collection of Vygotsky's articles that can be viewed as a finished work, unified by a consistent set of problems, methods, and findings. The article "The Genetic Roots of Thinking and Speech (see *Estestvoznanie i Marksizm* [Natural Science and Marxism], 1929, No. 2) was the first in the collection to be written and constitutes the fourth chapter of *Thinking and Speech.* It focuses on Kohler's positions and their relationship to cultural-historical theory, a question that was very important to Vygotsky. An article first published as an introduction to Piaget's book *Rech' i Myshlenie Rebenka* [The Speech and Thinking of the Child] and titled "The Problem of the Speech and Thinking of the Child in Piaget's Theory" constitutes the second chapter of *Thinking and Speech.* This analysis of Piaget's theory was no less significant for Vygotsky than his analysis of Kohler's theory. The fifth chapter of the book,

"The Experimental Investigation of Concept Development," was closely related to the work of Vygotsky's student Sakharov (i.e., "Methods of Investigating Concepts") and to Vygotsky's report to the Leningrad Pedagogical Institute on the 20th of May in 1933, "The Development of Everyday and Scientific Concepts in the School Age" (see L.S. Vygotsky, *Umstvennoe Razvitie Detei v Protsesse Obucheniiia* [The Intellectual Development of Children in the Process of Education], Moscow-Leningrad, 1935).

As Vygotsky notes in the introduction, the remaining chapters of *Thinking and Speech* were written especially for this book, which was completed in 1934. It was reprinted in 1956 in: L.S. Vygotsky, *Izbrannye Psikhologicheskie Issledovaniia* [Selected Psychological Investigations], Moscow. In 1962, it was translated into English and published in the United States, with an introduction by Jerome Bruner and an afterward by Jean Piaget. It has since been published in many foreign languages. For our "Collected Works," we have taken the 1956 edition. This edition was prepared by Leont'ev and Luria with the help of Vygotsky's daughter, G.L Vygodskaya.

1. *The Wurzburg school*—a tradition in the study of the psychology of thinking that developed in the beginning of the 20th century in the psychological institute in Wurzburg, Germany with Kulpe as its founder and Ach and Buhler as its most prominent members. Philosophically, the school relied on the phenomenology of Brentano and Husserl. In its psychology, the school opposed concepts dominating associative psychology at the end of the 19th century that reduced thinking to the combination of representations in accordance with the laws of association. The Wurzburg school argued that imageless thinking is possible. What the individual experiences is not images, but relationships and integral sets. The school developed a series of methods (all forms of refined self observation) for studying of thinking and gathered a large amount of data. The Wurzburg school was very different from Vygotsky both philosophically and methodologically. Their concrete research methods, however, had a unmistakable influence on him. This was particularly true of Ach's research methods (see Chapters 5 and 7 for more detail).

2. This concept of two methods of analysis in accordance with "units" and "elements" was one of Vygotsky's favorite notions. With his example of the isolation of the molecule of water into atoms of hydrogen and oxygen, he first expressed it in *Psikhologii Iskusstva* [The Psychology of Art) in 1923.

3. *Associative psychology* or associationism is a tradition that dominated philosophy and psychology in Europe between the 17th and 19th centuries (T. Hobbes, Spinoza, Locke, Berkeley, Hartley, Mill, Bain, and others). There were a multitude of different schools and varieties of associationism. Hartley's materialistic associationism and Berkeley's idealistic associationism were particularly significant. Associationism began to develop as a tradition of scientific psychology in the 19th century. The presence of the single principle of association is the common feature of all varieties of associationism. All the mental processes (i.e., memory, attention, thinking, and so on) are explained in terms of this single principle. Several different kinds of associations were proposed, association in accordance with contiguity, similarily, and so forth. The 20th century began as a century of crisis for associative psychology, with several new traditions emerging as alternatives. By the time that Thinking arid Speech was written, associative psychology had been completely undermined.

4. *Phonology*—a discipline within linguistics that studies the structure and function of phonemes. Phonology differs from phonetics in that it views phonemes not in physical terms but with respect to their role as components of morphemes or syllables. The emergence of phonology was influenced by the works of de Saussure, Baudouin de Courtenay, and Buhler. As a developed research tradition, phonology emerged in the 1920's and 1930's in the Prague linguistic circle (Trubetzkoy, Jacobson, and others).

5. *Robert Yerkes* (1876–1956)—American psychologist and behaviorist who was a specialist in zoopsychology, comparative psychology, and, in particular, studies of the apes.

6. *Henri Bergson* (1859–1941)—French philosopher, writer, and psychologist who was a member of the French Academy and a Nobel Prize laureate in literature. Bergson was one of the creators of intuitivism and the philosophy of life and had a substantial influence on existentialism. According to Bergson, the primary reality is life, a reality which differs from both matter and spirit. For Bergson, the latter are the product of the disintegration of life. The essence of life can be comprehended only intuitively. In psychology, he created an original conception of memory.

7. *Edward Thorndike* (1874–1949)—American psychologist and the first behaviorist. Specialist in comparative psychology and the psychology of learning. Thorndike formulated a law in accordance with which learning occurs through trial and error and developed a method of studying animal behavior by using a "problem-box" (i.e., a box with a secret mechanism which the animal himself had to "discover").

8. *Vladimir Aleksandrovich Vagner* (1849–1934)—Russian biologist, zoologist, and psychologist and founder of comparative psychology in Russia. Vagner developed the idea of evolution along pure and mixed lines. This idea had a tremendous influence on Vygotsky in the later period of *his* life, with the creation of his conception of functional systems.

9. *Vladimir Makshnovich Borovskii* (1882–?)—Russian psychologist and specialist in animal psychology who later abandoned scientific psychology and took up zoology.

10. *Leonard Hobhouse* (1864–1929)—English zoologist and philosopher who attempted to apply anthropological and physiological data in social research.

11. *Karl Von Frisch* (born 1886)—Austrian physiologist, ethologist, and Nobel Prize laureate who deciphered the mechanism through which bees transmit information.

12. *Charlotte Buhler* (born 1893)—Austrian psychologist, wife and coauthor of Karl Buhler, who was a specialist in child psychology.

13. *Georgii Valentinovich Plekhanov* (1856–1918)—Russian Marxist philosopher and one of the founders of the #RSDRP. In the 1920s, *Plekhanov's* works were extremely popular and were particularly widely used in attempts to construct a Marxist psychology. Vygotsky used them in this connection (see: "The Historical Significance of the Psychological Crisis," *Problems of the Theory and History of Psychology*).

14. *Hellen Keller* (1880–?)—American deaf and blind woman who became a writer.

15. *Rene Descartes* (1596–1650)—French philosopher, psychologist, mathematician, and physiologist. Vygotsky analyzed Descartes' theories in his last unfinished manuscript *"The* Theory of Emotions" *("The* Theory of Spinoza and Descartes on the Passions in Light of Contemporary Psychoneurology," in *Scientific Archive*, also in the Russian Edition of the *Collected Works*, Volume 6).

16. *Ludwig Uhland* (1787–1862)—German romantic poet. The reference here is to the prologue to Uland's historical drama "Ernst, the Duke of Shvabskii" (1818).

17. *Herman Paul* (1846–1921)—German philologist and one of the leaders of what is called the young grammatical or rico-grammatical tradition in philology.

18. *Wilhelm Humboldt* (1767–1835)—German philologist, philosopher, and political activist who founded a school of historical linguistics which, through A. A. Potebnia, had a great influence on Vygotsky.

19. *Vladimir Mikhailovich Bekhterev* (1857–1927)—Russian psychologist, psychiatrist, neuropathologist, physiologist, morphologist and founder of reflexology.

20. *Ivan Mikhailovich Sechenov* (1829–1905)—Russian physiologist and psychologist who developed the theory of interiorization. Vygotsky, like most psychologists of the 1920's, underestimated the significance of Sechenov's ideas for psychology, though he was familiar with his basic works.

21. *Kurt Goldstein* (1878–1965)—German neurologist specializing in aphasia and disturbances in the optical sphere.

22. *Lev Petrovich Yakubinskii* (1892–1945)—Russian linguist and specialist in literature.

23. *Evgenii Dmitrievich Polivanov* (1891–1938)—Russian orientalist and linguist.

24. *Gabriel Tarde* (1843–1904)—French sociologist and criminologist who developed one of the first social-psychological conceptions that placed the individual at the center. According to Tarde, the basic law of social life is imitation.

25. *Fedor Mikhailovich Dostoevskii* (1821–1881)—Russian writer whose work had an extremely strong influence on Vygotsky from his youth (see: *Psikhologiia Iskusstva* [The Psychology of Art], 1968. "Commentary"). Vygotsky wrote a paper on Dostoevskii's work in 1913–1914, but the manuscript has been lost.

26. Vygotsky borrowed the example from Dostoevskii, as he did the following example from Uspenskii, from A.G. Gorifel'd's book The *Torment of the Word* SPB (1906), a book Vygotsky studied in working on his *Psychology of Art*.

27. *Lev Vladimirovich Shcherba* (1880–1944)—Soviet linguist, specialist in literature, and academic who specialized in general linguistics and the Slavic and Romance languages. Shcherba was the founder of the Leningrad phonological school and a student of Baudouin de Courtenay.

28. *Apperception* is a term introduced by Leibnitz. For him, it designated conscious awareness that had still not attained consciousness of impressions. For Kant, it designated the unity of representations in consciousness. In psychology, the concept of apperception occupied a central place in Wundt's system, for which it designated conscious awareness of the perceived, its integral nature, and its dependence on previous experience. In this conception, the idea is related to ideas such as Gestalt and set.

29. *Frederick Paulhan* (1856–1931)—French psychologist who studied issues related to the psychology of the cognitive processes (in particular, thinking, memory, and speech) as well as the psychology of affects. Vygotsky used Polan's work on the psychology of speech.

30. *Gleb Uvanovich Uspenskii* (1843–1902)—Russian writer and revolutionary democrat.

31. The citation, introduced from the poems of A. A. Feta, is an example of secondary citation from the volume: V. N. Voloshinov (1930). *Marxism and the Philosophy of Language*. Moscow.

32. The citation is from N. Gumilev's poem "Word."

33. *Velomir (Viktor Vladimirovich) Kidebnikov* (1885–1922)—Russian futurist poet who coined many new words (in particular, the word "letchik" (i.e. pilot or flyer).

34. *Behaviorism* is a term introduced by James Watson which literally means the "science of behavior." Behaviorism has been an important tradition in American psychology. It emerged in the beginning of the 20th century (with a forefather in Thorndike) and has been dominant to the present time. Born of the struggle with subjective-empirical psychology, which recognized only the method of self observation, behaviorism placed itself in opposition to this tradition as an approach striving to study objective processes (i.e., behavior) through objective methods. Vygotsky was familiar only with the classic Watsonian model of behaviorism, which included the familiar "stimulus-reaction" scheme. In the 1920's, the influence of behaviorism in Soviet psychology was very strong. Vygotsky was therefore frequently obliged to cloth his ideas in behavioristic terminology, in spite of the internal contradictions between his theory and behaviorism. Thus, in his work of 1930, Vygotsky developed a three member scheme that he compared directly with the two member scheme of classic behaviorism (see: "The Instrumental Method in Psychology," *Problems of tlze Theory and History of Psyclzology).* After several years, the neobehaviorism of Tolman and Hull began to be recognized. Here, the two member scheme of classical *behaviorism* was replaced with a three member scheme that included a middle link reflecting the subject's internal state. In spite of the significant external similarity between this and Vygotsky's three member scheme, there was a fundamental methodological difference between them.

35. This is a case of secondary citation. There is reason to think that Vygotsky took this citation not directly from the Gumileds poem but from Mandel'shtam's article "On the Nature of the Word." *This* citation served as the epigraph to the first publication of this article (1922) as a separate brochure, but was removed in latter editions.

36. "In the beginning was the word."—John 1:1.

37. "In the beginning was the deed."—Goethe, Faust, Chapter 1, Scene: "Faust's Workroom."

38. *Ludwig Feuerbach* (1804–1872)—German philosopher. Vygotsky was very familiar with his work, and valued it highly. He felt that Feuerbach's ideas could be used as a point of departure for the construction of a Marxist materialistic psychology (see: "The Historical Significance of the Psychological Crisis," Section III).

## Notes (from the Russian Edition) to pp. 111–138

1. This work is a stenogram of lectures read by Vygotsky in March and April of 1932 at the Leningrad Pedagogical Institute. Lecture 4 ("Emotions and Their Development in Childhood") was published in *Voprosy Psikhologii* [Issues in Psychology] (1959, No.3). All the lectures were published in the book: L. S. Vygotsky, *Razvitie Vysshikh Psikhicheskikh Funktsii* [*The Development of the Higher Mental Functions*], Moscow, 1960. Our edition is based on a collation of the A. I. Gertsen Leningrad Federal Pedagogical Institute [LGPI]. The lectures represent a complete course and can be viewed as a synopsis of Vygotsky's basic views as well as of

the findings obtained by Vygotsky and his colleagues within the framework provided by the cultural-historical theory.

2. Gestalt Psychology (Gestaltism, structural psychology). The term was introduced by Christian von Ehrenfels. A school of general psychology, Gestalt psychology initially emerged with an analysis of the processes of perception, where several new phenomena were discovered and explained with these theses (M. Wertheimer). Subsequently,the attempt was made to extend this explanatory scheme to the processes of problem solving (K. Duncker), the phytogenesis (Kohler) and ontogenesis (Koffka) of thinking, and the analysis of the psychology of personality and the motivational sphere (Lewin). In the 1930's, with the Nazi's rise to power in Germany, the leading figures in the school emigrated. This served as an external stimulus to the school's disintegration toward the end of the 1930's. Gestalt psychology (along with the French school) apparently had tremendous influence on Vygotsky. The most attractive aspect of Gestalt psychology for Vygotsky was its attempt to approach all mental phenomena with the assumption of their integral nature. In distinction from the Gestalt psychologists, however, Vygotsky always combined this view of the nature of mental phenomena as integral with a historical approach to the analysis of mind (it was, at any rate, always his intention to combine thses perspectives).

3. *Kurt Gottschaldht* (1902–?)—German psychologist specializing in child psychology.

4. *Hermann Helmholtz* (1821–1894)—German physiologist, anatomist, and psychologist who developed theories of vision and hearing.

5. *Ewald Hering* (1834–1918)—One of the founders of experimental physiological psychology who developed theories of vision and hearing in opposition to those of Helmholtz. Hering discovered an optical illusion known as "the Hering illusion."

6. *Herman Rorschach* (1884–1922)—Swiss psychologist and psychiatrist who developed a widely known projective test that is commonly called the "inkspot" or "Rorschach" test.

7. *Alfred Binet* (1857–1911)—French psychologist and one of the pioneers of experimental studies of the higher mental functions, in particular, thinking and memory. his later works had a special significance for Vygotsky (see: "The Problem of the Cultural Development of the Child." Pedalogiia [Pedagogy], 1928, No.1). Binet was a specialist in testing, working in the domain of measuring the level of mental development.

8. *Jean Demor* (1867–1941)—Belgian doctor and pedagogue specializing in the education of the mentally retarded.

9. *Herbert Spencer* (1920–1930)—English philosopher and sociologist and one of the founders of positivism. Spencer specialized in the study of primitive cultures.

10. *Theodule Ribot* (1839-1916)—French psychologist specializing in pathological and general psychology who worked in the domains of the psychology of memory and voluntary attention.

11. *Nikolai Nikolaevich Lange* (1858–1921)—Russian psychologist concerned with psychological methodology, general psychology, and the psychology of attention. His antidualistic tendencies were compatible with Vygotsky's views (see: "The Historical Significance of the Psychological Crisis," *Problems of the Theory and History of Psychology*)[1].

12. *Walter Cannon* (1871–1945)—American physiologist specializing in the mechanisms of emotional behavior who asserted the unity on neurohumoral regulation.

13. *Boris Mikhailovich Zavadovskii* (1895–1951)—Soviet biologist and academician. Zavadovskii was a specialist in Darwinism, the methodology of biology, and the internal secretion of the glands.

14. *Vladimir Leonidovich Durov* (1863–1934)—Russian circus artist, clown, wild animal trainer, and creator of the new Russian school of training. Durov was a practical specialist in zoopsychology.

15. *Alfred Adler* (1870–1937)—German doctor and psychologist who developed a system of individual psychology. Adler's interpretation of the role of inclinations in mental life was similar to that of Freud. The concept of compensation, understood as a universal mechanism in man's mental activity, had a central place in his psychological system.

16. *Paul Broca* (1824–1880)—French anatomist and one of the founders of modern anthropology—[Soviet anthropology corresponds essentially with American *physical* anthropology-Eds.]—who described speech disorders connected with disease in certain areas of the brain. (Broca's area).

17. *Carl Wernicke* (1848–1936)—German philosopher, musicologist, psychiatrist, neuropathologist, and neuroanatomist who developed the classic theory of aphasia. Wernicke also described the syndrome of alcoholic hallucinations.

## Notes (from the English Edition), pp. 33–141

The following notes, which are designated in the text by Arabic numerals between brackets (e.g.[ 1]), were provided by the translator and editors.

[1]. Western scholars seem to be at variance with our Soviet colleagues in believing that the Lange of the James-Lange theory was C. G. Lange, a Norwegian and not a Russian, as notes to the Russian edition suggest. See Boring, E. G. *A History of Experimental Psychology* (1929) New York, D. Appleton-Century, page 532 where a paper by Lange, "Concerning Emotion" (1885) in Norwegian which was translated into German is cited.

[3]. Vygotsky may have had in mind the experiments such as those by Jacobsson, L. E. "The Electrophysiology of Mental Activities." *American Journal of Psychology,* 1932, vol. 44, pp. 677–694. These experiments on imagining and verbal thinking were replicated and extended by Max, L. W. in, among others, "An Experimental Study of the Motor Theory of Consciousness. III. Action-current Responses in Deaf-mutes during Sleep, Sensory Stimulation and Dreams." *Journal of Comparative Psychology,* 1935, vol 1.9, pp. 469–486. (The editors' access to these references in through Crafts, L. W. Schneirla, T. C., Robinson, E. E., and Gilbert, R. W. (Editors) *Recent Experiments in Psychology* (1938) New York: McGraw-Hill, whence the foregoing references were obtained.

[4]. A thoroughgoing example of how such Hegelian-Marxist concepts as "the dialectial leap" can be appried to a wide range of natural phenomena is provided in Engels' The *Dialectics of Nature.* Though Vygotsky was not precisely an orthodox, doctrinaire Marxist this passage is one of many illustrating his creative use of the concepts of dialectical materialism and his unambiguously socialistic orientation in the formulation of his psychological, psycholinguistic, and educational concepts.

[9]. The term "speech" is used here in the sense discussed in our Preface. Speech for the structuralist linguist and, obviously for Vygotsky, was the primary form of language. As the passage continues it becomes quite clear that it is the special characteristics of speech as a method of thought and communication which Vygotsky has in mind and not the more circumscribed definition of which others might ascribe to; namely the motor acts of the vocal tract which accompany linguistic communication. The use of the word speech in the sense described leads to certain surprising results. Later in the present text it yields the expression "written speech," which is a literal rendering of pis'meny rech.' Vygotsky seems intentionally not to have used the word "writing," possibly because to him and to the early structuralist linguists, writing was regarded only as a form of notation for speech; not a form of communication in its own right. The concept of "written speech" which is developed in Chapter 7 as a special kind of mental formulation occurring when situational and expressive supports are lacking, i.e., the kind verbal thinking which is responsive to the pragmatic constraints imposed by the writing process is, clearly, to be distinguished from "writing" in the sense of notation for speech. Further, Vygotsky's understanding of the term "speech" leads to the suggestion that the function of speech can be assumed by other forms of communication. Thus Vygotsky in the present chapter clearly anticipates a series of experiments which followed some forty years later. In those studies, after Liberman's demonstration that the vocal tract of chimpanzees was not suited to the production of complex speech sounds, Gardner, Premak, Terrace, and others then attempted to discern and demonstrate that the functions of speech could be taken up by other organs (such as the hands using American sign language) or other devices (such as "joy sticks" or abstract tokens to which significanda were assigned) for communication. The reference, later in the chapter, to the sign language of the deaf follows the same vein and is equally contemporary in its outlook.

# II

# Fundamentals of Defectology (Abnormal Psychology and Learning Disabilities)

DAVID K. ROBINSON, *Truman State University*

*Defectology* is a word that does not fit the demands for euphemistic expressions that reign in the United States today. (Its more expansive cousin, *pedology*, sounds even worse!) In Russia and the Soviet Union, however, when the term *defectology* appeared early in the twentieth century, it represented quite a stride forward in scholarly study and humanitarian treatment of children (and others) who were suffering from learning disabilities. Although Vygotsky is remembered today mostly for his contributions to psycholinguistics and developmental psychology, his work in what we now call special education is also of great historical significance: it was the field of his most intensive activity when he first began his career in Moscow, and this work had important influences on the formation of his general theories. Jane E. Knox and Carol B. Stevens (1993), translators of Volume 2 of *Collected Works*, have made this argument persuasively.

After Vygotsky received his law degree in Moscow in 1917, he returned to his hometown of Gomel, Belarus, to teach psychology and literature in the normal school, which trained teachers. Some biographers credit him with opening a psychological laboratory there and working with handicapped students. Other writers note that Gomel actually had a home for the handicapped, not a very common institution in that part of the world at the time. There is, however, no direct evidence that Vygotsky took advantage of that resource in his studies, and Vygotsky did not publish on special education in the Gomel period, when his articles mostly concerned literature and, occasionally, psychology.

The problem of the handicapped had received little official attention during the imperial period of Russian history, but the ravages of the World War and its aftermaths burdened the young Soviet Union with up to seven million homeless children, many of whom were orphaned, disabled, and/or antisocial. At the end of the Civil War, therefore, as famine and disease still ravaged the cities and the countryside, the Commissariat of Education (NarKomPros, led by A. Lunacharsky) established the Section for Social and Legal Protection of Minors (SPON, in the Russian acronym) in 1923. Soon after Vygotsky joined the Moscow Institute of Psychology in 1924, he also joined SPON as head of a subsection devoted to the education of physically handicapped and otherwise "difficult" children. By all accounts Vygotsky was remarkably successful working with the children, as well as with his co-workers.

In 1925 or 1926, Vygotsky was able to organize a laboratory/clinic for the study of abnormal children at the Medical Pedagogical Station in Moscow, and later he was made associate director of the Defectological Section of the Pedagogical Faculty of the Second Moscow State University. Vygotsky's aggregation of titles might possibly indicate his rise to prominence (as it would have in the French academic system); more likely the plethora of titles was simply a symptom of the inspired, but chaotic, early Soviet expansion of institutions during the 1920s. Suffice it to say, Vygotsky was fully engaged with disabled children of various kinds, working closely with specialists who were devoted to educating and helping them, and this work began to influence his thinking about psychology in general. Veresov (1999) makes the case that studies in defectology, combined with his earlier engagement in literary studies, led Vygotsky to the theoretical breakthroughs in *Crisis* and later writings (see Section III of the present volume). So how does Vygotsky represent the learning problems (and indeed successes) of these special children, and how did this work contribute to his broader theories?

The articles on defectology included in this volume give a fair picture of Vygotsky's work in the field and of the theoretical background against which he developed it. (Extensive discussions of experiments, however, are not included here or anywhere else in *Collected Works*.) "Introduction: The Fundamental Problems of Defectology" is a programmatic report of the Defectological Section of the Second Moscow State University, published in 1929. The discussion highlights the approach of Vygotsky and his colleagues compared to prominent foreign theorists on education and child development, particularly the Germans, William Stern and Alfred Adler (famous for "inferiority complex"). However, the most interesting moments are revelations of the humanity and creativity of Vygotsky's approach, one that emphasized qualitative over quantitative measures. "The thesis holds that a child whose development is impeded by a defect is not simply a child less developed than his peers but is a child who has developed differently" (p. 31). "The course created by a defect—that of compensation—is the major course of development for a child with a physical handicap or functional disability" (p.34). "The history of cultural development in an abnormal child constitutes the most profound and critical problem in modern defectology. It opens up a completely *new line of development* in scientific research (p. 42 emphasis in original).

Vygotsky's optimistic approach makes it somewhat easier for the general reader to deal with the dreary classification of deficiencies that are discussed in the essay: mental retardation, deafness, blindness, etc., as well as some new categories, such as motor disability, moral insanity, and even a special Russian term, the "difficult" child. Vygotsky's attitude is even more impressive when the reader notices that he frequently draws a parallel between learning disabilities and a particular biological disease, tuberculosis—a person can live with it if the body can compensate. Of course, this is what Vygotsky himself had to do, and was able to do for a few years.

Vygotsky's report insists that special (auxiliary) schools are needed, where specially trained teachers can help the special children. The compensatory mechanisms can function in positive ways (progressive development) or in negative directions (heightened sensitivity, inferiority complex, antisocial behavior), and "more teaching" is needed to help the pupils along the positive track. Compensation can even lead to superior development, as in the case of Helen Keller. Nevertheless, the ways to help the child to compensate positively are not always obvious or directly intuitive. If the child is deficient in abstract thought, for example, his teachers would actually be wrong to rely too much on visual aids, as that method could hinder the needed development of abstract thought. The auxiliary school should have a "creative character"; it should be "a school of social compensation, of socialization" (p.50). Vygotsky's prescriptions for these schools give a flavor of the concepts for which he is now well known—the cultural–historical approach, scaffolding, the unity of affect and intellect, and the Zone of Proximal Development–though he did not yet use those exact terms.

The essays on educating blind, deaf-mute, and retarded children are all available in Volume 2 of *Collected Works;* in the present volume we reproduce the remarkable article "The Difficult Child" to illustrate the breadth of Vygotsky's conceptualization of disability. The Russian word *trudny* implies "hard to deal with" or "difficult to raise"–a child that imposes almost unexplainable difficulties on those who are involved with her. Vygotsky supposes that the origins of such a tendency could be anything, from subtle physical deficiencies (poor hearing, for example) to giftedness. By discussing giftedness as a kind of handicap, Vygotsky emphasizes that defectology is mainly about social problems within social environments, not so much about the handicaps themselves.

In "The Dynamics of Child Character" Vygotsky explores a common term that enjoyed little attention in psychological theory concerning pedagogical practice. Vygotsky understands character in terms of social process, rather than as a state or condition, and he compares his conception with those of Adler, Pavlov, Freud, and others. The final essay here in Section II, "The Collective as a Factor in the Development of the Abnormal Child," invokes a theme that was broadly advocated in Soviet ideology concerning work and education. Vygotsky explores collaboration between abnormal children, as well as their interaction with teachers and other caregivers. There is considerable discussion of Piaget's notion of egocentric speech, and Vygotsky's concept of inner speech, a distinction that is explored more fully in Section I of the present work. Again Vygotsky points toward the promise of improvement: " . . . unlike the defect itself, which is a factor in the failure of the elementary function's development, the collective, as a factor in the development of the higher psychological functions, is something that we can control" (p.199). It is important to educate the handicapped, but it is even more important to reeducate the broader society.

Vygotsky's program of defectology was surely one of the most impressive and promising parts of the wider Soviet program in pedology, which had aspirations to modernize society and sweep away many old problems and injustices. By 1931, however, Communist activists were demanding more doctrinaire adherence to Marxism and were less willing to tolerate constructive references to foreign "bourgeois" scholars. These Party loyalists grew impatient in the face of persistent problems, especially concerning education and other indicators of lagging progress that the specialists liked to discuss. Some charged that pedology's programs in educational testing were only producing new problems for children, problems that had not even existed before. In 1933 Lunacharsky was removed as Commissar of Education, replaced by someone with less interest in modernization, and by 1934 Stalin started purging his Party leadership. That was also the year that Vygotsky died of tuberculosis. In 1936, the Central Committee of the Communist Party decreed that pedology was a "pseudoscience." This work, whose experimental and observational techniques took account of both heredity and environment, and which derived so much from Western methods of social science and might well have contributed to them eventually, was officially and almost totally abolished in the Soviet Union. Leaders such as P. P. Blonsky and A. B. Zalkind paid for their advocacy with their lives. Others managed to move out of the way, to Ukraine or Uzbekistan. As part of the general pedological movement, defectology suffered too, in spite of Vygotsky's criticism of quantitative testing, and the Moscow Institute of Psychology took the full brunt of the purge. Only after Stalin's death did institutions devoted to psychological research begin slowly to reemerge in Moscow, where the Experimental Defectological Institute carried on Vygotsky's work in special education, at least in theory (Bein *et al.*, 1993).

Though Vygotsky was dead, his ideas certainly were not. The general psychological theories that arose in connection with the work in defectology have probably never been more influential than they are today. His characterization of how children learn, indeed how damaged and deficient children compensate to continue to develop their activities and build fulfilling lives, could also stand as a metaphor for Russian psychology, even for Russian society.

# References

Bein, E. S., Vlasova, T. A., Levina, R. E., Morozova, N. G., & Shif, Zh. I. (1993). Afterword. In *Collected works, Volume 2: The fundamentals of defectology (abnormal psychology and learning disabilities)* (R. W. Rieber & A. S. Carton, Eds.; pp. 302–314). New York: Kluwer Academic/Plenum.

Knox, J. E. (1989). The changing face of Soviet defectology: A study in rehabilitating the handicapped. *Studies in Soviet Thought, 37,* 217–236.

Knox, J. E., & Stevens, C. (1993). Vygotsky and Soviet Russian defectology: An introduction. In *Collected works, Volume 2: The fundamentals of defectology (abnormal psychology and learning disabilities)* (R. W. Rieber & A. S. Carton, Eds.; pp. 1–25). New York: Kluwer Academic/Plenum.

McCagg, W. O., & Siegelbaum, L. (Eds.) (1989). *The disabled in the Soviet Union: Past and present theory and practice.* Pittsburgh: University of Pittsburgh Press.

Veresov, N. N. (1999). *Undiscovered Vygotsky: Etudes on the pre-history of cultural-historical psychology.* European Studies in the History of Science and Ideas, vol. 8. Frankfurt-am-Main: Peter Lang.

Vygotsky, L. S. (1993). *Collected works, Volume 2: The fundamentals of defectology (abnormal psychology and learning disabilities)* (R. W. Rieber & A. S. Carton, Eds.). New York: Kluwer Academic/Plenum.

Yoo, Y. (Ed.). (1980) *Soviet education: An annotated bibliography and reader's guide to works in English.* Westport, CT: Greenwood Press.

# 6

# Introduction
## *The Fundamental Problems of Defectology*

### 1

Only recently, the entire field of theoretical knowledge and practical scientific work, which we conveniently call by the name of "defectology," was viewed as a minor part of pedagogy, not unlike how medicine views minor surgery. All the problems in this field have been posed and resolved as quantitative problems. Entirely accurately, M. Kruenegel states that the prevailing psychological methods for studying an abnormal child (A. Binet's metric scale or G. I. Rossolimo's profile) are based on a purely quantitative conception of childhood development as impeded by a defect (M. Kruenegel, 1926). These methods determine the degree to which the intellect is lowered, without characterizing either the defect itself or the inner structure of the personality created by it. According to O. Lipmann, these methods may be called measurement, but not an examination of ability, *Intelligenzmessungen* but not *Intelligenzpruefungen* (O. Lipmann, H. Bogen, 1923), since they establish the degree, but neither the kind nor the character of ability (O. Lipmann, 1924).

Other pedological methods for studying the handicapped child are also correct and relevant—not only psychological methods, but also those encompassing other sides of a child's development (anatomical and physiological). And here, scale and measure have become the basic categories of research, as if all problems of defectology were but problems of proportion, and as though all the diverse phenomena studied in defectology could be encompassed by a single scheme: "more versus less." In defectology, counting and measuring came before experimentation, observation, analysis, generalization, description, and qualitative diagnosis.

Practical defectology likewise chose the simplest course, that of numbers and measures, and attempted to realize itself as a minor pedagogical field. If, in theory, the problem was reduced to a quantitatively limited, proportionally retarded development, then, in practice, the idea of simplified and decelerated instruction naturally was advanced. In Germany, the very same Kruenegel, and in our country A. S. Griboedov, rightly defend the notion: "A reexamination of the curriculum and methods of instruction used in our auxiliary schools is essential" (A. S. Griboedov, 1926, p. 28), since "a reduction of educational material and a prolongation of its study time" (ibid.)—that is, purely quantitative indicators-have constituted until this time the only distinctive features of the special school.

Originally appeared in English translation as Introduction to Part I in *The Collected Works of L.S. Vygotsky, Volume 2: The Fundamentals of Defectology (Abnormal Psychology and Learning Disabilities)* (Robert W. Rieber and Aaron S. Carton, Eds.; Jane E. Knox and Carol B. Stevens, Trans.) (pp. 29–51). New York: Plenum Press, 1993.

A purely arithmetical conception of a handicapped condition is characteristic of an obsolete, old-school defectology. Reaction against this quantitative approach to all theoretical and practical problems is the most important characteristic of modern defectology. The struggle between these two attitudes toward defectology—between two antithetical ideas, two principles—is the burning issue in that positive crisis which this area of scientific knowledge is presently undergoing.

Viewing a handicapped condition as a purely quantitative developmental limitation undoubtedly has the same conceptual basis as the peculiar theory of preformed childhood operations, according to which post-natal childhood development is reduced exclusively to quantitative growth and to the expansion of organic and psychological functions. Defectology is currently undertaking a theoretical task which is analogous to the one once performed by pedology and child psychology, when both defended the position that a child is not simply a small adult. Defectology is now contending for a fundamental thesis, the defense of which is its sole justification for existence as a science. The thesis holds that a child whose development is impeded by a defect is not simply a child less developed than his peers but is a child who has developed differently.

If we subtract visual perception and all that relates to it from our psychology, the result of this subtraction will not be the psychology of a blind child. In the same way, the deaf child is not a normal child minus his hearing and speech. Pedology has long ago mastered the idea that if viewed from a qualitative perspective, the process of child development is, in the words of W. Stern, "a chain of metamorphoses" (1922). Defectology is currently developing a similar idea. A child in each stage of his development, in each of his phases, represents a qualitative uniqueness, i.e., a specific organic and psychological structure; in precisely the same way, a handicapped child represents a qualitatively different, unique type of development. Just as oxygen and hydrogen produce not a mixture of gases, but water, so too, says Guertler, the personality of a retarded child is something qualitatively different than simply the sum of underdeveloped functions and properties.

The specific organic and psychological structure, the type of development and personality, and not qualitative proportions, distinguish a retarded child from a normal one. Did not child psychology long ago grasp the deep and true similarities between the many developmental processes in a child and the transformation of a caterpillar first into a chrysalis and from a chrysalis into a butterfly? Now, through Guertler, defectology has voiced the view that a child's retardation is a particular variety or special type of development, and not a quantitative variant of the normal type. These, he states, are different organic forms, not unlike a tadpole and a frog (R. Guertler, 1927).

There is, actually, complete correspondence between the particular characteristic of each age-level in the development of a child and the particular characteristics of different types of development. Just as the transition from crawling to walking, and from babble to speech, is a metamorphosis (i.e., a qualitative transformation from one form into another) in the same way, the speech of a deaf-mute child and the thought processes of an imbecile are functions qualitatively different from the speech and thought processes of normal children. Only with this idea of qualitative uniqueness (rather than the overworked quantitative variations of separate elements) in the phenomena and processes under examination, does defectology acquire, for the first time, a firm methodological basis. But no theory is possible if it proceeds from exclusively negative premises, just as no educational practice can be based on purely negative definitions and fundamentals. This notion is methodologically central to modern defectology, and one's attitude toward this notion determines the exact position of a particular, concrete problem. Defectology acquires, with this idea, a whole system of positive tasks, both theoretical and practical. The field of defectology becomes viable as a science because it has assumed a particular method and defined its object for research and understanding. As B. Schmidt [no ref.] put it, only "pedological anarchy" can follow from a purely quantitative conception of juvenile handicaps, and programs of treatment and remediation can be based only on uncoordinated compendia of empirical data and techniques and not upon systematic scientific knowledge.

It would be a great mistake, however, to think that with the discovery of this idea the methodological* formation of a new defectology is complete. On the contrary, it has only just begun. As soon as the possibility of a particular perspective on scientific knowledge is determined, then the tendency arises to search for its philosophical foundations. Such a search is extremely characteristic of modern defectology and is an indication of its scientific maturity. As soon as the uniqueness of the phenomena being studied by defectologists has been asserted, the philosophical questions immediately arise: that is, questions of principles and methods of knowledge and examination of this uniqueness. R. Guertler has attempted to establish a basis for defectology in an idealistic philosophy (R. Guertler, 1927). H. Noell based his discussion of the particular problem of vocational training for students in auxiliary schools on the modern "philosophy of value," developed by W. Stern, A. Messer (1906, 1908), Meinung,[†] H. Rickert, and others. If such attempts are still relatively rare, then the tendency toward some philosophical formulation is easily detected in almost any significant new scientific work on defectology.

Apart from this tendency toward philosophical formulations, absolutely concrete separate problems face defectology. Their solution constitutes the major goal of research projects in defectology.

Defectology has its own particular analytical objective and must master it. The processes of childhood development being studied by defectology represent an enormous diversity of forms, almost a limitless number of types. Science must master this particularity and explain it, as well as establish the cycles and transformations of development, its imbalances and shifting centers, and discover the laws of diversity. Further, there is the practical problem of how to master the laws of development.

This chapter attempts to outline critically the fundamental processes of defectology in their intrinsic relationship and unity from the point of view of those philosophical ideas and social premises, assumed to be the basis of our educational theory and practice.


2


The dual role of a physical disability, first in the developmental process and then in the formation of the child's personality, is a fundamental fact with which we must deal when development

---

* The term methodological means here a general method of inquiry and is closer to scientific epistemology. [Tr.]

† Possibly, a reference to Alexius Meinong (1853–1920), who was concerned with a theory of knowledge at Vienna and Graz. [Ed.]

is complicated by a defect. On the one hand, the defect means a minus, a limitation, a weakness, a delay in development; on the other, it stimulates a heightened, intensified advancement, precisely because it creates difficulties. The position of modern defectology is the following: Any defect creates stimuli for compensatory process. Therefore, defectologists cannot limit their dynamic study of a handicapped child to determining the degree and severity of the deficiency. Without fail, they must take into account the compensatory processes in a child's development and behavior, which substitute for, supersede, and overarch the defect. Just as the patient—and not the disease—is important for modern medicine, so the child burdened with the defect—not the defect in and of itself—becomes the focus of concern for defectology. Tuberculosis*, for example, is diagnosed not only by the stage and severity of the illness, but also by the physical reaction to the disease, by the degree to which the process is or is not compensated for. Thus, the child's physical and psychological reaction to the handicap is the central and basic problem—indeed, the sole reality—with which defectology deals.

A long time ago, W. Stern pointed out the dual role played by a defect. Thus, the blind child compensates with an increased ability to distinguish through touch—not only by actually increasing the stimulability of his nerves, but by exercising his ability to observe, estimate, and ponder differences. So, too, in the area of psychological functions, the decreased value of one faculty may be fully or partially compensated for by the stronger development of another. For example, the cultivation of comprehension may replace keenness of observation and recollection, compensating for a poor memory. Impressionability, the tendency to imitate, and so forth compensate for weakness of motivation and inadequate initiative. The functions of personality are not so exclusive that, given the abnormally weak development of one characteristic, the task performed by it necessarily and in all circumstances suffers. Thanks to the organic unity of personality, another faculty undertakes to accomplish the task (W. Stern, 1921).

In this way we can apply the law of compensation equally to normal and abnormal development. T. Lipps saw in this a fundamental law of mental life: if a mental event is interrupted or impeded, then an "overflow" (that is, an increase of psychological energy) occurs at the point of interruption or obstruction. The obstruction plays the role of a dam. This law Lipps named the law of psychological damming up or stowage *(Stauung)*. Energy is concentrated at that point where the process met with delay, and it may overcome the delay or proceed by roundabout ways. Thus, in place of delayed developmental processes, new processes are generated due to the blockage (T. Lipps, 1907).

A.Adler and his school posit as the basis of their psychological system the study of abnormal organs and functions, the inadequacy of which constantly stimulates an intensified (higher) development. According to Adler, awareness of a physically handicapped condition is, for the individual, a constant stimulation of mental development. If any organ, because of a morphological or functional deficiency, does not fully cope with its task, then the central human nervous and mental apparatus compensates for the organ's deficient operation by creating a psychological superstructure which shores up the entire deficient organism at its weakened, threatened point. Conflict arises from contact with the exterior milieu; conflict is caused by the incompatibility of the deficient organ or function and the task before it. This conflict, in turn, leads to an increased possibility of illness and fatality. The same conflict may also create greater potentialities and stimuli for compensation and even for over-compensation. Thus, defect becomes the starting point and the principal motivating force in the psychological development of personality. It establishes the target point, toward which the development of all psychological forces strive. It gives direction to the process of growth and to the formation of personality. A handicap creates a higher developmental tendency; it enhances such mental phenomena as foresight and presentiment, as well as their operational elements (memory, attention, intuition, sensibility, interest)—in a word, all supporting psychological features (A. Adler, 1928).

We may not and *ought* not agree with Adler when he ascribes to the compensatory process a universal significance for all mental development. But, there is no contemporary defectologist, it seems, who would not ascribe paramount importance to the effect of personality on a defect or to the adaptive developmental processes, i.e., to that extremely complex picture of a defect's positive effects, including the roundabout course of development with its complicated zigzags. This is a picture which we observe in every child with a defect. Most important is the fact that along with a physical handicap come strengths and attempts both to overcome and to equalize the handicap. These tendencies toward higher development were not formerly recognized by defectology. Meanwhile, precisely these tendencies give uniqueness to the development of the handicapped child; they foster creative, unendingly diverse, sometimes profoundly eccentric forms of development, which we do not observe in the typical development of the normal child. It is not necessary to be an Adlerite and to share the principles of his school in order to recognize the correctness of this position.

"He will want to see everything," Adler says about a child, "if he is nearsighted; to hear everything, if he is hearing impaired; he will want to say everything, if he has an obvious speech defect or a stutter. . . . The desire to fly will be most apparent in those children who experience great difficulty even in jumping. The contrast between the physical disability and the desires, fantasies, dreams, i.e., psychological drives to compensate, are so universal that one may base upon this *a fundamental law." Via subjective feelings of inadequacy, a physical handicap dialectically transforms itself into psychological drives toward compensation and overcompensation"* (1927, p. 57). Formerly, it was believed that the entire life and development of a blind child would be flamed by blindness. The new law states that development will go against this course. If blindness exists, then mental development will be directed away from blindness, against blindness. Goal-oriented reflexes, according to I. P. Pavlov, need a certain tension to achieve full, proper, fruitful development. The existence of obstacles is a principal condition for goal achievement (1951, p. 302). Modern psychotechnics is inclined to consider control [or self-direction] to be a function so central to the educational process and to the formation of personality as a special case of the phenomena of overcompensation (J. N. Spielrein, 1924).

The study of compensation reveals the creative character of development directed along this course. It is not in vain that such psychologists as Stern and Adler partly based the origins of giftedness on this understanding. Stern formulates the idea as follows: "What does not destroy me, makes me stronger; thanks to adaptation, strength arises from weakness, ability from deficiencies" (W. Stern, 1923, p. 145).

It would be a mistake to assume that the process of compensation always, without fail, ends in success, that it always leads from the defect to the formation of a new capability. As with every process of overcoming and struggle, compensation may also have two extreme outcomes—victory and failure—and between these two are all possible transitional points.

The outcome depends on many things, but basically, it depends on the relationship between (1) the severity of the defect and (2) the wealth of compensatory reserves. But whatever the anticipated outcome, *always and in all circumstances,* development, complicated by a defect, represents a creative (physical and psychological) process. It represents the creation and re-creation of a child's personality based on the restructuring of all the adaptive functions and on the formation of new processes—overarching, substituting, equalizing—generated by the handicap, and creating new, roundabout paths for development. Defectology is faced with a world of new, infinitely diverse forms and courses of development. The course created by a defect—that of compensation—is the major course of development for a child with a physical handicap or functional disability.

The positive uniqueness of the handicapped child is created not by the failure of one or another function observed in a normal child but by the new formations caused by this lapse. This uniquely individual reaction to a defect represents a continually evolving adaptive process. If a blind or deaf child achieves the same level of development as a normal child, then the child with a defect achieves this *in another way, by another course, by other means.* And, for the pedagogue, it is particularly important to know the *uniqueness* of the course, along which he must lead the child. The key to originality transforms the minus of the handicap into the plus of compensation.

### 3

There are limits to uniqueness in the development of handicapped children. The entire adaptive system is restructured on new bases when the defect destroys the equilibrium that exists among the adaptive functions; then, the whole system tends towards a new equilibrium. Compensation, the individual's reaction to a defect, initiates new, roundabout developmental processes—it replaces, rebuilds a new structure, and stabilizes psychological functions. Much of what is inherent in normal development disappears or is curtailed because of a defect. A new, special kind of development results. "Parallel to the awakening of my consciousness," A.M. Shcherbina tells us about himself, "was the gradual, organic elaboration of my psychic uniqueness. Under such conditions, I could not *spontaneously* sense my physical shortcomings" (1916, p. 10). But the social milieu in which the developmental process occurs place limits on organic uniqueness and on the creation of a "second nature." K. Buerklen formulated this idea beautifully as it applies to the psychological development of the blind. In essence, this idea may be extended to all of defectology. "They develop special features," he said about the blind, "which we cannot observe among the seeing. We must suppose that if the blind associated only with the blind and had no dealings with the seeing then a special kind of people would come into being" (K. Buerklen, 1924, p. 3).

Buerklen's views can be elaborated as follows: Blindness, as a physical handicap, gives impetus to compensatory processes. These, in turn, lead to the formation of unique features in a blind person's psychology and to the reformulation of all his various functions, when directed toward a basic, vital task. Each individual function of a blind person's neuropsychological apparatus has unique features, often very marked in comparison with those of a seeing person. In the event that a blind person were to live only among blind people, these biological processes, which formulate and accumulate special features and abnormal deviations, would, when left alone, inevitably lead to the creation of a new stock of people. Notwithstanding, under pressure from social demands, which are identical for the seeing and the blind, the development of these special features takes a form in which the structure of a blind person's personality *as a whole* will tend to achieve a specific, normal social type.

The compensatory processes which create unique personality features in a blind child do not develop freely. Rather, they are devoted to a specific end. Two basic factors shape this social conditioning of a handicapped child's development.

First, the effect of the defect itself invariably turns out to be secondary, rather than direct. As we have already said, the child is not directly aware of his handicap. Instead, he is aware of the difficulties deriving from the defect. The immediate consequence of the defect is to diminish the child's social standing; the defect manifests itself as a social aberration. All contact with people, all situations which define a person's place in the social sphere, his role and fate as a participant in life, all the social functions of daily life are reordered. As emphasized in Adler's school of thought, the organic, inherent (congenital) causes of this reordering operate neither independently nor directly, but indirectly, via their negative effect on a child's social position. All hereditary and organic factors must also be interpreted psychologically, so that their true role in a child's development can be taken into consideration. According to Adler, a physical disability which leads to adaptation creates a special psychological position for a child. It is through that special position, and only through it, that a defect affects a child's development. Adler calls the psychological complex, which develops as a result of the child's diminished social position due to his handicap, an "inferiority complex" *(Minderwertigkeitsgefuehl).* * This introduces a third, intermediate factor into the dyadic process of "handicap compensation" so that it becomes "handicap inferiority complex compensation." The handicap, then, evokes its compensation not directly but indirectly, through the feelings of inferiority which it generates. It is easy to illustrate, through examples, that an inferiority complex is a psychological evaluation of one's own social position. The question of renaming the auxiliary school has been raised in Germany. The name *Hilfsschule* seems degrading to both parents and children. It inflicts a stamp, as it were, of inferiority on the pupil. The child does not want to attend a "school for fools." The demeaning social status associated with a "school for fools" partially affects even the teachers. They are, somehow, on a lower level than teachers in a school for normal children. Ponsens and O. Fisher [no ref] propose names such as therapeutic, training, or special school *(Sonderschule),* school for the retarded, and other new names.

For a child to end up at a school for fools means to be placed in a difficult social position. Thus, for Adler and his followers, the first and basic point of the educational process is a struggle against an inferiority complex. It cannot be allowed to develop and possess the child or to lead him into unhealthy forms of compensation. The basic idea of individual-psychological therapeutic education, says A. Friedmann, is encouragement *(Ermutigung).* Let us assume that a physical handicap does not lead, for social reasons, to the generation of an inferiority complex—that is, to a low psychological estimation of one's own social standing.

---

\* The Russian text has *Minderwertigkeitsgefuehl.* Perhaps, however, the Adlerian term *Minderwertigkeitskomplex* was intended for insertion since that describes the *complex* of feelings interrelated with their attendant social status.

Thus, notwithstanding the presence of a physical handicap, there will be no psychological conflict. As a result, some people with, let us say, a superstitious, mystical attitude toward the blind have a specific conception of the blind, a belief in their spiritual insight. For them, a blind person becomes a soothsayer, a judge, a wise man. Because of his handicap, he holds a high social position. Of course, in such circumstances, there can be no question of an inferiority complex, feelings of disability, and so on. In the final analysis, what decides the fate of a personality is not the defect itself, but its social consequences, its socio-psychological realization. The adaptive processes, also, are not aimed directly at making up the deficiency, which is for the most part impossible, but at overcoming the difficulties which the defect creates. The development and education of a blind child have to do not so much with blindness itself as with the social consequences of blindness.

A. Adler views the psychological development of the personality as an attempt to attain social status with respect to the "inherent logic of human society," and with respect to the demands of daily life in society. Development unwinds like a chain of predetermined, even if unconscious, actions. And, in the end, it is the need for social adaptation which, by objective necessity, determines these actions. Adler (1928), with good reason, therefore, calls his psychology positional psychology, in contrast to dispositional psychology. The first derives psychological development from the personality's social position, the second from its physical disposition. If social demands were not placed upon a handicapped child's development, if these processes were at the mercy of biological laws only, if a handicapped child did not find it necessary to transform himself into an established social entity, a social personality type, then his development would lead to the creation of a new breed of human being. However, because the goals of development are set *a priori* (by the necessity of adapting to a sociocultural milieu based on the normal human type), even the adaptation process does not occur freely, but follows a definite social channel.

Thus, a handicapped child's developmental processes are socially conditioned in two ways. The social effect of the defect (the inferiority complex) is one side of the social conditioning. The other side is the social pressure on the child to adapt to those circumstances created and compounded for the normal human type. Within the context of final goals and forms, profound differences exist between the handicapped and the normal child in the ways and means of their development. Here, precisely, is a very schematic view of social conditioning in that process. Hence, there is a dual perspective of past and future in analyzing development that has been complicated by a defect. Inasmuch as both the beginning and the end of that development are socially conditioned, all its facets must be understood, not only with respect to the past, but also with respect to the future. Along with an understanding of compensation as the basic form of such development comes an understanding of a drive toward the future. The entire process, as a whole, is revealed as a unified one, as a result of objective necessity striving forward toward a final goal, which was established in advance by the social demands of daily life. The concept of unity and wholeness in a child's developing personality is connected to this. Personality develops as a united whole, with its own particular laws; it does not develop as the sum or as a bundle of individual functions, each developing on the basis of its particular tendency.

This law applies equally to somatics and physics, to medicine and pedagogy. In medicine, the belief is becoming more prevalent that the sole determinant of health or illness is the effective or ineffective functioning of the organs and that isolated abnormalities can be evaluated by the degree to which the other functions of the organism do or do not compensate for the abnormality.

W. Stern advances the following idea: Individual functions deviate from normality, while the whole personality or organism might still belong to an entirely normal type. A *child* with a defect is not necessarily a *defective child*. The degree of his disability or normality depends on the outcome of his social adaptation that is, on the final formation of his personality as a whole. In and of themselves, blindness, deafness, and other individual handicaps do not make their bearer handicapped. Substitution and compensation do not just occur randomly, sometimes assuming gigantic proportions and creating talents from defects. Rather, *as a rule,* they necessarily arise in the form of drives and idiosyncrasies at the point where the defect prevails. Stern's position supports the fundamental possibility of social compensation where direct compensation is impossible, i.e., it is the possibility in principle that the handicapped child can, in principle, wholly approximate a normal type that might enable winning full social self-esteem.

Compensation for moral defectiveness (moral insanity),* when it is viewed as a *special kind of organic handicap or illness,* can serve as the best illustration of secondary social complications and their role in a handicapped child's development. All consistent, intelligent psychologists proceed from a similar point of view. In part, in *our* country the reexamination of this question and the clarification of the falsity and scientific groundless of the very concept of moral disability as applied by P. P. Blonskii, A. B. Zalkind, and others has had great theoretical and practical significance. West European psychologists are coming to the same conclusions. What was taken to be a physical handicap or illness is, in fact, a complex of symptoms with a specific psychological orientation found in children who have been completely derailed socially; it is a socio and psychogenic phenomenon, not a biogenic disorder.

Anytime the erroneous recognition of certain *values* comes into question, as J. Lindworsky stated at the First Congress on Special Education [lit."Therapeutic Pedagogy"] in Germany, the reason for this should be sought, not in an inherent anomaly of the will, nor in specific distortions of individual functions. Rather, it should be sought in the view that neither the surrounding milieu nor the individual himself fostered recognition of those values. Probably, the notion of calling emotional illness *moral insanity* would never have been conceived, if first the attempt had been made to summarize all the shortcomings of values and motives met among normal people. Then, it might have been discovered that every individual has his own insanity. M. Wertheimer also comes to this conclusion. Wertheimer, citing F. Kramer [no ref] and V. K. Garis [no ref], the founder of Gestalt psychology in the United States,† asserts that if one examines the personality as a whole, in its interaction with the environment, the congenital psychopathic tendencies in a child disappear. He emphasizes the fact that a well-known type of

---

\* The text frequently writes "moral insanity" in Roman letters either as a gloss for the Russian term or even as a section heading.

† It is quite likely that Vygotsky intended to credit Wertheimer with founding American Gestalt psychology although the translation adheres closely to the Russian text. Of course the triumvirate which founded Gestalt psychology in Germany (Koehler, Koffka, and Wertheimer) all emigrated to the United States at about the same time (see E. Boring, *A History of Experimental Psychology,* second ed. Appleton-Century-Crofts, New York, 1950 [Ed.].)

childhood psychopathy exhibits the following symptoms' rude carelessness, egoism, and preoccupation with the fulfillment of elemental desires. Such children are unintelligent and weakly motivated, and their physical sensitivity (for example, pain sensitivity) is considerably lowered. In this, one sees a particular type which, from birth, is destined for asocial behavior, ethically handicapped with respect to inclinations, and so on. While the earlier term *moral insanity* implied an incurable condition, transferring these children into a different environment often shows that we are dealing with a particularly keen sensitivity and that the deadening this sensitivity is a means of self defense, of closing oneself off, and of surrounding oneself with a biological defensive armor against environmental conditions. In a new environment, such children display completely different characteristics. Such results occur when children's characteristics and activities are examined not in isolation, but in their relation to the whole, in the dynamics of their development *(Si duo paciunt idem non est idem)*. In theoretical terms, this example is indicative. It explains the emergence of alleged psychopathy, of an alleged defect (moral insanity), which was created in the imagination of the investigators. And this is why they were unable to explain the profound social unsuitability of the children's development in similar cases. The significance of sociopsychogenic factors in the child's development is so great that it could give the illusion of being a handicap, the semblance of illness, and an alleged psychopathy.

4

In the last two decades, scientific defectology has become aware of a new form of disability in children. In essence, it is a motor deficiency (M. O. Gurevich). Although oligophrenia (mental retardation) has always been characterized primarily by some mental defect or another, a new form of abnormal behavior—the underdevelopment of a child's motor apparatus—has recently become the object of intense study as well as of practical and therapeutic pedagogical activity. This form of disability in children has various names. Dupré calls it *debilité motrice* (i.e., motor disability, by analogy with mental disability). While T. Heller calls it motor delay, and in extreme forms, motor idiocy. K. Jacob and A[?]. Homburger (1926a, 1926b) label it motor infantilism and M. O. Gurevich calls it motor deficiency. The essence of this phenomenon, as implied by the various nomenclatures, is a more-or-less pronounced developmental motor deficiency, which is in many ways analogous to the mental disability of oligophrenia.

This motor disability, to a large extent, permits compensation, motor functions, and the equalization of the handicap (Homburger, M. Nadoleczny, Heller). Motor retardation often and easily responds, within certain limits, of course, to pedagogical and therapeutic influence. Therefore, taken alone, motor delay requires, as in the scheme, the dual characterization: defect—compensation. The dynamics of this form of disability, like those of any other form, can be ascertained only if one takes into account the organ's positive response stimuli, namely, those which compensate for the defect.

The introduction of this new form of deficiency into the inventory of science has had a fundamental and profound significance. This is not only because our definition of disability in children has broadened and been enriched by the knowledge of vitally important forms of abnormal development in a child's motor system and the compensatory processes created by it but also, and principally, because it has demonstrated the relationship between this new form and other forms which were already known to us. For defectology (both theoretical and practical), the fact that this form of disability is not necessarily connected to mental retardation is of fundamental importance. "A deficiency of this type," says Gurevich, "not infrequently coexists with mental deficiency. Sometimes, however, it may exist independently of it, just as mental deficiency may be present when the motor apparatus is well developed" (cf. *Questions of Pedology and Child Psychoneurology,* 1925, p. 316). Therefore, motor operations are of exceptional importance in the study of handicapped children. Motor delay may combine, in varying degrees, with all forms of mental retardation, thus creating a unique picture of childhood development and behavior. This form of disability can often be observed in deaf children. Naudacher [in a report in Gurevich, *op. cit.*] offers statistics for the frequency with which this form of deficiency combines with other forms: 75 percent of all idiots, 44 percent of the imbeciles, 24 percent of the debiles, and 2 percent of normal children that were studied were found to have a motor disability.

It is not the statistical computation that is fundamentally important and decisive. Rather, it is the unquestionable proposition that motor delay *can* occur independently of any mental disability. It may be absent in the case of mental retardation and may exist in the absence of any mental deficiency. In instances of combined motor and mental deficiencies, each form has its own dynamics. Compensation for operations in one sphere may occur at a different tempo, in a different direction, than in another sphere. As a result, an extremely interesting interrelationship between these spheres is created in the process of a handicapped child's development. Given the relative independence of the motor system from the higher mental functions and the fact that it is easily guided, it is often found to play a central role in compensating for mental defects and in equalizing behavior. Therefore, when studying a child we must not demand only a twofold characterization (motor and mental) but must also establish the relation between the two spheres of development. Very frequently this relation may be the result of compensation.

In many cases, according to K. Birnbaum's view [no ref.], even real defects, embedded organically in cognitive behavior, can be compensated for, within certain limits, by training and through development of substitutional function; "motor training" which is now so highly valued. Experimental investigations and practical experience in school corroborate this. M. Kruenegel, who has most recently conducted experimental research on the motor skills of mentally retarded children (M. Kruenegel, 1927), applied N.I. Ozeretskii's metric scale of motor skills. Ozeretskii set himself the task of creating a method for determining motor development graduated by age level. Research has shown that motor skills are more highly developed than mental capabilities from one to three years, for 60 percent of all the children studied. In 25 percent of cases, motor skills coincided with cognitive development and they lagged behind in 15 percent. This means that motor development in a mentally retarded child most frequently outstrips his intellectual development at one to three years and only in one quarter of the cases coincides with it. On the basis of his experiments, Kruenegel comes to the conclusion that about 85 percent of all mentally retarded children in auxiliary schools, with the appropriate education, are capable of work (trade, industrial, technical, agricultural, and so forth). It is easy to imagine the great practical significance that the development of motor skills can have in compensating, to a certain degree, for mental defects in mentally retarded children. M. Kruenegel, along with

K. Bartsch, demands the creation of special classes for vocational training and for the development of motor skills for mentally retarded children (ibid.).

The problem of motor disability is a wonderful example of that unity in diversity which can be seen in the development of a handicapped child. Personality develops as a single entity, and as such, it reacts to the defect and to the destruction of equilibrium caused by the defect. It works out a new system of adaptation and a new equilibrium in place of the one destroyed. But precisely because personality represents a unit and acts as a single entity, its development involves the advances of a variety of functions which are diverse and relatively independent of each other. These hypotheses—the diversity of relatively developmentally independent functions, and the unity of the entire progress in personality development—not only do not contradict each other, but, as Stern has shown, reciprocally condition each other. The compensatory reaction of the entire personality, stimulated by the defect in another sphere, finds expression in intensified and increased development of some single function as, for example, motor skills.

## 5

The notion, expressed in the study of motor skills, that the separate functions of the personality are diverse and complex in structure, has recently pervaded all areas of development. When carefully analyzed, not only personality as a whole, but also its separate aspects reveal the same unity in diversity, the same complicated structure, and the same interrelationship of separate functions. One might say, without fear of error, that the development and expansion of scientific ideas about personality at the present time are moving in two, seemingly opposing directions: (1) discovery of its unity and (2) discovery of its complicated and diverse structure. In part, the new psychology moving in this direction has almost destroyed, once and for all, former notions about the unity and homogeneity of the intellect and that function which the Russians, not altogether accurately, call "giftedness" and which the Germans call Intelligenz.*

Intellect, like personality, undoubtedly represents a single entity but is neither uniform nor simple. Rather, it is a diverse and complicated structural unity. Thus, Lindworsky reduces the intellect to the function of perceiving relationships, a function, which in his eyes, distinguishes humans from animals, and which gives thought unto thought. This function (the so-called intellect) is no more inherent in Goethe than to an idiot and the enormous difference which we observe in the thought processes of various people can be reduced to the life of ideas and memory (J. Lindworsky, 1923). We will return later to this paradoxically expressed, but profound idea of Lindworsky. Now, what is important to us is the conclusion which the author drew from his understanding of the intellect at the Second German Congress on Therapeutic Pedagogy. Any mental defect, Lindworsky affirmed, is based in the final analysis on one or another of the factors used in perceiving relationships. A mentally retarded child can never be presented simply as mentally retarded. It is always necessary to ask what constitutes the intellect's deficits, because there are no possibilities for substitution, and they must be made

---

\* N. E. Rumiatsev translates this word as intelligence [intellegentnost']. Hereafter, we will use the less-than-accurate term intellect for this sense. [Transl.]

available to the mentally retarded. In this formulation we already find the notion absolutely clearly expressed that various factors must enter into the composition of such a complicated education; that, corresponding to the complexity of its structure, there is not one but many qualitatively different types of mental disability; and finally, that because the intellect is so complex, its structure permits broad compensation of its separate functions.

This doctrine now meets with general agreement. O. Lipmann systematically traces the steps through which the development of the idea of overall ability has passed. In the beginning, it was identified with any single given function, for example, memory; the next step was the recognition that ability appears in an entire group of psychological functions (attention, synthesis, discrimination and so forth). C. Spearman distinguishes two factors in any rational activity: one is the factor specific to the given type of activity and the other is the general one, which he considers to be ability. A. Binet finally reduced the determination of ability to the mean of an entire series of heterogeneous functions. Only recently the experiments of R. Yerkes and W. Koehler on monkeys, and those of E. Stern and H. Bogen [no ref.] on normal and retarded children have established that not just one ability but many types of ability exist. Specifically, rational cognition coincides with a rational operation. For one and the same person, a certain type of intellect may be well developed and, simultaneously, another type may be very weak. There are two types of mental retardation—one affects cognition and the other operation; they do not necessarily coincide. ("There is," says Lipmann, "a mental retardation of cognition and a mental retardation of operations.")* Similar formulations by Kenman, M. N. Peterson, P. Pinter, G. Thompson, E. Thorndike and others more or less recognize this (O. Lipmann, 1924). E. Lindemann applied the methods of W. Koehler, which were developed for experiments on monkeys, to severely retarded children. Among them, there appeared a group of severely retarded children who turned out to be capable of rational activity. Only their ability to remember new operations was extremely weak (E. Lindeman, 1926). This means that the ability to devise tools, to use them purposefully, to select them, and to discover alternate methods—that is, of rational activity—was found to occur in severely retarded children. Therefore, we must select, as a separate sphere of research, practical intellect; namely, the ability for rational, purposeful activity *(praktische, natuerliche Intelligenz)*. By its psychological nature, rational activity is different from motor ability and from theoretical intellect.

Lipmann and Stern's suggested profiles of practical intellect are based on the criteria of practical intellect, laid out by Koehler, namely the ability to use tools purposefully. This ability undoubtedly has played a deciding role in the transition from monkey to man and which appeared as the first precondition of labor and culture.

A special qualitative type of rational behavior, relatively independent of other forms of intellectual activity, practical intellect may be combined in varying degrees with other forms, each time creating a unique picture of the child's development of behavior. It may appear as the fulcrum of compensation, as the means of equalizing other mental defects. Unless this factor is counted, the entire picture of development, diagnosis, and prognosis will certainly be incomplete. Let us leave for a moment these questions of how many major types of intellectual activity can be discerned—two, three or more—of what the qualitative characteristics of

* *Es gibt ein Schwachsinn des Erkennens und einen Schwachsinn des Handelns.*

each type are, and of which criteria allow one to distinguish one given type from another. Let us limit ourselves to pointing out the profoundly qualitative distinctions between practical and theoretical (problematic) intellect, which have been established by a series of experimental studies. In particular, the brilliant experiments by Bogen on normal and mentally retarded (feebleminded) children without doubt revealed that the aptitude for rational, practical functioning represents a special and independent type of intellect; the differences in this area between normal and disabled children, established by the author, are very interesting (O. Lipmann and H. Bogen, 1923).

Studies on practical intellect have played and will long continue to play a revolutionizing role in the theory and practice of defectology. They raise the question of a qualitative study of mental retardation and its compensation, and of the qualitative determination of intellectual development in general. For example, by comparison with a blind child, a deaf-mute, whether mentally retarded or normal, turns out to be different in terms not of degree, but of type, of intellect. Lipmann speaks about the essential difference in origin and type of intellect and when one type prevails in one individual and another in another (O. Lipmann, 1924). Finally, even the idea of intellectual development has changed. Intellectual development is no longer characterized by merely quantitative growth, by a gradual strengthening and heightening of mental activity; rather, it boils down to the notion of transition from one qualitative type to another, to a chain of metamorphoses. In this sense, Lipmann brings up the profoundly important problem of qualitative characteristics of age, by analogy with the phases of speech development established by Stern (1922): the stages of speech about objects, actions, relationships, and so forth. The problem of complexity and heterogeneity in the intellect demonstrates new possibilities for compensating within the intellect itself. The fact that aptitude for rational performance is present in profoundly retarded children reveals vast and absolutely new perspectives for the education of such a child.

6

The history of cultural development in an abnormal child constitutes the most profound and critical problem in modern defectology. It opens up a completely *new line of development in* scientific research.

A normal child's socialization is usually fused with the processes of his maturation. Both lines of development—natural and cultural—coincide and merge one into the other. Both series of changes converge, mutually penetrating each other to form, in essence, a single series of formative socio-biological influences on the personality. Insofar as physical development takes place in a social setting, it becomes a historically conditioned biological process. The development of speech in a child serves as a good example of the fusion of these two lines of development—the natural and the cultural.

This fusion is not observed in a handicapped child. Here the two lines of development usually diverge more or less sharply. The physical handicap causes this divergence. Human culture evolved in conditions of a certain stability and consistency in the human biological type. Therefore, its material tools and contrivances, its sociopsychological apparatuses and institutions are all intended for a normal psychophysiological constitution. The use of these tools and apparatuses presupposes, as necessary prerequisites, the presence of innate human intellect, organs, and functions. The creation of conformable functions and apparatuses conditions a child's socialization; at a certain stage, if his brain and speech apparatus develop normally, he masters language; at another, higher stage of intellectual development, the child masters the decimal system of counting and arithmetic operations. The gradual and sequential nature of the socialization process is conditioned by organic development.

A defect creates a deviation from the stable biological human type and provokes the separation of individual functions, deficiencies or damage to the organs. It thereby generates a more or less substantial reorganization of the entire development on new bases and according to a new type: in doing all this, it naturally disturbs the normal course of the child's acculturation. After all, culture has adapted to the normal typical human being and accommodates his constitution. Atypical development (conditioned by a defect) cannot be spontaneously and directly conditioned by culture, as in the case of a normal child.

From the point of view of the child's physical development and formation, deafness, as a physical handicap, appears not to be a particularly severe disability. For the most part, deafness remains more or less isolated and its direct influence on development as a whole is comparatively small. It does not usually create any particularly severe damage or delays in overall development. But the muteness which results from this defect, the absence of human speech, creates one of the most severe complications of all cultural development. The entire cultural development of a deaf child will proceed along a different channel from the normal one. Not only is the quantitative significance of the defect different for both lines of development, but, most importantly, the qualitative character of development in both lines will be significantly different. A defect creates certain difficulties for physical development and completely *different ones* for cultural development. Therefore, the two lines of development will diverge substantially from one another. The degree and character of the divergence will be determined and measured in each case by the different qualitative and quantitative effects of the defect on each of the two lines.

Frequently, unique, specially created cultural forms are necessary for cultural development in the handicapped child. Science is aware of a great number of artificial cultural systems of theoretical interest. Parallel to the visual alphabet used by all humanity is a specially created tactile alphabet for the blind—Braille. Dactylology, (i.e., the finger alphabet) and the gesticulated, mimed speech of the deaf-mute have been created alongside the phonetic alphabet of the rest of mankind. By comparison with the use of the usual cultural means, the process of acquiring and using these auxiliary cultural systems is distinguished by profoundly distinctive features. To read with the hand, as blind children do, and to read with the eye are different psychological processes, even if they fulfill one and the same cultural function in the child's behavior and have similar physiological mechanisms at their base.

To formulate the problem of cultural development in a handicapped child as a particular line of development, governed by special laws, with its own particular difficulties and means of overcoming them, represents a serious goal for modem defectology. The notion of primitivism in a child is basic here. At the moment, it seems as though singling out a special type of psychological development among children, namely, *the development pattern of the primitive child,* meets with no objections from any direction, although there is still some controversy about the content of this idea. The meaning of the concept of primitivism is defined by its opposite—acculturation. Just as being handicapped is the polar opposite of ability, so *primitiveness* is the polar opposite of *cultural development*.

A primitive child is a child who has not completed cultural development. The primitive mind is a healthy one. In certain conditions the primitive child completes normal cultural development, and achieves the intellectual level of a cultured person. In this respect, primitivism is distinct from mental retardation. The latter is a result of a physical handicap; the mentally retarded are limited in their natural intellectual development and *as a result of this* do not usually attain full cultural development. With respect to natural development, on the other hand, a "primitive child" does not deviate from the norm. His practical intellect may reach a very high level, but he still remains outside cultural development. A "primitive" is an example of pure, isolated *natural development*.

For a long time, primitivism in a child was considered to be a pathological form of childhood development and was confused with mental retardation. In fact, the outward appearances of these two phenomena are often extremely similar. Limited psychological activity, stunted intellectual development, deductive inaccuracy, conceptual absurdity, impressionability, and so forth, can be symptoms of either. Because of the research methods currently available (Binet and others), the primitive child may be portrayed in a way that is similar to the portrayal of the mentally retarded. Special research methods are necessary to discover the true cause of unhealthy symptoms and to distinguish between primitivism and mental retardation. In particular, the methods for analyzing practical, natural intellect *(natuerliche Intelligenz)* may easily reveal primitivism with a completely healthy mind. A. E. Petrova, in giving us an excellent study of childhood primitivism and outlining its most important types, demonstrated that primitivism may equally combine with an exceptional, an average, and a pathological child's mind ("Children Are Primitives," in Gurevich (Ed.), *Questions of Pedology and Childhood Psycho-neurology.* Moscow, 1925).

Instances in which primitivism combines with certain pathological forms of development are particularly interesting for the study of defects, since such instances occur most frequently in the histories of handicapped children's cultural development. For example, psychological primitivism and delays in cultural development may very often be combined with mental retardation. It would be more accurate to say that delays in the cultural development of a child occur as a result of mental retardation. But in such mixed forms, primitivism and mental retardation remain two *different* natural phenomena. It is in just such a way that congenital or early childhood deafness usually combines with a primitive type of childhood development. But primitivism may occur without a defect. It may even coexist with a highly gifted mind. Similarly, a defect does not necessarily lead to primitivism but may also coexist with a highly cultured type of mind. A defect and psychological primitivism are two different things, and when they are found together, they must be separated and distinguished from one another.

An issue of particular theoretical interest is alleged pathology in a primitive individual. When analyzing a primitive little girl who spoke Tatar and Russian simultaneously and who was acknowledged to be psychologically abnormal, Petrova demonstrated that the entire complex of symptoms, implying illness, stemmed in fact from primitivism, which, in turn, was conditioned by the lack of command of either language. "Our numerous observations prove," Petrova says, "that complete substitution of one poorly grasped language for another, equally lacking in fluency, does not occur without psychological repercussions. This *substitution of one form of thought for another diminishes mental activity particularly when it is already not abundant*" (ibid., p. 85). This conclusion permits us to establish *precisely* what constitutes cultural development from a psychological point of view and what, if missing, causes primitivism in a child. In the given example, primitivism is created by an imperfect command of language. But more generally, the process of cultural development basically depends on acquiring cultural psychological tools, which were created by mankind during its historical development and which are analogous to language from a psychological perspective. Primitiveness boils down to the inability to use such tools and to the natural forms in which psychological operations appear. Like all other higher psychological operations, all the higher forms of intellectual activity become possible only when given the use of similar kinds of cultural tools. "Language," says Stern, "becomes a tool of great power in the development of his [the child's—L.V.] life, his ideas, emotions and will; it alone ultimately makes possible any real thought, generalization and comparison, synthesis and comprehension" (W. Stern, 1923, p. 73).

These artificial devices, which by analogy with technology are sometimes called psychological tools, are directed toward mastering behavioral processes–someone else's or one's own—in the same way that technology attempts to control the processes of nature. In this sense, T. Ribot (1892) has called reflex attention natural and conscious attention artificial, seeing in it a product of historical development. The use of psychological tools modifies the whole course and structure of psychological function, giving them a new form.

During childhood, the development of many natural psychological functions (memory, attention) either are not observable to any significant degree or take place in insignificant quantities. There is no way, therefore, that the development of these functions atone can account for the enormous difference in the corresponding activities of children and adults. In the process of development, a child is armed and rearmed with the most varied of tools. A child in the more advanced stages is as different from a child in the younger stages as an adult is from a child—not only in the greater development of functions, but also in the degree and character of cultural preparedness, in the tools at his disposal, that is, in the degree and means he has of controlling the activity of his psychological functions. Thus, older children are distinguished from the younger ones in the same way adults are distinguished from children, and normal children are distinguished from the handicapped ones. They are distinguished not only by a more developed memory, but also by the fact that they remember *differently*, in different manners, by different methods; they use memory to a different degree.

The inability to use natural psychological functions and to master psychological tools in the most basic sense determines the kind of cultural development a handicapped child will attain. Mastering a psychological tool and, by means of it, one's own natural psychological functions generates an *artificial development*, as it were; that is, it raises a given function to a higher level, increases and expands its activity. Binet explained experimentally the significance of making use of a psychological function with the help of a tool. In analyzing the memory of individuals with exceptional computational skills, he happened upon one individual with an average memory, but armed with a *skill in remembering* equal to and, in many respects, superior to that of those with exceptional computational skills. Binet called this phenomenon a simulated exceptional memory. "The majority of psychological operations can be simulated," he says, "that is, they can be replaced by others, which are similar to them in externals alone, but which are different in nature" (A. Binet, 1894, p. 155). In the given case a difference was discovered between natural memory and artificial or technical mnemonic memory, that is, a difference between two ways of *using* memory. Each of them, in Binet's opinion, possesses its own kind of rudimentary and instinctive technical mnemonics. Technical mnemonics should be introduced in schools along with mental arithmetic and stenography—not in order to develop the intellect, but to make available a way of using memory (ibid., p. 164). It is easy to see in this example how natural development and the use of some functions as tools may not coincide.

There are three fundamental points which define the problem of cultural development for an abnormal child: *the degree of primitivism in the childhood mind; the nature of his adoption of cultural and psychological tools; and the means by which he makes use of his own psychological functions.* The primitive child is differentiated not by a lesser degree of accumulated experience, but by the different (natural) way in which it was accumulated. It is possible to combat primitivism by creating new cultural tools, whose use makes culture accessible to the child. Braille's script and finger spelling (dactylology) are most powerful methods of overcoming primitivism. We know how often mentally retarded children are found to have not only a normal, but a highly developed, memory. Its use, however, almost always remains at the lowest level. Evidently, the degree of development of memory is one thing, and the degree of its use quite another.

The first experimental research into the use of psychological tools in handicapped children was recently carried out by followers of N. Ach. Ach himself, having created a method for analyzing functional word use as a means, or as a tool, for elaborating conceptualization, pointed out the fundamental similarity between this process and the process by which the deaf acquire language (1932 [sic], but probably 1921). Bacher (1925) applied this method to an investigation of learning disabled children *(debiles)* and showed that this is the best method for analyzing mental retardation qualitatively. The correlation between theoretical and practical intellect turned out to be insignificant, and mentally retarded children (to the extent of their debilitation) could apply their practical intellect much better than their theoretical intellect. The author sees in this a correspondence with similar results achieved by Ach in his experiments with brain-damaged individuals. Because the mentally retarded do not use words as tools for working out ideas, higher forms of intellectual activity based on the use of abstract concepts are impossible for them (ibid.). How the mastering of one's own psychological activity influences the execution of intellectual operations was discovered at the time of Bacher's research. But this is precisely the problem. Stern considers these two means of using language as different stages in speech development. He said: ". . . But subsequently a decisive turnabout in speech development occurs again, *a vague awareness of the meaning of language and the will to conquer it awakens*" (1922, p. 89). The child makes the most important discovery of his life, that *"everything has a name"* (ibid.); that *words are signs*—they are the means of naming and communicating. It is this *full*, conscious, voluntary use of speech that a mentally retarded child apparently does not attain. As a result, higher intellectual activity remains inaccessible to him. F. Rimat was completely justified in selecting this method as a test for examining mental ability; the ability or inability to use words is a decisive criterion of intellectual development (F. Rimat, 1925). The fate of all cultural development depends on whether children themselves make the discovery about which Stern speaks. Do they master words as fundamental psychological tools?

Studies of primitive children reveal *literally the same thing*. "How do a tree and a log differ?" Petrova asks one such child. "I haven't seen a tree, I swear I haven't seen one." (There is a linden tree growing in front of the window). In response to the question (while pointing to the linden tree) "And what is this?" comes the answer: "It's a linden." This is a primitive answer, in the spirit of those primitive people whose language has no word for "tree;" it is too abstract for the concrete nature of the boy's mind. The boy was correct: none of us has seen a tree. We've seen birches, willows, pines and so forth, that is, specific species of trees (A.E. Petrova, in Gurevich (Ed.), 1925, p. 64). Or take another example. A girl "with two languages" was asked: "In one school some children write well, and some draw well. Do all the children in this school write and draw well?. . . . How should I know? *What I haven't seen with my own eyes, I cannot explain it* as if I had seen with my own eyes . . ." (a primitive visual response) (ibid., p. 86). This nine-year old girl is absolutely normal, but she is primitive. She is totally unable to use words as a means of solving mental tasks, although she *talks;* she knows how to use words as a means of communication. She can explain only what she has seen with her own eyes. In the very same way, a "debile" draws conclusions from concrete object to concrete object. His inadequacy for higher forms of abstract thought is not a direct result of an intellectual defect; he is completely capable of other forms of logical thinking, of operations governed by common sense and so forth. He simply has not mastered the use of words as tools for abstract thinking. This incapacity is a result and a symptom of his primitivism, but not of his mental retardation.

Kruenegel (1926) is fully justified when he states that G. Kerschensteiner's basic axiom does not apply to cultural development in a mentally retarded child. That axiom says that the congruence of one or another cultural form with the psychological structures of a child's personality lies at the base of cultural development: the emotional structure of cultural forms should be entirely or partially adequate to the emotional structure of individuality (G. Kerschensteiner, 1924). The fundamental problem in a handicapped child's cultural development is inadequacy, the incongruence between his psychological structure and the structure of cultural forms. What remains is the necessity of creating special cultural tools suitable to the psychological make-up of such a child, or of mastering common cultural forms with the help of special pedagogical methods, *because the most important and decisive condition of cultural development—precisely the ability to use psychological tools—is preserved in such children.* Their cultural development is, in principle, completely possible. In the use of artificial means *(Hilfer)* aimed at overcoming a defect, W. Eliasberg justifiably perceived a symptom which is differential, which allows us to distinguish mental retardation *(demenz)* from aphasia (W. Eliasberg, 1925). The use of psychological tools is, indeed, the most essential aspect of a child's cultural behavior. It is totally lacking only in the mentally retarded.

7

We have taken a theoretical cross section of the most important problems of modern defectology noted above because a theoretical approach to the problem provides the most comprehensive, the most concise view, exposing the very essence, the nucleus, of the question. In fact, however, each of the issues merges with a series of practical-pedagogical, and concrete-methodological problems or, more precisely, boils down to a series of separate concrete questions. In order to tackle these issues, special considerations of each question would have been necessary. By limiting ourselves to the most general formulation of the problems, we will concisely indicate the presence of concrete, practical tasks in each problem. Thus, the problem of motor skills and motor deficiency is directly connected to the questions of physical training, and vocational and professional education for handicapped children. The problem of practical intellect is as closely connected with vocational training and with practical experience in acquiring daily living skills, the crux of all education for handicapped children. The problem of cultural development embraces all major questions of academic instruction. The problem of the analytical and artificial methods used in teaching speech to the deaf, which is particularly worrisome to defectologists, can be formulated with the following question: Should children be mechanically drilled in the simplest elements of speech skills, in the same fashion in which fine motor skills are cultivated? Or should children first and foremost be taught the ability to use speech, in other words, be taught the functional use of words as "intellectual tools," as J. Dewey put it? The problem of compensation in a handicapped child's development and the problem of social conditioning in this development includes all the issues involved in organizing communal living for children, in a children's social movement, in socio-political education, in personality formation, and so forth.

Our account of the basic problems of being handicapped would stop short of its most essential point if we did not attempt to project a base line in practical defectology, which inevitably derives from this formulation of theoretical problems. What we have designated in theory as the transition from a quantitative understanding of a disability corresponds completely with the primary feature of practical defectology; the formulation of positive tasks confronting special schools. In special schools we can no longer be satisfied with simply a limited version of the public school curriculum or with the use of modified and simplified methods. The special schools confront the task of positive activity, of creating forms of work which meet the special needs and character of its pupils. Among those who have written on this question, A. S. Griboedov has expressed this thought most concisely, as we have already observed. If we reject the idea that a handicapped child is a lesser likeness of a normal child, then, unavoidably, we must also reject the view that special schools are prolonged versions of public schools. Of course, it is extremely important to establish with the greatest possible accuracy the qualitative differences between handicapped and normal children, but we cannot stop here. For example, we learn from numerous contemporary observations of the mentally retarded that these children have smaller cranial circumferences, smaller stature, smaller chest size, less muscle strength, reduced motor ability, lowered resistance to negative influences, delayed associations, and decreased attention and memory span, and that they are more prone to fatigue and exhaustion, less able to exert their will, and so forth (A. S. Griboedov, 1926). But we still know nothing about positive characteristics, about the children's uniqueness: such is the research of the future. It is only half true to characterize such children as developmentally delayed in physical and psychological terms, weakened, and so forth; such negative characteristics in no way exhaust these children's positive and unique features. It is not the individual fault of one researcher or another that positive material is lacking. Rather, it is a calamity shared by all of defectology, which is just beginning to reorganize its principal bases and thus to give new direction to pedological research. In any case, Griboedov's basic conclusion formulates precisely this view: "In studying the pedology of retarded children, we can clearly see that the differences between them and normal children are not only quantitative, but also qualitative, and that consequently they *need not stay longer in school nor attend smaller classes, nor even associate with those who have similar levels and tempo of psychological development. Rather, they need to attend special schools, with their own programs, with unique methodologies and special pedagogical personnel"* (1927, p. 19).

There is, however, a serious danger in formulating the question this way. It would be a theoretical mistake to make an absolute concept out of the developmental uniqueness of a child with one kind of defect or another, while forgetting that there are limits to this uniqueness prescribed by the social conditioning of the development. It is equally inaccurate to forget that the parameters of the special school's uniqueness are described by the common social goals and tasks confronting both public and special schools. Indeed, as has already been said, children with a defect do not constitute "a special breed of people," in K. Buerklen's phrase. Instead, we discover that all developmental uniqueness tends to approximate determined, normal, social types. And, the school must play a decisive role in this "approximation." The special school can set a general goal for itself; after all, its pupils will live and function not as "a special breed of people," but as workers, craftspeople, and so forth, that is, as specific social units. *The greatest difficulty and profoundest uniqueness of the special schools (and of all practical defectology is precisely to achieve these common goals, while using unusual means to reach them.* Similarly, the most important feature for the handicapped child is the final point, one held in common with normal children, but attained through unique developmental processes. If special means (a special school) were used to attain special goals, this would not warrant being called a problem; the entire issue stems from the apparent contradiction of special means to achieve precisely the same goals, which the public schools also set themselves. This contradiction is really only an apparent one: it is *precisely in order that* handicapped children achieve the same things as normal children that we must employ utterly different means.

"The goal of unified vocational schools is to create builders of a new life of communist principles," says Griboedov. "The goal of the auxiliary school cannot be the same since the mentally retarded, although they have been educated and molded to fit the society around them, and armed with the means of survival, cannot be builders, or creators of a new life; we demand from them only that they not keep others from building" (1926, p. 99). Such a formulation of the practical problems of therapeutic pedagogy seems to us unsound from a sociopedagogical and psychological point of view.

Can pedagogy, in fact, base its work on such a purely negative goal ("not hinder others from building")? Such problems are solved not through pedagogy, but by completely different means.

An educational system without definite, positive societal goals is impossible; similarly, one cannot admit that a child, on completion of an auxiliary school, must limit his role in social life to staying out of the way! According to the data introduced by Griboedov himself (1926), more than 90 percent of the mentally retarded children who have received an education are capable of working and undertaking craft-related, industrial or agricultural labor. Can it be that a conscientious worker—in industry, agriculture or handicrafts—is not also a builder, or a creator of new life? After all, one must understand this "building" as a collective social effort, in which each worker participates according to his strengths. Data from German and American statistics about occupational distribution among the mentally retarded tells us that those who have completed an auxiliary school may be builders and are not all doomed to the role of not hindering others as they build." From a psychological perspective, it is equally false to deny that there are creative processes present in mentally retarded children. Retarded children often register higher than normal children, not in productivity, but in the intensity with which these creative processes run their course. In order to accomplish the same things that a normal child does, the retarded child must display greater creativity. For example, to master the four arithmetic operations is a more creative process for the mentally retarded than for the normal school child. Griboedov sympathetically introduces Kruenegel's opinion of therapeutic pedagogy, which can be reduced primarily to (1) the exercise of residual psychological functions and (2) the development of compensatory operations (ibid.). But after all, this really means basing pedagogy on the principle of compensation, i.e., constructive development. This view suggests that illness (in general) should be reevaluated on the basis of our overall understanding of development in mentally retarded children. "The therapeutic factor must saturate and leave its imprint upon all the work in the school," Griboedov demands (ibid., p. 98), agreeing completely with the common view of a mentally retarded child as a *sick child*.

Still, P. Ia. Troshin cautioned against the view which "sees in abnormal children only disease, forgetting that, in addition to illness, they have normal psychological lives" (1915, p. 2). Therefore, the principles embodied in the auxiliary school program of the People's Commissariat of Enlightenment* seems to us to be more correct: "The common goals and tasks, confronting any single vocational school also represent the goals and tasks of the auxiliary school" *(Programs of the Auxiliary School,* 1927, p. 7). Actual formation of programs on the same basis as the GUS† program for public schools is an expression of the school's fundamental goal: the closest possible approach of the retarded child to the norm. To construct a plan for an auxiliary school "independently of the plans for the common vocational schools," as Griboedov demands (1926, p. 99), means, in essence, to exclude the practice of therapeutic pedagogy from the sphere of social education. After all, even foreign schools are coming around to the idea of complexes‡ (combined programs), as Griboedov himself indicated (ibid.). R. Guertler's "Lesson with a Handkerchief" represents an incidental and primitive "complex," whereas what is basically proposed

---

* The People's Commissriat of Enlightenment (NARKOMPROS), the equivalent of a "ministry of education," was founded November 9, 1917. The first Commissar of Enlightenment was A. Lunacharskii. [Transl.]

† *GUS* stands for Gosudarstvennyi Uchennyi Soviet, or State Council of Scholars. This division of NARKOMPROS existed from 1919 to 1933. Its first chair, Pokrovskii, was Lunacharskii's second in command. [Transl.]

‡ Vygotsky referred here to Soviet reforms which made broad curriculum changes. The reformed curriculum rejected the division of schoolwork into "subjects;" instead it taught pupils to work together under a single broad theme.

by the GUS "complex" is "a reflection of connections between fundamental, vital phenomena (nature, labor, society)" *(Programs of the Auxiliary School,* 1927, p. 8).

The mentally retarded child needs to have these links disclosed in the process of academic instruction *more than a normal child does.* Circumstances where this "complex" is more difficult than the "handkerchief" should be a positive strength in such programs, because raising surmountable obstacles also means carrying out the creative goals of education with respect to development. The statement of Eliasberg, who has worked so hard on problems of the psychology and pathology of abstraction and against the exclusive dominance of visual aids in auxiliary schools, we consider to be both sympathetic and profoundly just. Precisely because the retarded child is so dependent on his experience with visual, concrete impressions and develops abstract thinking to such a small degree when left to his own devices, the school must free itself from the abundant use of visual aids, which serve as an obstacle to the development of abstract thought. In other words, a school must not only adapt to the disabilities of such a child but also must fight these disabilities and overcome them. This constitutes the third fundamental characteristic of practical problems in defectology. There are, first, common goals, which confront both normal and special schools, and, second, the special features and uniqueness of means used in special schools. But apart from both of these, there exists the creative character of the entire school, which makes it a school of social compensation, of socialization, and not "a school for the weakminded," and which forces it not to conform to a defect, but to conquer it. That creative character emerges as the necessary feature in issues of practical defectology. These three points define the parameters of practical defectology.

As has been mentioned above, we have limited ourselves here to posing problems in their most general form. We have indicated that these are problems for which defectology is only beginning to approach solutions. They are aimed toward the future more than toward the past or the present of our discipline. We have tried to demonstrate that defectology studies development—a development which has its own laws, its own tempo, its own cycles, its own imbalances, its own metamorphoses, its own shifts from the center, its own structure—and that this is a special and relatively independent area of knowledge about a profoundly unique subject. In practical terms and in education, as we have attempted to show, defectology faces tasks the solution of which demands creative work and the introduction of special forms. To solve these and other problems of defectology it is necessary to find a solid foundation for both theory and practice. In order not to build on sand, to avoid the eclectic and superficial empiricism which characterized it in the past, in order to shift from a clinical-therapeutic approach to a positive, creative pedagogy, defectology must rest on the same philosophical dialectics and materialistic foundation and be guided by our pedagogy in general, that is, by the social foundation which determines our social education. These are the issues facing defectology as we know it today.

# 7

# The Difficult Child

The psychology of a difficult child* presents a most crucial problem for investigation from various angles, because the notions of "difficult child" and "hard-to-raise child" are very broad, Here, in fact, we confront categories of children who differ greatly from one another, who are united by one negative attribute: they all present difficulties in terms of upbringing. Therefore, the terms "difficult child" or "hard to raise child" are not scientific terms and do not represent any definite psychological or pedagogical content. It is a general label for huge groups of children who differ from one another; it is a prefatory term, advanced out of practical convenience.

The scientific study of these forms of childhood development has still not reached the point of enabling us to have more definitions at our disposal. It has been justifiably pointed out, particularly in recent times, that the problem of the difficult-to-raise category should not be limited only to the age of childhood. In fact we often confront in the behavior of adults forms which represent a direct analogy with childhood difficulties, and if one cannot call adults hard-to-bring-up because we do not bring them up, then in any case these people are difficult to handle. In past attempts to shed light on this concept, cases were cited where adults in a family have turned out to be the difficult family members or problem workers in a production line or in a social activity. It has been successfully shown in concrete terms that from a psychological point of view these adults exhibit precisely the same displays of difficult character and other symptoms as do children. In other words, what was at issue were those forms of character or degree of personal capabilities which led to a series of difficulties and deficits in social adaptation, activity, and behavior. The problem is becoming more and more widespread, and the most authoritative American psychologists working in this area propose isolating the problem in a special branch of psychological knowledge which they preliminarily call "psychology of border-line phenomena." With this label, they had in mind not only the impairment of nervous processes, which assumes neuropathological or psychological forms, but activity which, while remaining within the boundaries of the norm, nevertheless presents very serious problems, interrupting the correct course of a person's upbringing, social and work activities, personal life, and family life.

---

Originally appeared in English translation in Part II of *The Collected Works of L.S. Vygotsky, Volume 2: The Fundamentals of Defectology (Abnormal Psychology and Learning Disabilities)* (Robert W. Rieber and Aaron S. Carton, Eds.; Jane E. Knox and Carol B. Stevens, Trans.) (pp. 139–149). New York: Plenum Press, 1993.
\* The term is a strict translation of the Russian *trudnye*. Perhaps a more idiomatic, if somewhat outdated, English expression, would be "problem child." It seemed advisable to retain a strict translation leaving the interpretation of the term to the reader. [Ed.]

In view of the unusual complexity and breadth of this theme, allow me to dwell only on two basic points which have pivotal meaning: the problem of the formation of a child's character and the problem of his natural talents. An enormous number of difficult children present problems primarily in these two areas. We usually have before us either a child who is difficult to educate because of few or very low natural capabilities or a child who is difficult to manage because of those tendencies in his behavior and character which make him difficult to live with. It is difficult to handle him, he does not submit to school discipline, and so forth. Let us turn to the problem of a difficult character and the problem of a child's character formation.

1

In psychology, the problem of character has recently undergone revision and reexamination. It is not my task to describe the full scope of this problem: I am interested only in the aspect connected with the problem of a difficult-to-raise child.

In modern doctrines on character research, investigators have been conducting work in two opposite directions. Some psychologists are investigating the biological basis of what we call human character or, more accurately, the humanizing temperament [or "human-guiding" temperament]. They study the interrelationships of organic systems which correlate with one or another behavior pattern. E. Kretschmer's well-known doctrine may serve as the most striking example of research based on knowledge of the human body. Other investigators study not merely the biological character but also how it develops in various conditions of the social environment in which the child must build his character. In other words, these researchers are dealing with character in the fill sense of the word, and not with temperament. They have in mind those tendencies in a person's behavior which are not so much inherent at birth, as cultivated on the basis of qualities acquired during the process of upbringing, of development, of adaptation to one or another environment. Research of the second order presents the greatest interest because, as I will try to show, it more closely approaches the problem of the formation of deviations in a child's character or a difficult character.

I permit myself to begin with a concrete example which will clarify how modern psychologists are inclined to picture the formation of certain character traits, or a certain behavioral tendency. Let us say that we have before us a child who is afflicted with a hearing loss as a result of one or another cause. It is easy to imagine that this child will experience a series of difficulties in adapting to his surroundings. During play, other children will leave him in the background; he will lag behind on walks; he will be eliminated from active participation in children's festivities and conversations. In a word, a child with a hearing impairment will be placed, because of his simple organic deficiency, in a lower social position than other children. We want to say, that in the process of adapting to the social milieu, this child will run up against more obstacles than will a normal child. How will this circumstance affect the formation of the child's character? I think that the development of a child's character will proceed along the following fundamental lines: As a result of poor hearing, he will confront difficulties; therefore, a heightened sensitivity, attentiveness, curiosity, distrustfulness with respect to his environment will develop. Perhaps he will cultivate still another series of particular psychological traits, the appearance of which is understandable if we take into account that these character traits are the child's response to the difficulties encountered on his path. The child who, as a result of his deficiency, becomes the object of derision among his comrades will develop increased suspicion, curiosity, and caution, and an entire complex psychological superstructure, We understand this complex system of attitudes and behavioral modes to be a reaction, or response to the difficulties the child encounters in the process of adapting to his social environment.

We are able to note three basic types of such forms of reaction in the child. One of these is well known in psychiatry; in medicine, it is called the delirium of the hard of hearing. This group is so different from others that psychiatrists long ago singled it out. Those forms of response mentioned above begin to occur in the hard of hearing. Suspicion, distrust, over-anxiety, and caution develop in the person who is beginning to lose his hearing. Each word from those surrounding him gives him cause for strong anxiety; it seems to him that people are thinking something bad about him. He loses sleep and begins to feel that he will be killed. He is ready to accuse others of conspiring against him. Each new face arouses suspicions in him. In the final analysis, he develops a persecution mania.

Are these character traits the same, according to my psychological nature, as those with which I was born? I propose that a given formation appears in response to difficulties arising in the course of adaptation to the environment. If a hearing defect did not cut this person off from his surrounding environment, and normal relations with other people continued, then there would not be anything particular about his behavior. Although we have the right to say that this is simply a case of a response formation, suspicion, and caution, it is, however, a well-known behavioral way of relating to the environment, a mode cultivated in response to those difficulties which a person confronts. But this is a fictitious condition does not stem from reality, inasmuch as close friends and relations do not wish him evil. Further, those means of behavior cultivated by a sick person in response to difficulties do not really overcome them. The difficulties themselves arise on the basis of ideas which are divorced from reality and on the basis of the unreal means used by the afflicted person in his struggle with these phantoms. Modern psychologists suggest that such a system of character formation be called fictitious compensation. They say that this attitude of caution, suspicion and overanxiety arises as a form of compensation when a person tries to defend himself in some way in the face of difficulties. If we turn to the example with which I began, then we see that the two opposing lines of character development are also possible in the case of a hard-of-hearing child. The first (which we can call real compensation) occurs in response to more or less realistically accountable difficulties. Thus. if a hard of hearing child develops a heightened sensitivity, keenness of observation, curiosity, attentiveness, and sharpness and learns to recognize by vague signs that which other children learn by means of auditory perception, he does so because he has a healthy regard for his difficulties. He will not leave his watch post lest he miss something. This is called real compensation. We have already discussed fictitious compensation.

Finally, the last type of compensation. It may assume the most diverse forms. Here, we do not encounter the two types of compensation already identified (hallucinatory and real compensation). The third type—the most difficult to define—is so multifarious, so far removed from external unity, that it is difficult to define with one word. Here, however, is a rough explanation. Imagine that a child experiences a certain weakness. Under certain conditions, this weakness can become a strength. The child may cover up his weakness. He is weak and hears poorly. This lowers his responsiveness to other children and elicits a greater solicitude on the part of others. And he begins to cultivate an illness within himself in order to obtain the right to have more attention. He seems in devious ways to reward himself for the difficulties he experiences. Adults know what kind of advantages can be made of illness: when responsiveness on the child's part is lowered, he can place himself in an exceptional position. A child takes particular advantage of this position within the family where, because of his illness, he suddenly becomes the center of the attention of all surrounding him. This example of withdrawal into illness for the sake of camouflaging one's weakness represents the third type of compensation. It is difficult to determine whether or not it is real. It is real in the sense that the child achieves certain advantages; it is fictitious because not only does he not rid himself of his difficulties but, on the contrary, he accentuates them even more. We have in mind the child who makes his deficit into a burden. When exposed to sound, he is apt to make his loss appear far greater than it is in reality because it is more-or-less advantageous for him to do so.

A reaction of a different nature can, however, occur. A child may compensate for his difficulties by exhibiting responsive, aggressive actions with respect to his social environment (his peers, his parents, the school). In other words, a child may take compensatory action of yet another kind. Allow us to illustrate with the concrete example of this deaf child. He may exhibit an increased irritability, stubbornness, and aggressiveness toward other children; he will attempt to eradicate by practical means the deprivation caused by his defect. Holding last place in any game, this child will, as a consequence of his hearing loss, try to play a greater role. He will always gravitate toward younger children. Such a course of compensation is very distinctive. Here we find the cultivation of certain character traits, which we conventionally would call love of power, a tendency toward "autocracy," stubbornness, that is, the tendency to insist without fail on one's own way, although what was suggested in no way runs counter to the child's desires. What links this last case of a child's character development with the previous example of a child who withdraws into illness and cultivates his defect? To a certain degree, this third type of compensation is real because the child achieves by other means what his defect has denied him, and at the same time, of course, it is also fictitious compensation because although he gets what he wants in a collective of younger children by stubbornness, he does not really overcome the difficulties confronting him.

On the basis of these examples, we are able to say that a child's character development is based on the mechanism of compensatory reaction; the child responds by trying to overcome the difficulties confronting him. This reaction can occur in three different forms: the real, the fictitious or the average type of compensation, already mentioned by us. From the examples introduced, it is absolutely clear that we have entered the area of the psychology of a hard-to-raise child because, even in the case of real compensation, we will encounter difficulties in cultivating the child's character. In an attempt to surmount the unhappiness caused by the degradation of his real position, the child who develops quick-wittedness and other positive qualities will also develop certain deficits caused by those aspects which cannot be compensated for. This will be an undesirable process and, to a significant degree, harmful. We cannot call it an unhealthy process because it leads to health. Still one cannot call it healthy because it occurs in an unhealthy fashion.

When the child encounters difficulties inherent in the environment itself, he collides with uncontrollable phenomena which affect the formation of his character. As a result, the child forms a conflicting character, wherein the emotional qualities are intermixed and you can never assuredly say what is going on inside the child. Instead, you say, "I do not even know what to say; he was thoroughly out of hand, and now you can't praise him enough," or on the contrary, "He was well behaved and now is unmanageable."

If you take other cases of compensation, then you will have before you a difficult child in the complete sense of the word. You will have before you character traits with which pedagogues must carry on a long struggle and which interfere with the normal development necessary for special situations.

## 2

I shall allow myself to devote a few words to a discussion of some of the effective means which such a psychological understanding of childhood personality problems suggests. Nowhere has this new system for educating a difficult child been formulated into a developed program (nor has it had its last say) although attempts are being made in various countries including ours. I should only like to illustrate for you the psychological principle which one should use as the basis for educating such a child. The Viennese pedagogue A. Friedmann* calls this principle "methodological dialectics." It is an approach in which we find it necessary to use the opposite of the direct goal in order to achieve the necessary result. Friedmann tells us about a nervous, excitable child, who, with his nervous fits, could hold everyone around in fear and submission. During a lesson he runs up to the window with his knapsack and shouts, "I will throw it out the window." The teacher says, "As you wish," and the child stops in bewilderment because, as the teacher explains, she outwardly yields to the child in order to gain the upper hand over him, in order to be on the offensive. The teacher understands that the boy wants to fling the knapsack out the window because he wants to frighten her and not because he is fed up with the lesson. With her answer, as if yielding to the child, the teacher immediately nips this reaction at the root, thereby putting the boy in a difficult position. And each such example of upbringing, each such move, made with an understanding of the psychological roots of one or another of the boy's reaction or condition, is calculated to adjust externally to his defect while taking the upper hand over him. In other words, to yield to him in order to advance. This is what Friedman calls the principle of "methodological dialectics." We use this principle in a situation where we refuse by direct intervention to suppress certain reactions in the child.

If we begin to understand the causes which provoked various difficulties, and if those difficulties, leading to negative character traits, had been eradicated in the beginning, and not upon their manifestation, then we would be able to use the defect to transform those character

---

* Designated as a German pedagogue in a note above.

traits into positive ones. This combination of actions will be called the principle of methodological dialectics. For example, within any group of children, there is always one disorganizer, a child who disrupts other children at work, who violates group discipline. We will try to influence this child in the following way: We offer him the role of class organizer; we make him the leader of the group, and then relative harmony will prevail within the group. Relative harmony, because such a course of action is very dangerous, if we do not get the upper hand over this leader in time. Otherwise, as Friedman says, the best you're doing is posting a thief to guard your amber jewelry. But if you don't put in this role the child who is striving to attain a certain position within the group and who expresses this desire by disrupting classes in this role, then his desire will find another outlet. If, however, you curb his autocratic obstinacy, he will proceed along the channel which is advantageous for you. In this case you will gain a transformation in the child's attitudes and a conversion of his weakness and negative traits into pluses, into strengths, and into what may lead to the development of positive character traits.

As a conclusion to our discussion of the first problem, I would like to point out what a critical psychological problem the difficult child poses, what minuses and pluses are interlaced, how in this case one contradiction supersedes another and how those same difficulties which trip up a child may further develop both positive and negative character traits.

An old observation tells us that a hard-to-handle child is frequently gifted, although in this instance one has to confront childish illusions, stubbornness, and the like. It is hard to admit that all this psychological energy, this entire direction of behavior could not be deflected from certain paths of development and redirected along others. I cannot say that this problem is easily solved or that solving it theoretically will suffice to change everything in practice and provide some means whereby suddenly all of what the child has already developed will swing from left to right and vice versa. In fact, this problem is infinitely difficult because, if development has proceeded along the wrong path, then an entire series of organic and external forces and circumstances, including incidental occurrences, promote development precisely in this direction. It is far more complicated and difficult to purposefully guide development. In this case, an all-encompassing and captivating influence is needed. More-or-less external means often turn out to be very effective when we speak about a child who does not display great resistance. However, all these means, as wonderful as they may be in and of themselves, may turn out to be ineffective when you confront fierce resistance on the part of the child. Such resistance really represents enormous strength because the child resists not because he wants to be obstinate but because certain causes determining his character development have, from the outset cultivated this stubbornness. We are beginning to find only the most general techniques for our very time-consuming and complicated task of remolding the child.

### 3

Allow me to dwell on another psychological problem, very closely connected to unmanageability, namely, the problem of giftedness. There are those gifted children who present difficulty with respect to upbringing as a result of certain character defects and there is also another large group of children with learning problems related to one or another defect of giftedness;

that is to say, there is a lag in the general reserve of their psychological development which inter-feres with learning in school and with the acquisition of the knowledge which other children acquire. It goes without saying that I have chosen questions concerning only the crudest traits and am omitting overlapping cases where a difficult-to-educate child may also be difficult to handle. I am omitting border-line cases and those which do not come under the already indi-cated headings. The problem of giftedness is also being reexamined much more intensely than the problem of character development. If in theories on character we see the continuation of two fundamental lines well known since the times of ancient psychology—the theories link-ing character either with physical features or with the social circumstances of one's upbring-ing—then in regard to the problem of giftedness, modern psychology is making a complete turn around (in the full sense of the word).

It is very difficult to lay out the problem of giftedness systematically. As with the ques-tion of character, I again permit myself to touch on only one side of the problem. The question of unity in plurality has direct bearing on the question of the education and development of a difficult-to-educate child. This question can be phrased as follows: Does giftedness represent a single, homogeneous, integrated factor or function of a specific nature, or are many forms concealed behind this one general label? The question has passed through many stages, and in the history of the doctrine of giftedness few chapters as extensive as this one are to be found.

Allow me to dwell on the aspect of giftedness as it is directly connected with the prob-lem of a difficult child. All psychological investigations address the fact that, rather than con-stituting a single function, giftedness comprises a series of various functions which are united in one whole. In conjunction with this, we conceive of giftedness as a shaped function. In particular, the definition for "a debilitated childhood" indicates that our conception of gifted-ness is not precise enough. We call a child with negative qualities a *debile*. Any child who accepts disciplinary instruction in school with great difficulty is seen in our country as a hard-to-edu-cate child. When a certain function is measured, attention, for example, and it turns out to be lower in a mentally retarded child than in a normal child then what has been pointed out is what the mentally retarded child lacks but not what he possesses.

It turns out that children with similarly impaired functions possess different additional capabilities which normal children do not have. Therefore O. Lipmann is absolutely correct when he says that no psychologist should resolve to define a feebleminded child solely as fee-bleminded. A psychologist must not do this precisely for the same reason that a modern doc-tor cannot diagnose a patient only by the degree of his illness. When a child is taken to a doc-tor, the doctor determines not only the negative but also the positive aspects of his health that compensate for his physical state. In precisely the same way, a psychologist must differentiate a child's delay and analyze its essence.

I shall point out basic combined forms of retardation and development in children who have been studied by modern psychologists. I must add the reservation that the question will not be totally exhausted by the forms mentioned below. Still, these forms should show the com-plex state which the psychology of a mentally retarded child has reached and the difficulty posed by a solution which indicates only a retarded child's deficiencies,

In initiating a discussion of this problem, it is necessary to say at the outset that the iden-tification of motor deficiency is very important. Various authors have begun to observe this particular form of childhood delay, which was labeled in various ways: *motor debility, motor idiocy,* and so forth. Yet, however we label it, we are essentially dealing with one and the same thing. We have before us a child who does not have an obvious, severe impairment of his motor apparatus; nevertheless the child exhibits a delay in the character of his movements. This may be analyzed in two different ways: First, either by using an elaborated scale which notes the type of movements delayed at six, seven, eight, nine, and ten years of age and to determine the delay over a two to three-year period or, second, by putting together with the help of R. I. Rossolimo's scale, the components of mental retardation and by pointing out the fact that the child does not have sufficient coordination between the left and the right hand so that the child proves to have difficulty in combining the movements of his hands, and so forth. The former distinction between mental and motor retardation has broken down. More often than not, they go hand in hand, but sometimes, and frequently enough, a motor delay is not accompanied by an intellectual delay, and, vice versa, an intellectual delay does not necessarily accompany a motor delay.

Kruedelen's latest research in Germany has shown that the vast majority of debiles have motor capabilities which are lower than their age levels. This fact has enormous fundamental meaning both for the theory of childhood retardation and for practical work with children: If the two links of development can flow independently of each other, then it is clear that the very word retardation is in need of further elaboration. This is my first point. Second, as research has already shown, one developmental link may serve in relation to the other as the central link of compensation; that is, it is possible to augment what the child already possesses. Independently of his circumstances a child will develop either his motor abilities intensely or, vice versa, his cognitive abilities, and the intellectual side of his development will be strengthened. This fact has enormous significance for the psychological theory of giftedness. Tested on the basis of broad material, it would support the view that a tendency toward heightened development in some areas assumes the possibility of a developmental deficiency in other areas where the child comes up against difficulty. This fact has been corroborated statistically. But even if we were not dealing here with definite mathematical values, the psychological significance of the indicated fact is in no way diminished; it is important that such a correlation is possible and that motor development in delayed children leads to positive results. Precisely on this basis we can explain why 90 percent of the children who are not able to learn in public schools are able to perform complicated forms of work above the level of those elementary tasks prescribed for imbeciles.

Mental retardation is in itself diverse. Thus, one may speak of a mild mental retardation. In this case, retardation and compensation may occur independently of one another and even proceed to an antithesis in as much as one link serves as compensation for the other damaged link. This will be called practical intellect.

Contemporary psychologists conventionally call the ability of an animal or a child to act rationally *practical* intellect. W. Koehler's research on apes has shown that the ability to act purposefully is not necessarily connected with the ability to make rational arguments. His observations tell us that the child who, in a theoretical aspect seems severely retarded, turns out to be significantly advanced with respect to practical intellect and practical activity. The child has advanced the area of his practical, purposeful activity much further than his theoretical development. Lipmann used Koehler's method to study imbeciles and found that in the case of extensive intellectual retardation practical sense proved to be considerably higher than intellectual reasoning. A whole group of these children proved to be capable of rational activity. Lipmann set up an extremely interesting experiment: He asked his test subjects to solve one and the same problem, first by action, and then theoretically. The task consisted of grabbing an object from a swinging pedestal. When the test subject approached the object and attempted to get it, we have one result; when he began reasoning, the nature of his reasoning yielded quite another result. The test subject could not solve the puzzle theoretically, whereas practically he did a good job solving it. Long ago study of the intellect in mentally retarded children already showed that very often the child is much more resourceful in practice than in theory; that he knows how to act purposefully and "thinks" much better with his hands than with his head. Several investigations have shown that practical and theoretical intellect may exist in reverse ratio to each other and that, precisely because of a weakness in abstract thinking, the development of a child's practical thinking is intensified and vice versa.

I permit myself to explain this in relation to cultural development. Both cultural development and practical development are connected with the use of cultural means of thinking, in particular verbal thinking. In recent times, psychologists have discerned a form of child thought which sheds light on the problem of cultural development; this is *child primitiveness* where the degree of cultural development is minimal. Allow me to introduce an example of child primitiveness, which we have borrowed from A. E. Petrova, who analyzed this phenomenon in the clinic of M. O. Gurevich. A child severely delayed in her adaptive reactions was analyzed. The child had lived in many institutions and was then sent to the psychiatric hospital because of suspected mental illness. In the hospital, no mental illness was discovered and the child ended up in Gurevich's experimental clinic. The child—a Tatar girl—who in early childhood exchanged one not yet firmly established language for another, learned to understand those who spoke in that language but was absolutely untrained to think in it. The girl had not become accustomed to the fact that, on the basis of words alone, one could draw a conclusion. The psychologist gave her a series of intellectual tasks requiring practical activity in some and words in others. When faced with practical activity, the test subject produced positive results. She reacted to the verbal tasks with incomprehension and inability to think. For example, the girl is told, "My aunt is taller than me, and my uncle is still taller than my aunt. Is my uncle taller than me?" The little girl responded, "I don't know. How can I tell you whether your uncle is taller, if I have never seen him?" She responded to all questions in the same manner: If she had not seen with her own eyes, then she could not tell you anything. She could not imagine that on the basis of two verbal sentences she could use words to come up with a third sentence. This was impossible for her. The child was delayed in her cultural development, in the development of verbal thinking, but she was not a *debile,* she was not feebleminded, although on the surface she was similar to a debile: Her reasoning was weak, she gave nonsensical answers, and she refused to complete the simplest reflective operation. But we have made a gross error if we think that the girl did not know how to draw a conclusion on the basis of practical data.

Allow me to sum up: There is now under way an extensive reexamination of old conceptions in the area of understanding child giftedness and the negative aspects linked with it such as learning problems and abnormal behavior.

The old conception of giftedness as a single function has given way and in its place there has arisen a position based on the functional complexity of its individual forms, Therefore, I think that it is most appropriate to finish this discussion by pointing out which form of psychological investigation one should select when studying learning problems. A child is brought for consulting because the suspicions of the pedagogues indicate that he appears to be mentally retarded. Previously, they would usually be convinced that the child is not performing as he should, that he does not orient himself in the simplest surroundings, and the result would already have been predetermined. The first demand that modern psychology has placed before us is never to identify with only the child's negative characteristics because this still says decisively little about the child's positive traits. The child, let's say, does not possess certain knowledge; he does not, for example, have any conception of the calendar, but we do not know definitely what he can do and does know. The present research study can be summed up with the statement that the characteristics of a retarded child must necessarily be twofold. Similarly, modern medicine gives a twofold classification of tuberculosis: On the one hand, it characterizes the stage of the disease's development, and on the other it indicates the degree of the compensating process. Indications 1, 2, and 3 show the gravity of the illness, while A, B, and C show compensation for the disease. Only the combined data give a complete picture of the person's illness because, although one patient may have been much more deeply infected with the disease than another, his process of compensation may be greater. A person may be in the third stage of tuberculosis, but his compensation may be such that he finds himself completely able to work, while another, suffering from a far milder infection, may also exhibit less compensation so that the development of the disease plays a more destructive role.

In an analysis of an abnormal child, the defect alone tells the psychologist nothing unless he determines the degree of compensation for the defect, until he shows what lines of counterbalancing behavior will form and what attempt the child will make to compensate for those difficulties which he encounters. In practice, this dual character has become a typical phenomenon almost everywhere. In fact, we may even have defect and compensation of a triple character. Those who have had the occasion to study children closely, know how frequently one or another function in a retarded child—let's say, memory—may prove in and of itself to be rather highly developed. The trouble, however, lies in the fact that the child's ability to control it may be weak. Precisely the same was true of the primitive girl about whom we have already spoken in this discussion. The girl reasons well. In her reasoning there is contained a complete syllogism, but her inability to include it in a verbal chain of reasoning leads to her apparent severely retarded appearance.

We often encounter types in whom the levels of the organic basis for memory is in and of itself very high, or significantly departs from the average level, or surpasses it, yet the ability to remember and to use this ability for the performance of higher cultural processes proves to be minimal. I will introduce a case of a severely retarded child whose visual memory was developed to such a degree that he, not being able to read, proved able to execute the following tests: Before him were arranged notes with names and a rather large number of faces pictured on cards. A note lay before each image. Subsequently, the notes were reshuffled and the child, according to the inscription, again laid them out as they should be. And still, in spite of a colossal visual memory, this child could not learn to read, because the task of remembering, and mastering letters and connecting them with sounds, and so forth, turned out to be beyond his power. His capacity for acquisition was minimal.

A new idea has arisen in current research—to give double, even triple characteristics: the characteristics of practical intellect, practical knowledge, and its practical use. In a word, in place of the general definition of feeblemindedness or a learning disability, there is an attempt, first of all, to determine how it is expressed; secondly, to examine how the child himself attempts to cope with this phenomenon; and third, to learn which path the school must take in order to overcome the defects afflicting the given child.

What kind of pedagogical inferences dictate a new approach to research? Allow me to demonstrate this with a concrete example. We well know that mildly retarded children are distinguished by insufficient development of abstract thinking, and therefore, their education is based on visual aids. Visual education, however, develops in the child only visual thinking and cultivates his weaknesses. Not one contemporary pedagogue will dispute the fact that the visual method of education can occupy a central place in the auxiliary school, but when taking into account the child's mental weakness, it is necessary to form in him a certain basis for abstract thought, using visual material as auxiliary means. In other words, it is necessary to advance the mentally retarded child's overall line of development. In modern pedagogy (even in those countries less inclined toward a revolutionary pedagogy), a certain principle has begun to make headway: It is necessary to develop thinking in children in the auxiliary school and to cultivate in them social concepts, and the use of visual material is the basis for doing this. Thus, if we summarize our practical deductions from all that has been reported here, then it is possible to say the following: The entire difference between the new and the old practice is that the new negates old suppositions but goes further. If we earlier understood a child's unmanageability only as a complex of deficits, then modern psychology tries to show what is concealed behind the minuses. If the old upbringing was inclined to yield to the defect, to follow along behind it, then today's training takes into account the deficit and yields in order to take the upper hand over it and to overcome the defect that has made the child hard-to-handle or difficult educate.

# 8

# The Dynamics of Child Character

Because of the very way in which the question was formulated, room has not been left in psychological theory and pedagogical practice for the study of child character nor for the examination of its development and formation. The question has been approached statistically, so that character has been viewed as a steady and constant entity, always internally consistent, present, and seen as a given. Character has been understood as a status, not as a process; as a condition, and not as a formation. The classical formula of this traditional view was given by T. Ribot, who set forth two necessary and sufficient conditions for establishing an understanding of character: unity and stability. With this formula he implied a unity across time. The true sign of character, according to Ribot, is that which appears in early childhood and remains constant throughout the course of life; genuine character is innate.

Recently, the statistical view of character found complete and total expression in the theory of E. Kretschmer, for whom character is connected with the structure of the body; a psychological mental construction side by side with a somatic construction. In his opinion, both the former and the latter—body structure and character structure—are defined in the final analysis by the innate endocrine system. Kretschmer makes a distinction between two large, complex biotypes, the schizothymic and the cyclothymic. From these two types, a great many normal shades of temperament are formed in a widely varying mixture. These extreme biological types are connected with two basic forms of mental illness: schizophrenia and manic-depressive psychosis (cyclical). This doctrine, as A. B. Zalkind justly points out, has strongly affected child psychology (1926).

We find that P. P. Blonskii has extended and developed, or rather, transformed Kretschmer's viewpoint into a science about the child. "One of the merits of Kretschmer," Blonskii states, "is the establishment of the connection between the structures of body and of character. I go further and assert that different temperaments distinguish not only different individuals, but also different ages. In particular, a cyclothymic temperament is characteristic of the baby-tooth stage of childhood" (1925, p. 182). Adolescence replaces the cyclothymic temperament with the schizoid temperament (ibid., p. 227). The only change that the static conception of character has undergone with reference to the child is that it replaces a unified type of character, predetermined and fatally conditioned by the endocrine system, with a sequence of changes as one type follows another. The very principle of stability which Ribot enunciated remains inviolable here. Character type, it turns out, takes hold only at a certain age, and not accord-

Originally appeared in English translation in Part II of *The Collected Works of L.S. Vygotsky, Volume 2: The Fundamentals of Defectology (Abnormal Psychology and Learning Disabilities)* (Robert W. Rieber and Aaron S. Carton, Eds.; Jane E. Knox and Carol B. Stevens, Trans.) (pp. 153–163). New York: Plenum Press, 1993.

ing to an established constitution. The chain of stable types through which the child consecutively passes is still a static, not a dynamic, series. This is the fundamental distinction of both doctrines, resembling, in this respect, the majority of characterological theories. As we have noted, A. B. Zalkind justifiably calls this trend an absolute, *biological, static* approach to character (1926). According to his assessment of it, "The development of human character is merely a passive unfolding of that biological type which is inherent in the person." (ibid., p. 174).

Kretschmer's scheme does not work for the division of characterological traits by age. None of this, however, prohibits us from attempting to elucidate the prevailing predominant specific content of each stage in development. This specific content, not now taken into consideration by any of the existing characterological systems, undergoes extraordinary changes under environmental influences. This is why it is dangerous to attach rigid "labels" to any systems *in the given state of science.* The incompleteness of this viewpoint, like all static, non-dynamic views, lies in the fact that it is powerless to solve questions of origin, development, and growth. Such a view is necessarily limited, therefore, to a theoretical statement and generalizations and to the collection, correlation and classification of empirical data without insight into the true [underlying] nature of the studied phenomena. "If the outward forms of things coincided directly with their essence, then every science would be superfluous," wrote K. Marx (K. Marx, F. Engels, *Collected Works*, vol. *25,* Part II p. 384). Thus, this viewpoint, which is satisfied with the form of the "appearance of things"—that is, with bare empirical data, without an analysis of their "essence"—is an unscientific point of view. Such a theory starts in a fatal manner from the conclusion. This is why characterology, from Hippocrates to Kretschmer, has struggled in vain with classification as the fundamental problem of character. Classification can be scientifically substantial and productive only when it is based on an essential indication of phenomena dispersed among various classes, that is, when it presupposes an earlier knowledge of the essence of things. Otherwise, classification will necessarily be a scholastic division of empirical data. And such will be almost all classifications of character. The essence of things, however, is a dialectic and is revealed in the dynamics of a process in motion, change, formation, and distinction, that is, in the study of genesis and development.

Characterology—historical and contemporary—recalls the condition of the biological sciences before C. Darwin. Scientific thought tried to take into consideration, to regulate, and to introduce a system and sense into the great diversity of vegetable and animal forms. But it did not possess the key to understanding this diversity of forms, accepting it as fact, as data, and as immutable evidence of the creation of all being. The key to biology was found in evolution, in the idea of the natural development of living forms. Just as biology began with *the origin of forms* so, too, psychology should begin from *the origin of individuals;* the key to the origin of individuals is the conditional reflex. If Darwin gave us the biology of forms, then Pavlov gives the biology of individuals, the biology of personality. The mechanism of the conditional reflex reveals the dynamics of personality; it shows that personality arises on the basis of the organism like a complex superstructure, created by the external *conditions* of an individual life. It is namely this doctrine that ultimately resolves the ancient argument between nativism and empiricism. It shows that *everything* in personalities is built on an inherited, innate basis and, at the same time, that everything in them is superorganic, conditioned, that is, *social.*

The doctrine of conditional reflexes does not simply render what is God's to God and what is Caesar's to Caesar. It shows us that, precisely in those conditions which restructure inherited experience, there is a fundamental motive force which pushes development ahead and causes change. The innate reaction is only the material: Its fate depends on the formative conditions in which it is destined to emerge. An unending number and great variety of things can be created on this innate foundation. One can hardly find a better illustration for proof of what is almost an absolute—the reeducability of human nature—than the conditioned salivary response to the debilitating painful irritation caused by a strong electrical current. Placed under appropriate conditions, (i.e., being fed at the time of painful shock) a dog begins to respond to induced bums and pains with a positive reaction, which in the language of subjective psychology is called *joyful anticipation,* and in the language of objective psychology *a digestive reflex.* The dog not only does not guard itself from pain but actually is drawn to it. On viewing the experiment, C. Sherrington, as J. Bon [no ref.] reports, exclaimed: "Now I understand the joy of the martyrs as they climbed onto the pyres" (cited in Iu. P. Frolov, 1925, p. 155). Thus, the biological, by means of social factors, melds into the social; the biological and organic into the personal; the "natural," "absolute," and unconditioned into the conditioned. This is the true material of psychology.

C. Sherrington recognized an enormous psychological future in this experiment with the dog; he saw the key to the solution of the origin of higher forms of human psychology. In essence, he stated what can be translated and interpreted for our purposes as the following: In order to understand the character of the martyr who climbs joyfully onto the fire, we must ask from what are the *conditions* from which this character will necessarily arise. What causes the martyr to enjoy this? What is the history, that is to say, the dynamics and conditioning (or conditionality), of this joy. Character is conditioned (or conditional); such is its dynamic formula. Static character is equal to a sum of certain basic signs of personality and behavior. It is a diametric cross-section of personality, in its unchanging status, and its ready condition. To understand character *dynamically,* however, means to translate it into the language of a fundamental whole within its entire social environment, to understand it in its struggle to overcome obstacles, *in the necessity of its emergence and unfolding,* in the internal logic of its development.

## 2

The logic of character development is the same as the logic of any development. All that develops, develops by necessity. Nothing is perfected or goes forward from the internal "vital impulse" which H. Bergson proposes in his philosophy. It would be a miracle if character developed when not under the pressure of necessity which commands and pushes it toward development. What is the necessity in which the motive forces of character development are embedded? To this question, there is only one answer: the fundamental and definitive necessity of all human life-the necessity to live in a historical, social environment and to reconstruct all organic functions in agreement with the demands set forth by this environment. Only in the capacity of a defined social unit can the human organism exist and function.

This position serves as the point of departure for A. Adler's system of individual psychology (the social psychology of personality). We set aside here the question of the relationship between this doctrine and Marxist philosophy. This is a complex question, which can be debated and, above all, demands particular and special research. Adler's basic philosophical positions are distorted by metaphysical elements. The characterological interest is limited to Adler's practice. With good reason, Adler calls this doctrine "positional psychology" in the profoundest sense of the word and in contrast to dispositional psychology. For the former, psychological development proceeds from the social position which the personality has attained; for the latter—from the organic disposition, that is, predisposition. Here the original meaning is returned to the concept of character. *Character* means an *engraving* in Greek.

Character is the social imprint on personality. It is the hardened, crystallized, typical behavior of personality; it is the struggle for social position. It is a secession from the primary line, the leading line of development, the unconscious plan of life, from the integral course of development of all psychological acts and functions. In connection with this, it becomes absolutely necessary for the psychologist to understand each psychological act and the person's character as a whole, not only with respect to the person's past but also with respect to his future. This can be called the ultimate direction of behavior. Just as in a film, a framesequence representing one moment of motion remains incomprehensible without the subsequent moments, outside the motion as a whole, similarly the trajectory of a bullet is defined by the final point or gun sight. In precisely the same way, every act and every feature of character raises the following questions: Toward what is it striving? What is its goal? Into what is it transformed? Toward what does it gravitate? In essence, this understanding of psychological phenomena—not only from the past, but also from the future—does not designate anything other than the dialectical necessity of accepting phenomena in unending motion, of disclosing the future-oriented tendency ofphenomena, determined by the present. As, in the historical sphere, we shall never understand fully the essence of the capitalist system if we look at it statically, outside the tendencies of its development, outside its necessary connection with the future system maturing in its womb, so, too, in the sphere of psychology, we shall never understand fully the human personality if we are to look at it statically as a sum ofphenomena, of acts, and the like, without an integral biographical plan of personality, without a main line of development which transforms the history of a man's life from a row of disconnected and separate episodes into a connected, integral, life-long process.

## 3

No one instinctive action of an animal can be understood and interpreted by us if we do not know its final "goal," the point at which it is aimed. Imagine the behavior of an animal before sexual unification. It may be understood only if taken as a whole, only if seen from the final act, the last link at which all the preceding links on this chain are directed. The motions of a tiger, lying in wait for its prey, will be completely meaningless if we do not have in mind the final act of this drama, when the tiger devours its prey. We could go down the evolutionary ladder to the very lowest organic functions, and everywhere we would find the very same trait: the final character, the ultimate direction of the biological reaction. If the teeth of an animal masticate and grind food, this can be understood only in connection with (the fact) that the food will be digested and assimilated by the organism, that is, in connection with the whole process of digestion and nourishment. A general biological formulation of the very same idea is, essentially, what is usually conditionally called the immanent teleology of the organism, or that methodological principle according to which we view parts of the animal body as organs, and their activity as organic functions acquiring meaning and sense only in relation to the organism as a whole.

Thus, the final character of psychological acts, or their future-oriented tendency, appears already in the most elementary forms of behavior. As we have seen, not one instinctive action can be understood fully if not examined from a future perspective. I. P. Pavlov confirmed this fundamental fact in the brilliant term *goal reflex*. Studying the simplest and most basic forms of innate activity of the nervous system, Pavlov came to the conclusion that a unique unconditional reflex should be formulated—the goal reflex. By using a paradoxical term, Pavlov from the first glance underlines the uniqueness of this reflex: It is directed at the attainment of a *goal*, and may be understood only from the viewpoint of the future. At the same time, this form of activity is not a particular exception, but rather the most normal reflex. Precisely because of this, Pavlov replaces here the term *instinct* with the preferred term *reflex*. "This term clarifies the idea of determinism; the connection between stimulus and effect, cause and result becomes more self-evident" (1951, p. 306).

It is curious that Adler, when expounding on this notion of the future-oriented tendency of behavior, calls to mind Pavlov's experiments in training a conditional, signal reflex (A. Adler, 1927). And it is all the more curious that Pavlov's explanation of a goal-reflex mechanism is similar to the doctrine of compensation. He saw in this reflex "life's most important factor," which is particularly indispensable for a most crucial area: education. The mechanism for training a goal reflex by means of the presence of obstacles was established in both Pavlovian and Adlerian psychology. T. Lipps called it the law of *damming up* and saw in it a common law of psychological activity, concluding that energy, when concentrated at a given point, is increased and may overcome the restraint, and even flow in a *roundabout* way. This already contains the idea of compensation. In general, Lipps explains any drive as a result of this law; he thought that all purposeful activity was achieved precisely at the time when an obstacle arises in the path of preceding aimless or automatic events. Only thanks to the dam, the restraint, the obstacle, does a "goal" become possible for any mental process. The point of interruption or disruption of any automatically operating functions becomes the "goal" for other functions, which aim at this point and, therefore, have the appearance of purposeful activity. Thus, the "goal" is a given beforehand; in essence, it only appears to be a goal but, in fact, constitutes the primary cause of all development.*

---

*   There has been extensive comment on the notion that behavior could be accounted for because motive forces or psychic energy were conserved and re-directed. Despite disputes among advocates who explored the notion from a variety of philosophical vantages, Vygotsky's Marxist treatment of the theme here reveals its prevalence in the *Zeitgeist* of the early 20th century. The list of Freudian mechanisms *(displacement, suppression, repression, sublimation,* and so on) may be read as a detailed elaboration of the ways in which Lipp's *Stauungen* are re-directed. A relatedness between the Freudian and Pavlovian approach has later been noted among students of instinct (see, for example,

The dynamic theory cannot be limited to a statement about the factual existence of a goal-oriented reflex, that is, of a fatalistic psychology. This theory strives to learn how this goal reflex arises, that is, what constitutes the causal conditionality and determination of these forms of future-oriented behavior. The answer to this question lies in Pavlov's formula for the existence of obstacles. The existence of obstacles (as psychology showed even before Pavlov) is not only the main condition for the *attainment of a goal* but also the indispensable condition for the very *emergence* and *existence of the goal*.

The two basic psychological assumptions on which the dynamic theory of character rests—clarification of the future-oriented mind set and the principle of compensation in psychological development—are therefore, inwardly connected. One is essentially the dynamic continuation of the other. The existence of obstacles creates a "goal" for mental acts, that is, it introduces into development a future-directed mentality. The presence of this "goal" creates a stimulus for compensatory tendencies. These are two moments of one and the same psychodynamic process. We note in passing that, in order to completely understand the internal logic of the views presented here, one must bear in mind a third basic assumption: the principle of social conditionality in developmental processes. This principle is intrinsically connected with the first two assumptions for the reason that it forms, in causal sequence, the first, all-defining principle and that in inverse causality or goal-directed order it contains the ultimate, or final, moment of the very same integral process: *development out of necessity.*

The social conditions in which a child should take root comprise, on the one hand, the entire scope of a child's unadapted state and serve as the genesis of his developmental creative forces; the obstacles which thrust a child forward developmentally are rooted in those conditions of the social milieu in which he *is supposed* to grow. On the other hand, the child's whole development is oriented toward achieving a necessary social level. Here, we have the start and the finish, the alpha and omega of his development. Chronologically, the three moments in this process can be explained as follows: (1) a child's unsocialized, unacculturated nature places powerful obstacles in the path of psychological growth (the principle of social conditionality for development); ( 2 ) these obstacles serve as stimuli for compensatory development and become the final goal, determining the whole process (the principle of future-oriented psychology); and (3) the presence of obstacles augments the operation of certain functions and forces their perfection. This results in triumph over these obstacles and hence in adaptability or assimilation (the principle of compensation). The fact that personal interaction with the environment stands at the beginning (1) and at the end (3) of the process,

---

Lorenz. K., *On Aggression.* New York: Harcourt Brace Jovanovich, 1966.) Interestingly, Vygotsky does not acknowledge the degree to which Adler's formulations are derivative from Freud's. Instead they are presented in a context which would make them appear to be essentially related to the Pavlovian view although he asks whether Adler's view are thoroughly Marxist (Section 2 of this chapter) and concludes that they are and they are not (see the Concluding Section of this chapter). In the passage here, Vygotsky provides a remarkable clarification of the degree to which the Pavlokian system and its kindred systems are teleological in their formulation although he associates teleology with idealism, which he eschews. Later in the chapter, overlooking Freud's therapeutic ambitions, he denies that this teleology may be available in the Freudian system. Throughout, Vygotsky, the optimistic Marxist and educator, favors the theory which provides the latitude for environmental manipulations and the greatest possibilities for the amelioration of defects. [Ed.]

gives the process a closed, circular form and allow us to examine the process in its direct (casual) and inverted (goal-oriented) aspect.

4

If we understand, however, how strength arises from weakness and how capabilities arise from defects, then we hold in our hands the key to a child's "giftedness." The dynamic theory of giftedness is, of course, still a matter for future discussion; until now, and even now, this problem has been resolved purely statically. Researchers have approached child giftedness as a fact, as a given, and have asked only one question: "What is the numerical score?" They are interested only in the numerical points and not the actual components of aptitude. In the dynamic theory of child character, prerequisites are given for the creation of a new, dialectic doctrine about the plus and minus of a child's aptitude, i.e., about the child's talents and handicaps, The former atomistic and quantitative point of view immediately reveals complete theoretical bankruptcy. Let us imagine a man with a poor memory. Suppose that he knows about his shortcoming, and examination has shown a poor recall of meaningless syllables. According to established *use* in psychology—which we should more appropriately call *abuse*—we should conclude that this man's inadequate memory is due to hereditary causes, or illness. Strictly speaking, in this manner of research the conclusion usually contains what has already been expressed in different words in the premise. For example, in the given case, if someone has a poor memory or somebody remembers few words, then he supposedly has little capacity for retention. The question should be put differently: "To what purpose is a memory weak? What necessitates it?" We can establish this purpose only from an intimate knowledge of the individual as a whole; our understanding of this component arises from an understanding of the whole.

The dynamic point of view allows us to see giftedness and deficiency as two different results of one and the same process of compensation. Only scientifically unwarranted optimism would assume that the mere presence of a defect or handicap is sufficient to cause compensation and to transform the defect into a strength. Overcompensation would be a magical process, and not a biological one, if it transformed all types of shortcomings into merits, irrespective of the internal-biological and external conditions in which the process occurs. We could not make a more implausible and absurd caricature of this idea than if we were to go to extremes by saying that any defect facilitates higher development. It would be very easy to live if this were really the case. But in fact, compensation is a battle, and every battle can result in two completely opposite outcomes: victory or defeat. Like all battles, the result depends on the relative strength of the fighting sides. In the given case, it depends on the severity of the defect and on the strength of the compensating reserves. If compensation successfully overcomes a defect, then we have a picture of a fully developed child with superior abilities. If compensation is not successful, we have primitive, incomplete, delayed, and malformed development. One pole of this process borders on genius; the other, on neurosis.

Neurosis, a retreat into illness, and the totally asocial nature of this psychological position, all testify to a *fictitious* goal which directs the lifelong course along a false path, distorting the mainline of development and the child's character. Thwarted compensation turns into a defensive battle, with the help of illness; the conqueror defends himself by building on his weakness. Between these two poles, these two extreme cases, falls an entire gradation of compensation—from minimal to maximal. This is the definition of child giftedness (aptitude), to which we are accustomed—the definition most often stated and encountered by us in practice. The uniqueness of the dynamic approach does not lie in a change in the quantitative analysis of aptitude and its special forms, but in the refusal to attribute to this appraisal a self-contained significance. By itself, the defect says nothing about development as a whole. A child with a particular defect is still not a defective child. Along with a defect come stimuli for overcoming it. The development of giftedness, similar to the development of character, is dialectical and evolves by contradiction.

An internal contradiction guides character development along a path of "psychophysical contrast," as Adler literally named the antithesis between organic deficiency and psychological compensation.

S. Freud advanced a well-known thesis on a characterological triad (accuracy, stinginess, and obstinacy) and on its connection with anal eroticism. Or consider yet another Freudian thesis: "Subjects suffering from enuresis are noted for their excessive, ardent ambition" (S. Freud, 1923, p. 23). "The internal necessity of similarly connected phenomena" (ibid., p. 20) is far from completely clear and comprehensible even to the author of this theory himself. We are justified in asking what significance for future life these character traits can have. What is the connection between this triad and anal eroticism? Why is *life-long* behavior defined by this trait? What keeps it from atrophy? What nourishes it? On the contrary, if, as in the case of a child's impaired hearing ability, we are shown how *greater* sensitivity, suspiciousness, anxiety, curiosity, and other similar functions strive to compensate for a hearing impairment by means of reaction formations and compensations, and in order to construct a defensive psychological superstructure over the defect, and if we are shown how these develop, then the logic of character, its social and psychological conformity to laws becomes intelligible and understandable.

For Freud, "initial inclinations which persist unfailingly" come to light in character traits. Character is rooted in the *distant past.* For Adler character is the side of personality which is future-oriented. Freud, in his dream interpretations, proceeds from remnants of the past and remote childhood experiences, while Adler views a dream as a military reconnaissance, a sounding out of the future, and a preparation for future activity. This latter approach may be taken toward the doctrine of personality structure and character. This new doctrine introduces a future-oriented perspective, a highly valuable perspective for the psychologist. This perspective frees us from the inertia of conservative and backward theories. Indeed, for Freud, a man is chained to his past, like a convict to his wheelbarrow; all of life is determined in early childhood from elementary combinations and, without exception, boils down to living out childhood conflicts. It remains incomprehensible how all subsequent conflicts, traumas, and experiences could constitute only outer layers encrusted on remote infantile experiences, which constitute the trunk and core of one's entire life. In the new doctrine, the revolutionary future-oriented perspective allows us to understand the development and life of a personality as an integral process which *struggles forward* with objective necessity toward an ultimate goal, toward a finale, projected by the demands of social existence.

The psychological perspective of the future offers theoretical possibilities for education. By nature, a child always appears inferior or "unfinished" in a society of adults; from the beginning, his very position gives grounds for the development of feelings of inferiority, insecurity, and embarrassment. For years on end, a child remains unfit for independent existence, and in his inadequacy and childhood awkwardness lie the seeds of his development. Childhood is a period of social ineptness, "inferiority," as well as a time for compensation by taking advantage of one's strength; a time for the conquest of position in relation to the social whole. In the process of this conquest, a human being as a specific biotype is transformed into a human being as a sociotype; an animal organism becomes a human personality. *The societal mastery of this natural process is called education.* It would be impossible, if a future-oriented perspective, defined by the demands of social existence, were not impregnated in the most natural processes of child development and formation. The very possibility of an integral plan in education and its future-oriented attitude testifies to the presence of such a plan in the developmental process which strives to master education. Essentially, this means only one thing: *Child development and character formulation are socially oriented processes.* O. Ruele says the following about this lifelong line of development: "It is his {the child's—L.V,} thread of Ariadne, which leads him to the goal. Insofar as all mental functions proceed in time in a selected direction and all mental processes acquire their own typical expression there will result an aggregate of forms of tactical devices, aspirations, and capabilities overlaying and outlining life's determined plan. This is what we call character" (1926, p, 12).

Many important scientific discoveries about the child have been made along these lines. Thus, despite S . Hall and his biogenetic theory, the excellent classic investigations of K. Groos have shown us that play, as a fundamental form of natural training for young animals and small children, can be understood and explained not by its connection with the past, but by its future-oriented tendencies. For the child, play arises as a result of the insufficiency of his natural abilities to cope with life's difficult tasks resulting from his impracticality. Childhood is a biological time for the "acquisition of skills, required by life, but not developed directly from natural abilities" (1916, p.71). It is a time for compensating for underdevelopment. Play is the natural means of a child's self-education, an exercise oriented toward the future. Recently, a new point of view in regard to the psychological nature of exercising has been advanced and strengthened. It is, essentially, a further development of Groos's idea. In accordance with this view exercise which is, generally speaking, most important in the developmental process of education is a compensatory process in the process of cultivating the functions of personality.

Only in the light of Groos's theory of play and the new theory of exercise can one really understand and appraise the significance of a child's movement and its educational sense. A child's movement (in certain components) must be analyzed as an experience in the rationalization and organization of group play among children on an international scale. That is, play in a revolutionary era, which, like any game, prepares the child for the future implants the fundamental lines of his future behavior. The very idea and practical application of such play would be impossible if the development of personality were a passive unfolding of innate primary abilities. The idea of consciously stretching out all human life from childhood on and directing it along one continuous straight line, demarcated by history, may be well substantiated but only on the condition that character is not born, but created. The correct name for the process of emergence of character is not *unfolding,* but *enculturation* Precisely this viewpoint gives us the key to understanding personality in its social aspect, the key to understanding its class-oriented character, not in a literal-metaphorical sense, but in the real, concrete sense of an imprint made by social class on the biological structure of personality. A.B. Zalkind points out that the basic failing of static theories of character is an inherent contradiction: these theories are based on the fundamental fact that every human being is not only a biological, but also a historical unit, whose character bears historical traits.

"Can class position (the position of the exploiter or the exploited), or a historical epoch (revolution, reaction) instigate one character type or another?" (A. B. Zakind, 1926, p. 188). With this question, the difference between these two ways of interpreting character is brought into sharp focus. One approach adheres to the biological determination of character; the other approaches character as a historical form of personality. The first view was explicated in the famous thesis of G. Kompeire who examined character as a completed totality of signs, fixed from the moment of birth. "Without lapsing into paradox," he states, "one might say that a child who subsequently will be industrious will exhibit this inclination by the manner in which he seizes and holds the feeding bottle"(in *Mental Life of the Child,* 1916, p. 261) [Ref not provided but see Kompeire, 1910,1912]. In other words,character is born with the human being and is already present in the manner in which the newborn seizes and holds the bottle. In contrast to this view, Groos sees the enormous biological significance of play as a natural means of formatting features which lead us away from inherent nature to a new, "acquired" human nature, or, "using (an old expression) here, in a certain sense from the old Adam toward a new Adam" (K. Groos, 191 6, p. 72). But character is the new Adam, the new second nature of man.

\* \* \*

In recent years Adler's doctrine, particularly his applied and practical pedagogical views, have exerted a great influence on the theory and practice of social education in Germany and Austria. Pedagogy is the most important area of this psychological doctrine. In the words of 0. F. Kanitz, this doctrine already has, therefore, great significance for the socialist workers' movement, which puts primary importance on the influence of environment and education: "This gives a psychological foundation to the words of Marx; our social being determines our consciousness" (0. F. Kanitz, 1926, p. 165). In particular, Kanitz insists that the practical yield from Adler's work, the application of this theory to education, is at variance with a capitalistic system and its cultural environment. *"In a word, once individual psychology is put into practice it shatters the framework of the capitalist social order* and in this way a bourgeois psychologist of this particular bent will sometime and somewhere experience his Damascus"(ibid., p. 164). In 1925, at the Congress on Individual Psychology in Berlin, Kanitz put forward the following thesis: "Individual psychology will penetrate the masses only when it is guided by the world view of the masses" (ibid.).

As has already been said, we will leave aside the complex question of the interrelationship of individual psychology and Marxism. We do consider it necessary, however, to point out the presence of two opposite tendencies intrinsic in this doctrine in order to shed light on the factual status of this question.

A. Adler's doctrine is supported by a mixed, complex basis. On the one hand, it affirms that the ideas of K. Marx, more than anyone else's, can have significance for individual psychology. On the other hand, he avidly absorbs the ideas of H. Bergson, W. Stern, and other idealists and notes the concurrence of many of his ideas with the basic points of their philosophy. With complete justification, Adler states that the intention of establishing a relationship between individual psychology and philosophy entered neither his thoughts nor his work. Adler, who tries to give a gnoseological basis to this theory, was right when he says that separate elements of this doctrine have associations, which were found by purely empirical means, that is, this theory does not have its own philosophically consistent methodology.

*Precisely because of this*, it absorbs philosophical elements of the most irreconcilable nature. All of contemporary psychology is undergoing a crisis, in the sense that there exists not one but two psychologies. Until now, both have been developing side by side as a materialistic psychology based on the natural sciences and an idealistic, teleological psychology. This idea has been expressed in the works of modern psychologists such as F. Brentano, H. Muensterberg, W. Dilthey, E. Husserl, P. Nathorp and many others. Adler's psychology, like all other forms of modern psychology, contains in undeciphered form the principles of these two completely incompatible, directly opposing scientific systems. Hence arises the methodological struggle within this direction of psychology, accompanied by attempts to formulate this trend methodologically with the help of one or the other system.*

---

* The Russian text ends this chapter with an ellipsis. In this passage Vygotsky seems to re-iterate thoughts which appeared in his Questions *of Theory and the History of Psychology : Historical Significance of the Crisis in Psychology.* (Voprosy teorii i istorii psikhologii: Istoricheskii smysl psikhologicheskogo krizisa) in [Rus ] Volume 1 of the *Collected Works.*

# 9

# The Collective as a Factor in the Development of the Abnormal Child

## 1

Contemporary scientific research, occupied with the problem of comparative research into the development of normal and abnormal children, proceeds from the general assumption that the laws governing the development of normal and abnormal children alike are basically the same. In the same way, the laws governing vital activity remain fundamentally the same, whether for normal or ill-functioning conditions in an organ or organism of the body. The task of comparative psychology is precisely to find the general laws which characterize the normal and abnormal development of a child and which wholly encompass all areas of child development.

Recognizing the general applicability of the laws of development to the normal and pathological spheres is the cornerstone of the comparative study of children. But these broad regularities find their own concrete manifestations in one situation or another. When dealing with normal development, these regularities are realized in one complex of conditions. Where something atypical unfolds before us, something which deviates from the norms of development, those same regularities, now appearing in an entirely different complex of conditions, take on a qualitatively individual, specific appearance, one which is not an absolute copy or photographic replica of childhood development. Thus, comparative research must always maintain dual tasks in its field of vision: (1) establishment of general laws and (2) uncovering their specific manifestations in the different variants of child development. Thus, we must start out from the general laws of child development and then study their peculiarities as they apply to abnormal children. This should be the path of our research even now, in examining the problem which interests us, the problem of the collective as a factor in the development of an abnormal child.

Obviously, we will limit ourselves to only summary and abstract statements of those positions in the light of which we are intending to investigate the development of the abnormal child. The basic proposition which interests us can be formulated in the following manner: Research on the development of higher psychological functions persuades us that both their phylogenesis and ontogenesis have social origins.

As far as phylogenesis goes, this proposition has hardly ever met with serious opposition because it is entirely clear that the higher psychological functions (that is, thinking in concepts, reasoning, speech logical memory, voluntary attention and so on) coalesced in the historical

Originally appeared in English translation in Part III of *The Collected Works of L.S. Vygotsky, Volume 2: The Fundamentals of Defectology (Abnormal Psychology and Learning Disabilities)* (Robert W. Rieber and Aaron S. Carton, Eds.; Jane E. Knox and Carol B. Stevens, Trans.) (pp. 191–208). New York: Plenum Press, 1993 period of human and anthropoid development. These functions arose not in the biological evolution of a human bio-type, but through the historical development as a social creature. Only collective social life developed and elaborated all those higher forms of intellectual activity, which are characteristic of humans.

As for ontogenesis, only recently have the results of a series of studies on child development made it possible to establish that the building and formation of higher forms of psychological activity are completed in the process of a child's social development, in the process of a child's relationships, and in his cooperation with the surrounding social sphere. On the basis of some of our own work and work of our collaborators, we have elsewhere formulated this proposition in the following way: Observation of the development of the higher functions shows that the construction of each of them is clearly subsumed under one or another lawful regularity. Specifically, every higher psychological function occurs twice during the process of behavioral development: first, as a function of collective behavior, as a form of cooperation or cooperative activity, as a means of social accommodation (i.e., on an interpsychological plane) and, again, a second time, as a means of a child's individual behavior, as a means of individual adaptation, as an inner process; that is, on an intrapsychological plane.

In order to follow the transition from the collective form of "working together" to the individual form of a child's behavior, we must understand the principle for building the higher mental functions in the making.

In order that this overly general and abstract proposition about the collective origins of the higher psychological functions not remain simply an unclear verbal formulation, in order to fill it with concrete contents, we must clarify by using practical examples to show, in the words of P. Janet [1930?], how this important basic law of psychology works in the psychological development of a child. By the way, examples can help us significantly in studying the results of the application of these laws to abnormal child development. The examples serve as a bridge, tying together concrete facts, linking the laws of normal development and abnormal development.

We could take the process of speech development as the first and simplest example illustrating the general law. It is sufficient to compare the beginning and final moments in speech development; then, one can see to what extent the formulation we have just addressed is justified. In fact, in the beginning, speech appears in a child in the role of communication, that is, as a means of communicating, of influencing the surroundings, of linking up with it, as a form of working with other children or adults, as a process of working with others and of cooperation. But it is worth comparing the beginning moment of speech development with more than just its final stage, namely, the speech function in an adult. It is also worth comparing the first moment with one of the following stages of development—for example, with the fate of the function of speech at school age or at an interim stage—to see how speech at that point becomes one of the most important means of thought, one of the most important and leading inner psychological processes of a child.

This first stage of speech in the process of thought formation led many researchers to reach an entirely false conclusion. They concluded that thinking is nothing other than soundless, mute, inner speech; thinking is speech without sound. This extreme perspective equated the processes of thought with inner speech. No matter how false this equation may be, it is deeply significant: The mistake, which led to this inaccurate identification, would not have arisen if the speech processes were not indeed so close to the thought process and so deeply and intimately intertwined with it that only special and subtle analysis can reveal the inaccuracy which lies at the basis of that understanding.

If we glance at the entire cycle of speech development, seeing it as a psychological function from its beginning to its final moments, then it is easy to understand that the cycle wholly conforms to that very important fundamental rule in psychology mentioned above. This rule shows how the path from outer speech to inner speech goes through a whole series of changes during a child's development, how the most important form of collective behavior—social cooperation with others—becomes an inner form of psychological activity for the personality itself. Let us briefly take note of the most significant moments in the process of transformation from outer to inner speech.

The first turning point and a decisive stage in the subsequent development of child thought is that form of speech which contemporary psychology often calls *egocentric speech*. When studying child speech from the functional perspective at the early, preschool age, we can easily establish that speech activity takes two basic forms. On one hand, there is socialized speech. The child asks questions and answers questions put to him, voices objections, makes requests, informs or tells something. In a word, he uses speech as a form of working with the people around him. On the other hand, there is egocentric speech; the child speaks, as it were, to himself aloud, and for himself. For example, while busy at some activity such as drawing, playing with a toy, or manipulating subjects, he carries on a dialogue, as it were, with himself; he does not enter into cooperative speech with those around him. This form of speech may be called *egocentric*, since it performs an entirely different function from verbal communication. Still, since egocentric speech was first studied, a correct psychological understanding of it has run into a number of difficulties.

J. Piaget was first among Contemporary researchers to study, describe, and measure in sufficient detail the phenomenon of egocentric speech in children of various ages. He was inclined to attribute no very real meaning to this form of speech as far as the subsequent fate of a child's thought was concerned. For Piaget, the fact that a child accompanies his own activity with spoken utterances is just an expression of that general law of child activity according to which a child still does not distinguish some forms of activity from others. That is to say, a child becomes involved in the process of activity with his whole being. That general, discerning. undifferentiated activity appears not only in a child's motor functions but in his egocentric speech. Thus, egocentric speech appears to be something like an extra, peripheral function, which accompanies the child's basic activity like the accompaniment of any basic melody. But this accompanying activity, this egocentric speech, fulfills no independent psychological function; it has no reason to be there. Nothing essential would be changed in a child's behavior if that accompaniment disappeared.

Indeed, according to Piaget's observations and very careful measurements, egocentric speech does not develop; rather, it is curtailed with the child's progressive development. Its most luxurious flowering occurs at an early age. As early as mid and pre-school years, it takes a turn which is not a sharp nor abrupt but still decisive. It experiences a breaking point after which its development begins constantly, though slowly, to decline. At the beginning of the school years, according to Piaget's research, the coefficient of egocentric speech (a numerical indicator of diffusion and frequency in the behavior of a child of a given age) falls to zero. Thus, the functional and genetic evaluation of egocentric speech speaks to the fact that it is a product of insufficiently developed child behavior, stemming from the idiosyncratic set of the early childhood years and disappearing as the child's behavior reaches a higher level of development. In other words, egocentric speech, in Piaget's opinion, is an incidental product of child activity, an epiphenomenon, some kind of free supplement to other kinds of activity, an expression of the incomplete nature of a child's behavior. Functionally, it is not necessary to anything, and nothing essentially changes in the behavior of the child; genetically, it makes no contribution to development; rather it is fated to slow disappearance and curtailment.

In light of new and more profound research, we feel it must, however, be recognized that this evaluation of egocentric speech does not correspond to reality from either a functional or a genetic perspective. With special research devoted to studying the functional role of egocentric speech, we have been able to establish that it begins to play a unique and altogether specific function in a child's behavior, even early on—and that it cannot be regarded as a by-product of childish activity. Egocentric speech, as our research showed, is not included in the process of a child's behavior as an accompaniment, going along with the basic melody of one activity or another. Speech is not simply added to basic activity, more-or-less indistinguishably in step; rather, it becomes involved in the flow of that activity, and actively restructures it, changing the appearance of its structure, composition, and manner of functioning. Thus, by measuring the coefficient of egocentric speech in a child, we have been able to establish that this coefficient almost doubles in situations which are linked with troubling conditions.

Analysis of that same fact led us inescapably to a reevaluation of the functional role of egocentric speech. This means that a child reacts by using egocentric speech above all when his basic activity runs into an obstacle, a difficulty, which diverts the activity from its usual flow. From the psychology of thought, however, we know that it is precisely in circumstances linked with such difficulties that intellectual reaction occurs. The psychological function of the intellect arises precisely in the process of adapting to new circumstances and different conditions—thinking means overcoming difficulties.

Thus, the link between egocentric speech and problems in and of itself leads to the notion that egocentric speech in a child's behavior begins very early to fulfill intellectual functions—that is, it begins to serve as a means of thought. But decisive confirmation does not come from the mere fact of more frequent egocentric speech in the face of difficulties. Rather it comes from an analysis of the forms of egocentric speech which appear in a child's behavior in response to obstacles. Analysis shows that a greater part of a child's egocentric speech under such circumstances acquires an intellectual character. Speech does not just reflect the confusion arising from some activity; the child, as it were, asks himself questions, formulates his problem in words, as he gropes about for solutions.

Let us give the simplest of examples from our own experiments, showing clearly what we have in mind when we speak about the intellectual function of egocentric speech. The child is drawing a tram car. When outlining the last wheel, he presses down hard on the pencil so that the lead breaks, bouncing off to the side, and the wheel is left unfinished. The child first tries to complete the circle he has begun with a broken pencil, but nothing is left on the paper except impressed outlines. The child stops, looks at the paper, and pronounces "broken"—and then goes on to a different part of the picture, exchanging the pencil for paints. From this, it is clear that the word "broken," uttered by the child to himself, without reference to anyone present, was indeed a decisive moment in his activity. At first, it seemed that the word referred to the pencil and simply stated the fact that it was broken. Further observation revealed that this was not so. We can imagine the detailed sequence of the child' s behavior more or less in the following manner: The child tried to finish drawing the last wheel; he didn't succeed and found a way out of the difficulty by changing the theme of the picture. The unfinished wheel came to represent a broken wheel, and the entire picture began to unfold further, not according to the earlier model of an already finished drawing, but in a completely different direction. In the final version, the picture depicted a broken tram car, which had been in an accident, and which had been removed for repairs onto a side track.

One might ask: Can such an egocentric utterance in a child, concentrated in one word, be defined as simply accompaniment, going along with the basic activity—the drawing—and can one see in that one word only a by-product of the child's activity? On the contrary. It is clear that this word and its communication represent a key moment, a turning point, in the child's activity. Like a plan, that word contains within it, in condensed form, the entire further behavior of the child; it signifies a resolution discovered for a difficult situation, an expressed purpose, a sketch for future action. That word is the key to the entire future behavior of the child. In particular, the word became the solution of the problem which confronted the child at that moment when the pencil broke. That which was formulated in the word was then carried out in action. These new, complete relations between a child's words and actions (which we observed, admittedly, in the most primitive form) already fully merit being called an intellectual function of egocentric speech. A child resolves a problem in words; with the help of egocentric speech, he identifies the path of his actions; consequently, he is thinking in words, even if in a very primitive and extremely elementary form. An analysis of similar facts is also in accord, showing that egocentric speech fulfills an intellectual function and becomes a primitive method of children's thinking out loud in a difficult situation.

We will not discuss further the changes in composition, structure, and method of children's actions which take place in connection with the appearance of primitive verbal thought in the shape of egocentric speech. We will only say that these changes are, in the highest degree, serious and significant. This is understandable; if speech is included in a child's behavior as more than a second, parallel-moving kind of reaction, then attaching words does not represent merely an accompaniment with respect to the fate of basic activities. Rather, it represents the molding of the most basic melody of children's activities. Thus, we can conclude from this that egocentric speech fulfills an important function in children's behavior; it acts as the child's first, most initial verbal thought.

But, if this is the case, then one must anticipate in advance that the genetic fate of egocentric speech, and its role and function in the developmental process have been falsely evaluated in earlier research. In fact, if egocentric speech changes nothing in behavior—if it is merely a by-product and does not fulfill any function—it is completely natural that, with age and with the development of the child, it should disappear, vanish from behavior. But if it is by nature nothing other than the first stage in the development of children's thought, then it would be difficult to anticipate anything other than its being a close, internally inseparable link to the next stage in the development of a child's verbal thought processes. And, in fact, a variety of research allows us to conclude these things: We have, in egocentric speech, one of the most important moments in the transition from outer to inner speech; it is only the first step in the formation of inner speech and, consequently, in the verbal thought process of a child.

Egocentric speech (according to results we have formulated elsewhere) is still, physiologically speaking, outer speech. It still can be heard; the word occurs outside; the child is thinking out loud; his thoughts are not far from conversation. Outer speech still displays all the characteristics of an ordinary monologue, a conversation out loud with oneself. However, psychologically, inner speech is already there; that is, we have before us speech which basically, fundamentally, and decisively changes its function, transforming itself into a way of thinking, into an internal way of behaving, into a specific form of activity in a child's intellect.

We will not now discuss in detail all the factors that are said to be useful in recognizing egocentric speech as a first step in the development of inner speech in a child. Let us say only that the disappearance of egocentric speech by school age is further accompanied by other factors which show that the formation and development of inner speech occurs specifically during early school age. But, on the basis of this and many other facts, we have developed the hypothesis which states: Egocentric speech does not disappear entirely from a child's behavior; instead it changes its character and transforms itself into inner speech. This transformation is prepared for fully by the development of egocentric speech and is completed on the borderline between pre-school and school years. We have followed one of the most important transformations from outer to inner speech, and we could say that, in essence, the function of verbal thought develops in the following way: The child absorbs social forms of behavior, which he begins to apply to himself just as others earlier applied this method to him or as he himself applied them to other people.

Thus, to the question "Where do the higher processes of child thought come from? How are they built up, and through what means do they develop?" we should answer: "They arise during the process of a child's social development by means of the transferral to himself of those forms of cooperation which the child absorbs in the process of interaction with the surrounding social environment." We see that collective forms of cooperative work precede individual forms of behavior, grow out of their foundation, and act as the direct roots and sources of their appearance. It is in this basic sense that we formulated the law about the dual appearance of the higher psychological functions in the history of a child's development. Thus, the higher functions of intellectual activity arise out of collective behavior, out of cooperation with the surrounding people, and from social experience.

We can offer a few more examples which demonstrate the interdependence between the development of collective forms, on the one hand, and individual methods of behavior with respect to the higher psychological functions, on the other. First of all, let us mention argument. In their time, J. Baldwin [1904?, 1911?] and E. Rignano [no ref.] expressed the idea, that true thought is nothing other than discussion or argument carried on within an individual. Piaget was able to substantiate this idea genetically and to show that a conflict of opinions, an argument, should arise early in a children's collective, so that thought might later develop among children of that collective as a special process in inner activity which would be unknown to a child of an earlier age. The development of reflection is begun in argument, in the conflict of ideas; such is the fundamental conclusion of this research.

And, in fact, as Piaget has very wisely expressed it, we readily take ourselves at our own word. In the process of individual thought, the very task of checking, demonstrating, disproving a known position, and motivating confirmation cannot take place. Demonstrating the accuracy of one's thoughts, raising objections, presenting reasons—all of this occurs through a task of adaptation and can arise only in the process of children arguing with each other. "This is my spot," said a child whom Piaget observed. "You must give it to me, because I always sit there." "No, it's mine," objected the other, "because I got here first and took it."

The seeds of future reflection man understanding of justifications, proof, and so on—are already contained in the most primitive of children's quarrels.

In the history of a child's reflection, itself closely linked to argument, we can observe the genetic interdependence between collective forms of cooperation and individual methods of behavior with respect to the development of intellect. If so, then, based on the example of a game with rules, we can also observe (as a number of researchers have shown) the same genetic dependence in connection with the development of a child's volition. The ability to direct one's own behavior, to restrain and even replace spontaneous, impulsive actions with those that do not stem from the spontaneous influence of an external situation but which arise instead in the attempt to subordinate one's behavior to the rules and tasks of a specific game—the ability to coordinate one's actions with those of one's companions (in a word, all of the elements of the earliest stage of self-direction which merit the name of *voluntary processes*)—first emerges and appears in some collective form of activity.

A game with rules here again serves as an example of this. Later, these forms of cooperation, which led to the subordination of behavior to a given game's rules, become internalized forms of a child's activity, voluntary processes. A game with rules, consequently, occupies the same place in the history of a child's will as arguments and discussions occupy in the history of the development of reflection.

If the theme of this work permitted us to examine in detail each of the higher psychological functions, we would be able to demonstrate that the rules we formulated above equally include such functions as attention, memory, the practical intellect of a child, his education, and so forth. The development of a child's personality is seen in all cases as a result of the development of his collective behavior; everywhere we can observe one and the same law of shifting social forms of behavior into the sphere of individual adaptation.

We have already said that this law has special meaning for an accurate understanding of the development and underdevelopment of the higher mental functions of an abnormal child. Defects and lack of development of the higher psychological functions are related to one another in a different way than defects and lack of development are related in the elementary functions. This distinction must be mastered in order to unlock the whole enigma of the psychologically abnormal child. Although underdevelopment of the elementary functions is often the direct result of one defect or another (for example, motor underdevelopment due to blindness, underdevelopment in speech because of deafness, underdevelopment of thought due to feeblemindedness, and so forth), underdevelopment of higher functions in an abnormal child usually arises as a result of additional, secondary phenomena, which compound with his primary characteristics.

All contemporary psychological research on abnormal children is permeated with the basic idea that the image of mental retardation and other forms of abnormal development in a child represents a structure that is in the highest degree complex. It is a mistake to think that from the defect itself all the criterial symptoms and a complete characterizing picture can be derived immediately and decisively as though it were the fundamental nucleus. In fact, it turns out that those particularities which constitute the picture have a very complex structure. They display extremely intricate structural and functional interconnections and, along with the primary characteristics of the child stemming directly from the defect, they show also secondary, tertiary, and other complications which derive not from the defect itself but from the defect's primary symptoms. Thus, additional syndromes arise in an abnormal child, like a complex superimposition upon the basic picture of development. The ability to distinguish between what is basic and supplementary—what is primary and secondary in an abnormal child's development—is a requisite condition not only for an accurate theoretical understanding of the problems which interest us, but also for practical actions.

However paradoxical it may seem, all the scientific tendencies of contemporary defectology (if one takes its practical conclusions) orient us in a direction that is most unexpected from the point of view of traditional praxis. These tendencies teach us that the greatest possibilities for the development of the abnormal child most likely lie in the higher, rather than the lower, functions. For a long time, the laws of T. Ribot, H. Jackson, and others have been tacitly recognized as the basic premises in defectology. These laws say that the order of pathological destruction is opposite of the order of the construction of the functions. That which appears latest in the developmental process suffers first in the process of destruction. The processes of development and destruction are linked but in an inverse relationship.

From this perspective, it seems natural that, when a series of pathological processes are present, disintegration begins with the higher, most recent, most complex functions, leaving the primary ones alone and not touching the lowest functions. The application of this law to underdevelopment might be understood as follows: The sphere of higher psychological functions has always been considered to be close and beyond the ability of the abnormal child. Thus all pedagogical efforts have been directed at the advancement and perfection of the lower, more elementary processes. More clearly, the doctrine affected sensorimotor education in both theory and practice, inasmuch as in training and education that doctrine dealt with distinct sensations, different movements, separate elementary processes. The mentally retarded child was not taught to think, but to distinguish among smells, among nuances of color, among sounds, and so on. And it was not only sensorimotor training but the entire rearing process of the abnormal child that was oriented toward alignment of the elementary and the lower functions.

Current scientific research demonstrates that this perspective is mistaken. Precisely because of the theoretical bankruptcy of this pedagogical system, the approach described above has turned out to be of so little value and of such little practical usefulness that it has developed into the deep and serious crisis which has, at the moment, overtaken the whole field of education for abnormal children. In truth, as research shows the lower, elementary processes are, on the one hand, the least susceptible to training, the least dependent on external events, on the social development of the child. On the other hand, since they become the first symptoms, flowing directly from the very nucleus of the defect, they are closely tied to that nucleus that they cannot be defeated until the defect itself has been eliminated. And, since the elimination of the defect is impossible, it is natural that the struggle with the primary symptoms has been doomed beforehand to futility and failure. Both these instances taken together have meant that the development and training of the elementary lower functions have confronted almost insurmountable obstacles at every step.

Moreover, the dialectic of development in an abnormal child and his training is such, that his development and training must be completed not by direct but by indirect means. As we have already stated, the mental functions arose during humanity's historical development and depend in their structure on the collective behavior of the child; they represent an area which, in greater measure than the others, allows for leveling and a smoothing over of the effects of a defect and offers greater possibilities for the influence of education. Still, it would be erroneous to think that an abnormal child's higher processes are better developed than his elementary processes. With the exception of a small number of cases (such as, for example, the underdeveloped elementary motor processes of the blind or the deaf), the higher processes usually suffer more than the elementary ones. This should not discourage us. It is true that the underdevelopment of the higher processes is not primarily, but secondarily conditioned by the defect. And, consequently, they represent the weakest link in an abnormal child' s chain of symptoms. Therefore, this is where all educational efforts should be directed, in order to break the chain at its weakest point.

Why do the higher functions fail to develop in an abnormal child? Not because the defect directly impedes them or makes their appearance impossible. On the contrary, experimental research has now demonstrated without a doubt that it is theoretically possible to develop those modes of activity which lie at the base of the higher functions. Thus, the underdevelopment of the higher functions is a secondary structure on top of the defect. Underdevelopment springs from what we might call the isolation of an abnormal child from his collective. This process proceeds in approximately the following manner. Any given defect in a child produces a series of characteristics which impedes the normal development of his collective relations, cooperation, and interaction with others. Isolation from the collective or difficulty in social development, in its turn, conditions underdevelopment of higher mental functions which would, otherwise arise naturally, in the course of normal affairs, linked to the development of the child's collective activities.

Below, we will clarify this with a simple example. For the moment, let us simply say that the difficulties which an abnormal child experiences in collective activity become the reasons for underdevelopment of his higher functions. This is the fundamental conclusion to which our reexamination of the question has brought us. But unlike the defect itself, which is a factor in the failure of the elementary function's development, the collective, as a factor in the development of the higher psychological functions, is something which we can control. As hopeless as it is in practical terms to battle with the defect and its natural consequences, it is valid, fruitful, and promising to struggle with difficulties in collective activities.

In other words, when elementary functions fail to develop, we often are powerless to eliminate the cause leading to their underdevelopment. Consequently, we struggle with the symptoms rather than with the causes of retardation. With the development of higher mental functions we can affect not only the manifestations but the very cause; we struggle not just against the symptoms but with the illness itself. In the same way that medicine employs as its basic method causal therapy—rather than symptom therapy—in order to eliminate the reason for disease—and not only its particular burdensome effects—so, too, must curative pedagogy strictly distinguish between causal and symptomatic educational activity.

Precisely this possibility of eliminating even the most proximate reason for the underdevelopment of the higher psychological functions puts the problem of the abnormal child's collective activity at the forefront and opens up absolutely invaluable opportunities for the pedagogy of abnormal children.

Before us remains the task of briefly reviewing the concrete expression of these general propositions as they are applied to the feebleminded [retarded], the blind, and the deafmute child.

2

Research on collectives of feebleminded [retarded] children has begun relatively recently. It has led to the establishment of extraordinarily interesting regularities about the formation of collectives. We have, for example, the published observations of V. S. Krasusskii [no ref.], which show that very feebleminded [retarded] children enter into the formation of a collective with a variety of levels of mental development. This is one of the basic conditions for the existence of a collective. Yet in the majority of cases, the persistent and long-lasting collectives are made up of children who are at different levels of mental retardation.

One of the traditional methods of our pedagogical practice is the method of recruiting or selecting school-groups on the basis of equal levels of mental development. This assumes that children at the same level of mental retardation make up the best collectives. Research shows that feebleminded [retarded] children, when left to themselves, never group according to this principle. More exactly, they always violate this law.

Analysis of the [available] data, says our author, permits us to arrive at only one conclusion. The most desirable social combinations to which children are attracted are idiots and imbeciles and imbeciles and debiles. What happens in terms of social relations is a kind of mutual catering to one another. The intellectually more gifted have the opportunity to demonstrate social activeness with respect to the less gifted and less active. The latter, in their turn, get what they lack from social interaction with more active children; not infrequently, this becomes an unrecognized ideal to which the intellectually deficient child aspires. The most frequent age difference in unhampered social groupings of children is from three to four years. It is as though these data repeat the principles which apply variability in the intellectual development in normal children.

Let us not dwell on the details of that observation. Let us say only that there are other features which are characteristic of the life of collectives and which demonstrate that the same mixing of intellectual levels in a collective is the most dynamic.

Let us look at the following material as an example. When imbeciles are put with imbeciles, the number of people per group averages 2.6, and the average length of time that the collective lasts is 6–7 minutes. Similarly, when debiles are put with other debiles, their numbers averaged 2.0 people with an average duration of 9.2 minutes. On the other hand, when imbeciles and debiles were put together, their collectives averaged 5.2 members and the duration was 12.8 minutes. Unfortunately, most research on the problem of collectives among mentally retarded children studies the external, formal features, such as numbers, the collective's duration in existence, and so on but not the interstructure of each child's behavior nor the structural changes in the collective. Thus there seems to be a formal bias toward limiting observation to activities in which there is movement, to points of cessation of activities, to redistributions, and the like. If we moved from these formal features to the more profound changes which the personality of the feebleminded [retarded] child undergoes and which are hidden beneath this formal features, we would see that each of the children who made up the collective acquired a new quality and specialness by assimilating himself into some kind of [larger] entity. The study of unimpeded social life among severely retarded children will uncover a whole new side to the biological incompleteness of an idiot's or imbecile's personality; it will offer the opportunity to approach the problem of mental retardation from the perspective of social accommodation for the child. This area must be made the focus of attention in pedagogical work with severely retarded children. It will, of course, also place in our hands the key to the complex problem of recruitment into groups of severely retarded children.

The formulation offered by V. S. Krasusskii seems to us to be entirely justified. He says we must have an exhaustive and well-rounded understanding of the unencumbered social life of the children we are studying. Only then can the question of social compensation for a defect be discovered and detailed for each concrete circumstance.

Let us finish with these data. Although in itself true, it seems to us that it would be inappropriate to say simply that new sides to the personality of a severely mentally retarded child are revealed in open children's collectives; it would be more correct to speak of the fact that, in these collectives, the personality of the severely retarded child truly finds a dynamic source of development, and that, in the process of collective activity and cooperation, he is lifted to a higher level.

It is now clear how profoundly antipedagogical is the rule of using sameness as the basis for choosing collectives for retarded children. In doing this, we not only go against the natural tendency in the development of children; what is more important, we aggravate rather than ameliorate the most immediate cause of increased underdevelopment of higher functions when we deprive the mentally retarded child of collective cooperation and relations with others who stand higher than he does. Left to himself, the severely retarded child is drawn to the less retarded one—the idiot to the imbecile, the imbecile to the debile. This difference in intellectual level is an important condition of collective activity. The idiot who finds himself among other idiots, or the imbecile among other imbeciles, is deprived of this dynamic source of development. P. P. Blonskii, although he may have given an excessively paradoxical form to his ideas, nonetheless noticed that an idiot deprived of the right education suffers more from this than a normal child. And this is indeed the case.

It is therefore not difficult to imagine that the effects of the wrong education retard real possibilities much more in the case of a feebleminded [retarded] child than they do for a normal one. And everyone well knows to what degree a normal child who is deprived of the appropriate educational conditions shows the effects of pedagogical neglect and that these effects are almost indistinguishable from actual feeblemindedness. If one bears in mind that we are talking about severely retarded children, who are generally more narrow and limited in development than mildly retarded children, then the degree to which everything said above applies to even the mildly retarded child becomes clear. E. DeGreef approached the problem which interests us from the internal, qualitative side, and he demonstrated the following simple fact.

If one asks a feebleminded [retarded] child to evaluate his own mind and that of his comrade and of an adult educator (as that researcher did in his experiments), the mentally retarded child will habitually rank himself first, then his friend (also a retarded child), and in third place, the normal adult. The complex question of the exaggerated self-image of the mentally retarded child does not interest us for the moment and we leave it aside. That problem is, in itself, in the highest degree important, but peculiar. Let us focus on something else. Let us ask ourselves why, in the eyes of the mentally retarded child, the other feebleminded child is wiser than the normal adult. Because, DeGreef answers, the mentally retarded child understands his comrade better, because between them there is the possibility of cooperation, relations, and coactivity. On the other hand, an understanding the complex intellectual life of an adult is unattainable by the mentally retarded child. This is why, in paradoxical form, Blonskii, like DeGreef, formulates this absolutely accurate idea: Genius, from an imbecile's perspective, lies within the limits of psychological debility.

We should stop here and draw some conclusions. We see that the pedagogy of the collective is of the first order of importance in the whole structure of education for a feebleminded [retarded] child. We can see what value general collectives of normal and retarded children have, what importance the selection of the group and the distribution of intellectual levels has. In these conditions, we find a basic pedagogical norm, which is all but a general law for the education of all abnormal children.

When we compare the pedagogy of the collective for retarded children with that for normal children and ask ourselves what they have in common and what differences exist, we get the same answer we always get when we talk about a comparison of the different pedagogical measures used for normal and abnormal children: We see the same pedagogical aims with distinctive ways of attaining those goals, goals which are unattainable by abnormal children using the direct path. Thus, the general formula for comparing the pedagogy of normal and abnormal children is entirely appropriate for the problem at hand: the pedagogy of the child collective.

# 3

For a blind child, the same problem of under development of the higher functions occurs with respect to collective activity; this problem takes concrete form in an entirely different field of behavior and thought. However, if one investigates this problem accurately, its roots reveal a resemblance to those basics which we have already examined with respect to mentally retarded children. For ease and simplicity's sake, let us begin with a pedagogical statement of the problem. A blind child is immediately deprived of visual perceptions of visual forms. A question arises from that situation: How can this deficient activity be replaced for him?

Until now, this has been the key question in the pedagogy of the blind. Thus far, people in this area of pedagogy have come up against the same difficulties that have been encountered in the pedagogy of the feebleminded [retarded] child. Pedagogy has attempted to attack the question head on. Traditional psychology answers the question of how to struggle against the effects of blindness and psychological underdevelopment by cultivating sensorimotor activity, training the senses of touching and hearing, and using the so-called sixth sense of the blind (or the methods which blind people somehow detect large objects in a space directly in front of them using a method or sense which is unknown to seeing people). Traditional pedagogy also insists on the importance of visual aids in teaching the blind, on the necessity of filling up the meager reserve of impressions about external activities from other sources. It is just possible that if this problem were soluble, then such efforts might be crowned with complete success. That is to say, if we were to find some equivalent or some surrogate for the spatial and visual impressions of a seeing person, then, as W. Steinberg says, with the aid of that surrogate, we could compensate to a known degree for those omissions in a child's experience which result from blindness. But as far as concrete ideas and perceptions go, this task is insoluble. The whole difficulty consists precisely in the fact that no training of the sense of touch, no sixth sense, no extremely refined development of one or several of the usual methods of perception, and no auditory impressions—none of these things can act as a true equivalent or prove to be a substitute of equal value—to those visual images which are missing.

The pedagogue therefore embarks on an effort to replace visual images through other senses without understanding that the very nature of perception conditions the immediate character of activity. It also causes the impossibility of concretely replacing visual images. Thus, as far as the elementary processes go, we can never create a real possibility of concrete substitution for insufficient spatial images in the spheres of perception and performance.

Nevertheless, it is perhaps not useless to attempt to transmit perceptions of a visual form, or even the aesthetics of architectural perceptions, by using pictures made up of raised dots. Still, whenever the attempt to create surrogates for the visual perceptions of the sighted is made (this is especially the case for raised-dot pictures), it reminds one of a famous tale about a blind man which A. A. Potebnia [1922?] uses to show that a single generalization is far from knowledge. A blind man asks his guide: "Where have you been?"—"I wanted a drink of milk."—"What is milk like?"—"It is white."—"What is white?"—"Like a goose."—"And what is a goose like?"—"It is like my elbow." The blind man felt the guide's elbow and said, "Now I know what milk is like!"

Meanwhile, psychological research on the personality of a blind child demonstrates more and more clearly that perception and representation are not the natural sphere of compensation for the effects of blindness; compensation occurs not in the realm of elementary processes, but in the realm of concepts, that is, in the higher functions.

A. Petzeld, in his famous proposition, formulated this theoretical possibility of unlimited knowledge for a blind person. In his research, he showed that, although a blind person's impressions are extremely limited, he is in no way limited in abstract knowledge. The basic conclusion of his work—and it is a conclusion of profound practical and theoretical substance—is that a blind person has the possibility, in principle, of knowing everything even though he may lack identifiable impressions.

An analogous question has often been put with respect to humanity as a whole. It is asked, in a critique of the sensualists: If a person possessed not five, but four, senses, how could his mental and cognitive development take place? From the sensualist perspective, one might expect that the absence of one of the five senses would lead to the construction of an entirely different picture of reality and would bring about an entirely different direction in human psychological development, from the one which is realized on the basis of five senses. Still, we must answer the question in a slightly unexpected way.

We propose that, with only four senses, nothing essential would change in human cognition, and thought (that is, the method of reworking given experiences) would remain exactly the same in principle. However, our image of the realities surrounding us would be composed not only on the basis of immediate impressions, but also on the basis of experience, and rational reevaluation. Consequently, both the blind man and the seeing man, in principle, know much more than they imagine; they know much more than they can absorb with the help of their five senses. If we really knew as much as we could absorb directly through our five senses, then not a single science (in the true sense of that word) would be possible. For the links, dependencies, and relationships among things which are the content of our scientific knowledge are not the visually perceivable qualities of things; rather, they come to light through thought. This is also the way it works for a blind child. Thought is the basic area in which he compensates for the inadequacy of his visual perceptions.

The developmental limitations in higher knowledge go beyond the sensorimotor training which is possible in the elementary processes. *Thought is the highest form of compensation for the insufficiencies of visual perceptions.*

Overcompensation in thought leads to two dangers which we would like briefly to mention. The first and basic danger is verbalism, and it is widespread among blind children. Verbalism is the use of words for which no meaning can be found, the content of which remains empty. The blind person, using the same speech as the sighted, intersperses it with a series of words whose meanings are inaccessible to him. When the blind man says "I saw him yesterday," or "Today is a bright day," he is using words in each of these cases the direct meaning of which is inaccessible to him. Using empty words with no content is the basis of verbalism.

Such verbalism becomes a false, fictive compensation for the inadequacy of perceptions.

Nevertheless, if the word in question corresponds to some meaning based in the experience of the blind person, even though the direct visual meaning of that word is a subject inaccessible to him, what we have is not verbalism, not fictive, but true compensation—the working out of an understanding relative to a subject, which is otherwise unattainable through perception and representation. As Petzeld correctly formulated his position, a black table is as black for a blind person as for a sighted one. Proof of this lies in a daily fact from the lives of the blind, something they themselves carefully recount. For example, N. Saunderson, blind from birth, wrote a famous geometry text, and the blind A. M. Shcherbina, according to his own testimony, explained optics to her seeing comrades as they studied it in a high school physics class. The fact that the blind can work out entirely concrete comprehensions, on a par with the sighted, about subjects which they cannot absorb through sight is a factor of first-rate importance in the psychology and pedagogy of the blind.

The danger of verbalism brings us to the second danger—the danger of false understanding. Formal logic and the history of psychology have explained the process of forming understanding thus: First the child acquires a series of concrete perceptions and images; from mixing and superimposing separate representations one over the other, gradually general outlines are composed from a series of different impressions; the outlines from various sources are erased or suppressed, and a general understanding dawns, very like F. Galton's collective photographs.

If this path corresponded to reality, then the law Petzeld formulated about the possibility of unlimited knowledge for the blind would be impossible. If the path to the formation of a concept lay only through perceptions, then a blind person would be unable to arrive at an understanding of the color black which is adequate for our comprehension. The understanding held by the blind would necessarily be a false understanding and would represent, in the sphere of thought, something analogous to what we call verbalism, that is, the use of empty words. Here is the difference between formal and dialectical logic in studying a concept. For formal logic, a concept is nothing other than a general representation. It arises as a result of a series of many broad indications. The fundamental law, to which the movement of a concept belongs, is formed in logic as a law of inverse proportionality between the extent and the content of a concept. The broader the extent of any concept (that is, the more general an understanding and the broader the group of examples to which it applies), the weaker its content, (that is the number of indications of the concept which we hold in our minds). The path to generalization is thus a path which leads away from the riches of concrete reality toward the world of concepts, the kingdom of empty abstractions, tar from living life and from living knowledge.

In dialectical logic, it is quite the opposite: A concept seems richer in content than does a presentation. Thus the path to generalization is not a path formally divided into separate indications. Rather, it is an uncovering of the links of the relationship of a given matter with another. If the subject becomes truly intelligible, not through immediate experience, but in all the many links and relationships which define its place in the world and its connection to the rest of reality, then one's understanding is a deeper, more real, truer, and more complete reflection than the envisaged one.

But, and this is the most important thing that we have said so far, understanding, like all the higher psychological processes, develops in no other way than in the process of collective actions by the child. Only cooperation brings a child's logic to fruition; only socialization of a child's thought, as Piaget formulated it, leads to the formations of concepts.

This is why the pedagogy of the blind must participate here in studying the issue of cooperation with the sighted, as a basic pedagogical and methodological problem in teaching the blind. Collective thinking is the fundamental source of compensation for the effects of blindness. In developing collective thinking, we are eliminating the secondary effect of blindness; we are breaking through at the weakest point in the chain created around the defect; and *we are eliminating the very reason for the underdevelopment of psychological functions in a blind child,* opening up before him uncharted and unlimited possibilities.

4

Nowhere does the role of the collective as a factor in the abnormal child's development appear in the foreground with such clarity as in the development of a deaf child. Here, it is entirely clear that all the difficulties and limitations created by the defect are encompassed, not in the handicap itself, but in the effects, the secondary complications, called forth by that handicap. In itself, deafness might not be such a burdensome obstacle to intellectual development in a deaf-mute child, but for the absence of speech, called forth by his muteness, which becomes an enormous obstacle along that same path. Thus, all the individual problems in a deaf-mute child's development are united, focused, on the problem of speech.

This is the problem of problems for all pedagogues for the deaf.

Above, we have discussed the development of higher forms of thought and logic in a child with respect to the socialization of those functions. In that context, it should be absolutely clear that the absence of speech in a deaf-mute child complicates his full participation in the collective, tears him out of the collective, and becomes one of the fundamental obstacles to the development of his higher mental functions. Experimental research demonstrates this at every step: whatever we take away from a deaf-mute child in social relations, he later lacks in thought. A vicious circle has developed around this question; practical pedagogy has not yet found an exit.

On one hand, the fight against artificial speech, against phraseology, and the attempt to teach live, active speech, which offers the opportunity of social relations rather than just intelligible pronunciation of sounds—all this requires a reexamination of the role played by speech in the traditional education of deaf-mute children. If, in the traditional education, speech totally consumes all other aspects of education and becomes an end in itself, then it loses its vitality for that very reason. The deaf-mute child is taught to pronounce words, but he is not taught to speak, that is, to use speech as a means of communicating and thinking. Therefore, along with artificially inculcated speech, he more willingly uses his own language of mimicry, which fulfills for him the dynamic function of speech. The struggle between oral speech and mimicry (sign language), in spite of the good intentions on the part of the pedagogues, ends, as a rule, in the victory of sign language, not because mimicry is a psychologically natural speech for the deaf-mute, but because it is authentic speech with all the riches of functional meaning. The artificial addition of pronouncing words out loud lacks life's richness and is only a dead imitation of living speech.

Thus, the task that now stands before pedagogy is that of returning the life to spoken speech; making that speech necessary, understandable, and natural for a child; and restructuring the whole system for educating him. The following proposition is of primary focus: The deaf-mute child is a child first of all—and only afterwards deaf and mute. This means that the child must first of all grow, develop, and be educated, following the general interests, inclinations, and rules of the child's age; during the process of development he should master speech. The problems of education in general—the problems of socio-political education—are now arising as the foci in educating deaf-mute children. It seems entirely justifiable that, by inculcating collectivism, social behavior, and cooperative work habits in deaf children, we are creating the only real foundation on which speech can grow. And, indeed, pedagogy has attained striking successes by following this path, a path which one can say without exaggeration is radically changing the character of our schools.

It quickly becomes clear that this is only one side of the question. The other side lies precisely in the inadequate speech development of these children and serves as a colossal obstacle in their sociopolitical education. If, at first, it seemed that social education was a prerequisite for the natural development of live speech, then later, it appeared that socio-political education itself is absolutely necessary as one of the basic psychological requirements in the development of speech.

As a result, pedagogues had to turn to mimicry as the only language through which deaf-mute children could absorb a series of thoughts, positions, and information without which the content of their sociopolitical education would be absolutely dead and lifeless. Thus, simply because our school has begun a radical reexamination of the question of the relationship between speech training and other aspects of education for deaf-mutes, and because it has answered that question in a diametrically opposite fashion from the way it was resolved in traditional education, the problem of speech now looms before us with more pungency than in any European or American country.

Everything depends on which demands are placed on the education of a deaf-mute child and which goals are expected of that upbringing. If we require only external mastery of speech and an elementary adaptation to independent life, then the question of speech training will be resolved relatively easily and satisfactorily. If, however, the demand is for a limitless broadening of goals, as they are extended here—if the goal of the deaf-mute child is to approach the fullest possible self-worth in all ways except in hearing, if we strive to bring a deaf-mute school as near as possible to a normal school—then this will create an agonizing discrepancy between speech development and overall development for the deaf-mute child.

The vicious circle is closed permanently, when we arrive at the third and final consideration, namely the exclusion of the deaf-mute child from the general collective, the limitation of deaf-mute children to their own society, and likewise the rupture in relations and cooperation with the hearing. Thus, the whole circle consists of three intertwined factors. Social education is based on the underdevelopment of speech; the underdevelopment of speech leads to exclusion from the collective; and exclusion from the collective stalls both social education and speech development.

We have been unable here to indicate a radical solution to this question. Most important of all, we think, is the fact that contemporary pedagogy and the contemporary state of science about speech education for deaf-mute children, in both theoretical and practical guises, will unfortunately not allow us to break down this resistance with a single blow. The path toward overcoming these difficulties is much more tortuous and roundabout than one might hope. This path, in our opinion, will prompt development in deaf-mute children and in part in normal children as well; this path consists of polyglossia, that is multiple paths for the development of speech in deaf-mute children.

In connection with this, it becomes necessary to reevaluate traditional and practical attitudes toward the various forms of speech for the deaf-mute, and, first of all, of mimicry and written speech.

Psychological research, both experimental and clinical, agree in their demonstrations that polyglossia (that is, the mastery of several forms of speech) is an unavoidable and fruitful method of speech development and education for the deaf-mute child, given the current state of pedagogy for the deaf. In connection with this, radical changes should be made in the traditional view about the competition among a variety of forms of speech and about their mutually restrictive nature on the development of the deaf-mute child. We must also pose the theoretical and practical question concerning their coordination and structural composition at various stages of learning.

This latter question, in turn, demands a complex, differentiated approach to speech development and to the education of a deaf-mute child. The experience of the most advanced European and American pedagogues, especially the Scandinavians and Americans, testifies to the presence of a complex structure for combining different forms of speech, as well as a differentiated approach to speech education for the deaf-mute child. Rather than being simply acceptable, all this suggests in turn a whole series of problems and questions for the theoretical and practical pedagogy of the deaf. These might jointly be resolved, not at the level of methods, but at the level of the methodology of speech education. Their resolution absolutely demands an elaboration of the psychology of the deaf-mute child.

Only a serious investigation of the laws of speech development and a radical reform in the method of speech education can bring our schools to a real, rather than a minimal, victory over muteness in deaf children. This means that, in practice, we must make use of all possibilities for speech activity for a deaf-mute child. We must not approach mimicry with condescension and scorn, treating it as an enemy. Rather we must understand that different forms of speech do not only compete with one another or disrupt one another's development, but that they can also serve as steps on which the deaf-mute child climbs to the mastery of speech.

In any case, pedagogy cannot close its eyes to the fact that expelling mimicry from the domain of speech communication permitted to deaf-mute children also eliminates a major part of their collective life and activity, and consolidates, exaggerates, and expands the fundamental obstacle to their development—their difficulties in forming collective activity. Therefore, research on the collective of deaf-mute children, on the possibility of collective cooperation with hearing children, and on the maximal use of all kinds of speech that are accessible to the deaf-mute child—all these are necessary conditions for a radical improvement in the education of deaf-mute children.

Traditional pedagogy for deaf children is based on individual lip-reading in front of a mirror. But conversation with a mirror is bad conversation, and therefore, instead of speech, one gets a lifeless, mechanical imitation of it. Speech that is severed from collective activity with other children, becomes dead speech. At first, our pedagogy moved the center of gravity to the social collective education of a deaf-mute child. But, then it severed speech from that education in the collective and so very soon it felt the painful gap between social demands and speech potentials in the deaf-mute child. Only by linking the two together, only by introducing the collective as the basic factor in speech development, only *speech in the collective* can decisively break out of this vicious circle.

\* \* \*

With our discussion of deaf-mute children, we have finished our exposition of the basic features which make up the themes of this chapter.

In conclusion, we should like to indicate that our aim has by no means been some sort of exhaustive and final resolution of the questions we have posed. Rather, this is simply an introduction to boundless areas of research—and only that. The basic principal and fulcrum for all our pedagogy for the abnormal child requires us now to be able to understand anew, in the light of real, natural phenomena, the links between cooperation [collective activity] and the development of higher mental functions; between the development of the collective and the abnormal child's personality.

—Communist pedagogy is the pedagogy of the collective.

# III

## Problems of the Theory and History of Psychology
### Crisis in Psychology

ROBERT W. RIEBER, *City University of New York* and
DAVID K. ROBINSON, *Truman State University*

The Russian edition of Vygotsky's collected works actually began with this volume, probably in keeping with Russian/Soviet assumption that fundamental theoretical issues should come first. Characteristic Western interests in practical problems, it would seem, demanded earlier publication of the volumes on psycholinguistics and "defectology" (special education), and they brought out the writings on history and theory as the third volume.

The complete Volume 3 of Vygotsky's *Collected Works* (1997) contains many of his articles on theory and history of psychology, as well as some prefaces to works written by others, and these prefaces are all devoted to theoretical matters. The very first article, though not included in the present volume, is worthy of some comment, because it foreshadows issues that emerged in the fuller work that we reproduce here, *The Historical Meaning of the Crisis in Psychology.* That first article is the published version of what is often called Vygotsky's debut, his celebrated talk at the Combined Session of the Psychological and Neurological Sections of the Second All-Russian Congress on Psychoneurology in Petrograd (Leningrad), January 6, 1924 (published 1926). Entitled "The Methods of Reflexological and Psychological Investigation," it was apparently the vehicle that carried the young provincial scholar to the high stage of Soviet scholarship, because it caught the attention of K. N. Kornilov. (Veresov and others argue that this was probably not a debut, that as a university student Vygotsky was already well known to Moscow psychologists.) In the year previous to the Petrograd conference, Kornilov had started agitating for a Marxist psychology, and by November of 1923, G. I. Chelpanov, the founding director of the Psychological Institute of Moscow University, was ordered to turn the leadership over to Kornilov, whose program of "reactology" attempted to represent such a Marxist approach.

One thing that must have impressed Kornilov was Vygotsky's courage, there on the spot, to criticize the Petersburg school of reflexology (Bekhterev and Pavlov) and to call for a new, unified psychology to investigate consciousness. Actually, Vygotsky's comments show appreciation of the achievements of reflexology (he is more complimentary to Pavlov than to Bekhterev), but he insisted that the reflexological approach did not provide sufficient foundation for psychology, the study of both mind and behavior. A fundamental dualism in psychological thought was the major problem of the moment, Vygotsky asserted: "Psychology is experiencing a most serious crisis both in the West and in the USSR". Whether Kornilov imagined that this brilliant young Jew from Belarus could help him promote the Moscow program in reactology is not clear. In any case, it did not happen that way.

Once he arrived at Moscow, Vygotsky hit the ground running, starting many projects with a group of collaborators who soon became his adoring disciples. His earliest research and publications concentrated on "defectology" (see the introduction to the previous section), but he was moving on all possible fronts and did not neglect the broad theoretical issues that had marked his entrance to the center of Soviet psychology. In fact, his first full-length book, though he could not publish it, was *The Historical Meaning of the Crisis in Psychology: A Methodological Investigation*, written 1926–1927, when the tuberculosis that eventually killed him flared up and forced him to bedrest. Unable to continue the clinical and educational work, he still could not waste his time, so he deepened his reading from the Institute's library. The present volume offers this book in full for several reasons.

First, this important book was almost doomed to oblivion. *Crisis in Psychology* has a curious publication history, mostly a history of nonpublication. Vygotsky was a young man in a hurry and was usually not shy about publishing as quickly as possible. Yet this completed manuscript, apparently ready for publication, did not appear in print until the Russian edition of *Collected Works* in 1982, fifty-five years later. The delay surely resulted from the political climate, and that climate may even have altered the text. David Joravsky (1987, 1989) has argued that the original manuscript must have included quotations of Trotsky, Bukharin, and Kautsky. Soviet editors in the early 1980s may have purposefully omitted those references, and Joravsky suspects that they even fiddled the text some. Vygotsky's critical discussions of Marxist writers are still extensive, though critical notes by the Soviet editors correct the author whenever he ventures outside the realm of Soviet orthodoxy. Since Vygotsky composed this theoretical work during the period from 1924 (when Lenin died) to 1927 (when Trotsky was exiled), it makes sense that publication at the end of that period would have been problematic at best, and likely it was simply repressed. Sheila Fitzpatrick (1978) has called the period 1928–1931 a "cultural revolution" in Soviet history, indicating that Marxist enthusiasts suddenly became very tough with anyone who would compromise with non-Soviet philosophy, even though full Stalinist repression was still a few years away.

A second reason for including the *Crisis* in full is that it is the one writing in which Vygotsky fully exercises his impressive powers as reviewer and critic. Although all six volumes of *Collected Works* contain prefaces, critiques, and other review writings, no other single work of his addresses so many authors, psychological doctrines, and philosophical positions as *Crisis* does. The most wide-ranging access to Vygotsky's own reading material is found in *The Historical Meaning of the Crisis in Psychology*, although this work is certainly no easy key to Vygotsky's thought and its development. Scholars will argue the details for many years, and this may be one case where an authoritative text will really be needed, one that has been verified with original manuscripts.

One intriguing analysis, an interpretation of the overall development of Vygotsky's thought, is offered by Veresov, who calls *Crisis* "one of the most important and most significant works by Vygotsky." This work, he insists, "presents Vygotsky not only as founder of a certain psychological theory, but as a methodologist of science" (1999, p. 145). It was in this theoretical work, coming after several years of practical work with learning-impaired children, that Vygotsky made the crucial steps toward his famous cultural–historical theory of psychological development. *Crisis* is "the watershed between early Vygotsky and Vygotsky the creator of the cultural-historical theory" (p. 29). Before Vygotsky wrote this work, Veresov claims, he was using reflexological and structuralist assumptions in psychology and even behaviorist methods while working with the children he studied, although he was characteristically critical of all these methods.

Looking for some way to overcome dualism in psychological theory (and occasionally even bewildering pluralism), Vygotsky was impressed by the German Gestaltists. He was not impressed enough, however, to be satisfied with their approach. (Nor were the Gestaltists all that impressed with Vygotsky's work when they visited him in Moscow. See Scheerer, 1980; Harrower, 1983, pp. 135–137, 144–145.) Vygotsky continued to search for his own solution to the dualism that had precipitated the crisis, and the result of that search was his book on the subject. At the same time, interestingly, the Gestaltists paralleled Vygotsky's book with their better-known publications (especially Koffka, 1926; Buehler, 1927/28). Even Ash's monumental work (1995) on German Gestalt has not accounted for the broader impact of this crisis outside of Germany. A contemporary observer (Hartmann, 1935, Chap. 17) put his finger on the reason why Gestalt failed to unify psychology. The Gestaltists who were best known in the United States turned toward a physiological theory of perception based on isomorphic correlations between mind and brain. As Kurt Goldstein and Martin Scheerer continued their work, a schism in Gestalt occurred. In America they found that the classic position by Wolfgang Köhler and Kurt Koffka had given short schrift to issues that now concerned them, the role of the individual in society and theories of personality, as well as psychopathology in the individual. Vygotsky, in his time and place, was still concerned with all of these issues, although it is true that he often had difficulty knowing the place of the individual in his system. Out of the philosophical foundations of Marxism, Vygotsky finally steered toward his own celebrated theory.

Although Veresov's account of Vygotsky's development will seem too discontinuous to many readers of Vygotsky (whose own theory emphasized "emerging" and "development" rather than abrupt turns), most will probably agree with the emphasis that Veresov gives to the period during which Vygotsky wrote *Crisis.* It was an important time for Vygotsky and for the history of psychology.

A third reason for careful consideration of this work is that it is probably the best place for scholars, even if the text has suffered some tampering, to gain insight into what everyone agrees was Vygotsky's main effort: to create a Marxist science of psychology appropriate to the new Soviet society. Although Lenin and Trotsky had not shirked from dictatorial tactics during the Revolution and Civil War, for a few precious years in the mid-1920s, young Soviet intellectuals felt as if they were free to explore possibilities for the new world in front of them, a world with few limits, where lives that had long been miserable could be made anew and for the better. For Vygotsky and psychology, as for similar young leaders of literature, arts, architecture, medicine, science, and nearly every other facet of intellectual activity not too closely identified with the Tsarist regime (religion, for example), Marxism continued to be the doctrine of open possibilities, of a new life unfolding. The interesting thing is that Vygotsky could include such appreciative considerations of "bourgeois" and foreign work in psychology, even as he admitted that he still had only vague outlines of what Marxist psychology should be.

A fourth and final reason to read and think about "crisis" is that many critical observers of the profession of psychology still invoke the term to describe today's situation. Indeed, Rieber and Wollock (1997) introduce Volume 3 of *Collected Works* with a discussion of this very issue, and David Bakan (1996) tries to get a handle on just what kind of crisis psychology is facing. The crisis today–similar to the one addressed by Vygotsky, in that it is an identity crisis–manifests itself in even more complications in the evolution of its development. For example, many psychologists are currently defecting to the newly emerging fields of neuroscience and cognitive science, notwithstanding the schism between clinical and experimental academic psychologists in the last decades of the twentieth century. The tendency to overspecialize is now the runaway choice. Within that move is a paradox. Psychology as a profession is bigger and more popular than ever, and yet quality control sometimes boils down to a corrupt Darwinian principle of the "survival of the most vulgar." In the long run this is surely a misdirected solution to the general problems of psychology. Vygotsky, if he were still with us, would surely agree.

The fourteen chapters of *Crisis* are a rich field to mine for illumination of all these issues. In the first two parts, Vygotsky surveys psychologists' definitions of psychology and its purview, arguing that a unified theory is absolutely necessary for further development of the field. Parts 3 and 4 assess recent efforts for unification (psychoanalysis, reflexology, Gestalt, and William Stern's personalism) and survey some attempts to establish psychology based on Marxism. Parts 5 through 11 review many psychological and philosophical writers, particularly Germans and Russians. Part 12 tries to explain why the crisis was occurring at that particular time, as psychotechnics and other applications of psychology raced on, but without firm theoretical foundations for the underlying science. Part 13 is the key one, and the longest one; it shows Vygotsky struggling to determine what kind of Marxist approach would eventually fill the need for a unified theory of psychology. He is very critical of those Marxist writers who would take the easy way out, simply using quotations from Marxism's founders, who were really discussing other things. Part 14, the final one, admits that the task is as yet unfinished, that the needed Marxist psychology is only just developing. As Vygotsky puts it in the final paragraph:

> In the future society, psychology will indeed be the science of the new man. Without this the perspective of Marxism and the history of science would not be complete. But this science of the new man will still remain psychology. Now we hold its thread in our hands. There is no necessity for this psychology to correspond [any closer to] the present one as–in the words of Spinoza–the constellation Dog corresponds to a dog, a barking animal.

## References

Ash, M. G. (1995). *Gestalt psychology in German culture, 1890–1967: Holism and the quest for objectivity.* Cambridge: Cambridge University Press.

Bakan, D. (1996) The crisis in psychology. *Journal of Social Distress and the Homeless, 5,* 335–342.

Buehler, K. (1927/28). *Die Krisis in der Psychologie.* Frankfurt-am-Main: Ullstein.

Fitzpatrick, S. (Ed.) (1978). *The cultural revolution in Russia, 1928–1931.* Bloomington: Indiana University Press.

Harrower, M. (1983). *Kurt Koffka: An unwitting self-portrait.* Gainsville: University of Florida Press.

Hartmann, George W. (1935). *Gestalt psychology: A survey of the facts and principles.* New York: Roland Press.

Joravsky, D. (1987). L. S. Vygotskii: The muffled deity of Soviet psychology. In *Psychology in twentieth-century thought and society* (M. G. Ash & W. R. Woodward, Eds.; pp. 189–211). Cambridge: Cambridge University Press.

Joravsky, D. (1989). *Russian psychology: A critical history.* Oxford: Blackwell.

Koffka, K. (1926). Die Krisis in der Psychologie. *Die Naturwissenschaften, 14,* 581–586.

Kozulin, A. (1990). *Vygotsky's psychology: A biography of ideas.* Cambridge: Harvard University Press.

Rieber, R. W., & Wollock, J. (1997). Prologue: Vygotsky's "Crisis" and its meaning today. In *The collected works of L. S. Vygotsky, Volume 3: Problems of the theory and history of psychology* (R. W. Rieber & J. Wollock, Eds.; pp. vii–xii). New York: Kluwer Academic/Plenum.

Scheerer, E. (1980). Gestalt psychology in the Soviet Union: The period of enthusiasm. *Psychological Research, 41,* 113–132.

Veresov, N. N. (1999). *Undiscovered Vygotsky: Etudes on the pre-history of cultural-historical psychology.* European Studies in the History of Science and Ideas, vol. 8. Frankfurt-am-Main: Peter Lang.

Vygotsky, L. S. (1997). *The collected works, Volume 3: Problems of the theory and history of psychology* (R. W. Rieber & J. Wollock, Eds.). New York: Kluwer Academic/Plenum.

Wozniak, R. H. (1996). Qu'est-ce que l'intelligence? Piaget, Vygotsky, and the 1920s crisis in psychology. In *Piaget–Vygotsky: The social genesis of thought* (A. Tryphon & J. Vonèche, Eds.; pp. 11–24). Hove, UK: Psychology Press.

# 10

# The Historical Meaning of the Crisis in Psychology
## *A Methodological Investigation*

The stone which the builders rejected is become the head stone of the corner [1]

PSALMS 18, VERSE 22

1

Lately more and more voices are heard proclaiming that the problem of general psychology is a problem of the first order. What is most remarkable is that this opinion does not come from philosophers who have made generalization their professional habit, nor even from theoretical psychologists, but from the psychological practitioners who elaborate the special areas of applied psychology: psychiatrists and industrial psychologists, the representatives of the most exact and concrete part of our science. The various psychological disciplines have obviously reached a turning point in the development of their investigations, the gathering of factual material, the systematization of knowledge, and the statement of basic positions and laws. Further advance along a straight line, the simple continuation of the same work, the gradual accumulation of material, are proving fruitless or even impossible. In order to go further we must choose a path.

Out of such a methodological crisis, from the conscious need for guidance in different disciplines, from the necessity—on a certain level of knowledge—to critically coordinate heterogeneous data, to order uncoordinated laws into a system, to interpret and verify the results, to cleanse the methods and basic concepts, to create the fundamental principles, in a word, to pull the beginnings and ends of our knowledge together, out of all this, a general science is born.

This is why the concept of a general psychology does not coincide with the concept of the basic theoretical psychology that is central to a number of different special disciplines. The latter, in essence the psychology of the adult normal person, should be considered one of

Originally appeared in English as Chapter 15 in *The Collected Works of L.S. Vygotsky, Volume 3: Problems of the History and Theory of Psychology* (Robert W. Rieber and Jeffrey Wollock, Eds.; Rene van der Veer, Trans.) (pp. 233–343). New York: Plenum Press, 1997. This document had not been previously published. It is based on a manuscript found in Vygotsky's private archives.

the special disciplines along with zoopsychology and psychopathology. That it has so far played and in some measure still plays the role of a generalizing factor, which to a certain extent forms the structure and system of the special disciplines, furnishes their main concepts, and brings them into line with their own structure, is explained by the historical development of the science, rather than by logical necessity. This is the way things have been and to some extent still are, but they should not and will not remain this way since this situation does not follow from the very nature of the science, but is determined by external, extraneous circumstances. As soon as these conditions change, the psychology of the normal person will lose its leading role. To an extent we are already beginning to see this happen. In the psychological systems that cultivate the concept of the unconscious, the role of such a leading discipline, the basic concepts of which serve as the starting points for the related sciences, is played by psychopathology. These are, for example, the systems of Freud, Adler, and Kretschmer.

In the latter, this leading role of psychopathology is no longer connected with the central concept of the unconscious, as in Freud and Adler, i.e., not with the actual priority of the given discipline in the elaboration of the basic idea, but with a fundamental methodological view according to which the essence and nature of the phenomena studied by psychology can be revealed in their purest form in the extreme, pathological forms. We should, consequently, proceed from pathology to the norm and explain and understand the normal person from pathology, and not the other way around, as has been done until now. The key to psychology is in pathology, not only because it discovered and studied the root of the mind earlier than other branches, but because this is the internal nature of things, and the nature of the scientific knowledge of these things is conditioned by it. Whereas for traditional psychology every psychopath as a subject for study is more or less—to a different degree—a normal person and must be defined in relation to the latter, for the new systems each normal person is more or less insane and must be psychologically understood precisely as a variant of some pathological type. To put it in more straightforward terms, in certain systems the normal person is considered as a type and the pathological personality as a variety or variant of this main type; in others, on the contrary, the pathological phenomenon is taken as a type and the normal as one of its varieties. And who can predict how the future general psychology will decide this debate?

On the basis of such dual motives (based half on facts, half on principle) still other systems assign the leading role to zoopsychology. Of this kind are, for example, the majority of the American courses in the psychology of behavior and the Russian courses in reflexology, which develop their whole system from the concept of the conditional reflex and organize all their material around it. A number of authors propose that animal psychology, apart from being given the actual priority in the elaboration of the basic concepts of behavior, should become the general discipline with which the other disciplines should be correlated. As the logical beginning of a science of behavior, the starting point for every genetic examination and explanation of the mind, and a purely biological science, it is precisely this science which is expected to elaborate the fundamental concepts of the science and to supply them to kindred disciplines.

This, for example, is the view of Pavlov. What psychologists do can in his opinion have no influence upon animal psychology, but what zoopsychologists do determines the work of psychologists in a very essential way. The latter build the superstructure, but the former lay the foundation [Pavlov, 1928/1963, p. 113]. And indeed, the source from which we derive all our basic categories for the investigation and description of behavior, the standard we use to verify our results, the model according to which we align our methods, is zoopsychology.

Here again the matter has taken a course opposed to that of traditional psychology. There the starting point was man; one proceeded from man in order to get an idea of the mind of the animal. One interpreted the manifestations of its soul by analogy with ourselves. In so doing, the matter was by no means always reduced to a crude anthropomorphism. Serious methodological grounds often dictated such a course of research: with subjective psychology it could not be otherwise. It regarded man as the key to the psychology of animals; always the highest forms as the key to the lower ones. For, the investigator need not always follow the same path that nature took; often the reverse path is more advantageous.

Marx [1978, p. 636] referred to this methodological principle of the "reverse" method when he stated that "the anatomy of man is the key to the anatomy of the ape."

> The allusions to a higher principle in lower species of animals can only be understood when this higher principle itself is already known. Thus, bourgeois economy gives us the key to antique economy etc., but not at all in the sense understood by the economists who slur over all historical differences and see bourgeois forms in all forms of societies. We can understand the quitrent, the tithe, etc., when we are acquainted with the ground rent, but we must not equate them with the latter.

To understand the quitrent on the basis of the ground rent, the feudal form on the basis of the bourgeois form-this is the same methodological device used to comprehend and define thinking and the rudiments of speech in animals on the basis of the mature thinking and speech of man. A certain stage of development and the process itself can only be fully understood when we know the endpoint of the process, the result, the direction it took, and the form into which the given process developed. We are, of course, speaking only of the methodological transference of basic categories and concepts from the higher to the lower, not of the transference of factual observations and generalizations. The concepts of the social category of class and class struggle, for instance, are revealed in their purest form in the analysis of the capitalist system, but these same concepts are the key to all pre-capitalist societal formations, although in every case we meet with different classes there, a different form of struggle, a particular developmental stage of this category. But those details which distinguish the historical uniqueness of different epochs from capitalist forms not only are not lost, but, on the contrary, can only be studied when we approach them with the categories and concepts acquired in the analysis of the other, higher formation.

Marx [1978, p. 636] explains that

> bourgeois society is the most developed and diverse historical organization of production. The categories which express its relationships and an understanding of its composition yield therefore at the same time an insight into the composition and the productive relations of all societal forms which have disappeared. Bourgeois society was built with the rubbish and elements of these societies, parts of which have not been fully overcome and still drag on and the mere indications of which have developed into full-fledged meanings.

Having arrived at the end of the path we can more easily understand the whole path in its entirety as well as the meaning of its different stages.

This is a possible methodology; it has been sufficiently vindicated in a whole number of disciplines. But can it be applied to psychology? It is precisely on methodological grounds that Pavlov rejects the route from man to animal. He defends the reverse of the "reverse," i.e., the direct path of investigation, repeating the route taken by nature. This is not because of any factual difference in the phenomena, but rather because of the inapplicability and epistemic barrenness of psychological categories and concepts. In his words,

> it is impossible by means of psychological concepts, which are essentially nonspatial, to penetrate into the mechanism of animal behavior, into the mechanism of these relations [Pavlov, 1928/1963, p. 192].

Thus it is not a matter of facts but of concepts, that is, the way one conceives of these facts. He [ibid., p. 113] says that

> Our facts are conceived of in terms of time and space; they are purely scientific facts; but psychological facts are thought of only in terms of time.

The issue is about different concepts, not different phenomena. Pavlov wishes not only to win independence for his area of investigation, but to extend its influence and guidance to all spheres of psychological knowledge. This is clear from his explicit references to the fact that the debate is not only about the emancipation from the power of psychological concepts, but also about the elaboration of a psychology by means of new spatial concepts.

In his opinion, science, "guided by the similarity or identity of the external manifestations" [ibid., p. 59], will sooner or later apply to the mind of man the objective data obtained. His path is from the simple to the complex, from animal to man. He says [ibid., p. 113] that

> The simple, the elementary is always conceivable without the complex, whereas the complex cannot be conceived of without the elementary.

These data will become "the basis for psychological knowledge." And in the preface to the book in which he presents his twenty years of experience with the study of animal behavior, Pavlov [ibid., p. 41] declares that he

> is deeply and irrevocably convinced that along this path [we will manage] to find the knowledge of the mechanisms and laws of human nature [ibid., p. 41].

Here we have a new controversy between the study of animals and the psychology of man. The situation is, in essence, very similar to the controversy between psychopathology and the psychology of normal man. Which discipline should lead, unify, and elaborate the basic concepts, principles, and methods, verify and systematize the data of all other areas? Whereas previously traditional psychology has considered the animal as a more or less remote ancestor of man, reflexology is now inclined to consider man, with Plato, as a "featherless biped." Formerly the animal mind was defined and described in concepts and terms acquired in the study of man, Nowadays the behavior of animals gives "the key to the understanding of the behavior of man," and what we call "human" behavior is understood as the product of an animal which, because it walks and stands erect, has a developed thumb and can speak.

And again we may ask: which discipline other than general psychology can decide this controversy between animal and man in psychology; for, on this decision will rest nothing more and nothing less than the whole future fate of this science.

2

From the analysis of the three types of psychological systems we have considered above, it is already obvious how pressing is the need for a general psychology with the boundaries and approximate content partially outlined here. The path of our investigation will at all times be as follows: we will proceed from an analysis of the facts, albeit facts of a highly general and abstract nature, such as a particular psychological system and its type, the tendencies and fate of different theories, various epistemological methods, scientific classifications and schemes, etc. We will examine these facts not from the abstract-logical, purely philosophical side, but as particular facts in the history of science, as concrete, vivid historical events in their tendency, struggle, in their concrete context, of course, and in their epistemological-theoretical essence, i.e., from the viewpoint of their correspondence to the reality they are meant to cognize. We wish to obtain a clear idea of the essence of individual and social psychology as two aspects of a single science, and of their historical fate, not through abstract considerations, but by means of an analysis of scientific reality. From this we will deduce, as a politician does from the analysis of events, the rules for action and the organization of scientific research. The methodological investigation utilizes the historical examination of the concrete forms of the sciences and the theoretical analysis of these forms in order to obtain generalized, verified principles that are suitable for guidance. This is, in our opinion, the core of this general psychology whose concept we will attempt to clarify in this chapter.

The first thing we obtain from the analysis is the demarcation between general psychology and the theoretical psychology of the normal person. We have seen that the latter is not necessarily a general psychology, that in quite a number of systems theoretical psychology itself turns into one of the special disciplines, defined by another field; that both psychopathology and the theory of animal behavior can and do take the role of general psychology. Vvedensky (1917, p. 5) assumed that general psychology

> might much more correctly be called basic psychology, because this part lies at the basis of all psychology.

Høffding [1908, p. 37] who assumed that psychology "can be practiced in many modes and ways," that "there is not *one*, but *many* psychologies," and who saw no need for unity, was nevertheless inclined to view subjective psychology "as the basis and the *center*, around which the contributions of the other approaches should be gathered." In the present case it would indeed be more appropriate to talk about a basic, or central, psychology than about a general one; but to overlook the fact that systems may arise from a completely different basis and center, and that what the professors considered to be the basis in those systems, by the very nature of things, drifts to the periphery, would be more than a little dogmatic, and naively complacent. Subjective psychology was basic or central in quite a number of systems, and we must understand why. Now it loses its importance, and again we must understand why. In the present case it would be terminologically most correct to speak of theoretical psychology, as opposed to applied psychology, as Münsterberg [1920] does. Applied to the adult normal person it would be a special branch alongside child psychology, zoopsychology, and psychopathology.

Theoretical psychology, Binswanger [1922, p. 5] notes, is not general psychology, nor a part of it, but is itself the object or subject matter of general psychology. The latter deals with the questions whether theoretical psychology is in principle possible and what are the structure and suitability of its concepts. Theoretical psychology cannot be equated with general psychology, if only for the reason that precisely the matter of building theories in psychology is a fundamental question of general psychology.

There is a second thing that we may reliably infer from our analysis. The very fact that theoretical psychology, and later other disciplines, have performed the role of a general psychology, is conditioned by, on the one hand, the absence of a general psychology, and on the other hand, the strong need for it to fulfill its function temporarily in order to make scientific research possible. Psychology is pregnant with a general discipline but has not yet delivered it.

The third thing we may gather from our analysis is the distinction between two phases in the development of any general science, any general discipline, as is shown by the history of science and methodology. In the first phase of development the general discipline is only quantitatively distinct from the special one. Such a distinction, as Binswanger [1922, p. 3] rightly says, is characteristic of the majority of sciences. Thus, we distinguish general and special botany, zoology, biology, physiology, pathology, psychiatry, etc. The general discipline studies what is common to all subjects of the given science. The special discipline studies what is characteristic of the various groups or even specimens from the same kind of objects. It is in this sense that the discipline we now call differential psychology was called special. In the same sense this area was called individual psychology. The general part of botany or zoology studies what is common to all plants or animals, the general part of psychology what is common to all people. In order to do this the concept of some trait common to most or all of them was abstracted from the real diversity and in this form, abstracted from the real diversity of concrete traits, it became the subject matter studied by the general discipline. Therefore, the characteristic and task of such a discipline was seen to be the scientific study of the facts common to the greatest number of the particular phenomena of the given area [Binswanger, 1922, p. 3].

This stage of searching and of trying to apply an abstract concept common to all psychological disciplines, which forms the subject matter of all of them and determines what should be isolated from the chaos of the various phenomena and what in the phenomena has epistemic value for psychology—this stage we see vividly expressed in our analysis. And we may judge what significance these searches and the concept of the subject matter of psychology looked for and the desired answer to the question what psychology studies may have for our science in the present historical moment of its development.

Any concrete phenomenon is completely inexhaustible and infinite in its separate features. We must always search in the phenomenon what makes it a scientific fact. Exactly this distinguishes the observation of a solar eclipse by the astronomer from the observation of the same phenomenon by a person who is simply curious. The former discerns in the phenomenon what makes it an astronomic fact. The latter observes the accidental features which happen to catch his attention.

What is most common to all phenomena studied by psychology, what makes the most diverse phenomena into psychological facts—from salivation in a dog to the enjoyment of a tragedy, what do the ravings of a madman and the rigorous computations of the mathematician share? Traditional psychology answers: what they have in common is that they are all psychological phenomena which are nonspatial and can only be perceived by the experiencing subject himself. Reflexology answers: what they share is that all these phenomena are facts of behavior, correlative activity, reflexes, response actions of the organism. Psychoanalysts answer: common to all these facts, the most basic factor which unites them is the unconscious which is their basis. For general psychology the three answers mean, respectively, that it is a science of (1) the mental and its properties; or (2) behavior; or (3) the unconscious.

From this it is obvious that such a general concept is important for the whole future fate of the science. Any fact which is expressed in each of these three systems will, in turn, acquire three completely different forms. To be more precise, there will be three different forms of a single fact. To be even more precise, there will be three different facts. And as the science moves forward and gathers facts, we will successively get three different generalizations, three different laws, three different classifications, three different systems—three individual sciences which, the more successfully they develop, the more remote they will be from each other and from the common fact that unites them. Shortly after beginning they will already be forced to select different facts, and this very choice of facts will already determine the fate of the science as it continues. Koffka [1924, p. 149] was the first to express the idea that introspective psychology and the psychology of behavior will develop into two sciences if things continue as they are going. The paths of the two sciences lie so far apart that "it is by no means certain whether they will eventually lead to the same end."

Pavlov and Bekhterev share essentially the same opinion. They accept the existence of two parallel sciences—psychology and reflexology—which study the same object, but from different sides. In this connection Pavlov [1928/1963, p. 3291] said that "certainly psychology, insofar as it concerns the subjective state of man, has a natural right to existence." For Bekhterev, reflexology neither contradicts nor excludes subjective psychology but delineates a special area of investigation, i.e., creates a new parallel science. He talks about [Bekhterev, 1932, p. 380] the intimate interrelation of both scientific disciplines and even about subjective reflexology as an inevitable future development. Incidentally, we must say that in reality both Pavlov and Bekhterev reject psychology and hope to understand the whole area of knowledge about man by exclusively objective means, i.e., they only envision the possibility of one single science, although by word of mouth they acknowledge two sciences. In this way the general concept predetermines the content of the science.

At present psychoanalysis, behaviorism, and subjective psychology are already operating not only with different concepts, but with different facts as well. Facts such as the Oedipus complex, indisputable and real for psychoanalysts, simply do not exist for other psychologists; for many it is wildest phantasy. For Stern [1913, p. 73], who in general relates favorably to psychoanalysis, the psychoanalytic interpretations so commonplace in Freud's school and as far beyond doubt as the measurement of one's temperature in the hospital, and consequently the facts whose existence they presuppose, resemble the chiromancy and astrology of the 16th century. For Pavlov as well, it is pure phantasy to claim that a dog remembers the food on hearing the bell. Likewise, the fact of muscular movements during the act of thinking, posited by the behaviorist, does not exist for the introspectionist.

But the fundamental concept, the primary abstraction, so to speak, that lies at the basis of a science, determines not only the content, but also predetermines the character of the unity of the different disciplines, and through this, the way to explain the facts, i.e., the main explanatory principle of the science.

We see that a general science, as well as the tendency of various disciplines to develop into a general science and to spread their influence to adjacent branches of knowledge, arise out of the need to unify heterogeneous branches of knowledge. When similar disciplines have gathered sufficient material in areas that are relatively remote from each other, the need arises to unify the heterogeneous material, to establish and define the relation between the different areas and between each area and the whole of scientific knowledge. How to connect the material from pathology, animal psychology, and social psychology? We have seen that the substrate of the unity is first of all the primary abstraction. But the heterogeneous material is not united merely by adding one kind of material to another, nor via the conjunction "and," as the Gestalt psychologists say, nor through simply joining or adding parts so that each part preserves its balance and independence while being included into the new whole. Unity is reached by subordination, dominion, through the fact that different disciplines renounce their sovereignty in favor of one single general science. The various disciplines do not simply co-exist within the new whole, but form a hierarchical system, which has primary and secondary centers, like the solar system. Thus, this unity determines the role, sense, meaning of each separate area, i.e., not only determines the content, but also the way to explain things, the most important generalization, which in the course of the development of the science becomes its explanatory principle.

To take the mind, the unconscious, or behavior as the primary concept implies not only to gather three different categories of facts, but also to offer three different ways of explaining these facts.

We see that the tendency to generalize and unite knowledge turns or grows into a tendency to explain this knowledge. The unity of the generalizing concept grows into the unity of the explanatory principle, because to explain means to establish a connection between one fact or a group of facts and another group, to refer to another series of phenomena. For science to explain means to explain causally. As long as the unification is carried out within a single discipline, such an explanation is established by the causal linkage of the phenomena that lie within a single area. But as soon as we proceed to the generalization across different disciplines, the unification of different areas of facts, the generalization of the second order, we immediately must search for an explanation of a higher order as well, i.e., we must search for the link of all areas of the given knowledge with the facts that lie outside of them. In this way the search for an explanatory principle leads us beyond the boundaries of the given science and compels us to find the place of the given area of phenomena amidst the wider circle of phenomena.

This second tendency, which is the basis of the isolation of a general science, is the tendency toward a unified explanatory principle and toward transcending the borders of the given science in the search for the place of the given category of being within the general system of being and the given science within the general system of knowledge. This tendency can already be observed in the competition of the separate disciplines for supremacy. Since the tendency of becoming an explanatory principle is already present in every generalizing concept, and since the struggle between the disciplines is a struggle for the generalizing concept, this second tendency must inevitably appear as well. And in fact, reflexology advances not only the concept of behavior, but the principle of the conditional reflex as well, i.e., an explanation of behavior on the basis of the external experience of the animal. And it is difficult to say which of these two ideas is more essential for the current in question. Throw away the principle and you will be left with behavior, that is, a system of external movements and actions, to be explained from consciousness, i.e., a conception that has existed within subjective psychology for a long time. Throw away the concept of behavior and retain the principle, and you will get sensationalist associative psychology. About both of these we will come to speak below. Here it is important to establish that the generalization of the concept and the explanatory principle determine a general science only together, as a unified pair. In exactly the same way, psychopathology does not simply advance the generalizing concept of the unconscious, but also interprets this concept causally, through the principle of sexuality. For psychoanalysis to generalize the psychological disciplines and to unite them on the basis of the concept of the unconscious means to explain the whole world, as studied by psychology, through sexuality.

But here the two tendencies—towards unification and generalization—are still merged and often difficult to distinguish. The second tendency is not sufficiently clear-cut, and may even be completely absent at times. That it coincides with the first tendency must again be explained historically rather than by logical necessity. In the struggle for supremacy among the different disciplines, this tendency usually shows up; we found it in our analysis. But it may also fail to appear and, most importantly, it may also appear in a pure form, unmixed and separate from the first tendency, in a different set of facts. In both cases we have each tendency in its pure form.

Thus, in traditional psychology the concept of the mental may be explained in many ways, although admittedly not just any explanation is possible: associationism, the actualistic conception, faculty theory, etc. Thus the link between generalization and unification is intimate, but not unambiguous. A single concept can be reconciled with a number of explanations and the other way around. Further, in the systems of the psychology of the unconscious this basic concept is not necessarily interpreted as sexuality. Adler and Jung use other principles as the basis of their explanation. Thus in the struggle between the disciplines, the first tendency of knowledge—the tendency towards unification—is logically necessary, while the second tendency is not logically necessary but historically determined, and will be present to a varying degree. That is why the second tendency can be most easily and comfortably observed in its pure form—in the struggle between the principles and schools within one and the same discipline.

### 3

It can be said of any important discovery in any area, when it transcends the boundaries of that particular realm, that it has the tendency to turn into an explanatory principle for all psychological phenomena and lead psychology beyond its proper boundaries into broader realms of knowledge. In the last several decades this tendency has manifested itself with such amazing strict-ness and consistency, with such regular uniformity in the most diverse areas, that it becomes absolutely possible to predict the course of development of this or that concept, discovery, or idea. At the same time this regular repetition in the development of widely varying ideas evi-dently—and with a clarity that is seldom observed by the historian of science and methodolo-gist—points to an objective necessity underlying the development of the science, to a necessity which we may observe when we approach the facts of science from an equally scientific point of view. It points to the possibility of a scientific methodology built on a historical foundation.

The regularity in the replacement and development of ideas, the development and down-fall of concepts, even the replacement of classifications etc.—all this can be scientifically explained by the links of the science in question with (1) the general socio-cultural context of the era; (2) the general conditions and laws of scientific knowledge; (3) the objective demands upon the scientific knowledge that follow from the nature of the phenomena studied in a given stage of investigation (in the final analysis, the requirements of the objective reality that is studied by the given science). After all, scientific knowledge must adapt and conform to the particularities of the studied facts, must be built in accordance with their demands. And that is why we can always show how the objective facts studied by a certain science are involved in the change of a scientific fact. In our investigation we will try to take account of all three viewpoints.

We can sketch the general fate and lines of development of such explanatory ideas. In the beginning there is some factual discovery of more or less great significance which reforms the ordinary conception of the whole area of phenomena to which it refers, and even transcends the boundaries of the given group of phenomena within which it was first observed and formulated.

Next comes a stage during which the influence of these ideas spreads to adjacent areas. The idea is stretched out, so to speak, to material that is broader than what it originally cov-ered. The idea itself (or its application) is changed in the process, it becomes formulated in a more abstract way. The link with the material that engendered it is more or less weakened, and it only continues to nourish the cogency of the new idea, because this idea accomplishes its cam-paign of conquest as a scientifically verified, reliable discovery. This is very important.

In the third stage of development the idea controls more or less the whole discipline in which it originally arose. It has partly changed the structure and size of the discipline and has itself been to some extent changed by them. It has become separated from the facts that engen-dered it, exists in the form of a more or less abstractly formulated principle, and becomes involved in the struggle between disciplines for supremacy, i.e., in the sphere of action of the tendency toward unification. Usually this happens because the idea, as an explanatory principle, man-aged to take possession of the whole discipline, i.e., it in part adapted itself, in part adjusted to itself the concept on which the discipline is based, and now acts in concert with it. In our analysis, we have found such a mixed stage in the existence of an idea, where both tendencies help each other. While it continues expanding due to the tendency toward unification, the idea is easily transferred to adjacent disciplines. Not only is it continually transformed, swelling from ever new material, but it also transforms the areas it penetrates. In this stage the fate of the idea is completely tied to the fate of the discipline it represents and which is fighting for supremacy.

In the fourth stage the idea again breaks away from the basic concept, as the very fact of the conquest—at least in the form of a project defended by a single school, the whole domain of psychological knowledge, or all disciplines—this very fact pushes the idea to develop further. The idea remains the explanatory principle until the time that it transcends the boundaries of the basic concept. For to explain, as we have seen, means to transcend one's proper boundaries in search of an external cause. As soon as it fully coincides with the basic concept, it stops explaining anything. But the basic concept cannot develop any further on logical grounds without contradicting itself. For its function is to define an area of psychological knowledge. By its very essence it cannot transcend its boundaries. Concept and explanation must, consequently, separate again. Moreover, unification logically presupposes, as was shown above, that we establish a link with a broader domain of knowledge, transcend the proper boundaries. This is accomplished by the idea that separates itself from the concept. Now it links psychology with the broad areas that lie outside of it, with biology, physics, chemistry, mechanics, while the basic concept separates it from these areas. The functions of these temporarily co-operating allies have again changed. The idea is now openly included in some philosophical system, spreads to the most remote domains of being, to the whole world—while transforming and being transformed—and is formulated as a universal principle or even as a whole world view.

This discovery, inflated into a world view like a frog that has swollen to the size of an ox, a philistine amidst the gentry, now enters the fifth and most dangerous stage of development: it may easily burst like a soap-bubble. In any case it enters a stage of struggle and negation which it now meets from all sides. Admittedly, there had been a struggle against the idea in the previous stages as well. But that was the normal opposition to the expansion of an idea, the resistance of each different area against its aggressive tendencies. The initial strength of the discovery that engendered it protected it from a genuine struggle for life just like a mother protects her young. It is only now, when the idea has entirely separated itself from the facts that engendered it, developed to its logical extremes, carried to its ultimate conclusions, generalized as far as possible, that it finally displays what it is in reality, shows its real face. However strange it may seem, it is actually only now, reduced to a philosophical form, apparently obscured by many later developments and very remote from its direct roots and the social causes that engendered it, that the idea reveals what it wants, what it is, from which social tendencies it arose, which class interests it serves. Only having developed into a world view or having become attached to it, does the particular idea change from a scientific fact into a fact of social life again, i.e., it returns to the bosom from which it came. Only having become part of social life again, does it reveal its social nature, which of course was present all the time, but was hidden under the mask of the neutral scientific fact it impersonated.

And in this stage of the struggle against the idea, its fate is approximately as follows. Just like a new nobleman, the new idea is shown in light of its philistine, i.e., its real, origin. It is confined to the areas from which it sprang. It is forced to go through its development backwards. It is accepted as a particular discovery but rejected as a world view. And now new ways are being proposed to interpret this particular discovery and the related facts. In other words, other world views which represent other social tendencies and forces even reconquer the idea's original area, develop their own view of it—and then the idea either withers away or continues to exist more or less tightly integrated in some world view amidst a number of other world views, sharing their fate and fulfilling their functions. But as an idea which revolutionizes the science it ceases to exist. It is an idea that has retired and has received the rank of general from its department.

Why does the idea as such cease to exist? Because operating in the domain of world views is a law discovered by Engels, a law that says that ideas gather around two poles—those of idealism and materialism, which correspond to the two poles of social life, the two basic classes that fight each other. The idea reveals its social nature much more readily as a philosophical fact than as a scientific fact. And this is where its role ends—it is unmasked as a hidden, ideological agent dressed up as a scientific fact and begins to participate in the general, open struggle of ideas. But exactly here, as a small item within an enormous sum, it vanishes like a drop of rain in the ocean and ceases to exist independently.

## 4

Every discovery in psychology that has the tendency to turn into an explanatory principle follows this course. The ascent of such ideas itself may be explained by the presence of an objective scientific need, rooted in the final analysis in the nature of the studied phenomena, as it is revealed in the given stage of knowledge. It can be explained, in other words, by the nature of the science and thus, in the final analysis by the nature of the psychological reality studied by this science. However, the history of the science can only explain why, in a given stage of its development, the need for the ideas developed, why this was impossible a hundred years before. It cannot explain more. Exactly which ideas turn into world views and which not; which ideas are advanced, which path they cover; what is their fate—this all depends upon factors that lie outside the history of the science and determine this very history.

We may compare this with Plekhanov's (1922) theory of art. Nature has provided man with an aesthetic need, it enables him to have aesthetic ideas, tastes, and feelings. But precisely which tastes, ideas, and feelings a given person in the society of a given historical period will have cannot be deduced from man's nature; only a materialistic conception of history can give the answer. Actually, this argument is not even a comparison, nor is it a metaphor. It literally falls under the same general law which Plekhanov specifically applied to matters of art. Indeed, the scientific acquisition of knowledge is one type of activity of societal man amongst a number of other activities. Consequently, scientific knowledge acquisition, viewed as the acquisition of knowledge about nature and not as ideology, is a certain type of labor. And as with any labor, it is first of all a process between man and nature, in which man himself confronts nature as a natural force. This process is determined in the first place by the properties of the nature which is being transformed and the properties of the natural force which is transforming, i.e., in the present case, by the nature of the psychological phenomena and the epistemic conditions of man. But precisely because they are natural, i.e., immutable, these properties cannot explain the development, movement, and change in the history of a science. This is generally known. Nevertheless, in each stage of the development of a science we may distinguish, differentiate, or abstract the demands put forward by the very nature of the phenomena under investigation as they are known in the given stage, a stage determined, of course, not by the nature of the phenomena, but by the history of man. Precisely because the natural properties of mental phenomena at a certain level of knowledge are a purely historical category—for the properties change in the process of knowledge acquisition—and because the sum total of known properties is a purely historical quantity, they can be considered as the cause or one of the causes of the historical development of the science.

To illustrate the model for the development of general ideas in psychology just described, we will examine the fate of four ideas which have been influential in the last few decades. In doing so our sole interest will be the fact that made the development of these ideas possible, rather than the ideas in themselves, i.e., a fact rooted in the history of the science, not outside of it. We will not investigate why it is precisely these ideas and their history that is important as a symptom or indication of the stage that the history of the science is going through. At the moment we are interested not in a historical but a methodological question: to what extent are the psychological facts elicited and known at the moment, and what changes in the structure of the science do they require in order to make possible the further acquisition of knowledge on the basis of what is already known? The fate of the four ideas must bear witness to the need of the science at the present moment, to the content and dimensions of this need. The history of the science is important for us insofar as it determines the degree to which psychological facts are cognized.

These four ideas are: psychoanalysis, reflexology, Gestalt psychology, and personalism.

The idea of psychoanalysis sprang from particular discoveries in the area of neuroses. The unconscious determination of a number of mental phenomena and the hidden sexuality of a number of activities and forms, until then not included in the field of erotic phenomena, were established beyond doubt. Gradually this discovery, corroborated by the success of therapeutic measures based on this conception, i.e., sanctioned by practice, was transferred to a number of adjacent are as the psychopathology of everyday life and child psychology—and it conquered the whole field of the theory of neuroses. In the struggle between the disciplines this idea brought the most remote branches of psychology under its sway. It has been shown that on the basis of this idea a psychology of art and an ethnic psychology can be developed. But psychoanalysis at the same time transcended the boundaries of psychology: sexuality became a metaphysical principle amidst all other metaphysical ideas, psychoanalysis became a world view, psychology a metapsychology. Psychoanalysis has its own theory of knowledge and its own metaphysics, its own sociology and mathematics. Communism and totem, the church and Dostoyevsky's creative work, occultism and advertising, myth and Leonardo da Vinci's inventions—it is all disguised and masked sex and sexuality, and that is all there is to it.

The idea of the conditional reflex followed a similar course. Everybody knows that it originated in the study of mental salivation in dogs. But then it was extended to a number of other phenomena as well. It conquered animal psychology. In Bekhterev's system it is applied and used in all domains of psychology and reigns over them. Everything—sleep, thought, work, and creativity—turns out to be a reflex. It ended up dominating all psychological disciplines: the collective psychology of art, industrial psychology and pedology, psychopathology, even subjective psychology. And at the moment reflexology only rubs shoulders with universal principles, universal laws, first principles of mechanics. Just as psychoanalysis grew into a metapsychology via biology, reflexology via biology grows into a world view based on energy. The table of contents of a textbook in reflexology is a universal catalogue of global laws. And again, just as with psychoanalysis, it turned out that everything in the world is a reflex. Anna Karenina and kleptomania, the class struggle and a landscape, language and dream are all reflexes (Bekhterev, 1921; 1923).

Gestalt psychology also originally arose in the concrete psychological investigation of the processes of form perception. There it received its practical christening; it passed the truth test. But, as it was born at the same time as psychoanalysis and reflexology, it covered the same path with amazing uniformity. It conquered animal psychology, and it turned out that the thinking of apes is also a Gestalt process. It conquered the psychology of art and ethnic psychology, and it turned out that the primitive conception of the world and the creation of art are Gestalten as well. It conquered child psychology and psychopathology and both child development and mental disease were covered by the Gestalt. Finally, having turned into a world view, Gestalt psychology discovered the Gestalt in physics and chemistry, in physiology and biology, and the Gestalt, withered to a logical formula, appeared to be the basis of the world. When God created the world he said: let there be Gestalt—and there was Gestalt everywhere (Koffka, 1925; Köhler, 1917, 1920; Wertheimer, 1925).

Finally, personalism originally arose in differential psychological research.[10] Being an exceptionally valuable principle of personality in the theory of psychometrics and in the theory of occupational choice, etc., it migrated first to psychology in its entirety and then crossed its boundaries. In the form of critical personalism it extended the concept of personality not only to man, but to animals and plants as well. One more step, well known to us from the history of psychoanalysis and reflexology, and everything in the world is personality. The philosophy which began by contrasting the personality with the thing, by rescuing the personality from the power of things, ended up by accepting all things as personalities. The things disappeared altogether. A thing is only a part of the personality: it does not matter whether we are dealing with the leg of a person or the leg of a table. But as this part again consists of parts etc. and so on to infinity, it—the leg of a person or a table—again turns out to be a personality in relation to its parts and a part only in relation to the whole. The solar system and the ant, the tram-driver and Hindenburg, a table and a panther—they are all personalities (stern, 1924).

These fates, similar as four drops of the same rain, drag the ideas along one and the same path. The extension of the concept grows and reaches for infinity and according to the well-known logical law, its content falls just as impetuously to zero. Each of these four ideas is extremely rich, full of meaning and sense, full of value and fruitful in its own place. But elevated to the rank of universal laws, they are worthy of each other, they are absolutely equal to each other, like round and empty zeros. Stern's personality is a complex of reflexes according to Bekhterev, a Gestalt according to Wertheimer, sexuality according to Freud.

And in the fifth stage of development these ideas meet with exactly the same criticism, which can be reduced to a single formula. To psychoanalysis it is said: the principle of unconscious sexuality is indispensable for the explanation of hysterical neuroses, but it can explain neither the composition of the world nor the course of history. To reflexology it is said: we must not make a logical mistake, the reflex is only one single chapter of psychology, but not psychology as a whole and even less, of course, the world in its entirety (Vagner, 1923; Vygotsky, 1925a). To Gestalt psychology it is said: you have found a very valuable principle in your own area. But if thinking consists of no more than the aspects of unity and the integrated whole, i.e., of no more than the Gestalt formula, and this same formula expresses the essence of each organic and even physical process, then the picture of the world becomes, of course, amazingly complete and simple—electricity, gravity, and human thinking are reduced to a common denominator. We must not throw both thinking and relation into one single pot of structures: let it first be shown that it belongs in the same pot as structural functions [Strukturfunktionen]. The new factor guides a broad though limited area. But as a universal principle it does not stand up to critique. Let the thinking of bold theoreticians in their attempts to explain be characterized by the motto "it's all or nothing." But as a sound counterpoise the cautious investigator should take account of the stubborn opposition of the facts. After all, to try and explain everything means to explain nothing.

Doesn't this tendency of each new idea in psychology to turn into a universal law show that psychology really should rest upon universal laws, that all these ideas wait for a master-idea which comes and puts each different, particular idea in its place and indicates its importance? The regularity of the path covered with amazing constancy by the most diverse ideas testifies, of course, to the fact that this path is predetermined by the objective need for an explanatory principle and it is precisely because such a principle is needed and not available that various special principles occupy its place. Psychology, realizing that it is a matter of life or death to find a general explanatory principle, grabs for any idea, albeit an unreliable one.

Spinoza [1677/1955, p. 5] in his "Treatise on the improvement of the understanding" describes a similar state of knowledge:

> A sick man struggling with a deadly disease, when he sees that death will surely be upon him unless a remedy is found, is compelled to seek such a remedy with all his strength, inasmuch as his whole hope lies therein.

## 5

We have traced a distinct tendency towards explanation—which already took shape in the struggle between disciplines for supremacy—in the development of particular discoveries into general principles. But in so doing we already proceeded to the second phase of development of a general science which we have mentioned in passing above. In the first phase, which is determined by the tendency towards generalization, the general science is at bottom quantitatively different from the special ones. In the second phase—the phase in which the tendency towards explanation predominates—the internal structure of the general science is already qualitatively distinct from the special disciplines. Not all sciences, as we will see, go through both phases in their development. The majority knows only a general science in its first phase. The reason for this will become clear as soon as we carefully state the qualitative difference of the second phase.

We have seen that the explanatory principle carries us beyond the boundaries of a given science and must interpret the whole unified area of knowledge as a special category or stage of being amidst a number of other categories, i.e., at stake are highly generalized, ultimate, essentially philosophical principles. In this sense the general science is the philosophy of the special disciplines.

In this sense Binswanger [1922, p. 3] says that a general science such as, for example, general biology elaborates the foundations and problems of a whole area of being. Interestingly, the first book that lay the foundation of general biology was called "The philosophy of zoology" (Lamarckal). The further a general investigation penetrates, continues Binswanger, the larger the area it covers, the more abstract and more remote from directly perceived reality the subject matter of such an investigation will become. Instead of living plants, animals, persons, the subject matter of science becomes the manifestations of life and, finally, life itself, just as in physics force and matter replaced bodies and their changes. Sooner or later for each science the moment comes when it must accept itself as a whole, reflect upon its methods and shift the attention from the facts and phenomena to the concepts it utilizes. But from this moment on the general science is distinct from the special one not because it is broader in scope, but because it is organized in a qualitatively different way. No longer does it study the same objects as the special science; rather, it investigates the concepts of this science. It becomes a critical study in the sense Kant used this expression. No longer being a biological or physical investigation, the critical investigation is concerned with the concepts of biology or physics. Consequently, general psychology is defined by Binswanger as a critical reflection upon the basic concepts of psychology, in short, as "a critique of psychology." It is a branch of general methodology, i.e., of the part of logic that studies the different applications of logical forms and norms in the various sciences in accordance with the formal and material reality of the nature of their objects, their procedures, and their problems.

This argumentation, based on formal logical premises, is only half true. It is correct that the general science is a theory of ultimate foundations, of the general principles and problems of a given area of knowledge, and that consequently its subject matter, methods of investigation, criteria and tasks are different from those n the special disciplines. But it is incorrect to view it as merely a part of logic, as merely a logical discipline, as if general biology is no longer a biological discipline but a logical one, as if general psychology stops being psychology but becomes logic. it is incorrect to view it as merely critique in the Kantian sense, to assume that it rely studies concepts. It is first of all incorrect historically, but also according to the essence of the matter and the inner nature of scientific knowledge.

It is incorrect historically, i.e., it does not correspond with the actual state of affairs in any science. There does not exist a single general science in the form described by Binswanger. Not even general biology in the form in which it actually exists, the biology whose foundations were laid by the works of Lamarck and Darvin, the biology which is until now the canon of genuine knowledge of living matter, is, of course, part of logic, but a natural science, albeit of the highest level. Of course, it does not deal with living, concrete objects such as plants and animals, but with abstractions such as organism, evolution of species, natural selection and life, but in the final analysis it nevertheless studies by means of these abstractions he same reality as zoology and botany. It would be as much a mistake to say that it studies concepts and not the reality reflected in these concepts, as it would to say of an engineer who is studying a blueprint of a machine that he is studying a blueprint and not a machine, or of an anatomist studying an atlas that he studies a drawing and not the human skeleton. For concepts as well are no more than blueprints, snapshots, schemas of reality and in studying them we study models of reality, just as we study a foreign country or city on the plan or geographical map.

When it comes to such well-developed sciences as physics and chemistry, Binswanger [1922, p. 4] himself is compelled to admit that a broad field of investigations developed in between the critical and empirical poles and that this area is called theoretical, or general, physics, chemistry, etc. He remarks that natural-scientific theoretical psychology, which in principle wishes to be like physics, acts likewise. However abstractly theoretical physics may formulate its subject of study, for example as "the theory of causal dependencies between natural phenomena," it nevertheless studies real facts. General physics studies the concept of the physical phenomenon itself, of the physical causal link, but not the various laws and theories on the basis of which the real phenomena may be explained as physically causal. The subject matter of investigation of general physics is rather the physical explanation itself.

As we see, Binswanger himself admits that his conception of the general science diverges in one point from the actual conception as it is realized in a number of sciences. They are not differentiated by a greater or lesser degree of abstraction of the concepts—what can be further from the real, empirical things than causal dependency as the subject matter of a whole science?—but by their ultimate focus: general physics, in the end, focuses on real facts which it wishes to explain by means of abstract concepts. The general science is in principle not focused on real facts, but on the concepts themselves and has nothing to do with the real facts.

Admittedly, when a debate between theory and history arises, when there is a discrepancy between the idea and the fact, as in the present case, the debate is always solved in favor of history or fact. The argument from the facts may itself not always be appropriate in the area of fundamental research. Then to the reproach that the ideas and facts do not correspond we are fully justified to answer: so much the worse for the facts. In the present case, so much the worse for the sciences when they find themselves in a phase of development in which they have not yet attained the stage of a general science. When a general science in this sense does not yet exist, it does not follow that it will never exist, that it should not exist, that we cannot and must not lay its foundations. We must therefore examine the essence, the logical basis of the problem, and then it will also become possible to clarify the meaning of the historical deviation of the general science from its abstract idea.

It is important to make two points.

1. Every natural-scientific concept, however high the degree of its abstraction from the empirical fact, always contains a clot, a sediment of the concrete, real and scientifically known reality, albeit in a very weak solution, i.e., to every ultimate concept, even to the most abstract, corresponds some aspect of reality which the concept represents in an abstract, isolated form. Even purely fictitious, not natural-scientific but mathematical concepts ultimately contain some echo, some reflection of the real relations between things and the real processes, although they did not develop from empirical, actual knowledge, but purely a priori, via the deductive path of speculative logical operations. As Engels demonstrated, even such an abstract concept as the series of numbers, or even such an obvious fiction as zero, i.e., the idea of the absence of any magnitude, is full of properties that are qualitative, i.e., in the end they correspond in a very remote and dissolved form to real, actual relations. Reality exists even in the imaginary abstractions of mathematics.

> 16 is not only the addition of 16 unities, it is also the square of 4 and the biquadrate of 2. . . . Only even numbers can be divided by two. . . . For division by 3 we have the rule of the sum of the figures. . . . For 7 there is a special law. . . . Zero destroys any other number by which it is multiplied; when it is made divisor or dividend with regard to some other number, this number will in the first case become infinitely large, in the second case infinitely small [Engels, 1925/1978, pp. 522/524].

About both concepts of mathematics one might say what Engels, in the words of Hegel, says about zero: "The non-existence of something is a *specific* non-existence" [ibid., p. *525*], i.e., in the end it is a real non-existence. But maybe these qualities, properties, the *specificity* of concepts as such, have no relation whatsoever to reality?

Engels [ibid., p. 530] clearly rejects the view that in mathematics we are dealing with purely free creations and imaginations of the human mind to which nothing in the objective world corresponds. Just the opposite is the case. We meet the prototypes of each of these imaginary quantities in nature. The molecule possesses exactly the same properties in relation to its corresponding mass as the mathematical differential in relation to its variable.

> Nature operates with these differentials, the molecules, in exactly the same way and according to the same laws as mathematics with its abstract differentials [ibid., p. 531].

In mathematics we forget all these analogies and that is why its abstractions turn into something enigmatic. We can always find

> the real relations from which the mathematical relation . . . was taken . . . and even the natural analogues of the mathematical way to make these relations manifest [ibid., p. 534].

The prototypes of mathematical infinity and other concepts lie in the real world.

> The mathematical infinite is taken, albeit unconsciously, from reality, and that is why it can only be explained on the basis of reality, and not on the basis of itself, the mathematical abstraction (ibid., p. 534).

If this is true with respect to the highest possible, i.e., mathematical abstraction, then how much more obvious it is for the abstractions of the real natural sciences. They must, of course, be explained only on the basis of the reality from which they stem and not on the basis of themselves, the abstraction.

2. The second point that we need to make in order to present a fundamental analysis of the problem of the general science is the opposite of the first. Whereas the first claimed that the highest scientific abstraction contains an element of reality, the second is the opposite theorem: even the most immediate, empirical, raw, singular natural scientific fact already contains a first abstraction. The real and the scientific fact are distinct in that the scientific fact is a real fact included into a certain system of knowledge, i.e., an abstraction of several features from the inexhaustible sum of features of the natural fact. The material of science is not raw, but logically elaborated, natural material which has been selected according to a certain feature. Physical body, movement, matter—these are all abstractions. The fact itself of naming a fact by a word means to frame this fact in a concept, to single out one of its aspects; it is an act toward understanding this fact by including it into a category of phenomena which have been empirically studied before. Each word already is a theory, as linguists have noted for quite some time and as Potebnya [1913/1993] has brilliantly demonstrated.

Everything described as a fact is already a theory. These are the words of Goethe to which Münsterberg refers in arguing the need for a methodology. When we meet what is called a cow and say: "This is a cow," we add the act of thinking to the act of perception, bringing the given perception under a general concept. A child who first calls things by their names is making genuine discoveries. I do not see that this is a cow, for this cannot be seen. I see something big, black, moving, lowing, etc., and understand that this is a cow. And this act is an act of classification, of assigning a singular phenomenon to the class of similar phenomena, of systematizing the experience, etc. Thus, language itself contains the basis and possibilities for the scientific knowledge of a fact. The word is the germ of science and in this sense we can say that in the beginning of science was the word.

Who has seen, who has perceived such empirical facts as the heat itself in steam-generation? It cannot be perceived in a single real process, but we can infer this fact with confidence and to infer means to operate with concepts.

In Engels we find a good example of the presence of abstractions and the participation of thought in every scientific fact. Ants have other eyes than we have. They see chemical beams that are invisible to us. This is a fact. How was it established? How can we know that "ants see things that are invisible to us"? Naturally, this is based on the perceptions of our eye, but in addition to that we have not only the other senses but the activity of our thinking as well. Thus, establishing a scientific fact is already a matter of thinking, that is, of concepts.

> To be sure, we will never know *how* these chemical beams look to the ants. Who deplores this is beyond help [Engels, 1925/1978, p. 507].

This is the best example of the non-coincidence of the real and the scientific fact. Here this non-coincidence is presented in an especially vivid way, but it exists to a certain degree in each fact. We never saw these chemical beams and did not perceive the sensations of ants, i.e., that ants see certain chemical beams is not a real fact of immediate experience for us, but for the collective experience of mankind it is a scientific fact. But what to say, then, about the fact that the earth turns around the sun? For here in the thinking of man the real fact, in order to become a scientific fact, had to turn into its opposite, although the earth's rotation around the sun was established by observations of the sun's rotations around the earth.

By now we are equipped with all we need to solve this problem and we can go straight for the goal. If at the root of every scientific concept lies a fact and, vice versa, at the basis of every scientific fact lies a concept, then from this it inevitably follows that the difference between general and empirical sciences as regards the object of investigation is purely quantitative and not fundamental. It is a difference of degree and not a difference of the nature of the phenomenon. The general sciences do not deal with real objects, but with abstractions. They do not study plants and animals, but life. Their subject matter is scientific concepts. But life as well is part of reality and these concepts have their prototypes in reality. The special sciences have the actual facts of reality as their subject matter, they do not study life as such, but actual classes and groups of plants and animals. But both the plant and the animal, and even the birch tree and the tiger, and even *this* birch tree and *this* tiger are already concepts. And scientific facts as well, even the most primitive ones, are already concepts. Fact and concept form the subject matter of all disciplines, but to a different degree, in different proportion. Consequently, general physics does not cease being a physical discipline and does not become part of logic because it deals with the most abstract physical concepts. Ultimately, even these serve to know some part of reality.

But perhaps the nature of the objects of the general and the special disciplines is really the same, maybe they differ only in the proportion of concept and fact, and the fundamental difference which allows us to count the one as logic and the other as physics lies in the direction, the goal, the point of view of both investigations, so to speak, in the different role played by the same elements in both cases? Could we perhaps put it like this: both concept and fact participate in the development of the subject matter of any science, but in one case—the case of empirical science—we utilize concepts to acquire knowledge about facts, and in the second—general science—we utilize facts to acquire knowledge about concepts? In the first case the concepts are not the subject matter, the goal, the objective of knowledge, but its tools, means, auxiliary devices. The goal, the subject matter of knowledge are the facts. As a result of the growth of knowledge the number of known facts is enhanced, but not the number of concepts. Like any tool of labor the concepts, in contrast, suffer wear and tear in their use, become worn down, in need of revision and often of replacement. In the second case it is the other way around; we study the concepts themselves as such, their correspondence with the facts is only a means, a way, a method, a verification of their suitability. As a result we do not learn of new facts, but acquire either new concepts or new knowledge about the concepts. After all, we can look twice at a drop of water under the microscope and this will be two completely distinct processes, although both the drop and the microscope will be the same both times: the first time we study the composition of the drop of water by means of the microscope; the second time we verify the suitability of the microscope itself by looking at a drop of water—isn't it like that?

But the whole difficulty of the problem is exactly that it is not like that. It is true that in a special science we utilize concepts as tools to acquire knowledge of facts. But using tools means at the same time to test them, to study and master them, to throw away the ones that are unfit, to improve them, to create new ones. Already in the very first stage of the scientific processing of empirical material the use of a concept is a critique of the concept by the facts, the comparison of concepts, their modification. Let us take as an example the two scientific facts mentioned above, which definitely do not belong to general science: the earth's rotation around the sun and the vision of ants. How much critical work on our perceptions and, thus, on the concepts linked with them, how much direct study of these concepts—visibility, invisibility, apparent movement—how much creation of new concepts, of new links between concepts, how much modification of the very concepts of vision, light, movement etc. was needed to establish these facts! And, finally, does not the very selection of the concepts needed to know these facts require an analysis of the concepts in addition to the analysis of the facts? After all, if concepts, as tools, were set aside for particular facts of experience in advance, all science would be superfluous: then a thousand administrator-registrators or statistician counters could note down the universe on cards, graphs, columns. Scientific knowledge differs from the registration of a fact in that it selects the concept needed, i.e., it analyzes both fact and concept.

Any word is a theory. To name an object is to apply a concept to it. Admittedly, by means of the word we wish to comprehend the object. But each name, each application of the word, this embryo of science, is a critique of the word, a blurring of its form, an extension of its meaning. Linguists have clearly enough demonstrated how words change from being used. After all, language otherwise would never be renewed, words would not die, be born, or become obsolete.

Finally, each discovery in science, each step forward in empirical science is always at the same time an act of criticizing the concept. Pavlov discovered the fact of conditional reflexes. But didn't he really create a new concept at the same time? Did we really call a trained,

well-learned movement a reflex before? And it cannot be otherwise: if science would only discover facts without extending the boundaries of its concepts, it would not discover anything
new. It would make no headway in finding more and more new specimens of the same concepts. Each tiny new fact is already an extension of the concept. Each newly discovered relation
between two facts immediately requires a critique of the two corresponding concepts and the
establishment of a new relation between them. The conditional reflex is a discovery of a new
fact by means of an old concept. We learned that mental salivation develops directly from the
reflex, more correctly, that it is the same reflex, but operating under other conditions. But at
the same time it is a discovery of a new concept by means of an old fact: by means of the fact
"salivation occurs at the sight of food," which is well known to all of us, we acquired a completely new concept of the reflex, our idea of it diametrically changed. Whereas before, the reflex
was a synonym for a pre-mental, unconscious, immutable fact, nowadays the whole mind is
reduced to reflexes, the reflex has turned out to be a most flexible mechanism, etc. How would
this have been possible if Pavlov had only studied the fact of salivation and not the concept of
the reflex? This is essentially the same thing expressed in two ways, for in each scientific discovery knowledge of the fact is to the same extent knowledge of the concept. The scientific investigation of facts differs from registration in that it is the accumulation of concepts, the circulation of concepts and facts with a conceptual return.

Finally, the special sciences create all the concepts that the general science studies. For the
natural sciences do not spring from logic, it is not logic that provides them with ready-made
concepts. Can we really assume that the creation of ever more abstract concepts proceeds completely unconsciously? How can theories, laws, conflicting hypotheses exist without the critique
of concepts? How can we create a theory or advance a hypothesis, i.e., something which transcends the boundaries of the facts, without working on the concepts?

But perhaps the study of concepts in the special sciences proceeds in passing, accidentally
as the facts are being studied, whereas the general science studies only concepts? This would not
be correct either. We have seen that the abstract concepts with which the general science operates possess a kernel of reality. The question arises what science does with this kernel—is it
ignored, forgotten, covered in the inaccessible stronghold of abstractions like pure mathematics? Does one never in the process of investigation, nor after it, turn to this kernel, as if it did
not exist at all? One only has to examine the method of investigation in the general science and
its ultimate result to see that this is not true. Are concepts really studied by pure deduction,
by finding logical relations between concepts, and not by new induction, by new analysis, the
establishing of new relations, in a word—by work on the real contents of these concepts? After
all, we do not develop our ideas from specific premises, as in mathematics, but we proceed by
induction—we generalize enormous groups of facts, compare them, analyze and create new
abstractions. This is the way general biology and general physics proceed. And not a single general science can proceed otherwise, since the logical formula "A is B" has been replaced by a definition, i.e., by the real A and B: by mass, movement, body, and organism. And the result of an
investigation in a general science is not new forms of interrelations of concepts, as in logic, but
new facts: we learn of evolution, heredity, inertia. How do we learn of this, how do we reach
the concept of evolution? We compare such facts as the data of comparative anatomy and physiology, botany and zoology, embryology and photo- and zootechnics etc., i.e., we proceed as we

proceed with the individual facts in a special science. And on the basis of a new study of the facts elaborated by the various sciences we establish new facts, i.e., in the process of investigation and in its result we are constantly operating with facts.

Thus, the difference between the general and the special science as concerns their goal, orientation, and the elaboration of concepts and facts, again appears to be only quantitative. It is a difference of degree of one and the same phenomenon and not of the nature of two sciences. It is not absolute or fundamental.

Finally, let us proceed to a positive definition of the general science. It might seem that if the difference between general and special science as to their subject matter, method, and goal of study is merely relative and not absolute, quantitative and not fundamental, we lose any ground to distinguish them theoretically. It might seem that there is no general science at all as distinct from the special sciences. But this is not true, of course. Quantity turns into quality here and provides the basis for a qualitatively distinct science. However the latter is not torn away from the given family of sciences and transferred to logic. The fact that at the root of every scientific concept lies a fact does not mean that the fact is represented in every scientific concept in the same way. In the mathematical concept of infinity reality is represented in a way completely different from the way it is represented in the concept of the conditional reflex. In the concepts of a higher order with which the general science is dealing, reality is represented in another way than in the concepts of an empirical science. And the way, character, and form in which reality is represented in the various sciences in every case determines the structure of every discipline.

But this difference in the way of representing reality, i.e., in the structure of the concepts, should not be understood as something absolute either. There are many transitional levels between an empirical science and a general one. Binswanger [1922, p. 4] says that not a single science that deserves the name can "leave it at the simple accumulation of concepts, it strives rather to systematically develop concepts into rules, rules into laws, laws into theories." The elaboration of concepts, methods, and theories takes place within the science itself during the whole course of scientific knowledge acquisition, i.e., the transition from one pole to the other, from fact to concept, is accomplished without pausing for a single minute. And thereby the logical abyss, the impassable line between general and special science is erased, whereas the factual independence and necessity of a general science is created. Just like the special science itself internally takes care of all the work of funneling facts via rules into laws and laws via theories into hypotheses, general science carries out the same work, by the same method, with the same goals, but for a number of the various special sciences.

This is entirely similar to Spinoza's argumentation about method. A theory of method is, of course, the production of means of production, to take a comparison from the field of industry. But in industry the production of means of production is no special, primordial production, but forms part of the general process of production and itself depends upon the same methods and tools of production as all other production.

Spinoza [1677/1955, pp. 11–12] argues that

> We must first take care not to commit ourselves to a search going back to infinity, that is, in order to discover the best method for finding the truth, there is no need of another method to

discover such method; nor of a third method for discovering the second, and so on to infinity. By such proceedings, we should never arrive at the knowledge of the truth, or, indeed, at any knowledge at all. The matter stands on the same footing as the making of material tools, which might be argued about in a similar way. For, in order to work iron, a hammer is needed, and the hammer cannot be forthcoming unless it has been made; but in order to make it, there was need of another hammer and other tools, and so on to infinity. We might thus vainly endeavor to prove that men have no power of working iron. But as men at first made use of the instruments supplied by nature to accomplish very easy pieces of workmanship, laboriously and imperfectly, and then, when these were finished, wrought other things more difficult with less labor and greater perfection; and so gradually mounted from the simplest operations to the making of tools, and from the making of tools to the making of more complex tools, and fresh feats of workmanship, till they arrived at making, with small expenditure of labor, the vast number of complicated mechanisms which they now possess. So, in like manner, the intellect, by its native strength, makes for itself intellectual instruments, whereby it acquires strength for performing other intellectual operations, and from these operations gets again fresh instruments, or the power of pushing its investigations further, and thus gradually proceeds till it reaches the summit of wisdom.

The methodological current to which Binswanger belongs also admits that the production of tools and that of creative work are, in principle, not two separate processes in science, but two sides of the same process which go hand in hand. Following Rickert, he defines each science as the processing [Bearbeitung] of material, and therefore for him two problems arise in every science—one with respect to the material and the other concerning its processing. One cannot, however, draw such a sharp dividing line, since the concept of the object of the empirical science already contains a good deal of processing. And he (Binswanger, 1922, pp. 7–8) distinguishes between the raw material, the real object [wirklichen Gegenstand] and the scientific object [wissenschaftlichen Gegenstand]. The latter is created by science from the real object via concepts. When we raise a third cluster of problems—about the relation between the material and its processing, i.e., between the object and the method of science—the debate must again focus on what is determined by what: the object by the method, or vice versa. Some, like Stumpf, suppose that all differences in method are rooted in differences between the objects. Others, like Rickert, are of the opinion that various objects, both physical and mental, require one and the same method. But, as we see, we do not find grounds for a demarcation of the general from the special science here either.

All this only indicates that we can give no absolute definition of the concept of a general science and that it can only be defined relative to the special science. From the latter it is distinguished not by its object, nor by the method, goal, or result of the investigation. But for a number of special sciences which study related realms of reality from a single viewpoint it accomplishes the same work and by the same method and with the same goal as each of these sciences accomplish for their own material. We have seen that no science confines itself to the simple accumulation of material, but rather that it subjects this material to diverse and prolonged processing, that it groups and generalizes the material, creates a theory and hypotheses which help to get a wider perspective on reality than the one which follows from the various uncoordinated facts. The general science continues the work f the special sciences. When the material is carried to the highest degree of generalization possible in that science, further generalization is possible only beyond the boundaries of the given science and by comparing it with the material of a number of adjacent sciences. This is what the general science does. Its single difference from the special sciences is that it carries out its work with respect to a number of sciences. If it carried out the same work with respect to a single science it would never come to the fore as an independent science, but would remain a part of that single science. The general science can therefore be defined as a science that receives its material from a number of special sciences and carries out the further processing and generalization of the material which is impossible within each of the various disciplines.

The general science therefore stands to the special one as the theory of this special science to the number of its special laws, i.e., according to the degree of generalization of the phenomena studied. The general science develops out of the need to continue the work of the special sciences where these end. The general science stands to the theories, laws, hypotheses and methods of the special sciences as the special science stands to the facts of the reality it studies. Biology receives material from various sciences and processes it in the way each special science does with its own material. The whole difference is that [general] biology begins where embryology, zoology, anatomy etc. stop, that it unites the material of the various sciences, just as a [special] science unites various materials within its own field.

This viewpoint can fully explain both the logical structure of the general science and the factual, historical role of the general science. If we accept the opposite opinion that the general science is part of logic, it becomes completely inexplicable why it is the highly developed sciences, which already managed to create and elaborate very refined methods, basic concepts and theories, which produce a general science. It would seem that new, young, beginning disciplines are more in need of borrowing concepts and methods from another science. Secondly, why does only a group of adjacent disciplines lead to a general science and not each science on its own- why do botany, zoology and anthropology lead to biology? Couldn't we create a logic of just zoology and just botany, like the logic of algebra? And indeed such separate disciplines can exist and do exist, but this does not make them general sciences, just as the methodology of botany does not become biology.

Like the whole current, Binswanger proceeds from an idealistic conception of scientific knowledge, i.e., from idealistic epistemic premises and a formal logical construction of the system of sciences. For Binswanger, concepts and real objects are separated by an unbridgeable gap. Knowledge has its own laws, its own nature, its *a priori*, which it projects unto the reality that is known. That is why for Binswanger these a *priori*, these laws, this knowledge, can be studied separately, in isolation from what is cognized by them. For him a critique of scientific reason in biology, psychology, and physics is possible, just like the critique of pure reason was possible for Kant. Binswanger is prepared to admit that the method of knowing determines reality, just as in Kant reason dictated the laws of nature. For him the relations between sciences are not determined by the historical development of these sciences and not even by the demands of scientific experience, i.e., in the final analysis they are not determined by the demands of the reality studied by this science, but by the formal logical structure of the concepts.

In another philosophical system such a conception would be unthinkable, i.e., when we reject these epistemological and formal logical premises, the whole conception of the general science falls immediately. As soon as we accept the realistic, objective, i.e., the materialistic viewpoint in epistemology and the dialectical viewpoint in logic and in the theory of scientific knowledge, such a theory becomes impossible. With that new viewpoint we must immediately accept that reality determines our experience, the object of science and its method and that it is entirely impossible to study the concepts of any science independent of the realities it represents.

Engels [1925/1978, p. 514] has pointed out many times that for dialectical logic the methodology of science is a reflection of the methodology of reality. He says that

> *The classification of sciences* of which each analyzes a different form of movement, or a number of movements that are connected and merge into each other, is at the same time a classification, an ordering according to the inherent order of these forms of movement themselves and in this resides their importance.

Can it be said more clearly? In classifying the sciences we establish the hierarchy of reality itself.

> The so-called *objective* dialectic reigns in all nature, and the so-called subjective dialectic, dialectical thinking, is only a reflection of the movement by opposition, that reigns in all nature [ibid., p. 481].

Here the demand to take account of the objective dialectic in studying the subjective dialectic, i.e., dialectical thinking in some science, is clearly expressed. Of course, by no means does this imply that we close our eyes to the subjective conditions of this thinking. The same Engels who established a correspondence between being and thinking in mathematics says that "all laws of number are dependent upon and determined by the system that is used. In the binary and ternary system 2 x 2 does not = 4, but = 100 or = 11" [ibid., p. 523]. Extending this, we might say that subjective assumptions which follow from knowledge will always influence the way of expressing the laws of nature and the relation between the different concepts. We must take them into account, but always as a reflection of the objective dialectic.

We must, therefore, contrast epistemological critique and formal logic as the foundations of a general science with a dialectic "which is conceived of as the science of the most general laws of *all* movement. This implies that its laws must be valid for both movement in nature and human history and movement in thinking" [ibid., p. 530]. This means that the dialectic of psychology—this is what we may now call the general psychology in opposition to Binswanger's definition of a "critique of psychology"—is the science of the most general forms of movement (in the form of behavior and knowledge of this movement), i.e., the dialectic of psychology is at the same time the dialectic of man as the object of psychology, just as the dialectic of the natural sciences is at the same time the dialectic of nature.

Engels does not even consider the purely logical classification of judgments in Hegel to be based merely on thinking, but on the laws of nature. This he regards as a distinguishing characteristic of dialectical logic.

> What in Hegel seems a development of the judgment as a category of thinking as such, now appears to be a development of our knowledge of the nature of movement based on *empirical* grounds. And this proves that the laws of thinking and the laws of nature correspond necessarily with each other as soon as they are known properly [ibid., p. 493].

The key to general psychology as a part of dialectics lies in these words: this correspondence between thinking and being in science is at the same time object, highest criterion, and even method, i.e., general principle of the general psychology.


6


General psychology stands to the special disciplines as algebra to arithmetic. Arithmetic operates with specific, concrete quantities; algebra studies all kinds of general forms of relations between qualities. Every arithmetical operation can, consequently, be considered as a special case of an algebraic formula. From this it obviously follows that for each special discipline and for each of its laws the question as to which general formula they form a special case of is not at all indifferent. The general science's fundamentally guiding and supreme role, so to speak, does not follow from the fact that it stands above the sciences, it does not come from above, from logic, i.e., from the ultimate foundations of scientific knowledge, but from below, from the sciences themselves which delegate the authorization of truth to the general science. The general science, consequently, develops from the special position it occupies with regard to the special ones: it integrates their sovereignties, forms their representative. If we graphically represent the system of knowledge which covers all psychological disciplines as a circle, general science will correspond to the center of the circumference.

Now let us suppose that we have various centers as in the case of a debate between separate disciplines that aspire to become the center, or in the case of different ideas claiming to be the central explanatory principle. It is obvious that to these will correspond different circumferences and each new center will at the same time be a peripheral point on the former circumference. Consequently, we get several circumferences that intersect with each other. In our example this new position of each circumference graphically represents the special area of knowledge that is covered by psychology depending on the center, i.e., the general discipline.

Whoever takes the viewpoint of the general discipline, i.e., deals with the facts of the special disciplines not on a footing of equality, but as the material of a science, just as these disciplines themselves deals with the facts of reality, will immediately change the viewpoint of critique for the viewpoint of investigation. Criticism is on the same level as what is being criticized; it proceeds fully within the given discipline; its goal is exclusively critical and not positive; it wishes to know only whether and to what extent some theory is correct; it evaluates and judges, but does not investigate. A criticizes B, but both occupy the same position as to the facts. Things change when A begins to deal with B as B does with the facts, i.e., when he does not criticize B, but investigates him. The investigation already belongs to general science, its tasks are not critical, but positive. It does not wish to evaluate some theory, but to learn something new about the facts themselves which are represented in the theory. While science uses critique as a means, the course [of the investigation, Russian eds.] and the result of this process nevertheless differ fundamentally from a critical examination. Critique, in the final analysis, formulates an opinion about an opinion, albeit a very solid and well-founded opinion. A general investigation establishes, ultimately, objective laws and facts.

Only he who elevates his analysis from the level of the critical discussion of some system of views to the level of a fundamental investigation by means of the general science will understand the objective meaning of the crisis that is taking place in psychology. He will see the lawfulness of the clash of ideas and opinions that is taking place, which is determined by the development of the science itself and by the nature of the reality it studies at a given level of knowledge. Instead of a chaos of heterogeneous opinions, a motley discordance of subjective utterances, he will see an orderly blueprint of the fundamental opinions concerning the development of the science, a system of the objective tendencies which are inherent in the historical tasks brought forward by the development of the science and which act behind the backs of the various investigators and theorists with the force of a steel spring. Instead of critically discussing and evaluating some author, instead of establishing that this author is guilty of inconsistency and contradictions, he will devote a positive investigation to the question what the objective tendencies in science require. And as a result, instead of opinions about an opinion he will get an outline of the skeleton of the general science as a system of defining laws, principles and facts.

Only such an investigator realizes the real and correct meaning of the catastrophe that is taking place and has a clear idea of the role, place, and meaning of each different theory or school. Rather than by the impressionism and subjectivism inevitable in each criticism, he will be led by scientific reliability and veracity. For him (and this will be the first result of the new viewpoint) the individual differences will vanish-he will understand the role of personality in history. He will understand that to explain reflexology's claims to be a universal science from the personal mistakes, opinions, particularities, and ignorance of its founders is as impossible as to explain the French revolution from the corruption of the king or court. He will see what and how much in the development of science depends upon the good and bad intention of its practitioners, what can be explained from their intentions and what from this intention itself should, on the contrary, be explained on the basis of the objective tendencies operative behind the backs of these practitioners. Of course, the particularities of his personal creativity and the entire weight of his scientific experience determined the specific form of universalism which the idea of reflexology acquired in the hands of Bekhterev. But in Pavlov [1928/1963, p. 41] as well, whose personal contribution and scientific experience are entirely different, reflexology is the "ultimate science," "an omnipotent method," which brings "full, true and permanent human happiness." And in their own way behaviorism and Gestalt theory cover the same route. Obviously, rather than the mosaic of good and evil intentions among the investigators we should study the unity in the processes of regeneration of scientific tissue in psychology, which determines the intention of all the investigators.

## 7

Precisely what the dependency of each psychological operation upon the general formula means can be illustrated with any problem that transcends the boundaries of the special discipline that raised it.

When Lipps [1897, p. 146] says about the unconscious that it is less a psychological problem than *the* problem for psychology, he has in mind that the unconscious is a problem of general psychology. By this he wished *to* say, of course, no more than that this question will be answered not as a result of this or that particular investigation, but as a result of a fundamental investigation by means of the general science, i.e., by comparing the widely varying data of the most heterogeneous areas of science; by correlating the given problem with several of the basic premises of scientific knowledge, on the one hand, and with several of the most general results of all sciences, on the other; by finding a place for this concept in the system of the basic concepts of psychology; by a fundamental dialectical analysis of the nature of this concept and the features of being that it corresponds to and reflects. This investigation logically precedes any concrete investigation of particular questions of subconscious life and determines the very formulation of the problem in such investigations.

As Münsterberg [1920, p. v], defending the need for such an investigation for another set of problems, splendidly put it: "In the end it is better to get an approximately exact preliminary answer to a question that is stated correctly than to answer with a precision to the last decimal point a question that is stated inaccurately." A correct statement of a question is no less a matter of scientific creativity and investigation than a correct answer—and it is much more crucial. The vast majority of contemporary psychological investigations write out the last decimal point with great care and precision in answer to a question that is stated fundamentally incorrectly.

Whether we accept with Münsterberg [1920, pp. 158–163] that the subconscious is simply physiological and not psychological; or whether we agree with others that the subconscious consists of phenomena that temporarily are absent from consciousness, like the whole mass of potentially conscious reminiscences, knowledge and habits; whether we call those phenomena subconscious that do not reach the threshold of consciousness, or those of which we are minimally conscious, which are peripheral in the field of consciousness, automatic and unnoted; whether we find a suppression of the sexual drive to be the basis of the subconscious, like Freud, or our second ego, a special personality; finally, whether we call these phenomena un-, sub-, or superconscious, or like Stern accept all of these terms—it all fundamentally changes the character, quantity, composition, nature, and properties of the material which we will study. The question partially predetermines the answer.

It is this feeling of a system, the sense of a [common] style, the understanding that each particular statement is linked with and dependent upon the central idea of the whole system of which it forms a part, which is absent in the essentially eclectic attempts at combining the parts of two or more systems that are heterogeneous and diverse in scientific origin and composition. Such are, for instance, the synthesis of behaviorism and Freudian theory in the American literature; Freudian theory without Freud in the systems of Adler and Jung; the reflexological Freudian theory of Bekhterev and Zalkind; finally, the attempts to combine Freudian theory and Marxism (Luria, 1925; Fridman, 1925). So many examples from the area of the problem of the subconscious alone! In all these attempts the tail of one system is taken and placed against the head of another and the space between them is filled with the trunk of a third. It isn't that they are incorrect, these monstrous combinations, they are correct to the last decimal point, but the question they wish to answer is stated incorrectly. We can multiply the number of citizens of Paraguay with the number of kilometers from the earth to the sun and divide the product by the average life span of the elephant and carry out the whole operation irreproachably, without a mistake in any number, and nevertheless the final outcome might mislead someone who is interested in the national income of this country. What the eclectics do, is to reply to a question raised by Marxist philosophy with an answer prompted by Freudian metapsychology.

In order to show the methodological illegitimacy of such attempts, we will first dwell upon three types of combining incompatible questions and answers, without thinking for one moment that these three types exhaust the variety of such attempts.

The first way in which any school assimilates the scientific products of another area consists of the direct transposition of all laws, facts, theories, ideas etc., the usurpation of a more or less broad area occupied by other investigators, the annexation of foreign territory. Such a politics of direct usurpation is common for each new scientific system which spreads its influence to adjacent disciplines and lays claim to the leading role of a general science. Its own material is insufficient and after just a little critical work such a system absorbs foreign bodies, submits them, filling the emptiness of its inflated boundaries. Usually one gets a conglomerate of scientific theories, facts, etc. which have been squeezed into the framework of the unifying idea with horrible arbitrariness.

Such is the system of Bekhterev's reflexology. He can use anything: even Vvedensky's theory about the unknowability of the external ego, i.e., an extreme expression of solipsism and idealism in psychology, provided that this theory clearly confirms his particular claim about the need for an objective method. That it breaches the general sense of the whole system, that it undermines the foundations of the realistic approach to personality does not matter to this author (we observe that Vvedensky, too, fortifies himself and his theory with a reference to the work of . . . Pavlov, without understanding that by turning for help to a system of objective psychology he extends a hand to his grave-digger). But for the methodologist it is highly significant that such antipodes as Vvedensky-Pavlov and Bekhterev-Vvedensky do not merely contradict each other, but necessarily presuppose each other's existence and view the coincidence of their conclusions as evidence for "the reliability of these conclusions." For this third person [the methodologist, Russian eds.] it is clear that we are not dealing here with a coincidence of conclusions which were reached fully independently by representatives of different specialties, for example the philosopher Vvedensky and the physiologist Pavlov, but with a coincidence of the basic assumptions, starting-points and philosophical premises of dualistic idealism. This "coincidence" is presupposed from the very start: Bekhterev presupposes Vvedensky—when the one is right, the other is right as well.

Einstein's principle of relativity and the principles of Newtonian mechanics, incompatible in themselves, get on perfectly well in this eclectic system, In Bekhterev's "Collective reflexology" he absolutely gathered a catalogue of universal laws. Characteristic of the methodology of the system is the way imagination is given free reign, the fundamental inertia of the idea which by direct communication, omitting all intermediate steps, leads us from the law of the proportional correlation of the speed of movement with the moving force, established in mechanics, to the fact of the USA'S involvement in the great European war, and back again—from the experiment of a certain Dr. Schwarzmann on the frequency limits of electro-cutaneous irritation leading to an association reflex to the "universal law of relativity which obtains everywhere and which, as a result of Einstein's brilliant investigations, has been finally demonstrated in regard to heavenly bodies."

Needless to say, the annexation of psychological areas is carried out no less categorically and no less boldly. The investigations of the higher thought processes by the Würzburg school, like the results of the investigations of other representatives of subjective psychology, "may be harmonized with the scheme of cerebral or association reflexes." Never mind that this very phrase strikes out all the fundamental premises of his own system: for if we can harmonize everything with the reflex schema and everything "is in perfect accord" with reflexology—even what has been discovered by subjective psychology—why take up arms against it? The discoveries made in Würzburg were made with a method which, according to Bekhterev, cannot lead to the truth. However, they are in complete harmony with the objective truth. How is that?

The territory of psychoanalysis is annexed just as carelessly. For this it suffices to declare that "in Jung's doctrine of complexes we find complete agreement with the data of reflexology." But one passage higher it was said that this doctrine was based on subjective analysis, which Bekhterev rejects. No problem: we live in the world of pre-established harmony, of the miraculous correspondence, of the amazing coincidence of theories based on false analyses and the data of the exact sciences. To be more precise, we live in the world—according to Blonsky (1925a, p. 226)—of "terminological revolutions."

Our whole eclectic epoch is filled with such coincidences. Zalkind, for example, annexes the same areas of psychoanalysis and the theory of complexes in the name of the dominant. It turns out that the psychoanalytic school developed the same concepts about the dominant completely independently from the reflexological school, but "in our terms and by another method." The "complex orientation" of the psychoanalysts, the "strategical set" of the Adlerians, these are dominants as well, not in general physiological but clinical, general therapeutic formulations. The annexation—the mechanical transposition of bits of a foreign system into one's own—in this case, as always, seems almost miraculous and testifies to its truth. Such an "almost miraculous" theoretical and factual coincidence of two doctrines, which work with totally different material and by entirely different methods, forms a convincing confirmation of the correctness of the principal path that contemporary reflexology is following. We remember that Vvedensky too saw in his coincidence with Pavlov a testimony of the truth of his statements. And more: this coincidence testifies, as Bekhterev more than once showed, to the fact that we may arrive at the same truth by entirely different methods. Actually, this coincidence testifies only to the methodological unscrupulousness and eclecticism of the system within which such a coincidence is observed. "He that toucheth pitch shall be defiled," as the saying goes. He who borrows from the psychoanalysts—Jung's doctrine of complexes, Freud's catharsis, Adler's strategical set—gets his share of the "pitch" of these systems, i.e., the philosophical spirit of the authors.

Whereas the first method of transposition of foreign ideas from one school into another resembles the annexation of foreign territory, the second method of comparing foreign ideas is similar to a treaty between two allied countries in which both retain their independence, but agree to act together proceeding from their common interests. This method is usually applied in the merger of Marxism and Freudian theory. In so doing the author uses a method that by analogy with geometry might be called the method of the logical superposition of concepts. The system of Marxism is defined as being monistic, materialistic, dialectic etc. Then the monism, materialism etc. of Freud's system is established; the superimposed concepts coincide and the systems are declared to have fused. Very flagrant, sharp contradictions which strike the eye are removed in a very elementary way: they are simply excluded from the system, are declared to be exaggerations, etc. Thus, Freudian theory is de-sexualized as pan-sexualism obviously does not square with Marx's philosophy. No problem, we are told—we will accept Freudian theory without the doctrine of sexuality. But this doctrine forms the very nerve, soul, center of the whole system. Can we accept a system without its center? After all, Freudian theory without the doctrine of the sexual nature of the unconscious is like Christianity without Christ or Buddhism with Allah.

It would be a historical miracle, of course, if a full-grown system of Marxist psychology were to originate and develop in the West, from completely different roots and in a totally different cultural situation. That would imply that philosophy does not at all determine the development of science. As we can see, they started from Schopenhauer and created a Marxist psychology! But this would imply the total fruitlessness of the attempt itself to merge Freudian theory with Marxism, just as the success of Bekhterev's coincidence would imply the bankruptcy of the objective method: after all, if the data of subjective analysis fully coincide with the data of objective analysis, one may ask in what sense subjective analysis is inferior, If Freud, without knowing it himself, thinking about other philosophical systems and consciously siding with them, nevertheless created a Marxist doctrine of the mind, then in the name of what, may one ask, is it necessary to disturb this most fruitful delusion: after all, according to these authors, we need not change anything in Freud. Why, then, merge psychoanalysis with Marxism? In addition, the following interesting question arises: how is it possible that this system which entirely coincides with Marxism logically led to making the idea of sexuality, which is obviously irreconcilable with Marxism, into its cornerstone? Is not the method to a large extent responsible for the conclusions arrived at with its help? And how could a true method which creates a true system, based on true premises, lead its authors to a false theory, to a false central idea? One has to dispose of a good deal of methodological carelessness not to see these problems which inevitably arise in each mechanical attempt to move the center of any scientific system—in the given case, from Schopenhauer's doctrine of the will as the basis of the world to Marx's doctrine about the dialectical development of matter.

But the worst is still to come. In such attempts one often simply must close one's eyes to the contradictory facts, pay no attention to vast areas and main principles, and introduce monstrous distortions in both of the systems to be merged. In so doing, one uses transformations like those with which algebra operates, in order to prove the identity of two expressions. But the transformation of the systems to be merged operates with unities that are absolutely different from the algebraic ones. In practice, it always leads to the distortion of the essence of these systems.

In the article by Luria [1925, p. 55], for example, psychoanalysis is presented as "a system of monistic psychology," whose methodology "coincides with the methodology" of Marxism. In order to prove this a number of most naive transformations of both systems are carried out as a result of which they "coincide." Let us briefly look at these transformations. First of all, Marxism is situated in the general methodology of the epoch, alongside Darwin, Comte, Pavlov, and Einstein,[12] who together create the general methodological foundations of the epoch [ibid., p. 47], The role and importance of each of these authors is, of course, deeply and fundamentally different, and by its very nature the role of dialectical materialism is totally different from all of them. Not to see this means to deduce methodology from the sum total of "great scientific achievements" [ibid., p. 47]. As soon as one reduces all these names and Marxism to a common denominator it is not difficult to unite Marxism with any "great scientific achievement," because this was presupposed: the "coincidence" looked for is in the presupposition and not in the conclusion. The "fundamental methodology of the epoch" consists of the sum total of the discoveries made by Pavlov, Einstein, etc. Marxism is one of these discoveries, which belong to the "group of principles indispensable for quite a number of closely-related sciences" [ibid., p. 47]. Here, on the first page, that is, the argumentation might have ended: after Einstein one would only have to mention Freud, for he is also a "great scientific achievement" and, thus, a participant in the "general methodological foundations of the epoch." But one must have much uncritical trust in scientific reputation to deduce the methodology of an epoch from the sum total of famous names!

There is no unitary basic methodology of the epoch. What we have is a system of fighting, deeply hostile, mutually exclusive, methodological principles and each theory—whether by Pavlov or Einstein—has its own methodological merit. To distill a general methodology of the epoch and to dissolve Marxism in it means to transform not only the appearance, but also the essence of Marxism.

But also Freudian theory is inescapably subjected to the same type of transformations. Freud himself would be amazed to learn that psychoanalysis is a system of monistic psychology and that "methodologically he carries on . . . historical materialism" [Fridman, 1925, p. 159]. Not a single psychoanalytic journal would, of course, print the papers by Luria and Fridman. That is highly important. For a very peculiar situation has evolved: Freud and his school have never declared themselves to be monists, materialists, dialecticians, or followers of historical materialism. But they are told: you are both the first, and the second, and the third. You yourselves don't know who you are. Of course, one can imagine such a situation, it is entirely possible. But then it is necessary to give an exact explanation of the methodological foundations of this doctrine, as conceived of and developed by its authors, and then a proof of the refutation of these foundations and to explain by what miracle and on what foundations psychoanalysis developed a system of methodology which is foreign to its authors. Instead of this, the identity of the two systems is declared by a simple formal-logical superposition of the characteristics—without a single analysis of Freud's basic concepts, without critically weighing and elucidating his assumptions and starting-points, without a critical examination of the genesis of his ideas, even without simply inquiring how he himself conceives of the philosophical foundations of his system.

But, maybe, this formal-logical characterization of the two systems is correct? We have already seen how one distills Marxism's share in the general methodology of the epoch, in which everything is roughly and naively reduced to a common denominator: if both Einstein and Pavlov and Marx belong to science, then they must have a common foundation. But Freudian theory suffers even more distortions in this process. I will not even mention how Zalkind (1924) mechanically deprives it of its central idea. In his article it is passed over in silence, which is also noteworthy. But take the monism of psychoanalysis—Freud would contest it. The article mentions that he turned to philosophical monism, but where, in which words, in connection with what? Is finding empirical unity in some group of facts really always monism? On the contrary, Freud always accepted the mental, the unconscious as a special force which cannot be reduced to something else. Further, why is this monism materialistic in the philosophical sense? After all, medical materialism which acknowledges the influence of different organs etc. upon mental structures is still very far from philosophical materialism. In the philosophy of Marxism this concept has a specific, primarily epistemological sense and it is precisely in his epistemology that Freud stands on idealist philosophical grounds. For it is a fact, which is not refuted and not even considered by the authors of the "coincidences," that Freud's doctrine of the primary role of blind drives, of the unconscious as being reflected in consciousness in a distorted fashion, goes back directly to Schopenhauer's idealistic metaphysics of the will and the idea. Freud [1920/1973, pp. 49–50] himself remarks that in his extreme conclusions he is in the harbor of Schopenhauer. But his basic assumptions as well as the main lines of his system are connected with the philosophy of the great pessimist, as even the simplest analysis can demonstrate.

In its more "concrete" works as well, psychoanalysis displays not dynamic, but highly static, conservative, anti-dialectic and anti-historical tendencies. It directly reduces the higher mental processes—both personal and collective ones—to primitive, primordial, essentially prehistorical, prehuman roots, leaving no room for history. The same key unlocks the creativity of a Dostoyevsky and the totem and taboo of primordial tribes; the Christian church, communism, the primitive horde—in psychoanalysis everything is reduced to the same source. That such tendencies are present in psychoanalysis is apparent from all the works of this school which deal with problems of culture, sociology and history. We can see that here it does not continue, but contradicts, the methodology of Marxism. But about this one keeps silent as well.

Finally, the third point. Freud's whole psychological system of fundamental concepts goes back to Lipps [1903]: the concepts of the unconscious, of the mental energy connected with certain ideas, of drives as the basis of the mind, of the struggle between drives and repression, of the affective nature of consciousness, etc. In other words, Freud's psychological roots lead back to the spiritualistic strata of Lipps' psychology. How is it possible to disregard this when speaking about Freud's methodology?

Thus, we see where Freud and his system have come from and where they are heading for: from Schopenhauer and Lipps to Kolnay and mass psychology. But to apply the system of psychoanalysis while saying nothing about metapsychology, social psychology and Freud's theory of sexuality is to give it a quite arbitrary interpretation. As a result, a person not knowing Freud would get an utterly false idea of him from such an exposition of his system. Freud himself would protest against the word "system" first of all. In his opinion, one of the greatest merits of psychoanalysis and its author is that it consciously avoids becoming a system. Freud himself rejects the "monism" of psychoanalysis: he does not demand that the factors he discovered be accepted as exclusive or primary. He does not at all attempt to "give an exhaustive theory of the mental life of man," but demands only that his statements be used to complete and correct the knowledge which we have acquired through whatever other way. In another place he says that psychoanalysis is characterized by its technique and not by its subject matter, in a third that psychological theory has a temporary nature and will be replaced by an organic theory.

All this may easily delude us: it might seem that psychoanalysis really has no system and that its data can serve to correct and complete any system of knowledge, acquired in whatever way. But this is utterly false. Psychoanalysis has no a *priori*, conscious theory-system. Like Pavlov, Freud discovered too much to create an abstract system. But like Molière's hero who, without suspecting it, spoke prose all his life, Freud, the investigator, created a system: introducing a new word, harmonizing one term with another, describing a new fact, drawing a new conclusion, he created, in passing and step by step, a new system. This implies that the structure of his system is unique, obscure, complex and very difficult to grasp. It is much easier to find one's way in methodological systems which are deliberate, clear, and free from contradictions, which acknowledge their teachers and are unified and logically structured. It is much more difficult to correctly evaluate and reveal the true nature of unconscious methodologies which evolved spontaneously, in a contradictory way, under various influences. But it is precisely to the latter that psychoanalysis belongs. For this reason psychoanalysis requires a very careful and critical methodological analysis and not a naive superposition of the features of two different systems.

Ivanovsky (1923, p. 249) says that "For a person who is not experienced in matters of scientific methodology all sciences seem to share the same method." Psychology suffered most of all from such a misunderstanding. It was always counted as either biology or sociology and rarely were psychological laws, theories, etc., judged by the criterion of psychological methodology, i.e., with an interest in the thought of psychological science as such, its theory, its methodology, its sources, forms and foundations. That is why in our critique of foreign systems, in the evaluation of their truth, we lack what is most important: after all, it is only from an understanding of its methodological basis that we can correctly assess the extent to which knowledge has been corroborated and established beyond doubt (Ivanovsky, 1923). And the rule that one must doubt everything, take nothing on trust, ask each claim what it rests on and what is its source, is, therefore, the first rule and methodology of science. It safeguards us against an even grosser mistake—not only to consider the methods of all sciences to be equal, but to imagine that the structure of each science is uniform.

> The inexperienced mind imagines each separate science, so to speak, in one plane: given that science is reliable, indisputable knowledge, everything in it must be reliable. Its whole content must be obtained and proven by one and the same method which yields reliable knowledge. In reality this is not true at all: each science has its different facts (and groups of analogous facts) which have been established beyond doubt, its irrefutably established general claims and laws, but it also has pre-suppositions, hypotheses which sometimes have a temporary, provisional character and sometimes indicate the ultimate boundaries of our knowledge (at least for the given epoch); there are conclusions which follow more or less indisputably from firmly established theses; there are constructions which sometimes broaden the boundaries of our knowledge, sometimes form deliberately introduced 'fictions'; there are analogies, approximate generalizations etc., etc. Science has no homogeneous structure and the understanding of this fact is of the greatest significance for a person's understanding of science. Each different scientific thesis has its own individual degree of reliability depending upon the way and degree of its methodological foundation, and science, viewed methodologically, does not represent a single solid uniform surface, but a mosaic of theses of different degrees of reliability" (ibid., p. 250).

That is why (1) merging the method of all sciences (Einstein, Pavlov, Comte, Marx) and (2) reducing the entire heterogeneous structure of the scientific system to one plane, to a "single solid uniform surface," compromise the main mistakes of the secongd way of fusing two systems. To reduce personality to money; cleanliness, stubborness and a thousand other, heterogeneous things to anal erotics (Luria, 1925), is not yet monism. And with regard to its nature and degree of reliability it is a fundamental error to mix up this thesis with the principles of materialism. The principle that follows from this thesis, the general idea behind it, its methodological meaning, the method of investigation prescribed by it, are deeply conservative: like the convict to his wheelbarrow, the character is psychoanalysis is chained to childhood erotics. Human life is in its inner essence predetermined by childhood conflicts. It is all the overcoming of the Oedipal conflict, etc. Culture and the life of mankind are again brought close to primitive life. [But] it is a first indispensable condition for analysis to be able to distinguish the first apparent meaning of a fact from its real meaning. By no means do I want to say that everything in psychoanalysis contradicts Marxism. I only want to say that I am in principle not dealing with this question at all. I am only pointing out how we should (methodologically) and should not (uncritically) fuse two systems of ideas.

With an uncritical approach, everbody sees what he want to see and not what is: the Marxist finds monism, materialism, and dialectics in psychoanalysis, which is not there; the physiologist, like Lenz (1922, p. 69), holds that "psycho-physiological in his conception, i.e., the anti-physiological, constitutes Freud's merit in psychiatry. But he adds [1922, p. v] that "this knowledge does not know itself yet, i.e., it has no insight into its own conceptual foundations, its logos."

That is why it is especially difficult to study knowledge that has not yet become aware of itself and its logos. This does by no means imply, of course, that Marxists should not study the unconscious because Freud's basic concepts contradict dialectical materialism. On the contrary, prcisely because the area elaborated by psychoanalysis is elaborated with inadequate means it must be conquered for Marxism. It must be elaborated with the means of a genuine methodolgy, for otherwise, if everything in psychoanalysis would coincide with Marxism, psychologists might develop it in their quality as psychoanalysts and not as Marxists. And for the elaboration one must first take account of the methodological nature of each idea, each thesis. And under this condition the most metapsychological ideas can be interesting and instructive, for example, Freud's doctrine of the death drive.

In the preface which I wrote for the translation of Freud's book on this theme, I attempted to show that the fictitious construct of a death drive—despite the whole speculative nature of this thesis, the not very convincing nature of the factual confirmations (traumatic neurosis and the repetition of unpleasant experiences in children's play), its giddy paradoxical nature and the contradiction of generally accepted biological ideas, its conclusions which obviously coincide with the philosophy of the Nirvana, despite all this and despite the whole artificial nature of the concept—satisfies the need of modern biology to master the idea of death, just like mathematics in its time needed the concept of the negative number. I adduced the thesis that the concept of life has been carried to great clarity in biology, science has mastered it, it knows how to work with it, how to investigate and understand living matter. But it cannot yet cope with the concept of death. Instead of this concept we have a gaping hole, an empty spot. Death is merely seen as the contradictory opposite if life, as not-life, in short, as non-being. But death is a fact that has its positive sense as well, it is a special type of being and not merely non-being. It is a specific something and not absolutely nothing. And biology does not know this positive sense of death. Indeed, death is a universal law for living cannot imagine that this phenomenon would in no way be represented organism, i.e., in the processes of life. It is hard to believe that death would sense or just a negative sense.

Engels [1925/1978, p. 554] expresses a similar opinion. He refers to Hegel's opinion that only that philosophy can count as scientific that considers death to an essential aspect of life and understands that the negation of life is essential contained in life itself, so that life can be understood in relation to its inevitable result which is continually present in embryonic form: death. The dialectical understanding of life entails no more than that. "To live means to die."

It was precisely this idea that I defended in the mentioned preface to Freud's book: the need for biology to master the concept of death from a fundamental viewpoint and to designate this still unknown entity which no doubt exists—let it be with the algebraic "x" or the paradoxical "death drive"—and which represents the tendency towards death in the processes of the organism. Despite this I did not declare Freud's solution to this equation to be a highway in science or a road for all of us, but an Alpine mountain track above the precipice for those free of vertigo. I stated that science needs such books as well: they do not reveal the truth, but teach us the search for truth, although they have not yet found it. I also resolutely said that the importance of this book does not depend upon the factual confirmation of its reliability: in principle it asks the right question. And for the statement of such questions, I said, one needs sometimes more creativity than for the umpteenth standard observation in whatever science [see pp. 13–15 of Van der Veer and Valsiner, 1994].

And the judgment of one of the reviewers of this book showed a complete lack of understanding of the methodological problem, a full trust in the external features of ideas, a naive and uncritical fear of the physiology of pessimism. He decided on the spot that if it is Schopenhauer, it must be pessimism. He did not understand that there are problems that one cannot approach flying, but that one must approach on foot, limping, and that in such cases it is no shame to limp, as Freud [1920/1973, p. 64] openly says. But he, who only sees lameness here, is methodologically blind. For it would not be difficult to show that Hegel is an idealist, it is proclaimed from the housetops. But it needed genius to see in this system an idealism that stood materialism on its head, i.e., to distinguish the methodological truth (dialectics) from the factual falsehood, to see that Hegel went limping towards the truth.

This is but a single example of the path towards the mastery of scientific ideas: one must rise above their factual content and test their fundamental nature. But for this one needs to have a buttress outside these ideas. Standing upon these ideas with both feet, operating with concepts gathered by means of them, it is impossible to situate oneself outside of them. In order to critically regard a foreign system, one must first of all have one's own psychological system of principles. To judge Freud by means of principles obtained from Freud himself implies a vindication in advance. And such an attempt to appropriate foreign ideas forms the third type of combining ideas to which we will now turn.

Again it is easiest to disclose and demonstrate the character of the new methodological approach with a single example. In Pavlov's laboratory it was attempted to experimentally solve the problem of the transformation of trace-conditional stimuli and trace-conditional inhibitors into actual conditional stimuli. For this one must "banish the inhibition" established through the trace reflex. How to do this? In order to reach this goal, Frolov resorted to an analogy with some of the methods of Freud's school. Trying to destroy the stable inhibitory complexes, he exactly recreated the situation in which these complexes were orginally established. And the experiment succeeded. I consider the methodological technique at the basis of his experiment to be an example of the right approach to Freud's theme and to claims by others in general. Let us try to describe this technique. First of all, the problem was raised in the course of Pavlov's own investigations of the nature of internal inhibition. The task was framed, formulated, and understood in the light of his principles. The theoretical theme of the experimental work and its significance were conceived of in the concepts of Pavlov's school. We know what a trace reflex is and we also know what an actual reflex is. To transform the one into the other means to banish inhibition etc., i.e., the whole mechanism of the process we understand in entirely specific and homogeneous categories. The value of the analogy with catharsis was merely heuristic: it shortened the path of Pavlov's experiments and led to the goal in the shortest way possible. But it was only accepted as an assumption that was immediately verified experimentally. And after the solution of his own task the author came to the third and final conclusion that the phenomena described by Freud can be experimentally tested upon animals and should be analyzed in more detail via the method of conditional salivary reflexes.

To verify Freud via Pavlov's ideas is totally different from verifying them via his own ideas; and this possibility as well was established not through analysis, but through the experiment. What is most important is that the author, when confronted with phenomena analogous to those described by Freud's school, did not for one moment step onto foreign territory, did not rely on other people's data, but used them to carry through his own investigation. Pavlov's discovery has its significance, value, place and meaning in his own system, not in Freud's. The two circles touch at the point of intersection of both systems, the point where they meet, and this one point belongs to both at the same time. But its place, sense and value is determined by its position in the first system. A new discovery was made in this investigation, a new fact was found, a new trait was studied—but it was all in the [framework of the] theory of conditional reflexes and not in psychoanalysis. In this way each "almost miraculous" coincidence disappeared!

One has only to compare this with the purely verbal way Bekhterev [1932, p. 413] comes to a similar evaluation of the idea of catharsis for the system of reflexology, to see the deep difference between these two procedures. Here the interrelation of the two systems is also first of all based on catharsis, i.e.,

> discharge of a 'strangulated' affect or an inhibited mimetic-somatic impulse. Is not this the discharge of a reflex which, when inhibited, oppresses the personality, shackles and diseases it, while, when there is discharge of the reflex (catharsis), naturally the pathological condition disappears? Is not the weeping out of a sorrow the discharge of an impeded reflex?

Here every word is a pearl. A mimetic-somatic impulse—what can be more clear or precise? Avoiding the language of subjective psychology, Bekhterev is not squeamish about philistine language, which hardly makes Freud's term any clearer. How did this inhibited reflex "oppress" the personality, shackle it? Why is the wept out sorrow the discharge of an *inhibited* reflex? What if a person weeps in the very moment of sorrow? Finally, elsewhere it is claimed that thought is an inhibited reflex, that concentration is connected with the inhibition of a nervous current and is accompanied by conscious phenomena. Oh salutary inhibition! It explains conscious phenomena in one chapter and unconscious ones in the next!

All this clearly indicates the theme with which we started this section: in the problem of the unconscious one must distinguish between a methodological and an empirical problem, i.e., between a psychological problem and *the* problem for psychology. The uncritical combination of both problems leads to a gross distortion of the whole matter. The symposium on the unconscious showed fundamental solution of this matter transcends the boundaries of empirical psychology and is directly tied to general philosophical convictions. Whether we accept with Brentano that the unconscious does not exist, or with Münsterberg that it simply physiology, or with Schubert-Soldern that it is an epistemologically indispensable category, or with Freud that it is sexual—in all these cases our argumentation and conclusions transcend the boundaries of empirical psychology.

Among the Russian authors it is Dale who emphasizes the epistemological motives which led to the formation of the concept of the unconscious. In his opinion it is precisely the attempt to defend the independence of psychology as an explanatory science against the usurpation of physiological methods and principles that is the basis of this concept. The demand to explain the mental from the mental, and not from the physical, that psychology in the analysis and description of the facts should stay itself, within its own boundaries, even if this implied that one had to enter the path of broad hypotheses—this is what gave rise to the concept of the unconscious. Dale observes that psychological constructions or *hypotheses* are no more than the theoretical continuation of the description of *homogeneous* phenomena in one and the same independent system of reality. The tasks of psychology and theoretical-epistemological demands require that it fight the usurpationist attempts of physiology by means of the unconscious. Mental life proceeds with interruptions, it is full of gaps. What happens with consciousness during sleep, with reminiscences that we do not now recollect, with ideas of which we are not consciously aware at the moment? In order to explain the mental from the mental, in order not to turn to another domain of phenomena—physiology— to fill the pauses, gaps and blanks in mental life, we must assume that they continue to exist in a special form: as the unconscious *mental.* Stern [1919, pp. 241–243] as well develops such a conception of the unconscious as both an essential assumption and a hypothetical continuation and complement to mental experience.

Dale distinguishes two aspects of the problem: the factual and the hypothetical or methodological, which determines the epistemological or methodological value of the category of the unconscious for psychology. Its task is to clarify the meaning of this concept, the domain of phenomena it covers, and its role for psychology as an explanatory science. Following Jerusalem, for the author it is first of all a category or a way of thinking which is indispensable in the explanation of mental life. Apart from that, it is also a specific area of phenomena. He is completely right in saying that the unconscious is a concept created on the basis of indisputable mental experience and its necessary hypothetical completion. Hence the very complex nature of each statement operating with this concept: in *each* statement one must distinguish what comes from the data of indisputable mental experience, what comes from the hypothetical completion, and what is the degree of reliability of both. In the critical works examined above, the two things, both sides of the problem, have been mixed up: hypothesis and fact, principle and empirical observation, fiction and law, construction and generalization—it is all lumped together.

Most important of all is the fact that the main question was left out of consideration. Lenz and Luria assure Freud that psychoanalysis is a physiological system. But Freud himself belongs to the opponents of a physiological conception of the unconscious. Dale is completely right in saying that this question of the psychological or physiological nature of the unconscious is the *primary,* most important phase of the whole problem. Before we describe and classify the phenomena of the unconscious for psychological purposes, we must know whether we are operating with something physiological or with something mental. We must prove that the unconscious in fact is a mental reality. In other words, before we turn to the solution of the problem of the unconscious as a psychological problem, we must first solve it as *the* problem for psychology.

8

The need for a fundamental elaboration of the concepts of the general science—this algebra of the particular sciences—and its role for the particular sciences is even more obvious when we borrow from the area of *other* sciences. Here, on the one hand, it would seem that we have the best conditions for transferring results from one science into the system of another one, because the reliability, clarity and the degree to which the borrowed thesis or law have been fundamentally elaborated are usually much higher than in the cases we have described. We may, for example, introduce into the system of psychological explanation a law established in physiology or embryology, a biological principle, an anatomical hypothesis, an ethnological example, a historical classification etc. The theses and constructions of these highly developed, firmly grounded sciences are, of course, methodologically elaborated in an infinitely more precise way than the theses of a psychological school which by means of newly created and not yet systematized concepts is developing completely new areas (for example, Freud's school, which does not yet know itself). In this case we borrow a more elaborated product, we operate with better-defined, exact, and clear unities; the danger of error has diminished, the likelihood of success has increased.

On the other hand, as the borrowing here comes from other sciences, the material turns out to be more foreign, methodologically heterogeneous, and the conditions for appropriating it become more difficult. This fact, that the conditions are both easier and more difficult compared with what we examined above, provides us with an essential method of variation in theoretical analysis which takes the place of real variation in the experiment.

Let us dwell upon a fact which at first sight seems highly paradoxical and which is therefore very suitable for analysis. Reflexology, which in all areas finds such wonderful coincidences of its data with the data of subjective analysis and which wishes to build its system on the foundation of the exact natural sciences, is, very surprisingly, forced to protest precisely against the transfer of natural scientific laws into psychology.

After studying the method of genetic reflexology, Shchelovanov—with an indisputable thoroughness quite unexpected for his school—rejected the imitation of the natural sciences in the form of a transfer of its basic methods into subjective psychology. Their application in the natural sciences has produced tremendous results, but they are of little value for the elaboration of the problems of subjective psychology.* Herbart and Fechner mechanically transferred mathematical analysis and Wundt the physiological experiment into psychology. Preyer raised the problem of psychogenesis by analogy with biology and then Hall and others borrowed the Müller-Haeckel principle from biology and applied it in an uncontrolled way not only as a methodological principle, but also as a principle for the explanation of the "mental development" of the child. It would seem, says the author, that we cannot object to the application of well-tried and fruitful methods. But their use is only possible when the problem is correctly stated and the method corresponds to the nature of the object under study. Otherwise one only gets the illusion of science (the characteristic example is Russian reflexology). The veil of natural science which was, according to Petzoldt, thrown over the most backward metaphysics, saved neither Herbart nor Wundt: neither the mathematical formulas nor the precision equipment saved an imprecisely stated problem from failure.

We are reminded of Münsterberg and his remark about the last decimal point given in the answer to an incorrectly stated question. In biology, clarifies the author, the biogenetic law is a theoretical generalization of masses of facts, but its application in psychology is the result of superficial speculation, exclusively based upon an analogy between different domains of facts (Does not reflexology do the same? Without investigation of its own it borrows, using similar speculations, the readymade models for its own constructions from the living and the dead— from Einstein and from Freud). And then, to crown this pyramid of mistakes, the principle is not applied as a working hypothesis, but as an established theory, as if it were scientifically established as an explanatory principle for the given area of facts.

We will not deal with this matter, as does the author of this opinion, in great detail. There is abundant, including Russian, literature on it. We will examine it to illustrate the fact that many questions which have been incorrectly stated by psychology acquire the outward appearance of science due to borrowings from the natural sciences. As a result of his methodological analysis, Shchelovanov comes to the conclusion that the genetic method is in principle impossible in empirical psychology and that because of this the relations between psychology and biology become changed. But why was the problem of development stated incorrectly in child psychology, which led to a tremendous and useless expenditure of effort? In Shchelovanov's opinion, child psychology can yield nothing other than what is already contained in general psychology. But general psychology as a unified system does not exist, and these theoretical contradictions make a child psychology impossible. In a very disguised form, imperceptible to the investigator himself, the theoretical presuppositions fully determine the whole method of processing the empirical data. And the facts gathered in observation, too, are interpreted in accordance with the theory which this or that author holds. Here is the best refutation of the sham natural-science empiricism. Thanks to this, it is impossible to transfer facts from one theory to another. It would seem that a fact is always a fact, that one and the same subject matter—the child—and one and the same method—objective observation—albeit combined with different objectives and starting points, allow us to transfer facts from psychology to reflexology. The author is mistaken in only two respects.

His first mistake resides in the assumption that child psychology got its positive results only by applying general biological, but not psychological principles, as in the theory of play developed by Groos [1899]. In reality, this is one of the best examples not of borrowing, but of a purely psychological, comparative-objective study. It is methodologically impeccable and transparent, internally consistent from the first collection and description of the facts to the final theoretical generalizations. Groos gave biology a theory of play created with a psychological method. He did not take it from biology; he did not solve his problem in the light of biology, i.e., he did not set himself general psychological goals as well. Thus, exactly the opposite is correct: child psychology obtained valuable theoretical results precisely when it did not borrow, but went its own way. The author himself is constantly arguing against borrowing. Hall, who borrowed from Haeckel, gave psychology a number of curious topics and far-fetched senseless analogies, but Groos, who went his own way, gave much to biology—not less than Haeckel's law. Let me also remind you of Stern's theory of language, Bühler's and Koffka's theory of children's thinking, Bühler's theory of developmental levels, Thorndike's theory of training: these are all psychological theories of the purest water. Hence the mistaken conclusion: the role of child psychology cannot be reduced, of course, to the gathering of factual data and their preliminary classification, i.e., to the preparatory work. But the role of the logical principles developed by Shchelovanov and Bekhterev can and must precisely be reduced to this. After all, the new discipline has no idea of childhood, no conception of development, no research goal, i.e., it does not state the problem of child behavior and personality, but only disposes of the principle of objective observation, i.e., a good technical rule. However, using this weapon nobody has drawn out any great truths.

The author's second mistake is connected with this. The lack of understanding of the positive value of psychology and the underestimation of its role results from the most important and methodologically childish idea that one can study only what is given in immediate experience. His whole "methodological" theory is built upon a single syllogism: (1) psychology studies consciousness; (2) given in immediate experience is the consciousness of the adult; "the empirical study of the phylogenetic and ontogenetic development of consciousness is impossible"; (3) therefore, child psychology is impossible.

But it is a gross mistake to suppose that science can only study what is given in immediate experience. How does the psychologist study the unconscious; the historian and the geologist, the past; the physicist-optician, invisible beams, and the philologist-ancient languages? The study of traces, influences, the method of interpretation and reconstruction, the method of critique and the finding of meaning have been no less fruitful than the method of direct "empirical" observation. Ivanovsky used precisely the example of psychology to explain this for the methodology of science. Even in the experimental sciences the role of immediate experience becomes smaller and smaller. Planck says that the unification of the whole system of theoretical physics is reached due to the liberation from anthropomorphic elements, in particular from specific sense perceptions. Planck [1919/1970, p. 118] remarks that in the theory of light and in the theory of radiant energy in general, physics works with such methods that

> the human eye is totally excluded, it plays the role of an accidental, admittedly highly sensitive but very limited reagent; for it only perceives the light beams within a small area of the spectrum which hardly attains the breadth of one octave. For the rest of the spectrum the place of the eye is taken by other perceiving and measuring instruments, such as, for example, the wave detector, the thermo-element, the bolometer, the radiometer, the photographic plate, the ionization chamber. The separation of the basic physical concept from the

specific sensory sensation was accomplished, therefore, in exactly the same way as in mechanics where the concept of force has long since lost its original link with muscular sensations.

Thus, physics studies precisely what cannot be seen with the eye. For if we, like the author, agree with Stern [1914, p. 7] that childhood is for us "a paradise lost forever," that for us adults it is impossible to "fully penetrate in the special properties and structure of the child's mind" as it is not given in direct experience, we must admit that the light beams which cannot be directly perceived by the eye are a paradise lost forever as well, the Spanish inquisition a hell lost forever, etc., etc. But the whole point is that scientific knowledge and immediate perception do not coincide at all. We can neither experience the child's impressions, nor witness the French revolution, but the child who experiences his paradise with all directness and the contemporary who saw the major episodes of the revolution with his own eyes are, despite that, farther from the scientific knowledge of these facts than we are. Not only the humanities, but the natural sciences as well, build their concepts in principle independently from immediate experience. We are reminded of Engels' words about the ants and the limitations of our eye.

How do the sciences proceed in the study of what is not immediately given? Generally speaking, they reconstruct it, they re-create the subject of study through the method of interpreting its traces or influences, i.e., indirectly. Thus, the historian interprets traces—documents, memoirs, newspapers, etc.—and nevertheless history is a science about the past, reconstructed by its traces, and not a science about the traces of the past, it is about the revolution and not about documents of the revolution. The same is true for child psychology. Is childhood, the child's mind, really inaccessible for us, does it not leave any traces, does it not manifest or reveal itself? It is just a matter of how to interpret these traces, by what method. Can they be interpreted by analogy with the traces of the adult? It is, therefore, a matter of finding the right interpretation and not of completely refraining from any interpretation. After all, historians too are familiar with more than one erroneous construct based upon genuine documents which were falsely interpreted. What conclusion follows from this? Is it really that history is "a paradise forever lost"? But the same logic that calls child psychology a paradise lost would compel us to say this about history as well. And if the historian, or the geologist, or the physicist were to argue like the reflexologist, they would say: as we cannot immediately experience the past of mankind and the earth (the child's mind) and can only immediately experience the present (the adult's consciousness)—which is why many falsely interpret the past by analogy with the present or as a small present (the child as a small adult)—history and geology are subjective, impossible. The only thing possible is a history of the present (the psychology of the adult person). The history of the past can only be studied as the science of the traces of the past, of the documents etc. as such, and not of the past as such (through the methods of studying reflexes without any attempt at interpreting them).

This dogma—of immediate experience as the single source and natural boundary of scientific knowledge—in principle makes or breaks the whole theory of subjective and objective methods. Vvedensky and Bekhterev grow from a single root: both hold that science can only study what is given in self-observation, i.e., in the immediate perception of the psychological, Some rely on the mental eye and build a whole science in conformity with its properties and the boundaries of its action. Others do not rely on it and only wish to study what can be seen with the real eye. This is why I say that reflexology, methodologically speaking, is built entirely according to the principle that history should be defined as the science of the documents of the past. Due to the many fruitful principles of the natural sciences, reflexology proved to be a highly progressive current in psychology, but as a theory of method it is deeply reactionary, because it leads us back to the naive sensualistic prejudice that we can only study what can be perceived and to the extent we perceive it.

Just as physics is liberating itself from anthropomorphic elements, i.e., from specific sensory sensations and is proceeding with the eye fully excluded, so psychology must work with the concept of the mental: direct self-observation must be excluded like muscular sensation in mechanics and visual sensation in optics. The subjectivists believe that they refuted the objective method when they showed that genetically speaking the concepts of behavior contain a grain of self-observation—cf. Chelpanov (1925), Kravkov (1922), Portugalov (1925). But the genetic origin of a concept says nothing about its logical nature: genetically, the concept of force in mechanics also goes back to muscular sensation.

The problem of self-observation is a problem of technique and not of principle. It is an instrument amidst a number of other instruments, as the eye is for physicists. We must use it to the extent that it is useful, but there is no need to pronounce judgments of principle about it—e.g., about the limitations of the knowledge obtained with it, its reliability, or the nature of the knowledge determined by it. Engels demonstrated how little the natural construction of the eye determines the boundaries of our knowledge of the phenomena of light. Planck says the same on behalf of contemporary physics. To separate the fundamental psychological concept from the specific sensory perception is psychology's next task. This sensation itself, self-observation itself, must be explained (like the eye) from the postulates, methods, and universal principles of psychology. It must become one of psychology's particular problems.

When we accept this, the question of the nature of interpretation, i.e., the indirect method, arises. Usually it is said that history interprets the traces of the past, whereas physics observes the invisible as directly as the eye does by means of its instruments. The instruments are the extended organs of the researcher. After all, the microscope, telescope, telephone etc. make the invisible visible and the subject of immediate experience. Physics does not interpret, but sees.

But this opinion is false. The methodology of the scientific instrument has long since clarified a new role for the instrument which is not always obvious. Even the thermometer may serve as an example of the introduction of a fundamentally new principle into the method of science through the use of an instrument, On the thermometer we read the temperature. It does not strengthen or extend the sensation of heat as the microscope extends the eye; rather, it totally liberates us from sensation when studying heat. One who is unable to sense heat or cold may still use the thermometer, whereas a blind person cannot use a microscope. The use of a thermometer is a perfect model of the indirect method. After all, we do not study what we see (as with the microscope)—the rising of the mercury, the expansion of the alcohol—but we study heat and its changes, which are indicated by the mercury or alcohol. We interpret the indications of the thermometer, we reconstruct the phenomenon under study by its traces, by its influence upon the expansion of a substance. All the instruments Planck speaks of as means to study the invisible are constructed in this way. To interpret, consequently, means to re-create a phenomenon from its traces and influences relying upon regularities established before (in the present case—the law of the extension of solids, liquids, and gases during heating). There is no fundamental difference whatsoever between the use of a thermometer on the one hand and interpretation in history, psychology, etc. on the other. The same holds true for any science: it is not dependent upon sensory perception.

Stumpf mentions the blind mathematician Saunderson who wrote a textbook of geometry; Shcherbina (1908) relates that his blindness did not prevent him from explaining optics to sighted people. And, indeed, all instruments mentioned by Planck can be adapted for the blind, just like the watches, thermometers, and books for the blind that already exist, so that a blind person might occupy himself with optics as well. It is a matter of technique, not of principle.

Kornilov (1922) beautifully demonstrated that (1) disagreement about the procedural aspect of the design of experiments makes for conflicts which lead to the formation of different currents in psychology, just as the different philosophies about the chronoscope—which resulted from the question as to in which room this apparatus should be placed during the experiments—determined the question of the whole method and system of psychology and divided Wundt's school from Külpe's; and (2) the experimental method introduced nothing new into psychology. For Wundt it is a correction of self-observation. For Ach the data of self-observation can only be checked against other data of self-observation, as if the sensation of heat can be checked only against other sensations. For Deichler the quantitative estimations give a measure for the correctness of introspection. In sum, experiment does not extend our knowledge, it checks it. Psychology does not yet have a methodology of its equipment and has not yet raised the question of an apparatus which would—like the thermometer—liberate us from introspection rather than check or amplify it. The philosophy of the chronoscope is a more difficult matter than its technique. But about the indirect method in psychology we will come to speak more than once.

Zelenyj (1923) is right in pointing out that in Russia the word "method" means two different things: (1) the research methods, the technology of the experiment; and (2) the epistemological method, or methodology, which determines the research goal, the place of the science, and its nature. In psychology the epistemological method is subjective, although the research methods may be partially objective. In physiology the epistemological method is objective, although the research methods may be partially subjective as in the physiology of the sense organs. Let us add that the experiment reformed the research methods, but not the epistemological method. For this reason, he says that the psychological method can only have the value of a diagnostic device in the natural sciences.

This question is crucial for all methodological and concrete problems of psychology. For psychology the need to fundamentally transcend the boundaries of immediate experience is a matter of life and death. The demarcation, separation of the scientific concept from the specific perception, can take place only on the basis of the indirect method. The reply that the indirect method is inferior to the direct one is in scientific terms utterly false. Precisely because it does not shed light upon the plentitude of experience, but only on one aspect, it accomplishes scientific work: it isolates, analyzes, separates, abstracts a single feature. After all, in immediate experience as well we isolate the part that is the subject of our observation. Anyone who deplores the fact that we do not share the ant's immediate experience of chemical beams is beyond help, says Engels, for on the other hand we know the nature of these beams better than ants do. The task of science is not to reduce everything to experience. If that were the case it would suffice to replace science with the registration of our perceptions. Psychology's real problem resides also in the fact that our immediate experience is limited, because the whole mind is built like an instrument which selects and isolates certain aspects of phenomena. An eye that would see everything, would for this very reason see nothing. A consciousness that was aware of everything would be aware of nothing, and knowledge of the self, were it aware of everything, would be aware of nothing. Our knowledge is confined between two thresholds, we see but a tiny part of the world. Our senses give us the world in the excerpts, extracts that are important for us. And in between the thresholds it is again not the whole variety of changes which is registered, and new thresholds exist. Consciousness follows nature in a saltatory fashion as it were, with blanks and gaps. The mind selects the stable points of reality amidst the universal movement. It provides islands of safety in the Heraclitean stream. It is an organ of selection, a sieve filtering the world and changing it so that it becomes possible to act. In this resides its positive role—not in reflection (the non-mental reflects as well; the thermometer is more precise than sensation), but in the fact that it does not always reflect correctly, i.e., subjectively distorts reality to the advantage of the organism.

If we were to see everything (i.e,, if there were no absolute thresholds) including all changes that constantly take place (i.e., if no relative thresholds existed), we would be confronted with chaos (remember how many objects a microscope reveals in a drop of water). What would be a glass of water? And what a river? A pond reflects everything; a stone reacts in principle to everything. But these reactions equal the stimulation: *causa aequat effectum*. The reaction of the organism is "richer": it is not like an effect, it expends potential forces, it selects stimuli. Red, blue, loud, sour—it is a world cut into portions. Psychology's task is to clarify the advantage of the fact that the eye does not perceive many of the things known to optics. From the lower forms of reactions to the higher ones there leads, as it were, the narrowing opening of a funnel.

It would be a mistake to think that we do not see what is for us biologically useless. Would it really be useless to see microbes? The sense organs show clear traces of the fact that they are in the first place organs of selection. Taste is obviously a selection organ for digestion, smell is part of the respiratory process. Like the customs checkpoints at the border, they test the stimuli coming from outside. Each organ takes the world *cum grano salis*—with a coefficient of specification, as Hegel says, [and] with an indication of the relation, where the quality of one object determines the intensity and character of the quantitative influence of another quality. For this reason there is a complete analogy between the selection of the eye and the further selection of the instrument: both are organs of selection (accomplish what we accomplish in the experiment). So that the fact that scientific knowledge transcends the boundaries of perception is rooted in the psychological essence of knowledge itself.

From this it follows that as methods for judging scientific truth, direct evidence and analogy are in principle completely identical. Both must be subjected to critical examination; both can deceive and tell the truth. The direct evidence that the sun turns around the earth deceives us; the analogy upon which spectral analysis is built, leads to the truth. On these grounds some have rightly defended the legitimacy of analogy as a basic method of zoopsychology. This is fully acceptable, one must only point out the conditions under which the analogy will be correct. So far the analogy in zoopsychology has led to anecdotes and curious incidents, because it was observed where it actually cannot exist. It can, however, also lead to spectral analysis. That is why methodologically speaking the situation in physics and psychology is in principle the same. The difference is one of degree.

The mental sequence we experience is a fragment: where do all the elements of mental life disappear and where do they come from? We are compelled to continue the known sequence with a hypothetical one. It was precisely in this sense that Høffding [1908, p. 92/114] introduced this concept which corresponds with the concept of potential energy in physics. This is why Leibnitz introduced the infinitely small elements of consciousness [cf. Høffding, 1908, p. 108].

> We are forced to continue the life of consciousness into the unconscious in order not to fall into absurdities [ibid., p. 286].

However, for Høffding (ibid., p. 117) "the unconscious is a boundary concept in science" and at this boundary we may "weigh the possibilities" through a hypothesis, but

> a real extension of our factual knowledge is impossible . . . . Compared to the physical world, we experience the mental world as a fragment; only through a hypothesis can we supplement it.

But even this respect for the boundary of science seems to other authors insufficient. About the unconscious it is only allowed to say that it exists. By its very definition it is not an object for experimental verification. To argue its existence by means of observations, as Høffding attempts, is illegitimate. This word has two meanings, there are two types of unconscious which we must not mix up—the debate is about a twofold subject: about the hypothesis and about the facts that can be observed.

One more step in this direction, and we return to where we started: to the difficulty that compelled us to hypothesize an unconscious.

We can see that psychology finds itself here in a tragicomic situation: I want to, but I cannot. It is forced to accept the unconscious so as not to fall into absurdities. But accepting it, it falls into even greater absurdities and runs back in horror. It is like a man who, running from a wild animal and into an even greater danger, runs back to the wild animal, the lesser danger—but does it really make any difference from what he dies? Wundt views in this theory an echo of the mystical philosophy of nature [Naturphilosophie] of the early 19th century. With him Lange (1914, p. 251) accepts that the unconscious mind is an intrinsically contradictory concept. The unconscious must be explained physically and chemically and not psychologically, else we allow "mystical agents," "arbitrary constructions that can never be verified," to enter science.

Thus, we are back to Høffding: there is a physico-chemical sequence, which in some fragmentary points is suddenly *ex nihilo* accompanied by a mental sequence. Please, be good enough to understand and scientifically interpret the "fragment." What does this debate mean for the methodologist? We must psychologically transcend the boundary of immediately perceived consciousness and continue it, but in such a way as to separate the concept from sensation. Psychology as the science of consciousness is in principle impossible. As the science of the unconscious mind it is doubly impossible. It would seem that there is no way out, no solution for this quadrature of the circle. But physics finds itself in exactly the same position. Admittedly, the physical sequence extends further than the mental one, but this sequence is not infinite and without gaps either. It was science that made it in principle continuous and infinite and not immediate experience. It extended this experience by excluding the eye. This is also psychology's task.

Hence, interpretation is not only a bitter necessity for psychology, but also a liberating and essentially most fruitful method of knowledge, a *salto vitale*, which for bad jumpers turns into a *salto mortale*. Psychology must develop its philosophy of equipment, just as physics has its philosophy of the thermometer. In practice both parties in psychology have recourse to interpretation: the subjectivist has in the end the words of the subject, i.e., his behavior and mind are interpreted behavior. The objectivist will inevitably interpret as well. The very concept of reaction implies the necessity of interpretation, of sense, connection, relation. Indeed, *actio* and *reactio* are concepts that are originally mechanistic—one must observe both and deduce a law. But in psychology and physiology the reaction is not equal to the stimulus. It has a sense, a goal, i.e., it fulfills a certain function in the larger whole. It is qualitatively connected with its stimulus. And this sense of the reaction as a function of the whole, this quality of the interrelation, is not given in experience, but found by inference. To put it more easily and generally: when we study behavior as a system of reactions, we do not study the behavioral acts in themselves (by the organs), but in their relation to other acts—to stimuli. But the relation and the quality of the relation, its sense, are never the subject of immediate perception, let alone the relation between two heterogeneous sequences—between stimuli and reactions. The following is extremely important: the reaction is an answer. An answer can only be studied according to the quality of its relation with the question, for this is the sense of answer which is not found in perception but in interpretation.

This is the way everybody proceeds.

Bekhterev distinguishes the creative reflex. A problem is the stimulus, and creativity is the response reaction or a symbolic reflex. But the concepts of creativity and symbol are semantic concepts, not experiential ones: a reflex is creative when it stands in such a relation to a stimulus that it creates something new; it is symbolic when it replaces another reflex. But we cannot see the symbolic or creative nature of a reflex.

Pavlov distinguishes the reflexes of freedom and purpose, the food reflex and the defense reflex. But neither freedom nor purpose can be seen, nor do they have an organ like, for example, the organs for nutrition; nor are they functions. They consist of the same movements as the other ones. Defense, freedom, and purpose—they are the meanings of these reflexes.

Kornilov distinguishes emotional reactions, selective, associative reactions, the reaction of recognition, etc. It is again a classification according to their meaning, i.e., on the basis of the interpretation of the relation between stimulus and response.

Watson, accepting similar distinctions based on meaning, openly says that nowadays the psychologist of behavior arrives by sheer logic at the conclusion that there is a hidden process of thinking. By this he is becoming conscious of his method and brilliantly refutes Titchener, who defended the thesis that the psychologist of behavior, exactly because of being a psychologist of behavior, cannot accept the existence of a process of thinking when he is not in the situation to observe it immediately and must use introspection to reveal thinking. Watson demonstrated that he in principle isolates the concept of thinking from its perception in introspection, just like the thermometer emancipates us from sensation when we develop the concept of heat. That is why he [1926, p. 301] emphasizes:

> If we ever succeed in scientifically studying the intimate nature of thought . . . then we will owe this to a considerable extent to the scientific apparatus.

However even now the psychologist

> is not in such a deplorable situation: physiologists as well are often satisfied with the observation of the end results and utilize logic. . . . The adherent of the psychology of behavior feels that with respect to thinking he must keep to exactly the same position [ibid., p. 302].

Meaning as well is for Watson an experimental problem. We find it in what is given to us through thinking.

Thorndike (1925) distinguishes the reactions of feeling, conclusion, mood, and cunning. Again [we are dealing with] interpretation.

The whole matter is simply *how* to interpret—by analogy with one's introspection, biological functions, etc. That is why Koffka [1925, pp. 10/13] is right when he states: There is no objective criterion for consciousness, we do not know whether an action has consciousness or not, but this does not make us unhappy at all. However, behavior is such that the consciousness belonging to it, if it exists at all, must have such and such a structure. Therefore behavior must be explained in the same way as consciousness. Or in other words, put paradoxically: if everybody had only those reactions which can be observed by all others, nobody could observe anything, i.e., scientific observation is based upon transcending the boundaries of the visible and upon a search for its meaning which cannot be observed. He is right. He was right [Koffka, 1924, pp. 152/160] when he claimed that behaviorism is bound to be fruitless when it will study only the observable, when its ideal is to know the direction and speed of the movements of each limb, the secretion of each gland, resulting from a fixed stimulation. Its area would then be restricted to the physiology of the muscles and the glands. The description "this animal is running away from some danger," however insufficient it may be, is yet a thousand times more characteristic for the animal's behavior than a formula giving us the movements of all its legs with their varying speeds, the curves of breath, pulse, and so forth.

Köhler (1917) demonstrated in practice how we may prove the presence of thinking in apes without any introspection and even study the course and structure of this process through the method of the interpretation of objective reactions. Kornilov (1922) demonstrated how we may measure the energetic budget of different thought operations using the indirect method: the dynamoscope is used by him as a thermometer. Wundt's mistake resided in the *mechanical* application of equipment and the mathematical method to check and correct. He did not use them to extend introspection, to liberate himself from it, but to tie himself to it. In most of Wundt's investigations introspection was essentially superfluous. It was only necessary to single out the unsuccessful experiments. In principle it is totally unnecessary in Kornilov's theory. But psychology must still create its thermometer. Kornilov's research indicates the path.

We may summarize the conclusions from our investigation of the narrow sensualist dogma by again referring to Engels' words about the activity of the eye which in combination with thinking helps us to discover that ants see what is invisible to us.

Psychology has too long striven for experience instead of knowledge. In the present example it preferred to share with the ants their visual experience of the sensation of chemical beams rather than to understand their vision scientifically.

As to the methodological spine that is supporting them there are two scientific systems. Methodology is always like the backbone, the skeleton in the animal's organism. Very primitive animals, like the snail and the tortoise, carry their skeleton on the outside and they can, like an oyster, be separated from their skeleton. What is left is a poorly differentiated fleshy part. Higher animals carry their skeleton inside and make it into the internal support, the bone of each of their movements. In psychology as well we must distinguish lower and higher types of methodological organization.

This is the best refutation of the sham empiricism of the natural sciences. It turns out that nothing can be transposed from one theory to another. It would seem that a fact is always a fact. Despite the different points of departure and the different aims one and the same object (a child) and one and the same method (objective observation) should make it possible to transpose the facts of psychology to reflexology. The difference would only be in the interpretation of the same facts. In the end the systems of Ptolemy and Copernicus rested upon the same facts as well. [But] It turns out that facts obtained by means of different principles of knowledge are *different* facts.

Thus, the debate about the application of the biogenetic principle in psychology is not a debate about facts. The facts are indisputable and there are two groups of them: the recapitulation of the stages the organism goes through in the development of its structure as established by natural science and the indisputable traits of similarity between the phylo- and ontogenesis of the mind. It is particularly important that neither is there any debate about the latter group. Koffka [1925, pp. 32], who contests this theory and subjects it to a methodological analysis, resolutely declares that the analogies, from which this false theory proceeds, exist beyond any doubt. The debate concerns the *meaning* of these analogies and it turns out that it cannot be decided without analyzing the principles of child psychology, without having a general idea of childhood, a conception of the meaning and the biological sense of childhood, a certain theory of child development. It is quite easy to find analogies. The question is *how* to search for them. Similar analogies may be found in the behavior of adults as well.

Two typical mistakes are possible here: one is made by Hall. Thorndike and Groos have brilliantly exposed it in critical analyses. The latter [Groos, 1904/1921, p. 7] justly claims that the purpose of any comparison and the task of comparative science is not only to distinguish similar traits, but even more to search for the differences within the similarity. Comparative psychology, consequently, must not merely understand man as an animal, but much more as a non-animal.

The straightforward application of the principle led to a ubiquitous search for similarity. A correct method and reliably established facts led to monstrously strained interpretations and distorted facts when applied uncritically. Children's games have indeed traditionally preserved many echoes of the remote past (the play with bows, round dances). For Hall this is the repetition and expression in innocent form of the animal and pre-historic stages of development.

Groos considers this to show a remarkable lack of critical judgment. The fear of cats and dogs would be a remnant of the time when these animals were still wild. Water would attract children because we developed from aquatic animals. The automatic movements of the infant's arms would be a remnant of the movements of our ancestors who swam in the water, etc.

The mistake resides, consequently, in the interpretation of the child's whole behavior as a recapitulation and in the absence of any principle to verify the analogy and to select the facts which must and must not be interpreted. It is precisely the play of animals which cannot be explained in this way. "Can Hall's theory explain the play of the young tiger with its victim?"—asks Groos [1904/1921, p. 73]. It is clear that this play cannot be understood as a recapitulation of past phylogenetic development. It foreshadows the future activity of the tiger and not a repetition of his past development. It must be explained and understood in relation to the tiger's future, in the light of which it gets its meaning, and not in the light of the past of his species. The past of the species comes out in a *totally* different sense: through the individual's *future* which it predetermines, but not directly and not in the sense of a repetition.

What are the facts? This quasi-biological theory appears to be untenable precisely in *biological* terms, precisely in comparison with the nearest homogeneous analogue in the *series of homogeneous phenomena* in other stages of evolution. When we compare the play of a child with the play of a tiger, i.e., a higher mammal, and consider not only the similarity, but the *difference* as well, we will lay bare *their common* biological essence which resides exactly in their *difference* (the tiger plays the chase of tigers; the child that he is a grown-up; both practice necessary functions for their life to come—Groos' theory). But despite all the seeming similarity in the comparison of *heterogeneous* phenomena (play with water—aquatic life of the amphibian-man) the theory is biologically meaningless.

Thorndike [1906] adds to this devastating argument a remark about the different order of the *same biological principles* in onto and phylogenesis. Thus, consciousness appears very early in ontogenesis and very late in phylogenesis. The sexual drive, on the other hand, appears very early in phylogenesis and very late in ontogenesis. Stern [1927, pp. 266–267], using similar considerations, criticizes the same theory in its application to play.

Blonsky (1921) makes another kind of mistake. He defends—and very convincingly—this law for embryonic development from the viewpoint of biomechanics and shows that it would be miraculous if it did not exist. The author points out the hypothetical nature of the considerations ("not very conclusive") leading to this contention ("it may be like this"), i.e., he gives arguments for the methodological possibility of a working hypothesis, but then, instead of proceeding to the investigation and verification of the hypothesis, follows in Hall's footsteps and begins to *explain* the child's behavior on the basis of very intelligible analogies: he does not view the climbing of trees by children as a recapitulation of the life of apes, but of primitive people who lived amidst rocks and ice; the tearing off of wallpaper is an atavism of the tearing off of the bark of trees etc. What is most remarkable of all is that the error leads Blonsky to the same conclusion as Hall: to the *negation of play.* Groos and Stern have shown that exactly where it is easiest to find analogies between onto and phylogenesis is this theory untenable. And neither does Blonsky, as if illustrating the irresistible force of the methodological laws of scientific knowledge, search for new terms. He sees no need to attach a "new term" (play) to the child's activity. This means that on his methodological path he first lost its *meaning* and then—

with creditable consistency—refrained from the term that expresses this meaning. Indeed, if the activity, the child's behavior, is an atavism, then the term "play" is out of place. This activity has nothing in common with the play of the tiger as Groos demonstrated. And we must translate Blonsky's declaration "I don't like this term" in methodological terms as "I lost the understanding and meaning of this concept."

Only in this way, by following each principle to its ultimate conclusions, by taking each concept in the extreme form toward which it strives, by investigating each line of thinking to the very end, at times completing it for the author, can we determine the methodological nature of the phenomenon under investigation. That is why a concept that is used deliberately, not blindly, in the science for which it was created, where it originated, developed, and was carried to its ultimate expression, *is blind*, leads nowhere when transposed to another science. Such *blind* transpositions of the biogenetic principle, the experiment, the mathematical method from the natural sciences, created the appearance of science in psychology which in reality concealed a total impotence in the face of the studied facts.

But to complete the sketch of the circle described by the meaning of a principle introduced into a science in this way, we will follow its further fate. The matter does not end with the detection of the fruitlessness of the principle, its critique, the pointing out of curious and strained interpretations at which schoolboys poke their finger. In other words, the history of the principle does not end with its simple expulsion from the area that does not belong to it, with its simple rejection. After all, we remember that the foreign principle penetrated into our science via a *bridge of facts*, via really existing analogues. Nobody has denied this. While this principle became strengthened and reigned, the number of facts upon which its false power rested increased. They were partially false and partially correct. In its turn the critique of these facts, the critique of the principle itself, draws still other new facts into the scope of the science. The matter is not confined to the facts: the critique must provide an explanation for the colliding facts. The theories assimilate each other and on this basis the *regeneration* of a new principle takes place.

Under the pressure of the facts and foreign theories, the newcomer changes its face. The same happened with the biogenetic principle. It was reborn and in psychology it figures in two forms (a sign that the process of regeneration is not yet finished): (1) as a theory of utility, defended by neo-Darwinism and the school of Thorndike, which finds that individual and species are subject to the same laws—hence a number of coincidences, but also a number of non-coincidences. Not everything that is useful for the species in its early stage is useful for the individual as well; (2) as a theory of synchronization, defended in psychology by Koffka and the school of Dewey, in the philosophy of history by Spengler. It is a theory which says that all developmental processes have some general stages, some successive forms, in common— from elementary to more complex and from lower to higher levels.

Far be it from us to consider any of these conclusions the right one. We are in general still far from a fundamental examination of the question. For us it is important to follow the dynamics of the spontaneous, blind reaction of a scientific body to a foreign, inserted object. It is important for us to trace the forms of scientific inflammation relative to the kind of infection in order to proceed from pathology to the norm and to clarify the normal functions of the different composite parts—the organs of science. This is the purpose and meaning of our analyses, which seemingly sidetrack us, but although we make no mention of it we continually hold to the comparison (prompted by Spinoza) of the psychology of our days to a severely diseased person. If we wish to formulate the aim of our last digression from this viewpoint, the positive conclusion which we have reached, the result of the analysis, we must determine it as follows: previously—on the basis of the analysis of the unconscious—we studied the nature, the action, the manner of the spreading of the infection, the penetration of the foreign idea after the facts, its lording over the organism, the disturbance of the organism's functions; now—on the basis of the analysis of the biogenesis—we were able to study the counter-action of the organism, its struggle with the infection, the dynamic tendency to resolve, throw out, neutralize, assimilate, degenerate the foreign body, to mobilize forces against the contagion. We studied—to stick to medical terms—the elaboration of antibodies and the development of immunity. What remains is the third and final step: to distinguish the phenomena of the disease from the reactions, the healthy from the diseased, the processes of the infection from the recovery. This we will do in the analysis of scientific terminology in the third and final digression. After that we will directly proceed to the statement of a diagnosis and prognosis for our patient—to the nature, meaning and outcome of the present crisis.


# 9


If one would like to get an objective and clear idea of the contemporary state of psychology and the dimensions of its crisis, it would suffice to study the psychological *language,* i.e., the nomenclature and terminology, the dictionary and syntax of the psychologist. Language, scientific language in particular, is a tool of thought, an instrument of analysis, and it suffices to examine which instruments a science utilizes to understand the character of its operations. The highly developed and exact language of contemporary physics, chemistry, and physiology, not to speak of mathematics where it plays an extraordinary role, was developed and perfected during the development of science and far from spontaneously, but deliberately under the influence of tradition, critique, and the direct terminological creativity of scientific societies and congresses. The psychological language of contemporaneity is first of all terminologically insufficient: this means that psychology does not yet have its *own* language. In its dictionary you will find a conglomerate of words of three kinds: (1) the words of everyday language, which are vague, ambiguous, and adapted to practical life (Lazursky leveled this criticism against faculty psychology; I succeeded in showing that it is more true of the language of empirical psychology and of Lazursky himself in particular; see Preface to Lazursky in this volume). Suffice it to remember the touchstone of all translators—the visual *sense* (i.e., sensation) to realize the whole metaphorical nature and inexactness of the practical language of daily life; (2) the words of philosophical language. They too pollute the language of psychologists, as they have lost the link with their previous meaning, are ambiguous as a result of the struggle between the various philosophical schools, and are abstract to a maximal degree. Lalande (1923) views this as the main source of the vagueness and lack of clarity in psychology. The tropes of this language favor vagueness of thought. These metaphors are valuable as illustrations, but dangerous as formulas. It also leads to personifications through the ending -ism, of mental facts, functions, systems and theories, between which small mythological dramas are invented; (3) finally, the words and ways of speaking taken from the natural sciences which are used in a figurative sense bluntly serve deception. When the psychologist discusses energy, force, and even intensity, or when he speaks of excitation etc., he always covers a non-scientific concept with a scientific word and thereby either deceives, or once again underlines the whole indeterminate nature of the concept indicated by the exact foreign term.

Lalande [1923, p. 52] correctly remarks that the obscurity of language depends as much upon its syntax as upon its dictionary. In the construction of the psychological phrase we meet no fewer mythological dramas than in the lexicon. I want to add that the *style,* the manner of expression of a science is no less important. In a word, all elements, all functions of a language show the traces of the age of the science that makes use of them, and determine the character of its workings.

It would be mistaken to think that psychologists have not noticed the mixed character, the inaccuracy, and the mythological nature of their language. There is hardly any author who in one way or another has not dwelt upon the problem of terminology. Indeed, psychologists have pretended to describe, analyze and study very subtle things, full of nuances, they have attempted to convey the unique mental experience, the facts *sui generis* which occur only once, when science wished to convey the experience itself, i.e., when the task of its language was equal to that of the word of the artist. For this reason psychologists recommended that psychology be learned from the great novelists, spoke in the language of the impressionistic fine literature themselves, and even the best, most brilliant stylists among the psychologists were unable to create an exact language and wrote in a figurative-expressive way. They suggested, sketched, described, but did not record. This was the case for James, Lipps, and Binet.

The 6th International Congress of psychologists in Geneva (1909) put this question on its agenda and published two reports—by Baldwin and Claparade—on this topic, but did no more than establishing rules for linguistical possibilities, although Claparade tried to give a definition of 40 laboratory terms. Baldwin's dictionary in England and the technical and critical dictionary of philosophy in France have accomplished much, but despite this the situation becomes worse every year and to read a new book with the help of the above-mentioned dictionaries is impossible. The encyclopedia from which I take this information views it as one of its tasks to introduce solidity and stability into the terminology, but gives occasion to new instability as it introduces a new system of terms [Dumas, 1923].

The language reveals as it were the molecular changes that the science goes through. It reflects the internal processes that take shape—the tendencies of development, reform, and growth. We may assume, therefore, that the troubled condition of the language reflects a troubled condition of the science. We will not deal any further with the essence of this relation. We will take it as our point of departure for the analysis of the contemporary molecular terminological changes in psychology. Perhaps, we will be able to read in them the present and future fate of the science. Let us first of all begin with those who are tempted to deny any fundamental importance to the language of science and view such debates as scholastic logomachy. Thus, Chelpanov (1925) considers the attempt to replace the subjective terminology by an objective one as a ridiculous pretension, utter nonsense. The zoopsychologists (Beer, Bethe, Von Uexktill) have used "photoreceptor" instead of "eye," "stiboreceptor" instead of "nose," "receptor" instead of "sense organ" etc. (Chelpanov, 1925).

Chelpanov is tempted to reduce the whole reform carried out by behaviorism to a play of words. He assumes that in Watson's writings the word "sensation" or "idea" is replaced by the word "reaction." In order to show the reader the difference between ordinary psychology and the psychology of the behaviorist, Chelpanov (1925) gives examples of the new way of expressing things:

> In ordinary psychology it is said: 'When someone's optical nerve is stimulated by a mixture of complementary light waves, he will become *conscious* of the white color.' According to Watson in this case we must say: 'He *reacts* to it as if it were a white color.'

The triumphant conclusion of the author is that the matter is not changed by the words used. The whole difference is in the words. Is this really true? *For a psychologist of Chelpanov's kind it is definitively true.* Who does not investigate nor discover anything new cannot understand why researchers introduce new terms for new phenomena. Who has no view of his own about the phenomena and accepts indifferently both Spinoza, Husserl, Marx, and Plato, for such a person a fundamental change of words is an empty pretension. Who eclectically—in the order of appearance—assimilates all Western European schools, currents and directions, is in need of a vague, undefined, levelling, everyday language—"as is spoken in ordinary psychology." For a person who conceives of psychology only in the form of a textbook it is a matter of life and death to preserve everyday language, and as lots of empiricist psychologists belong to this type, they speak in this mixed and motley jargon, in which the *consciousness of the white color* is simply a fact which is in no need of any further critique.

For Chelpanov it is a caprice, an eccentricity. But why is this eccentricity *so regular?* Doesn't it contain something essential? Watson, Pavlov, Bekhterev, Kornilov, Bethe and Von Uexkiill (Chelpanov's list may be continued *ad libitum* from any area of science), Köhler, Koffka and others and still others demonstrated this eccentricity. This means that there is some objective necessity in the tendency to introduce new terminology.

We can say in advance that *the word that refers to a fact at the same time provides a philosophy of that fact,* its theory, its system. When I say: "the consciousness of the color" I have scientific associations of a *certain* kind, the fact is included in a *certain* series of phenomena, I attach a *certain* meaning to the fact. When I say: "the reaction to white" everything is wholly *different.* But Chelpanov is only pretending that it is a matter of words. For him the thesis "a *reform of terminology is not needed"* forms the conclusion from the thesis "a *reform of psychology is not needed."* Never mind that Chelpanov gets caught in contradictions: on the one hand Watson is only changing words; on the other hand behaviorism is *distorting* psychology. It is one of two things: either Watson is playing with words—then behaviorism is a most innocent thing, an amusing joke, as Chelpanov likes to put it when he reassures himself; or behind the change of words is concealed a change of the matter then the change of words is not all that funny. A revolution always tears off the old names of things—both in politics and in science.

But let us proceed to other authors who do understand the importance of new words. It is clear to them that new facts and a new viewpoint necessitate new words. Such psychologists fall into two groups. Some are pure eclectics, who happily mix the old and new words and view this procedure as some eternal law. Others speak in a mixed language out of necessity. They do not coincide with any of the debating parties and strive for a unified language, for the creation of their own language.

We have seen that such outspoken eclectics as Thorndike equally apply the term "reaction" to temper, dexterity, action, to the objective and the subjective. As he is not capable of solving the question of the nature of the studied facts and the principles of their investigation, he simply deprives both the subjective and the subjective terms of their meaning. "Stimulus-reaction" is for him simply a convenient way to describe the phenomena. Others, such as Pillsbury [1917, pp. 4–14], make eclecticism their principle: the debates about a general method and viewpoint are of interest for the technically-minded psychologist. Sensation and perception he explains in the terms of the structuralists, actions of all kinds in those of the behaviorists. He himself is inclined towards functionalism. The different terms lead to discrepancies, but he prefers the use of the terms of many schools to those of a single specific school. In complete accordance with this he explains the subject matter of psychology with illustrations from everyday life, in vague words, instead of giving formal definitions. Having given the three definitions of psychology as the science of mind, consciousness, or behavior, he concludes that they may very well be neglected in the description of the mental life. It is only natural that terminology leaves our author indifferent as well.

Koffka (1925) and others try to realize a fundamental synthesis of the old and the new terminology. They understand very well that the word is a theory of the fact it designates and, therefore, they view behind two systems of terms two systems of concepts. Behavior has two aspects—one that must be studied by natural scientific observation and one that must be experienced and to these correspond functional and descriptive concepts. The functional objective concepts and terms belong to the category of natural scientific ones, the phenomenal descriptive ones, es are absolutely foreign to it (to behavior). This fact is often obscured by the language which does not always have separate words for this or that kind of concept, as everyday language is not scientific language.

The merit of the Americans is that they have fought against subjective anecdotes in animal psychology. But we will not fear the use of descriptive concepts when describing animal behavior. The Americans have gone too far, they are too objective. What is again highly remarkable: Gestalt theory, which is internally deeply dualistic, reflecting and uniting two contradictory tendencies which, as will be shown below, currently determine the whole crisis and its fate, wishes in principle to preserve this *dual* language forever, for it proceeds from the *dual* nature of behavior. However, sciences do not study what is closely related in nature, but what is conceptually homogeneous and similar. How can there be *one* science about two absolutely different kinds of phenomena, which evidently require *two* different methods, *two* different explanatory principles, etc.? After all, the unity of a science is guaranteed by unity of the viewpoint on the subject. How then can we build a science with two viewpoints? Once again a contradiction in terms corresponds to a contradiction in principles.

Matters are slightly different with another group of mainly Russian psychologists, who use various terms but view this as the attribute of a period of transition. This "demi-saison", as one psychologist calls it, requires clothes that combine the properties of a fur coat and a summer dress, warm and light at the same time. Thus, Blonsky holds that it is not important how we designate the phenomena under study but how we understand them. We utilize the ordinary vocabulary for our speech but to these ordinary words we attach a content that corresponds to the science of the 20th century. It is not important to avoid the expression "The dog is angry."

What is important is that this phrase is not the explanation, but the problem (Blonsky, 1925). Strictly speaking, this implies a complete condemnation of the old terminology: for there this phrase was the explanation. But this phrase must be formulated in an appropriate way and not with the ordinary vocabulary. This is the main thing required to make it a scientific problem. And those whom Blonsky calls the pedants of terminology appreciate much better than he does that the phrase conceals a content given by the history of science. However, like Blonsky many utilize two languages and do not consider this a question of principle. This is the way Kornilov proceeds, this is what I do, repeating after Pavlov: what does it matter whether I call them mental or higher nervous [processes]?

But already these examples show the *limits* of such a bilingualism. The limits themselves show again most clearly what our whole analysis of the eclectics showed: bilingualism is the external sign of dual thinking. You may speak in two languages as long as you convey dual things or things in a dual light. Then it really does not matter what you call them.

So, let us summarize. For empiricists it is necessary to have a language that is colloquial, indeterminate, confused, ambiguous, vague, in order that what is said can be reconciled with whatever you like—today with the church fathers, tomorrow with Marx. They need a word that neither provides a clear philosophical qualification of the nature of the phenomenon, nor simply its clear description, because the empiricists have no clear understanding and conception of their subject. The eclectics, both those that are so by principle and those that adhere to eclecticism only for the time being, are in need of two languages as long as they defend an eclectic point of view. But as soon as they leave this viewpoint and attempt to designate and describe a newly discovered fact or explain their own viewpoint on a subject, they lose their indifference to the language or the word.

Kornilov (1922), who made a new discovery, is prepared to turn the *whole* area to which he assigns this phenomenon from a chapter of psychology into an independent science—reactology. Elsewhere he contrasts the reflex with the reaction and views a fundamental difference between the two terms. They are based on wholly different philosophies and methodologies. Reaction is for him a biological concept and reflex a strictly physiological one. A reflex is only objective, a reaction is subjective objective. This explains why a phenomenon acquires one meaning when we call it a reflex and another when we call it a reaction.

Obviously, it makes a difference how we refer to the phenomena and there is a reason for pedantry when it is backed by an investigation or a philosophy. A wrong word implies a wrong understanding. It is not for nothing that Blonsky notices that his work and the outline of psychology by Jameson (1925)—this typical specimen of philistinism and eclecticism in science—overlap. To view the phrase "the dog is angry" as the problem is wrong if only because, as Shchelovanov (1929) justly pointed out, the finding of the term is the end point and not the starting point of the investigation. As soon as one or the other complex of reactions is referred to with some psychological term all further attempts at analysis are finished. If Blonsky would leave his eclectic stand, like Kornilov, and acknowledge the value of investigation or principle, he would find this out. There is not a single psychologist with whom this would not happen. And such an ironic observer of the "terminological revolutions" .as Chelpanov suddenly turns out to be an astonishing pedant: he objects to the name "reactology." With the pedantry of one of Chekhov's gymnasium teachers he preaches that this term causes misunderstanding, first etymologically and second theoretically. The author declares with aplomb that etymologically speaking the word is entirely incorrect—we should say "reactiology" [reaktsiologija]. This is of course the summit of linguistic illiteracy and a flagrant violation of all the terminological principles of the 6th Congress on the international (Latin-Greek) basis of terms. Obviously, Kornilov did not form his term from the home-bred "reaktsija," but from *reactio* and he was perfectly right in doing so. One wonders how Chelpanov would translate "reactiology" into French, German, etc. But this is not what it is all about. It is about something else: Chelpanov declares that this term is inappropriate in Kornilov's system of psychological views. But let us speak to the point. The important thing is that *the meaning of a term is accepted in a system of views*. It turns out that even reflexology *conceived of in a certain way* has its raison d'etre.

Let people not think that these trifles have no importance, because they are too obviously confused, contradictory, incorrect, etc. Here there is a difference between the scientific and the practical points of view. Münsterberg explained that the gardener loves his tulips and hates the weeds, but the botanist who describes and explains loves or hates nothing and, from his point of view, cannot love or hate. For the science of man, he says, stupidity is of no less interest than wisdom. It is all indifferent material that merely claims to exist as a link in the chain of phenomena. As a link in the chain of causal phenomena, this fact—that terminology suddenly becomes an urgent question for the eclectic psychologist who does not care about terminology unless it touches his position—is a valuable methodological fact. It is as valuable as the fact that other eclectics *following the same path* come to the same conclusion as Kornilov: neither the conditional nor the correlative reflexes appear sufficiently clear and understandable. Reactions are the basis of the new psychology, and the whole psychology developed by Pavlov, Bekhterev and Watson is called neither reflexology nor behaviorism, but 'psychologie de reaction,' i.e., reactology. Let the eclectics come to opposite conclusions about a specific thing. They are still related by the method, the process by which they arrive at their conclusions.

We find the same regularity in all reflexologists—both investigators and theoreticians. Watson [1914, p. 9] is convinced that we can write a course in psychology without using the words "consciousness," "content," "introspectively verified," "imagery" etc. And for him this is not a terminological matter, but one of principle: just as the chemist cannot use the language of alchemy nor the astronomer that of the horoscope. He explains this brilliantly with the help of one specific case: he regards the difference between a visual reaction and a visual image as extremely important because behind it lies the difference between a consistent monism and a consistent dualism [1914, pp. 16–20]. A word is for him the tentacle by which philosophy comprehends a fact. Whatever is the value of the countless volumes written in the terms of consciousness, it can only be determined and expressed by translating them into objective language. For according to Watson consciousness and so on are no more than undefined expressions. And the new textbook breaks with the popular theories and terminology. Watson condemns "half-hearted psychology of behavior" (which brings harm to the whole current) claiming that when the theses of the new psychology will not preserve their clarity its framework will be distorted, obscured, and it will lose its genuine meaning. Functional psychology perished from such half-heartedness. If behaviorism has a future then it must break completely with the concept of consciousness. However, thus far it has not been decided whether behaviorism will become the dominating *system* of psychology or simply remain a methodological approach. And therefore

Watson (1926) too often takes the methodology of common sense as the basis of his investigations. In the attempt to liberate himself from philosophy he slips into the viewpoint of the "common man," understanding by this latter not the basic feature of human practice but the common sense of the average American businessman. In his opinion the common man must welcome behaviorism. Ordinary life has taught him to act that way. Consequently, when dealing with the science of behavior he will not feel a change of method or some change of the subject (ibid.). This [viewpoint] implies the verdict on all behaviorism. Scientific study absolutely requires a *change* of the subject (i.e., its treatment in concepts) and the *method*. But behavior itself is understood by these psychologists in its everyday sense and in their arguments and descriptions there is much of the philistine way of judgment. Therefore, neither radical nor half-hearted behaviorism will ever find—either in style and language, or in principle and method—the *boundary* between everyday and philistine understanding. Having liberated themselves from the "alchemy" in language, the behaviorists have polluted it with everyday, non-terminological speech. This makes them akin to Chelpanov: the whole difference can be attributed to the life style of the American or Russian philistine. The reproach that the new psychology is a philistine psychology is therefore partially justified.

This vagueness of language in the Americans, which Blonsky considers a lack of pedantry, is viewed by Pavlov [1928/1963, pp. 213–214] as a failing. He views it as a

> gross defect which prevents the success of the work, but which, I have no doubt, will sooner or later be removed. I refer to the application of psychological concepts and classifications in this essentially objective study of the behavior of animals. Herein lies the cause of the fortuitous and conditional character of their complicated methods, and the fragmentary and unsystematic character of their results, which have no well planned basis to rest on.

One could not express the role and function of language in scientific investigation more clearly. And Pavlov's entire success is first of all due to the enormous consistency in his language. His investigations led to a theory of higher nervous activity and animal behavior, rather than a chapter on the functioning of the salivary glands, exclusively because he lifted the study of salivary secretion to an enormously high theoretical level and created a transparent system of concepts that lies at the basis of the science. One must marvel at Pavlov's principled stand in methodological matters. His book introduces us into the laboratory of his investigations and teaches us how to create a scientific language. At first, what does it matter what we call the phenomenon? But gradually each step is strengthened by a new word, each new principle requires a term. He clarifies the sense and meaning of the use of new terms. The selection of terms and concepts predetermines the outcome of an investigation:

> I cannot understand how the non-spatial concepts of contemporary psychology can be fitted into the material structure of the brain [ibid., p. 224].

When Thorndike speaks of a mood reaction and studies it, he creates concepts and laws that lead us away from the brain. To have recourse to such a method Pavlov calls cowardice. Partly out of habit, partly from a "certain anxiety," he resorted to psychological explanations.

> But soon I understood that they were bad servants. For me there arose difficulties when I could see no natural relations between the phenomena. The succor of psychology was only

in words (the animal has 'remembered,' the animal 'wished,' the animal 'thought'), i.e., *it was only a method of indeterminate thinking, without a basis in fact* (italics mine, L. V.) [ibid., p. 237].

He regards the manner in which psychologists express themselves as an insult against serious thinking.

And when Pavlov introduced in his laboratories a penalty for the use of psychological terms this was no less important and revealing for the history of the theory of the science than the debate about the symbol of faith for the history of religion. Only Chelpanov can laugh about this: the scientist does not fine for [the use of] an incorrect term in a textbook or in the exposition of a subject, *but in the laboratory—in the process of the investigation.* Obviously, such a fine was imposed for the non-causal, non-spatial, indeterminate, mythological thinking that came with that word and that threatened to blow up the whole cause and to introduce—as in the case of the Americans—a fragmentary, unsystematic character and to take away the foundations.

Chelpanov (1925) does not suspect at all that new words may be needed in the laboratory, in an investigation, that the sense [and] meaning of an investigation are determined by the words used. He criticizes Pavlov, stating that "inhibition" is a vague, hypothetical expression and that the same must be said of the term "disinhibition." Admittedly, we don't know what goes on in the brain during inhibition, but nevertheless it is a brilliant, transparent concept. First of all, it is well defined, i.e., exactly determined in its meaning and boundaries. Secondly, it is honest, i.e., it says no more than is known. Presently the *processes* of inhibition in the brain are not wholly clear to us, but the *word* and the *concept* "inhibition" are wholly clear. Thirdly, it is principled and scientific, i.e., it includes a fact into a system, underpins it with a foundation, explains it hypothetically, but causally. Of course, we have a clearer image of an eye than of an analyzer. Exactly because of this the word "eye" doesn't mean anything in science. The term "visual analyzer" says both less and more than the word "eye." Pavlov revealed a new function of the eye, compared it with the function of other organs, connected the whole sensory path from the eye to the cortex, indicated its place in the system of behavior—and all this is expressed by the new term. It is true that we must think of visual sensations when we hear these words, but the genetic origin of a word and its terminological meaning are two absolutely different things. The word contains *nothing* of sensations; it can be adequately used by a blind person. Those who, following Chelpanov, catch Pavlov making a slip of the tongue, using fragments of a psychological language, and find him guilty of inconsistency, do not understand the heart of the matter. When Pavlov uses [words such as] happiness, attention, idiot (about a dog), this only means that the mechanism of happiness, attention etc. *has not yet been studied,* that these are the as yet obscure spots of the system; it does not imply a fundamental concession or contradiction.

But all this may seem incorrect as long as we do not take the opposite aspect into account. Of course, terminological consistency may become pedantry, "verbalism," commonplace (Bekhterev's school). When does that occur? When the word is like a label stuck on a finished article and is not born in the research process. Then it does not define, delimit, but introduces vagueness and shambles in the system of concepts.

Such a work implies the pinning on of new labels which explain absolutely nothing, for it is not difficult, of course, to invent a whole catalogue of names: the reflex of purpose, the reflex of God, the reflex of right, the reflex of freedom, etc. A reflex can be found for everything. The problem is only that we gain nothing but trifles. This does not refute the general rule, but indirectly confirms it: new words keep pace with new investigations.

Let us summarize. We have seen everywhere that the word, like the sun in a drop of water, *fully* reflects the processes and tendencies in the development of a science, A certain fundamental unity of knowledge in science comes to light which goes from the highest principles to the selection of a word. What guarantees this *unity* of the whole scientific system? The fundamental methodological skeleton. The investigator, insofar as he is not a technician, a registrar, an executor, is always a philosopher who during the investigation and description is *thinking* about the phenomena, and his way of thinking is revealed in the words he uses. A tremendous discipline of thought lies behind Pavlov's penalty. A discipline of mind similar to the monastic system which forms the core of the religious world view is at the core of the scientific conception of the world. He who enters the laboratory with his own word is deemed to repeat Pavlov's example. The word is a philosophy of the fact; it can be its mythology and its scientific theory. When Lichtenberg said: "Es denkt, sollte man sagen, so wie man sagt: es blitzt," he was fighting mythology in language. To say "cogito" is saying too much when it is translated as "I think." Would the physiologist really agree to say "I conduct the excitation along my nerve"? To say "I *think*" or "It *comes to my mind*" implies two opposite theories of thinking. Binet's whole theory of the mental poses requires the first expression, Freud's theory the second and Külpe's theory now the one, now the other, Høffding [1908, p. 106, footnote 2] sympathetically cites the physiologist Foster who says that the impressions of an animal deprived of [one of] its cerebral hemispheres we must "either call sensations, or we must *invent an entirely new word for them,*" for we have stumbled upon a *new* category of facts and must choose a way to think about it—whether in connection with the old category or in a new fashion.

Among the Russian authors it was Lange (1914, p. 43) who understood the importance of terminology. Pointing out that there is no shared system in psychology, that the crisis shattered the whole science, he remarks that

> Without fear of exaggeration it can be said that the description of any psychological process becomes different whether we describe and study it in the categories of the psychological system of Ebbinghaus or Wundt, Stumpf or Avenarius, Meinong or Binet, James or G. E. Müller. Of course, the purely factual aspect must remain the same. However, in science, at least in psychology, to separate the described fact from its theory, i.e., from those scientific categories by means of which this description is made, is often very difficult and even impossible, for in psychology (as, by the way, in physics, according to Duhem) each description is always already a certain theory investigations, in particular those of an experimental character, seem to the superficial observer to be free from those fundamental disagreements about basic scientific categories which divide the different psychological schools.

But the very statement of the questions, the use of one or the other psychological term, always implies a certain way of understanding them which corresponds to some theory, and consequently the whole factual result of the investigation stands or falls with the correctness or falsity of the psychological system. Seemingly very exact investigations, observations, or measurements may, therefore, prove false, or in any case lose their meaning when the meaning of the basic psychological theories is changed. Such crises, which destroy or depreciate whole series of facts, have occurred more than once in science. Lange compares them to an earthquake that arises due to deep deformations in the depths of the earth. Such was [the case with] the fall of alchemy. The dabbling that is now so widespread in science, i.e., the isolation of the technical executive function of the investigation—chiefly the maintenance of the equipment according to a well-known routine—from scientific thinking, is noticeable first of all in the breakdown of scientific language. In principle, all thoughtful psychologists know this perfectly well: in methodological investigations the terminological problem which requires a most complex analysis instead of a simple note takes the lion's share. Rickert regards the creation of unequivocal terminology as the most important task of psychology which precedes any investigation, for already in primitive description we must select word meanings which "by generalizing simplify" the immense diversity and plurality of the mental phenomena [Binswanger, 1922, p. 26]. Engels [1925/1978, p. 553] essentially expressed the same idea in his example from chemistry:

> In organic chemistry the meaning of some body and, consequently, its name are no longer simply dependent upon its composition, but rather upon its place in the *series* to which it belongs. That is why its old name becomes an obstacle for understanding when we find that a body belongs to such a series and must be replaced by *a name that refers to this series* (paraffin, etc.).

What has been carried to the rigor of a chemical rule here exists as a general principle in the whole area of scientific language.

Lange (1914, p. 96) says that

> Parallelism is a word which seems innocent at first sight. It conceals, however, a terrible idea—the idea of the secondary and accidental nature of technique in the world of physical phenomena.

This innocent word has an instructive history. Introduced by Leibniz it was applied to the solution of the psychophysical problem which goes back to Spinoza, changing its name many times in the process. Høffding [1908, p. 91, footnote 1] calls it the identity hypothesis and considers that it is the

> only precise and opportune name. . . . The frequently used term 'monism' is etymologically correct but inconvenient, because it has often been used vague and inconsistent conception. Names such as 'parallelism' and 'dualism' are inadequate, because they . . . smuggle in the idea that we must conceive of the mental and the bodily as two completely separate series of developments (almost as a pair of rails) which is exactly what the hypothesis does *not* assume.

It is Wolff's hypothesis which must be called dualistic, not Spinoza's.

Thus, a *single* hypothesis is now called (1) monism, now (2) dualism, now (3) parallelism, and now (4) identity. We may add that the circle of Marxists who have revived this hypothesis (as will be shown below)—Plekhanov, and after him Sarab'janov, Frankfurt and others-view it precisely as a *theory of the unity but not identity* of the mental and the physical. How could this happen? Obviously, the hypothesis itself can be developed on the basis of different more general views and may acquire different meanings depending on them: some emphasize its dualism, others its monism etc. Høffding [1908, p. 96] remarks that it does not exclude a deeper metaphysical hypothesis, in particular idealism. In order to become a philosophical world view, hypotheses must be elaborated anew and this new elaboration resides in the emphasis on now this and now that aspect. Very important is Lange's (1914, p. 76) reference:

> We find psychophysical parallelism in the representatives of the most diverse philosophical currents—the dualists (the followers of Descartes), the monists (Spinoza), Leibnitz metaphysical idealism), the positivists-agnostics (Bain, Spence), Wundt and Paulsen (voluntaristic metaphysics).

Høffding [1908, p. 117] says that the unconscious follows from the hypothesis of identity:

> In this case we act like the philologist who via conjectural critique *[Konjekturulkritik]* supplements a fragment of an ancient writer, Compared to the physical world the mental world is for us a fragment; only by means of a hypothesis can we supplement it.

This conclusion follows inevitably from [his] parallelism.

That is why Chelpanov is not all that wrong when he says that before 1922 he called this theory parallelism and after 1922 materialism. He would be entirely right if his philosophy had not been adapted to the season in a slightly mechanical fashion. The same goes for the word "function" (I mean function in the mathematical sense). The formula "consciousness is a function of the brain" points to the theory of parallelism; "physiological sense" leads to materialism. When Kornilov (1925) introduced the concept and the term of a functional relation between the mind and the body, he regarded parallelism as a dualistic hypothesis, but despite this fact and *without noticing it himself, he introduced this theory,* for although he rejected the concept of function in the physiological sense, its second sense remained.

Thus, we see that, beginning with the broadest hypotheses and ending with the tiniest details in the description of the experiment, the word reflects the general disease of the science. The specifically new result which we get from our analysis of the word is an idea of the molecular character of the processes in science. Each cell of the scientific organism shows the processes of infection and struggle. This gives us a better idea of the character of scientific knowledge. It emerges as a deeply unitary process. Finally, we get an idea of what is healthy or sick in the processes of science. What is true of the word is true of the theory. The word can bring science further, as long as it (1) occupies the territory that was conquered by the investigation, i.e., as long as it corresponds to the objective state of affairs; and (2) is in keeping with the right basic principles, i.e., the most general formulas of this objective world.

We see, therefore, that scientific research is at the same time a study of the fact and of the methods used to know this fact. In other words, methodological work is done in science itself insofar as this science moves forward and reflects upon its results. The choice of a word is already a methodological process. That methodology and experiment are worked out simultaneously can be seen with particular ease in the case of Pavlov. Thus, science is philosophical down to its ultimate elements, to its words. It is permeated, so to speak, by methodology. This coincides with the Marxist view of philosophy as "the science of sciences," a synthesis that penetrates science. In this sense Engels [1925/1978, p. 480] remarked that

Natural scientists may say what they want, but they are ruled by philosophy. . . . Not until natural science and the science of history have absorbed dialectics will all the philosophical fuss . . . become superfluous and disappear in the positive science.

The experimenters in the natural sciences imagine that they free themselves from philosophy when they ignore it, but they turn out to be slaves of the worst philosophy, which consists of a medley of fragmentary and unsystematic views, since investigators cannot move a single step forwards without thinking, and thinking requires logical definitions. The question of how to deal with methodological problems—"separately from the sciences themselves" or by introducing the methodological investigation in the science itself (in a curriculum or an investigation)—is a matter of pedagogical expediency. Frank (1917/1964, p. 37) is right when he says that in the prefaces and concluding chapters of all books on psychology one is dealing with problems of philosophical psychology. It is one thing, however, to explain a methodology—"to establish an understanding of the methodology"—this is, we repeat, a matter of pedagogical technique. It is another thing to carry out a methodological investigation. This requires special consideration.

Ultimately the scientific word aspires to become a mathematical sign, i.e., a pure term. After all, the mathematical formula is also a series of words, but words which have been very well defined and which are therefore conventional in the highest degree. This is why all knowledge is scientific insofar as it is mathematical (Kant). But the language of empirical psychology is the direct antipode of mathematical language. As has been shown by Locke, Leibnitz and all linguistics, *all words* of psychology are metaphors taken from the spatial world.


## 10

We proceed to the positive formulations. From the fragmentary analyses of the separate elements of a science we have learned to view it as a complex whole which develops dynamically and lawfully. In which stage of development is our science at this moment, what is the meaning and nature of the crisis it experiences and what will be its outcome? Let us proceed to the answer to these questions. When one is somewhat acquainted with the methodology (and history) of the sciences, science loses its image of a dead, finished, immobile whole consisting of ready-made statements and becomes a living system which constantly develops and moves forward, and which consists of proven facts, laws, suppositions, structures, and conclusions which are continually being supplemented, criticized, verified, partially rejected, interpreted and organized anew, etc. Science commences to be understood *dialectically* in its movement, i.e., from the perspective of its dynamics, growth, development, evolution. It is from this point of view that we must evaluate and interpret each stage of development. Thus, the first thing from which we proceed is the acknowledgement of a *crisis*. What this crisis signifies is the subject of different interpretations. What follows are the most important kinds of interpretation of its meaning.

First of all, there are psychologists who totally deny the existence of a crisis. Chelpanov belongs among them, as do most of the Russian psychologists of the old school in general (only Lange and Frank have seen what is being done in science). In the opinion of such psychologists everything is all right in our science, just as in mineralogy. The crisis came from outside. Some persons ventured to reform our science; the official ideology required its revision. But for neither was there any objective basis in the science itself. It is true, in the debate one had to admit that a scientific reform was undertaken in America as well, but for the reader it was carefully—and perhaps sincerely-concealed that not a single *psychologist* who left his trace in science managed to avoid the crisis. This first conception is so blind that it is of no further interest to us. It can be fully explained by the fact that psychologists of this type are essentially eclectics and popularizers of other persons' ideas. Not only have they never engaged in the research and philosophy of their science, they have not even critically assessed each new school. They have accepted everything: the Würzburg school and Husserl's phenomenology, Wundt's and Titchener's experimentalism and Marxism, Spencer and Plato. When we deal with the great revolutions that take place in science, such persons are outside of it not only theoretically. In a practical sense as well they play no role whatever. The empiricists betrayed empirical psychology while defending it. The eclectics assimilated all they could from ideas that were hostile to them. The popularizers can be enemies to no one, they will popularize the psychology that wins. Now Chelpanov is publishing much about Marxism. Soon he will be studying reflexology, and the first textbook of the victorious behaviorism will be compiled by him or a student of his. On the whole they are professors and examiners, organizers and "Kulturträger," but not a single investigation of any importance has emerged from their school.

Others see the crisis, but evaluate it very subjectively. The crisis has divided psychology into two camps. For them the borderline lies always between the author of a specific view and the rest of the world. But, according to Lotze, even a worm that is half crushed sets off its reflection against the whole world. This is the official viewpoint of militant behaviorism. Watson (1926) thinks that there are two psychologies: a correct one—his own—and an incorrect one. The old one will die of its halfheartedness. The biggest detail he sees is the existence of half-hearted psychologists. The medieval traditions with which Wundt did not want to break ruined the psychology without a soul. As you see, everything is simplified to an extreme. There is no particular problem in turning psychology into a natural science. For Watson this coincides with the point of view of the ordinary person, i.e., the methodology of common sense. Bekhterev, on the whole, evaluates the epochs in psychology in the same way: everything before Bekhterev was a mistake, everything after Bekhterev is the truth. Many psychologists assess the crisis likewise. Since it is subjective, it is the easiest initial naive viewpoint. The psychologists whom we examined in the chapter on the unconscious also reason this way: there is empirical psychology, which is permeated by metaphysical idealism—this is a remnant; and there is a genuine methodology of the era, which coincides with Marxism. Everything which is not the first must be the second, as no third possibility is given.

Psychoanalysis is in many respects the opposite of empirical psychology, This already suffices to declare it to be a Marxist system! For these psychologists the crisis coincides with the struggle they are fighting. There are allies and enemies, other distinctions do not exist.

The objective-empirical diagnoses of the crisis are no better: the severity of the crisis is measured by the number of schools that can be counted. Allport, in counting the currents of American psychology, defended this point of view (counting schools): the school of James and the school of Titchener, behaviorism and psychoanalysis. The units involved in the elaboration of the science are enumerated *side by side,* but not a single attempt is made to penetrate into the objective meaning of what each school is defending and the dynamic relations between the schools.

The error becomes more serious when one begins to view this situation as a fundamental characteristic of a crisis. Then the boundary between *this* crisis and any other, between the crisis in *psychology* and any *other science,* between every particular disagreement or debate and a crisis, is erased. In a word, one uses an anti-historical and anti-methodological approach which usually leads to *absurd results.*

Portugalov (1925, p. 12) wishes to argue the incomplete and relative nature of reflexology and not only slips into agnosticism and relativism of the purest order, but ends up with obvious nonsense. "In the chemistry, mechanics, electrophysics and electrophysiology of the brain everything is changing dramatically and nothing has yet been clearly and definitely demonstrated." Credulous persons believe in natural science, but "when we stay in the realm of medicine, do we really believe, with the hand on our heart, in the unshakable and stable force of natural science . . . and does natural science itself , . .believe in its unshakable, stable, and genuine character?"

There follows an enumeration of the theoretical changes in the natural sciences which are, moreover, lumped together. A sign of equality is put between the lack of solidity or stability of a particular theory and the whole of natural science, and what constitutes the foundation of the truth of natural science—the change of its theories and views—is passed off as the proof of its impotence. That this is agnosticism is perfectly clear, but two aspects deserve to be mentioned in connection with what follows: (1) in the whole chaos of views that serve to picture the natural sciences as lacking a single firm point, it is only . . . subjective child psychology based upon introspection which turns out to be unshakable; (2) amidst all the sciences which demonstrate the unreliability of the natural sciences, geometry is listed alongside optics and bacteriology. It so happens that

> Euclid said that the sum of the angles of a triangle equals two right angles; Lobachevsky dethroned Euclid and demonstrated that the sum of the angles of a triangle is less than two right angles, and Riemann dethroned Lobachevsky and demonstrated that the sum of the angles of a triangle is more than two right angles (ibid., p. 13).

We will still have more than one occasion to meet the analogy between geometry and psychology, and therefore it is worthwhile to memorize this model of a-methodological thinking: (1) geometry is a natural science; (2) Linné, Cuvier, and Darwin "dethroned" each other in the same way as Euclid, Lobachevsky, and Riemann did; finally (3) Lobachevsky *dethroned* Euclid and demonstrated that . . . But even people with only elementary knowledge of the subject know that here we are not dealing with the knowledge of *real* triangles, but with *ideal* forms in mathematical, *deductive* systems, that these *three* theses follow from *three* different assumptions and do not contradict each other, just like other arithmetical counting systems do not contradict the decimal system. They *co-exist* and this determines their whole meaning and methodological nature. But what can be the value for the diagnosis of the crisis in an inductive science of a viewpoint which regards each two consecutive names as a crisis and each new opinion as a refutation of the truth?

Kornilov's (1925) diagnosis is closer to the truth. He views a struggle between two currents—reflexology and empirical psychology and their synthesis—Marxist psychology.

Already Frankfurt (1926) had advanced the opinion that reflexology cannot be viewed as a united whole, that it consists of contradictory tendencies and directions. This is even more true of empirical psychology. A unitary empirical psychology does not exist at all. In general, this simplified schema was created more as a program for operations, critical understanding, and demarcation than for an analysis of the crisis. For the latter it lacks reference to the causes, tendency, dynamics, and prognosis of the crisis. It is a logical classification of viewpoints present in the USSR and no more than that.

Thus, there has been no *theory of the crisis* in anything so far discussed, but only subjective communiqués compiled by the staffs of the quarreling parties. Here what is important is to beat the enemy; nobody will waste his time studying him.

Still closer to a theory of the crisis comes Lange (1914, p. 43), who already presents an embryonic description of it. But he has more feeling for than understanding of the crisis. Not even his historical information is to be trusted. For him the crisis commenced with the fall of associationism, i.e., he takes an accidental circumstance for the cause. Having established that "presently some general crisis is taking place" in psychology, he continues: "It consists of the replacement of the previous associationism by a new psychological theory." This is incorrect if only because associationism never was a generally accepted psychological system which formed the core of our science, but *to the present day remains* one of the fighting currents which has become much stronger lately and has been revived in reflexology and behaviorism. The psychology of Mill, Bain, and Spencer was never more than what it is now. It has fought faculty psychology (Herbart) like it is doing now. To *see* the root of the crisis in associationism is to give a very subjective assessment. Lange himself views it as the root of the rejection of the sensualistic doctrine. But today as well Gestalt theory views associationism as the main flaw of *all* psychology, including the newest.

In reality, it is not the adherents and opponents of this principle who are divided by some basic trait, but groups that evolved upon much more fundamental grounds. Furthermore, it is not entirely correct to reduce it to a struggle between the views of individual psychologists: it is important to lay bare what is shared and what is contradictory behind these various opinions. Lange's false understanding of the crisis ruined his own work. In defending the principle of a realistic, biological psychology, he fights Ribot and relies upon Husserl and other *extreme* idealists, who reject the possibility of psychology as a natural science. But some things, and not the least important ones, he established correctly. These are his correct propositions:

(1)  There is no generally accepted system of our science. Each of the expositions of psychology by eminent authors is based upon an entirely different system. All basic concepts and categories are interpreted in various ways. The crisis touches upon the very foundations of the science.

(2)  The crisis is destructive, but wholesome. It reveals the growth of the science, its enrichment, its force, not its impotence or bankruptcy. The serious nature of the crisis is caused by the fact that the territory of psychology lies between sociology and biology, between which Kant wanted to divide it.

(3)  Not a single psychological work is possible without first establishing the basic principles of this science. One should lay the foundations before starting to build.

(4) Finally, the common goal is to elaborate a new theory—a "renewed system of the science." However, Lange's understanding of this goal is entirely incorrect. For him it is "the critical evaluation of all contemporary currents and the attempt to reconcile them" (Lange, 1914, p. 43). And he tried to reconcile what cannot be reconciled: Husserl and biological psychology; together with James he attacked Spencer and with Dilthey he renounced biology. For him the idea of a possible reconciliation followed from the idea that "a revolution took place" *"against associationism* and physiological psychology" (ibid., p. 47) and that all new currents are connected by a common starting point and goal. That is why he gives a global characteristic of the crisis as an earthquake, a swampy area, etc. For him "a period of chaos has commenced" and the task is reduced to the "critique and logical elaboration" of the various opinions engendered by a common cause. This is a picture of the crisis as it was sketched by the participants in the struggle of the 1870s. Lange's personal attempt is the best evidence for the struggle between the real operative forces which determine the crisis. He regards the combination of subjective and objective psychology as a necessary *postulate of psychology,* rather than as a topic of discussion and *a problem.* As a result he introduces this dualism into his *whole* system. By contrasting his realistic or biological understanding of the mind with Natorp's [1904] idealistic conception, he in fact accepts the existence of two psychologies, as we will see below.

But the most curious thing is that Ebbinghaus, whom Lange considers to be an associationist, i.e., a pre-critical psychologist, defines the crisis more correctly. In his opinion the relative imperfection of psychology is evident from the fact that the debates concerning almost all of the most general of its questions have never come to a halt. In other sciences there is unanimity about all the ultimate principles or the basic views which must be at the basis of investigation, and if a change takes place it does not have the character of a crisis. Agreement is soon reestablished. In psychology things are entirely different, in Ebbinghaus' [1902, p. 9] opinion. Here these basic views are constantly subjected to vivid doubt, are constantly being contested.

Ebbinghaus considers the disagreement to be a chronic phenomenon. Psychology lacks clear, reliable foundations. And in 1874 the same Brentano, with whose name Lange would have the crisis start, demanded that instead of the many psychologies, one psychology should be created. Obviously, already at that time there existed not only many currents instead of a single system, but *many psychologies.* Today as well this is a most accurate diagnosis of the crisis. Now, too, methodologists claim that we are at the same point as Brentano was [Binswanger, 1922, p. 6]. This means that what takes place in psychology is not a struggle of views which may be reconciled and which are united by a common enemy and purpose. It is not even a struggle between currents or directions within a single science, but a *struggle between different sciences.* There are many psychologies—this means that it is different, mutually exclusive and really existing types of science that are fighting. Psychoanalysis, intentional psychology, reflexology—all these are *different types of science,* separate disciplines which tend to turn into a *general psychology,* i.e., to the subordination and exclusion of the other disciplines. We have seen both the meaning and the objective features of this tendency toward a general science. There can be no bigger mistake than to take this struggle for a struggle of views. Binswanger (1922, p. 6) begins by mentioning

Brentano's demand and Windelband's remark that with each representative psychology begins anew. The cause of this he sees neither in a lack of factual material, which has been gathered in abundance, nor in the absence of philosophical—methodological principles, of which we also have enough, but in the lack of *cooperation* between philosophers and empiricists in psychology: "There is hardly a single science where theorists and practitioners took such diverse paths." Psychology lacks a methodology—this is the author's conclusion, and the main thing is that we *cannot* create a methodology now. We cannot say that general psychology has already fulfilled its duties as a branch of methodology. On the contrary, wherever you look, imperfection, uncertainty, doubt, contradiction reign. We can only talk of the *problems* of general psychology and not even of that, but of an introduction to the problems of general psychology [ibid., p. 5]. Binswanger sees in psychologists a "courage and will toward (the creation of a new) psychology." In order to accomplish this they must break with the prejudices of centuries, and this shows one thing: that to this day, the general psychology has not been created. We must not ask, with Bergson, what would have happened if Kepler, Galileo, and Newton had been psychologists, but what can still happen *despite* the fact that they were mathematicians [ibid., p. 21].

Thus, it may seem that the chaos in psychology is entirely natural and that the meaning of the crisis which psychology became aware of is as follows: *there exist many psychologies which have the tendency to create a single psychology by developing a general psychology.* For the latter purpose it is not enough to have a Galileo, i.e., a genius who would create the foundations of the science. This is the general opinion of European methodology as it had evolved toward the end of the nineteenth century. Some, mainly French, authors hold this opinion even today. In Russia, Vagner (1923)—almost the only psychologist who has dealt with methodological questions—has always defended it. He expresses the same opinion on the occasion of his analysis of the *Annés Psychologiques*, i.e., a synopsis of the international literature. This is his conclusion: *thus, we have quite a number of psychological schools, but not a unified psychology as an independent area of psychology* [sic]. From the fact that it doesn't exist does not follow that it cannot exist (ibid.). The answer to the question where and how it may be found can only be given by the history of science.

This is how biology developed. In the seventeenth century two naturalists lay the foundation for two areas of zoology: Buffon for the description of animals and their way of life, and Linné for their classification. Gradually, both sections engendered a number of new problems, morphology appeared, anatomy, etc. The investigations were isolated from each other and represented as it were different sciences, which were in no way connected but for the fact that they both studied animals. The different sciences were at enmity, attempted to occupy the prevailing position as the mutual contacts increased and they *could not* remain apart. The brilliant Lamarck succeeded in integrating the uncoordinated pieces of knowledge into one book, which he called "Philosophy of Zoology." He united his investigations with those of others, Buffon and Linné included, summarized the results, harmonized them with each other, and created the area of science which Treviranus called general biology. A single and abstract science was created from the uncoordinated disciplines, which, since the works of Darwin, could stand on its own feet. It is the opinion of Vagner that what was done with the disciplines of biology before their combination into a general biology or abstract zoology at the beginning of the nineteenth century is now taking place in the field of psychology at the beginning of the twentieth century. This belated synthesis in the form of a *general psychology* must repeat Lamarck's synthesis, i.e., it must be based on an analogous principle. Vagner sees more than a simple analogy in this. For him psychology must traverse *not a similar, but the same path.* Biopsychology is *part* of biology. It is an abstraction of the concrete schools or their synthesis, the *achievements of all of these schools* form its content. It cannot have, and neither has general biology, its own special method of investigation. Each time it makes use of the method of a science that is its composite part. It takes account of the achievements, *verifying them from the point of view of evolutionary theory and indicating their corresponding places in the general system* (Vagner, 1923). This is the expression of a more or less general opinion.

Some details in Vagner call forth doubt. In his understanding, general psychology (1) now forms a *part* of biology, is based upon the theory of evolution (its basis) etc. Consequently, it is in no need of its *own* Lamarck and Darwin, or their discoveries, and can realize its synthesis on the basis of already present principles; (2) now still must develop in the same way as general biology developed, which is not included in biology as its part, but exists side by side with it. Only in this way can we understand the *analogy,* which is possible between two similar independent wholes, but not between the fate of a *whole* (biology) and its *part* (psychology).

Vagner's (ibid., p. 53) statement that biopsychology provides "exactly what Marx requires from psychology" causes another embarrassment. In general it can be said that Vagner's *formal* analysis is, evidently, as irreproachably correct as his attempt to solve the essence of the problem, and to outline the *content* of general psychology is methodologically untenable, even simply underdeveloped (part of biology, Marx). But the latter does not interest us now. Let us turn to the formal analysis. Is it correct that the psychology of our days is going through the same crisis as biology before Lamarck and is heading for the same fate?

To put it this way is to keep silent about the *most important and decisive aspect* of the crisis and to present the whole picture in a false light. Whether psychology is heading for agreement or rupture, whether a general psychology will develop from the combination or separation of the psychological disciplines, depends on what these disciplines bring with them—parts of the future whole, like systematics, morphology and anatomy, or mutually exclusive principles of knowledge. It also depends on what is the nature of the *hostility* between the disciplines—whether the contradictions which divide psychology are soluble, or whether they are irreconcilable. And it is precisely this analysis of the specific conditions under which psychology proceeds to the creation of a general science that we do not find in Vagner, Lange and the others. Meanwhile, European methodology has already reached a much higher degree of understanding of the crisis and has shown *which* and *how many* psychologies exist and *what* are the possible outcomes. But before we turn to this point we must first quit radically with the misunderstanding that psychology is following the path biology already took and in the end will simply be attached to it as its part. To think about it in this way is to fail to see that sociology edged its way between the biology of man and animals and tore psychology into two parts (which led Kant to divide it over two areas). We must develop the theory of the crisis in such a way as to be able to answer *this question.*

## 11

There is one fact that prevents all investigators from seeing the genuine state of affairs in psychology. This is the empirical character of its constructions. It must be torn off from psychology's constructions like a pellicle, like the skin of a fruit, in order to see them as they really are. Usually empirism is taken on trust, without further analysis. Psychology with all its diversity is treated as some fundamental scientific unity with a common basis. All disagreements are viewed as secondary phenomena which take place within this unity. But this is a false idea, an illusion. In reality, empirical psychology as a science of general principle—even *one* general principle—does not exist, and the attempts to create it have led to the defeat and bankruptcy of the very idea of creating an empirical psychology. The same persons who lump together many psychologies according to some common feature which contrasts with their own, e.g., psychoanalysis, reflexology, behaviorism (consciousness the unconscious, subjectivism—objectivism, spiritualism—materialism), do not see that *within such an* empirical psychology *the same* processes take place which take place between it and a branch that breaks away. They do not see that the development of *these branches themselves* is subject to more *general tendencies* which are being operative in and can, in consequence, only be properly understood on the basis of the whole field of science. It is the *whole of psychology* which should be lumped together. What does the *empiricism* of contemporary psychology mean? First of all, it is *a purely negative* concept both according to its historical origin and its methodological meaning, and this is not a sufficient basis to unite something. Empirical means first of all "psychology without a soul" (Lange), psychology without any metaphysics (Vvedensky), psychology based on experience (Høffding). It is hardly necessary to explain that these are *essentially* negative definitions as well. They do not say a word about *what psychology is dealing with,* what is its positive meaning.

However, the objective meaning of this negative definition is now completely different from what it used to be. Once it concealed nothing—the task of the science was to liberate itself from *something,* the term was a slogan for that. Now it *conceals* the positive definitions (which each author introduces in his science) and the genuine processes taking place in the science. It was a temporary slogan and could not be anything else in principle. Now the term "empirical" attached to psychology designates the *refusal* to select a certain philosophical principle, the refusal to clarify one's ultimate premises, to become aware of one's own scientific nature. As such this refusal has its historical meaning and cause—we will dwell upon it below—but about the nature of the science it says essentially nothing, it conceals it. The Kantian thinker Vvedensky (1917, p. 3) expressed this most clearly, but *all* empiricists subscribe to his formula. Høffding, in particular, says the same. All more or less lean towards one side—Vvedensky provides the ideal balance: *"Psychology must formulate all its conclusions in such a way that they will be equally acceptable and equally binding for both materialism, spiritualism, and psychophysical monism."*

From this formula alone it is evident that empiricism formulates its tasks in such a way as to reveal their *impossibility.* Indeed, on the basis of empiricism, i.e., completely discarding basic premises, no scientific knowledge whatever is logically and historically possible. Natural science, which psychology wishes to liken through this definition, was by its nature, its undistorted essence, always *spontaneously materialistic.* All psychologists agree that natural science, like, of course, all human praxis, does not solve the problem of the essence of matter and mind, but starts from a certain solution to it, namely the assumption of an objective reality which exists outside of us, in conformity with certain laws, and which can be known. And this is, as Lenin has frequently pointed out, the very *essence* of materialism. The existence of natural science *qua* science is due to the ability to distinguish in our experience between what exists objectively and independently and what exists subjectively. This is not at variance with the different philosophical interpretations or whole schools in natural science which think idealistically. Natural science *qua* science is in itself, and independently from its proponents, materialistic. Psychology proceeded as spontaneously, despite the different ideas of its proponents, from an idealistic conception.

In reality, *there is not a single* empirical system of psychology. All transcend the boundaries of empiricism and this we can understand as follows: from a purely negative idea one can deduce nothing. Nothing can be born from "abstinence," as Vvedensky has it. In reality, all the systems were rooted in metaphysics and their conclusions were overstated. First Vvedensky himself with his theory of solipsism, i.e., an extreme manifestation of idealism.

Whereas psychoanalysis openly speaks about metapsychology, each psychology without a soul concealed its soul, the psychology without any metaphysics—its metaphysics. The psychology based on experience included what was not based on experience. In short, each psychology had its metapsychology. It might not consciously realize it, but this made no difference. Chelpanov (1924), who more than anyone else in the current debate seeks shelter under the word "empirical" and wants to demarcate his science from the field of philosophy, finds, however, that it must have its philosophical "superstructure" and "substructure." It turns out that there are philosophical concepts which must be examined *before one turns to the study of psychology* and a study which prepares psychology he calls the substructure. This does not prevent him from claiming on the next page that psychology must be freed from all philosophy. However, in the conclusion he once more acknowledges that it is precisely the *methodological problems which are the most acute problems* of *psychology.*

It would be wrong to think that from the concept of empirical psychology we can learn nothing but negative characteristics. It also points to positive processes which take place in our science and which are concealed by this name. With the word "empirical" psychology wants to join the natural sciences. Here all agree. But it is a very specific concept and we must examine what it designates when applied to psychology. In his preface to the encyclopedia, Ribot [1923, p. ix] says (heroically trying to accomplish the agreement and unity of which Lange and Vagner spoke and in so doing showing its impossibility) that psychology forms part of biology, that it is neither materialistic nor spiritualistic, else it would lose all right to be called a science. In what, then, does it differ from other parts of biology? *Only* in that it deals with phenomena which are 'spirituels' and not physical.

What a trifle! Psychology wanted to be a natural science, but one that would deal with things of a very different nature from those natural science is dealing with. But doesn't the nature of the phenomena studied determine the character of the science? Are history, logic, geometry, and history of the theater really possible as natural sciences? And Chelpanov, who insists that psychology should be as empirical as physics, mineralogy etc., naturally does not join Pavlov but immediately starts to vociferate when the attempt is made to realize psychology as a genuine natural science. What is he hushing up in his comparison? He wants psychology to be a natural science about (1) phenomena which are completely different from physical phenomena, and (2) which are conceived in a way that is completely different from the way the objects of the natural sciences are investigated. One may ask what the natural sciences and psychology can have in common if the subject matter and the method of acquiring knowledge are different. And Vvedensky (1917, 300 Chapter 15 p. 3) says, after he has explained the meaning of the empirical character of psychology: "Therefore, contemporary psychology often characterizes itself as a *natural science about mental phenomena or a natural history* of *mental phenomena.*" But this means that psychology wants to be a natural science about unnatural phenomena. It is connected with the natural sciences by a purely *negative* feature—the rejection of metaphysics—and not by a single *positive* one.

James explained the matter brilliantly. Psychology is to be treated as a natural science—that was his main thesis. But no one did as much as James to prove that the mental is "not natural scientific." He explains that all the natural sciences accept some assumptions on faith—natural science proceeds from the materialistic assumption, in spite of the fact that further reflection leads to idealism. Psychology does the same—it accepts other assumptions. Consequently, it is similar to natural science only in that it uncritically accepts some assumptions; the assumptions themselves are contrary [see pp. 9–10 of Burkhardt, 1984].

According to Ribot, this tendency is the main trait of the psychology of the 19th century. Apart from this he mentions the attempts to give psychology its own principle and method (which it was denied by Comte) and to put it in the same relation to biology as biology occupies with respect to physics. But in fact the author acknowledges that what is called psychology consists of several categories of investigations which differ according to their goal and method. And when the authors, in spite of this, attempted to beget* a system of psychology and included Pavlov and Bergson, they demonstrated that this task cannot be realized. And in his conclusion Dumas [1924, p. 1121] formulates that the unity of the 25 authors consisted in the *rejection* of ontological speculation.

It is easy to guess what such a viewpoint leads to: the rejection of ontological speculations, empirism, *when it is consistent,* leads to the rejection of *methodologically constructive principles* in the creation of a system, to eclecticism; insofar as *it is inconsistent,* it leads to a hidden, uncritical, vague methodology. Both possibilities have been brilliantly demonstrated by the French authors. For them Pavlov's psychology of reactions is just as acceptable as introspective psychology if only they are in different chapters of the book. In their manner of describing the facts and stating the problems, even in their vocabulary, the authors of the book show tendencies of associationism, rationalism, Bergsonism, and synthesism. It is further explained that Bergson's conception is applied in some chapters, the language of associationism and atomism in others, behaviorism in still others, etc. The "Traité" wants to be impartial, objective, and complete. If it has not always been successful, Dumas [1924, p. 1156] concludes, at least the difference of opinion testifies to intellectual activity and ultimately in that sense it represents its time and country. We couldn't agree more.

This disagreement—we have seen how far it goes—only convinces usof the fact that an impartial psychology is impossible today, leaving aside the fatal dualism of the "Traité de psychologie" for which psychology is now part of biology, now stands to it as biology itself stands to physics.

Thus, the concept of empirical psychology contains an insoluble methodological contradiction. It is a natural science about unnatural things, a tendency to develop with the methods of natural science, i.e., proceeding from totally opposite premises, a system of knowledge which is contrary to them. This had a fatal influence upon the methodological construction of empirical psychology and broke its back.

*Two psychologies exist*—a natural scientific, materialistic one and a spiritualistic one. This thesis expresses the meaning of the crisis more correctly than the thesis about the existence of *many* psychologies. For *psychologies* we have *two*, i.e., two different, irreconcilable types of science, *two* fundamentally different constructions of systems of knowledge. All the rest is a difference in views, schools, hypotheses: individual, very complex, confused, mixed, blind, chaotic combinations which are at times very difficult to understand. But the real struggle only takes place between two tendencies which lie and operate behind all the struggling currents.

That this is so, that two psychologies, and not many psychologies, make up the meaning of the crisis, that all the rest is a struggle *within* each of these two psychologies, a struggle which has quite another meaning and operational field, that the creation of a general psychology is not a matter of agreement, but of a rupture—all this methodology realized long ago and *nobody contests it.* (The difference of this thesis from Kornilov's three directions resides *in the whole range of the meaning of the crisis:* (1) the concepts of materialistic psychology and reflexology do not coincide (as he says); (2) the concepts of empirical and idealistic psychology do not coincide (as he says), (3) our evaluation of the role of Marxist psychology differs.) Finally, here we are dealing with two tendencies which show up in the struggle between the multitude of concrete currents and within them. Nobody contests that the general psychology will not be a third psychology added to the two struggling parties, but one of them.

That the concept of empiricism contains a methodological conflict which a self-reflective theory must solve in order to make investigation possible—this idea was made well known by Münsterberg [1920]. In his capital methodological work he declared that this book does not conceal the fact that it wants to be a militant book, it defends idealism against naturalism. It wants to guarantee an unlimited right for idealism in psychology. He lays the theoretical epistemological foundations of empirical psychology and declares that this is the most important thing the psychology of our day needs. Its main concepts have been gathered haphazardly, its logical means of acquiring knowledge have been left to the instinct. Münsterberg's theme is the synthesis of Fichte's ethical idealism with the physiological psychology of our day, for the victory of idealism does not reside in its dissociating itself from empirical investigation, but in finding a place for it in its own area. Münsterberg showed that naturalism and idealism are irreconcilable, that is why he talks about a book of militant idealism, says of general psychology that it is bravery and a risk—and not about agreement and unification. And Münsterberg [ibid., p. 10] openly advanced the idea of the existence of two sciences, arguing that psychology finds itself in the strange position that we know incomparably more about psychological facts than we ever did, but much less about the question as to what psychology actually is.

The unity of external methods cannot conceal from us that the different psychologists are talking about a totally different psychology. This internal disturbance can only be understood and overcome in the following way.

> The psychology of our day is struggling with the prejudice that only one type of psychology exists. . . . The concept of psychology involves two totally different scientific tasks, which must be distinguished in principle and for which we can best use special designations since, in reality, there are two kinds of psychology [ibid., p. 10].

In contemporary science all sorts of forms and types of mixing two sciences into a seeming unity are represented. What these sciences have in common is their object, but this does not say anything about these sciences themselves. Geology, geography, and agronomics all study the earth, but their construction, their principle of scientific knowledge differs. We may through description change the mind into a chain of causes and actions and may picture it as a combination of elements—objectively and subjectively. If we carry both conceptions to the extreme and give them a scientific form we will get two "fundamentally different theoretical disciplines. . . . One is causal, the other is teleological and intentional psychology" [ibid., pp. 12–13].

The existence of two psychologies is so obvious that it is accepted by all. The disagreement is only about the precise definition of each science. Some emphasize some nuances, others emphasize others. It would be very interesting to follow all these oscillations, because each of them testifies to some objective tendency, to a striving toward one or the other pole, and the scope, the range of contradictions shows that both types of science, like two butterflies in one cocoon, still exist in the form of as yet undifferentiated tendencies.

But now we are not interested in the contradictions, but in the common factor that lies behind them.

We are confronted with two questions: what is the common nature of both sciences and what are the causes which have led to the *bifurcation* of *empiricism into naturalism and idealism?*

*All agree* that precisely these two elements lie at the basis of the two sciences, that, consequently, one is natural scientific psychology, and the other is idealistic psychology, whatever the different authors may call them. Following Münsterberg all view the difference not in the material or subject matter, but in the way of acquiring knowledge, in the principle. The question is whether to understand the phenomena in terms of causality, in connection with and having fundamentally the same meaning as all other phenomena, or intentionally, as spiritual activity, which is oriented towards a goal and exempt from all material connections. Dilthey [1894/1977, pp. 37–41], who calls these sciences explanatory and descriptive psychology, traces the bifurcation to Wolff, who divided psychology into rational and empirical psychology, i.e., to the very origin of empirical psychology. He shows that the division has always been present during the whole course of development of the science and again became explicit in the school of Herbart (1849) and in the works of Waitz. The method of explanatory psychology is identical to that of natural science, Its postulate—there is not a single mental phenomenon without a physical one—leads to its bankruptcy as an independent science and its affairs are transferred into the hands of physiology (ibid.). Descriptive and explanatory psychology do not have the same meaning as systematics and explanation—its two basic parts according to Binswanger (1922) as well—have in the natural sciences.

Contemporary psychology—this doctrine of a soul without a soul—is intrinsically contradictory, is divided into two parts. Descriptive psychology does not seek explanation, but description and understanding. What the poets, Shakespeare in particular, presented in images, it makes the subject of analysis in concepts. Explanatory, natural scientific psychology cannot lie at the basis of a science about the mind, it develops a deterministic criminal law, does not leave any room for freedom, cannot be reconciled with the problem of culture. In contrast, descriptive psychology will become the foundation of the human studies, as mathematics is that of the natural sciences [Dilthey, 1894/1977, p. 74].

Stout [1909, pp. 2–6] openly refuses to call analytic psychology a physical science. It is a positive science in the sense that it investigates matter of fact, reality, what is and is not a norm, not what ought to be. It stands next to mathematics, the natural sciences, theory of knowledge. But it is not a physical science. Between the mental and the physical there is such a gulf that there is no means of tracing their connections. No science of matter stands to psychology in a relation analogous to that in which chemistry and physics stand to biology, i.e., in a relation of more general to more special, but in principle homogeneous, principles.

Binswanger [1922, p. 22] divides *all* problems of methodology into those due to a natural scientific and those due to a non-natural scientific concept of the mind. He openly and clearly explains that there are two radically different psychologies, Referring to Sigwart he calls the struggle against natural psychology the source of the split. This leads us to the phenomenology of experiencing, the basis of Husserl's pure logic and empirical, but non-natural scientific psychology (Pfänder, Jaspers).

Bleuler defends the opposite position. He rejects Wundt's opinion that psychology is not a natural science and, following Rickert, he calls it a generalizing psychology, although he has in mind what Dilthey called explanatory or constructive psychology.

We will not thoroughly examine the question as to *how* psychology as a natural science is possible and the concepts by means of which it is constructed—all this belongs to the debate *within one* psychology and it forms the subject of the positive exposition in the next part of our work. What is more, we also leave open another question—whether psychology really is a natural science in the exact sense of the word. Following the European authors we use this word to designate the materialistic nature of this kind of knowledge as clearly as possible. Insofar as Western European psychology did not know or hardly knew the problems of social psychology, this kind of knowledge was thought to coincide with natural science. But to demonstrate that psychology is possible as a materialistic science is still a special and very deep problem, which does not, however, belong to the problem of the meaning of the crisis as a whole.

Almost all Russian authors who have written anything of importance about psychology accept the division—from hearsay, of course—which shows the extent to which these ideas are generally accepted in European psychology. Lange (1914), who mentions the disagreement between Windelband and Rickert on the one hand (who regard psychology as a natural science) and Wundt and Dilthey on the other, is inclined with the latter authors to distinguish two sciences. It is remarkable that he criticizes Natorp as an exponent of the idealistic conception of psychology and contrasts him with a realistic or biological understanding. However, according to Münsterberg, Natorp has from the very beginning demanded the same thing he did, i.e., a subjectivating and an objectivating science of the mind, i.e., two sciences.

Lange merged both viewpoints into a single postulate and expounded both irreconcilable tendencies in his book, considering that the meaning of the crisis resides in the struggle with associationism. He explains Dilthey and Münsterberg with real sympathy and states that "two different psychologies resulted." Like Janus, psychology showed two different faces: one turned to physiology and natural science, the other to the sciences of the spirit, history, sociology; one science about causal effects, the other about values (ibid., p. 63). It would seem that what remains is to opt for *one of the two,* but Lange unites them.

Chelpanov proceeded in the same way. In his current polemics he implores us to believe him that psychology is a materialistic science, refers to James as his witness and does not with a single word mention that in the Russian literature the idea of two sciences belongs to *him.* This deserves further reflection.

Following Dilthey, Stout, Meinong, and Husserl he explains the idea of the analytic method. Whereas the inductive method is distinctive of natural scientific psychology, descriptive psychology is characterized by the analytic method which leads to the knowledge of *a priori* ideas. Analytic psychology is the *basic* psychology. It must precede the development of child psychology, zoopsychology, and objective experimental psychology and provide the foundation for all types of psychological investigation. This does not look like the relation of mineralogy to physics, or like the complete separation of psychology from philosophy and idealism.

To show *what kind* of jump Chelpanov made in his psychological views since 1922, one must not dwell upon his general philosophical statements and accidental phrases, but upon his theory of the analytic method. Chelpanov protests against mixing the tasks of explanatory psychology with those of descriptive psychology and explains that they are absolutely contradictory. In order not to leave any doubt about the question as to which psychology he regards as of primary importance, he connects it with Husserl's phenomenology, with his theory of ideal essences, and explains that Husserl's *eidos* or essence is basically equivalent to Plato's ideas. For Husserl, phenomenology stands to descriptive psychology as mathematics does to physics. Phenomenology and mathematics are, like geometry, sciences about essences, about ideal possibilities; descriptive psychology and physics are about facts. Phenomenology makes explanatory and descriptive psychology possible.

Despite Husserl's opinion, for Chelpanov phenomenology and analytic psychology partially overlap and the phenomenological method is completely identical with the analytic method. Chelpanov explains Husserl's refusal to regard eidetic psychology and phenomenology as being identical in the following way. By contemporary psychology he understands only empirical, i.e., inductive psychology, despite the fact that it also contains phenomenological truths. Thus, there is no need to separate phenomenology from psychology. The phenomenological method must be laid at the basis of the objective experimental methods, which Chelpanov timidly defends against Husserl. This is the way it was, this is the way it will be, the author concludes.

How can we square this with his claim that psychology is only empirical, excludes idealism by its very nature and is independent from philosophy?

We can summarize. Whatever the division in question is called, whatever shades of meaning in each term are emphasized, the basic essence of the question remains the same and it can be reduced to two propositions.

1. In psychology empiricism indeed proceeded just as spontaneously from idealistic premises as natural science did from materialistic ones, i.e., empirical psychology was idealistic in its foundation.

2. For certain reasons (to be considered below), in the era of the crisis empiricism split into idealistic and materialistic psychology. Münsterberg (1920, p. 14), too, interprets

the difference in terminology as unity of meaning. We can speak of causal and intentional psychology, or about the psychology of the spirit and the psychology of consciousness, or about understanding and explanatory psychology. But the only thing of principal importance is that we recognize the dual nature of psychology. Elsewhere Münsterberg [1920, pp. vii–viii] contrasts the psychology of the contents of consciousness with the psychology of the spirit, the psychology of contents with the psychology of acts, and the psychology of sensations with intentional psychology.

We have basically reached an opinion which established itself in our science long ago: psychology has a deeply dualistic nature which pervades its whole development. We have, thus, arrived at an indisputably historic situation. The history of the science does not belong to our tasks and we may leave aside the question as to the historical roots of dualism and confine ourselves to pointing out this fact and explaining the proximate causes which led to the exacerbation and bifurcation of dualism in the crisis. It is, essentially, the fact that psychology is attracted to two poles, this intrinsic presence of a "psychoteleology" and a "psychobiology," which Dessoir [1911, p. 230] called the singing in two voices of contemporary psychology, and which in his opinion will never cease.

12

Now we must briefly dwell upon the proximate causes or driving forces of the crisis.

Which factors lead us to the crisis, the rupture, and which passively *experience* it as an inevitable evil? Naturally, we will dwell here only upon the driving forces *within* our science, leaving all others aside. We are justified in doing so, because the external—social and ideological—causes and phenomena are, one way or the other, represented in the final analysis by forces within the science, and they act through them. It is our intention, therefore, to analyze the proximate causes lying within the science and to refrain from a deeper analysis.

Let us say right away that *the main driving force of the crisis in its final phase is the development of applied psychology as a whole.*

The attitude of academic psychology toward applied psychology has up until not remained somewhat disdainful as if it had to do with a semi-exact science. Not everything is well in this area of psychology, there is no doubt about that, but nevertheless there can be no doubt for an observer who takes a bird-eye's view, i.e., the methodologist, that the leading role in the development of our science belongs to applied psychology. It represents everything of psychology which is progressive, sound, which contains a germ of the future. It provides the best methodological works. It is only by studying this area that one can come to an understanding of the meaning of what is going on and the possibility of a genuine psychology.

The center has shifted in the history of science: what was at the periphery became the center of the circle. One can say about applied psychology what can be said about philosophy which was rejected by empirical psychology: "the stone which the builders rejected is become the head stone of the corner."

We can elucidate this by referring to three aspects. The first is *practice*. Here psychology was *first* (through industrial psychology, psychiatry, child psychology, and criminal psychology) confronted with a highly developed—industrial, educational, political, or military—practice. This confrontation compels psychology to reform its principles so that they may withstand the highest test of practice. It forces us to accommodate and introduce into our science the supply of practical psychological experiences and skills which has been gathered over thousands of years; for the church, the military, politics, and industry, insofar as they have consciously regulated and organized the mind, base themselves on an experience which is enormous, although not well ordered from the scientific viewpoint (every psychologist experienced the reforming influence of applied science). For the development of psychology, applied psychology plays the same role as medicine did for anatomy and physiology and technique for the physical sciences. The importance of the new practical psychology for the *whole* science cannot be exaggerated. The psychologist might dedicate a hymn to it.

A psychology which is called upon to confirm the truth of its thinking in practice, which attempts not so much to explain the mind but to understand and master it, gives the practical disciplines a fundamentally different place in the whole structure of the science than the former psychology did. There practice was the colony of theory, dependent in all its aspects on the metropolis. Theory was in no way dependent on practice. Practice was the conclusion, the application, an excursion beyond the boundaries of science, an operation which lay outside science and came after science, which began after the scientific operation was considered completed. Success or failure had practically no effect on the fate of the theory. Now the situation is the opposite. Practice pervades the deepest foundations of the scientific operation and reforms it from beginning to end. Practice sets the tasks and serves as the supreme judge of theory, as its truth criterion. It dictates how to construct the concepts and how to formulate the laws.

This leads us directly to the *second aspect, to methodology.* However strange and paradoxical it may seem at first glance, it is precisely practice as the constructive principle of science which requires a philosophy, i.e. a methodology of science. This does not in any way contradict the frivolous, "lighthearted" (in the words of Münsterberg) relation of psychotechnics to its principles. In reality, both the practice and the methodology of psychotechnics are often amazingly helpless, weak, superficial, and at times ludicrous. Psychotechnic diagnoses are vacuous and remind us of the physicians's reflections about medicine in Molière. The methodology of psychotechnics is invented *ad hoc* each time and lacks critical sense. It is often called picnic psychology, i.e., it is something light, temporary, half-serious. All this is true. But it does not for one moment change the fundamental state of affairs, that it is exactly this psychology which will create an iron methodology. As Münsterberg [1920, p. v] says, not only the general part, but also the examination of particular questions will force us time and again to investigate the principles of psychotechnics.

That is why I assert: despite the fact that it has compromised itself more than once, *that its practical meaning is very close to zero and the theory often ludicrous, its methodological meaning is enormous.* The principle and philosophy of practice is—once again—the stone which the builders rejected and which became the head stone of the corner. Here we have the whole meaning of the crisis.

Binswanger [1922, p. 50] says that we do not expect to get the solution to the most general question—the supreme question of all psychology, the problem which includes all problems of psychology, the question of subjectivating and objectivating psychology-from logic, epistemology, or metaphysics, but from methodology, i.e., the theory of scientific method. We would say: from the methodology of psychotechnics, i.e., the *philosophy* of *practice*. The practical and theoretical value of Binet's measuring scale or other psychotechnic tests may be obviously insignificant, the test bad in itself, but as an idea, a methodological principle, a task, a perspective it is enormous. The most complex contradictions of psychological methodology are transferred to the grounds of practice and only there can they be solved. There the debate stops being fruitless, it comes to an end. "Method" means "way," we view it as a means of knowledge acquisition. But in all its points the way is determined by the goal to which it leads. That is why practice reforms the whole methodology of the science.

The *third aspect* of the reforming role of psychotechnics may be understood from the first two. It is that psychotechnics *is a one-sided* psychology, it instigates a rupture and creates a real psychology. Psychiatry too transcends the boundaries of idealistic psychology. One cannot treat or cure relying on introspection. One can hardly carry this idea to a more absurd consequence than when applying it to psychiatry. Psychotechnics also realized, as was observed by Spiel'rejn, that it cannot separate psychological functions from physiological ones, and it is searching for an integral concept. About psychologists who demand inspiration from teachers, I have written that hardly any one of them would entrust the control of a ship to the captain's inspiration or the management of a factory to the engineer's enthusiasm. Each of them would select a professional sailor and an experienced technician. And these highest possible requirements for the science, this most serious practice, will revive psychology. Industry and the military, education and treatment will revive and reform the science. Husserl's eidetic psychology, which is not interested in the truth of its claims, is not fit for the selection of tram-drivers. Neither is the contemplation of essences fit for that goal, even values are without interest. But all this will not in the least protect it against a catastrophe. The goal of such a psychology is not Shakespeare in concepts, as it was for Dilthey, but *in one word psychotechnics,* i.e., a scientific theory which would lead to the subordination and mastery of the mind, to the artificial control of behavior.

And it is Münsterberg, this militant idealist, who lays the foundations for psychotechnics, i.e., a materialistic psychology in the highest sense of the word. Stern, no less enthusiastic about idealism, is elaborating a methodology for differential psychology and reveals with fatal precision the untenability of idealistic psychology.

How could it happen that extreme idealists play into the hands of materialism? It shows that the two struggling tendencies are deeply and with objective necessity rooted in the development of psychology; how little they coincide with what the psychologist says about himself, i.e., with his subjective philosophical convictions; how inexpressibly complex the picture of the crisis is; in what mixed forms both tendencies meet; what tortuous, unexpected, paradoxical zigzags the front line in psychology makes, frequently *within* one and the same system, frequently *within* one term. Finally, it shows that *the struggle between the two psychologies does not coincide with the struggle between the many conceptions and psychological schools, but stands behind them and determines them.* It shows how deceptive the external forms of the crisis are and that we need to take account of the genuine meaning behind them.

Let us turn to Münsterberg [1920, p. ix]. The question of causal psychology's legitimacy is of decisive importance for psychotechnics.

> This one-sided causal psychology only now comes into its own . . . explanatory psychol-
> ogy is the answer to an unnatural, artificial question; mental life requires understanding, not
> explanation. Psychotechnics, however, which can only work with a causal psychology, tes-
> tifies to the necessity of such an artificial statement of the question and legitimatizes it. The
> genuine meaning of explanatory psychology is only revealed in psychotechnics and, thus,
> the whole system of the psychological sciences culminates in it.

It is difficult to demonstrate the objective force of this tendency and the non-coincidence of the
philosopher's convictions with the objective meaning of his work more clearly: materialistic psychology is unnatural, says the idealist, but *I am forced* to work with precisely *such a psychology*.

Psychotechnics is oriented toward action, practice—and there we act in a way which is
fundamentally different from purely theoretical understanding and explanation. That is why
psychotechnics *cannot* hesitate in the selection of the psychology it needs (not even when it is
elaborated by consistent idealists). It is dealing exclusively with causal, objective psychology.
Non-causal psychology plays no role whatsoever for psychotechnics.

It is precisely this situation that is of decisive importance for all psychotechnical sciences. It
is consciously one-sided. It is the only empirical science in the full sense of the word. It is-inevitably—
a comparative science. The link with physical processes is for this science so fundamental that it
is a physiological psychology. It is an experimental science. And its general formula is

> We proceeded from the assumption that the only psychology relevant for psychotechnics
> must be a descriptive-explanatory science. We may now add that, on top of that, it must be
> an empirical, comparative science which takes physiology into account, and which, finally,
> is experimental [Münsterberg, 1920, p. 18].

This means that psychotechnics introduces a revolution in the development of the science
and marks an era in its development. From this viewpoint Münsterberg [ibid., p. 19] says
that empirical psychology hardly *originated* before the second half of the 19th century. Even in
the schools which rejected metaphysics and studied the facts research was guided by another
interest. Application [of the experiment; Soviet eds.] was impossible as long as psychology did
not become a natural science, But along with the introduction of the experiment there evolved
a paradoxical situation which would be unthinkable in the natural sciences: equipment equivalent to the first steam engine or the telegraph was well known in the laboratories, but not
applied in practice. Education and law, trade and industry, social life and medicine were
uninfluenced by this movement. To this very day it is considered a profanation of the investigation to connect it with practice and it is advised to wait until psychology has completed its
theoretical system. But the experience of the natural sciences tells us another story. Medicine
and technique did not wait until anatomy and physics celebrated their ultimate triumphs. It
is not only that life needs psychology and practices it in different forms everywhere: we must
also expect an upsurge in psychology from this contact with life.

Of course, Münsterberg would not be an idealist if he accepted this situation as it is and did
not retain a special area for the unlimited rights of idealism. He merely transfers the debate to another
area when he accepts the untenability of idealism in the area of a causal psychology that feeds on
practice. He explains this "epistemological tolerance" [ibid., p. 31] and deduces it from an idealistic understanding of the essence of science which does not seek for the distinction "between true

and false concepts, but between those suited or not suited for certain ultimate hypothetical [gedankliche] goals" [ibid., p. 29]. He believes that a temporary truce between psychologists can be established as soon as they leave the battlefield of psychological theory [ibid., p. 31].

Münsterberg's work is a striking example of the internal discord between a methodology determined by science and a philosophy determined by a world view, precisely because he is a methodologist who is consistent to the very end and a philosopher who is consistent to the very end, i.e., a contradictory thinker to the very end. He understands that in being a materialist in causal psychology and an idealist in teleological psychology he arrives at some sort of double-entry bookkeeping which inevitably must be unscrupulous, because the entries on the one side are different from those on the other side. For in the end only one truth is conceivable. But for him the truth is not life itself, but the logical elaboration of life, and the latter can vary, as it is determined by many viewpoints [ibid., pp. 42–43]. He understands that empirical science does not require the rejection of an epistemological point of view, but a *certain theory*, but in various sciences different epistemological viewpoints are possible. In the interest of practice we express the truth in one language, in another in the interests of the mind [Geist].

When natural scientists have differences of opinion these do not touch upon the fundamental assumptions of the science.

> It is no problem at all for a botanist to communicate about his subject with all other plant researchers. No botanist bothers to stop to answer the question what it actually means that plants live in space and time and are ruled by causal laws [ibid., p. 28].

But the nature of psychological material does not allow us to separate the psychological propositions from philosophical theories to the extent that other empirical sciences have managed to do that.

> The psychologist fundamentally deceives himself when he imagines that his laboratory work can lead him to the solution of the basic questions of his science; they belong to philosophy. The psychologist who does not want to join the philosophical debate about fundamental questions must simply tacitly accept one or the other epistemological theory as the basis of his particular investigations [ibid., p. 29].

It was exactly epistemological tolerance and not a rejection of epistemology which led Münsterberg to the idea of two psychologies, one of which contradicts the other, but both of which can be accepted by the philosopher. After all, tolerance does not stand for atheism. In the mosque he is a Mohammedan, but in the cathedral a Christian.

There is only one fundamental misunderstanding that may arise: that the idea of a dualistic psychology leads to the *partial* acceptance of the rights of causal psychology, that the dualism is transferred into psychology itself, which is divided into two phases; that *Münsterberg proclaimed tolerance also within* causal psychology. *But this is absolutely not the case.* This is what he [ibid., p. 15] says:

> The fundamental question as to whether a psychology that thinks along teleological lines may really exist alongside a causal psychology, whether in scientific psychology we can and should deal with apperception, task awareness, affect, will, or thought in a teleological fashion, does not concern the psychotechnician, for he knows that we can always somehow

handle these events and mental performances in the language of causal psychology and that psychotechnics can only deal with this causal conception.

Thus, the two psychologies do not overlap, do not supplement each other, but they serve *two* truths, one in the interest of practice, the other in the interest of mind *[Geist]*. Double-entry bookkeeping is practiced in Münsterberg's world view, but not in psychology. The materialist will *fully* accept Münsterberg's conception of causal psychology and will reject dualism in science. The idealist will reject dualism as well and will *fully* accept the conception of a teleological psychology. Münsterberg himself proclaims epistemological tolerance and accepts both sciences, but elaborates one of them as materialist and the other as idealist. Thus, the debate and the dualism exist beyond the boundaries of causal psychology. It is not part of anything and *in itself* does not form part of any science.

This instructive example of the fact that in science idealism is *forced* to find its grounds in materialism is fully confirmed by the example of *any* other thinker.

Stern followed the same path. He was led to objective psychology through the problems of differential investigation, which is likewise one of the main reasons for the new psychology. We do not investigate thinkers, however, but their fate, i.e., the objective processes that stand behind them and control them. And these are not revealed through induction, but through analysis. In the words of Engels [1925/1978, p. 496] one steam engine demonstrates the law of transformation of energy no less convincingly than 100,000 engines. We add as a mere curiosity that in the preface to the translation of Münsterberg the Russian idealistic psychologists list among his merits that he meets the aspiration of the psychology of behavior and the requirements of an integral approach of man without pulverizing man's psychophysical organization into atoms. What the great idealists accomplish as a tragedy, the small ones repeat as a farce.

We can summarize. We view the cause of the crisis as its driving force, which is therefore not only of historical interest, but also of primary—methodological—importance, as it not only led to the development of the crisis, but continues determining its further course and fate. This cause lies in the development of applied psychology, which has led toward the reform of the whole methodology of the science on the basis of the principle of practice, i.e., towards its transformation into a natural science. This principle is pressing psychology heavily and pushing it to split into two sciences. It guarantees the right development of materialistic psychology in the future. Practice and philosophy are becoming the head stone of the corner.

Many psychologists have viewed the introduction of the experiment as a fundamental reform of psychology and have even equated experimental and scientific psychology. They predicted that the future would belong solely to experimental psychology and have viewed this epithet as a most important methodological principle. But in psychology the experiment remained on the level of a technical device, it was not utilized in a fundamental way and it led, in the case of Ach for instance, to its own negation. Nowadays many psychologists see a way out *in methodology,* in the correct formation of principles. They expect salvation from the other end. But their work is fruitless as well. Only a fundamental rejection of the blind empiricism which is trailing behind immediate introspectional experience and which is internally split into two parts; only the emancipation from introspection, its exclusion just like the exclusion of the eye in physics; only a rupture and the selection of a single psychology will provide the way out of the crisis. The dialectic unity of methodology and practice, applied to psychology from two sides, is the fate and destiny of one of the psychologies. A complete severance from practice and the contemplation of ideal essences is the destiny and fate of the other. A complete rupture and separation is their common destiny and fate. This rupture began, continues, and will be completed along the lines of *practice*.

## 13

However obvious the historical and methodological dogma about the growing gap between the two psychologies as the formula for the dynamics of the crisis may seem after our analysis, it is disputed by many. In itself this is of no concern to us. The tendencies we found seem to us to express the truth, because they exist objectively and do not depend on the views of some author. On the contrary, they themselves determine these views insofar as they become psychological views and are involved in the process of the science's development.

That is why we should not be surprised to find that different views exist on this account. From the very beginning we have not set ourselves the task to investigate views, but what these views are aimed at. It is this that distinguishes a critical investigation of the views of some author from the methodological analysis of the problem itself. But we must nevertheless pay attention to one thing: we are not entirely indifferent as to views; we must be able to *explain* them, to lay bare their objective, their inner logic. To put it more simply, we must be able to present each struggle between views as a complex expression of the struggle between the two psychologies. On the whole, this is a critical task which should be *based* on the present analysis and it should show for the most important psychological currents *what* the dogma found by us can yield toward understanding them. But to show its *possibility*, to establish the fundamental course of the analysis, forms part of our present task.

This can be done most easily by analyzing those systems which openly side with one or the other tendency or even merge them. But it is much more difficult and therefore more attractive to demonstrate it for those systems which in principle place themselves *outside* the struggle, outside these two tendencies, which seek a way out in a third tendency and seemingly reject our dogma about the existence of only two paths for psychology. They say there is a third way: the two struggling tendencies may be merged, or one of them may be subjected to the other, or both may be totally removed and a new one created, or both may be subjected to a third one, etc. For the confirmation of our dogma it is in principle extremely important to show *where* this third way leads, as the dogma stands or falls with it.

Following the method we adopted we will examine how both objective tendencies operate in the conceptual systems of the adherents of a third way. Are they bridled or do they remain masters of the situation? In short, who is leading, the horse or the horseman?

First of all, we will clearly distinguish between conceptions and tendencies. A conception may identify itself with a certain tendency and nevertheless not coincide with it. Thus, behaviorism is right when it asserts that a scientific psychology is only possible as a natural science. This does not mean, however, that it has *realized* psychology as a natural science, that it has not compromised this idea. For each conception the tendency is a *task* and not something given. To realize what the task is does not yet imply the ability to solve it. Different conceptions may exist on the basis of one tendency, and in one conception both tendencies may be represented to different degrees.

With this precise demarcation in mind we may proceed to the systems which advocate a third way. Very many of them exist. However, the majority belong either to blind men who unconsciously mix the two ways up, or to deliberate eclectics who run from path to path. Let us pass them by; we are interested in principles, not in their distortions. There are three of these fundamentally pure systems: Gestalt theory, personalism, and Marxist psychology. Let us examine them from the point of view that fits our goal. All three schools share the conviction that psychology as a science is neither possible on the basis of empirical psychology, nor on the basis of behaviorism and that there is a third way which stands above these two ways and which allows us to realize a scientific psychology which does not reject either of the two approaches but unites them into a single whole. Each system solves this task in its own way and each has its own fate, but together they exhaust *all* logical possibilities of a third way, as if it were a methodological experiment especially designed for this purpose.

Gestalt theory solves this problem by introducing the basic concept of structure (Gestalt), which combines both the functional and the descriptive side of behavior, i.e., it is a *psychophysical* concept. To combine both aspects in the subject matter of one science is only possible if one finds something fundamental which both have *in common* and makes this *common factor* the subject of study. For if we accept mind and body as two different things which are separated by an abyss and do not coincide in a single aspect, then, naturally, a single science about these two absolutely distinct things will be impossible. This is the crux of the whole methodology of the new theory. The Gestalt principle is equally applicable *to the whole of nature*. It is not only a property of the mind; the principle has a psychophysical character. It is applicable to physiology, physics and in general to all real sciences. Mind is only *part* of behavior, conscious processes are part-processes of larger wholes [Koffka, 1924, p. 160]. Wertheimer (1925, p. 7) is even clearer about this. The formula of the whole Gestalt theory can be reduced to the following: *what takes place in a part of some whole is determined by the internal structural laws of this whole.* "This is Gestalt theory, no more and no less." The psychologist Köhler [1920] showed that in principle the same processes take place in physics. *Methodologically* this is a striking fact and for Gestalt theory it is a decisive argument. The investigative principle is identical for the mental, organic, and non-organic. This means that psychology is connected with the natural sciences, that psychological investigation is possible on the basis of physical principles. Gestalt theory does not view the mental and physical as absolutely heterogenous things which are combined in a meaningless way, but instead asserts their connection. They are parts of one whole. Only persons belonging to recent European culture can divide the mental and the physical as we do. A person is dancing. Do we really have a sum-total of muscular movements on the one hand and joy and inspiration on the other? The two sides are structurally similar. Consciousness brings nothing fundamentally new which would require other investigative methods. Where is the boundary between materialism and idealism? There are psychological theories and even many textbooks which, despite the fact that they only talk about the elements of consciousness, are more devoid of mind and sense and are more torpid and materialistic than a growing tree.

What does all this mean? Only that Gestalt theory realizes a materialistic psychology insofar as it fundamentally and methodologically consistently lays down its system. This is *seemingly* in contradiction with Gestalt theory's doctrine about phenomenal reactions, about introspection, but only seemingly, because for these psychologists the mind is the phenomenal *part of behavior,* i.e., in principle they choose *one of the two ways* and not a third one.

Another question is whether this theory advances its view consistently, whether it does not run against contradictions in its conceptions, whether the means to realize this third way have been chosen correctly. But this does not interest us here, only the methodological system of principles. And we can add to this that everything in the conceptions of Gestalt theory which does not coincide with this tendency is a manifestation of the other tendency. When the mind is described in the same concepts as physics we have the way of natural scientific psychology.

It is easy to show that Stern [1919] in his theory of personalism follows the opposite path of development. In his wish to avoid the two ways and to defend a third, he in reality also defends *only one of the two ways:* the way of idealistic psychology. He proceeds from the assumption that we do not have a psychology, but many psychologies. In order to preserve the subject of psychology in the perspective of both tendencies he introduces the concept of psychophysically neutral acts and functions and ends up with the following hypothesis: the mental and the physical go through identical levels of development. The division is secondary, it arises from the fact that the personality may appear before itself and before others. The basic fact is the existence of the psychophysically neutral person and his psychophysically neutral acts. Thus, unity is reached by the introduction of the concept of the psychophysically neutral act.

Let us consider what is in reality hidden behind this formula. It turns out that Stern follows a road opposite to the one known to us from Gestalt theory. For him the organism and even an organic systems are also psychophysical neutral persons. Plants, the solar system, and man must in principle be understood identically, by extending the teleological principle to the non-mental world. We are faced with a teleological psychology. Once again a third way proved to be *one of the two* well-known ways. Once again we are talking about personalism's methodology; about the question what a psychology created according to these principles would look like. What it is in reality is another question. In reality, Stern is forced, like Münsterberg, to be an adherent of causal psychology in differential psychology. In reality, he provides a materialist conception of consciousness, i.e., within his system that same struggle is still going on which is well known to us and which he, unsuccessfully, wished to overcome.

The third system which attempts to defend a third way is the system of Marxist psychology which is developing before our eyes. It is difficult to analyze, because it does not yet have its own methodology and attempts to find it ready-made in the haphazard psychological statements of the founders of Marxism, not to mention the fact that to find a ready-made formula of the mind in the writings of others would mean to demand "science before science itself." It must be remarked that the heterogeneity of the material, its fragmentary nature, the change of meaning of phrases taken out of context and the polemical character of the majority of the pronouncements—correct in their contradiction of a false idea, but empty and general as a positive definition of the task—do not allow us to expect of this work anything more than a pile of more or less accidental citations and their Talmudic interpretation. But citations, even when they have been well ordered, never yield systems.

Another formal shortcoming of such work is the mixing up of two goals in these investigations. For it is one thing to examine the Marxist doctrine from the historical-philosophical point of view and quite another one to investigate the problems themselves which these thinkers stated. If they are combined, a double disadvantage results: some particular author is used to solve the problem, the problem is stated only on a scale and in a context which fits this author, who is dealing with it *in passing* and for quite another reason. The distorted statement of the question deals with its accidental aspects, does not touch on its core, does not develop it *in a way* which the essence of the question requires.

The fear of verbal contradiction leads to a confusion of epistemological and methodological viewpoints, etc.

But neither can the second goal—the study of the author—be attained via this road, because the author is willy-nilly being modernized, is drawn into the present debate, and, most importantly, is grossly distorted by arbitrarily combining into a system citations found in different places. We might put it as follows: they are looking, firstly, *in the wrong place;* secondly, *for the wrong thing;* thirdly, *in the wrong manner.*

*In the wrong place,* because neither in Plekhanov nor in any of the other Marxists can one find *what one is looking for,* for not only do they not have an accomplished methodology of psychology, they do not even have the beginnings of one. For them this problem never arose, and their utterances concerning this theme have first of all a nonpsychological character. They do not even have an epistemological theory about the way to know the mental. As if it were really such a simple matter to create so much as a hypothesis about the psychophysical relation! Plekhanov would have inscribed his name in the history of philosophy next to that of Spinoza had he himself created some psychophysical theory. He could not do that, because he himself never dealt with psychophysiology and science could not yet give occasion to the construction of such a hypothesis.

Behind Spinoza's hypothesis was the whole of Galileo's physics. Translated into philosophical language, it expressed the whole fundamentally generalized experience of physics which first discovered the unity and regularity of the world. And what in psychology might have engendered such a theory? Plekhanov and others were always interested in their local goals: polemics, explanation, in general, a goal tied to a specific context, not an independent, generalized idea elevated to the level of a theory.

*For the wrong thing,* because what is needed is a methodological system of principles by means of which the investigation can be started and what they are looking for is a fundamental answer, the still vague scientific end point of many years of joint research. If we already had the answer, there would be no need to build a Marxist psychology. The external criterion for the formula we seek must be its methodological suitability. Instead, they are looking for a pompous ontological formula which is as empty and cautious as possible and avoids any solution. What we need is a formula which *would serve us* in research. What they are searching for is a formula which we must serve, which we must prove. As a result they stumble upon formulas—such as negative concepts, etc.—which *paralyze* the investigation. They do not show how we can realize a science proceeding from these accidental formulas.

*In the wrong manner,* because their thinking is fettered by authoritarian principles. They study not methods but dogmas. They do not come any further than stating that two formulas are logically equivalent. They do not approach the matter in a critical, free and investigative way.

But all these three flaws follow from a common cause: a misunderstanding of the historical task of psychology and the meaning of the crisis. The next section is specially dedicated to this matter. Here I state everything necessary to make the boundary between conceptions and a system clearer, to relieve the system from the responsibility for the sins of the conceptions. We will call it a falsely understood system. We are all the more justified in doing this as this understanding itself did not realize where it would lead to.

The new system lays the concept of reaction—as distinct from the reflex and the mental phenomenon—at the basis of the third way in psychology. The integral act of the reaction includes both the subjective and the objective aspect. However, in contrast with Gestalt theory and Stern, the new theory refrains from methodological assumptions which unite both parts of the reaction into one concept. Neither viewing fundamentally the same structures in the mind as in physics, nor finding goals, entelechy and personality in anorganic nature, e.g., neither the way of Gestalt theory, nor the way of Stern, lead to the goal.

Following Plekhanov, the new theory accepts the doctrine of psychophysical parallelism and the complete irreducibility of the mental to the physical. Such a reduction it regards as crude, vulgar materialism. But how can there be one science about *two* categories of being which are fundamentally, qualitatively heterogeneous and irreducible to each other? How can they merge into the integral act of the reaction? We have two answers to these questions. Kornilov, by seeing a functional relation between them, immediately destroys any *unity:* it is two *different* things that can stand in a functional relation to each other. Psychology cannot be studied with the concepts of reaction, for *within* the reaction we find two functionally independent elements which cannot be unified. This is not solving the psychophysical problem, but moving it into each element. Therefore it makes any research impossible, just as it has impeded psychology as a whole. At the time it was the relation of the whole area of the mind to the whole area of physiology which was unclear. Now the same insolubility is entangled in each separate reaction. What does this solution of the problem offer, *methodologically speaking?* Instead of solving it problematically (hypothetically) at the start of the investigation one must solve it experimentally, empirically in each separate case. But this is impossible. And how can there be one science with two fundamentally different methods of knowledge acquisition (not research methods: Kornilov regards introspection as the only adequate way to know the mind and not just as a technical device)? It is clear that methodologically the integral nature of the reaction remains a *pia desiderata* and in reality such a concept leads to two sciences with two methods which study two different aspects of reality.

Frankfurt (1926) provides a different answer. Following Plekhanov, he becomes entangled in a hopeless and insoluble contradiction. He wishes to prove the material nature of the nonmaterial mind and to link two ways of science for psychology which cannot be linked. The outline of his argumentation is as follows: the idealists view matter as another form of existence of the mind; the mechanistic materialists view the mind as another form of being of matter. The dialectical materialist preserves both parts of the antinomy. For him the mind is (1) a special property amidst *many* other properties which is irreducible to movement; (2) an internal state of moving matter; (3) the subjective side of a material process. The contradictory nature and the heterogeneity of these formulas will be revealed in the systematic exposition of the concepts of psychology. There I hope to show how the juxtaposition of ideas plucked from absolutely

different contexts distorts their meaning. Here we deal exclusively with the *methodological* aspect
of the question: can there be *one* science about two fundamentally different kinds of being?
They have nothing in common, cannot be unified. But perhaps there is an unequivocal link
between them that allows us to combine them? No. Plekhanov (cf. Frankfurt, 1926, p. 51)
clearly says that Marxism does not accept "the possibility of explaining or describing one kind
of phenomenon by means of ideas or concepts 'developed' to explain or describe another kind."
Frankfurt (ibid., pp. 52–53) says that "Mind is a *special* property which we can describe or
explain by means of *special* concepts or ideas." Once again the same—*different* concepts. But
this means that there are two sciences, one about behavior as a unique form of human movement, the other about the mind as non-movement. Frankfurt also talks about physiology in a
narrow and a broad sense—including the mind. But will this be physiology? Is our wish sufficient to make a science appear according to our *fiat?* Let them show us so much as a single example of *one* science about *two* different kinds of being which are being explained and described
by means of different concepts, or let them show us the possibility of such a science.

There are two points in this argumentation which categorically show that such a science is *impossible.*

1. Mind is a special quality or property of matter, but a quality is not part of a thing, but
a special capacity. But matter has many qualities, mind is *just one of them.* Plekhanov compares
the relation between mind and movement with the relations between the properties of growth
and combustibility of wood, with the hardness and shine of ice. But why, then, are there only
two parts in the antinomy? There should be as many as there are qualities, i.e., many, infinitely
many. Obviously, notwithstanding Chernychevsky, all qualities have something in common.
There is a *general concept* under which all the qualities of matter can be subsumed: both the
shine of ice and its hardness, both the fact that wood is easy to burn and the way it grows. If
not, there would be as many sciences as there are qualities: one science about the shine of ice,
another about its hardness. What Chernychevsky says is *simply absurd* as a methodological principle. After all, also within the mind we find different qualities: pain resembles lust in the same
way as shine resembles hardness—once again a special property.

The whole matter is that Plekhanov is operating with a general concept of the mind under
which a multitude of the most heterogeneous qualities are subsumed, and that movement, under
which all other qualities are subsumed, is also such a general concept. Obviously, mind stands
in principle in another relation to movement than qualities do to each other: both shine and
hardness are in the end movement; both pain and lust are in the end mind. Mind is not one of
many properties, but one of two. But this means that in the end there are *two* principles and
not one or many. Methodologically this means that the dualism of the science is completely
preserved. This becomes particularly clear from the second point.

2. The mental does not influence the physical, according to Plekhanov (1922). Frankfurt
(1926) clarifies that it influences itself mediately, via physiology, it exerts its influence in a peculiar way. If we combine two right-angled triangles, their forms will combine into a new form—
a square. The forms themselves do not exert influence "as a second, 'formal' aspect of the
combination of our material triangles." We observe that this is an exact statement of the famous
*Schattentheorie,* the theory of shadows: two men shake hands and their shadows do the same.
According to Frankfurt the shadows "influence" each other via the body.

But this is not the methodological problem. Does the author understand that, for a materialist, he arrived at a monstrous formulation of the nature of our science? Really, what sort of science about shadows, forms and mirror reflections is this? The author half understands what he arrived at, but does not see what it implies. Is a natural science about forms as such really possible, a science which uses induction, the concept of causality? It is only in geometry that we study abstract forms. The final word has been said: psychology is possible as geometry. But exactly this is the highest expression of Husserl's eidetic psychology. Dilthey's descriptive psychology as mathematics of the spirit is like that and so are Chelpanov's phenomenology, Stout's, Meinong's, and Schmidt-Kovazhik's analytic psychology. What unites them all with Frankfurt is the whole fundamental structure. They are using the same analogy.

1. The mind must be studied as geometrical forms, *outside causality*. Two triangles do not engender a square, the circle knows nothing of the pyramid. No relation of the real world may be transferred to the ideal world of forms and mental essences: they can only be described, analyzed, classified, but not explained. Dilthey [1894/1977, p. 93] regards it as the main property of the mind that its parts are not linked by the law of causality:

> Representations contain no sufficient ground for going over into feelings; one could imagine a purely representational creature who would be, in the midst of a battle's tumult, an unconcerned spectator indifferent about his own destruction. Feelings contain no sufficient ground for being transformed into volitional processes. One could imagine the same creature whose awareness of the surrounding combat would be accompanied by feelings of fear and terror, yet without movements of defense resulting from these feelings.

*Precisely because* these concepts are a-deterministic, noncausal and nonspatial, precisely because they have been formed like geometrical abstractions, Pavlov rejects their suitability for science: they are incompatible with the material construction of the brain. Following Pavlov, we say that, precisely because they are geometrical, they are not fit for real science.

But how can there be a science which combines the geometrical method with the scientific-inductive one? Dilthey [ibid., p. 46] understood perfectly well that materialism and *explanatory* psychology presuppose each other. Materialism is "in all its nuances, an explanatory psychology. Every theory which depends on the system of physical processes and merely incorporates mental facts into that system, is a materialism." Exactly the wish to defend the independence of the mind and all the sciences of the mind, the fear of transferring to this world the causality and necessity which reign in nature, leads to the fear of explanatory psychology. "No explanatory psychology . . . is capable of serving as the basis of the human studies" [ibid., p. 73]. This signifies that the sciences of the mind must not be studied materialistically. Oh, if Frankfurt only understood what it really implies to demand a psychology as geometry! To accept a special link—"efficacy"—instead of the physical causality of the mind, to reject explanatory psychology, means no more and no less than *to reject the concept of regularity in the whole field of the mind. This is what the debate is about.* The Russian idealists understand this perfectly well. For them Dilthey's thesis about psychology is a thesis that contrasts with the mechanistic conception of the historical process.

2. The second feature of the psychology at which Frankfurt arrived resides in its method, in the nature of the knowledge of this science. If the mind cannot be linked with natural processes, if it is noncausal, then it cannot be studied inductively, by observing real facts and generalizing

them. It must be studied by the method of speculation, through the direct contemplation of the truth in these Platonic ideas or mental essences. There is no place for induction in geometry; what has been proved for one triangle, has been proved for all of them. It does not study real triangles, but ideal abstractions—the different properties which have been abstracted from things are carried to the extreme and studied in their ideally pure form. For Husserl, phenomenology stands to psychology as mathematics to natural science. But according to Frankfurt it would be impossible to realize geometry and psychology as natural sciences. Their method is different. Induction is based on the repeated observation of facts and their empirically-based generalization. The analytical (phenomenological) method is based on a single immediate contemplation of the truth. This deserves reflection. We must know exactly with which science we want to break all ties. This theory about induction and analysis involves an essential misunderstanding which we must lay bare.

Analysis is applied entirely systematically in both causal psychology and the natural sciences. And there we often *deduce a general regularity from a single observation.* The domination of induction and mathematical elaboration and the underdevelopment of analysis substantially damaged the case of Wundt and experimental psychology as a whole.

What is the difference between one analysis and the other, or, not to make a mistake, between the analytical method and the phenomenological one? When we know this we can add to our map the last characteristic distinguishing the two psychologies.

The method of analysis in the natural sciences and in causal psychology consists of the study of a *single* phenomenon, a typical representative of a whole series, and the deduction of a proposition *about the whole series* on the basis of that phenomenon. Chelpanov (1917) clarifies this idea by giving the example of the study of the properties of different gases. Thus, we assert something about the properties of all gases after we conducted an experiment with only one type of gas. When we arrive at such a conclusion we assume that the gas we experimented upon has the same properties as all other gases. According to Chelpanov, in such an inference the inductive and the analytical method are simultaneously present.

Is this really true, i.e., is it really possible to merge the geometrical method with the natural scientific one, or do we have here a simple mixture of terms, with Chelpanov using the word *analysis* in two entirely distinct senses? The question is too important to ignore. We must not only distinguish the two psychologies, we must set apart their methods as deeply and as far as possible as they *cannot have* methods in common. Apart from the fact that we are interested in that part of the method which after the separation falls to the lot of descriptive psychology, because we want to know it exactly—apart from all this, *we do not wish to concede one bit* of the territory that belongs to us in the process of division. As we will see below, the analytical method is in principle too important for the development of the whole of social psychology, to render it without striking a blow.

When our Marxists explain the Hegelian principle in Marxist methodology they rightly claim that each thing can be examined as a microcosm, as a universal measure in which the whole big world is reflected. On this basis they say that to study one single thing, one subject, one phenomenon *until the end,* exhaustively, means to know the world in all its connections. In this sense it can be said that each person is to some degree a measure of the society, or rather class, to which he belongs, for the whole totality of social relationships is reflected in him.

From this alone we see that knowledge gained on the path from the special to the general is the key to all social psychology. We must reconquer the right for psychology to examine what is special, the individual as a social microcosm, as a type, as an expression or measure of the society. But about this we must only speak when we are face to face with causal psychology. Here we must exhaust the theme of the division.

What is undoubtedly correct in Chelpanov's example is that analysis in physics does not contradict induction, since it is precisely due to analysis that a single observation can lead to a general conclusion. Indeed, what justifies us in extending our conclusion about one gas to all others? Obviously, it is only because we elaborated the concept of gas *per se* through previous inductive observations and established the extension and content of this concept. Further, because we study the given particular gas *not as such*, but from a special viewpoint. We study the general *properties of a gas* realized in it. It is exactly this possibility, i.e., this viewpoint that in the particular, the special can be separated from the general, which we owe to analysis.

Thus, analysis is in principle not opposed to induction, but related to it. It is its highest form which contradicts its essence (repetition). It rests on induction and guides it. It states the question. It *lies at the basis of each experiment. Each experiment is an analysis in action, as each analysis is an experiment in thought.* That is why it would be correct to call it an *experimental method.* Indeed, when I am experimenting, I am studying A, B, C. . . . i.e., a number of concrete phenomena, and I assign the conclusions to different groups: to all people, to school-aged children, to activity, etc. The analysis suggests to what extent the conclusions may be generalized, i.e., it distinguishes in A, B, C . . . the characteristics that a given group has in common. But even more: in the experiment I always observe just one feature of a phenomenon, and this is again the result of analysis.

Let us now turn to the inductive method in order to clarify the analysis. Let us examine a number of applications of this method.

Pavlov is studying the activity of *the salivary gland in dogs.* What gives him the right to call his experiments the study of the higher nervous activity of *animals?* Perhaps, he should have verified his experiments on horses, crows, etc., on all, or at least the majority of animals, in order to have the right to draw these conclusions? Or, perhaps, he should have called his experiments "a study of salivation in dogs"? But it is precisely the salivation of dogs *per se* which Pavlov did not study and his experiments have not for one bit increased our knowledge of dogs as such and of salivation as such. In the dogs he did not study the dog, but *an animal in general,* and in salivation *a reflex in general,* i.e., in this animal and in this phenomenon he distinguished what they have in common with all homogeneous phenomena. That is why his conclusions do not just concern all animals, but the whole of biology as well. The established fact that Pavlov's dogs salivated to signals given by Pavlov immediately became a general biological principle—the principle of the transformation of inherited experience into personal experience. This proved possible because Pavlov *maximally abstracted* the phenomenon he studied from the specific conditions of the particular phenomenon. He brilliantly *perceived the general in the particular.*

What did the extension of his conclusions rest upon? Naturally, on the following: we extend our conclusions to something which has to do *with the same elements* and we rely upon similarities established in advance (the class of hereditary reflexes in all animals, the nervous system, etc.). Pavlov discovered a *general biological* law while studying *dogs*. But in the dog he studied what forms the basis of any animal.

This is the methodological path of any explanatory principle. In essence, Pavlov did not extend his conclusions, and the degree of their extension was determined in advance. It was implied in the very statement of the problem. The same is true for Ukhtomsky. He studied several preparations of frogs. If he had generalized his conclusions to all frogs this would have been induction. But he talks about the dominant as a principle of psychology applicable to the heroes of "War and Peace," and this he owes to analysis. Sherrington studied the scratching and flexive reflexes of the hind leg in many cats and dogs, but he established the principle of the struggle for the motor path which lies at the basis of the personality. But neither Ukhtomsky nor Sherrington added anything to the study of frogs or cats as such.

It is, of course, a very special task to find *the precise factual boundaries* of a general principle in practice and the *degree* to which it can be applied to different species of the given genus. Perhaps the conditional reflex has its highest boundary in the behavior of the human infant and its lowest in invertebrates and is found in absolutely different forms beyond these extremes. Within these limits it is more applicable to the dog than to a chicken and to what extent it is applicable to each of them can be exactly ascertained. But all this is already induction, the study of the specifically particular in relation to a principle and on the basis of analysis. There is no end to this process. We can study the application of a principle to different breeds, ages, sexes of the dog; further, to an individual dog, still further, to a particular day or hour of the dog's life, etc. The same is true of the dominant and the general motor path.

I have tried to introduce such a method into conscious psychology and to deduce the laws of the psychology of art on the basis of the *analysis* of one fable, one short story, and one tragedy. In doing so I proceeded from the idea that the well-developed forms of art provide the key to the underdeveloped ones, just as the anatomy of man provides the key to the anatomy of the ape. I assumed that Shakespeare's tragedy explains the enigmas of primitive art and not the other way around. Further, *I talk about all art* and do not verify my conclusions on music, painting, etc. What is even more: I do not verify them on *all* or the majority of the *types* of literature. I take *one* short story, *one* tragedy. Why am I entitled to do so? I have not studied the fable, the tragedy, and still less a *given* fable or a *given* tragedy. I have studied in them what makes up the basis of all art—the nature and mechanism of the aesthetic reaction. I relied upon the general elements of form and material which are inherent in any art. For the analysis I selected the most difficult fables, short stories and tragedies, precisely those in which the general laws are particularly evident. I selected the monsters among the tragedies etc. The analysis presupposes that one abstracts from the concrete characteristics of the fable as such, as a specific genre, and concentrates the forces upon the essence of the aesthetic reaction. That is why I say *nothing* about the fable as such. And the subtitle 'An analysis of the aesthetic reaction" itself indicates that the goal of the investigation is not a systematic exposition of a psychological theory of art in its entire volume and width of content (all types of art, all problems, etc.) and not even the inductive investigation of a specific number of facts, but precisely *the analysis of the processes in their essence*.

The objective-analytical method, therefore, is similar to the experiment. Its meaning is broader than its field of observation. Naturally, the principle of art as well is dealing with a reaction which in reality *never manifested itself* in a pure form, but always with its "coefficient of specification."

To find the factual boundaries, levels and forms of the applicability of a principle is a matter of factual research. Let history show *which* feelings in *which* eras, via *which* forms have been expressed in art. My task was to show *how* this proceeds in general. And this is the common methodological position of contemporary art theory: it studies the essence of a reaction knowing that it will never manifest itself in exactly that form. But the type, norm or limit will always be part of the concrete reaction and determine its specific character. Thus, a purely aesthetic reaction never occurs in art. In reality it will be combined with the most complex and diverse forms of ideology (morals, politics, etc.). Many even think that the aesthetic aspects are no more essential in art than coquetry in the reproduction of the species. It is a facade, *Vorlust*, a lure, and the meaning of the act lies in something else (Freud and his school). Others assume that historically and psychologically art and aesthetics are two intersecting circles which have a common and a separate surface (Utitz). This is all true, but it does not change the veracity of a principle, because it is *abstracted* from all this. It only says that the *aesthetical reaction is like this*. It is another matter to find the boundaries and sense of the aesthetic reaction itself within art.

Abstraction and analysis does all this. The similarity with the experiment resides in the fact that here, too, we have an artificial combination of phenomena in which the action of a specific law must manifest itself in the purest form. It is like a snare for nature, an analysis in action. In analysis we create a similar artificial combination of phenomena, but then through abstraction in thought. This is particularly clear in its application to art constructions. They are not aimed at scientific, but at practical goals and rely upon the action of some specific psychological or physical law. Examples are a machine, an anecdote, lyrics, mnemonics, a military command. Here we have a practical experiment. The analysis of such cases is an experiment with finished phenomena. Its meaning comes close to that of pathology—this experiment arranged by nature itself—to its own analysis. The only difference is that disease causes the loss or demarcation of superfluous traits, whereas we here have the presence of necessary traits, a selection of them—but the result is the same.

Each lyrical poem is such an experiment. The task of the analysis is to reveal the law that forms the basis of nature's experiment. But also when the analysis does not deal with a machine, i.e., a practical experiment, but with any phenomenon, it is in principle similar to the experiment. It would be possible to prove how infinitely much our equipment complicates and refines our research, how much more intelligent, stronger and more perspicuous it makes us. Analysis does the same.

It may seem that analysis, like experiment, distorts reality by creating artificial conditions for observation. Hence the demand that the experiment should be realistic and natural. If this idea goes further than a technical demand—not to scare off what we are searching for—it leads to absurdity. The strength of analysis is in abstraction, just as the strength of experiment is in its artificiality. Pavlov's experiments are the best specimen: for the dogs it is a *natural* experiment—they are fed etc.; for the scientist it is the summit of artificiality—salivation takes place when a specific area is scratched, which is an unnatural combination. Likewise, we need destruction in the analysis of a machine, mental or real damage to the mechanism, and in the [analysis of the] aesthetic form we need deformation.

If we remember what was said above about the indirect method, then it is easy to observe that analysis and experiment presuppose *indirect* study. From the analysis of the stimuli we infer the mechanism of the reaction, from the command, the movements of the soldiers, and from the form of the fable the reactions to it.

Marx [1867/1981, p. 12] says essentially the same when he compares abstraction with a microscope and chemical reactions in the natural sciences. The whole of *Das Kapital* is written according to this method. Marx analyzes the "cell" of bourgeois society—the form of the commodity value—and shows that a mature body can be more easily studied than a cell. He discerns the structure of the whole social order and all economical formations in this cell. He says that "to the uninitiated its analysis may seem the hair-splitting of details. We are indeed dealing with details, but such details as microscopic anatomy is also dealing with." He who can decipher the meaning of the cell of psychology, the mechanism of one reaction, has found the key to all psychology.

That is why analysis is a most potent tool in methodology. Engels [1925/1978, p. 496] explains to the "all-inductionists" that "no induction whatever might ever explain the *process* of induction. This could only be accomplished by the *analysis* of this process." He further gives mistakes of induction which are frequently encountered. Elsewhere he compares both methods and finds in thermodynamics an example which shows that the pretensions of induction to be the only or most fundamental form of scientific discovery are ill-founded.

> The steam engine formed the convincing proof of the fact that one can use heat to accomplish mechanical movements. One hundred thousand steam engines would not prove this more convincingly than a single engine . . . Sadi Carnot was the first to study it seriously. But not through induction. He studied the steam engine, analyzed it, found that the relevant process does not appear in it in a *pure* form but was concealed by all sorts of incidental processes, removed these inessentials which are indifferent for the essential process, and construed an ideal steam engine . . . which, to be sure, is as imaginary as, for example, a geometrical line or plane, but fulfills the same service as these mathematical abstractions: it represents the process in a pure, independent, and undistorted form [ibid., pp. 496–497].

It would be possible to show how and when such an analysis is possible in the methods of investigation of this applied branch of methodology. But we can also generally say that analysis is the application of methodology to the knowledge of a fact, i.e., it is an evaluation of the method used and of the meaning of the obtained phenomena. In this sense it can be said that analysis is *always* inherent in investigation, otherwise induction would turn into registration.

How does this analysis differ from Chelpanov's analysis? By four characteristics: (1) the analytical method is aimed at the knowledge of realities and strives for the same goal as induction. The phenomenological method does not at all presuppose the existence of the essence it strives to know. Its subject matter can be pure phantasy, deprived of any existence; (2) the analytical method studies facts and leads to knowledge which has the trustworthiness of a fact. The phenomenological method obtains apodictic truths which are absolutely trustworthy and universally valid; (3) the analytical method is a special case of empirical knowledge, i.e., factual knowledge, according to Hume. The phenomenological method is *a priori*, it is not a kind of experience or factual knowledge; (4) via the study of new special facts the analytical method, which relies on facts which have been studied and generalized before, ultimately leads to new relative and factual generalizations which have a boundary, a variable degree of applicability, limitations and even exceptions. The phenomenological method does not lead to knowledge of the general, but of the idea, the essence. The general is known through induction, the essence by intuition. It exists outside time and reality and is not related to any temporal or real thing.

We see that the difference is as big as a difference between two methods can be. One method—let us call it the analytical method—is the method of the real, natural sciences, the other—the phenomenological, *a priori* one—is the method of the mathematical sciences and of the pure science of the mind.

Why does Chelpanov call it the analytical method and assert that it is identical to the phenomenological one? Firstly, it is a plain *mistake* which the author himself tries to sort out several times. Thus, he points out that the analytical method is not identical to normal analysis in psychology. It yields knowledge of another kind than induction—we are reminded of the precise distinctions, all of them established by Chelpanov. Thus, there are *two types of induction* which have nothing in common but their name. This general term is confusing and we must distinguish its two meanings.

Further, it is clear that the analysis in the case of a gas, which the author adduces as a possible counterargument against the theory which says that the main feature of the "analytical" method is that it examines phenomena just once, is a natural scientific and not a phenomenological analysis. The author is simply *mistaken* when he sees a combination of analysis and induction here. It is analysis, but of another kind. Not one of the four points distinguishing both methods leaves any doubt about the fact that: (1) it is aimed at real facts, not at "ideal possibilities"; (2) it has only factual and not apodictic validity; (3) it is *a posteriori;* (4) it leads to generalizations which have boundaries and degrees, not to the contemplation of essences *[Wesensschau]*. In general, it results from experience, from induction and not from intuition.

That we are dealing with a mistake and a mixture of terms is absolutely clear from the absurd attempt to combine the phenomenological and the inductive method in one experiment. This is what Chelpanov does in the case of gases. It is as if we partly tried to prove Pythagoras' theorem and partly completed it with the study of real triangles. It is absurd. But behind the mistake is some dimension: the psychoanalysts have taught us to be sensitive to and suspicious about mistakes. Chelpanov belongs to the harmonizers: he sees the dualism of psychology, but unlike Husserl he does not accept psychology's complete separation from phenomenology. For him psychology is partly phenomenology. Within psychology there are phenomenological truths and they are the fundamental core of the science. But at the same time Chelpanov sympathizes with the experimental psychology which Husserl slighted with contempt. Chelpanov wishes to *combine what cannot be combined* and his story about the gases is the only one where he combines the analytical (phenomenological) method with induction in physics in the study of real gases. And this mixture he conceals with the general term "analytical."

The split of the dual analytical method into a phenomenological and an inductive-analytical one leads us to the ultimate points upon which the bifurcation of the two psychologies rests—their epistemological premises. I attach great importance to this distinction, see it as the crown and center of the whole analysis, and at the same time for me it is now as obvious as a simple scale. Phenomenology (descriptive psychology) proceeds from a radical distinction between physical nature and mental being. In nature we distinguish phenomena in being. "In other words, in the mental sphere there is no distinction between phenomenon *[Erscheinung]* and being *[Sein]*, and while nature is existence *[Dasein]* which manifests itself in the phenomena," this cannot be asserted about mental being (Husserl, 1910/1965, p. 35). Here *phenomenon and being coincide.* It is difficult to give a more precise formulation of psychological idealism. And this is the epistemological formula of psychological materialism: "The difference between *thinking* and *being* has not been destroyed in psychology. Even concerning thinking one must distinguish the thinking of thinking and the thinking as such" [Feuerbach, 1971, p. 127]. *The whole debate is in these two formulas.*

We must be able to state the epistemological problem *for the mind* as well and to find the distinction between being and thinking, as materialism teaches us to do in the theory of knowledge of the external world. The acceptance of a radical difference between the mind and physical nature conceals the identification of *phenomenon* and *being*, mind and matter, within *psychology*, the solution of the antinomy by removing one part—matter—in psychological knowledge. This is Husserl's idealism of the purest water. Feuerbach's whole materialism is expressed in the distinction of phenomenon and being within psychology and in the acceptance of being as the real object of study.

I venture to prove for the whole council of philosophers—idealists as well as materialists—that the essence of the divergence of idealism and materialism in psychology lies precisely here, and that only Husserl's and Feuerbach's formulas give consistent solution of the problem in the two possible variants and that the first is the formula of phenomenology and the second that of materialistic psychology. I venture, proceeding from this comparison, to cut the living tissue of psychology, cutting it as it were into two heterogeneous bodies which grew together by mistake. This is the only thing which corresponds with the objective order of things, and *all* debates, *all* disagreements, *all* confusion merely result from the absence of a clear and correct statement of the epistemological problem.

From this it follows that by only accepting from empirical psychology its *formal* acceptance of the mind, Frankfurt also accepts its whole epistemology and all its conclusions—he is forced to resort to phenomenology. It follows that by demanding a method for the study of the mind which corresponds to its qualitative nature, he is demanding a phenomenological method, although he does not realize it himself. His conception is the materialism of which Høffding [1908, p. 86, footnote 1] is entirely justified in saying that it is "a miniature dualistic spiritualism." Precisely *"miniature,"* i.e., with the attempt to reduce, quantitatively diminish the reality of the nonmaterial mind, to leave 0.001 of influence for it. But the fundamental solution *in no way* depends on a quantitative statement of the question. It is one of two things: either god exists, or he does not; either the spirits of dead people manifest themselves, or they do not; either mental (spiritistic—for Watson) phenomena are nonmaterial, or they are material. Answers which have the form "god exists, but he is very small," or "the spirits of dead people do not manifest themselves, but tiny parts of them very rarely visit spiritists," or "the mind is material, but distinct from all other matter," are humorous. Lenin wrote of the "bogostroiteli" ["God-builders"] that they differ little from the "bogoiskateli" ["God-seekers"]: what is important is to either accept or reject deviltry in general; to assume either a blue or a yellow devil does not make a big difference.

*When one mixes up the epistemological problem with the ontological one* by introducing into psychology not the whole argumentation but its final results, this leads to the distortion of *both*. In Russia the subjective is identified with the mental and later it is proved that the mental cannot be objective. Epistemological consciousness as part of the antinomy "subject-object" is confused with empirical, psychological consciousness and then it is asserted that consciousness cannot be material, that to assume this would be Machism. And as a result one ends up with neoplatonism, in the sense of infallible essences for which being and phenomenon coincide. They flee for idealism only to plunge into it headlong. They dread the identification of being with consciousness more than anything else and end up in psychology with their perfectly Husserlian identification. We must not mix up the relation between subject and object with the relation between mind and body, as Høffding [1908, p. 298, footnote 1] splendidly explains. The distinction between mind *[Geist]* and matter is a distinction in the content of our knowledge. But the distinction between subject and object manifests itself independently from the content of our knowledge.

> Both mind and body are for us objective, but whereas mental objects *[geistigen Objekte]* are by their nature related to the knowing subject, the body exists *only* as an object for us. The relation between subject and object is an epistemological problem *[Erkenntnisproblem]*, the relation between mind and matter is an ontological problem *[Daseinsproblem]*.

This is not the place to give both problems a precise demarcation and basis in materialistic psychology, but to indicate the possibility of two solutions, the boundary between idealism and materialism, the existence of a materialistic formula. For distinction, distinction to the very end, is psychology's task today. After all, many "Marxists" are not able to indicate the difference between theirs and an idealistic theory of psychological knowledge, because it does not exist. Following Spinoza, we have compared our science to a mortally ill patient who looks for an unreliable medicine. Now we see that it is only the surgeon's knife which can save the situation. A bloody operation is immanent. Many textbooks we will have to rend in twain, like the veil in the temple, many phrases will lose their head or legs, other theories will be slit in the belly. We are only interested in the border, the line of the rupture, the line which will be described by the future knife.

And we assert that this line will lie in between the formulas of Husserl and Feuerbach. The thing is that in Marxism the problem of epistemology with regard to psychology has not been stated at all and the task of distinguishing the *two* problems about which Høffding is talking did not arise. The idealists, on the other hand, elaborated this idea with great clarity. And we claim that the viewpoint of our "Marxists" is *Machism in psychology*: it is the identification of being and consciousness. *It is one of two things:* either the mind is directly given to us in introspection, and then we side with Husserl; or we must distinguish subject and object, being and thinking in it, and then we side with Feuerbach. But what does this imply? It implies that my joy and my introspectional comprehension of this joy are different things.

There is a citation from Feuerbach that is very popular in Russia: "what *for me* [or *subjectively*] is a [purely] mental, nonmaterial, supra-sensory act, is *in itself* [or *objectively*] a material, sensory act" [Feuerbach, *1971*, p. *125*]. It is usually cited in confirmation of subjective psychology. But this speaks *against it* . One may wonder what we must study: this act as such, as it is, or as it appears to me? As with the analogous question about the objective existence of the world, the materialist does not hesitate and says: the objective act *as such*. The idealist will say: my perception. But then one and the same act will turn out to be different depending on whether I am drunk or sober, whether I am a child or an adult, whether it is today or yesterday, whether it regards me or you. What is more, it turns out that in introspection we cannot directly perceive thinking, comparison—these are unconscious acts and our introspectional comprehension of them is not a functional concept, i.e., it is not deduced from objective experience. What must we, what can we study: thinking as such or the thinking of thinking? There can be no doubt whatsoever about the answer to this question. But there is one complication which prevents us from reaching a clear answer. *All* philosophers who have attempted to divide psychology have stumbled upon this complication. Stumpf distinguished mental functions from phenomena and asked who, which science, will study the phenomena rejected by physics and psychology. He assumed that a *special science* would develop which is neither psychology nor physics. Another psychologist (Pfänder, *1904*) refused to accept sensations as the subject matter of psychology for the sole reason that physics refuses to accept them. What place is left for them? *Husserl's phenomenology is the answer to this question.*

In Russia it is also asked: if you will study thinking as such and not the thinking of thinking; the act as such and not the act for me; the objective and not the subjective—who, then, will study the subjective itself, the subjective distortion of objects? In physics we try to eliminate the subjective factor from what we perceive as an object. In psychology, when we study perception it is again required to separate perception as such, as it is, from how it seems to me. Who will study what has been eliminated both times, this *appearance?*

But the problem of appearance is an apparent problem. After all, in science we want to learn about the *real* and not the *apparent* cause of appearance. This means that we must take the phenomena as they exist independently from me. The appearance itself is an illusion (in Titchener's [1910/1980, pp. 333–335] basic example: Müller-Lyer's lines are physically equal, psychologically one of them is longer). This is the difference between the viewpoints of physics and psychology. It *does not exist in reality,* but results from two non-coincidences of two really existing processes. If I would know the physical nature of the two lines and the objective laws of the eye, as they are in themselves, I would get the explanation of the appearance, of the illusion as a result. The study of the subjective factor in the knowledge of this illusion is a subject of logic and the historical theory of knowledge: just like being, the subjective is the result of two processes which are objective in themselves. The mind is not always a subject. In introspection it is split into object and subject. The question is whether in introspection phenomenon and being coincide. One has only to *apply* the epistemological formula of materialism, given by Lenin [1975, p. 260] (a similar one can be found in Plekhanov) *for the psychological subject-object,* in order to see what is the matter:

> the only 'property' of matter connected with philosophical materialism is the property of being an objective reality, of existing outside of our consciousness. . . . Epistemologically the concept of matter means *nothing* other than objective reality, existing independently from human consciousness and reflected by it.

Elsewhere Lenin says that this is, essentially, the principle of *realism,* but that he avoids this word, because it has been captured by inconsistent thinkers.

Thus, this formula *seemingly* contradicts our viewpoint: it cannot be true that consciousness exists outside our consciousness. But, as Plekhanov has correctly established, self-consciousness is the consciousness of consciousness. And consciousness *can* exist without self-consciousness: we become convinced of this by the unconscious and the relatively unconscious. I can see not knowing that I see. That is why Pavlov [1928/1963, p. 219] is right when he says that we can live according to subjective states, but that we cannot analyze them.

*Not a single science is possible* without separating direct experience from knowledge. It is amazing: only the psychologist-introspectionist thinks that experience and knowledge coincide. If the essence of things and the form of their appearance directly coincided, says Marx [1890/1981b, p. 825], all science would be superfluous. If in psychology appearance and being were the same, then *everybody would be a scientist-psychologist* and science would be impossible. Only registration would be possible. But, obviously, it is *one thing* to live, to experience, and *another* to analyze, as Pavlov says.

A most interesting example of this we find in Titchener [1910/1980, pp. 38–39]. This consistent adherent of introspection and parallelism arrives at the conclusion that mental phenomena can only be described, but not explained. He asserts that

> If, however, we attempted to work out a merely descriptive psychology, we should find that there was no hope in it of a true science of the mind. A descriptive psychology would stand to scientific psychology very much . . . as the view of the world which a boy gets from his cabinet of physical experiments stands to the trained physicist's view . . . there would be no unity or coherence in it In order to make psychology scientific we must not only describe, we must also explain mind. We must answer the question 'why.' But here is a difficulty. It is clear that we cannot regard one mental process as the cause of another mental process Nor can we, on the other hand, regard nervous processes as the cause of mental processes. . . . The one cannot be the cause of the other.

This is the real situation in which descriptive psychology finds itself. The author finds a way out in a purely *verbal subterfuge:* mental phenomena can only be explained in relation to the body. Titchener [ibid., pp. 39–40] says that

> The nervous system does not cause, but it does explain mind. It explains mind as the map of a country explains the fragmentary glimpses of hills and rivers and towns that we catch on our journey through it. . . . Reference to the body does not add one iota to the data of psychology. . . . It does furnish us with an explanatory principle for psychology.

If we refrain from this, only two ways to overcome the fragmentary nature of mental life remain: either the purely descriptive way, the rejection of explanation, or to assume the existence of the unconscious.

> Both courses have been tried. But, if we take the first, we never arrive at a science of psychology; and if we take the second, we voluntarily leave the sphere of fact for the sphere of fiction. These are scientific alternatives [ibid., p. 40].

This is perfectly clear. But is a science possible with the explanatory principle which the author has selected? Is it possible to have a science about the *fragmentary glimpses of hills, rivers, and towns,* with which in Titchener's example the mind is compared? And further: how, why does the map explain these views, how does the map of a country help to explain its parts? The map is a copy of the country, it explains insofar as the country is reflected upon it, i.e., similar things explain each other. A science based on such a principle is impossible. In reality, the author reduces everything to *causal explanation,* as for him both causal and parallelistic explanation are defined as the indication of "proximate circumstances or conditions under which the described phenomenon occurs" [ibid., p. 41]. But, after all, this way will not lead to science either. Good "proximate conditions" are the ice age in geology, the fission of the atom in physics, the formation of planets in astronomy, evolution in biology. After all, "proximate conditions" in physics are followed by other "proximate conditions" and the causal chain is *infinite in principle,* but in parallelistic explanations the matter is hopelessly limited to merely *proximate* causes. Not without reason the author [ibid., p. 41] confines himself to comparing his explanation with the explanation of dew in physics. It would be a nice physics which did not go farther than pointing out the proximate conditions and similar explanations, It would simply cease to exist as a science.

Thus, we see that for psychology as a field of knowledge there are two alternatives: either the way of science, in which case it must be able to explain, or the knowledge of fragmentary visions, in which case it is impossible as *science.* For the use of the geometrical analogy deludes us. A geometrical psychology is absolutely impossible, for it lacks the basic characteristic: being an ideal abstraction it nevertheless refers to real objects. In this respect we are first of all reminded of Spinoza's attempt to investigate human vices and stupidities by means of the geometrical method and to examine human actions and drives exactly as if they were lines, surfaces, and bodies. This method is suitable for descriptive psychology and not for any other approach. For it takes from geometry only its verbal style and the outward appearance of irrefutability of its proofs, and all the rest—its core included—is based upon a nonscientific way of thinking.

Husserl bluntly states the difference between phenomenology and mathematics: mathematics is an exact science and phenomenology a descriptive one. Neither more nor less: phenomenology cannot be apodictic for lack of such a trifle as exactitude! Try and imagine inexact mathematics and you will get geometrical psychology.

In the end, the question can be reduced, as has already been said, to the differentiation of the ontological and the epistemological problem. In epistemology *appearance* exists, and to assert that it is being is false. In ontology *appearance* does not exist at all. Either mental phenomena exist, and then they are material and objective, or they do not exist, and then they do *not* exist and cannot be studied. No science can be confined to the subjective, to *appearance,* to phantoms, to what does not exist. What does not exist, *does not exist at all* and it is not half-nonexistent, half-existent. This must be understood. We cannot say: in the world there exist real and *unreal* things—the unreal does not exist. The unreal must be explained as the non-coincidence, generally as the relation of two real things; the subjective as the corollary of two objective processes. The subjective is apparent and therefore it does *not exist.*

Feuerbach [1971, p. 125] comments upon the distinction between the subjective and the objective [factor] in psychology: "In a similar way, for me my body belongs to the category of imponderabilia, it does not have weight, although in itself or for others it is a heavy body."

From this it is clear what kind of reality he ascribed to the subjective. He openly says that "Psychology is full of godsends; only the conclusions are present in our consciousness and feeling, but not the premises, only the results, but not the processes of the organism" [ibid., p. 124] But can there really be a science about results without premises?

Stern [1924, p. 143] expressed this well when he said, following Fechner, that the mental and the physical are the concave and the convex. A single line can represent now this and now that. But in itself it is neither concave nor convex, but round, and it is precisely as such that we want to know it, independently from how it may appear.

Høffding compares it with the same content expressed in two languages which we do not manage to reduce to a common protolanguage. But we want to know the *content* and not the *language* in which it is expressed. In physics we have freed ourselves from language in order to study the content. We must do the same in psychology.

Let us compare consciousness, as is often done, with a mirror image. Let the object A be reflected in the mirror as A. Naturally, it would be false to say that *a* in itself is as real as A. It is real *in another way*. A table and its reflection in the mirror are not equally real, but real in a different way. The reflection as reflection, as an image of the table, as a second table in the mirror is not real, it is a phantom. But the reflection of the table as the refraction of light beams on the mirror surface-isn't that a thing which is equally material and real as the table? Everything else would be a miracle. Then we might say: there exist things (a table) and their phantoms (the reflection). But *only* things exist—(the table) and the reflection of light upon the surface. The phantoms are just *apparent* relations between the things. That is why no science of mirror phantoms is possible. But this does not mean that we will never be able to explain the reflection, the phantom. When we know the *thing* and the *laws* of *reflection of light*, we can always explain, predict, elicit, and change the phantom. And this is what persons with mirrors do. They study not mirror reflections but the movement of light beams, and explain the reflection. A science about mirror phantoms is impossible, but the theory of light and the things which cast and reflect it fully explain these "phantoms."

It is the same in psychology: the subjective itself, as a phantom, must be understood as a consequence, as a result, as a godsend of *two* objective processes. Like the enigma of the mirror, the enigma of the mind is not solved by studying phantoms, but by studying the two series of objective processes from the cooperation of which the phantoms as apparent reflections of *one thing in the other* arise. In itself the appearance does not exist.

Let us return to the mirror. To identify A and *a*, the table and its mirror reflection, would be idealism: *a* is nonmaterial, it is only A which is material and its material nature is a synonym for its existence independent of *a*. But it would be exactly the same idealism to identify *a* with X—with the processes that take place in the mirror. It would be wrong to say: being and thinking do not coincide *outside* the mirror, in nature (there A is not *a*, there A is a thing and *a* a phantom); being and thinking, however, do coincide inside the mirror (here *a* is X, *a* is a phantom and X is also a phantom). We cannot say: the *reflection* of a table is a table. But neither can we say: the *reflection* of a table is the refraction of light beams and *a* is neither A nor X. Both A and X are real processes and *a* is their apparent, i.e., unreal *result*. The reflection does not exist, but both the table and the light exist. The reflection of a table is identical neither with the real processes of the light in the mirror nor with the table itself.

Not to mention the fact that otherwise we would have to accept the existence in the world of both things and phantoms. Let us remember that the mirror itself is, after all, *part of the same nature as the thing outside the mirror*, and subject to all of its laws. After all, a cornerstone of materialism is the proposition that consciousness and the brain are a product, a part of nature, which reflect the rest of nature. And, therefore, the objective existence of X and A independent of *a* is a dogma of materialistic psychology.

Here we can end our protracted argumentation. We see that the third way of Gestalt psychology and personalism was, essentially, both times one of the two ways already known. Now we see that the third way, the way of so-called "Marxist psychology," is an attempt to combine both ways. This attempt leads to their renewed separation within one and the same scientific system: one who combines them is, like Münsterberg, following two different roads.

Like the two trees in the legend which were tied up in their tops and which tore apart the ancient knight, so any scientific system will be torn apart if it binds itself to two different trunks. Marxist psychology can only be a natural science. Frankfurt's way leads to phenomenology. Admittedly, in one place he himself consciously denies that psychology can be a natural science (Frankfurt, 1926). But, firstly, he mixes up the natural sciences with the biological ones, which is not correct. Psychology can be a natural science without being a biological science. Secondly, he understands the concept "natural" in its proximate, factual meaning, as a reference to the sciences about organic and non-organic nature and not in its fundamental methodological sense.

Such a usage of this term, which had long since been accepted in Western science, has been introduced into the Russian literature by Ivanovsky (1923). He says that mathematics and applied mathematics must be strictly distinguished from the sciences which deal with things, with "real" objects and processes, with what "actually" exists, or *is*. That is why these sciences can be called *real* or *natural* (in the broad sense of this word). In Russia the term "natural sciences" is usually used in a more narrow sense as merely designating the disciplines which study non-organic and organic nature. It does not cover the social and conscious nature which in such a usage of the word frequently appears different from "nature" as something which is "unnatural," or "supernatural," if not "contra-natural," I am convinced that the extension of the term "natural" to everything which really exists is entirely rational.

Whether psychology is possible as a science is, above all, a methodological problem. In no other science are there so many difficulties, insoluble controversies and combinations of incompatible things as in psychology. The subject matter of psychology is the most complicated of all things in the world and least accessible to investigation. Its methods must be full of special contrivances and precautions in order to yield what is expected of them.

All the time I am speaking about precisely this latter thing—the principle of a science about [what is] the real. In this sense Marx [1890/1981a, p. 161 studies, in his own words, the process of the development of economic formations as a *natural-historical process*.

Not a single science represents such a diversity and plentitude of methodological problems, such tightly stretched knots, such insoluble contradictions, as ours. That is why we cannot take a single step without thousands of preparatory calculations and cautions.

Thus, it is acknowledged all the same that the crisis gravitates toward the creation of a methodology, that the struggle is for a general psychology. Anyone who attempts to skip this problem, to jump over methodology in order to build some special psychological science right away, will inevitably jump over his horse while trying to sit on it. This has happened with Gestalt theory and Stern. Starting from universal principles which are equally applicable in physics and psychology but which have not been made concrete in methodology, we cannot proceed to a particular psychological investigation. That is why these psychologists are accused of knowing just one predicate and thinking it equally applicable to the whole world. We cannot, as Stern does, study the psychological differences between people with a concept that covers both the solar system, a tree, and man. For this we need another scale, another measure. The whole problem of the general and the special science, on the one hand, and methodology and philosophy, on the other, is a problem of scale. We cannot measure human height in miles, for this we need a tape-measure. And while we have seen that the special sciences have a tendency to transcend their boundaries towards the struggle for a common measure, a larger scale, philosophy is going through the opposite tendency: in order to approximate science it must narrow, decrease the scale, make its theses more concrete.

Both tendencies—of philosophy and of the special science—lead equally to methodology, to the general science. But this idea of scale, the idea of a general science, is so far foreign to "Marxist psychology" and this is its weak spot. It attempts to find a direct measure for psychological elements—the reaction—in universal principles: the law of the transition of quantity into quality and "the forgetting of the nuances of the gray color" according to Lehmann and the transition from thrift into stinginess; Hegel's triad and Freud's psychoanalysis. Here the absence of a measure, scale, an intermediate link between the two, makes itself clearly felt. That is why the dialectical method will fall with fatal inevitability into the same category as the experiment, the comparative method, and the method of tests and surveys. A feeling for hierarchy, the difference between a technical research method and a method by which to know "the nature of history and thinking," is missing. The direct frontal collision of particular factual truths with universal principles; the attempt to decide the matter-of-fact debate about instinct between Vagner and Pavlov by references to quantity-quality; the step from dialectics to the survey; the criticism of irradiation from the epistemological viewpoint; the use of miles where a tape-measure is needed; the verdicts of Bekhterev and Pavlov from the height of Hegel; these attempts to swat a fly with a sledgehammer, have led to the false idea of a third way.

Binswanger [1922, p. 107] reminds us of Brentano's words about the amazing art of logic which makes *one* step forward with a thousand steps forward in science as a result. This strength of logic they do not want to know in Russia. According to the apt expression, methodology is the linchpin through which philosophy guides science. The attempt to realize such a guidance without methodology, the direct application of force to the point of application without a linchpin—from Hegel to Meumann—makes science impossible.

I advance the thesis that the analysis of the crisis and the structure of psychology indisputably testifies to the fact that no philosophical system can take possession of psychology directly, without the help of methodology, i.e., without the creation of a general science. The only rightful application of Marxism to psychology would be to create a general psychology—its concepts are being formulated in direct dependence upon general dialectics, for it is the dialectics of psychology. Any application of Marxism to psychology via other paths or in other points outside this area, will inevitably lead to scholastic, verbal constructions, to the dissolution of dialectics into surveys and tests, to judgment about things according to their external, accidental, secondary features, to the complete loss of any objective criterion and the attempt to deny all historical tendencies of the development of psychology, to a terminological revolution, in sum to a gross distortion of both Marxism and psychology. This is Chelpanov's way.

Engels' [1925/1978, p. 348] formula—not to foist the dialectical principles on nature, but to find them in it—is changed into its opposite here. The principles of dialectics are introduced into psychology from outside. The way of Marxists should be different. The *direct* application of the theory of *dialectical materialism* to the problems of natural science and in particular to the group of biological sciences or psychology *is impossible,* just as *it is impossible to apply it directly* to history and sociology. In Russia it is thought that the problem of "psychology and Marxism" can be reduced to creating a psychology which is up to Marxism, but in reality it is far more complex. Like history, sociology is in need of the intermediate *special theory* of historical materialism which explains the *concrete* meaning, for the given group of phenomena, of the abstract laws of dialectical materialism. In exactly the same way we are in need of an as yet undeveloped but inevitable theory of biological materialism and psychological materialism as an intermediate science which explains the concrete application of the abstract theses of dialectical materialism to the given field of phenomena.

Dialectics covers nature, thinking, history—it is the most general, maximally universal science. The theory of the psychological materialism or dialectics of psychology is what I call general psychology.

In order to create such intermediate theories—methodologies, general sciences—we must reveal the *essence* of the given area of phenomena, the laws of their change, their qualitative and quantitative characteristics, their causality, we must create categories and concepts appropriate to it, in short, we must create our *own Das Kapital.* It suffices to imagine Marx operating with the general principles and categories of dialectics, like quantity-quality, the triad, the universal connection, the knot [of contradictions], leap etc.—without the abstract and historical categories of value, class, commodity, capital, interest, production forces, basis, superstructure etc.—to see the whole monstrous absurdity of the assumption that it is possible to create any Marxist science while bypassing by *Das Kapital.* Psychology is in need of its own *Das Kapital*—its own concepts of class, basis, value etc.—in which it might express, describe and study its object, And to discover a confirmation of the law of leaps in Lehmann's statistical data of the forgetting of the nuances of the grey color means not to change dialectics or psychology one jot. This idea of the need for an intermediate theory without which the various special facts cannot be examined in the light of Marxism has long since been realized, and it only remains for me to point out that the conclusions of our analysis of psychology match this idea.

Vishnevsky develops the same idea in his debate with Stepanov (it is clear to anyone that historical materialism is not dialectical materialism, but its application to history. Therefore, only the social sciences which have their general basis in the history of materialism can, strictly speaking, be called Marxist; other Marxist sciences do not yet exist), "Just as historical materialism is not identical with dialectical materialism, the latter is not identical with specifically natural scientific theory, which, incidentally, is still in the process of being born" (Vishnevsky, 1925, p. 262). But Stepanov (1924) identifies the dialectical-materialist understanding of nature with th the mechanistic one and finds that it is given and can already be found in the mechanistic conception of the natural sciences. As an example the author mentions the debate in psychology about the question of introspection.

Dialectical materialism is a most abstract science. The direct application of dialectical materialism to the biological sciences and psychology, as is common nowadays, does not go beyond the formal logical, scholastic, verbal subsumption of particular phenomena, whose internal sense and relation is unknown, under general, abstract, *universal* categories. At *best* this leads to an accumulation of *examples* and illustrations. But not more than that. Water—steam—ice and natural economy—feudalism—capitalism are one and the same, one and the same process from the viewpoint of *dialectical materialism*. But historical materialism would lose much qualitative wealth in such a generalization!

Marx called his *Das Kapital* a critique of political economy. Such a critique of psychology one wants to skip today. "A *textbook* of psychology, explained from the viewpoint of dialectical materialism," must sound essentially like "a textbook of mineralogy, explained from the viewpoint of formal logic." After all, this goes without saying—to reason logically is not a property of the given textbook or mineralogy as a whole. And dialectics is not logic, it is broader. Or: "a textbook of sociology, from the viewpoint of dialectical materialism" instead of "historical." We must develop a theory of psychological materialism. We cannot yet create textbooks of dialectical psychology.

But we would lose our main criterion in critical judgment as well. The way one now determines, as in the assay office, whether a given theory is in accord with Marxism, can be understood as a method of "logical superposition," i.e., one checks whether the forms, the logical features coincide (monism, etc.). It should be known what can and must be looked for in Marxism. Man is not made for the sabbath, but the sabbath is made for man. We must find a theory which would help us to know the mind, but by no means the solution of the question of the mind, not a formula which would give the ultimate scientific truth. We cannot find it in the citations from Plekhanov for the simple reason that it is not there. Neither Marx, nor Engels, nor Plekhanov possessed such a truth. Hence the fragmentary nature, the brevity of many formulations, their rough character, their meaning which is strictly limited to the context. Such a formula can in principle not be given in advance, before the scientific study of the mind, but develops as the result of the scientific work of centuries. What can be searched for in the teachers of Marxism beforehand is not a solution of the question, not even a working hypothesis (as these are developed on the basis of the given science), but the method to develop it [the hypothesis; Russian eds.]. I do not want to learn what constitutes the mind for free, by picking out a couple of citations, I want to learn from Marx's whole method how to build a science, how to approach the investigation of the mind.

That is why Marxism is not only applied in the wrong place (in textbooks instead of a general psychology), but why one takes the wrong things from it. We do not need fortuitous utterances, but a method; not dialectical materialism, but historical materialism. *Das Kapital* must teach us many things—both because a genuine social psychology begins *after Das Kapital* and because psychology nowadays is a psychology *before Das Kapital*. Struminsky is fully right when he calls the very idea of a Marxist psychology as a synthesis of the thesis "empirism" with the antithesis "reflexology" a scholastic construction. After a real path has been found, one may for clarity's sake signal these three points, but to search for real paths by means of this schema would mean taking the road of speculative combination and dealing with the dialectics of ideas rather than the dialectics of facts or being. Psychology has no independent paths of development; we must find the real historical processes behind them, which condition them. He is only wrong when he asserts that to select the paths of psychology on the basis of the contemporary currents in a Marxist fashion is impossible in principle (Struminsky, 1926).

The idea he develops is right, but it only concerns the historical analysis of the development of science and not the methodological one. Because the methodologist takes no interest in what *really* will take place in the process of development of psychology tomorrow, he also ignores factors outside of psychology. But he is interested in the kind of disease psychology is suffering from, what it lacks in order to become a science, etc. After all, the external factors as well push psychology along the road of its development and can neither abolish the work of centuries nor make it skip a century. The logical structure of knowledge grows organically.

Struminsky is also right when he points out that the new psychology virtually came so far as to frankly accept the position of the older subjective psychology. But the trouble is not that the author fails to take account of the external, real factors of the development of the science he attempts to take account of; the trouble is that he does not take the methodological nature of the crisis into account. The course of development of each science has its *own* strict sequence. External factors can speed up or slow down this course, they may sidetrack it, and finally, they can determine the qualitative character of each stage, but to change the sequence of these stages is impossible. Using the external factors we can explain the idealistic or materialistic, religious or positive, individualistic or social, pessimistic or optimistic character of the stage, but no external factors can establish that a science which finds itself in the stage of gathering raw material can proceed straight to the creation of technical, applied disciplines, or that a science with well—developed theories and hypotheses, with well—developed technique and experimentation will start dealing with the gathering and description of primary material.

Thanks to the crisis, the division into two psychologies through the creation of a methodology has been put on the agenda. How it will turn out depends on external factors. Titchener and Watson in their American and socially different way, Koffka and Stern in a German and again socially different way, Bekhterev and Kornilov in their Russian and again different way—they all *solve one problem*. What this methodology will be and how fast it will be there we do not know, but that psychology does not move any further as long as the methodology has not been created, that the methodology will be the first step forward, is beyond doubt.

The fundamental stones have in principle been laid correctly. The general way, which will take decades, has also been indicated correctly. The goal is also correct, as is the general plan. Even the practical orientation in contemporary currents is correct, though incomplete. But the next path, the next steps, the plan of action, suffer from deficits: they lack an analysis of the crisis and a correct orientation on methodology. The works of Kornilov are the beginning of this methodology, and anyone who wants to develop the idea of psychology and Marxism further will be forced to repeat him and to continue his road. As a road this idea is unequalled in strength in European psychology. If it does not lose itself in criticism and polemics, if it does not turn into a paper war [war with pamphlets] but rises to a methodology, if it does not search for ready-made answers, and if it understands the tasks of contemporary psychology, then it will lead to the creation of a theory of psychological materialism.


## 14


We have finished our investigation. Did we find everything we were looking for? In any case, we have come quite close. We have prepared the ground for research in the field of psychology and, in order to justify our argumentation, we must test our conclusions and construct a model of general psychology. But before that we would like to dwell on one more aspect which, admittedly, is of more stylistic than fundamental importance. But the stylistic completion of an idea is not totally irrelevant to its complete articulation.

We have split the tasks and method, the area of investigation and the principle of our science. What remains is to split its name. The processes of division which became evident in the crisis have also influenced the fate of the name of our science. Various systems have half broken with the old name and use their own to designate the whole research area. In this fashion one sometimes speaks of behaviorism as the science of behavior as a synonym for psychology and not for one of its currents. Psychoanalysis and reactology are often mentioned in this way.

Other systems break completely with the old name as they see the traces of a mythological origin in it. Reflexology is an example. This latter current emphasizes that it rejects the tradition and builds on a new and vacant spot. It cannot be disputed that such a view has some truth to it, although one must look at science in a very mechanical and unhistorical manner not to understand the role of continuity and tradition at all, even during a revolution. Watson, however, is partly right when he demands a radical rupture with the older psychology, when he points to astrology and alchemy and to the danger of an ambiguous psychology. Other systems have so far remained without a name—Pavlov's is an example. Sometimes he calls his area physiology, but by terming his work the study of behavior and higher nervous activity he has left the question of the name open. In his early works Bekhterev openly distinguished himself from physiology; for Bekhterev reflexology is not physiology. Pavlov's students set forth his theory under the name "science of behavior." And indeed, two sciences which are so different should have two different names. Münsterberg [1922, p. 13] expressed this idea long ago:

> Whether the intentional understanding of inner life should really be called psychology is, of course, still a question that can be debated. Indeed, much speaks in favor of keeping the name psychology for the *descriptive* and *explanatory* science, excluding the science of the understanding of mental experiences and inner relations from psychology [emphasis by Vygotsky].

However, this knowledge nevertheless exists under the name of psychology; "It is true that it seldom appears in pure and consistent form. It is mostly somehow superficially connected with elements of causal psychology" [ibid., p. 13]. But as we know the author's opinion that the whole confusion in psychology is due to this mixture, the only conclusion is to select another name for intentional psychology. In part this is how it goes. Right before our eyes phenomenology is producing a psychology which is "necessary for certain logical goals" [ibid., p. 13] and instead of a division into two sciences by means of adjectives, which cause enormous confusion . . . , it begins to introduce various substantives. Chelpanov observes that "analytical" and "phenomenological" are two names for one and the same method, that phenomenology partially coincides with analytical psychology, that the debate as to whether the phenomenology of psychology exists or not is a terminological matter. If we add to this that the author considers this method and this part of psychology to be basic, then it would be logical to call analytical psychology phenomenology. Husserl himself prefers to confine himself to an adjective in order to preserve the purity of his science and he talks about "eidetic psychology." But Binswanger [1922, p. 135] openly writes: we must distinguish "between pure phenomenology and . . . empirical phenomenology (descriptive psychology)" and bases this on the adjective "pure" introduced by Husserl himself. The sign of equality is written down in a highly mathematical fashion. If we recall that Lotze called psychology applied mathematics; that Bergson in his definition almost identified empirical metaphysics with psychology; that Husserl wishes to regard pure phenomenology as a metaphysical theory about essences (Binswanger, 1922), then we will understand that idealistic psychology itself has both a tradition and a tendency to abandon a decrepit and compromised name. And Dilthey explains that explanatory psychology goes back to Wolff's rational psychology, and descriptive psychology, to empirical psychology.

It is true, some idealists are against attaching this name to natural scientific psychology. Thus, Frank [1917/1964, pp. 15–16] uses harsh words to point out that two different sciences are living under a single name, writing that

> It is not at all a matter of the more or less scientific nature of two different methods of a single science, but of simply supplanting one science *by* a totally different one, which though it has retained some weak traces of kinship with the first, has essentially a totally different subject . . . Present-day psychology declares itself to be a natural science. . . . This means that contemporary so-called psychology is not at all psycho-logy, but physio-logy . . . The excellent *term* "psychology"—theory of t h e soul—was simply illegally stolen and used as a title for a completely different scientific field. It has been stolen so thoroughly that when you now think about the nature of you are doing something which is destined to remain nameless or for which one must invent some new term.

But even the current *distorted* name "psychology" does not correspond to its essence for three quarters of it—it is psychophysics and psychophysiology. And the new science he wants to call philosophical psychology in order to "revive the real meaning of the term 'psychology' and give it back to its legitimate owner after the theft mentioned before, which already cannot be redeemed directly" [ibid., p. 36].

We see the remarkable fact that reflexology, which strives to break with "alchemy," and philosophy, which wishes to contribute to the resurrection of the rights of *psychology* in the old, literal and precise meaning of this word, are both looking for a new term and remain nameless. What is even more remarkable is that their motives are identical. Some fear the traces of its materialistic origin in this name, others fear that it lost its old, literal and precise meaning. Can we find a—stylistically—better manifestation of the dualism of contemporary psychology? However, Frank also agrees that natural scientific psychology has stolen the name irredeemably and thoroughly. And we propose that it is the materialistic branch which must call itself psychology. There are two important considerations which speak in favor of this and against the radicalism of the reflexologists. Firstly, it is exactly the materialistic branch which forms the crown of *all genuinely scientific tendencies, eras, currents, and authors which are represented in the history of our science, i.e., it is indeed psychology according to its very essence.* Secondly, by accepting this name, the new psychology does not at all 'steal' it, does not distort its meaning, nor does it commit itself to the mythological traces which are preserved in it, but, on the contrary, it retains a vivid historical reminder of its whole development from the very starting point.

Let us start with the second consideration.

Psychology as a science of the soul, in Frank's sense, in the precise and old sense of the word, *does not exist.* He himself is forced to ascertain this after he convinced himself with amazement and almost despair that such literature is virtually *nonexistent.* Further, empirical psychology as a complete science *does not exist at all.* And what is going on now is at bottom not a revolution, not even a reform of science and not the completion through synthesis of some foreign reform, but the *realization* of psychology and the *liberation* of what is capable of growing in science from what is not capable of growth. Empirical psychology itself (incidentally, it will soon be 50 years since the name of this science has not been used at all, since each school adds its own adjective) is as dead as a cocoon left by the butterfly, as an egg deserted by the nestling. James says that

> When, then, we talk of 'psychology as a natural science' we must not assume that that means a sort of psychology that stands at last on solid ground. It means just the reverse; it means a psychology particularly fragile, and into which the waters of metaphysical criticism leak at every joint, a psychology all of whose elementary assumptions and data must be reconsidered in wider connections and translated into our terms. It is, in short, a phrase of diffidence, and not of arrogance; and it is indeed strange to hear people talk of 'the New Psychology,' and write 'Histories of Psychology,' when into the real elements and forces which the word covers not the first glimpse of clear insight exists. A string of raw facts; a little gossip and wrangle about opinions; a little classification and generalization on the mere descriptive level; a strong prejudice that we *have* states of mind, and that our brain conditions them: but not a single law in the sense in which physics shows us laws, not a single proposition from which any consequence can causally be deduced. We don't even know the terms between which the elementary laws would obtain if we had them. This is no science, it is only the hope of a science [see pp. 400–401 of Burkhardt, 1984].

James gives a brilliant inventory of what we inherit from psychology, a list of its possessions and fortune. It gives us a string of raw facts and the hope of a science.

How are we connected with mythology through this name? Psychology, like physics before Galileo or chemistry before Lavoisier, is not yet a science which may somehow influence the future science. But have the circumstances perhaps fundamentally changed since James wrote this? At the 8th Congress of Experimental Psychology in 1923, Spearman repeated James' definition and said that psychology was still not a science but the hope for a science. One must have a considerable amount of philistine provincialism to represent the matter as Chelpanov did. As if there exist unshakable truths which are accepted by everybody, which have been corroborated over the centuries and which some wish to destroy for no reason at all. The other consideration is even more serious. In the final analysis we must openly say that psychology does not have two, but only one heir, and that there can be no serious debate about its name.

The second psychology is impossible as a science. And we must say with Pavlov that from the scientific viewpoint we consider the position of this psychology to be hopeless. As a real scientist, Pavlov [1928/1963, p. 77] does not ask whether a mental aspect exists, but how we can study it. He says:

> How must the physiologist treat these psychical phenomena? *It is impossible to neglect them, because they are closely bound up with purely physiological phenomena and determine the work of the whole organ.* If the physiologist decides to study them, he must answer the question, How?

Thus, in this division we *do not yield a single phenomenon* to the other side. We study everything on our path that exists and explain everything that [merely] seems [to exist].

For how many thousands of years has man elaborated psychical facts pages have been written to describe the internal world of the human being, but with what result? Up to the present we have no laws of the psychic life of man [ibid., p. 114].

What is left after the division, will go to the realm of art. Already now Frank [1917/1964, p. 16] calls the writers of novels the teachers of psychology. For Dilthey [1894/1977, p. 36] psychology's task is to catch in the web of its descriptions what is hidden in King Lear, Hamlet, and Macbeth as he saw in them "more psychology than in all the manuals of psychology together." It is true, Stern laughed maliciously at such a psychology procured from novels and said that you cannot milk a painted cow. But in contrast with his idea and in accordance with Dilthey's, descriptive psychology is *really* developing into fiction. The first congress on individual psychology, which regards itself as this second psychology, heard Oppenheim's paper, who seized in the web of his concepts what Shakespeare gave in images—exactly what Dilthey wanted. The second psychology becomes metaphysics whatever it is called. It is precisely the impossibility of such knowledge as *science* which determines our choice.

Thus, there is only one heir for the name of our science. But, perhaps, it should decline the heritage? Not at all. We are dialecticians. We do not at all think that the developmental path of science follows a straight line, and if it has had zigzags, returns, and loops we understand their historical significance and consider them to be necessary links in our chain, inevitable stages of our path, just as capitalism is an inevitable stage on the road toward socialism. We have set store by each step which our science has ever made toward the truth. We do not think that our science started with us. We will not concede to anyone Aristotle's idea of association, nor the theory about the subjective illusions of sensations by him and the skeptics, nor J. Mill's idea of causality, nor J. S. Mill's idea of psychological chemistry, nor the "refined materialism" of Spencer which Dilthey [1924, p. 45] viewed not as a "sure foundation, but a danger." In a word, we will not concede to anyone this whole line of materialism in psychology which the idealists sweep aside so carefully. We know that they are right in one thing: "The hidden materialism of [Spencerian] explanatory psychology has played a disintegrating role in the economic and political sciences and in criminal law" (ibid., p. 45).

Herbart's idea of a dynamic and mathematical psychology, the works of Fechner and Helmholtz, Taine's idea about the motor nature of the mind as well as Binet's theory of the mental pose or internal mimics, Ribot's motor theory, the James-Lange peripheral theory of emotions, even the Würzburg school's theory of thinking and of attention as activity—in one word, every step toward truth in our science, belongs to us. After all, we did not choose one of the two roads because we liked it, but because we consider it to be the right one.

Consequently, this road encompasses absolutely everything which was scientific in psychology. The attempt itself to study the mind *scientifically*, the effort of free thought to master the mind, however it became obscured and paralyzed by mythology, i.e., the very idea of a *scientific* conception of the soul, contains the whole future path of psychology. For science is the path to truth, even if by way of delusion. But this is precisely the road of our science: we struggle, we overcome errors, via incredible complications, in a superhuman fight with age-old prejudices. We do not want to deny our past. We do not suffer from megalomania by thinking that history begins with us. We do not want a brand-new and trivial name from history. We want a name covered by the dust of the centuries. We regard this as our historical right, as an indication of our historical role, our claim to realize psychology as a science. We must view ourselves in connection with and in relation to the past. Even when denying it we rely upon it.

It might be said that in its literal sense this name is not applicable to our science now, as it changes its meaning in every epoch. But be so kind as to mention a single word that has not changed its meaning. Don't we make a logical mistake when we talk of blue ink or a pilot's art? But on the other hand we are loyal to another logic—the logic of language. If the geometer even today calls his science with a name which means "measuring the earth," then the psychologist can refer to his science by a name which once meant "theory of the soul." Whereas the concept of measuring the earth is now too narrow for geometry, it was once a decisive step forward, to which the whole science owes its existence. Whereas the idea of the soul is now reactionary, it once was the first scientific hypothesis of ancient man, an enormous achievement of thought to which we owe the existence of our science now. Animals probably do not have the idea of the soul, nor do they have psychology. We understand that, historically, psychology had to begin with the idea of the soul. We are as little inclined to view this as simply ignorance and error as we consider slavery to be the result of a bad character. We know that science on its path toward the truth inevitably involves delusions, errors and prejudices. Essential for science is not that these exist, but that they, being errors, nevertheless lead to the truth, that they are overcome. That is why we accept the name of our science with all its age-old delusions as a vivid reminder of our victory over these errors, as the fighting scars of wounds, as a vivid testimony of the truth which develops in the incredibly complicated struggle with falsehood.

All sciences essentially proceed this way. Do the builders of the future really start from scratch, aren't they those who complete and follow all that is genuine in human experience? Do they really not have allies and forebears in the past? Let us be shown but a single word, a single scientific name, which can be applied in a literal sense. Or do mathematics, philosophy, dialectics and metaphysics signify what they once signified? Let it not be said that two branches of knowledge about a single object must absolutely carry the same name. Let logic and the psychology of thinking be remembered. Sciences are not classified and named according to their object of study, but according to the principles and goals of the study. Does Marxism really not want to know its ancestors in philosophy? *Only unhistorical and uncreative minds* are inventive with respect to new names and sciences. Such ideas do not become Marxism. Chelpanov comes with the information that during the French revolution the term "psychology" was replaced by the term "ideology," since for that era psychology was the science about the soul. But ideology formed part of zoology and was divided into physiological and rational ideology. This is correct, but what incalculable harm results from such unhistorical word usage can be seen from the difficulty which we now have in deciphering different loci about ideology in Marx's texts, how ambiguous this term sounds. It gives occasion to such "investigators" as Chelpanov to claim that for Marx ideology signified psychology. This terminological reform is *partly* responsible for the fact that the role and meaning of the older psychology is undervalued in the history of our science. And finally, it leads to a clear rupture with its genuine descendants, it severs the vivid line of unity. Chelpanov, who declared (1924, p. 27) that psychology has nothing in common with physiology, now vows for the Great Revolution. Psychology has always been physiological and "contemporary scientific psychology is the child of the psychology of the French revolution." Only *extreme ignorance* or the expectation that *others would be so ignorant* can have dictated these phrases. Whose *contemporary* psychology? Mill's or Spencer's, Bain's or Ribot's? Correct. But that of Dilthey and Husserl, Bergson and James, Münsterberg and Stout, Meinong and Lipps, Frank and *Chelpanov*? Can there be a bigger untruth? After all, all of these builders of the new psychology advanced another system as the *foundation* of science, a system which was hostile to Mill and Spencer, Bain, and Ribot. The same name which Chelpanov uses as a shelter they slighted "like a dead dog." But Chelpanov shelters behind names which are foreign and hostile to him and speculates on the ambiguity of the term "contemporary psychology." Yes, in contemporary psychology there is a branch which can regard itself as the child of revolutionary psychology. But during his entire life (and today) Chelpanov has done nothing but attempt to chase this branch into a dark corner of science, to separate it from psychology.

But once again: how dangerous is a common name and how unhistorically did the psychologists of France act who betrayed it!

This name was first introduced into science in 1590 by Goclenius, professor in Marburg, and accepted by his student Casmann in 1594. It was not introduced by Christian Wolff around the mid-eighteenth century and is not found for the first time in Melanchthon, as is usually incorrectly thought. It is mentioned by Ivanovsky as a name to indicate part of anthropology, which together with somatology formed one science. That this term is ascribed to Melanchthon is based on the preface of the publisher to the 13th volume of his writings, in which Melanchthon is incorrectly indicated as the first author of psychology. This name was quite rightly retained by Lange, the author of the psychology without a soul. But isn't psychology called the theory of the soul?, he asks. How can we conceive of a science which doubts whether it has a subject matter to study at all? However, he found it pedantic and unpractical to throw away the traditional name once the subject matter of the science had changed, and called for the unwavering acceptance of a psychology without a soul.

The endless fuss about psychology's name started precisely with Lange's reform. This name, taken in itself, ceased to mean anything. Each time one had to add: "without a soul," "without any metaphysics," "based on experience," "from an empirical viewpoint," etc. Psychology *per se* ceased to exist. Here resided Lange's mistake. Having accepted the old name he did not embrace it *fully*, completely, did not distinguish, separate it from tradition. Once psychology is without a soul, then with a soul we do not have psychology, but something else. But here, of course, he did not so much lack good intentions, as strength. The time was not yet ripe for a division.

We, too, must now face this terminological matter which belongs to the theme of the division into two sciences.

How will we call natural scientific psychology? It is now often called objective, new, Marxist, scientific, the science of behavior. Of course, we will reserve the name psychology for it. But what kind of psychology? How do we distinguish it from every other system of knowledge which uses the same name? We only have to sum up a small part of the definitions which are now being applied to psychology in order to see that there is no logical unity at the basis of these divisions. Sometimes the epithet designates the school of behaviorism, sometimes Gestalt psychology; sometimes the method of experimental psychology, psychoanalysis; sometimes the principle of construction (eidetic, analytical, descriptive, empirical); sometimes the subject matter of the science (functional, structural, actual, intentional); sometimes the area of investigation *(Individualpsychologie);* sometimes the world view (personalism, Marxism, spiritualism, materialism); sometimes many things (subjective-objective, constructive-reconstructive, physiological, biological, associative, dialectical, etc. etc.). On top of that one talks about historical and understanding, explanatory and intuitive, scientific (Blonsky) and "scientific" (used by the idealists in the sense of natural-scientific) psychology.

What does the word "psychology" signify after this? Stout [1909, p. ix] says that "The time is rapidly approaching when no one will think of writing a book on Psychology in general, anymore than of writing a book on Mathematics in general." All terms are unstable, they do not logically exclude each other, are not well-defined, are vague and obscure, ambiguous, accidental, and refer to secondary features, which not only does not facilitate the understanding, but hampers it. Wundt called his psychology "physiological," but later he repented and regarded this as an error and reasoned that the same work should be called "experimental." This illustrates best how little all these terms mean. For some, "experimental" is a synonym for "scientific," for others, it is only the designation of a method. We will only point out the epithets which are most widely used in psychology, considered in the light of Marxism.

I consider it inexpedient to call it "objective." Chelpanov correctly pointed out that in foreign psychology this term is used in most diverse senses. In Russia as well it engendered many ambiguities and furthered confusion in the epistemological and methodological problem of mind and matter. The term promoted the confusion of method as a technical procedure and as a method of knowledge. This resulted in the treatment of the dialectical method alongside the survey method as equally objective, and in the conviction that the natural sciences have done away with all use of subjective indicators, subjective (in their genesis) concepts and divisions. The term "objective" is often vulgarized and equated with "truthful," while the term "subjective" is equated with "false" (the influence of the common use of these words). Further, it does not express the crux of the matter at all. It expresses the essence of the reform only in a conditional sense and concerning one aspect. Finally, a psychology which also wishes to be a theory about the subjective or also wishes to explain the subjective on its paths, must not falsely call itself "objective."

It would also be incorrect to call our science "the psychology of behavior." Apart from the fact that this new epithet, like the preceding one, does not distinguish us from quite a number of currents and, therefore, does not reach its goal; apart from the fact that it is false, for the new psychology wants to know the mind as well; it is a philistine, everyday term, which is why it attracted the Americans. When Watson equates "the concept of personality in the science of behavior and in common sense" (1926, p. 355), when he sets himself the task of creating a science so that the "ordinary man" "who takes up the science of behavior would not feel a change of method or some change of the object" (ibid., p. ix); a science which among its problems also has the following one: "Why George Smith left his wife" (ibid., p. 5); a science which begins with the exposition of everyday methods; which cannot formulate the difference between them and scientific methods and views the *whole* difference in the study of those cases which are of no interest for everyday life, which do not interest common sense—then the term "behavior" is the most appropriate one. But if we become convinced, as will be shown below, that it is logically unten-able and does not provide a criterion by which we might decide why the peristalsis of the intes-tine, the excretion of urine, and inflammation should be excluded from the science; that it is ambiguous and undefined and means very different things for Blonsky and Pavlov, Watson and Koffka; then we will not hesitate to throw it away.

I would, further, consider it incorrect to define psychology as "Marxist." I have already said that it is unacceptable to write textbooks from the viewpoint of dialectical materialism (Struminsky, 1923; Kornilov, 1925); but also "Outline of Marxist Psychology," as Rejsner trans-lated the title of Jameson's booklet, I regard as improper word usage. Even such word combi-nations as "reflexology and Marxism," when one is dealing with different concrete currents within physiology, I consider to be incorrect and risky. Not because I doubt the possibility of such an evaluation, but because one takes incommensurable quantities, because the intermedi-ate terms which alone make such an evaluation possible are missing. The scale is lost and dis-torted. After all, the author passes judgment upon the *whole* of reflexology not from the view-point of the *whole* of Marxism, but on the basis of different pronouncements by different groups of Marxists-psychologists. It would not be correct, for instance, to raise the problem of the dis-trict soviet and Marxism, although the theory of Marxism has undoubtedly no fewer resources to shed light upon the question of the district soviet than upon reflexology and although the district soviet is a directly Marxist idea which is logically connected with the entire whole. And nevertheless we make use of other scales, we utilize intermediate, more concrete and less universal concepts. We talk about the Soviet power and the district soviet, about the dictator-ship of the proletariat and the district soviet, about class struggle and the district soviet. Not everything which is connected with Marxism should be called Marxist. Often this goes with-out saying. When we add to this that what psychologists usually appeal to in Marxism is dialec-tical materialism, i.e., its most universal and generalized part, then the disparity of the scales becomes still clearer.

Finally, there is a special difficulty in the application of Marxism to new areas. The present concrete state of this theory, the enormous responsibility in using this term, the polit-ical and ideological speculation with it—all this prevents good taste from saying "Marxist psychology" *now*. We had better let others say of our psychology that it is Marxist than call it that ourselves. We put it into practice and wait a little with the term. In the final analysis, Marx-ist psychology *does not yet exist*. It must be understood as a historical goal, not as something already given. And in the contemporary state of affairs it is difficult to get rid of the impression that this name is used in an unserious and irresponsible manner.

An argument against its use is also the circumstance that a synthesis between psychology and Marxism is being accomplished by more than one school and that this name can easily give rise to confusion in Europe. Not many people know that Adler's individual psychology links itself to Marxism. In order to understand what kind of psychology this is, we should remem-ber its methodological foundations. When it argued its right to be a science it referred to Rick-ert, who says that the word "psychology" applied by the natural-scientist and the historian has two different meanings and therefore distinguishes natural-scientific and historical psychology. If one would not do this, then the psychology of the historian and the poet could not be called psychology, because it has nothing in common with psychology. And the theorists of the new school assumed that Rickert's historical psychology and individual psychology were one and the same thing [of. Binswanger, 1922, p. 333].

Psychology has been divided into two parts and the debate is only about the name and the theoretical possibility of the new independent branch. Psychology is impossible as a natural science, the individual factor cannot be subsumed under any law; it does not want to explain, but to understand (ibid.). This division was introduced into psychology by Jaspers, but by understanding psychology he meant Husserl's phenomenology. As the basis of any psychology it is very important, even irreplaceable, but it is not itself and does not want to be, individual psychology. Understanding psychology can only proceed from teleology. Stern founded such a psychology; personalism is but another name for understanding psychology. But he attempts to study the personality in differential psychology with the means of experimental psychology, of the natural sciences: both explanation and understanding remain equally unsatisfactory. Only intuition and not discursive-causal thinking can lead to the goal. The title "philosophy of the ego" it considers to be honorary. It is no psychology at all, but philosophy, and wishes to be so. And *such* a psychology, about whose nature there can be no doubt, refers in its constructions, for example in the theory of mass psychology, to Marxism, to the theory of the base and superstructure, as to its natural foundation. In *social* psychology it has yielded the hitherto best and most interesting project of a synthesis of Marxism and individual psychology in the theory of class struggle: Marxism and individual psychology must and are called upon to extend and impregnate each other. The Hegelian triad is applicable to both mental life and economics (just as in Russia). This project evoked an interesting polemic which showed in the defense of this idea a sound, critical and—in a number of questions—entirely Marxist approach. While Man taught us to understand the economic foundations of the class struggle, Adler did the same for its psychological foundations.

This not only illustrates the entire complexity of the current situation in psychology, where the most unexpected and paradoxical combinations are possible, but also the danger of this epithet (incidentally, talking about paradoxes: this very psychology contests Russian reflexology's right to a theory of relativity). When the eclectic and unprincipled, superficial and semi-scientific theory of Jameson is called Marxist psychology, when also the majority of the influential Gestalt psychologists regard themselves as Marxists in their scientific work, then this name loses precision with respect to the beginning psychological schools which have not yet won the right to "Marxism." I remember how extremely amazed I was when I realized this during an informal conversation. I had the following conversation with one of the most educated psychologists:

> What kind of psychology do you have in Russia? That you are Marxists does not yet tell what kind of psychologists you are. Knowing of Freud's popularity in Russia, I at first thought of the Adlerians. After all, these are also Marxists. But you have a totally different psychology. We are also social-democrats and Marxists, but at the same time we are Darwinists and followers of Copernicus as well.

I am convinced that he was right because of one, in my view decisive, consideration. After all, we would indeed not call our biology "Darwinian." This is included in the concept of *science* itself. It implies the acceptance of all great conceptions. A Marxist historian would never use the title "A Marxist History of Russia." He would regard this as self-evident. "Marxist" is for him synonymous with "truthful" and "scientific." Another *history* than a Marxist one he does not acknowledge. And for us it should be the same. Our science will become Marxist to the degree that it becomes truthful and scientific. And we will work precisely on making it truthful and to make it agree with Marx's theory. According to the very meaning of the word and the essence of the matter we cannot use "Marxist psychology" in the sense we use associative, experimental, empirical, or eidetic psychology. Marxist psychology is not a school amidst schools, but the only genuine psychology as a science. A psychology other than this cannot exist. And the other way around: *everything* that was and is genuinely scientific belongs to Marxist psychology. This concept is broader than the concept of school or even current. It coincides with the concept *scientific* per se, no matter where and by whom it may have been developed.

Blonsky (1921) uses the term "scientific psychology" in this sense. And he is entirely right. What we wanted to do, the meaning of our reform, the crux of our divergence with the empiricists, the basic character of our science, our goal and the size of our task, its content and the method of its fulfillment—is all expressed by this epithet. It would fully satisfy me if only it were not unnecessary. Expressed in its most correct form it clearly revealed that it cannot express anything more than is already contained in the word it predicates. After all, "psychology" is the name of a *science and not of a theaterpiece or a movie.* It cannot be anything other than scientific. Nobody would call the description of the sky in a novel "astronomy." The name "psychology" is as little suited for the description of the thoughts of Raskol'nikov or the ravings of Lady Macbeth. Whatever describes the mind in a nonscientific way is not psychology, but something else—whatever you like: advertising, review, chronicle, fiction, lyric poetry, philosophy, philistinism, gossip and a thousand other things besides. After all, the epithet "scientific" is not only applicable to Blonsky's outline, but also to Müller investigations of memory, Köhler's experiments with apes, Weber-Fechner's theory about thresholds, Groos' theory of play, Thorndike's theory of training, Aristotle's association theory, i.e., to *everything* in history and contemporaneity which belongs to science. I would be prepared to argue that theories which are known to be incorrect, which have been falsified or are doubtful, can also be scientific, for being scientific is not the same as being valid. A ticket for the theater can be absolutely valid and nonscientific. Herbart's theory about feelings as the relations between ideas is absolutely false, but equally absolutely scientific. The goal and means determine whether a theory is scientific and no other factors. That is why to say "scientific psychology" is equal to saying nothing or, more correctly, to saying simply "psychology."

It remains for us to accept this name. It perfectly well stresses what we want the size and the content of our task. And it does not reside in the creation of a school next to other schools; it does not cover some part or aspect, or problem, or method of interpretation of psychology alongside analogous parts, schools, etc. We are talking about *all* of psychology, *in its full capacity;* about the only psychology which does not admit of another one. We are talking about the realization of psychology as a science.

That is why we will simply say: psychology. We will do better to explain other currents and schools with epithets and to distinguish what is scientific from what is nonscientific in them, psychology from empirism, from theology, from *eidos* and from everything which has stuck to it in the centuries of its existence as to the side of an ocean-going ship.

Epithets we need for other things: for the systematic, *consistently logical, methodological division* of disciplines within psychology. Thus, we will speak about general and child psychology, zoo and pathopsychology, differential and comparative psychology. Psychology will be the common name for an entire family of sciences. After all, our task is not at all to *isolate* our work from the general psychological work of the past, but to *unite* our work with all the scientific achievements of psychology into one whole, and on a new basis. We do not want to distinguish our school from science, but science from nonscience, psychology from nonpsychology. The psychology about which we are talking does not yet exist. It still has to be created—and by more than one school. Many generations of psychologists will still work on it, as James said [see p. 401 of Burkhardt, 1984]. Psychology *will have* its geniuses and its ordinary investigators. But what will emerge from the joint work of the generations, of both the geniuses and the simple skilled workmen of science, will be psychology. With this name our science will enter the new society on the threshold of which it begins to take shape. Our science could not and cannot develop in the old society, We cannot master the truth about personality and personality itself so long as mankind has not mastered the truth about society and society itself. In contrast, in the new society our science will take a central place in life. "The leap from the kingdom of necessity into the kingdom of freedom" inevitably puts the question of the mastery of our own being, of its subjection to the self, on the agenda. In this sense Pavlov is right when he calls our science the last science about man himself. It will indeed be the last science in the historical or prehistorical period of mankind. The new society will create the new man. When one mentions the remolding *of* man as an indisputable trait of the new mankind and the artificial creation of a new biological type, then this will be the only and first species in biology which will create itself . . .

In the future society, psychology will indeed be the science of the new man. Without this the perspective of Marxism and the history of science would not be complete. But this science of the new man will still remain psychology. Now we hold its thread in our hands. There is no necessity for this psychology to correspond as little to the present one as—in the words of Spinoza [1677/1955, p. 611—the constellation Dog corresponds to a dog, a barking animal.

# IV

# The History of the Development
# of Higher Mental Functions

JOSEPH GLICK, *City University of New York,
Graduate School and University Center*

In his seminal book, *The History of the Development of Higher Mental Functions*, L. S. Vygotsky sets out some of the key terms basic to his conception of psychology. The key feature of his conceptualization is the distinction between "lower" and "higher" mental functions. A psychologically adequate analysis must not confuse the higher with the lower, and Vygotsky claims that this was a characteristic mistake made by other broad approaches to psychology that were in vogue at the time. Associationism (reflexology) reduced the higher to the more elementary, and Gestalt psychology, while focusing on higher forms of behavior, treated the higher in the same ahistorical and acultural terms as the lower. Vygotsky argues that any approach to thinking–particularly any approach to understanding higher mental functions–must understand those functions in terms of their unique and integral qualities and, in particular, in terms of their origins in historical and cultural development. He sets forth his theoretically revolutionary agenda as follows:

> . . . elucidation of this subject requires a basic change in the traditional view of the process of mental development. . . . the one-sidedness and erroneousness of the traditional view of the facts on development of higher mental functions consist primarily and mainly in an inability to look at these facts as facts of historical development (Vygotsky, 1997, p. 1–2).

As Vygotsky sees it, his contemporaries' search for basic elements and processes, or for autochthonous (nonhistorical) laws, amounts to ripping qualitatively distinct behaviors from the contexts that would allow us to see their essential qualities; thus those contemporaries obscure the essential differences between "natural" and "cultural" lines of development. Vygotsky insists on the necessity to understand higher mental functions in terms of their cultural and historical origins.

However, as Scribner (1985) has pointed out, Vygotsky's uses of the concept of history, and of history as an analytic tool, are complex and multilayered, with several different referents. So too with ideas of culture: the different meanings can only be ferreted out by means of a close examination of Vygotsky's texts and a close reading of the use made of these concepts in the construction of inquiries, in the analyses of behaviors, and in the theoretical accounts that accompany the analyses.

This introduction to readings from *The History of the Development of Higher Mental Functions* follows Vygotsky's own methodological logic by focusing on the place of this work within his own history, within the history of the field at the time, and within the culture where it is now being received (here and now, in English, by us and our interpretive community). As we try to understand Vygotsky's work, we discover that this historically oriented mode of analysis is made compelling by the circumstances of the way his thinking came to be known by English-speaking audiences and by the twists and turns of the languages and the dates of the initial publications of his work.

As we search for one 'authoritative' text that reflects Vygotsky's thinking, we should always remember that we are always dealing with at least four texts: (1) the text as a text, considered as far as possible in terms internal to itself (the text as written); (2) the text as an argument addressed to the author's contemporary audience (the text as argument); (3) the text as encountered in the context of other texts–the intertextual text that will be eternally evolving as new texts are added to the interpretive world and to the frames of interpretation of the reader (the text as intertextually read); and finally, (4) the text as resurrected from the past and as used for contemporary purposes (the political text). The student of Vygotsky should be aware of all of these senses of what an authoritative text is: it is alive as a part of ever-changing interpretive communities and theoretical purposes.

In the same way that Vygotsky claims that a phenomenon cannot be understood without seeing it as a part of a cultural—historical formation, likewise a text cannot be understood when it is ripped out of the cultural—historical formulation within which it was generated, with respect to the audience to which it was addressed, and within which it is read and reread by different audiences with different frames of reference. Texts transform. Reading transforms texts.

Even more central to this understanding is the recognition that texts do not stand on their own, as self-evidently authentic. Readers read texts, and they do so while making use of the background of other texts that they have read. Thus, the examination of a text cannot be sufficient without simultaneously recognizing the relations of that text to other texts that surround it and to the readers who are reading it with still other texts in mind.

The recognition of this intertextuality is critical to reading and understanding Vygotsky, as is an understanding of the historical period within which he wrote, and the historical processes by which his written texts became known to us. We must factor these considerations in along side of our attempts to understand his meanings. Vygotsky wrote, not in all finality but in a particular place: living in the new Soviet Union, he addressed himself to the psychological literature of his time and to the field, as he knew it. Similarly we come to read him in the framework of our own theoretical interests, and in a field that is considerably different from the one that was known to Vygotsky.

Rather than thinking of Vygotsky as an individual, a theorist, and a genius whose individual mind speaks to us across the years, and as someone whose true meaning can be 'uncovered' by proper study, it is more instructive to think of Vygotsky in social terms, as a producer of texts, addressed to specific audiences, engaging the texts of others of the same and the preceding historical period. We, from our own vantage point, try to understand Vygotsky's text. Indeed, in this process we recreate the text in a context different from the context in which it was generated. This text, created as much in the reading as in the writing of it, is a text that necessarily addresses the concerns of the reader as much as the concerns of the writer.

The selections in this volume, bearing a very modern publication date (this essay was written in 2003), are translations from the six-volume Russian-language edition of Vygotsky's writings that appeared in 1982—1984, approximately half a century after the author's death. For some, this delay equals a lifetime, and, in Vygotsky's case it was longer than his lifetime. He was born in 1896 and died in 1934 at the age of thirty-seven.

It is, in part, a tribute to his genius that Vygotsky's work still has relevance, reference, and a lively intellectual viability today. He is taken not simply as an historical figure whose theoretical thinking should be a part of every well-read psychologist's repertoire; he is also an essentially contemporary voice, very much addressing the concerns of today. That relevance is not simply a product of Vygotsky's genius; it is also a part of the intertextual field within which his works–dislocated in time and intertextual reference–appeared, at least to the English-speaking world, but to some extent in Russian psychology as well. These dislocations in time are not simple historical or political accidents; indeed the discovery and rediscovery of Vygotsky relate to developments in contemporary psychology, not only to the vagaries governing the publication of his works. Indeed, the *Collected Works* are not the *complete* works; the origins of some of the writings are obscure; and the Vygotsky manuscripts, at this publication time, are mostly in private hands and are not available in any archive. There is much scholarly work to do before the Vygotsky corpus can be considered to be complete or secure.

Few of Vygotsky's important writings were published until well after his death. Only then did his publications reach an audience wider than the circle of brilliant colleagues who worked with him in Moscow and Kharkov (A. N. Leontiev and A. R. Luria particularly notable among them). Vygotsky's texts now reach across historical periods to address the concerns of audiences who are significantly "displaced" in time and history.

As an example, the text of this section was authored in 1931 but did not see partial publication in Russian until 1960 (Chaps. 1–5), and the full text was only published in the Russian *Collected Works* in 1982–1984. English-speaking audiences had their first glimpses of it with the publication of an edited compilation and resynthesis of some key Vygotsky texts with the publication of *Mind in Society* in 1978 (Cole, Scribner, John-Steiner, & Souberman). Similarly, one of the critically important works in Vygotsky's oeuvre *Tool and Symbol* was originally written in 1930 in collaboration with Luria for the English-language *Carmichael's Manual of Child Psychology,* which appeared in 1932. But *Tool and Symbol* did not make it into this volume or to the English-language audience until portions of it appeared in *Mind in Society,* carrying only Vygotsky's name as author; the full version was included in Van der Veer and Valsiner's *Vygotsky reader* in 1994, with the senior authorship of A. R. Luria restored (Luria & Vygotsky, 1930/1994).

What would the relationship be between texts produced during different historical periods? And what would be the interpretive relationship between a text that was authored at one particular time and the same work published many years later, in a very different historical setting? Is this history relevant, or are we to understand such texts to be 'free-standing' and self-evident?

To try to anticipate Vygotsky's answers to such questions, we consider his criticism of Jean Piaget's work, as he knew it in 1931:

> Everything is taken outside the historical aspect. The concepts of the world and of causality of a modern European child from an educated milieu and the same concepts of a child of any primitive tribe, the worldview of a child of the stone age, the middle ages and the 20th century, all of these are basically the same, identical, equivalent to each other.

> Cultural development is as if isolated from history, and considered as a self-satisfying process governed by internal, self-contained forces, subject to its own immanent logic. Cultural development is considered to be [i.e., is not separable from] self-development (Vygotsky, 1997, p. 9).

As with child development, so goes the development of our understanding. The best approach to reading Vygotsky is to suspend attempts to offer a "true" and "eternal" approach to the "real meaning" of his texts. At best, we can attempt to render the spirit of his method as revealed in the writing that is accessible to us, and to understand that we read that writing through the lens of a very different context than the context that Vygotsky immediately addressed. Considered in intertextual terms, thousands of texts have appeared to fill the referential spaces, minds, and perspectives of students who encounter Vygotsky's writings that appeared from 1930 to more than seventy years later.

Throughout this work Vygotsky sharply criticizes the psychology of his day for being reductionist, for not recognizing the sharp distinctions that must be made between lower (natural) and higher (cultural–historical) mental processes. He argues against the methodological regimes that seek to decompose mind into analytic "elements" that do not reflect the qualities that are specific to each level or type of functioning. He argues for analysis that is historical and not simply experimental, analytic, and positivist. In the spirit of this method of scholarship, we can "locate" Vygotsky's texts, as they have become known to us, within the dynamics of the history of developmental psychology in the English-speaking world, particularly in the United States.

## Vygotsky and the History of
## Developmental Psychology, 1962–1997

The first major presentation of Vygotsky's thinking in English was the 1962 publication of *Thought and Language*, translated by Eugenia Hanfmann and Gertrude Vakar, and introduced by Jerome Bruner. While serious students of developmental psychology read the book and were impressed, it did not "take off." Very little work in the "Vygotskian mode" followed that publication. It seemed to be a one-time event, the discovery of a refreshing historical root. Even those who would later help bring Vygotsky to prominence in the United States, Michael Cole and Sylvia Scribner, made scant reference to Vygotsky in 1974, in their seminal book, *Culture and Thought: A Psychological Introduction*. Vygotsky's name appeared only in reference to Luria, and only then in the narrow context of some cross-cultural studies that Vygotsky and Luria had performed.

Sixteen years after the first book-length publication of Vygotsky in English and four years after *Culture and Thought*, came the publication of *Mind in Society*, carrying Vygotsky's name as author, but carefully composed from many separate writings (including selections from *The History of The Development of Higher Mental Functions*). That publication, edited by Cole, Scribner, John-Steiner, and Souberman, was a hallmark event in Vygotsky studies.

The Vygotsky of *Mind in Society* really took off, spawning many publications that dwelt on and expanded his basic concepts and led to many more publications by and about Vygotsky. In 1982–1984, six volumes of Vygotsky's collected works appeared in Russian. Kluwer Academic/Plenum later published a translation of these six volumes, under the general editorship of Robert Rieber, and the present volume is a selection from them. In 1985, Wertsch published his scholarly exegesis of Vygotsky's thought in *Vygotsky and the Social Formation of Mind*, and in the same year a collection of papers, edited by Wertsch, was devoted to Vygotskian topics: *Culture, Communication, and cognition: Vygotskian Perspectives*. The year 1986 saw a retranslation of *Thought and Language* by Kozulin, and in the very next year came the first volume of the Kluwer Academic/Plenum translation of Vygotsky's *Collected Works*, led off by Minick's retranslation of the same work, now entitled *Thinking and Speech*. Kozulin followed in 1990 with an intellectual biography of Vygotsky, and, in 1991, Wertsch integrated Vygotskian and Bakhtinian perspectives in *Voices of the Mind*. In 1991, Van der Veer and Valsiner produced another Vygotsky biography, *Understanding Vygotsky: A Quest for Synthesis*. Later, in 1994, they published *The Vygotsky Reader*, which contains many complete texts (for example, "Tool and Symbol") and other theretofore unpublished articles. The list could go on, easily containing hundreds of Vygotsky-related or Vygotsky-inspired publications.

Something obviously happened between 1962 and 1978, something that effected an interest in and a fascination with Vygotsky's ideas, or at least what were taken to be Vygotsky's ideas. In 1962,, the publication of *Thought and Language* seemed a one-time event. In 1978 *Mind in Society* spawned a generation of scholarship. It is unlikely that we can find the difference by looking at the development of Vygotsky's own ideas. Vygotsky actually wrote *Thought and Language* after he wrote the pieces that were assembled into *Mind in Society*. The reasons for the different reception lay elsewhere. As we will see, an examination of those reasons leads one to be cautious about any attempt at a contemporary exegesis of Vygotsky. It is likely that what anyone takes to be the core Vygotskian ideas are precisely those ideas that address a contemporary theoretical need, and which do not reflect the full scope of Vygotsky's thinking in its own terms.

### Behaviorism, Piaget, and Vygotsky

In the United States, positivism and a theoretical and methodological behaviorism dominated psychological thinking from the 1920s until the early 1960s. For a number of reasons, the constraints imposed by this narrow conception of psychological processes began to be recognized, and a new discipline–cognitive psychology–began to emerge.

Chomsky's (1959/64) review of Skinner's behaviorist account of language was a hallmark event, as was Neisser's 1967 publication of *Cognitive Psychology*. Both Chomsky and Neisser reviewed studies that, even in narrow experimental terms, seemed to necessitate a more complicated psychological architecture than behaviorism invited, and so Piaget was discovered by mainstream developmental psychology.

This discovery of Piaget began in 1962 with the publication of a monograph by the Society for Research in Child Development (SRCD), edited by Kessen and Kuhlman: *Thought in the Young Child.* Clearly, something was happening in the 1960s; it was a rediscovery of "structure" and the placing of structural issues at the core of psychological inquiry. The essence of the cognitive movement was to recognize that there were, in fact, structural aspects of behavior and thinking that necessitated a form of theorizing that went beyond the element-oriented metaphors of the behaviorist canon.

Recognition of these structural aspects further indicated that treatments of human learning and development must take into account such structural limitations. The shift involved a refocusing from "learning" to structure-dependent "development." Since structure-dependent development was of central concern to Piaget, he quickly came into the focus of cognitive-developmental psychology. Flavell's 1963 distillation of Piagetian theory for English-speaking audiences was followed by a steady stream of translations of Piaget's books. From the mid-1960s to the late 1970s, Piagetian concepts and their verification or refutation occupied center stage.

It was against this backdrop that the initial English-language publication of Vygotsky's *Thought and Language* appeared in 1962. While Vygotsky focused on a number of deep developmental problems, the emphasis of his work, as known through the early translation of *Thought and Language,* did not hit the dead center of psychologists' interest, which was still fascinated with structure. From the early 1960s through the late 1970s, many aspects of the Piagetian paradigm were battered from a number of directions, not all of which were very relevant to core Piagetian ideas. At issue was not so much Piagetian theory as intended by Piaget, but rather the way in which Piagetian theory was being consumed by the English-speaking psychological establishment.

There were three foci of concern with received Piagetian theory, and all were related to the underlying problematic implications of the structure-dependency idea. In the American context these amounted to:

- An attempt to escape the inherently conservative and limiting aspects of the structure-dependency position, which saw possible future developments as constrained by initial conditions. Studies were conducted to show the limits of such structure dependency by showing that what Piaget treated as developmentally constraining factors could be overcome by "training" that could show accelerated acquisition.

- A rejection of the "universalism" associated with the structure-dependency idea. Studies were designed to test the limits of the notion of structure, by examining whether supposedly common, underlying structures showed up in different content areas (the problem of horizontal décalage) or by comparing differing populations to see if they attained the same structural landmarks at approximately the same developmental age.

- A questioning of the "processes" presumed to underlie development. For Piaget, constrained developmental structures resulted from the dynamics of a "constructive" process that depended heavily on initial states in interaction with a physically constrained world. The constructive idea was challenged from three different directions: (1) by an emerging "nativism" which, expanding on the structural aspect of Piaget's theory, saw many aspects of that structure as "in-built" and not constructed; or, alternatively and from another direction, (2) by a shift from the consideration of construction as an intra-individual process to an exploration of processes of social structuring; and (3) by focusing on the "knowledge base" and strategies that characterize particular domains, which were seen as defined "expertise" in an area–a more relevant factor than structural constraints.

Clearly, Piaget was under frontal attack from a number of directions. It was during this attack that Vygotsky was reintroduced to the English-speaking audience via the publication of *Mind in Society* in 1978. In contrast to the earlier introduction of Vygotsky in *Thought and Language*, the Vygotsky of *Mind in Society* proved to be fruitful and inspirational to further work.

This publication came at the point of disenchantment with the Piagetian treatment of structure and hence seemed to be an answer to the problems encountered over a two-decade involvement with Piaget. Moreover and not incidentally, the 'rediscovered' Vygotsky seemed to be more compatible with the stress on learning that behaviorism had championed before being driven into retreat by the Piagetian onslaught. However, this treatment of Vygotsky, within the context of reaction to Piagetian theory, highlighted only certain aspects of Vygotsky's approach, either not recognizing or ignoring other, perhaps more central, aspects.

## The Vygotskian Approach

Many of the main tenets of Vygotsky's approach, as understood by modern scholars, seemed particularly well suited as an answer to Piaget:

- The concept of the zone of proximal development (ZPD) was given center stage, since it was taken to mean that structure dependency was not an absolute limiting factor in development. Rather than following development and depending on it, learning could be seen actually to lead developmental change (Vygotsky, 1978, pp. 86–91).
- The concept of "mediation" similarly implied that factors external to the developing organism could influence its development (ibid., pp. 52–55). This promised the possibility of a "prosthetic" support for developmental change.
- Finally, the assertion of the social origins of development was given law-like status, asserting that every function appears twice, first in an interpersonal process and then as intra-personal process (ibid., pp. 56–57).

These three notions are now reasonably well understood and stand as the essential characteristics of the Vygotskian approach.

But things are not quite so simple. To a large extent the Vygotsky as received by the field of developmental psychology via *Mind in society* was a subtly different Vygotsky from the one introduced in 1962. Some of the topics now taken as central to a Vygotskian view are topics that underwent a slight alteration between *Thought and Language* and *Mind in Society*. In general, the shifts had to do with whether one sees the central concepts of Vygotsky as representing "laws of acquisition" of advanced behaviors, or as an attempt at "differential diagnosis" of differing developmental levels. The Vygotsky of *Mind in Society* was received as if his central concern was with acquisition, while the Vygotsky of *Thought and Language* seemed to be more concerned with the analytic problem of sorting out the compositional structure of various levels of behavioral development.

As an example of these shifts we can look at the treatment of the ZPD in the two volumes (and in much of the work that followed them). In *Thought and Language* (1962 translation), the ZPD is mentioned and discussed in two pages (pp. 103–105) and is not given an index entry. The discussion of the ZPD is framed within a treatment of a particular topic: the child's development of what Vygotsky termed the "scientific" concept (alternatively, the "academic" concept). Vygotsky's treatment here implies an interpretation of the ZPD in "diagnostic" terms. The basic idea of ZPD in *Thought and Language* concerned the issue of developmental assessment, and it is quite elegant in concept. Most tests of developmental level consider that the level is defined by the achievement of which the child is capable on her own, under some form of noninteractive and noninterventionist testing regime. Vygotsky argued that this only allows us to see the "completed" part of development and does not give us a view of developmental potential, which can be indicated by the degree to which a child can profit from external intervention. Vygotsky limits this discussion quite clearly to the development of school-related concepts, precisely those concepts which, incidentally, are not capable of being individually "constructed" and which were therefore not of particular interest to Piaget.

In *Mind in Society*, the concept of the ZPD reappears, but it is treated in a very different manner. Rather than being a subtopic within a discussion of the diagnosis of children's abilities and their readiness to profit from school-based instruction, the ZPD now appears as a topic in its own right, announced by a major heading: "The Zone of Proximal Development: A New Approach" (Vygotsky, 1978, p. 84). Along with this textual shift there is a shift to a law-like statement of the role and function of the ZPD in developmental analysis:

> ". . . what we call the Zone of Proximal Development . . . is the distance between the actual developmental level determined by individual problem solving and the level of development as determined through problem solving under guidance or in collaboration with more capable peers" (ibid., p. 86).

The specific bounding of the ZPD in issues of diagnosis and with respect to the effects of learning and instruction on a particular class of concepts has disappeared. The Vygotskian text of 1978 now addresses the issues with a new language, contrasting the "fruits of development" (p. 86) with the "buds and flowers" of development (p. 86), a botanical metaphor that is categorically rejected in the full-text version of "Tool and symbol" (included in Luria & Vygotsky, 1994).

A related interpretive shift occurs in the 1978 volume as well, one which fits in quite seamlessly with the generalized interpretation of the ZPD. In Chapter 4 of *Mind in Society* there is an extended discussion of processes of "internalization" which are given a "law-like" formulation, perhaps best summarized in the following language: "Every function in the child's cultural development appears twice: first, on the social level, and later, on the individual level; first, *between* people *(interpsychological)* and then *inside* the child *(intrapsychological)*" (Vygotsky, 1978, p. 57).

With these and similar moves of textual construction, the Vygotsky of the 1962 volume is transformed from merely an interesting new voice into a much more compelling voice that embodies the general reaction of the field to the Piagetian paradigm. By 1978, interest in Piaget was fading, and alternatives were being sought; the Vygotsky of 1978 was such an alternative. Where Piaget posed structural constraints, Vygotsky was taken to emphasize open possibilities. Where Piaget posed individual constructive processes that posed sharp limits on learning, Vygotsky posed internalization of interpersonal processes as the substrate of development.

The Vygotsky as presented in *Mind in Society* provided an interesting and appealing alternative to Piaget. Indeed, this Vygotsky could be construed to have a great deal in common with the behaviorism that had preceded the "discovery" of Piaget–a feature noticed by the editors of *Mind in Society*, who cautioned English-speaking readers that, though Vygotsky might look like a behaviorist at first glance, he really was not one. It seems that very few got the message.

## Constructing, Deconstructing, and Reconstructing Vygotsky

The gap between the reception of Vygotsky in 1962 and in 1978 by the English-speaking world and the relation between that differential reception to a growing unease with Piaget's theory both suggest that we are faced with a rather complex phenomenon when we read Vygotsky. We are reading a thinker whose ideas have been hidden too long, but we are also reading a thinker whose long-hidden ideas have been reintroduced, and perhaps have been changed by the contemporary context into which these ideas are introduced. That is, of necessity, a different context than the context within which the ideas were produced.

Such difference is more striking when we consider the manner in which Vygotsky's texts have been constructed for consumption by English-speaking audiences. The 1962 edition of *Thought and Language* is not simply a translation of the *Thought and Language* that appeared in Russian shortly after Vygotsky's death in 1934. As explained in the translator's introduction:

> Perhaps because the book [Vygotsky's original] was prepared in haste, it is not very well organized and its essential inner unity is not readily apparent. . . . It was agreed that excessive repetition and certain polemical discussions of little interest to the contemporary reader [i.e., Marxist rhetoric] should be eliminated, in favor of a more straightforward exposition. In translating the book, we have simplified and clarified Vygotsky's involved style, while striving always to render his meaning exactly (E. Hanfmann and G. Vakar, translators' introduction to *Thought and Language*, 1962, pp. xi–xii).

Nor was *Mind in Society* quite the newly unearthed Vygotsky as Vygotsky's name on the title page might indicate. The editors' preface makes the principle of construction quite clear:

> We have constructed the first four chapters of this volume from *Tool and symbol*. The fifth chapter summarizes the major theoretical and methodological points made in *Tool and*

> *symbol* and applies them to a classic problem in cognitive psychology, the nature of choice
> reactions. This chapter was taken from section 3 of the *The history of the development of higher
> psychological functions*. . . . At several places we have inserted material from additional sources
> in order to more fully explicate the meaning of the text. In most cases these importations
> are from sections of *The history of the development of higher psychological functions* other than
> the one included here. In putting several essays together we have taken significant liber-
> ties. The reader will encounter here not a literal translation of Vygotsky but rather our edited
> translation of Vygotsky, from which we have omitted material that seemed redundant and
> to which we have added material that seemed to make his points clearer" (Cole, Scribner,
> John-Steiner, & Souberman, editors' introduction to *Mind in Society*).

The processes of editing, clarifying, reducing seeming redundancies, eliminating polemical arguments of no contemporary interest, and constructing volumes out of other volumes must, almost
of necessity, mold an author into a contemporary voice. The judgments of what is dated, what
is redundant, what is unclear, and in what terms, are contemporary judgments; and, inevitably,
a contemporary construction addresses contemporary needs and understandings of what the core
problems are. The translation of the six volumes of his writings was an attempt to remedy
some of this distortion, as is this volume that samples a wide range of works by Vygotsky.

## The Vygotsky of *The History of the
Development of Higher Mental Functions*

The present volume includes two chapters (4 and 9) from *The History of the Development
of Higher Mental Functions* (other versions say "higher psychological functions"). In reading this
work, the modern reader will be immediately struck by two contradictory impulses. On the one
hand, many passages of the text may seem quite familiar. Given the appropriation of portions
of this manuscript and their incorporation into *Mind in Society*, this is to be expected. On the
other hand, these "familiar" passages occur in contexts of discussion that have not been previously exposed, alongside of concepts that probably have not even been encountered before (e.g.,
the discussion of establishing the "cultural age" of the child, in addition to the more familiar
"mental age" and "chronological age" measures that are used to define IQ). Some of these discussions will seem startlingly new, while others will seem dated or possibly "of no interest to
contemporary readers."

One might attempt to do an exegesis that will make clear what is new and to highlight
what has not been highlighted before. To do so, however, would probably violate the spirit and
the essential contribution of the monumental publishing effort, in both Russian and English,
that has attempted to present Vygotsky's full texts, polemical warts and all.

The main outlines of Vygotsky's theory are well known and have been given admirable
discussion by A. M. Matyushkin in his concluding remarks to Volume 4 of *Collected Works*.
However, the major task here is not to further identify and reinforce central Vygotskian constructs; the main task is rather to reconstruct the contexts within which they were framed,
and to sort out the concerns of Vygotsky himself as an inspirational but historically placed
figure, and to distinguish his constructs from the modern uses to which they have been put.

In *The History of the Development of Higher Mental Functions* Vygotsky fights against theoretical reductionism, attempting to understand development as a complexly woven tapestry of functions. The spirit of the enterprise is admirably expressed in an extended passage in Chapter 5:

> All psychological methods used thus far for studying the behavior of the normal and the abnormal child . . . have one common characteristic that links them in a certain respect . . . the negative description of the child that results from existing methods. All the methods speak of what the child does not have. . . . Such a picture tells us nothing about the positive uniqueness that distinguishes the child from the adult and the abnormal child from the normal child. . . . But a positive picture is possible only if we radically change our representation of child development and take into account that it is a complex dialectical process that is characterized by a complex periodicity, disproportion in the development of separate functions, metamorphoses or qualitative transformation of certain forms into others, a complex merging of the process of evolution and involution, a complex crossing of external and internal factors, a complex process of overcoming difficulties and adapting (Vygotsky, 1997, pp. 98–99).

Some of Vygotsky's ideas concerning these complexities are revealed in another passage that connects Vygotsky's thinking to other intellectual traditions with which he is generally not associated:

> Two completely equally tenable problems confront science: disclosing the lower in the higher and disclosing the development of the higher from the lower. . . . (Heinz) Werner maintains that the psychological structure is characterized by not one but by many genetic strata superimposed on one another. For this reason even a separate individual considered genetically displays in his behavior certain phases of developmental processes that are already genetically concluded. Only the psychology of elements represents human behavior as a single closed sphere. As distinct from this the new psychology establishes that man displays genetically different stages in his behavior (Vygotsky, 1997, p. 102).

The Vygotsky we encounter in these passages is a thinker enmeshed in the core issues of developmental analysis, as these issues were understood by traditions of thinking and research that were fundamentally opposed to the behaviorism ("psychology of elements" in the above passage) that had preceded the 'discovery' of Piaget in the English-speaking world.

As is amply clear in *The History of the Development of Higher Mental Functions*, Vygotsky as a thinker was deeply involved in developments within psychological theory on a wide number of fronts, in many different languages, and in a number of different analytic traditions. As such, his theoretical frame of reference was broader than the theoretical frame of reference within the English-speaking world at the time. In a very real sense he represented not only a Marxist approach to theorizing about development but a broadly European approach as well.

Within the European tradition of the time, the major analytic thrust was precisely to "diagnose differentially" and to examine the complex layering of different developmental strata underlying behavior. The analytic metaphors were geological. Methods had to be developed which would prove "differential," first showing the composition of behavior and then "testing its limits." For example, in one of the chapters reproduced in this section, "Mastering Attention," Vygotsky focuses on the differential diagnosis and the different structuring of basic cognitive functions. The focus is on distinguishing between the "higher" and the "lower" forms of a mental function, forms that were usually treated as unitary before. It is a mistake to measure development in terms of a system of measurement that does not take into account such changes in "interfunctional" relationships that are the hallmark of the differences between higher and lower forms. This critique can apply even to some of the work that has been done recently in the 'Vyogotskian tradition.'

Careful reading of *The History of the Development of Higher Mental Functions* will show that Vygotsky takes a similar tack throughout, often providing strikingly illuminating insights derived from an orientation derived from a complex developmental "geology." As is evident throughout this work, Vygotsky is centered on a core theme: to develop a theoretical and methodological approach that will differentiate higher mental functions from the more basic functions that many other theorists of his time were positing as the functions upon which the entire psychological apparatus is built. For Vygotsky, such reductive accounts, either in the direction of reducing thinking to perceptual structures (the tack that the Gestalt psychologists took, here represented by Koehler), or to elementary associations (the tack that many behaviorists took), or to maturational laws (asserted by other developmentalists) all missed the point of the specifically human form of adaptation that constituted the higher functions. For Vygotsky, the higher functions reflect a uniquely cultural form of adaptation that involves both an overlay on, and a reorganization of, more basic psychological functions. It was therefore of key theoretical concern for Vygotsky to engage in the sort of analytic enterprise that would allow for the identification of the differences between the higher and lower forms, since different developmental factors applied to each. Not all behaviors were of the higher form, and just as certainly were not all behaviors of the lower form. In any given instance the issue was to find ways to differentiate the two by close analysis. Only once this is accomplished could one speculate upon the means by which these behaviors developed.

There is pleasure to be derived from the intellectual adventure that we embark upon in this book. We can see Vygotsky reasoning through his positions, and developing them carefully. He discusses, with respect and interest, the work of his contemporaries and forebears. The modern reader would not be well served by an elision of these aspects of Vygotsky as thinker in process. She would not be well served by serving Vygotsky up as a finished product, with the answers to all of our questions. What others have taken to be disorganized and rambling and repetitive can be better seen as the essential process of working through a profound theoretical position. In this work, dated as it is, with its long, "polemical" discussions, "not of interest to contemporary readers," there is much to be discovered, not only about the past of the field of developmental psychology, but also about what its future ought to be.

## References

Chomsky, N. (1959/64). A review of B. F. Skinner's *Verbal behavior*. In *The structure of language: Readings in the philosophy of language* (J. A. Fodor & J. J. Katz, Eds.). Englewood Cliffs, NJ: Prentice-Hall. Original work published in *Language* 35 (1959).
Cole, M., & Scribner, S. (1974). *Culture and thought: A psychological introduction*. New York: Wiley.
Flavell, J. H. (1963). *The developmental psychology of Jean Piaget*. Princeton, NJ: Van Nostrand.

Kessen, W., & Kuhlman, C. (Eds.) (1962). Thought in the young child: Report of a conference on intellective development with particular attention to the work of Jean Piaget. *Monographs of Society for Research in Child Development*, Vol. 27.

Kozulin, A. (1990). *Vygotsky's psychology: A biography of ideas*. Cambridge: Harvard University Press.

Luria, A. R., & Vygotsky, L. S. (1930/1994). *Tool and symbol*. In *The Vygotsky reader* (R. Van der Veer & J. Valsiner, Eds.). Oxford: Blackwell.

Neisser, U. (1967). *Cognitive psychology*. New York: Appleton-Century-Crofts.

Scribner, S. (1985). Vygotsky's uses of history. In *Culture, communication, and cognition: Vygotskian perspectives* (J. Wertsch, Ed.). Cambridge: Harvard University Press.

Van der Veer, R. & Valsiner, J. (1991). *Understanding Vygotsky: A quest for synthesis*. Oxford: Blackwell.

Van der Veer, R. & Valsiner, J. (Eds.) (1994). *The Vygotsky reader*. Oxford: Blackwell.

Vygotsky, L. S. (1962). *Thought and Language* (E. Hanfmann & G. Vaker, Trans.). Cambridge: MIT Press.

Vygotsky, L. S. (1978). *Mind in Society: The development of higher psychological processes* (M. Cole, S. Scribner, V. John-Steiner, & E. Souberman, Eds.). Cambridge: Harvard University Press.

Vygotsky, L. S. (1986). *Thought and Language* (A. Kozulin, Trans.). Cambridge: MIT Press.

Vygotsky, L. S. (1997). *The collected works of L. S. Vygotsky, Volume 4: The History of the Development of Higher Mental Functions* (R. W. Rieber, Ed.). New York: Kluwer Academic/Plenum.

Wertsch, J. V. (Ed.) (1985). *Culture, communication, and cognition: Vygotskian-perspectives*. Cambridge: Harvard University Press.

Wertsch, J. V. (1985). *Vygotsky and the social formation of mind*. Cambridge: Harvard University Press.

Wertsch, J. V. (1991). *Voices of the mind: A sociocultural approach to meditated action*. Cambridge: Harvard University Press.

# 11

## The Structure of Higher Mental Functions

The conception of psychological analysis that we tried to develop in the preceding chapter leads us to a new representation relative to the mental process as a whole and its nature. The most substantial change that occurred in psychology recently is that an analytical approach to the mental process was replaced by a holistic or structural approach. The most influential representatives of modern psychology advanced the holistic point of view and placed it at the base of all psychology. The essence of the new point of view is that the significance of the whole, which has its own specific properties and determines the properties and functions of the parts that constitute it, is foremost. In contrast to the old psychology, which represented the process of the formation of a complex form of behavior as a process of mechanical summation of separate elements, the new psychology places at its center the study of the whole and such of its properties as cannot be deduced from the sum of the parts. The new point of view has accumulated much experimental evidence that confirms its correctness.

For dialectical thinking, there is nothing new in the position that the whole does not arise mechanically by means of a sum of separate parts, but has specifically unique properties and qualities which cannot be deduced from a simple combining of the qualities of the parts.

In the history of the cultural development of the child, we find the concept of a twofold structure. First, this concept arose at the very beginning of the history of cultural development of the child and formed the initial moment of the point of origin of the whole process; second, the process of cultural development itself must be understood as a change in the basic original structure and the development of new structures on its base that are characterized by a new relation of the parts. We will term the first structures primitive; this is a natural psychological whole that depends mainly on the biological features of the mind. The second, arising in the process of cultural development, we will term higher structures since they represent a genetically more complex and higher form of behavior.

The main feature of primitive structures is that the reaction of a subject and all stimuli are at the same level and belong to one and the same dynamic complex which, as research demonstrates, has an extremely clear affective tinge. Many authors see the major capacity of the mind in the primacy of the whole over the parts, in the holistic character of primitive

Originally appeared in English as Chapter 4 in *The Collected Works of L.S. Vygotsky, Volume 4: The History of the Development of Higher Mental Functions* (Robert W. Rieber, Ed., Marie J. Hall, Trans.) (pp. 83–96). New York: Kluwer Academic/Plenum, 1997.

forms of child behavior, tinged affectively. The traditional representation that the whole is comprised of parts is disproved here, and researchers demonstrate experimentally that the whole, perception and action, not differentiating separate parts, is genetically primary, most elementary and simple. The whole and the parts develop in parallel and together with each other. Depending on this, many authors assume that the problems of psycho logical study changed radically, especially where explaining higher forms of behavior is concerned.

In contrast to Wundt, who seemed to believe that to explain higher forms, the existence of creative syntheses that unite separate elements into new qualitatively unique processes must be assumed, Werner advanced another point of view stating that not creative syntheses, but creative analysis is the real path to the formation of higher forms of behavior. New whole processes do not come from elements of a complex mind, but, on the contrary, they come from the breakdown of the dynamic whole, which from the very beginning exists as a whole, and the parts and connections and their interrelations that are developing among them on the basis of this whole must be brought forward and understood. Psychology must proceed from living unities and, through analysis, make a transition to lower unities.

However, primitive structures, for which such a merging into a single complex of the whole situation and reaction to it is characteristic, are only a point of departure. Moving on from it, a disruption and reconstruction of the primitive structure and a transition to a higher type begins. The attempt to apply the meaning of the new principle to ever newer areas of psychology begins to attach a universal significance to the concept of structure. This concept, metaphysical in essence, be gins to signify something indivisible that comprises an eternal law of nature. Not in vain does Volkelt, speaking of their primary structures as the most important feature of the primitive mind of the child, call them "perpetually childlike." Actually, research shows that the "perpetual child" is as instantaneous, ephemeral, self-obliterating, and transitional to a higher form as all other forms of primitive behavior.

New structures that we contrast with lower or primitive structures differ mainly in that direct fusion of stimuli and reactions into a single complex seems to be disrupted. If we analyze thoroughly the unique forms of behavior that we had the opportunity to observe in the selection reaction, then we cannot help but note that in behavior, a seeming stratification of a primitive structure is occurring in this case. Between the stimulus to which behavior is directed and the person's reaction, a new intermediate member intervenes and the whole operation assumes the character of a mediated act. In connection with this, analysis develops a new point of view of the relation that exists between the behavioral act and external phenomena. We can distinguish clearly two orders of stimuli of which some are stimuli-objects and others, stimuli-means; each of these stimuli according to its relations uniquely determines and directs behavior. The uniqueness of the new structure is the presence in it of stimuli of both orders.

In our experiments, we were able to observe how the very structure of the whole process changes depending on a change in the position of the middle stimulus (sign)—the very structure of the whole process changes in behavior. Using words as a means of remembering was enough to make all the processes connected with remembering the instruction assume a single direction. But if only the words were replaced by meaningless geometrical figures, then the whole process took a different direction. Because of simpler experiments that were carried out, we believe it is possible to assume the following as a general rule: *in the higher structure, the sign and methods of its use are the functional, determining whole or focus of the whole process.*

Just as the use of one tool or another dictates the whole system of a work operation, the character of the sign used is the base on which the construction of the rest of the process depends. The same fundamental relation that lies at the base of the higher structure is the special form of organization of the whole process which consists of the process being constructed by involving certain artificial stimuli in the situation as signs. Thus, the functionally different role of two stimuli and their connection with each other serves as a base of the connections and relations that form the process itself.

The process of involving secondary stimuli in a situation which then acquires a certain functional meaning may be observed most easily in experiments when the child first makes the transition from a direct operation to using a sign. In our experimental studies, we placed the child in a situation in which he was presented with a problem of remembering, comparing, or selecting something. If the problem did not exceed the natural capacity of the child, he dealt with it directly or with the primitive method. In these cases, the structure of his behavior resembled completely the diagram drawn by Volkelt. The essential characteristic of the diagram is that the reaction itself constitutes a part of the situation and is inescapably included in the structure of the situation itself as a whole. This dominant whole of which Volkelt speaks predetermines the direction of the child's grasping movement. But the situation in our experiments was almost never like that. The problem confronting the child usually exceeded his capacity and seemed too difficult to solve with this kind of primitive method. At the same time, beside the child, there usually was some object that was completely neutral in relation to the whole situation, and in this case, under certain conditions, when the child was confronted by a problem he could not solve, we could observe how the neutral stimuli stopped being neutral and were drawn into the behavioral process, acquiring the function of a sign.

We could place this process in parallel with the process described by Köhler. As we know, the simian that once had the sense to use a stick as a tool began later to use as tools any objects that were somewhat outwardly similar to a stick. Köhler said that if we assume that a stick that caught the eye acquired a certain functional significance for certain situations and that this significance was extended to all other objects, whatever kind they may be, then we come directly to the one and only view that coincides with the observed behavior of animals.

We could say that when an obstacle arises, the neutral stimulus acquires the function of a sign and from that time, the structure of the operation takes on an essentially different aspect.

In this way, we make a transition to the other side of the problem closely connected with it. As we know, in organic nature, structure and function are very closely connected. They are a unit and mutually explain each other. Morphological and physiological phenomena, form and function, depend on each other. In the most general form, we could define the direction in which structure is changed: it is changed in the direction of greater differentiation of parts. The higher structure differs from the lower most of all in that it is a differentiated whole in which the separate parts fulfill different functions and in which a combination of the parts into a whole process occurs on a base of functional double connections and interrelations between functions. Werner cites the words of Goethe,[61] who said that the difference between lower and higher organism consists in the greater differentiation in the higher. The more developed an organism is, the less similar are its parts to one another. In the one case, the whole and the parts are more or less similar to each other; in the other, the whole differs substantially from the parts. The more similar the parts are to each other, the less they are subordinate one to another. Subordination signifies a more complex relation of the parts of an organism. In this connection, Werner sees the very essence of the process of development in progressive differentiation and centralization connected with it.

As applied to structure, we could say that it is specifically differentiation of the primitive whole and clear separation of the two layers (stimulus-sign and stimulus-object) that are the mark of the higher structure. But differentiation has another aspect that consists in the entire operation as a whole acquiring a new character and significance. We could not describe the new significance of the whole operation any better than to say that it represents *a mastery of the behavioral process itself.*

Actually, if we compare the diagram of the selection reaction as we drew it in the preceding chapter with the diagram that Volkelt provides, we can see that the most important difference of the one from the other lies in the character of the determination of the behavior as a whole. In the second case, the activity of the organism is determined by the total complex of the whole situation, the logic of the structure, and in the first case, man himself creates the connection and ways for his reacting; he reconstructs the natural structure; with the help of signs, he subordinates to his will processes of his own behavior.

The fact that traditional psychology did not at all note this phenomenon which we call mastery of one's own behavior seems surprising to us. In attempts to explain the fact of "will," psychology resorted to miracle, to intervention of a spiritual factor in the course of neural processes and, in this way, tried to explain the effect along the line of greatest resistance, as James had done, for example, in developing the teaching on the creative character of will.

But even in the psychology of recent times, which has begun gradually to introduce the concept of mastery of one's own behavior into the system of psychological concepts, there is still neither the necessary clarity in the concept itself nor an adequate evaluation of its true significance. Lewin is justified in noting that phenomena of mastery of one's own behavior have not yet appeared in all clarity in the psychology of the will. Conversely, in pedagogy, problems of mastery of one's own behavior have for a long time been considered as basic problems of education. In contemporary education, the will replaced the position of deliberate action. In place of external discipline, in place of compulsory training, independent mastery of behavior is promoted which does not propose suppressing the natural inclinations of the child, but has in mind his mastery of his own actions.

In this connection, obedience and good intentions are relegated to the background and the problem of mastery of oneself is moved to the forefront. This problem actually has much greater significance, since we have in mind the intention that controls the child's behavior. Moving the problem of intention to the background in relation to the problem of self mastery appears in the problem of obedience of the very small child. The child must learn obedience through self mastery. Self mastery is not constructed on obedience and intention, but, conversely, obedience and intention develop from self mastery. Analogous changes with which we are familiar from the pedagogy of the will are indispensable to the basic problem of the psychology of the will.

Together with an act of intention or decision, even more strongly must the problem of mastery of behavior be brought to the forefront in connection with the causal-dynamic problem of the will. However, regardless of ascribing such a central significance to the mastery of behavior, we do not find in Lewin any kind of clear determination or even a study of this process. Not once does Lewin return to it, and, as a result of research, arrives at distinguishing two basic forms of behavior. Since this distinction coincides closely with the distinction between the primitive and the higher structure which is where we begin, we will consider Lewin's remarks in somewhat greater detail.

With him, in the interests of a purer scientific formation of concepts, we agree to give up the term "will," and in its place to introduce the term "dependent actions and independent actions," or actions arising directly from forces within the situation itself. The latter seem to us to be especially important. According to Lewin, it is understood that controlled actions also are subject to determining forces of the general situation, but with this type of action, man usually does not feel that he is involved with his whole personality in that situation; to a certain degree, he remains outside the situation and owing to this, he holds the action itself firmly in hand. Delimitation of the psychological systems in this case is different from what it is in a simple action due to the greater independence or greater dominance of the system "I."

Regardless of this confused formulation of the whole problem, Lewin still arrives at establishing the fact that the formation of such ties, made with the help of an auxiliary action, is a feature of adult cultured man or, as we could say in other words, it is the product of cultural development. Lewin indicates that the basic problem arises relative to whether "any intentions" can be formed. In itself, most remarkable is the fact that man has exceptional freedom in the sense of intentional implementation of any action, even senseless action. This freedom is characteristic for civilized man. It is present in the child and probably in primitive peoples to a much lesser degree and, in all probability, distinguishes man from animals closest to him much more than his superior intellect. The difference, consequently, is reduced to the possibility of man's mastery of his own behavior.

In contrast to Lewin, we attempt to provide for the concept of mastery of one's own behavior a completely clear and precisely determined content. We proceed from the fact that the processes of behavior represent the same kind of natural processes subject to the laws of nature as all other processes. Neither is man, subjecting processes of nature to his will and intervening in the course of these processes, an exception in his own behavior. But a basic and very important question arises: how should he represent the mastery of his own behavior to himself?

Two basic facts were known to the old psychology. On the one hand, it recognized a hierarchical relation of higher and lower centers by which some processes regulate the course of others; on the other hand, psychology, coming to a spiritualistic interpretation of the problem of will, advanced the idea that mental forces act on the brain and through it on the whole body.

The structure we have in mind differs substantially from both the first and the second case. The differences are that we bring forward the problem of means by which behavior is mastered. Just as mastery of one process or another in nature, mastery of one's own behavior assumes not a change in basic laws that control these phenomena, but subjection to them. We know that the basic law of behavior is the law of stimulus-response; for this reason, we cannot master our behavior in any other way except through appropriate stimulation. The key to mastery of behavior is mastery of stimuli. Thus, *mastery of behavior is a mediated process* that is always accomplished through certain auxiliary stimuli. We tried to disclose the role of stimuli-signs in our experiments on the selection reaction.

Recently in child psychology, the idea of studying specific features of human behavior has been advanced a number of times. Thus, M. Ya. Basov advanced the concept of man as an active agent in the environment, contrasting his behavior with the passive form of adaptation typical of animals. This author maintains that as a subject for psychology, we have before us an organism as an agent in his environment and the activity he exhibits in interaction with his environment in various forms and processes of behavior.

However, even Basov, who came closest to the problem of the specific in human behavior, did not delimit in his research any distinctly active and passive form of adaptation.

We might summarize what our comparative consideration of higher and lower forms of behavior leads to and say: the unity of all the processes that constitute the higher form is formed on the basis of two instances: first, the unity of the problem confronting man, and second, as we have already said, the means that dictate the whole structure of the process of behavior.

As an example that will make it possible to distinguish clearly the features of the higher and lower forms and simultaneously disclose the major instances of this difference, we can use the primitive and cultured structure of children's speech.

As we know, the first word pronounced by the child is a whole sentence in meaning. And even more, it is sometimes complex speech. Thus, the external form of development of speech as it develops from the phenotypic aspect is deceptive. Actually, if we are to believe external consideration, we would have to conclude that the child is at first pronouncing separate sounds, then separate words, and later begins to unite the words in two's and three's and makes the transition to a simple sentence which later develops into a complex sentence and into a whole system of sentences.

This external picture, as we have already said, is deceptive. Research has shown definitively that the primary or original form of children's speech is a complex, affective and undifferentiated structure. When the child pronounces the first "Ma," Stern says, this word cannot be translated into the language of adults with the one word "Mama," but must be translated by a whole sentence such as "Mama, put me on the chair," etc. We will add that by no means is only the word "Ma" itself taken separately deserving of such an extended translation, but the entire situation as a whole: the child who wants to be placed on a chair, the toy which he wants to get by this operation, his unsuccessful attempt, the approaching proximity of the mother who is watching his behavior, and finally, his first exclamation—all of this, merged into a single whole complex could have been fully represented by Volkelt's diagram.

Let us compare this primitive undifferentiated structure with the structure of speech of this child at age three when he expresses the same desire in the developed form of a simple sentence. We ask, how is the new structure different from the earlier structure? We see that the new structure is differentiated. Here, the single word "Ma" is converted into four separate words of which each precisely indicates and signifies an object of action that constitutes the corresponding operation and grammatical relations that convey the relation between real objects.

Thus, the differentiation and subordination of separate members of the common whole distinguish the development of this speech structure from the primitive structure with which we compare it. But its most essential difference is that it does not represent action directed toward a situation. In contrast to the initial cry that is an integral part in the merged complex of the situation, the present speech of the child has lost the direct connection with action on objects. It is now only an influence on another person. And so these functions of influence on behavior which are divided here between two persons, between the child and the mother, are united in a single whole in the complex structure of behavior. The child begins to apply to himself those forms of behavior that adults usually apply to him, and this is the key to the fact of mastery of one's own behavior, the fact that interests us.

It still remains for us to elucidate the problem touched on earlier relative to what kind of distinguishing traits set the given structure apart from the more general type of structures that we, together with Köhler, could term detour structures. By this term, Köhler understands an operation that develops when attaining a goal by direct means is obstructed. Köhler has in mind two basic concrete forms in which such detour structures appear. The first are detours in the literal sense of the word when some physical barrier in the form of a road block stands between an animal and his goal and the animal moves toward the goal bypassing the obstacle in a roundabout way. The second concrete form consists in using tools, which, in a figurative sense, may also be termed detours or roundabout ways: when the animal cannot master something directly, cannot get it with his hand, the animal moves it closer with a developed operation and, as if in a roundabout way, attains his goal.

Of course, the structure we are considering belongs to a number of similar detours. However, there is a substantial difference that compels us to consider it as a structure of a special kind. The difference is in the direction of the whole activity and in the character of the detours. While a tool or a real detour is directed toward a change of something in the external situation, the function of a sign consists most of all in changing something in the reaction or in the behavior of man himself. The sign changes nothing in the object itself, it only gives a new direction or reconstructs the mental operation.

Thus, a tool directed outward and a sign directed inward fulfill technically different mental functions. Depending on this, the very character of the detours differs in an essential way. In the first case, we have certain objective detours consisting of material bodies; in the second case, detours of mental operations. These circumstances simultaneously indicate similarities and differences between the structures we are considering and the structures of detours.

What has been said allows us to approach still another essential problem. At present, we may consider as completely elucidated the formerly debatable question of the need to isolate a third step in the development of behavior, that is, to place intellectual reactions in a separate class on the basis of genetic, functional, and structural traits that preclude considering these reactions simply as complex habits. If we assume, with Bühler, that the indicated acts retain the character of "trials," then the trials themselves acquire a completely different character. They no longer have to do directly with the object; they have to do with the internal aspect of the process, becoming exceptionally complex and in this case indicating a new step in the development of behavior. Of course, this new step cannot be considered as being cut off from the preceding second step.

The connection between the two steps is the same as it is over the whole extent of development. The lower forms are not destroyed, but are incorporated into the higher and continue to exist in it as a subordinate instance. For this reason we believe that relative to the three steps in the development of behavior proposed by Bühler, Koffka is justified in saying that areas of behavior must not be considered as fixed, congealed, separated from one another by an impassable wall. They must rather be understood as forms of behavior special in structural and functional relation that are found in an exceptionally complex dependence on each other and that are included in various relations in one and the same process of behavior.

In this case, we are interested in another question, opposite in a certain sense to the question we have just been considering. For us, speaking of three steps in the development of behavior is undoubtedly the very first requisite of the researcher. But we will take the question further: can we limit ourselves to the three steps indicated and do we not make the same mistake in this way that Bühler tried to avoid when he separated the second and third steps, does not this teaching contain a further simplification of higher forms of behavior, and does not the present state of our science oblige us to speak of still another, in this case, a fourth step in the development of behavior that characterizes the higher forms of behavior in man?

Introducing the concept of a third step, Bühler maintains that it is necessary to reduce to a common denominator both the higher forms of human thinking and the more primitive forms with which we became familiar in the child and in the chimpanzee, and that, theoretically, their bases are identical. The problem of science is completely legitimate: to understand what is common, what unites higher and lower forms, since the seed of higher forms is contained in the lower. But it is exactly the reduction to a common denominator of higher and primitive forms of behavior that is the gross mistake based on an inadequate study of them, on the study only of the latter.

Actually, if we capture only what is identical in the higher and lower forms of behavior, we will do only half the job. In this case, we will never be able to describe adequately the higher forms with the whole specific quality that makes them what they in fact are. For this reason, the common denominator that Bühler sees in purposeful behavior accomplished with an object without repeated trials still does not disclose what is essential in higher forms, what they contain.

We will say outright: three steps in the development of behavior exhaust diagrammatically all the variety of forms of behavior in the animal world; in human behavior, they disclose what is identical with the behavior of animals; for this reason, the three-step diagram encompasses, more or less fully, only the common course of biological development of behavior. But it lacks what is the most essential, specifically, those unique forms of mental development that distinguish man. And if we want to be consistent in carrying out the trend that we termed the trend toward humanizing psychology, if we want separate out the human, and only the human, in the development of the child, we must go beyond the bounds of the diagram.

Actually, the common denominator assumes that all difference between the unique forms of human and animal behavior is removed. The fact that man builds new forms of action first mentally and on paper, stages battles on maps, works on mental models, in other words, everything that in human behavior is connected with the use of artificial means of thinking, with social development of behavior, and specifically, with the use of signs, is left beyond the bounds of the diagram. For this reason, together with the three-step diagram, we must isolate a special, new step in the development of behavior constructed above it, a step which may incorrectly be called a fourth step, since it stands in a somewhat different relation to the third than the third does to the second, but in any case, it would be more correct, moving from ordinal to cardinal numbers, to speak not of three, but of four steps in the development of behavior.

A fact of no small importance hides behind this position. We have only to recall how many arguments were caused by the discovery and recognition of the third step in the development of behavior to understand the enormous significance that adding a fourth step will have for all the prospects of genetic psychology.

As we know, recognizing intellectual reactions as a special class of reactions raised objections from two sides. Some found the introduction of a new concept to be superfluous and tried to demonstrate that intellectual reactions contain nothing basically new in comparison with habit, that they may be fully and completely adequately described in terms of the formation of conditioned reactions, that all behavior may be wholly exhausted with the two-step diagram that differentiated innate and acquired reactions.

Supporters of this view expressed misgivings that together with recognizing a third step which was still inadequately studied and insufficiently clear, the meta physical and speculative concept would once again be introduced into psychology, that behind the new terms, once again the road would be paved for a purely spiritualistic interpretation, that an anthropomorphic transfer of human methods of behavior to animals might once again fatally pervert all of the genetic perspectives of psychology. We note incidentally that the misgivings were to a certain degree justified. However, this does not seem to us to be evidence to any degree that its authors are right; from the position that any thing can serve as an object of abuse, it does not follow that the thing should not be used.

If adherents of the view under consideration assumed introducing a third step to be superfluous and criticized the new concept from below, from the aspect of biology, then it met with no less bitter attacks from the top, from the aspect of subjective psychology, which feared that with the introduction of the new concept the rights of the human intellect would be depreciated, that, as with Darwin, the divine nature of man would again be genetically linked to the chimpanzee. Psychologists of the Wurzburg school, being occupied with the study of thinking and considering it as a purely mental act, declared that contemporary psychology is again on the path to Platonic ideas. For this idealistic thinking, Köhler's discovery was a cruel blow showing as it did the root of human thinking in the primitive use of tools by the chimpanzee.

For us, this developing situation seems characteristic to a high degree since the discovery of the third step in the development of behavior evoked bitter attacks both from above and from below.

An analogous situation is also created when we attempt to introduce further complexity into psychology and speak not of three, but of four basic steps in the development of behavior. This is the basic and principal problem of all genetic psychology, and we must expect in advance that the new diagram will meet bitter opposition both from the aspect of biological psychology, which tries to reduce human thinking based on the use of signs and primitive thinking of the chimpanzee to a common denominator, as well as from the aspect of spiritualistic psychology, which must again see in the new diagram an attempt to expose higher forms of behavior and present them as natural and historical formations and in this way encroach again on Platonic ideas.

We can find comfort only in the fact that the criticism from above and the criticism from below cancel each other out, neutralize each other, in the fact that complication of the simple, initial diagram alone seems not to be justified, and in the fact that it will be accepted by others as an unnatural simplification.

Actually, we admit that in our new attempt, there is also more likely to be the danger of simplification and of extraordinary complication since only the first steps have been taken. Undoubtedly, consciously and unconsciously, we simplify the problem when we try to present it in a schematic form and again reduce to one denominator all that we conditionally designate as higher behavior. Undoubtedly, further research within human behavior will be able to distinguish the newer and newer epochs and steps when our attempts will also seem methodologically not final; they will actually seem a simplification of the problem and a reduction of heterogeneous things to one common denominator. But at present, we are speaking of gaining a new concept for science. We are speaking of moving psychology out of its biological captivity and into the area of historical human psychology.

Thus, our initial position is the recognition of the new, fourth step in the development of behavior. We have already said that it would be incorrect to call it a fourth step, and there is a basis for this. The new step is not built over the preceding three in exactly the same way that the preceding steps are built on one another. It signifies a change in the very type and direction in the development of behavior and it corresponds to the historical type of development of humanity. It is true that when we consider its relation to the first three steps, which we can call natural steps in the development of behavior, this relation seems similar to the one we have already mentioned. And here we note the unique geology in the development of genetically available layers in behavior. Similarly to the way in which instincts are not eliminated but merged with conditioned reflexes or in which habits continue to exist in an intellectual reaction, natural functions continue to exist within the cultural.

As we have seen from our analysis, every higher form of behavior is disclosed directly as a certain aggregate of lower, elementary, natural processes. Culture creates nothing, it only uses what is given by nature, modifies it, and places it at the service of man. If we use the terminology of the old psychology, analogously to intellect, we could term the fourth step in the development of behavior the will because specifically in the chapter on will, the old psychology occupied itself most of all with the study of those real foundations of higher forms of behavior that are the subject of our research.

It would be a mistake to think that, together with spiritualistic representations of the will, those real unquestionable phenomena and forms of behavior that the old psychology interpreted erroneously and sometimes described must also be discarded. With this in mind, Høffding said that involuntary activity forms a basis and content of voluntary activity. Nowhere does the will create, but it always only changes and selects. He said that the will intervenes in the course of other mental processes only according to the same laws that are present in the processes themselves. Thus, the old psychology had every basis for also distinguishing not only voluntary and involuntary activity but also voluntary and involuntary memory and voluntary and involuntary flow of ideas; Høffding also maintained that the action of the will is not primary in evoking appropriate ideas. He said that the will provides the first push and bores through, but when the opening is made, then the stream of water must pass through under its own force and then it remains for us only to compare what we are seeking with what has been established.

Thinking in the true sense, formation of concepts, judgment and conclusions are based on the intervention of will in a representation. But just as these words carry so many meanings that they do not give a clear representation of the basic relation between the fourth step of behavior and other steps, we prefer to use a different term for this new area of development of which we continue to speak. Using Bühler's comparison, we could say that we have noted yet another area of development which, in contrast to the first three, is not subject to the biological laws of the formula of selection. In it, selection ceases to be the main law of social adaptation and in this area of behavior all neutral forms of behavior have already been socialized. Admitting a conditional comparison, we might say that the new area relates to the other three areas as the process of historical development of humanity on the whole relates to biological evolution.

In preceding chapters, we have already noted the uniqueness of this area of development. Now it remains for us to consider briefly the character itself of development.

We must say that in contemporary psychology the very concept of cultural development has not been assimilated. Even now many psychologists are inclined to consider facts of cultural changes in our behavior from their natural aspect and think of them as facts of habit formation or as intellectual reactions directed toward a cultural content. Psychology is deficient with respect to understanding the independence and specific pattern in the movement of forms of behavior. Moreover, studies show that the structure of higher forms of behavior does not remain unchanged; it has its internal history that includes it in the whole history of the development of behavior as a whole. Cultural devices of behavior do not appear simply as external habit; they comprise an inalienable part of the personality itself, rooted in its new relations and creating their completely new system.

Considering the changes to which the new mode of behavior is subjected, we can in every case disclose with precision all the traits of development in the true sense of the word. This development, of course, is profoundly unique in comparison with organic development. Its uniqueness has thus far hindered psychologists from identifying these processes as a special type of development, seeing in them a completely new plan in the history of behavior. A. Binet discovered the fact that remembering based on signs leads to augmenting the function, that a mnemotechnique may attain better results than the most outstanding natural memory. This phenomenon Binet termed simulation of outstanding memory. As we know, by this he wished to express the idea that every mental operation may be simulated, that is, replaced by other operations that lead to the same results, but by a completely different path.

Binet's determination can scarcely be termed fortunate. It indicates correctly that in externally similar operations, some of them, in essence, simulated others. If Binet's designation had in view only the uniqueness of the second type of development of memory, one could not argue with him, but if it contains the idea that simulation, that is, deception, is occurring here, it leads to error. This practical point of view is prompted by the specific conditions of an appearance on a stage and for this reason is inclined toward illusion. It is, more likely, the point of view of a court investigator than of a psychologist. But, of course, as Binet also recognizes, such simulation is not illusion. Each of us has his own type of mnemotechnique, and mnemotechnique, in the author's opinion, should be taught in schools together with mental arithmetic. The author would not want to say that the art of simulation should be taught in schools.

Designating the type of development we are considering as fictive, that is, leading only to a fiction of organic development, seems to us just as inappropriate. Here again the negative aspect of the matter is correctly expressed, specifically, that in cultural development, the concept of function at a higher step, promoting its activity, is based not on organic, but on functional development, that is, on the development of the device itself.

However, the latter term hides the basic truth that in this case there is not a fictive, but a real development of a special type that governs special patterns. For this reason, we prefer to speak of cultural development of behavior as distinct from natural or biological development.

We now move to the problem of elucidating the genesis of cultural forms of behavior. We will present a short outline of this process as it was noted in our experimental studies. We shall try to show that cultural development of the child proceeds, if we can believe the artificial conditions of the experiment, through four basic stages or phases sequentially replacing each other and arising one from another. Taken as a whole, these stages describe the circle of cultural development of any mental function. Data obtained by nonexperimental means fully coincide with the pattern noted, beautifully fall in with it, expanding in it their own sense and their hypothetical elucidation.

We shall trace briefly the four stages of cultural development of the child since they sequentially replace each other in the process of a simple experiment. It is understood that the phases identified in the cultural development of the child are no more than an abstract outline that must be filled in with concrete content in subsequent chapters of the history of the cultural development of the child. Now, however, we believe it is necessary to dwell on one basic general problem; without this a transition from the abstract outline to a concrete history of separate mental functions would be impossible.

We would like to say that this outline, which we developed in the process of experimental study, cannot, of course, be considered as reflecting accurately the real process of development in all its complexity. In the best case, having unfolded a certain form of behavior as a process, it helps to note, in a condensed form, the more important instances of cultural development and to find their relation to each other. But it would be a major mistake to consider our diagrammatic representation, developed on the basis of the artificial conditions of an experiment, as something more than only an outline. The greatest difficulty in genetic analysis consists precisely in using experimentally elicited and artificially organized processes of behavior to penetrate into how the real, natural process of development occurs.

In other words, the enormous problem of transferring the experimental outline to real life always opens up before genetic research. If the experiment discloses for us a sequence of patterns or any specific type, we can never be limited by this and must ask ourselves how the process being studied occurs under conditions of actual real life, what replaces the hand of the experimenter who deliberately evoked the process in the laboratory. One of the most important supports in transferring the experimental outline into reality are the data obtained nonexperimentally. We have already indicated that we see in these data a valid confirmation of the correctness of our outline.

However, this is not everything. In true research, it is still necessary to trace the path along which the cultural forms of behavior develop. Here again the basic difficulty consists in overcoming the traditional prejudice closely linked with intellectualism which still continues its cryptic dominance in child psychology. The basis of the intellectualistic view of the process of development is the assumption that development occurs like a logical operation. To the question as to how conscious use of speech develops in the child, the intellectualistic theory replies that the child discovers the meaning of speech. It attempts to substitute a simple logical operation for the complex process of development, not noting that such an approach involves an enormous difficulty because it assumes as given that which requires explanation.

We tried to show the insupportability of this point of view using the development of speech as an example. Actually, it would be impossible to find a more striking example of the fact that cultural development is not a simple logical operation.

We are not at all inclined to reject the fact that in the process of cultural development, intellect, thinking, invention, and discovery in the true sense of the word play an enormous role. But the problem in genetic research is not to explain the origin of new forms of behavior through discovery, but, on the contrary, to demonstrate genetically the rise of this development itself, of the role we must ascribe to it in the process of the child's behavior, and of other factors that promote its appearance and action.

The role of the intellect in development is most easily elucidated if we point out another prejudice that is just as firmly rooted in psychology as the first. If Stern tried to explain the development of a child's speech as discovery, then contemporary reflexology wants to present this process exclusively as a process of developing a habit without indicating that it is singling out speech from the remaining mass of habits. It stands to reason that the process of speech development includes the development of a motor habit and that all the patterns present in the formation of a simple conditioned reflex can undoubtedly be found in the development of speech also. But this only means that all the natural, innate functions are found in speech and that we are still far from an adequate description of the process itself.

Thus, we must overcome both the intellectualistic view that takes culture out of the activity of the human intellect and the mechanistic view that considers the higher form of behavior exclusively from the point of view of its functional mechanism. Overcoming the one error and the other leads us directly to the point where we can conditionally identify the *natural history of signs*. The natural history of signs tells us that the cultural forms of behavior have natural roots in natural forms, that they are tied to them by a thousand threads, that they arise in no other way than on the base of the natural forms. Where researchers thus far saw either simple discovery or a simple process of the formation of a habit, a true study discloses a complex process of development.

We would like to promote to the first rank the significance of one of the basic paths of cultural development of the child, which we might call by the generally accepted word *imitation*. It may seem that in speaking of imitation as of one o f the basic paths of cultural development of the child, we are returning again to the prejudices of which we have just spoken. A supporter of the habit theory may say that imitation is, of course, a mechanical transfer from one already developed form of behavior to another, that it is a process of habit formation, and we know it very well from animal development. Against such a view, we could point to the break that occurs in contemporary psychology of imitation.

Actually, psychology thus far has no intellectually clear idea of the process of imitation. As a matter of fact, it seems that processes of imitation are much more complex than it would seem at first glance. Thus, it would seem that the aptitude for imitation is strictly limited in different animals and people so that, summarizing the new position of psychology in this area, we might say: *the circle of available imitation coincides with the circle of the actual developmental possibilities of the animal.*

For example, it was pointed out long ago that the development of speech in the child cannot be explained by the fact that he imitates the adult. It is true that an animal hears the sounds of a human voice and with a certain structure of the vocal apparatus, it can imitate it, but we all know from experiments on domestic animals how limited is the circle of their imitation of man. A dog, the most domesticated animal with almost unlimited possibilities of training, does not in any way imitate motions of human behavior, and not one researcher has yet established that any but instinctive imitation was possible here.

We must again voice a reservation: we do not want to say that imitation does not play a decisive role in the development of a child's speech. We want to say quite the opposite: imitation is one of the basic paths in cultural development of the child in general. We would only like to note that imitation cannot explain the development of speech and that imitation itself requires explanation. Köhler, considering the reproaches that might be raised against ascribing intelligent behavior to a chimpanzee, dwells especially on the problem of imitation. The question arises: could not the chimpanzee in certain experiments see similar solutions reached by man and could he not simply imitate man s action? Köhler says that this objection might be a strong reproach if we assume the existence of simple imitation without any intelligent participation, a mechanical transfer of the behavior of one man to another. There is no doubt that such a purely reflex imitation exists; however, we must establish its true boundary.

If we assume that imitation of another kind is occurring here, not simple mechanical transferring from one to another, but connected with a certain understanding of the situation, then that in itself gives a new interpretation to the really intelligent behavior of animals. Actually no one has ever observed that complex actions could at once be reproduced by simple reflex imitation. The process of imitation itself assumes a certain understanding of the significance of the action of another. Actually, the child who can understand, cannot imitate a writing adult. Animal psychology confirms that the matter of imitation in animals is in the same situation. Studies by American authors showed, in contrast to the results of E. Thorndike,[62] that imitation, although with difficulty and limited in scope, does occur in higher vertebrates. This discovery coincides with the assumption that imitation itself is a complex process that requires preliminary understanding.

To anyone who was engaged in animal research, Köhler could say in his own words: if an animal that sees a problem solved can actually by imitation arrive at the solution as he could not before, we would have to give that animal the highest mark. Unfortunately, we come across such cases very rarely in chimpanzees, and what is most important, only when a suitable situation and solution of it are within approximately the same boundaries that exist in the chimpanzee and are related to his spontaneous actions. Simple imitation is found in chimpanzees as it is in man, that is, when behavior produced by imitation is already common and understandable. Köhler assumes that the conditions are the same for imitation in higher animals and in man; man cannot simply imitate if he does not understand the process or the course of ideas well enough.

We would like to limit Köhler's position only to the area of natural imitation. As far as special or higher forms of imitation are concerned, we are inclined to say that they follow the same path of cultural development as all other functions. Specifically, Köhler says that under natural conditions, the chimpanzee is capable of imitating human behavior and he sees evidence in this for the intelligence of its behavior. Köhler stressed that, as a rule, the chimpanzee does not imitate human behavior. This is incorrect. There are cases in which even the greatest skeptic would have to admit that the chimpanzee imitates new methods of action not only similar to his own, but also those of man.

We could express this new evaluation of imitation another way by saying that imitation is possible only to the extent and in those forms in which it is accompanied by understanding. It is easy to see what enormous significance imitation acquires as a method of research that makes it possible to establish the limit and level of actions accessible to the intellect of the animal and the child. Roughly speaking, by testing the limits of possible imitation, we test the limits of the intellect of the given animal. For this reason, imitation is an exceptionally convenient methodological device for research, particularly in the genetic area. If we want to learn how much a given intellect has matured for one function or another, we can test this by means of imitation, and we consider an experiment with imitation that we developed to be one of the basic forms of the genetic experiment: a child is present when another solves a suitable problem, then he solves the same problem himself.

These considerations compel us to reject the opinion that reduces the essence of imitation to the simple formation of habits and to recognize imitation as a substantial factor in the development of higher forms of human behavior.

# 12

# Mastering Attention

The history of the child's attention is the history of the development of the organization of his behavior. This history begins at the moment of birth. Initial attention occurs through hereditary nerve mechanisms that organize the reflex processes according to the principle of the dominant that is familiar in physiology. This principle establishes that in the operation of the nervous system, the organizing point is a dominant focus of excitation that inhibits the process of other reflexes and is augmented at their expense. The dominant nerve process is the organic base of the process of behavior that we call attention.

The first chapter in the development of the child's attention is traced through the genetic study of the child's reflexes. The study establishes how new dominants appear sequentially in the child's behavior and how the formation of complex conditioned reflexes in the cortex of the brain begins on this basis. It is extremely important to note that the formation of conditioned reflexes depends on the development of an appropriate dominant. For example, genetic studies have demonstrated a definite dependence of the formation of an associative reflex on the development of dominant processes in the central nervous system, since an associative reflex, in the words of V. M. Bekhterev, can be formed only from the receptive surface from which a dominant functional affect arises in the central nervous system.

The newborn has only two dominants: the feeding dominant and the position dominant that is manifested by a change in position. Bekhterev says that with these dominants, only an association between them can be formed: a conditioned reflex in the form of a feeding reaction that arises when the child is placed in a position customary for breast feeding. Before corresponding dominants develop, no other conditioned reflexes related to other perceived surfaces can be formed. Gradually, the child develops visual, aural, and other dominants, and only with their development is the formation of new conditioned reflexes related to the eyes and ears possible.

Thus, the dominant process stands at the very beginning of the formation of new connections in the cortex of the child's brain and determines the character and direction of these connections. We term this period in the development of the child, which encompasses the natural maturation of separate dominants, the period of natural or primitive development of attention. This term is based on the fact that development of attention at this time is a function of a general organic development of the child and primarily of the structural and functional development of the central nervous system.

Originally appeared in English as Chapter 9 in *The Collected Works of L.S. Vygotsky, Volume 4: The History of the Development of Higher Mental Functions* (Robert W. Rieber, eds.; Marie J. Hall, Trans.) (pp. 153–177). New York: Plenum Press, 1997.

Consequently, a purely organic process of growth, maturation, and development of the nervous apparatus and functions of the child form the base of the development of attention during this period. This process is analogous to the process of evolutionary development of attention from lower to higher organisms where it can be observed with greatest clarity. We do not want to say that the organic development of attention in the child is parallel to the process of evolutionary development of attention or repeats it to any extent. However, we want to stress that these processes are similar with respect to type of development: in both cases, the base for development of attention as a specific function of behavior is the organic development or maturation of the corresponding nervous processes.

This process, which occupies a dominant place in the first year of the child's life, does not stop, does not end in later childhood or even in the subsequent life of the person. The relative equilibrium and stability that we observe in the adult in comparison with the child indicates essentially only an enormous retardation of the rate, and sometimes a change in direction of the processes, but not their cessation. These seemingly attenuated and retarded processes of organic change, however, affect the operation of our attention every day, and this dependency becomes especially perceptible and clear when these seemingly attenuated processes are revived when they change in morbidity.

The significance of the organic process that is the basis for development of attention moves to the background very early in comparison with the new processes of development of attention that are qualitatively different in type, specifically the processes of cultural development of attention. As cultural development of attention, we have in mind the evolution and change in the devices of control and the operation of attention, the mastery of these and their subjection to the will of the person, that is, processes analogous in type to the cultural development of other functions of behavior which we spoke of in preceding chapters.

Consequently, psychological study shows that in the development of attention we can also definitely see two basic lines with which we are already familiar. We can identify the line of natural development of attention and the line of cultural development of attention. We will not consider the relation that exists between the one line and the other in the development of attention because this problem has already been adequately elucidated in preceding chapters. Our task is to trace and graphically note the path of the second line, that is, the history of the cultural development of attention.

Strictly speaking, cultural development of attention also begins at a very early age, with the first social contact between the child and the adults around him. Like all cultural development, it is a social development.

The cultural development of any function, including attention, consists of a person's developing a series of artificial stimuli and signs in the process of mutual living and activity. The social behavior of the personality is directed by means of these and they form the basic means through which the personality masters its own processes of behavior.

In order to trace the history of the mechanisms of attention genetically, we proceeded in the same way as in the study of other processes described above. We tried to create a situation experimentally in which the child would be confronted with the task of mastering processes of his attention with the help of external stimuli-devices. Implementation of this can be found in the work of our colleague, A. N. Leont'ev, who developed a method of double stimulation applicable to the study of mediated processes of attention. The essence of the experiments consists of the child's being confronted with a problem that requires a long, exerted attention, a concentration on the given process.

The experimenter plays a game with the child, "Questions and Answers," a game of the "Forfeit" type, with the following stipulation" "You must not say 'yes' or 'no,' or 'black' or 'white.'" The child is asked questions to some of which he must respond by naming a certain color. For example: "Do you go to school? What color is the desk? Do you like to play? Were you ever in a village? What color is the grass? Were you ever in the hospital? Did you see a doctor? What color is his smock?" etc. The child must answer the questions as quickly as possible observing the instructions that he must not name the two forbidden colors, for example, black and white or red and blue, and not name the same color twice. The experiment is set up in such a way that meeting the requirements is quite possible but requires constant attentive effort on the part of the child. If the child breaks a rule and names a forbidden color or repeats the same color twice, he pays a forfeit or loses the game.

An experiment set up in this way demonstrated that the task is extremely difficult for a preschool child and quite difficult even for an eight or nine-year-old who cannot carry it out without error. Actually, the situation requires concentration of attention to an internal process on the part of the child. It requires him to control his internal attention and is beyond his ability. The course of the experiment changes radically when the child is given colored cards as an aid: black, white, cream, red, green, blue, yellow, brown, gray. The child immediately has an external auxiliary device for solving the internal problem of concentrating and intensifying attention, and he makes a transition from direct to mediated attention. As we have already said, the child must master his internal attention, but he works with external stimuli. Thus, the internal operation is carried out or at least connected with the external operation and presents us with the possibility of studying it objectively. A double-stimulus type of experiment unfolds before us.

Two series of stimuli confront the child. The first is the question of the experimenter, the second, the colored cards. The second series of stimuli is the device that helps fix attention on the correct response. The result of introducing the auxiliary series of stimuli usually is very quickly apparent and the number of incorrect responses decreases rapidly, which indicates the increased stability of attention and the fact that the child masters these processes with the help of the auxiliary stimuli.

Let us consider the development with age of both forms of concentration and the establishment of attention in the double-stimulus experiment. In the preschool child, both forms of attention are usually close to each other. Their divergence increases markedly during the first and especially during the second school year and becomes insignificant again in adults. Tracing the development of attention from the preschool child to the adult, we reach a basic conclusion. The difference in activity of mediated and direct attention increases beginning with preschool age, reaches a maximum during the second year of schooling, and then exhibits a tendency toward leveling off. Subsequently, we can easily see in the two curves that show the basic genetic law of development of attention, a picture that is essentially similar to the parallelogram of the development of memory, which we shall try to elucidate in the next chapter.

In order to explain the sequence in the development of mediated attention, we must briefly trace the course of the experiment at various age levels. Here we will note mainly that in the preschool child, the difference between the number of errors with the one method and the other of directing attention is negligible and the introduction of a new device does not essentially change the course of the whole process. The preschool child does not use the stimulus-device that he is given to any significant degree. He frequently plays with the cards as if they had no connection to the task at hand and sometimes selects one randomly and is guided in his response by the suggestive influence of the card. The child who carries out the task most successfully begins to make partial use of the auxiliary device. He isolates the forbidden colors, say white and black, puts them aside and uses the colors of the cards that he kept. But once the color has been named, the child does not remove that color from the cards that he has.

As a rule, it is only at school age that the child makes full use of the device he is given. The internal operation becomes external, and the child controls his attention with the help of the external stimuli-devices. The cards begin to be clearly differentiated into "possible" or "impossible" colors, as one of the subjects of the experiment put it; the used colors, those already named, are added to the forbidden colors. The school-age children clearly exhibit a dependence on the device by attempts to mechanize the whole operation, which frequently results in mindless responses since the children display a tendency toward being guided only by the color of the card but not by the sense of the question.

Thus, in the school-age child, resorting to the stimulus-device quickly increases efficiency of internal attention, but essentially reduces the quality of the response and moves in this way toward an inexpedient use of the device he is given. Older school children use external devices most fully and most adequately; they no longer exhibit complete dependence on the cards as do the younger children.

The number of errors decreases correspondingly. In the preschool child, mediated attention scarcely decreases the percentage of errors; in children in the lower grades, the percentage of errors drops by half, and in the older school children, by a factor of ten. Thus we have a seemingly sequential picture of the development of mediated attention: the processes are mastered gradually and attention is subjected to the will. Only in adults do we note again an extremely insignificant drop in number of errors when they resort to the cards.

To elucidate this fact, which plays a central role in the process of development of voluntary attention, we turn to experiments in a special series that show that in an individual child, the curves of development of both processes of developing attention are similar in form. If we continue these experiments with a preschool child for a long time, within the framework of this operation, the child generally follows the same course relatively quickly. The child's behavior during the experiment will pass through the following stages sequentially: (1) incomplete and inexpedient use of the cards; (2) transition to vigorous use of the cards and complete subjection to the external devices, (3) expedient use of the cards for solving the internal task with external devices, and finally, (4) transition to the type of behavior that adults exhibit.

As strange as this may seem at first glance, in our experiments, in the transition to using cards, the adult behaves very much like the preschool child if we are to judge by external appearance. The adult also makes little use of the cards; his operation has the character of using a semi-external device and he makes notes "in his mind" of the forbidden and already used colors, but does not touch the cards. Observing this behavior, which we saw in the long-term experiment with a child, we have a firm basis for assuming that this is due to a conversion of the processes, that is, to a transition from an externally to an internally mediated process.

In contrast to the preschool child, in the adult, the processes of voluntary attention are well developed and, in his mind, through words or through some other method, he can fix the forbidden or used colors; we can observe this same process in the child when the external auxiliary stimulus is replaced by an internal stimulus. In a corresponding experiment, together with a decrease and sometimes an extinction of the external operation, internal attention increases significantly in both the child and the adult, which is evident in objective results. On this basis, we conclude that the child experienced a reorganization of the internal processes as a result of the transition to the mediated form of attention and a conversion of the external device during which the external operation became an internal operation.

Data from analysis of the structure of the operation support this. They show that one and the same problem can be solved by different internal operations. In the expression of A. Binet, the child simulates attention when he isolates the forbidden colors from the field of vision and fixes his attention on the colors that remain before him. He replaces one operation with another that has the same effect but which essentially has nothing in common with the first. Again we see the deep difference between phenotypic and genotypic forms of the processes.

Sometimes the child solves the problem completely differently. He does not put the forbidden colors aside, but selects them and puts them before him and fixes his eyes on them. In these cases, the external device corresponds precisely to the internal operation, and we have before us the operation of mediated attention. With this operation the very process of searching for an answer is reorganized. The child must give a correct response, that is, a thoughtful response to the question posed and must observe the stated formal rules and not use certain colors. This unique purposefulness of attention transforms and reorganizes the process of seeking an answer; it directs thinking in a roundabout way. The child's responses become more and more qualitative. In place of a direct response to the question as to what color the grass is, the child who must not say "green" responds, "In the fall, the grass is yellow." To the question, "Are tomatoes red?" when red is a forbidden color, the child responds, "They're green when they're not ripe!" In this way, the subject resorts to new situations and makes a transition to a more difficult way of thinking.

In the most general outlines, such is the history of the development of attention. With T. Ribot, who was the first to connect the problem of voluntary attention with the problem of the cultural development of man, we can say that its genesis is very complex, but it corresponds to reality.

It seems that Ribot was the first psychologist to consider voluntary attention as a product of human cultural historical development. He called involuntary attention natural, and voluntary attention, cultivated. He said, "The cultivated uses natural strengths to accomplish its tasks and in this sense, I term such a form of attention cultivated" (1897, p. 30).

To the question as to how voluntary attention arose, he responds that the same progress that forced man to make a transition from primitive savagery to a state of organized society forced him to make a transition from the dominance of involuntary attention to the dominance of voluntary attention. "The latter serves simultaneously as a consequence and a cause of civilization" (ibid., p. 33).

Digressing at present from considering to what extent Ribot is historically correct in linking the development of voluntary attention with the development of society, we cannot help but note that Ribot's formulation of the question itself involves a colossal revolution in the views of attention and lays out the first path toward its historical elucidation.

According to Ribot's views, voluntary attention is a historical form of natural attention that arose under specific conditions of adaptation of social man to nature. Ribot says that as soon as man left his wild state for one reason or another (inadequate supply of game, population density, soil infertility, nearness of tribes that were better armed) and was confronted by either death or adaptation to more complex conditions of life, that is, work, voluntary attention became in its turn a factor of primary importance in this new form of struggling to live.

As soon as man had the capability of devoting himself to work that was essentially not attractive but necessary for living, voluntary attention came to be. It is easy to say that before the appearance of civilization, attention did not exist or appeared for an instant as a fleeting flicker of lightning.

Ribot, who was the first to point to the social nature of voluntary attention, also demonstrated that this form of attention develops and that, in general, the development proceeds from the external to the internal. Voluntary attention gradually is converted into an internal operation and, finally, at a certain period of development, the developed attention becomes second nature—the task of the cultivated is accomplished. It is enough to find oneself in familiar circumstances, in a familiar environment, for all the rest to follow.

But it seems to us that Ribot's theory does not explain the mechanism itself of the activity of voluntary attention or give any precise picture of its ontogenesis. Ribot's mechanism can frequently be reduced to training. As we would now say, it shows the emergence of voluntary attention as the emergence of a simple conditioned reflex to remote stimuli that signal another stimulus that elicits natural attention. Undoubtedly this mechanism is the basis of the transition from involuntary to voluntary attention, but it is not most characteristic or most essential for it; it plays a subordinate role and elucidates, in general, any transition from an innate to an acquired form of behavior.

From this point of view, as Ribot establishes, an animal also has voluntary attention. So it is not evident why voluntary attention is a product of civilization. Ribot says that there is no need to prove that a transition from involuntary to voluntary attention also occurs in animals as a result of rearing and training. Binet stresses only the limitation of means by which we affect animals, evidently due to not knowing a wide range of conditioned stimuli that can, as knowledge of conditioned reflexes shows, elicit conditioned attention in an animal.

Ribot fails to note the basic fact that an animal's attention, even with training, is not voluntary, that man, not the animal, controls this attention. In animals, there is no transition from being controlled by others to self-control, from being managed to managing, a transition that is the most characteristic trait in the development of voluntary attention in man. Ribot's error is due to the fact that he did not know the mechanism for the formation of voluntary attention and did not consider the means by which historical development of both attention and behavior in general is accomplished. Only by establishing the mechanism in which we can see control of behavior through signs can we understand how a child makes the transition from external actions to internal voluntary attention.

We attempted to trace this transition with experimentally established data on the genesis of voluntary attention.

Recently, P. P. Blonskii adopted Ribot's ideas, indicating that active voluntary attention is undoubtedly a late product of development. Primitive attention, which appears at the very beginning of a child's life and which Ribot was inclined to identify with maximum wakefulness, differs from involuntary attention in that the latter, in his opinion, is determined mostly by thinking and is the most developed form of attention.

Thus, the genetic approach to the problem of voluntary attention is noted with all clarity. However, even here no very clear genesis of this form of attention is presented, and what is the main thing, neither is any analysis of how it develops. It seems to us that in light of the data we have accumulated, the more important laws of the development of attention established by researchers, which are now accorded their place in the whole process of development of voluntary attention, could be elucidated.

The most fully developed positions of the genetic theory of attention were worked out by E. Titchener on the basis of the fact that the two forms of attention are distinguished in their popular meaning—specifically, passive or involuntary attention and active or voluntary attention are in reality characteristic for different stages of mental development. They differ from each other only in complexity as earlier and later forms and exhibit one and the same type of consciousness, but at different periods of our mental growth. Titchener tries to explain the difference and character of each of them on the basis of the conditions under which they appear.

Analysis brings the author to the conclusion that involuntary and voluntary attention are essentially primary and secondary attention and that primary attention represents a certain stage of development, specifically the earliest stage of development of voluntary attention. Characteristic for secondary attention is that the relation between the subject and the object changes substantially. In themselves impressions not only do not attract and do not hold our attention, but on the contrary: it seems that we pay attention to some impressions or others with the help of internal effort.

A problem in geometry does not leave as strong an impression as a clap of thunder. However, it can attract our attention and such attention Titchener terms secondary attention. In his opinion, secondary attention is the inescapable result of the complexity of nervous organization and is secondary or active as long as it retains a trace of conflict.* We could scarcely bring more weighty evidence for the origin of secondary attention from the primary than the fact from everyday experience that secondary attention is continuously converted into primary. Titchener calls this voluntary primary attention and in this way arrives at three stages in the development of attention and attempts to reduce the difference between them to a mainly genetic difference.

He says that on the whole, in the human mind, attention is found at three stages of development. Secondary attention is a transitional stage, a conflict stage, a stage of dissipating nervous energy, although this attention is an indispensable preliminary condition for the stage of subordinate voluntary attention. From Titchener's point of view, there are three stages of attention, but only a single type of mental process of attention. The three stages exhibit a change in complexity, but not in the character of the experience itself.

---

*    Editor's note: Conflict between the task and the impression made by the clap of thunder.

Here we see Titchener's attempt to define attention genetically; Titchener tries to apply his theory to different ages. Considering life as a whole, he believes we can say that the period of learning and education is a period of secondary attention and the period of mature and independent activity that follows it is the period of voluntary primary attention. It seems to us that Titchener's theory comes closest to the data that we established in our genetic studies.

We cannot help but see that three of the four main stages that we noted in the development of all cultural behavior are repeated in Titchener's stages. His primary attention corresponds to our primitive or natural attention; his secondary attention, to the stage of externally mediated attention; finally, his third stage, to the fourth stage of turning.* Lacking is only the second, transitional, naive-psychological stage which we were not able to trace precisely in our experiments, but which nevertheless was observed in clinical observations especially in abnormal children.

Moreover, Titchener established without a doubt that voluntary attention differs from involuntary attention only in the way it is generated, not in its method of functioning. In other words, the development of attention is accomplished not according to type of organic maturation and change, but according to type of evolution of the form of behavior itself. It seems to us, however, that Titchener's theory, although it approaches the problem of attention genetically, is still based on a purely external phenotypic description of a separate stage and does not demonstrate the mechanism of development and the mechanism of action of these separate processes. Thus, Titchener dwells on experiences and not on objective function of the process and does not demonstrate the uniqueness of the structure of secondary attention in contrast to the preceding stage. On the basis of his point of view, why derived primary attention is raised to a higher state in comparison with the point of departure remains unclear. Completely correctly he states that secondary attention originates from conflicts of initial forms of attention, from features of perception and from the struggle of incompatible motor acts. But, of course, such struggle occurs even when the child is very young. If in explaining the appearance of voluntary attention we do not involve the fact that together with natural stimuli and their interrelations, social stimuli that control his attention are also significant for the child, it still remains unclear why and how our attention is initially subject to external impressions or direct interests and later begins to subject these impressions or interests to itself.

This inadequacy of a purely empirical description of the transition of voluntary attention to involuntary without noting the genesis and mechanism of this transition, like the qualitative features of the second stage, is also evident in the statement of E. Meumann, who wrote that voluntary attention is gradually converted to involuntary. As we have already said, here we see experimental evidence that voluntary attention does not differ from involuntary in the mechanism of its organic basis, but in the structure of psychological behavior.

In his experiments, Meumann found an equally clearly expressed symptom for voluntary and involuntary attention—the slowing of the pulse, which probably can be explained by the following: in the subjects, voluntary attention consistently and very quickly turned into involuntary attention. But other researchers found the opposite symptoms for voluntary and

---

*    Editor's note: In the analysis of transitions from the primary to the secondary and then the tertiary stages of attention, Titchener proceeds from a different determination of attention and different conditions of transition.

involuntary attention: symptoms of involuntary attention are closer to the affects and coincide with the symptoms of amazement and fright, while voluntary attention is characterized by symptoms that are appropriate to willful acts.

We believe that this disagreement can be explained in the light of the genesis of attention that we noted. In the one case, we are speaking of the very moment of establishing attention which is the same voluntary process of controlling behavior as any other. In the other case, we are speaking of an already established and automatically working mechanism of attention. In other words, the difference in symptoms here is the difference in the stages of development of attention.

Now let us consider very briefly one complex phenomenon that is not clear in subjective analysis and which is termed the *experience of exertion*. Where does it originate in voluntary attention? It seems to us that it flows from the additional complex activity that we term *control of attention*. It is completely natural that this exertion is absent where the mechanism of attention begins to work automatically. Here we have additional processes, we have conflict and struggle, we have an attempt to direct the processes of attention along other lines, and it would be a miracle if all of this could be accomplished without exertion, without serious internal work on the part of the subject, work that can be measured by resistance met by voluntary attention.

The inadequacy of a purely subjective analysis also marks the work of Revault d'Allones; along the lines of Ribot, he was the first to propose differentiating attention according to structure as direct or indirect, i.e., mediated, and he perceived as an essential characteristic the fact that voluntary attention is directed toward some object by means of some kind of auxiliary device or stimulus, which in this case is used as an instrument. From this point of view, Revault d'Allones defines attention as an intellectual operation that considers things through the mediation or with the help of one or several other things. Understood in this way, attention is converted into a direct instrumental or intellectual operation and it places an auxiliary device between the object of attention and the subject.

The author identifies various forms depending on which auxiliary devices are used, to what extent and how for mediating attention. But all the time, he has in mind only internal devices and predominantly configurations with which we direct our attention to one object or another. Revault d'Allones does not suspect that the devices may be internal and that they are consistently internal initially, and for this reason he sees in the "configurations" (continuing the ideas of H. Bergson[91]) a certain primary fact of a purely intellectual order. It seems to us that this theory may also be turned upside down and probably elucidated if we note that in this case we are undoubtedly speaking of the fourth stage or of voluntary primary attention, as Titchener puts it.

As a point of departure, Revo d'Allon takes the final stage of development and without tracing the processes as a whole, comes to a postulate of a purely idealistic character, but does not show the real process of formation of these configurations.

On the basis of the analysis of the experiments presented above and the positions that were developed in psychology on this problem, we reached the following understanding of the processes of voluntary attention. These processes must be considered as a certain stage in the development of instinctive attention; the general laws and character of their development coincide completely with what we were able to establish for other forms of cultural development of behavior. For this reason, we can say that voluntary attention is a process of the turning inward of mediated attention; the process itself is wholly subordinate to the general laws of cultural development and formation of higher forms of behavior. This means that voluntary attention in composition and in structure and function is not simply the result of natural organic development of attention, but is the result of its change and reconstruction under the influence of external stimuli-devices.

In place of the position that states that voluntary and involuntary attention are related to each other in the same way as will and instinct (the observation is quite correct, but somewhat general), we would like to say that voluntary and involuntary attention are related to each other as logical memory is related to mnemonic functions or as thinking in concepts is related to syncretic thinking.

In order to reinforce the conclusions we reached and to make certain theoretical generalizations, we still needed to elucidate experimentally an exceptionally important point in our research. We proceeded from the proposition that the path from natural to voluntary attention consists of a transition from direct to mediated operations. This is a path that is generally familiar to us on the whole in all other mental processes. But the question arises: how does mediation of the process of attention occur?

We know very well that all mediation is possible only on the basis of using natural laws for this operation, which is the subject of cultural development. For example, in memory, the mnemotechnical operation, that is, the relation between the stimulus-sign and the stimulus-object, was created on the basis of well-known natural laws of formation of structures. Now with respect to attention, we needed to elucidate what kind of natural-mental connection must exist between two stimuli in order that one might play the role of an instrumental stimulus that calls attention to the other. What, in general, are the natural conditions required for mediating attention? What is the natural history of the laws of attention? The second and related question requires that research disclose how the actual transition from natural to instrumental occurs under certain natural conditions.

To answer these questions, which are of fundamental significance for the whole history of attention, we undertook quite complexly structured experimental studies. We shall now consider these in detail.

We proceeded from the fact that attention cannot be observed in its pure form. As we know, this caused some psychologists to use attention to explain all changes that occurred in processes of memory, thinking, perception, will, etc., and others, on the other hand, to deny completely the existence of attention as a separate mental function and to eliminate the word itself from the dictionary of psychology, as did Foucault, E. Rubin,[92] and others. Finally, a third group proposed speaking not of single attention, but of many attentions, having in mind the specificity of this function in each separate case. Actually psychology then took the path for dividing single attention into separate functions. We have a clear example of this in the work of German authors (N. Ach) and in the theory of attention of Revault d'Allones.

We know that the process of attention can occur in different ways and, as is clear from experiments cited above, we were dealing with different kinds of attention in different forms of activity. What remained was finding the most primitive and natural activity in which the role of attention could appear in the purest form and could facilitate the study of the culture of attention specifically. As such activity, we selected the reaction of selection of structural relations first used by W. Köhler in experiments with the domestic chicken, chimpanzee, and a child.

In Köhler's experiment, a chicken was presented with grain scattered on light gray and dark gray pieces of paper; the chicken was not allowed to peck at the light gray paper, but was shooed away, but it was allowed to peck freely at the dark gray paper. When this was repeated a great number of times, the chicken developed a positive reaction to the dark gray paper and a negative reaction to the light gray paper. Then in crucial experiments, the chicken was presented with a new pair of papers: one, white and the other, the light gray used in the first series. The chicken exhibited a positive reaction to the light gray paper, that is, to the same paper that elicited a negative reaction in the first pair. In the same way, when a new pair of papers was presented, the dark gray from the first series and black, the chicken exhibited a positive reaction to the black and a negative reaction to the dark gray, which elicited a positive reaction in previous experiments.

With certain changes, a similar experiment was carried out with a chimpanzee and a child. The results were even more significant. We were able to establish experimentally that under such circumstances, the animal and the child react to the structure, to the whole, to the relation between two colors and not to the absolute quality of the color. On this basis, a transfer of previous training to new conditions seems possible. In making the transfer, both the animal and the child exhibit very clearly the basic law of all psychological structure: psychological properties and functions of parts are determined by the properties of the whole. Thus, the light gray paper when included in a single whole elicited a negative reaction since in the given pair, it was the lighter of the two shades. Being included in a new pair, it elicited a positive reaction since it was the darker of the two. In the same way, the dark gray color changed from a positive to a negative reaction when it was included in a pair with black. Thus, the animal and the child reacted not to the absolute quality of the gray of one shade or another, but to the darker of the two shades.

Köhler indicates that for the experiments to be successful, very large colored surfaces with a significant difference in shades must be used and a set-up must be selected in which the relations of the colors are clearly evident. Köhler found that the difficulty with the selection reaction in previous experiments with monkeys was not in the formation of a connection between a familiar reaction and a familiar stimulus, but mainly with calling attention during the selection specifically to the given property of the visual field which must be used as a conditioned stimulus.

We must not forget that the researcher who wants to elicit and direct attention of the monkey is confronted with two completely different problems. One is calling the attention of the monkey to the experiment. If monkeys suddenly begin to relate to the conditions of the experiment apathetically, it is impossible to get the effect described. The first problem is solved fairly simply: in order to elicit the monkey s attention and direct it to the goal of the experiment, the goal selected must be obtaining food and everything startling, strong and attention-diverting must be removed from the set-up. Another more complex problem remains: directing the monkey's attention to the characteristic to which a connection must be formed. Köhler recommends selecting characteristics which in themselves attract the animal's attention, are fascinating to the animal or are eye-catching. Clearly obvious differences, large surfaces presented on a neutral background are required.

We introduced substantial changes into the experiment pertaining to attracting attention. Contrary to the advice of Köhler and using both normal and abnormal children, we presented the child with the following situation. The child was asked to select one of two cups standing before him, one of which contained a nut that he could not see and the other of which was empty. Both cups were covered with identical square lids of white cardboard to the top of which were fastened small light and dark gray squares taking up not more than one-quarter of the surface of the lid.

In this way, we purposely selected a trait that did not catch the eye in order to observe how attention is directed in this case. We made the change because the purpose of our experiment, comprising only the first link in a series, was the opposite of Köhler's purpose. Köhler was mainly interested in the formation of a connection and for this reason he wanted to create favorable conditions for creating this connection and especially for directing attention correspondingly. We already knew the process of formation of the connection from Köhler's experiments and we were interested only in the process in which we might trace the activity of attention.

We will present briefly a typical experiment with a three-year-old child. The whole attention of the child was directed toward the goal, and he did not at all understand the operation which he was asked to carry out. At the very beginning of the experiment and very frequently in its course, the child selected both cups and when he was asked to point to the one that he wanted to uncover, he stretched out both hands and had to be reminded that he must point to only one cup. Every time he was asked to indicate which of the two cups he wanted to uncover, he would repeatedly respond, "I want the one that has the nut," or he would point to both cups, saying, "I want the one that has the nut." When he won, he grabbed the nut greedily without paying attention to what the experimenter was doing; when he lost, he would say, "Wait, now I'll guess," or "Now I'll win." Soon after, when he selected the cup on the right three times in a row, he developed a reaction to place and when this rule was broken, he began to make random selections.

Because of alternation of success and failure, the most that could be elicited in a child of this age were certain vacillations before selection, but in the vacillations nothing indicated identification of a trait which the child might use in making his selection. After 30 experiments, the child seemed to be establishing a positive reaction to the dark gray and this persisted for a certain time, but this was not confirmed in critical experiments and neither was it confirmed in a return to the original situation. To the question as to why one cup or the other was selected, the reason given seemed independent of whether the cup was covered or uncovered: "Because the nut was here," or "I didn't want to lose any more," etc.

In the experiment described, winning and losing alternated frequently enough so that the child was satisfied with the situation. His attention was fixed on the goal the whole time. It is possible that very long training would have led to the same result that Köhler got, but we lost interest in the experiment since our purpose, let us repeat, was not to verify, confirm, or develop Köhler's facts further. Usually the child's attention was not directed to the gray paper, and perhaps a greater number of experiments would be required for success.

In the same situation, a child of five, winning or losing, will give this answer to the question as to reasons for his selection: "I took this cup because I wanted it." But after a certain point in the experiment, it was apparent that the child was reacting mainly by trial and error. He chose the cup with which he had just lost. By the 23rd experiment, the child refused to forfeit the nut, saying, "I won't give the last one, I'll keep it," and in the 24th experiment, he considered for a long time. By the 49th, after three losses in a row, the child cried, "I won't play with you any more, so there." When the experimenter calmed him and asked for the reasons for his selection, he responded, "The nut moves from cup to cup, it seems to me."

We proceeded as follows. We placed the nut into the cup as the child watched, then we pointed to the dark gray paper attached to the lid. With another movement, we pointed out the light gray paper attached to the lid of the empty cup.

By the 51st experiment, the child won and as a reason, he explained, "There is gray paper here and there is gray paper here." In critical experiments, he immediately transferred his device and explained his selection: "Because the gray paper is here and the black, there." In experiments with white and gray paper, he again transferred the rule immediately and said, "Aha, this is dark gray, the nut is where it is darker. I didn't know before how to win, I didn't know that the nut was where the dark paper was." The next day and for several days, the child won at once without errors, maintaining and transferring his device reliably.

For us, the most essential point in the experiments is the instant of pointing out, the instant of paying attention, the gesture which is sufficient as a supplementary stimulus to call the child's attention to the trait with which he must connect his reaction. A very small additional nudge is sufficient for the whole process that leads the child to affective outburst to be immediately and properly solved not only with respect to the given pair of colors, but also with respect to the critical experiment. For this reason we are reminded of Köhler's beautiful statement about the chickens that in his experiments fell to the ground in a stupor, sometimes fell into a swoon, and sometimes exhibited an explosive reaction when presented with new shades of gray.

We will say at once that in the experimental moment as a gesture that calls the child's attention to something, we see—what is first and most basic—the natural conditions for the appearance of voluntary attention. In contrast to us, Köhler made every effort to eliminate difficulties, to facilitate getting the attention of the animal, and to show that in that case, a conditional connection is formed instantaneously; he said that in this respect the monkey is much more convenient than other animals. A stick is placed in the monkey's paws with which it can point to the container instead of picking it up. The process of teaching is shortened due to the fact, as Köhler says, that he used all means to call the monkey's attention to the material that was the stimulus for selection, indicating that a banana had been put in exactly that place. We see an exceptionally important circumstance which, from Köhler's point of view, is yet another point of auxiliary significance. Köhler himself indicates that this kind of experimental set-up represents something on the order of a primitive explanation of his principle, not a literal explanation. We must note that this device led to a striking certainty on the part of the animal and to correctness of subsequent selections. In this circumstance, we see the primary function of language as a means of directing attention.

Bühler also believes that, in this case, pointing to both papers from the beginning vigorously directs the chimpanzee to the correct path: "Notice these objects. We only need to say to it: the food is in the cup with the lighter paper."

Consequently, in this experiment we see the natural roots of voluntary attention in the function of pointing, since Köhler had to create a kind of special mimic language for indicating to the monkey what it should pay attention to, and the monkey indicated to him which cup it was selecting. We, on the other hand, had to lower the child to a primitive pointing out, having excluded verbal instructions from our experiment. Actually, we could have told the child at the very beginning that the nut was in the cup with the dark lid and he would have solved the problem sooner. But the entire purpose of our experiment was the following: we were able to trace in an articulated and analyzed form what is merged and indivisible in verbal instruction and in this way to disclose genotypically the two most important elements that are represented phenotypically in a merged form in verbal instruction.

Actually, it was very clear to us even in Köhler's experiments and from our subsequent experiments that in the process of forming the selection reaction on the basis of the darker of two shades, there are two psychological points that Köhler also tried to separate. First, we have the instant of paying attention, that is, identifying the appropriate traits and settling on the gray paper without which the process itself of forming a connection is impossible; second, we have the formation itself of the connection. Verbal instruction includes both instants simultaneously. It also turns the child's attention to appropriate traits, that is, it creates the settling of attention and creates the required connection as well. The task of genetic study was to separate these instants in the instruction. Köhler carried out the first part of the genetic analysis: specifically, wishing to show that the chimpanzee can form structural connections very easily even with one trial, he tried to study the effect of the settling of attention from the beginning by introducing traits that were eye-catching and then, with a direct attempt to evoke the settling, by instruction. And actually after the instant of settling was identified, Köhler was able to study in a pure form the laws of formation of the structural connection and the selection reaction.

We attempted to carry out the second part of the genetic analysis, trying to present both collaborating processes, the settling of attention and the formation of the connection, in a separated form and to demonstrate the role of the settling or paying attention. In our experiment, the child did not form a natural connection, partly because of not paying attention to the colors (remember that we purposely made them unobtrusive) and partly because of the spurious paying attention to the game of guessing and the paying attention to how the nut passed from cup to cup.

So there is no doubt that the difficulties that the child experienced were difficulties related specifically to settling his attention. These were most clearly expressed in the child's affective agitation, in crying and in refusing to continue the experiment. Here we saw the instant that may be involved only in directing attention, but not in establishing the connection itself, and we traced further how, depending on this nudge, the process, confused and confronting an affective dead-end, begins to develop in all intellectual clarity and transparency and in all its purity.

The connection is established by itself and, as critical experiments show, the transfer is made with the first try, that is, subsequently it develops according to natural laws, as Köhler explained. In this way, the critical experiments have for us the nature of control experiments that confirm that our instructive gesture, our pointing, was directed only to the attention of the child, and the connection developed on this basis by direct observation of the relation in the structure of the perceived field although verbal formulation of the connection developed only at the end, after the third transfer, when the child realized the situation and thought it through. After our instruction (50th experiment), the child won (51st and 52nd experiments), still giving an incorrect reason: "Here is gray paper and here is gray paper"; he gave correct responses in experiments 53 and 54, giving the following reason at first: "Because here the paper is gray and here it is black"; and only in the end did he move to the form: "Aha, here it is dark gray and where it is darker, that's where the nuts are. I didn't know how to win before." But our confidence in the results obtained would be incomplete if we did not conduct another parallel experiment in which the formation of the connection would be impeded regardless of the set-up and where, consequently, the turning of attention in itself would not lead to the formation of the required connection.

The child with whom we began the parallel experiments was present the whole time; therefore he not only paid attention, but also heard the verbal formulation of the task. In the critical experiments immediately following, the child won and answered the question as to why he chose the cup as follows: "Because that's where the nut is. Here is the gray paper and here is the nut." The child did not react to losing as to his own error, he said, "Now I'll win." In the ninth experiment, the experimenter again turned the child's attention to the color by pointing, then the child in most cases won till the 20th experiment; nevertheless, in the interval, he lost several times (the 13th and 14th trials), explaining his selection thus: "Because you told me," "Because you put the nut in this cup twice," etc.

In the critical series, the child won most of the time, but he did lose occasionally. As a reason, he sometimes said, "This one is gray and this is black." We note that where the process of forming the connection is impeded, the turning of attention and the experimenter's instruction in themselves still do not lead to success. The next morning, after repeating the experiment with the same instruction, the child won immediately, and we are right in concluding that we were successful in creating a seeming experimental instruction and obtaining the instant in pure form that creates the settling of attention in the instruction, the instant that functions regardless of subsequent processes of forming a connection.

We shall consider this instant and analyze it. We cannot now determine more precisely the reason for the success than to say that the key instant of the experiment is the instruction. But the question arises as to how we might understand the role of the instruction physiologically. Unfortunately, we still have nothing but a hypothesis with respect to the physiological processes that are the basis of attention. But no matter how we might imagine these processes, the most probable physiological explanation of the phenomena of attention consists of the principle of the dominant, and its mechanism rests in the principle of the general motor rule as established by Titchener.

G. Müller[93] develops the catalyzing theory of attention and Hering speaks of the sensitization of nerve paths, but it seems to us that the position established by A. A. Ukhtomskii[94] is most important; he indicates that the essential property of the dominant is not its strength, but increased excitability and, what is the main thing, its capability for summarizing excitation. From this, Ukhtomskii concludes that the dominant reactions are analogous not to explosive reactions, as may seem at first glance, but to catalytic processes.

We must imagine in a general form that catalyzation of certain processes is achieved by way of instruction. The monkey or the child looking at the set-up of the experiment sees the gray color; but when we point to the gray color, we do not create new paths, but only sensitize or catalyze the appropriate nerve paths. In this way, with additional stimulation, we intrude on the intercentral relations being created in the cortex of the brain, in the relations that play a decisive role in the control of our behavior. Ukhtomskii says that the intercentral affects must be considered as most potent factors. Our intrusion causes a redistribution of energy in the nerve paths. We know, as Köhler established in his experiments, that in an affective state, both the monkey and man direct all their attention to the goal and do not divert it to auxiliary objects or tools.

I. P. Pavlov terms one of the innate reflexes the "What is it?" reflex. He says that the least change in the variation of the environment immediately evokes a disturbance of equilibrium in the state of the animal and immediately evokes the dominant reflex of alertness, expectation, and orientation toward change. Strictly speaking, we create the "What is it?" reflex with respect to the situation that the child looks at. It is as if we were putting an additional weight on the scale and disturbing the equilibrium that was being established and changing the inter-central relations that had developed.

Thus, we arrive at the following conclusion: the natural basis for the influence of signs on attention is not the creation of new paths as signs in memory, but a change in the intercentral relations that catalyze the respective processes and the evoking of additional "What is it?" reflexes. We assume that in the child, development of voluntary attention occurs in specifically this way. For the child, our initial words serve the function of instruction.

In addition, it seems to us that we approach the primary function of speech not developed by any researcher before us. The primary function of speech is not that words have meaning for the child, not that an appropriate new connection is created by the words, but that the initial word is an *instruction*. The word as instruction is the primary function in the development of speech from which all other functions are derived.

Thus, the development of attention in the child from the very first days of his life finds itself in a complex environment consisting of two kinds of stimuli. On the one hand, things, objects, and phenomena attract his attention in proportion to the strength of their properties; on the other hand, corresponding stimuli-catalyzers, specifically words, direct his attention. From the very beginning, the child's attention becomes directed attention. Initially, adults direct it, but together with gradual mastery of language, the child begins to direct his attention by the same means, first with respect to others and then with respect to himself. Using a comparison, we might say that the child's attention during the first period of life moves not like a ball that falls into the waves of the sea, depending on the strength of each separate wave that tosses it back and forth, but moves as if along separate, constructed canals, guided to the shore by their flow. From the very beginning, for the child, words are a kind of way out established along his path to be used for acquiring experience.

Whoever does not take into account this most important of the initial functions of speech will never understand how the whole higher psychological experience of the child is formed. But we already know the subsequent path. We know that the general sequence of the cultural development of the child is as follows: at first other people act on the child, then the child begins to interact with those around him, next he begins to act on others, and finally, he acts on himself.

This is how the development of speech, thinking, and all other higher processes of behavior occurs. The situation is the same with voluntary attention. At first, the adult directs the attention of the child with words creating as if additional pointers—arrows—to the things around the child and creates from the words potent stimuli-instructions. Then the child begins to participate actively in the instructions and himself begins to use a word or a sound as a means of indicating, that is, turning the attention of the adults to an object that interests him.

The stage of development of the child's language, which Meumann termed the willful, affective stage and which he believed to include only the subjective state of the child, is, in our opinion, the stage of speech as instruction. For example, the child's phrase "ma-ma," which W. Stern translates into our language as, "Mama, put me on the chair," is actually an instruction to his mother; it is turning her attention to the chair. If we should want to give a more precise and primitive con tent of "mama," we would have to translate it initially by a gesture of grasping or the child's turning his mother's head with his hand to call her attention to himself and then with an indicating gesture pointing to the chair. Agreeing with this, Bühler says that the first and main position in comparative study is the function of pointing without which there is no perception of relations; further, there is only one path to knowledge of relations: through signs; no more direct perception of relation exists. For this reason, all attempts to find such a path have been unsuccessful thus far.

Let us proceed to describing our subsequent experiments. In some children, as we noted above, the selection reaction was established to the darker of two shades. Now we will turn to the second part of the basic experiments, which may seem to divert us from the basic line, and fix a goal of tracing, as far as possible in pure form, the manifestation of another natural process in the child: the action of abstraction. That attention plays a decisive role in abstraction when a part of the general situation is isolated can be disputed only if under the word "attention," the concept of formation is not understood from the very beginning.

It is very convenient for us to trace the activity of attention in the processes of abstraction in a young child. To do this, we used the methodology of experiments developed by Eliasberg, which we modified somewhat in connection with other problems that we had. We again used the experiments of others only as material, since the basic operation in them was studied with adequate clarity and we tried to set a different goal for ourselves. In contrast to Eliasberg, we were not interested in the natural process of abstraction in itself and how it occurs in the child, but in the role of attention in the course of this process.

We placed the child in the following situation. He had before him several completely identical cups standing either in a row or randomly placed. Some of the cups were covered by cardboard lids of one color, some, of another. There were nuts under one set of lids, for example, the blue; there were no nuts under the others, red, for example. How would the child behave in such a situation? Eliasberg's experiment had shown and our experiments confirmed that the child would uncover one or two cups at random at first and then suddenly confidently begin to uncover only the cups with lids of a certain color. In our experiments, a five-year-old was initially tested in critical experiments (described earlier) with positive success. To the question as to why he selected the black paper, he responded irritably, "You explained it to me yesterday and we don't need to talk about it any more."

Thus, the result of preceding experiments was preserved. Convinced by this, we moved on. Eleven cups were placed in an arc before the child; of these five were covered with blue lids and the nuts were in these and the rest were covered with red and empty. The child immediately asked, "How do I win?" wanting an explanation. He took the blue lid and guessed, then he took all the blue ("There is always a nut under the blue lids.") A three-year-old present added, "And there aren't any under the red lids." The child did not touch the red lids but said, "Only the red are left."

In the second experiment, the white was negative and the orange positive. The child quickly picked up a white lid, turned it over, took an orange one and then uncovered all the orange lids leaving the white and adding: "There is nothing in the white ones." In the third experiment, the black was negative and the blue, positive. The child picked up the blue and left the black. To the suggestion of the experimenter: "Do you want to try the black?" he responded: "There is nothing there." Thus we can attest that the experiment proceeded normally and smoothly from the first abstraction as Eliasberg's experiment did.

We worked with a three-year-old. The orange color was negative and the blue, positive. The child uncovered the orange immediately, paid the forfeit, then opened a blue cup, then opened all the blue and said, "There is nothing in the reddish ones." Next we started to distract the child with conversation and the child began to open all the cups in succession, both the red and the white. The child had no idea of abstraction of the required trait nor did he see the required relation. The child distracted himself by distributing the cards and from a correct solution of the problem, he made a transition to uncovering all the cups. With further distraction of attention, the child proceeded as follows: he uncovered all the cups, lost all the nuts, and cried. His attention was severely distracted, and in the fourth experiment he again uncovered all the cups in succession with a slight variation. Besides the statement "They're not in the red ones," as he stated earlier, he only said, "Not here; here it is, I won," etc. Thus, we were able to establish that both children, to a different degree, it's true, exhibited a natural process of primary abstraction; in the younger child, the process was disturbed when his attention was distracted to the extent that the child stopped paying attention to the color and began to uncover all the cups in succession.

A very interesting situation developed. The basic attention that the child directed toward the game was scarcely decreased and he looked for the nuts with the same attention, won or lost with the same emotions, and only the color no longer had any significance in his reactions regardless of the fact that the child saw what the other child did, made correct choices himself, and even gave a tolerable account of what was needed to win. Thus, a slight distraction of attention, mainly diverting him from the colored lids, resulted in a completely new form of behavior on his part. Obviously, here we proceeded differently from the way we proceeded in the previous experiment: there we *called the child's attention* to the required point; here we *distracted his attention* from the required abstraction. There we catalyzed a weak process; here we provided a kind of negative catalysis. If there we could demonstrate experimentally how the addition of our slight nudge led to liberating the whole intellectual process, then here in the same way, we could demonstrate experimentally how distracting attention immediately demotes the operation to a lower level.

We have already said that in pointing we see the primary form of mediating attention with which we begin to control with additional stimuli. Here we have opposite evidence for the same thing and we can establish how the process changes when we subtract from it the attention that is directed to color. From being mediated, directed toward the trait, attention becomes nonmediated, directed specifically toward the goal. If this can be called a subtraction of attention, then in the preceding experiment we had an addition, augmentation of attention. There, owing to concentration of attention on the basic point, we immediately obtained an error-free transition from nonmediated attention directed toward the nut and the cup that contained it, to mediated attention, to a selection not of the nut and not of the cup, but of the indicating traits, the shades of color. In this we see two main forms of natural mediation of attention and transition from direct to indirect attention.

Let us move to outlining the next experiment. A child of five is placed in the same situation as in the preceding experiment but with the difference that now the subject is allowed to uncover only one cup. If he guesses right, he can then uncover another, etc., but if he uncovers an empty cup, he loses the whole game, that is, the child is confronted with the problem of solving which of the two colors is the right one without trials and errors. However, since the colors change in significance each time, the child has no chance of a solution in good time. For this reason, we combined both parts of the experiment as they proceeded thus far, the method of Köhler and the method of Eliasberg. Onto cards of different colors we pasted a thin band of black or white paper and in this way gave the child some indication as to how he should act. These bands provided instruction for the child which he had to deduce from the experiment itself. In our experiment, the black bands were pasted on orange lids. The child discovered the principle and immediately took the orange card on which the black paper was pasted; he chose all the orange, then stopped: "There are no more." To a question as to his choice, he responded, "I knew where they were, I wanted the red and I took the red."

In the next experiment, the white were positive and the red, negative. Gray paper was pasted on the red and black on the white. After thinking for a while, the child removed the red lid and lost the game. The experiment was continued with additional gray and white bands. The child lost again, and asked why he lost, replied, "Because that's what happened." We see that the two operations the child mastered completely are independent of each other: specifically, the operation of choosing between two shades of gray and the operation of choosing between two colors are separate operations. As a result, the process returns again to the first stage of blind attempts, trials and errors.

What inhibited the whole operation? Obviously the fact that in following our method, we placed the gray signs at the center of attention, but made them smaller. The child saw them, he even began selection specifically with the lids that were marked with the gray bands, but he did not pay attention to them, was not guided by them. For him, they were not signs showing the way regardless of the fact that the connection set up with them remained.

Now we have two possibilities that lead in the same way to the same result. In some cases, we replaced the small papers with the former ones, the ones from the old experiment, and pasted them in exactly the same way. The problem was solved correctly immediately. The child explained, "Now I understand: the nut is where the dark paper is. That's how I guessed this time," and even when he solved the problem when there was a change, he exclaimed, "Aha, there is the dark paper." However, the child can reach the same result by a different path, not by the path of renewing the old connection, but by the path of simple turning of attention. Distributing the cups for a new experiment, we again used the earlier paper-indicators, but reduced them to one-third the size, making them less eye-catching. Again seeing the child hesitatingly looking at the cups, we called his attention to one of the gray papers by pointing to it and again this slight nudge was enough for the child to solve the problem of choice that confronted him.

Because of our pointing, the child immediately perceived the instruction from experience and from the beginning, guided by the gray signs, made a choice between the two colors, the gray and the red, and then guided by the color, made a correct abstraction and selected all the proper cups.

Thus, the second operation of selection and abstraction occurred relatively smoothly due to the light and insignificant nudge to attract attention. In the last experiment, there are several very important points.

First, in this case the effect of attracting attention is absolutely equal to the act of direct regeneration of the old connection. When we used the same series of cards, regeneration of the old connection led to correct selection along the previously assimilated structural path. This same regeneration of the connection occurred with simply calling attention, which also led to reinforcement of the pertinent signal. The pointing finger guides the attention of the child, and guiding his attention, sets off and regenerates old conditioned connections and generates new processes of abstraction. We could have reminded the child with verbal instruction of the significance of the gray signs in the new set-up, but in this case, the child's experience and the instruction would have united two different operations, specifically, the operation of closure of the required connection and the operation of turning attention. We tried to separate the one from the other in two parallel experiments and to present both instances separately.

Second, the child finds the natural mediated processes to be very complex. His attention in this case is mediated twice. The basic direction of his attention remains the same throughout. The child seeks the nut according to a color trait he has abstracted and, consequently, turns his attention to the color. But in order to select the correct color of the two presented, he must be guided by two gray cards and in this way, all his attention becomes mediated. Here we have a natural, mediated process that, as we know, is found in studies of the development of memory. In this case, it is important for us to create this mediated operation for the child; we guide his initial attention and only later does the child himself begin to create the same thing for himself.

Finally, the third point, the gray cards acquired the functional meaning of signals for the child. In the first experiment, they were for him a trait according to which he chose a cup and now he is making a selection between colors. It would be a mistake to say that the gray shades play the role of words that mean "yes" and "no" or "+" and "−." However, they play the role of signs that turn the child's attention and guide him along a certain path, and at the same time acquire something like a common meaning. The combination of the two functions, the indicating sign and the memory sign, seems to us to be most characteristic in this experiment because we are inclined to understand the functions of the gray cards to be a model of the primary formation of meaning.

Let us recall that for a correct solution of the problem in the basic experiment, the child had to abstract correctly the trait of color, but the abstraction itself was made because of turning his attention with the help of indicating signs. Indicating which sets abstraction into motion is also, in our opinion, a psychological model of the first assigning of a certain meaning to a sign, in other words, it is a model of the first formation of a sign.

It seems that our experiments cast light on the processes of the formation of voluntary attention in this child and that the reaction is a process that results directly from directing attention correctly.

On this basis, Eliasberg defines attention as a function of pointing: he says that what is perceived becomes a pointer toward another perception, to the signal that did not previously appear as dominating or was not perceived. Signs and meanings can initially be completely independent of each other and in this case, pointing establishes their relation to each other. Eliasberg sees as the advantage of his experiments that they make it possible to observe the instant of attention without involving the hypothesis of nominative function. Comparing his experiments with the experiments of Ach, he indicates that in Ach's experiment the name was separated from other properties of the object, but by indicating the object with a word and pointing to it, we placed the word in a certain relation to the object.

Ach also stresses that the direction of attention leads to the formation of a concept. In the chapter on concepts, we shall see that the word that signifies the concept actually appears first in the role of an indicator that isolates some traits of an object, calls attention to these traits, and only then does the word become a sign that represents these objects. Ach says that words are the means of directing attention so that in a series of objects that have the same name, common properties are identified on the basis of the name which thus leads to the formation of a concept.

The name or the word is an indicator for attention and a nudge toward forming new ideas. If the verbal system is damaged, for example, in someone suffering brain damage, the whole function of using a word to call attention suffers.

Ach quite justifiably points out that, consequently, words are as if an outlet that forms the social experience of the child and directs his thought along already established paths. At a transitional age, as Ach believes, under the influence of speech, attention is directed more and more toward abstract relations and leads to the formation of abstract concepts. For this reason, the use of language as a means of directing attention and as a method of forming ideas is of very great significance for pedagogy. With complete validity, Ach indicates that with this understanding of directing attention with words, we move beyond the bounds of individual psychology and find ourselves in the area of social psychology.

From a different direction, we approached the statement of T. Ribot that voluntary attention is a social phenomenon. Thus, we see that the process of voluntary attention directed by language or speech is initially, as we have said, a process in which the child is more likely to be dependent on the adult than to manage his own perception. With language, adults direct the attention of the child and only on this basis does the child himself gradually begin to control his own attention. For this reason it seems to us that Ach is right when he understands the social moment of contact as being the functional action of the word.

Eliasberg correctly says that at this age, even in the youngest subjects that Ach studied, language had long since become the means of contact. It must be noted that only on the basis of the initial function of language, the function of contact, can its subsequent role, direction of attention, be formed.

On this basis, we can reach the conclusion that it is not apperceptive attention that determines mental processes, but that mental connections direct and distribute attention. The word "attention" in itself serves only to define the degree of clarity; the process itself of concentrating attention in thinking, Eliasberg proposes to explain by other volitional factors. In his work, the character of the primary factors that determine attention remain unknown. From our point of view, the primary condition that forms attention is not inner "volitional" function, but the cultural, historically developed operation that leads to the appearance of voluntary attention. Pointing lies at the beginning of directing attention, and it is remarkable that man created for himself a kind of special organ of voluntary attention in the pointing finger, which in most languages got its name from this function. The first pointing was a kind of artificial indication with the fingers and, in the history of the development of speech, we have seen that the initial words play the role of similar indications that call attention. For this reason, the history of voluntary attention must begin with the history of the pointing finger.

The history of the development of voluntary attention can be beautifully traced in the abnormal child. We have already seen (in the chapter on speech) to what degree the speech of the deaf-mute child, depending on gestures, is evidence of the primacy of the function of pointing. The deaf-mute child speaking of people or things that are before him points to them and calls attention to them. Specifically, in the language of the deaf-mute child we see how the function of pointing acquires an independent meaning. For example, in the language of the deaf-mute, a tooth may have four different meanings: (1) tooth, (2) white or (3) hard, and finally, (4) stone. For this reason, when a deaf-mute, in the course of conversation, points to a tooth, which is a conditioned symbol for each of the four enumerated concepts, he must make at least one more pointing gesture to indicate to which of the qualities of the tooth we must pay attention. The deaf-mute must give direction to our abstraction: he calmly makes a pointing gesture when the tooth must signify a tooth; he strikes the tooth gently when he uses the sign in the sense of "hard"; he moves his finger across the tooth when he is indicating the color white; finally, he makes a throwing gesture when the tooth signifies a stone. In the language of deaf-mute children, we see very clearly the conditioned functions of pointing and the function of remembering that is typical of the word. The separation of the one from the other indicates the primitive nature of the language of deaf-mutes.

As we have seen, the pointing finger stands at the beginning of the development of voluntary attention. In other words, at first adults begin to direct the attention of the child and control it. In the deaf-mute, contact by means of gestures appears exceptionally early, but without words he loses all the instructions for directing attention that are linked to words and for this reason his voluntary attention develops extremely slowly. The common type of his attention may be described as predominantly primitive or externally mediated.

Experiments with abstractions, about which we have just spoken, were set up with deaf-mute children. The experiments showed that in the deaf-mute child there are primitive processes of paying attention that are required for processes of abstraction. Gifted deaf-mute children age six to seven conducted themselves in the experiment like three-year-old normal children, that is, they quickly found the required abstraction of both the positive and negative connections between the color and success. They also succeeded in making the transition to a new pair of colors, but hardly ever without special auxiliary devices.

Eliasberg sees in this fact a confirmation of his ideas on the effect of speech on thinking. Primitive processes of attention in the deaf-mute are not disrupted, but the development of complex forms of attention organized with the help of thought are strongly inhibited. True, Eliasberg says that we must not forget that a six-year-old deaf-mute child has a different system of language, gestures with a primitive syntax that frequently cannot be expressed logically; for this reason, the very question on forms of organization of behavior of the child remains an open question for him.

We conducted special experiments with deaf-mute children which showed the following: actually with very little difficulty, the deaf-mute child resorts to an external auxiliary device which facilitates directing attention. It developed that regardless of the lesser development of voluntary attention in deaf-mute children and of the very primitive resources of this function, directing their attention was very much easier. The pointing gesture for a deaf-mute is all that he has at his disposal and in connection with this, his speech itself still remains at the primitive stage of pointing, and he always maintains a primitive mastery of operations. For this reason, for the deaf-mute child, an insignificant visual difference very soon becomes a directing sign that points to the path for his attention. However, it is difficult for the deaf-mute child to make any complex connection between the pointing function of the sign and its signifying function.

Thus at first glance, in the deaf-mute child we have a paradoxical, and for us a completely unexpected, combination of two symptoms. On the one hand, there is the lesser development of voluntary attention, its arrest at the stage of the external sign-indication resulting from absence of words and connecting the indicating gesture with its signifying function. This is responsible for the exceptional lack of significance of indicating with respect to objects not presented visually. This paucity of inner signs of attention is the most characteristic feature of the deaf-mute child. On the other hand, the direct opposite is characteristic for the deaf-mute child. Such a child exhibits a much greater tendency to use mediated attention than does the normal child. What for the normal child influenced by words became an automatic habit, for the deaf-mute child, was still a new process and for this reason, the child when faced with any difficulty very readily turns from the direct path of solving the problem toward mediated attention.

Eliasberg correctly notes as a general phenomenon, passing like a red thread through all his experiments with children, the use of auxiliary devices, that is, the transition from direct to mediated attention. As a rule, frequently this does not depend on speech. The child who does not say anything during the experiment, who generally speaks only of his needs with two-word sentences, immediately transfers his experience to any other pair of colors and, in the final analysis, experiments with him run the same course as if the child had formulated a rule: "Of two colors of any kind, only one is the trait." Conversely, the external verbal formulation appears only when the child is confronted by a difficult situation. Let us recall our experiments with the development of egocentric speech under difficult circumstances. In experiments with abstraction, we also see egocentric speech every time the child experiences difficulty. At the moment the difficulty arises, auxiliary devices enter—this is the general rule that we can deduce from all our experiments.

Whether the child resorts to mediated operations depends primarily on two factors: on the general mental development of the child and on mastery of such technical auxiliary devices as language, numbers, etc. It is very important that, in pathological cases, the extent to which a child applies auxiliary devices to compensate for the specific defect be considered as a criterion of intellect. As we have noted, children most retarded with respect to speech spontaneously resort to speech formulations when they encounter unavoidable difficulties. This is true even of three-year-olds. However, the significance of auxiliary devices becomes universal as soon as we move to pathological cases. Aphasics deprived of language, the most important organ of thinking, exhibit a tendency to using visual auxiliary stimuli and, specifically, the visual aspect of the stimuli may become devices for thinking. Thus, the difficulty consists not only in that thinking is deprived of most important devices, but also in that complex speech devices are replaced by other devices less expedient for establishing complex connections.

All aphasics, regardless of the fact that they have no direct intellectual defects, experience difficulty in separating the relation from its carriers. Comparing this characteristic with the behavior of children with poor speech development, Eliasberg reaches the conclusion that in itself the process of attention does not depend entirely on speech, but the complex development of thinking is seriously impeded by absence of speech. Finally, the general rule derived from the study of all the subjects: the method of using devices is of decisive significance. Eliasberg says that, as a rule, devices are directed toward minimizing a given defect. If we did not know about the defect beforehand, all of this could help us reach a conclusion about the defect itself.

Thus we see that a defect has a double effect: this is the position we proceed from in considering the development of the behavior of the atypical child. Eliasberg says, and we have established this in our experiments, that as a rule, the defect acts as difficulty does in a normal child. On the one hand, the defect decreases the level of execution of the operation: for the deaf-mute child, an identical problem is impossible or extremely difficult. This is the negative effect of the defect. However, like all difficulty, it nudges the subject onto the path of higher development, onto the path of mediated attention, to which, as we have seen, aphasic and deaf-mute children resort much more frequently than normal children.

For psychology and pedagogy of deaf-mute children, the double effect of the defect is of decisive importance, the fact that the defect creates simultaneously a tendency toward compensation, toward adjustment, and this compensation, or adjustment, is accomplished mainly along the paths of the cultural development of the child. The tragedy of the deaf-mute child, and specifically, the tragedy in the development of his attention, consists not in the fact that the child has by nature poorer attention than the normal child, but in his divergence from cultural development. While cultural development in the normal child is attained in the process of his growing into the speech of those around him, in the deaf-mute child, it is retarded. His attention is, in a way, neglected and not cultivated, is not taken over and directed as speech in adults, as is the attention of the normal child. It is not cultivated and for this reason, it remains for a very long time at the stage of the pointing finger, that is, within the bounds of external, elementary operations. But deliverance from this tragedy lies in the fact that the deaf-mute child is capable of the same kind of attention as the normal child. In principle, the deaf-mute child arrives at the same point, but does not have the appropriate technical devices. We believe that it would not be possible to express the difficulty in the development of the deaf-mute child any more clearly than to turn to the fact that in the normal child, assimilation of speech precedes the formation of voluntary attention, and in the normal child, speech because of its natural properties is a device for calling attention. In the deaf-mute child, conversely, the development of voluntary attention must precede speech, and for this reason, in him both appear to be inadequately developed. A retarded child differs from the normal most of all in the weakness of voluntary attention when it is directed toward the organization of internal processes, and for this reason, the higher processes of thinking and formation of concepts are difficult for him.

The path to development of attention lies in the general development of speech. This is why the trend in developing speech of the deaf-mute child that places all the stress on articulation, on the external aspect, when there is general retardation in the development of higher functions of speech, results in neglecting attention, as we said above.

P. Sollier was the first to try to base the psychology of mentally retarded children on the inadequacy of their attention. Following Ribot and making a distinction for this reason between spontaneous and voluntary attention, he selected specifically the latter as a criterion for dividing mentally retarded children according to various degrees of retardation. In his opinion, in the idiot, attention is impeded and weak in general; this is the essence of idiocy. In absolute idiots there is no voluntary attention at all; in representatives of the three other degrees of mental retardation, voluntary attention occurs rarely, periodically, or is easily but not stably elicited or acts only automatically.

According to Sollier, in imbeciles, the most characteristic trait is instability of attention. At present, Sollier's theory has lost its meaning and the criterion itself of reducing all symptoms of retardation to the dropping out of one function, specifically attention, is unsustainable, but undoubtedly, Sollier must be given credit for establishing how the inadequacy of voluntary attention creates a specific picture of the mentally retarded child. Regardless of the fact that Sollier argues with Seguin, whose position we are trying to establish, Sollier himself shares the point of view of Seguin since he always speaks of voluntary attention and for him, attention is, of course, a volitional act. For this reason, as Troshin correctly noted, Sollier's argument with Seguin seems a misunderstanding.

Binet, who disputed the point of view of Seguin and Sollier, called their work absurd, and rejected the idea that the retarded child's thinking was related to weakness of will, came to the same conclusions as a result of his own experiments. He actually used the same volitional acts, for example, a volitional glance, capability of expressing thought with gestures, etc., as a basis for dividing the severely mentally retarded into four levels. Binet can say that for him, these acts are not will alone, but an expression of will in the mind. But, of course, both Seguin and Sollier, in reducing the essence of development to the anomaly of will and attention, also understood the latter in a broad sense. Without a doubt, to reduce erroneously all underdevelopment to any one function, let alone a defect of the will as the most complex psychological phenomenon, may be the most characteristic aspect for mental underdevelopment. Not without reason did Seguin and Binet and Sollier essentially converge in this position regardless of their mutual contradiction. If we understand will in the genetic sense that we give this term, specifically as the stage of mastery of the processes of one's own behavior, then, of course, most characteristic in the mental underdevelopment of the atypical child, including the idiot, is, as we have already indicated, the divergence between his organic and his cultural development.

The same lines of development that coincide in the normal child diverge in the abnormal child. The means for cultural behavior have historically been devised in terms of normal psychophysiological organization of man. Specifically these means are not suitable for a child burdened with a defect. In the deaf-mute child, the divergence due to absence of hearing is consequently marked by a purely mechanical retardation along the path of speech development, but in the retarded child, the weakness is in the central apparatus: his hearing is preserved, but his intellect is so underdeveloped that the child does not have all the functions of speech and, consequently, the function of attention.

On the basis of the law of conformity between fixation and apperception, we can determine the capacity of the idiot to learn according to eye fixation on some object. On this basis, all idiots can be considered as being incapable of any education and completely not receptive to any therapeutic-pedagogical treatment. We have already seen that the capacity to pay attention requires a natural apparatus for catalyzing any perceived sign. If this process itself is absent, if visual dominants do not develop at all, then, as we have seen from the studies of V. M. Bekhterev, there can be no closure of any conditioned reflex from this organ. An imbecile who is capable of fixation on an object has passive attention and, consequently, is capable of training.

A further decisive step is the transition from passive to active attention; according to Heller, the difference between them is not in kind, but in degree. One differs from the other in that active apperception occurs in a field of attention containing several perceptions that conflict with each other and the child chooses among them. The presence of choice defines the instant of transition from passive to active attention. Only at this higher stage are volitional actions connected with choice in the true sense of the word possible. In this connection, Heller recommends training retarded children to apply the method of selection by presenting them with a number of objects and requiring them to choose and indicate an object named by the instructor.

We also ascribe great psychological significance to this method because we see in it only a continuation and augmentation of the indicating function of the word, which in the normal child occurs quite naturally. We would like to note the general artificiality and the child's lack of interest in this task. This point is more a technical than a basic difficulty. The selection reaction put into play becomes a potent means through which we begin to direct the attention of the child.

A further development of this method when it is applied in practice may be that the child says the appropriate word to himself and then selects the required object, in other words, the child learns to stimulate his active attention himself. From the outset, the imbecile has spontaneous attention directed to various objects, but in him this function is, as a rule, extremely weak and unstable, and for this reason the usual state which we call inattention or absentmindedness in the normal child is a characteristic trait of imbeciles. Finally, mild retardation, the least serious form of retardation, is characterized by underdevelopment of thinking in concepts, which we use to deduce abstractions from a concrete perception of things.

This defect may be established with experimental precision in the slightly retarded and may, in this way, indicate not only the incapacity for direct attention, but also the inability to form concepts. Let us recall, however, our experiments demonstrating how essentially significant directed attention is for processes of abstraction, and it will become clear that the mildly retarded find it impossible to form concepts mainly because of an inability to follow the course of their own attention along the very complex paths indicated for them by words. The higher function of the word, connected with development of concepts, is inaccessible for them mainly because their higher forms of voluntary attention are underdeveloped.

# V

## Child Psychology
### *Vygotsky's Conception of Psychological Development*

CARL RATNER, *Institute for Cultural Research and Education, Trinidad, California*

The central idea that informs all of Vygotsky's work on developmental psychology is that qualitatively new psychological phenomena arise over the life span. These phenomena consist of novel psychological operations, content, and relationships that are not continuous with previous ones. Consequently, perspectives and methods that are suitable to comprehending early behaviors are not necessarily suitable for comprehending mature psychology. Different concepts and methods must be devised to understand the different psychological stages.

The most fundamental qualitative change over the life span, as Vygotsky identified it, is from lower, elementary processes to higher, conscious, psychological processes. There is a transition from "direct, innate, natural forms and methods of behavior to mediated, artificial, mental functions that develop in the process of cultural development" (Vygotsky, 1998, p. 168). Lower, elementary processes are biologically programmed, natural behaviors that are immediate responses to stimuli. Sucking and rooting reflexes are examples. In lower processes, there is nothing mental, psychological, or conscious. By contrast, psychological processes are mental and conscious. Consciousness intervenes, or mediates, between a stimulus and the response. Consciousness comprises a "mental space" of psychological phenomena such as perception, emotions, memory, thinking, motivation, self, language, and accumulated learned information. These psychological phenomena "process" incoming stimuli and construct a response that is willful and intentional. Psychological processes are humanly created, mental phenomena. They are artifacts, not natural biological phenomena.

Vygotsky emphasizes this difference as follows:

> Higher mental functions are not simply a continuation of elementary functions and are not their mechanical combination, but a qualitatively new mental formation that develops according to completely special laws and is subject to completely different patterns. . . "In the thinking of the adolescent, not only completely new complex synthetic forms that the three-year-old does not know arise, but even those elementary, primitive forms that the child of three has acquired are restructured on new bases during the transitional age" (Vygotsky, 1998, pp. 34, 37).

The essence of psychological phenomena is that they are conscious, cognitive, and conceptual—that is to say, they are intellectual. It is only when the child has achieved these capacities that he develops a psychology:

> Development of thinking has a central, key, decisive significance for all the other functions and processes. We cannot express more clearly or tersely the leading role of intellectual development in relation to the whole personality of the adolescent and to all of his mental functions other than to say that acquiring the function of forming concepts is the principal and central link in all the changes that occur in the psychology of the adolescent. All other links in this chain, all other special functions, are intellectualized, reformed, and reconstructed under the influence of these crucial successes that the thinking of the adolescent achieves. . . . Lower or elementary functions, being processes that are more primitive, earlier, simpler, and independent of concepts in genetic, functional, and structural relations, are reconstructed on a new basis when influenced by thinking in concepts and . . . they are included as component parts, as subordinate stages, into new, complex combinations created by thinking on the basis of concepts, and finally . . . under the influence of thinking, foundations of the personality and world view of the adolescent are laid down (ibid., p. 81).

Since a fundamental criterion of psychological phenomena is that they rest upon cognitive concepts, knowledge, and schemas, psychological phenomena are all intellectualized. Vygotsky even refers to "intellectual perception" (ibid., pp. 290–291). He means that what we see is not simply a function of sensory impressions; rather, these impressions are themselves shaped by knowledge and concepts about things. Emotions are also shaped by knowledge and concepts (Ratner, 1991, Chaps. 1, 2, 5; Ratner, 2000). In cases of intellectualized psychological phenomena, the subject knows *what* he is seeing. He knows that the thing is a flower. Moreover, he knows *that* he is perceiving and feeling the thing. In contrast, elementary reactions are immediate responses to things and lack cognitive, intellectual, linguistic meaning.*

An example of the qualitative difference between a cognitively mediated psychological phenomenon and an elementary, natural, biological reaction is the difference between infantile sensory pleasure and psychological happiness. Psychological happiness is modulated by understandings and expectations. The happiness one experiences while gazing at a sunset over the ocean is different from the happiness one experiences when one's favorite basketball team wins the championship with a last-second basket, and from the warm glow that one feels when receiving a thoughtful present from a lover. These different forms of happiness entail, respectively, an appreciation of nature's grandeur and subtle richness; an identification with a group of players and even

---

* Vygotsky's view that human psychology has a cognitive basis stems from his rationalist view of man, which he derived from Spinoza's philosophy. This does not deny that human thoughts and actions can be irrational in the sense of being illogical, contradictory, careless, or impulsive. It simply means that there is a cognitive basis for irrationality as for all psychological functions (cf. Ratner, 1994). For instance, a man might compulsively gamble despite the high risk that it will bring financial ruin upon himself and his family because he believes he will beat the odds and win more than he loses. This belief in individual exceptionalism—the individual's ability to overcome a system stacked against him—is a cognition rooted in Western cultural ideology. The gambling compulsion is a need in addition to a belief. However, it is an intellectualized need where the gambler knows that he needs money, what money is, why he needs it, and how he will obtain it. Human psychological need is not a pure, blind impulse, as a fish needs food but has no awareness of the need, its basis, object, or means of fulfillment.

a city or country; and an appreciation of being wanted by and being together with a valued individual. The simple, inchoate pleasurable sensation that a neonate feels when fed and rested entails none of the foregoing cognitions and therefore none of the foregoing subtlety and richness. Vygotsky says that the young child can feel pleasure but he does not know he is happy; he does not know (conceptualize) what *happiness* is. In the same way, an infant feels hunger pangs, but he does not know he is hungry because he has no concept that identifies hunger as a phenomenon. "There is a great difference between feeling hunger and knowing that I am hungry. In early childhood, the child does not know his own experiences" (ibid., p. 291).

Vygotsky's emphasis on cognitive factors as basic to psychological development highlights the social organization of psychology, because cognition is socially organized. Thinking depends on social concepts objectified in language; it also depends on socially structured life activities. The cognitions that shape psychological phenomena therefore implant cultural concepts, linguistic terms, and social activities into those psychological phenomena. Vygotsky speaks of

> the law of sociogenesis of higher forms of behavior: speech, being initially the means of communication, the means of association, the means of organization of group behavior, later becomes the basic means of thinking and of all higher mental functions, the basic means of personality formation (ibid., p. 169). Thus, the structures of higher mental functions represent a cast of collective social relations between people (ibid.).

Vygotsky strongly believed that human psychology is a cultural phenomenon. It originates in cultural processes, embodies them, and perpetuates them. He speaks about "the central and leading function of cultural development" (ibid.) in psychological growth. Specifically, the content of thinking is related to one's position in societal production (ibid., p. 43). Vygotsky contrasts his cultural–cognitive psychological approach to other approaches that explain psychological development in terms of sexual maturation or emotional changes (ibid., p. 31).

In proposing that psychological phenomena are culturally and cognitively organized, Vygotsky denied any natural, "basic," or precultural form and content to psychological phenomena. The frequently noted distinction between basic psychological forms and cultural psychological content is false. All aspects of psychological functioning (both form and content) are cultural. As Vygotsky said, "Actually, the form and content of thinking are two factors in a single whole process, two factors internally linked to each other by an essential, not accidental, bond" (ibid., p. 38). He also noted that "deep, scientific studies show that in the process of cultural development of behavior, not only the content of thinking changes, but also its forms, new mechanisms, new functions, new operations, and new methods of activity arise that were not known at earlier stages of historical development" (ibid., p. 34).

Insisting that human psychology is fundamentally cultural, in both its form and content, and denying that there are natural, precultural aspects of psychology, Vygotsky founded a truly cultural psychology. If the structures of higher mental functions are "a transfer into the personality of an inward relation of social order" (ibid., p. 169), then this social order must be comprehensively understood in order to understand psychology. One must be well versed in the history, sociology, and politics of a culture in order to explain and describe a people's psychology (cf. Ratner, 1997, Chaps. 3, 4; Ratner, 2000; Ratner, 2002, for examples). Nebulous, superficial conceptions of culture obscure key processes and factors for understanding the formation and character of psychological phenomena (cf. Ratner & Hui, 2003, for examples).

Vygotsky's qualitative distinction between cognitive—cultural psychological phenomena and immediate, automatic, elementary biological responses (of animals and infants) is revolutionary because it undercuts all attempts at explaining psychological phenomena in terms of biological processes. Explanations of normal psychology in terms of genes, hormones, neurotransmitters, neuroanatomy, evolution, instincts, sensory processes, and infantile reactions are negated by Vygotsky's fundamental distinction.

Let us examine one popular developmental theory to demonstrate its implausibility and incongruence in light of Vygotsky's approach. One theory holds that infants possess emotions, perceptions, motives, intentionality, memory, will, personality, and social responsiveness that are quite similar to those of adults. For example, two-day-old infants are said to "prefer" their mothers' voices over other women's. This conclusion is based on an instrumental conditioning experiment where long sucks on a rubber nipple were rewarded by a tape-recorded story read by their mothers while short sucks were rewarded by a story read by another woman. (I have simplified the design in this discussion.) The infants produced more longer than shorter sucks.

However, this experiment does not demonstrate a psychological preference, certainly not according to Vygotsky. A psychological preference is cognitively mediated and bound up in psychological phenomena. A preference for Beethoven's music over Bartok's, for example, involves aesthetic criteria, emotional reactions, and recollections. Using Vygotsky's terminology, a psychological preference involves knowing that one prefers something to another thing and knowing something about the features that make it preferable. The response to sounds by the two-day-old does not entail such knowledge or any psychological elements.

It is likely that infants suck to elicit the mother's sound because it is a familiar stimulus (similar to sounds the infant heard while in the womb), not because it is their mother's voice (which they surely do not realize). Familiar stimuli may be positively rewarding because they have been proven safe to the neonate. Novel stimuli may be difficult for the immature neonate to cope with, so they are less rewarding. Such an automatic tendency to gravitate toward familiar stimuli, as a survival mechanism, would be as nonpsychological as the hummingbird's attraction to red flowers.

This interpretation is supported by evidence that even fetuses respond differently to familiar and unfamiliar sounds. Mothers recited a story to their fetuses from the 34th through 38th week of gestation. During the 38th week, each fetus heard either the familiar story or a novel one. Fetal heart rate was lower when the familiar story was presented and higher when the novel story was heard. This automatic reaction has nothing to do with an intentional preference. It is governed by the same biological mechanism that makes familiar sounds positively rewarding to the neonate (of. Cooper & Aslin, 1989; Ratner, 1991, Chap. 4).

Even though Vygotsky emphasizes an ontogenetic transformation from elementary biological reactions to higher, conscious psychological phenomena, he does not regard the infant as a blank slate. It is a misconception to hold that cultural psychology begins with an empty organism. Vygotsky clearly recognized that the infant comes equipped with numerous innate response tendencies that confront the caregiver. However, these natural responses gradually extinguish during childhood. The lower brain centers that control them become subsumed under developing cortical centers that enable learned, conceptually guided behavior to supercede reflexes.*

These maturational changes of the child determine his experience with the environment. Early on, when biological programs dominate behavior, behavior is an automatic, stereotyped, uncomprehending reaction to superficial features of the environment. The declining control of biology and the development of consciousness/cognitive understanding allows for increased sensitivity to the environment, better comprehension of it, and flexibility toward it (Vygotsky, 1998, pp. 293–295). "From the point of view of development, the environment becomes entirely different from the minute the child moves from one age level to another" (ibid., p. 293). Vygotsky urges adults to study this interaction and not to assume that the environment has an absolute effect independent of the child. Socialization becomes increasingly effective as the infant's biological reactions lose strength.

By seven years of age, most natural determinants of behavior have died out and the basis of behavior is overwhelmingly cultural. Vygotsky repeatedly stresses this qualitative transformation. There is no longer an interaction of biological and social determinants of behavior. At this point, the child's individuality is a function of her particular social experience, which has increased exponentially over the years (i.e., more in the later years, less in the early years). The manner in which others have reacted to her behavior and physical traits (such as beauty, gender, and skin color) replaces biological determinants of behavior.

The child's experience with others is her individualized *social experience.* Individual social experience filters, or mediates, experience with broad cultural factors such as school, movies, advertising, and political campaigns. Thus, two children who encounter the same movie, advertisement, or teacher may react differently because of their different individual social experiences. The individual's interaction with society is an interaction between broad cultural factors and accumulated particularized experience with society (individual social experience). Rather than personality being partly determined by biological mechanisms and partly determined by social experience, "personality is by nature social" (ibid., p. 170).

Every individual's unique social experience is a variation of broadly shared cultural elements. While every adolescent in the United States has a unique set of parents, for example, the interaction between most American adolescents and their parents manifests many

---

* The maturing cortex enables increasingly complex cognitive operations, as Piaget emphasized. However, the rigid, age-graded sequence of cognitive stages that Piaget attributed to biological epigenesis ("chreods") has been discredited. High-level cognitive operations High-level cognitive operations only appear during late childhood and adolescence in particular societies. This is due to different social stimulation and requirements in those societies. One's cognitive level also varies sonsiderably according to the familiarity of the task. Moreover, the fact that they only appear during late childhood and adolescence in particular societies is due to different social stimulation and requirements in those societies. One's cognitive level also varies considerably according to the familiarity of the task. Level of biological maturation does not dictate a uniform cognitive competence across tasks. Even biologically mature individuals utilize sensorimotor operations in certain situations. Furthermore, many of the specific sequences of cognitive development that Piaget proposed turn out to be culturally variable. Finally, many specific behaviors which Piaget attributed to biological mechanisms–such as animism, egocentrism, counting, adding, and subtracting–are due to social requirements, stimulation, and constructs (Ratner, 1991, pp. 108–111, 120–121, 124–127, 142).

similarities. Common experiences are necessary for organized, stable action and communication to occur.

Vygotsky's cultural psychology is not mechanical. The fact that a culture pre-exists the newborn, is external to him, and structures his life, does not mean that psychological development is a mechanical process of receiving inputs passively. Children actively strive, concentrate, learn, remember, figure out patterns, differentiate essential from nonessential issues, and identify with cultural events and figures (of. Bandura, 1986, on the active nature of human learning). Vygotsky prized children's activity and insisted that educators encourage independent activity in order to enhance learning. He despised autocratic pedagogy and rote learning of boring material (Vygotsky, 1926/1997).

At the same time, Vygotsky believed that educators should direct children's education, to ensure that children learn similar things and that they learn important information about their social and natural world. Vygotsky was by no means suggesting that children's activity should be highly personal, idiosyncratic, or only spontaneous.

## Contemporary Uses of Vygotsky's Approach

Quite a few contemporary researchers have supported Vygotsky's theories of child development (Ratner, 1991, Chap. 4). In particular, Bronfenbrenner has formulated an explanation for individual psychological differences that is consistent with Vygotsky's law of sociogenesis of psychological phenomena. Bronfenbrenner explains how biologically determined temperament relates to a child's particular social experiences. Instead of temperaments directly determining personality, they are "personal qualities that invite or discourage reactions from the environment of a kind that can disrupt or foster processes of psychological growth. Examples include a fussy vs. a happy baby; attractive vs. unattractive physical appearance; or social responsiveness vs. withdrawal." Gender, race, and birth order are other such qualities. "The effect of such characteristics on the person's development depends in significant degree on the corresponding patterns of response that they evoke from the person's environment" (Bronfenbrenner, 1989, pp. 218–225). The eminent child psychologist Jerome Kagan similarly wrote,

> Temperamental factors impose a slight initial bias for certain moods and behavioral profiles
> to which the social environment reacts. But the final behavior we observe at age 3, 13, or
> 33 years is a product of the experiences to which the changing temperamental surfaces have
> accommodated (cited in Ratner, 1997, p. 153).*

---

\*    A child's temperament may contribute to her reactions. A fragile, sensitive, intense child may be frightened by a harsh, critical parent more than a robust or distractible child would be. However, the effect that fear has on later psychology is itself a function of social experience. A frightened child may elicit patience or impatience from other people. The result affects whether the child becomes withdrawn, boastful, cooperative, aggressive, hopeless, careless, depressed, resentful, or forgiving. Temperament therefore does not determine mature behavior, motivation, personality, thinking, or memory (Ratner, 1991, Chap. 4).

This formulation generates a new interpretation of Lewin's formula that behavior is a function of the person and the environment: $B = f(P, E)$. It transforms how $P$ and $E$ are conceived and interrelated. One conception of Lewin's formula is that $P$ and $E$ are independent entities that each impart certain qualities to behavior or to psychology. $E$ is construed as generally homogeneous (imparting similar influences to everyone), while $P$ is construed as introducing personal variations into behavior. However, Bronfenbrenner and Kagan argue that the environment treats different attributes differently; therefore, $E$ also promotes behavioral diversity. In addition, the person and environment are not independent. What $P$ contributes to behavior/psychology is not an intrinsic characteristic of $P$, because $P$ is a function of $E$; $P$ contributes to behavior as $P$ has been affected by $E$. Therefore, $P$ is the accumulation of particular encounters with various environments; it is not the person's intrinsic character. The formula $B = f(P, E)$ could be written as $B = f(Ep, Eg)$ where $Ep$ is one's personal environment and $Eg$ is the general environment that most people confront.

The social treatment of natural characteristics organizes the child's personality. It even affects the individual's initiative and creativity.

> "It is true that individuals often can and do modify, select, reconstruct, and even create their environments. But this capacity emerges only to the extent that the person has been enabled to engage in self directed action as a joint function not only of his biological endowment but also of the environment in which he or she developed" (Bronfenbrenner, 1989, pp. 223–224; cf. Ratner, 2002, pp. 59–67).

Bronfenbrenner explicitly rejects the idea that individuals are the primary shapers of their own development, with the environment playing only a secondary role. The reverse is closer to the truth.

Cross-cultural research demonstrates how personality attributes are socially structured. Chen *et al.* (1995, 1998) found that shyness–inhibition can arise from social experience and be shaped by social experience to result in quite variable personalities. Shy-inhibited children are treated quite differently in China and the United States, and they develop corresponding psychological differences. In Western countries children are likely to become shy, reticent, and sensitive because they have been rejected by significant others. Inhibited children are then likely to be rejected or isolated by peers. They are regarded as incompetent and lacking in social assertiveness. These children experience difficulties in social adjustment and become withdrawn in the company of peers. They also experience academic difficulties and become lonely and depressed. In China, shyness–inhibition results from positive experiences with significant others who encourage it, not from negative experiences as in the West. Shy-inhibited children in China are more accepted by their caretakers and peers than their average counterparts are. They are considered more honorable, mature, competent, well behaved, and understanding. They receive higher scores on leadership than average children do. Finally, they are no more at risk for depression than other children.

Thus, personality attributes take quite different forms and have different social and psychological consequences, depending on how a culture treats them. Shyness that is fostered and valued, and shot through with competence, popularity, maturity, and decisive leadership is qualitatively different from shyness that stems from rejection, disappointment, embarrassment, unresponsiveness, insensitivity, and punishment, and is shot through with low confidence, dependence, immaturity, fear, withdrawal, and isolation.

## Criticism of Some Neo-Vygotskians

Vygotsky's central theme–that higher psychological processes are formed by cultural processes, including semiotic concepts, rather than by biological ones–is anathema to most mainstream psychologists today. They typically insist that psychological phenomena are either universal or individual phenomena–with biological origins in either case. Laws of perception, memory, learning, attitude change, and group process are construed as universal processes, while personality and mental illness are regarded as individual phenomena–and all of these are said to be rooted in human nature. According to this mainstream view, biology determines most of the form and content of psychological phenomena, and social processes have a marginal effect at best. Broad cultural factors and processes such as social institutions, legal systems, forms of government, social class, and prevalent ideologies are accorded virtually no role in mainstream psychology.

Although they claim to be inspired by his writings, some neo-Vygotskians also misunderstand and/or even reject his most important concepts. This is particularly true of the law of sociogenesis of psychological phenomena (the cultural organizing of psychology) and the distinction between early, simple, biological reactions and mature, complex psychological phenomena.

## Misunderstandings of Sociogenesis

Certain neo-Vygotskian cultural psychologists and activity theorists have repudiated the notion of an organized culture that is external to the individual and structures his psychology. They glorify the individual as the producer of his own psychology and even of culture at large. Each person is said to decide how to confront culture, how to behave in the culture, and what to accept and reject from culture. In other words, the individual appropriates culture (in the sense of taking it over for herself and making it her own) rather than internalizes culture (in the sense of incorporating culture into herself and being formed by it).

These neo-Vygotskians state that they are combining individual activity with culture, and sometimes employ the term "co-constructionism" to denote both elements. However, their writings emphasize the individual's construction of psychology and culture, and neglect the influence or even the existence of organized culture.* For instance, Valsiner claims that individuals do not simply synthesize culturally provided material; they reconstruct it to produce their own

---

\*    Co-constructionism, like all eclectic notions is a nebulous concept. Co-constructionists (i.e., individualistic neo-Vygotskians) never stipulate how the personal realm specifically interacts with culture, i.e., how much influence personal construction has vis-à-vis organized culture in generating psychological and social phenomena. No criteria are stipulated for distinguishing whether an individual act results from a personal choice, a biological abnormality, or particular social experiences that steer one in a particular direction. This makes research on the topic vulnerable to arbitrary interpretations that are difficult to validate.

material of a personal sort. He goes so far as to construe culture as a toxic milieu that individuals avoid by creating their own meanings (of. Ratner, 2002, Chap. 2, for documentation and discussion of Valsiner's position).

Wertsch, another influential writer on Vygotsky, similarly implies that individuals construct personal meanings about things rather than reflect social meanings. For example, consider the case offered by Rowe, Wertsch, and Kosyaeva (2002) of two patrons in a museum, looking at a painting that depicts the Winter Palace and its locale:

> K: See here? It's the Winter Palace, and in 1985 I lived in St. Petersburg for a summer with a friend in her apartment down this street here.

> S: You lived right there?

> K: Yes, well, not right in that building but down the street here a little way and I would walk down to the square everyday.

From this minimal interchange, the authors conclude that the two patrons have imbued the public painting with personal meaning (i.e., where one of them lived), and they have disregarded any historical—social significance:

> "Instead of bringing autobiographical narratives into contact with official culture as part of an attempt to enrich the latter, it seems to us that this [narrative] involves an escape from the public memory sphere . . . . These visitors are refusing to engage in the museum's public memory space. . . . It is meaning making on one's own terms (ibid., p.106)."

This conclusion diametrically opposes Vygotsky's emphasis on the social formation of psychology. Where Vygotsky emphasized that personal activity incorporates cultural factors, Wertsch et al., similar to Valsiner, propose that personal meanings refuse and escape from cultural life.

The claim that individuals continually displace, negate, escape, or reconstruct culture by creating personal meanings is an overstatement, one that is contradicted by massive standardization, monopolization, and conformity in society. It is also contradicted by the vast psychological literature on the power of modeling and referencing to mold behavior (of. Bandura, 1986). It is also contradicted by the uncanny ways that children's psychology recapitulates parents' psychology and by the enormous difficulty of breaking this pattern even with the aid of a therapist. In addition, social coordination, continuity, and communication require that individuals accept and abide by social conventions. Internalizing social values and norms is critical to preserving social life. If social conventions were continually being transformed into personal constructs, this would subvert social coordination, continuity, and communication. Freud, Hobbes, and all thoughtful social theorists have recognized this potential.

Of course, individuals do have personal ideas that color their sense of life. A child's sense of school is colored by her needs, desires, expectations, and fears. A factory worker may conjure up erotic thoughts to make his job bearable. Normally, these personal ideas are compatible with common social norms and pose no threat to them. Extreme personal experience, such as trauma, can radically distort one's behavior, and profound thinking by geniuses may also lead to novel behavior. Apart from these exceptions, personal thoughts do not usually displace, negate, escape, or transform the required regularity of social life.

To follow Vygotsky's intentions more closely, it can be noted that much of what appears to be personally invented meanings actually recapitulates the individual's social experience (how people have treated that person differently from the way they have treated others) or broadly shared social experiences and meanings that many individuals have internalized in similar fashion (the *Ep* and *Eg* in the earlier discussion of Lewin and Bronfenbrenner). In these cases, the individual cannot be said to have created meaning on his own terms. When a particular pupil fails in school, his behavior is often attributed to his own disinterest. However, his behavior is frequently characteristic of many children who have similar backgrounds and attributes (gender, ethnicity, socioeconomic status). Shared experiences with social institutions, and with similar physical infrastructures of their neighborhoods, lead these students to adopt common social meanings about formal education–that, for example, it is insignificant to their lives–and to lose their motivation to master it. The fact that an individual violates a particular set of social codes (e.g., the teacher's) does not mean he lives in a world of self-created, personal meanings. His action may be shaped by other social experiences, norms, meanings, and expectations, those of his own social group. Individualistic neo-Vygotskians are so intent on construing culture as a personal construct that they overestimate the presence and influence of personal constructs and underestimate the effect of organized culture on psychology.

K's casual remark that she lived on a street that appeared in the painting does not imply that she is escaping from the public memory sphere, refusing to engage in public memory, or regarding the painting entirely as a personal projection. If anything, the limited statements in the dialogue of S and K appear to be cultural responses rather than spontaneous, idiosyncratic ones. Making personal remarks about a historical artifact conforms to a prevalent tendency in modern society. The entertainment and news media often glamorize personal issues such as sex scandals over social, political, religious, and artistic issues. When S and K enact this pattern in the museum they are recapitulating culture, not refusing it (Ratner, 1993, 1999, 2002, Chap. 2). They are introducing one set of social norms (to personalize social issues) into a social domain that prescribes other social norms (to appreciate historical artifacts in museums). They are not really creating new values on their own terms. When neo-Vygotskians exaggerate the individualistic, personal basis of behavior they too are simply introducing a certain Western ideology into their study of psychology; they are not creating a new point of view.

## Elementary versus Higher Psychological Functions

Vygotsky's distinction between early, simple, biological reactions and mature, complex psychological phenomena has also been neglected, misunderstood, or rejected by mainstream psychologists who seek to reduce higher mental functions to lower explanatory constructs. The distinction has escaped some neo-Vygotskians as well.

Rogoff, for example, is sympathetic toward Vygotsky's sociocultural approach. Yet she maintains that biology and culture contribute equally to generating social—psychological phenomena. She believes that "gender roles can be seen as simultaneously biologically and culturally formed" (Rogoff, 2003, p. 76). According to Rogoff, certain specific features of gender roles spring from the genetic makeup of men and women (which is the result of phylogenetic evolution), and certain features spring from contemporary cultural factors. She claims that this in fact accords with Vygotsky's explanatory schema: "In Vygotsky's terms, evolutionary (biological) preparedness of gender roles involves phylogenetic development, and social learning of gender roles involves microgenetic and ontogenetic development of the current era's gender roles during the time frame of cultural-historical development" (ibid., p. 76).

Rogoff is not simply claiming that biology prepares gender roles in a general way by preparing humans to learn, speak, use tools, and think; she claims a much more specific role for biology. Rogoff (2003, pp. 71–73) claims that biological mechanisms prepare features of gender roles and personality as follows: a biological trait of women, which they share with many animals, is that they have to invest heavily in each child to reproduce their genes, whereas men need invest little time and effort. Women need to spend nine months pregnant, two to three years nursing, and more years protecting and teaching the child how to survive. In contrast, it is possible for men to father as many children as women allow, with very little time invested. Biological, reproductive processes of men and women are said to generate a social psychology wherein women are more attentive to and involved with children than men are.

Our discussion has emphasized that Vygotsky opposed biological explanation of social—psychological phenomena–even in combination with cultural explanations. He denied that biological mechanisms determine the form and content of higher, complex psychological phenomena; only cultural processes do. Biological mechanisms only determine simple reactions in animals and human infants. Biology enables psychology to develop, but it does not determine the specific features of psychology. *Vygotsky was not an interactionist*–he did not believe that biological mechanisms and cultural processes each contribute particular features to psychology. He believed that cultural processes *supercede* biological determinants of behavior. Vygotsky explains psychology in thoroughly sociocultural terms, not as something partitioned into biological features and cultural ones.

In *Studies on the History of Behavior: Ape, Primitive, and Child,* Vygotsky and Luria (1930/1993) specifically address the question of phylogenetic (evolutionary), ontogenetic, and cultural—historical processes in psychological development. They argue that human culture marks a qualitatively new stage in phylogeny. Culture *replaces* evolutionary, biological mechanisms as determinants of behavior:

> "The use and "invention" of tools by anthropoid apes *bring to an end the organic stage of behavioral development in the evolutionary sequence* and prepare the way for a transition of *all* development to a new path, creating thereby the main psychological prerequisite of historical development of behavior" (ibid., p. 37, my emphasis).

All human psychological development depends on cultural processes because organic, biological evolution has ceased determining human behavior.

Vygotsky and Luria adopted the dialectical philosophy of Marx, Engels, and Hegel to emphasize qualitative transformations in historical development. What is true of one stage and one species is not true of other stages and other species, because fundamentally new processes have arisen. In dialectical qualitative transformations, new processes are not added onto antecedent, "primitive" ones. Rather, a new integration occurs in which the older ones are subsumed within the new ones and alter their function to make way for them. For example, "primitive" parts of the human brain, which are vestiges from animals, are controlled by the neocortex, which transforms their functioning. They do not simply maintain their old functioning next to, or in addition to, cortical processes.

Human psychology, according to Vygotsky, does not consist of cultural behavior plus natural (evolutionary, biological) behavior. What is natural behavior in animals (and infants) is converted into cultural behavior in humans. "The development of man's behavior is always development conditioned primarily not by the laws of biological evolution, but by the laws of the historical development of society" (ibid., p. 78). Vygotsky and Luria rejected an eclectic combination of biological and cultural determinants in psychology, where both would have equal footing.

As behavior develops from natural to cultural—psychological, the role of biology changes. It strictly determines the behavior of infants and animals; however, it relaxes its control over adult behavior. Biology provides a potentiating substratum that allows a wide range of behaviors to be organized by cultural processes. Biology provides the energy, anatomical structure, physiology, and neuroanatomy that make psychological functioning possible, but biology itself does not make psychological functioning occur, nor does it determine what its specific form will be (cf. Ratner, 1991, Chaps. 1, 5; Ratner, 2000; Ratner, 2004). This perspective would interpret Rogoff's examples as being more culturally formed than she recognizes. Where she believes that biological mechanisms determine differential involvement of fathers and mothers with children, Vygotsky would argue that any such differences are due to different social roles that men and women occupy. Thus, male and female reproductive biology do not necessarily determine even a portion of gender roles and personality.*

Vygotsky's theories of psychological development are powerful tools for understanding human psychology. Psychologists would do well to read his ideas closely and follow his argument that human psychology arises out of a biological substrate but then develops into a qualitatively new (emergent) phenomenon that functions according to distinctive principles.

# References

Bandura, A. (1986). *Social foundations of thought and action: A social cognitive theory.* Englewood Cliffs, NJ: Prentice Hall.
Bronfenbrenner, U. (1989). Ecological systems theory. *Annals of Child Development, 6,* 187–249.
Chen, X., Rubin, K., & Li, B. (1995). Social and school adjustment of shy and aggressive children in China. *Development and Psychopathology, 7,* 337–349.

---

*   Rogoff recognizes cultural differences in the way mothers relate to their babies, and she realizes that these challenge the idea of innate, universal maternal roles (Rogoff, 2003, pp. 111—114). However, she holds to her incongruous mix of biological—phylogenetic and cultural explanations. She accepts the sociobiological explanation of psychological phenomena as having something to offer. This contradicts a coherent model of biological and cultural processes in psychological development (cf. Ratner & Hui, 2003, for examples of other failures to produce a coherent model). Vygotsky rejected eclectic combinations of theoretical constructs. He sought logically consistent integrations of concepts (cf. Vygotsky, 1987, pp. 243—246). Psychological phenomena cannot be partly conscious, conceptually organized, intellectualized, intentional, and culturally variable, and partly an automatic, stereotyped (fixed), nonconscious, immediate, natural response to a stimulus, as biological determinism would dictate.

Chen, X., Rubin, K., Cen, G., Hastings, P., Chen, H., & Stewart, S. (1998). Child-rearing attitudes and behavioral inhibition in Chinese and Canadian toddlers: A cross-cultural study. *Developmental Psychology, 34,* 677–686.

Cooper, R., & Aslin, R. (1989). The language environment of the young infant: Implications for early perceptual development. *Canadian Journal of Psychology, 43,* 247–265.

Ratner, C. (1991). *Vygotsky's sociohistorical psychology and its contemporary applications.* New York: Plenum.

Ratner, C. (1993). Review of D'Andrade & Strauss, *Human motives and cultural models. Journal of Mind and Behavior, 14,* 89–94.

Ratner, C. (1994). The unconscious: A perspective from sociohistorical psychology. *Journal of Mind and Behavior, 15,* 323–342.

Ratner, C. (1997). *Cultural psychology and qualitative methodology: Theoretical and empirical considerations.* New York: Kluwer/Plenum.

Ratner, C. (1999). Three approaches to cultural psychology: A critique. *Cultural Dynamics, 11,* 7–31.

Ratner, C. (2000). A cultural-psychological analysis of emotions. *Culture and Psychology, 6,* 5–39.

Ratner, C. (2002). *Cultural psychology: Theory and method.* New York: Kluwer Academic/Plenum.

Ratner, C. (2004, forthcoming). Genes and psychology in the news. *New Ideas in Psychology.*

Ratner, C., & Hui, L. (2003). Theoretical and methodological problems in cross-cultural psychology. *Journal for the Theory of Social Behavior, 33,* 67–94.

Rogoff, B. (2003). *The cultural nature of human development.* New York: Oxford University Press.

Rowe, S., Wertsch, J., & Kosyaeva, T. (2002). Linking little narratives to big ones: Narrative and public memory in history museums. *Culture and Psychology, 8,* 96–112.

Vygotsky, L. S. (1987). *Collected works, Volume 1: Problems of general psychology* (R. W. Rieber & A. S. Carton, Eds.). New York: Kluwer Academic/Plenum.

Vygotsky, L. S. (1997). *Educational psychology.* (V. V. Davydov, Intro.; R. Silverman, Trans.). Boca Raton: St. Lucie Press. (Originally published in Russian, 1926)

Vygotsky, L. S. (1998). *Collected works, Volume 5: Child psychology* (R. W. Rieber, Ed.). New York: Kluwer/Plenum.

Vygotsky, L. S., & Luria, A. (1993). *Studies on the history of behavior: Ape, primitive, and child.* (V. I. Golod & J. E. Knox, Eds. & Trans.). Hillsdale, NJ: Lawrence Erlbaum. (Originally published in Russian, 1930)

# 13

# Development of Thinking and Formation of Concepts in the Adolescent

## 1

The history of the development of thinking in the transitional age is itself undergoing a certain transitional stage from the old construction to a new understanding of maturation of the intellect. This understanding arises on the basis of new theoretical views of the psychological nature of speech and thinking, of development, and of the functional and structural interrelation of these processes.

In the area of the study of thinking in the adolescent, pedology is overcoming the basic and radical prejudice and a fateful error that stands in the way of developing a correct conception of the intellectual crisis and maturation that are the content of the development of thinking in the adolescent. This error is usually formulated as a conviction that there is nothing essentially new in the thinking of the adolescent compared with the thinking of the younger child. Some authors, defending thinking, come to the extreme view that the period of sexual maturation does not mark the appearance in the sphere of thinking of any kind of new intellectual operation that a child of three cannot already do.

From this point of view, development of thinking is not at all at the center of the processes of maturation. Substantial, violent shifts taking place during the transitional period in the whole organism and the personality of the adolescent, revelation of new, deep layers of personality, maturation of higher forms of organic and cultural life—all of this, from the point of view of these authors, does not affect the thinking of the adolescent. All changes occur in other areas and spheres of the personality. Thus, the intellectual changes in the whole process of crisis and maturation of the adolescent are diminished and reduced to almost zero.

On the one hand, if one holds this point of view, the process itself of intellectual changes that occur at this age can be reduced to a simple quantitative accumulation of characteristics already laid down in the thinking of a three-year-old ready for further purely quantitative increase to which, strictly speaking, the word *development* does not apply. Charlotte Bühler has expressed this point of view most consistently in the theory of the transitional age where, among other things, further uniform development of the intellect during the period of sexual maturation is setup. In the general system of changes and in the general structure of processes of which maturation is made up, C. Bühler ascribes an extremely insignificant role to intellect, not perceiving the enormous positive significance of intellectual development for the fundamental, most profound reconstruction of the whole system of the adolescent personality.

Originally appeared in English translation as Chapter 2 in *The Collected Works of L.S. Vygotsky, Volume 5: Child Psychology* (Robert W. Rieber, Ed.; Marie J. Hall, Trans.) (pp. 29–81). New York: Kluwer Academic/Plenum Publishers, 1998.

In general and on the whole, this author believes that during the time of sexual maturation, there is a very strong separation of dialectic and abstract thinking from visual thinking since the opinion that any one of the intellectual operations in general appears anew only at puberty is one of the tales that have long since been exposed by child psychology. Even in a three or four-year-old child, all potentials for later thinking are present. To support this thinking, the author cites the studies of Karl Bühler, which present the point of view that intellectual development in its most essential traits, in the sense of maturation of basic intellectual processes, is already set up in early childhood. According to Charlotte Bühler, the difference in the thinking of the young child and that of the adolescent is that in the child visual perception and thinking are usually much more closely connected.

She says that the young child seldom thinks purely verbally and purely abstractly. Even the most talkative and verbally gifted children always start from some concrete experience, and when they yield to the tendency to talk, they usually chatter without thinking. The mechanism is trained without pursuing any other function. The fact that children make deductions and judgments only within a circle of their concrete experiences and that the goals of their plans are contained in a tight circle of visual perception is well known and has provided grounds for the false conclusion that children cannot think abstractly at all.

C. Bühler believes that this opinion has long since been refuted since it has been established that a child perceives very early, abstracting and selecting, and fills in such concepts as "good," "evil," etc. with some vague, general content; the child forms other concepts by abstraction and makes judgments. But we must not deny that all of this is very dependent on the child's visual perceptions and representations. In the adolescent, on the contrary, thinking is freer of the sensible base and is less concrete.

Thus, we see that the denial of substantial changes that occur in the adolescent's intellectual development inevitably leads to admitting simple growth of the intellect during the years of maturation and greater independence from perceptible material. We might formulate the idea of C. Bühler thus: the thinking of the adolescent acquires a certain new quality in comparison with the thinking of the young child; it becomes less concrete and, in addition, "it becomes stronger and firmer," "grows and increases" in comparison with the thinking of the three-year-old, but not a single intellectual operation arises anew during the whole transition, and for this reason thinking itself during this period has no substantial or determining significance for the processes of development of the adolescent as a whole and occupies no more than a modest place in the general system of crisis and maturation.

This point of view should be considered as the traditional and, unfortunately, the most widespread and uncritically accepted of the contemporary theories on the transitional age. In light of contemporary scientific data on adolescent psychology, this opinion seems to us to be very wrong: its roots are in the old teaching that of all the mental changes that occur in the child that turn him into an adolescent, it noted the trait that is only the most external, superficial, and obvious, specifically the change in emotional state.

Traditional psychology of the transitional age is inclined to see the central nucleus and main content of the whole crisis in the emotional changes and to compare the development of the emotional life of the adolescent to the intellectual development of the schoolchild. We see this as everything being turned on its head; in light of this theory, everything seems to us to be turned inside out: specifically, the young child seems to be the most emotional being; in his general structure, emotion plays the pre-eminent role and the adolescent appears before us primarily as a thinking being.

The traditional point of view is expressed most fully, yet tersely, by E Giese. In his words, while the mental development of the child before sexual maturation involves primarily the functions of perception, a store of memory, intellect, and attention, emotional life is representative of the time of sexual maturation.

Subsequent development of this point of view leads to the banal view which is inclined to reduce all mental maturation of the adolescent to an increased emotionality and dreaminess, to outbursts and similar somnolent products of emotional life. The fact that the period of sexual maturation is a period of a powerful rise of intellectual development and that during this period, thinking moves to the forefront for the first time, not only remains unnoticed when the question is posed in this way, but is even completely enigmatic and unexplained from the point of view of this theory.

Other authors also express the same point of view, for example, O. Kroh, who, like C. Bühler, sees all differences between the thinking of the adolescent and the thinking of the young child in the fact that the visual base for thinking, which plays such a significant role in childhood, moves to the background during the period of maturation. Kroh diminishes the significance of this difference when he completely properly indicates that, between concrete and abstract forms of thinking, an intermediate step frequently appears in the process of development that is also characteristic of the transitional age. This author gives the most complete positive formulation to the theory, shared also by C. Bühler, who said that we must not expect the child of school age to make a transition in the area of judgment to completely new forms. Differentiation, appreciating nuances, great confidence and awareness in using forms available now and before must be considered here as the most essential tasks of development.

Generalizing the position that reduces development of thinking to further growth of forms already present, Kroh assumes that in both the area of processes that work on perception (selecting, directing, perception of categories, and reordering classification) and in the sphere of logical connections (understanding, judgment, deduction, criticism), during the on-going school age, no new forms of mental functions and acts arise. They all existed previously, but during school age, they undergo significant development that is apparent in their more differentiated and nuance-sensitive and frequently more conscious application.

If the content of this theory can be expressed in a single sentence, it might be said that the appearance of new shades or nuances, greater specialization, and conscious application is all that distinguishes thinking during the transitional age from the thinking of the young child.

In essence this same point of view is developed in our literature by M. M. Rubinstein, who considers sequentially all the changes that occur during the transitional age in the areas of thinking as further movement along the paths that were already in place in the thinking of the very young child. In this sense, the views of Rubinstein wholly agree with the views of C. Bühler.

Rejecting the position of E. Meumann, who finds that the ability to make deductions is formed entirely at age 14, Rubinstein asserts that not one of the forms of intellectual activity, including making deductions, appears initially during the transitional years. This author points

to the extreme error of the idea that childhood differs from youth in the area of mental development only in that the central act of thought—deduction—properly appears only during the transitional age. Actually, this is completely incorrect; there is absolutely no doubt that thought and
its central act—deduction—is present in children. For Rubinstein, the whole difference
between the thinking of the child and that of the adolescent is only the following: children accept
as essential traits what for us adults is objectively nonessential, accidental, and external. Rubinstein believes that, in general, in both determinations and judgments, only during adolescence
and youth does the major premise begin to be filled in by essential traits or, in any case, is a tendency to find specifically these and not to be guided by the first external trait clearly delineated.

The whole difference, it seems, can be reduced to the fact that these forms of thinking
are themselves filled in with different contents in the child and in the adolescent. Rubinstein
says the following about judgments: in the child, these forms are filled in with nonessential
traits, but in the adolescent a tendency develops to fill them in with essential traits. Thus, the
whole difference is in the material, in the content, in the filler. The forms remain the same and
at best undergo a process of further accumulation and strengthening. Among such new
shades or nuances, Rubinstein includes the ability to think in essentials and a significantly greater
stability in directed thought, a greater flexibility, greater extent, agility in thinking and similar
such traits.

The central idea of this theory can be understood easily from the objections that its author
addresses to those who are inclined to deny the sharp rise and intensification in mental development of the adolescent and youth. Defending the idea that intellectual development of the
adolescent is characterized by a sharp rise and intensification, Rubinstein writes that this is borne
out by the observation of facts and theoretical considerations; otherwise we would have to assume
that the inflow of new experiences, new content, and new interrelations contributes nothing:
the cause remains without effect. Thus, typical traits of increased mental development must be
sought not only in new interests and demands, but also in intensification and broadening of
the old, in their range, in the whole breadth of vital interestedness.

In this defense, Rubinstein reveals an internal contradiction that is equally present in all
theories that are inclined to deny the appearance of anything substantially new in thinking
during the period of sexual maturation. All authors who deny the appearance of new forms of
thinking during the transitional age agree, however, that filling in this thinking, its content,
the material with which it operates, the objects to which it is directed—all of this undergoes
a real revolution.

2

The break in the evolution of forms and content of thinking is very characteristic for any
dualistic and metaphysical system in psychology that does not know how to present them in
dialectical unity. Thus, it is deeply symptomatic that the most consistent, idealistic system of
the psychology of the adolescent, presented in Edward Spranger's book (1924), is silent on
the development of thinking during the transitional age. In this work, there is no chapter
devoted to this problem; moreover, all the chapters of the book, imbued with one common

idea, are devoted to disclosing the process which, in Spranger's opinion, is the basis of the whole process of maturation and which is termed the adolescent's growing into the culture of his time. Chapter after chapter considers how the content of adolescents' thinking changes, how the thinking is filled with completely new material, how it grows into completely new spheres of culture. The adolescent's growing into spheres of law and politics, professional life and morality, science and world view—for Spranger, all of this is the central nucleus of processes of maturation, but intellectual functions of the adolescent in themselves, the forms of his thinking, the composition and structure of his intellectual operations, remain unchanged, eternal.

If we think deeply about all these theories, we cannot dismiss the idea that at their base there is a serious, very simple, very elementary psychological conception of the forms and content of thinking. According to this conception, the relations between the form and content of thinking resemble the relation between a vessel and the liquid that fills it. This is the same mechanical filling of the form with sex, the same potential for filling this same unchangeable form with ever newer content, the same internal disconnectedness, mechanical contrasting of the vessel and the liquid, of the form and what fills it.

From the point of view of these theories, the most serious revolution in the completely reformed content of the adolescent's thinking is in no way connected with the development of the intellectual operations themselves, which are solely responsible for the appearance of one content of thinking or another.

This revolution, according to the conceptions of many authors, is derived either from outside in such a way that those same, unchangeable forms of thinking, always equal to each other at each new stage of development, depending on enrichment of experience and broadening of connections with the environment, are filled with ever newer content, or the flowing spring of this revolution is hidden in the wings of thinking in the emotional life of the adolescent. It mechanically turns on the processes of thinking in a completely new system and directs them, like simple acts, to a new content.

In both cases, evolution of the content of thinking seems to be an impassable chasm separated from the evolution of intellectual forms. Through the power of facts, every theory that consistently takes off in this direction comes up against this kind of an internal contradiction. This can be easily demonstrated with a simple example: not one of the theories cited above denies, nor can it deny, the very serious, fundamental revolution in the content of the thinking of the adolescent, the complete reformation of the whole material content that fills the empty forms. Thus C. Bühler, who finds in the three-year-old all the basic intellectual operations proper to the adolescent, limits her claim exclusively to the formal aspect of the problem under consideration. Bühler would, of course, call it a tale if someone should claim that there is essentially nothing new in the thinking of the adolescent in comparison with what is already present in the thinking of the three-year-old.

Bühler cannot deny the fact that only when adolescence is reached is there a transition to formally logical thinking. She cites the studies of H. Ormian (1926), who demonstrated that only at the age of approximately 11 is a turning to purely formal thinking noted. As to the content of thinking, she, like Spranger, devotes a significant part of the work to explaining new layers of the content of ethical, religious conceptions and the rudiments of a world view in the development of adolescents.

Precisely so, together with new nuances to which he reduces the development of thinking during school years, Kroh indicates that only in the adolescent does the possibility of operating logically with concepts arise. Citing the studies of E Berger, on the problem of perception of categories and its pedagogical significance, Kroh asserts that the perceiving and ordering function of psychological categories initially appears in all distinctness in experiences and memories during the period of sexual maturation.

Thus, all the authors agree that, while denying new formations in the area of intellectual forms, they must inevitably admit a complete reformation of the whole content of thinking during the transitional age.

We are considering the analysis and criticism of this point of view in such detail because without overcoming it decisively, without disclosing its theoretical bases, and without contrasting it with new points of view, we will not see any possibility of finding the methodological and theoretical key to the whole problem of the development of thinking during the transitional age. For this reason, it is very important for us to understand the theoretical bases on which all of these various theories, different in details, but similar in central nucleus, are constructed.

## 3

We have already said that the main root of all this theoretical blundering is the break between the evolution of form and content of thinking. The break in its turn is due to another basic defect of the old psychology, especially child psychology; specifically, child psychology until recently lacked a proper scientific conception of the nature of higher mental functions. The circumstance that higher mental functions are not simply a continuation of elementary functions and are not their mechanical combination, but a qualitatively new mental formation that develops according to completely special laws and is subject to completely different patterns, had still not been assimilated by child psychology.

Higher mental functions, the product of the historical development of humanity, have a special history in ontogenesis also. The history of the development of higher forms of behavior discloses a direct and close dependence on organic, bio logical development of the child and on the growth of his elementary psychophysiological functions. But the connection and dependence are not identity. For this reason, in research, we must identify the line of development of higher forms of behavior in ontogenesis also, tracing it in all its unique patterns, not forgetting for a moment its connection with the overall organic development of the child. We said at the beginning of the course that human behavior is not only the product of biological evolution that resulted in the appearance of a human type with all the psychophysiological functions proper to it, but also a product of historical or cultural development. The development of behavior did not stop with the beginning of the historical existence of humanity, but neither did it simply continue along the same paths along which biological evolution of behavior proceeded.

The historical development of behavior was carried out as the organic part of societal development of man, subject basically to all the patterns that determine the course of the historical development of humanity as a whole. Similarly to this, in ontogenesis also, we must distinguish both lines of development of behavior presented in an intertwined form, in a complex dynamic synthesis. But actually, a study that meets the true, real complexity of this synthesis, not intent on simplifying it, must take into account all the uniqueness of the formation of higher types of behavior that are the product of the cultural development of the child.

In contrast to Spranger, deep, scientific studies show that in the process of cultural development of behavior, not only the content of thinking changes, but also its forms; new mechanisms, new functions, new operations, and new methods of activity arise that were not known at earlier stages of historical development. Exactly so, the process of the cultural development of the child includes not only a growing into one area or another of culture, but also, step by step, together with the development of content, there is a development of forms of thinking and those higher, historically developed forms and abilities of activity whose development is the requisite condition for growing into a culture.

Actually, every really serious study teaches us to admit the unity and indivisibility of form and content, structure and function; it shows how every new step in the development of thinking is inseparably connected with the acquisition of new mechanisms of behavior and a rise to a higher step of intellectual operations.

A known content may be adequately represented only with the help of known forms. Thus, the content of our dreams cannot be adequately represented in the forms of logical thinking, in the forms of logical connections and relations; it is inseparably connected with the archaic, ancient, primitive forms or methods of thinking that are proper to it. And conversely: the content of one science or another, assimilation of a complex system, mastery, for example, of modern algebra, presupposes not simply filling with appropriate content the same forms that are already present in a three-year-old—new content cannot develop without new forms. The dialectical unity of form and content in the evolution of thinking is the alpha and omega of the modern scientific theory of speech and thinking. Actually, is it not enigmatic from the point of view of the theories set out above, which deny the development of new qualitative steps in the thinking of the adolescent, that modern studies have developed standards of mental development that require, for example, in the Binet-Simon tests (edited by C. Burt and P. P. Blonsky), a description and explanation of a picture from a 12-year-old, a solution to a life problem from a 13-year-old, defining abstract terms from a 14-year-old, indicating the difference between abstract terms from a 15-year-old, and catching the sense of a philosophical argument from a 16-year-old? Can these empirically established symptoms of intellectual development be understood from the point of view of a theory that admits only new nuances arising in the thinking of the adolescent? From the point of view of nuances, can we explain that the average 16-year-old adolescent attains a degree of mental development of which an indicative trait or symptom is capturing the sense of a philosophical argument?

Only a failure to distinguish between the evolution of elementary and higher functions of thinking, between biologically based and historically based forms of intellectual activity can lead to denying a qualitatively new stage in the development of the adolescent's intellect. Elementary new functions actually do not arise in the transitional age. This circumstance, as K. Bühler correctly indicates, agrees completely with biological data on the weight increase of the brain. L. Edinger, one of the eminent experts on the brain, established the following general position: who ever knows the structure of the brain in a living being will conclude that the appearance of new abilities is always connected with the appearance of new sections of the brain or with the growth of those that existed previously (1911).

This position, developed by Edinger with respect to phylogenesis of the mind, is now very frequently and readily applied to ontogenesis as well in an attempt to establish a parallel between the development of the brain, since this is evidenced by the increase in its weight, and the appearance of new abilities. Forgotten here is the fact that the parallel may be true only with respect to elementary functions and abilities that are, like the brain itself, the product of biological evolution of behavior; but the essence of historical development of behavior also consists specifically in the appearance of new abilities not connected with the appearance of new parts of the brain or with the growth of parts that are present.

There is every reason to assume that the historical development of behavior from primitive forms to the most complex and highest did not occur as a result of the appearance of new parts of the brain or the growth of parts already existing. This is the essence of both the transitional age and the age of cultural development or development of higher mental functions for the most part. P. P. Blonsky is absolutely right in thinking that the childhood of permanent teeth can be considered to be the time when the child becomes civilized, the time when he assimilates modern science, beginning with writing and modern technology. Civilization is a some what recent acquisition of humanity in order that it might convey itself by inheritance.

Thus, it is difficult to expect that evolution of higher mental functions would proceed parallel to the development of the brain, being accomplished mainly and specifically under the influence of inheritance. According to the data of O. Pfister, in the first three-quarters of a year, the brain doubles its original weight, by the end of the third year, it triples it; in all, in the process of development, there is a fourfold increase in the weight of the brain.

K. Bühler assumes that one of the phenomena of child psychology agrees completely with this. The child acquires all basic mental functions in the first three or four years of life and during all subsequent life, does not achieve such basic inner successes as he does, for example, at the time when he learns to speak.

This parallel, we repeat, may be valid only for maturation of elementary functions that are the product of biological evolution and develop together with the growth of the brain and its parts. For this reason, we must limit the position of Charlotte Bühler, who expects that sometime it may be possible to find physiological bases in the development of brain structure for each major shift in the inner life of the normal child.

We must limit her position: basically, it is applicable to shifts in mental development due to heredity, but the complex syntheses that arise in the process of the child's and the adolescent's cultural development are based on other factors—mainly on societal life, cultural development, and work activity of the child and adolescent.

True, there is the opinion that during the transitional age, the brain develops more intensively and owing to this development, the more serious intellectual shifts that are observed during the transitional time may occur. Blonsky developed the hypothesis that the phase of milk teeth in childhood, as distinct from the preceding and succeeding phases, is not a phase of intensive development of thinking and speech; more likely it is a phase of development of motor habits, coordinations, and emotions. Blonsky links this circumstance to the fact that during the milk teeth phase there is intensive growth of the spinal cord and the cerebellum in contrast to the toothless and school-age phase of childhood, which are mainly phases of intensive cortical (intellectual) development. Observation of the intensive transformation of the head during the prepuberty age leads the author to think that during the school age, there is mainly a development of the frontal part of the cortex. However, from the point of view of the data on which Blonsky relies and which he himself terms shaky and unreliable, we are justified in reaching conclusions only with respect to the prepuberty age, that is, early school age.

Regarding the transitional age, with respect to the adolescent, these hypotheses have no factual data. True, according to the reports of N. V. Vyazemskii, the whole brain increases quite significantly at age 14–15, then, after a certain pause and slowing down, makes a new slight rise at age 17–19 and 19–20. But according to newer data, during the whole period of development from age 14 to 20, the whole brain increases very insignificantly.

We must seek new ways to explain the intensive intellectual development that occurs during the period of sexual maturation.

Thus, the transition from research based on external manifestations, on phenotypic similarity, to a deeper study of the genetic, functional, and structural nature of thinking at different ages leads us inevitably to rejecting the established traditional view that is inclined to identify the thinking of the adolescent with the thinking of the three-year-old. Moreover, even in the part where these theories are ready to admit a qualitative difference between the thinking of a young child and of an adolescent, they erroneously formulate the positive achievement, the really new that occurs during this time.

As new studies show, the claim that the abstract thinking of the adolescent breaks away from the concrete, and the abstract from the visual, is incorrect: the movement of thinking during this period is characterized not by the intellect's breaking the connections to the concrete base which it is outgrowing, but by the fact that a completely new form of relation between abstract and concrete factors in thinking arises, a new form of their merging and synthesis, that at this time elementary functions long since established, functions such as visual thinking, perception, or the practical intellect of the child appear before us in a completely new form.

Thus, the theory of C. Bühler seems insupportable not only with respect to what it denies, but also with respect to what it claims, not only in its negative, but also in its positive part. And conversely, in the thinking of the adolescent, not only completely new complex synthetic forms that the three-year-old does not know arise, but even those elementary, primitive forms that the child of three has acquired are restructured on new bases during the transitional age. During the period of sexual maturation, not only new forms arise, but specifically due to their arising, the old are restructured on a completely new base.

Summarizing what has been set forth, we may say that the principal methodological obstacle for the traditional theory is the glaring internal contradiction between admitting a very serious revolution in the content of the adolescent's thinking and denying any substantial shift in the evolution of his intellectual operations, in the inability to correlate the changes in the development of the content and the form of thinking. As we tried to show, the break, in its turn, is due to the failure to distinguish the two lines in behavior—the development of elementary mental functions and the development of higher mental functions. On the basis of conclusions reached, we can now formulate the principal idea that always guides our critical research.

We might say that the fateful break between form and content flows inevitably from the fact that the evolution of content of thinking is always considered as a process of cultural development, primarily facilitated historically and socially, and development of the form of thinking is usually considered as a biological process due to organic maturation of the child and the parallel increase in brain weight. When we speak of the content of thinking and its changes, we have in mind a quantity historically changeable, socially facilitated, arising in the process of cultural development; when we speak of forms of thinking and their dynamics, we have in mind either the metaphysically fixed mental functions or biologically determined, organically arising forms.

Between the one and the other, a chasm develops. The historical and the biological in the child's development seem to be severed; no bridge exists between the one and the other that would enable us to unite the facts of the dynamics of form of thinking with the facts of the dynamics of the content that fills these forms. Only with the introduction of the teaching on the higher forms of behavior that are the product of historical evolution, only with the introduction of the special line of historical development or the development of higher mental functions in the ontogenesis of behavior does it become possible to fill this chasm, to throw a bridge across it, to approach the study of the dynamics of form and content of thinking in their dialectical unity. We can correlate the dynamics of content and form through the common factor of historicity that distinguishes equally both the content of our thinking and the higher mental functions.

Based on these views, which in their aggregate make up the teaching on the cultural development of the child, which we presented elsewhere, we find the key to the correct formulation, and consequently to the true solution of the problem of the development of thinking during the transitional age.

The key to the whole problem of development of thinking during the transitional age is the fact, established by a series of studies, that the adolescent masters for the first time the process of forming concepts, that he makes the transition to a new and higher form of intellectual activity—to thinking in concepts.

This is the central phenomenon of the whole transitional age, and underestimating the significance of intellectual development of the adolescent and the attempt of most modern theories on the transitional age to place changes of an intellectual nature in the background in comparison with emotional and other aspects of the crisis can be explained for the most part by the fact that the formation of concepts is a highly complex process and is not at all analogous to the simple maturation of elementary intellectual functions and for this reason cannot easily be subjected to external verification, to crude, visual determination. Changes that occur in the thinking of the adolescent who has mastered concepts are to the utmost degree changes of an internal, intimate, structural nature often not apparent externally, not hitting the eye of the observer.

If we limit ourselves to changes of an external nature only, we will have to agree with investigators who assume that nothing new arises in the thinking of the adolescent, that it grows evenly and gradually in a quantitative respect, being filled with always new content and becoming ever more correct, more logical, closer to actuality. But if we only move from purely external observations to deep internal investigation, this whole claim disintegrates to dust. As has already been said, the formation of concepts stands at the center of the development of thinking during the time of sexual maturation. This process signifies truly revolutionary changes both in the area of content and in the area of forms of thinking. We have said that from the methodological point of view, the break between the form and content of thinking, which is the tacit assumption at the base of most theories, is completely insupportable.

Actually, the form and content of thinking are two factors in a single whole process, two factors internally linked to each other by an essential, not accidental bond.

There is a certain content of thoughts that can be understood adequately only in certain forms of intellectual activity. There are other contents that may be adequately communicated in those same forms, but necessarily require qualitatively different forms of thinking that comprise an indissoluble whole with them. Thus, the content of our dreams cannot be adequately communicated within the system of logically structured speech, in forms of verbal, logical intellect; all attempts to communicate the content of graphic dream-thinking in the form of logical speech inevitably distorts the content.

The same is true of scientific knowledge. For example, mathematics and the natural and social sciences cannot be adequately communicated and presented other than in the form of logical verbal thinking. The content is closely connected with the form, and when we say that the adolescent rises to a higher level in thinking and masters concepts, by the same token, we indicate forms of intellectual activity that are actually new and content of thinking that is just as new opening before the adolescent at this time.

Thus, in the very fact of formation of concepts, we find a solution to the contradiction between the abrupt change in content of thinking and the immobility of its forms during the transitional time which flowed inevitably from the theories considered above. Many modern studies compel us to reach the incontrovertible conclusion that specifically the formation of concepts is the basic nucleus which is the center for all changes in the thinking of the adolescent.

N. Ach, the author of one of the most serious studies of the formation of concepts, whose book (1921) constituted an epoch in the study of this problem, in developing the complex picture of the ontogenesis of the formation of concepts, identifies the transitional age as this kind of crucial boundary that signifies a decisive qualitative turning point in the development of thinking.

In the words of Ach, we can establish yet another rapidly passing phase in the process of intellectualization of mental development. As a rule, it comes at the period bordering on sexual maturation. Before the onset of sexual maturity, the child has no potential for forming abstract concepts, as has been explained, for example, in the observations of H. Eng (1914), but due to the effect of training when educational material is assimilated that consists for the most part of general positions that express some law or rule, through the influence of speech, attention is diverted more and more in the direction of abstract relations and thus leads to the formation of abstract concepts.

N. Ach notes the influence of the content of assimilated knowledge on the one hand and the directing influence of speech on the attention of the adolescent on the other hand as two basic factors that lead to the formation of abstract concepts. He refers to the studies of A. Gregor (1915) that demonstrated the great influence of knowledge on the development of abstract thinking.

We see here an indication of the genetic role of the new content that is opened before the thinking of the adolescent and which of necessity requires his transition to new forms, and places before him problems that can be resolved only through the formation of concepts. At the same time, we can observe functional changes in the direction of attention made with the help of speech. The crisis in the development of thinking and the transition to thinking in concepts is thus prepared from both aspects: from the aspect of change in function and from the aspect of new problems that arise in the thinking of the adolescent relating to the assimilation of new material for thought.

In conjunction with the transition to a higher level, according to Ach, the process of intellectualization, like the transition to thinking in concepts, narrows more and more the circle of visual thinking in concepts and thinking in graphic representations. This leads to a demise of the method of thinking which the child uses, with which the child must part, and to the construction of a completely new kind or type of intellect in its place. To this, Ach links the problem to which we must turn in the following chapter. He asks whether the transition from graphic thinking to thinking in concepts is the basis of the fact that eidetic tendency, studied by E. Jaensch, is found significantly less frequently at this stage than in the child.

4

Thus, as a result of our studies, we have found that the adolescent makes a most important step along the path of intellectual development during the time of sexual maturation. He makes the transition from complex thinking to thinking in concepts. Forming concepts and operating with concepts—this is the essentially new ability that he acquires at this age. In concepts, the intellect of the adolescent finds not simply a continuation of preceding lines. A concept is not just an enriched and internally interconnected associative group. It is a qualitatively new formation that cannot be reduced to more elementary processes that characterize the development of the intellect at earlier stages. Thinking in concepts is a new form of intellectual activity, a new method of behavior, a new intellectual mechanism.

In this unique activity, the intellect finds a new, previously nonexistent *modus operandi* (mode of action—Ed.); a new function different in both composition and structure as well as in method of action develops in the system of intellectual functions.

The traditional view that is inclined to reject the appearance of essentially new formations in the intellect of the adolescent and strives to consider his thinking simply as a continuation, extension, and deepening of the thinking of the three-year-old, as is reflected most clearly in the work of C. Bühler, actually does not note the qualitative differences between concepts, complexes, and syncretic formations. This view is based on purely quantitative conceptions of the development of the intellect strangely similar to the theory of E. Thorndike, according to which higher forms of thinking differ from elementary functions only quantitatively according to the number of associative connections that enter into their composition. Specifically because this view prevails in traditional psychology of adolescence, we considered it necessary to trace carefully the whole course of the development of thinking and to show three different qualitative states through which it passes in all their uniqueness. The principal subject of our study was the thinking of the adolescent. However, we always used genetic sections in studying thinking just as an anatomist-investigator makes sections at various stages of development of any organ and compares these sections with each other and establishes the course of development from one stage to another.

In modern pedological studies, as A. Gesell correctly points out, the method of genetic sections is the central method for studying behavior and its development. The former method—describing characteristics of behavior according to age—was usually reduced to a static characterization, to enumerating a number of features, traits, different characteristics of thinking for a given stage of development. In this case, a static characterization usually substituted for a dynamic consideration of age. Development was lost from sight and the form, characteristic only for a given age, was assumed to be stable, immovable, always equal in itself. Thinking and behavior at each age stage was considered as a thing and not as a process, something at rest and not moving. In addition, the essence of each form of thinking can be disclosed only when we begin to understand it as a certain, organically in dispensable factor in a complex and merged process of development.

The only adequate method for disclosing this essence is the method of genetic sections for comparative genetic study of behavior at different stages of development.

This is the way we tried to proceed; we tried to disclose the uniqueness of the thinking of the adolescent. We were interested not simply in a cross section of the characteristics of thinking during the transitional age, an inventory of methods of intellectual activity found in the adolescent, and not in listing the forms of thinking in their quantitative relation to each other. We were interested primarily in establishing what is substantially new, in what the transitional age brings with itself to the development of thinking; we were interested in thinking and its coming into being. Our goal was to capture the process of crisis and maturation of thinking that is the basic content of this age.

To do this, we had to present the thinking of the adolescent in comparison with preceding stages, find the transition of one form of thinking to another and by comparison establish the decisive change, the fundamental reconstruction, the radical reorganization that occurs in the thinking of the adolescent. For this, we had to make as if sections of the process of the development of thinking at different stages and always following the comparative-genetic path, try to connect these sections with each other to establish the real process of movement that occurs in the transition of thinking from one stage to another.

In the future, we will proceed in precisely this way because the comparative-genetic method of examination, the method of genetic sections, is the basic and principal method of pedological research.

True, in subjecting the results of our comparative study to functional checking, we always brought in data not only on the ontogenesis of thinking, but also its phylogenetic development, data on the breakdown and involution of thinking in abnormal processes. Proceeding in this way, we were governed by the principle of unity of higher forms of intellectual activity no matter how various the processes in which this unity found its concrete expression. We assumed that the basic laws of structure and activity of thinking remain the same, the basic patterns directing them—the same in the normal and abnormal state, but only that these patterns acquire different concrete expression depending on different conditions.

Just as modern pathology considers illness as life in special, changed conditions, we are justified in considering the activity of thinking affected by one abnormality or another as a manifestation of general patterns of thinking under special conditions created by the abnormality.

In modern psychoneurology, the idea that development is the key to understanding the breakdown and involution of mental functions is firmly rooted, and the study of the breakdown and disintegration of these functions, the key to understanding their structure and development. Thus, general and pathological psychology mutually enlighten each other if they are constructed on a genetic base.

In comparing the data of onto- and phylogenesis, we did not for a moment take the point of view of biogenetic parallelism, intending to find in the history of the development of the child a repetition and recapitulation of those forms of thinking that prevailed at previous stages of human history. We followed the same comparative method by which K. Groos properly identified the task as consisting not only in finding similarity, but also in establishing differences; the word "comparison" here means not isolating only coinciding traits, but even more it means finding the differences in the similarity.

For this reason, we did not for a moment identify the process of concrete thinking of the child with the process of concrete thinking in the history of human development. We were always interested in the most complete elucidation of the nature of the phenomenon that was the object of our research. This nature is disclosed in the diverse connections and forms of manifestation of essentially one and the same type of thinking. Of course to say that logical thinking arises at a certain stage in the development of human history and at a certain stage in the development of the child is to claim an incontrovertible truth and at the same time not in any way to indicate that the one who claims this takes the point of view of biogenetic parallelism. Precisely so, comparative analysis of complex thinking in its phylogenetic and ontogenetic aspects does not in the least presuppose the idea of parallelism between the one process and the other or the idea of identity of the one form and the other.

We tried to emphasize one factor especially in the phenomenon that interests us, because it is preeminent in a comparative study of different manifestations of one and the same form of thinking. That factor is the unity of form and content in the concept. Specifically because of the fact that in the concept, form and content are given as a unity, the transition to thinking in concepts signified a real revolution in the thinking of the child.

## 5

Now it remains for us to consider what the basic traces are of the fact that the adolescent makes a transition to thinking in concepts. What we would like to bring to the forefront is the deep and fundamental changes in the content of the thinking of the adolescent. Without overstating, we could say that the whole content of thinking is reformed and reconstructed in conjunction with the formation of concepts. The content and form of thinking do not relate to each other as water does to a glass. The content and form are in an indissoluble relationship and mutual dependence.

If we understand content of thinking to be not simply the external data that comprise the subject of thinking at any given moment, but the actual content, we will see how, in the process of the child's development, it constantly moves inward, becomes an organic component part of the personality itself and of separate systems of its behavior. Convictions, interests, world view, ethical norms and rules of behavior, inclinations, ideals, certain patterns of thought—all of this is initially external, and becomes internal specifically because as the adolescent develops, in conjunction with his maturation and the change in his environment, he is confronted by the task of mastering new content, and strong stimuli are created that nudge him along the path of developing the formal mechanisms of his thinking as well.

The new content, which confronts the adolescent with a series of problems, leads to new forms of activity, to new forms of combining elementary functions, and to new methods of thinking. As we shall see, specifically during the transitional age, the new content itself creates new forms of behavior, mechanisms of a special type about which we will speak in a later chapter. Together with the transition to thinking in concepts, the adolescent is confronted by a world of objective, societal consciousness, a world of societal ideology.

Cognition in the true sense of that word, science, art, various spheres of cultural life may be adequately assimilated only in concepts. True, even the child assimilates scientific facts, and the child is imbued with a certain ideology, and the child grows into separate spheres of cultural life. But an inadequate, incomplete mastery of all of this is characteristic for the child, and for this reason, the child, perceiving the established cultural material, does not yet actively participate in its creation.

On the contrary, the adolescent, making the transition to an adequate assimilation of this content which can be presented in all its completeness and depth only in concepts, begins actively and creatively to participate in various spheres of cultural life that open before him. Without thinking in concepts there is no understanding of relations that underlie the phenomena. The whole world of deep connections that underlie external, outward appearances, the world of complex interdependencies and relations within every sphere of activity and among its separate spheres, can be disclosed only to one who approaches it with the key of the concept.

This new content does not enter mechanically into the thinking of the adolescent, but undergoes a long and complex process of development. Owing to this extension and deepening of the content of thinking, a whole world with its past and future, nature, history, and human life opens before the adolescent. Blonsky correctly states that the whole history of the child is a gradual broadening of his environment, beginning with the mother's womb and the crib and continuing with the room and the home with its immediate environment. Thus, by the extension of the environment, we can determine the development of the child in its onward course. The extension of the environment during the transitional age leads to the fact that for the adolescent, the world becomes the environment for thinking. As we know, E Schiller expressed this idea in a certain couplet where he compared the infant for whom his crib was boundless, with the youth whom the whole world could not contain.

Most of all, as Blonsky correctly notes, the basic change in the environment consists of the fact that it expands to participation in societal production. On this basis, in the content of thinking, societal ideology is represented most of all as connected with one position or another in societal production.

Blonsky says that we must also present class psychology not as suddenly arising, but as gradually developing. It is understood that we have its full development as early as during youth when a man already occupies or is preparing to occupy one position or another in societal production. The history of the school-age child and the youth is the history of very intensive development and formulation of class psychology and ideology.

In conjunction with this, Blonsky correctly indicates the widespread error concerning how class psychology and ideology arise and develop. Usually reference is made to the instinct of imitation as the basic mechanism for the origin and formulation of the content of thinking in the adolescent. Moreover, reference to the instinct of imitation, as the author correctly notes, undoubtedly obscures understanding of the formation of class psychology in the child.

Blonsky indicates that even authors who consider it possible to speak of class psychology of the child frequently present its formation thus: through imitation class psychology is created, class ideals are created, and class ethics are created. If we understand imitation as it is usually understood in psychology, then this claim is completely unwarranted.

Class psychology cannot, of course, be created by external imitation. The process of its formation is undoubtedly deeper. Class psychology in the child is created as a result of his working with those around him, or, stated more simply and directly, as a result of common life with them, common activity, common interests. Let us repeat, class cohesion is formed as a result not of external imitation, but by shared life, activity, and interests.

We agree completely that the process of formation of class psychology is incomparably deeper than authors who refer to instinct of imitation believe it to be. Further, we believe that we cannot argue with Blonsky's position that shared life, activity, and interests are the basic and central factor in this process. We think, however, that in this case an essential link in explaining the process as a whole has been omitted. For this reason, Blonsky's statement does not solve the problem, which remains open even after we reject the reference to the instinct of imitation.

It is understood that sharing of life, work, and interests places before the adolescent a number of problems; in the process of solving them, class psychology develops and takes shape. But we must not lose sight of that mechanism, those methods of intellectual activity that facilitate the completion of this process. In other words, we can never give a genetic explanation of the phenomenon of which Blonsky speaks specifically because the transitional age is a time of intensive development and formulation of class psychology and ideology. If we do not consider the formation of concepts as a basic intellectual function whose development opens a new content for the adolescent's thinking, we will not understand why shared life and interests do not result in such an intensive development in that area during the early or preschool age in which we are interested. Obviously, with genetic analysis of development of the content of thinking, we cannot for a moment lose sight of the connection between the evolution of content and the evolution of form of thinking. In particular, we cannot for a single moment forget the basic and central position of all of adolescent psychology: the function of formation of concepts lies at the base of all intellectual changes at this age.

In this sense, the attempt of some authors to ignore wholly the factor of formation of concepts in the development of forms of thinking and to proceed from direct analysis of content is of exceptional interest. Thus, W. Stern in his work on the development of the formation of ideals in the maturing youth comes to the conclusion that metaphysical world understanding instinctively becomes a part of the adolescent during sexual maturation, that it is as if hereditarily fixed at this age. We find similar attempts in the work of other authors who devote several pages or several lines to the development of thinking, and sometimes simply bypass it in silence, but instead try to reconstruct directly the structure of the content of thinking in various spheres of consciousness. It is natural that in this case the structure of thinking acquires a metaphysical character. In the exposition itself, in the characterization of the consciousness of the adolescent, they rush to idealization as the basic method of representation, and it is not surprising that for such authors as Stern and Spranger the adolescent seems to be a natural-born metaphysicist because where the deep changes and alterations in the content of his thinking originate, what moves the flood of his ideas, remains a mystery.

Moreover, if we do not follow the path of those authors who accept the metaphysics of their own constructs for the metaphysical structure of the thinking of the adolescent, we must consider, as we have already said, the evolution of the content of thinking in conjunction with the evolution of its form, and we must trace in detail the kind of changes in the content of thinking that formation of concepts elicits. We will see that the formation of concepts discloses before the adolescent a world of social consciousness and leads inevitably to intensive development and formulation of class psychology and ideology. For this reason it is not surprising that the adolescent that Stern and Spranger study stands before the investigators as a metaphysicist. The whole crux of the matter is that the metaphysical nature of thinking of the adolescent is not an instinctive peculiarity of the adolescent, but is the inevitable result of the formation of concepts within the sphere of a specific societal ideology.

Specifically the higher forms of thinking, especially logical thinking, open up before the adolescent in their significance. Blonsky says: if the child's intellect at the stage when teeth are replaced is still quite markedly eidetic, then the intellect of the adolescent is marked by a striving to be logical. This striving is manifested primarily in criticism and in greater demands that what is said be proven. The adolescent urgently requires proofs.

The mind of the adolescent is more likely to be burdened by the concrete, and concrete natural history, botany, zoology, and mineralogy (one of the favorite subjects in step I in school) take a secondary place for the adolescent, yielding to philosophical questions of natural history, the origin of the world, man, etc. In the same way, interest in the numerous historical concrete stories is also relegated to a secondary position. Their place is taken more and more by politics, which is of great interest to the adolescent. Finally, all of this is very closely connected to the fact that the average adolescent loses interest in art and drawing, which the child so loves during prepuberty. The most abstract art—music—is the greatest favorite of the adolescent.

The development of social-political world view does not account for all the changes that occur during the time of maturation of thinking in the adolescent. This is only one, perhaps the most clear and significant part of the changes that are occurring.

It is completely right that the decisive event in the life of the average adolescent is entry into societal production and by the same token, into full class self-determination. In Blonsky's opinion, the adolescent is not only the son of his social class, but is already himself an active member of that class. Correspondingly, the years of adolescence are the years of forming the adolescent, primarily his social-political world view. In these years, in their basic outlines, the views on life, people, and society are worked out, and one kind or another of social sympathies and antipathies are formed. The years of adolescence are the years of intensive racking of the brain over problems of life, as Blonsky maintains (1930, pp. 209–210). Problems that life itself poses for the adolescent and his decisive entry as an active participant into this life require for their solution the development of higher forms of thinking.

In describing the adolescent, we have thus far bypassed in silence a most essential trait that has been noted several times by investigators and which it would be strange to find at other stages of the child's development. It is typical and characteristic specifically for the adolescent. We have in view the contradictoriness that is the basic trait of that age, the contradictoriness that is expressed also in the content of the adolescent's thinking, specifically: the content of his thinking includes seemingly contradictory factors.

The intellect of the adolescent, according to Blonsky, is marked by an inclination toward mathematics. Although, according to a widespread point of view, adolescents are not very much in the habit of mastering mathematics, the author refers to school experience in defending his opinion. Blonsky believes that the interval from age 14 to 17 is usually the stage of maximally intensive mathematical formation in school practice and specifically during this time, a person usually acquires the greatest part of his mathematical baggage. In precisely the same way, there is an increased inclination toward physics. Finally, this is the age of philosophical interests and is logically sequential in tendencies toward argument. But how can love of mathematics, physics, and philosophy, love of logic, balance of judgment, and proof be reconciled with what E. Kretschmer terms "romanticism of thought," which also is undoubtedly present in the adolescent? Blonsky answers this contradiction with the words of Kretschmer: both complements of thinking, regardless of the external differences, are closely connected with each other in bio logical relation.

We think that the fact that Blonsky notes is pointed out quite correctly. The explanation, however, that he tries to give for the contradictoriness of intellectual tendencies and interests of the adolescent is essentially inadequate for solving the problem that confronts us. Blonsky explains the inclination toward mathematics, physics, and philosophy with characteristics of the schizothemic temperament for which a certain splitting between poles is characteristic: inordinate acuteness, increased impressionability, sensitivity, and excitability on the one hand and an affective dullness, coldness, and indifference, on the other.

We think, however, that the deep biological relationship between the two types of thinking to which Kretschmer refers can scarcely serve as a real base for the unique combination of "romanticism of thought" and excessive drive toward logic that is observed during the transitional age. We believe that specifically the genetic explanation will be the most correct in this case. If we take into account the great broadening of activity, the serious deepening in connection and relation between things and phenomena that the thinking of the adolescent masters for the first time, we will also understand the basis for the increased logical activity and the basis for the "romanticism of thought" that is present in the adolescent.

The fact of formation of concepts, novelty, and youth and the character of this new form of thinking, which is inadequately fixed, unstable, and underdeveloped, explain the contradiction that observers have noted. This contradiction is a contra diction of development, a contradiction of a transitional form, a contradiction of the transitional age.

We are inclined to use youth and the not yet fully established character of the new form of thinking to explain still another feature noted by Blonsky—the inadequate dialectics of the adolescent, his tendency to hone every question into the form of alternatives: either/or.

We think that here too what is at work primarily are not the characteristics of the temperament of the adolescent, but the simple circumstance that dialectical thinking is a higher level in the development of mature thinking and cannot, it is understood, become the property of the adolescent, who has just arrived at the formation of concepts. Moreover, with the formation of concepts, the adolescent enters the path of development that sooner or later will bring him to mastering dialectical thinking. But it would be improbable to expect that this necessary and higher level of development will already be present at the first steps that the adolescent takes who has just mastered a new method of intellectual activity.

The studies of Groos (1916) can be a good illustration of the radical change and the radical reconstruction in the content of thinking of the adolescent; these studies show in an isolated, pure form the effects of age on directedness of thinking, on the separate content of intellectual activity of the adolescent. Resorting to experiment, Groos attempted to explain what kind of questions arise at different age levels in the developing human being in connection with one process of thinking or another. The subjects were given different themes for consideration. After reading the themes, the subjects were asked each time: what would you want to learn most of all? The responses elicited in this way were recorded, collected, and classified with respect to logical interest that was evident in them. The study established the dominant logical interests in their age dynamics and in their increment.

One of the principal points of the study is an elucidation of whether interest of the thinking person is directed toward causes or effects. While in adult subjects of almost all ages, there is a predominance of movement of thought forward to consequences, in children questions relating to other circumstances predominate. Groos reached the conclusion that interest in consequences increases with growth in intellectual development (see Table 1).

In the data obtained, Groos is completely justified in seeing an important indication of the development of interests in the mind of the child and the youth because the relative growth of progressive and regressive positions at different ages while the themes remain identical undoubtedly indicates the role of age in the change of direction of logical interests in thinking.

TABLE 1.

| Age, years | Questions | | Ratio, % |
| --- | --- | --- | --- |
| | Regressive | Progressive | |
| 12–13 | 108 | 11 | 9.8 |
| 14–15 | 365 | 49 | 7.4 |
| 15–16 | 165 | 35 | 4.7 |
| 16–17 | 74 | 19 | 3.9 |
| Students | 46 | 36 | 1.3 |

Another study pertains to the nature of questions that arise in the thinking of the child and the adolescent. Groos assumes that judgment is always preceded by a state of uncertainty coupled with the need to know that we often express with a question even if we ask it of ourselves (we have in mind not a question asked aloud, but an internal question).

Groos believes that even in the internal, verbal formulation there are two kinds of questions corresponding to our motives of judging, specifically, questions of determination and questions of decision. The question of determination corresponds to simple not knowing with its complete uncertainty. It is similar to an empty vessel that may be filled only with the answer. For example: What is it? Where did it come from? Who was that? When? Why? Why was this done? Such a question cannot be answered with a simple "yes" or "no." On the other hand, questions of decision can be answered "yes" or "no," since the potential for decision is contained in the question itself. For example: Is this a rare plant? Was this rug brought from Persia? Such a question, especially if posed to oneself, is identical to the expression of a state of conscious expectation from which a hypothetical conclusion can be reached in some cases.

Since it is obvious that more mental activity is expressed in questions of decision than in questions of determination and since this division also masks a deeply rooted difference between the two motives of judgment, studying the results of our experiments directed toward eliciting questions from schoolchildren must be of interest. According to the data of Groos, as children grow, the number of questions of judgment increase more than the empty questions. Their ratio is presented in Table 2.

In the increase of progressive thinking as in the development of inherent assumptions and presuppositions internally related to it, the essential trait of the transitional age undoubtedly is apparent: not only an enormous enrichment of the content of thinking, but also new forms of movement, new forms of operating with this content. In this sense the decisive significance, it seems to us, is that of the unity of form and content as a basic trait in the structure of a concept. There are areas of reality, there are connections and phenomena that can be adequately rep resented only in concepts.

For this reason, those who consider abstract thinking as a removal from reality are wrong. On the contrary, abstract thinking primarily reflects the deepest and truest, the most complete and thorough disclosure of the reality opening up before the adolescent. Regarding the changes in content of the thinking of the adolescent, we cannot bypass one sphere that appears at this outstanding time of reconstruction of thinking as a whole. We are speaking of the awareness of one's own internal activity.

## TABLE 2.

| Age, years | Ratio, % |
|---|---|
| 11–13 | 2.0 |
| 14–15 | 13.0 |
| 15–16 | 12.0 |
| 16–17 | 42.0 |
| Students | 55.5 |

# 6

Kroh maintains that the mental world opens before the maturing adolescent, and his attention is initially directed toward other people to an ever increasing degree. The world of internal experiences, closed to the very young child, now opens before the adolescent and presents an extremely important sphere in the content of his thinking.

In the penetration into internal activity, into the world of his own experiences, the function of concept formation, which appears during the transitional age, again plays a decisive role. Just as the word is a means for understanding others, it is the means for understanding oneself. From birth, for the speaker, the word is a means for understanding himself, for the apperception of one's own perceptions. Because of this, only with the formation of concepts does an intensive development of self-perception, self-observation, intensive cognition of internal activity, the world of one's own experiences, occur. According to the correct note of W. Humboldt, thought becomes clear only in concepts, and only together with the formation of concepts does the adolescent begin to truly understand himself and his internal world. Lacking this, thought cannot attain clarity and cannot become concept.

Conception, being an important means of cognition and understanding, results in basic changes in the content of the adolescent's thinking. First, thinking in concepts leads to discovery of the deep connections that lie at the base of reality, to recognizing patterns that control reality, to ordering the perceived world with the help of the network of logical relations cast upon it. Speech is a powerful means of analysis and classification of phenomena, a means of ordering and generalizing reality. The word, becoming the carrier of the concept, is, as one of the authors correctly noted, the real theory of the object to which it refers. The general in this case serves as the law of the particular. Recognizing concrete reality with the help of words, which are signs for concepts, man uncovers in the world he sees connections and patterns that are confined in it.

In our experiments, we repeatedly found an extremely interesting close tie between different concepts. The mutual transition and linking of concepts, reflecting mutual transition and linking of phenomena of reality, means that every concept arises already connected with all others and, having arisen, seemingly determines its place in a system of previously recognized concepts.

In our experiments, the subject was confronted with the task of forming four different concepts. We saw how the formation of one concept was the key to the formation of the other three and how the latter three usually developed in the adolescent not in the same way as the first developed, but through the concept that had already been worked out and with its help. The course of thought in developing the second, third, and fourth concepts always differed profoundly from the course of thought in developing the first, and only in exceptional cases were the four concepts developed with the help of four identical operations. The mutual connection of concepts, their internal relation to one and the same system also make the concept one of the basic means of systematization and recognition of the external world. But the concept not only results in a system and serves as a basic means of recognizing external reality. It is also a basic means for understanding another, for adequate assimilation of the historically constituted social experience of humanity. Only in concepts does the adolescent systematize and comprehend the world of social consciousness for the first time. In this sense, Humboldt's definition is completely correct; he said that to think in words is to join one's own thinking to thought in general. Complete socialization of thought is contained in the function of concept formation.

Finally, the third sphere that arises anew in the adolescent's thinking in connection with the transition to forming concepts is the world of his own experiences, the systematization, cognition, and ordering of which becomes possible only at this point. On a firm basis, one of the authors says that consciousness is a phenomenon that is completely different from self-consciousness, which develops late in man, whereas consciousness is a normal attribute of his mental life.

"Self-consciousness is not given initially. It develops gradually to the extent that man, by using words, learns to understand himself. It is possible to understand oneself in various degrees. The child at an early stage of development understands himself very little."* His self-consciousness develops extremely slowly and in strict dependence on the development of thinking. But a decisive step along the path to understanding oneself, on the path toward the development and shaping of consciousness, is taken only during the transitional age together with the formation of concepts.

In this sense, completely consistent and justified is the analogy, made by thinking in concepts, between understanding and ordering things and the internal reality, an analogy cited by many authors. "Man subjects all his actions to such legislative plans. Strictly speaking, arbitrariness is possible only in deed and not in thought, not in words with which man explains his motives. The need to explain his behavior, to disclose it in words, to present it in concepts inevitably leads to subjecting his own actions to these legislative plans. A willful person summoned unexpectedly to account for the basis of his willfulness will say: 'That's what I want'; rejecting any measure of his actions, he cites his 'I' as law. But he himself is dissatisfied with his answer and only answered so because he had no other answer. It seems difficult to imagine *sic volo* (that's what I want—Ed.) said not as a joke but with no anger. Together with this attribute of self-consciousness, freedom and purpose are also established."

We will treat these complex problems in a subsequent chapter and will not discuss them in detail here. We will only say that, as we shall see later, separating the world of internal experiences from the world of objective reality is something that is constantly developing in the child, and we will not find this separation between self and the world in the child who is beginning to speak as we will in the adult. For the child in the first days of life, everything he senses and the whole content of his consciousness is still an undifferentiated mass. Self-consciousness is acquired only through development and is not given to us together with consciousness.

Thus, understanding reality, understanding others, and understanding oneself—this is what thinking in concepts brings with itself. This is the kind of revolution that occurs in the thinking and consciousness of the adolescent; this is what is new, what distinguishes the thinking of the adolescent from the thinking of the three-year-old.

---

* L. S. Vygotsky does not indicate the source of this and the following citation. We could not establish who the author was.—Editor's note.

We think that we shall express completely correctly the problem of studying thinking in concepts for the development of personality and its relation to the surrounding world if we compare it with the problem that confronts the history of language. A. A. Potebnya believed that showing the actual participation of the word in the formation of a sequential series of systems that encompass the relation of the personality to nature is the basic problem of the history of language. In general outline, we will truly understand the significance of this participation if we accept the basic premise that language is not the means to express an already prepared thought, but to create it, that it is not a reflection of world contemplation that has developed, but an activity that composes it. In order to perceive one's own mental movements, in order to interpret one's own internal perceptions, man must objectivize them in a word and must join this word to other words. For understanding even one's own external nature, it is not at all indifferent how this nature presents itself to us, by means of specifically which comparisons its separate elements are as perceptible to the mind as these same comparisons are real for us, in a word, Potebnya assumes that the primary property and degree of obliviousness of the internal form of the word are not indifferent for thought.

If we are speaking here of the formation of a number of systems that encompass the relation of the personality to nature mediated by speech, then together with this, we must not forget for a moment that both knowing nature and knowing personality is done with the help of understanding other people, understanding those around us, understanding social experience. Speech cannot be separated from understanding. This inseparability of speech and understanding is manifested identically in both social use of language as a means of communication and in its individual use as a means of thinking.

7

We elaborated material that was collected by our colleague, E. I. Pashkovskaya, which involved several hundred adolescents studying in a factory-trade apprenticeship school (FAS) and in the School for Christian Youth (SCY). The purpose of the study was to elucidate what in similar studies in younger children was called a study of the stock of ideas.

Actually in Pashkovskaya's studies more extensive problems were solved: we were interested here not so much in the stock of ideas, not so much in the inventory of the knowledge that an adolescent commands, not so much in a cross section of those points of which his thinking is made up—in general, not in the quantitative aspect of the stock of ideas as primarily in the structure of the content of thinking and the complex connections and relations established in the thinking of the adolescent between different spheres of experience. We were interested in elucidating the qualitative difference between the structure of one thought content or another in the adolescent and the corresponding idea of a child and how various spheres of reality are connected with each other in the thinking of the adolescent. On this basis, the word "idea" seems scarcely appropriate. We were not speaking of ideas at all in this case. If this word expresses more or less precisely the subject of study when it is directed toward the thinking of the young child, in applying it to an adolescent, it loses almost all meaning, all sense.

The unit (or the aggregate of units that comprise the content of the thinking during the transitional age), the simplest action with which the intellect of the adolescent operates, is, of course, not a representation, but a concept. Thus, Pashkovskaya's study encompassed the structure and connection of concepts pertaining to the various aspects of reality, external and internal, and formed as if a natural supplement to preceding research, the results of which we presented above. We were interested in the thinking of the adolescent from the aspect of content; we wanted to take a look at concept from the point of view of the content that it represented and to see whether the theoretical connection that we assumed between the development of a new form of thinking—the function of forming concepts—and a radical reconstruction of the whole content of intellectual activity of the adolescent really exists.

The research encompassed various spheres of experience of the adolescent and included a study of concepts that relate to phenomena of nature, technical processes and tools, phenomena of social life, and concepts related to abstract ideas of a psychological nature. Basically, the research confirmed the presence of connections that we expected and showed that together with functions of concept formation, the adolescent also acquires something completely new in structure and in method of systematization, in scope and depth of the content of the aspects of reality reflected in it. Because of this research, we can disclose how the content of his thinking is enriched and new forms are acquired.

In *this* we see the basic and central results of the whole work and the direct confirmation of the hypothesis which we mentioned above. We believe that one of the basic errors of modern psychology of concepts is not taking this circumstance into account, a failure that leads either to a purely formal consideration of concepts, ignoring the new areas and new system presented in the content of the concepts, or to a purely morphological phenomenological analysis of the content of thinking from the material aspect without taking into account the fact that morphological analysis alone is always insupportable and requires cooperation with functional and genetic analysis because the given content may be adequately presented only in a certain form, and mastery of the given content becomes possible only with the appearance of specific functions of thinking, specific methods of intellectual activity.

We have already indicated that the function of forming concepts during the transitional age is a young and unstable acquisition of the intellect. For this reason, it would be a mistake to imagine that all thinking of the adolescent is imbued with concepts. On the contrary, here we observe concepts only in the process of their being established; they will not be a dominant form of thinking until the very end of the transitional age, and the intellectual activity of the adolescent is still done for the most part in other, genetically earlier forms.

On this basis we tried to explain this inadequacy in the adolescent's thinking and the romanticism of his thinking which many investigators indicate. From the aspect of content, we find a complete parallel to this position. It is curious that a significant number of the adolescents studied, when confronted with the task of defining an abstract concept, respond on the basis of completely concrete determinations. Thus, to the question, what is good, they answer: "To buy the best, that is good" (14-year-old, FAS); "Good is when a man did something good for another man, this is good" (15-year-old, SCY). But even more often they give a worldly, practical definition of this term: "Good is what one acquires, for example, very good earrings, watches, trousers, etc." (13-year-old, SCY); "What you get, that is good" (13-year-old,

SCY); or even more concretely: "Finery when a girl is given in marriage, a hope chest" (13-year-old, SCY); "Good is what we have, that is, notebook, pen, ballpoint, etc." (14-year-old, FAS), or finally: "Valuable things" (13 year-old, SCY), etc.

If the subjects give other definitions for this concept based on its meaning as a certain psychological and moral quality, then the character of these definitions very often, especially at the beginning of the transitional age, remains just as concrete. They take the word in its worldly meaning and explain it with the help of the most concrete example. The definition of such concepts as "thought," "love," etc. have a similar character at the beginning of the transitional period. To the question, what is love, they answer: "love is that a person likes another person who touched his heart" (14-year-old, SCY); "Love is a name, a man loves a woman" (13-year-old, SCY); "Love is someone who wants to get married, then he sits with a girl and proposes that she marry him" (13-year-old, SCY); "Love happens between relations and acquaintances" (13-year-old, SCY).

Thus, even from the aspect of content of thinking at the beginning of the transitional age, we find the same predominance of the concrete, the same attempt to approach an abstract concept from the point of view of the concrete situation that manifests it. Essentially, these definitions differ in no way from the definition cited above from the material of A. Messer,[48] which is typical for early school age also. But here we must make an important reservation: what we have noted as a frequently encountered phenomenon in the first half of the transitional age is not an essential, not a specific, not a new, and for this reason from the genetic aspect, not a characteristic trait of the transitional age. It is a remnant of the old. Although this form of thinking now predominates, as the adolescent moves ahead, it will be involuted, curtailed, and will disappear.

There is a transition toward more abstract thinking; although it is not now a quantitatively dominant form, it is specific for the transitional age: as the adolescent moves ahead, it will develop. The past belongs to concrete thinking and most of the present, to the abstract— the smaller part of the present, but to make up for it, all of the future.

We will consider the studies of Pashkovskaya in detail on other pages. We will only say that two points are in the foreground in the analysis of the rich factual material. First, connection and relations that exist between concepts come through. Each of the 60 answers* was internally and organically linked with every other answer. The second point is that we observe how the content enters the internal com position of thinking, how it stops being its external, directing factor, how it begins to be expressed in the speaker's own name.

According to the Latin expression *communia proprio dicere* (literally: to express the general through the particular—Editor), the content of thinking becomes an internal conviction of the speaker, the directedness of his thoughts, his interest, the norm of his behavior, his desire and intention. This occurs especially markedly when we deal with the adolescents' answers to actual questions on contemporary events, politics, social life, plans for their own life, etc. It is characteristic that in the answers, the concept and the content reflected in it are not given as given by a child, as assimilated from outside, something completely objective; it is merged with

---

*     Each subject answered 60 questions, and the answers were analyzed.—Editor's note.

complex internal factors of the personality, and at this time it is difficult to determine where the objective statement ends and where the manifestation of personal interest, conviction, and direction of behavior begins.

In general, it would be difficult to find more distinct evidence for the position that content does not enter into thinking as a factor external and peripherally related to it, that it does not fill one form or another of intellectual activity the way water fills an empty glass, that it is organically connected with intellectual functions, that every sphere of the content has its specific functions and that content, becoming a property of the personality, begins to participate in the general system of movement of the personality, in the general system of its development as one of its internal factors.

Thought, clearly assimilated, being the personal thought of the adolescent, in addition to its own logic and its own movement, begins to be subject to the general patterns of development of the personal system of thinking in which it is included as a certain part, and the task of the psychologist is to trace this process exactly and know how to find the complex structure of the personality and its thinking, which includes clearly assimilated thought. Like a ball, which when thrown against the deck of a ship moves along the diagonal of a parallelogram of two forces, thought assimilated at this time moves along the diagonal of some kind of complex parallelogram reflecting two different forces, two different systems of movement.

8

Here we come close to establishing one of the central points that must be explained if we are to overcome the usual error relative to the break between form and content in the development of thinking. From formal logic, traditional psychology adopted the idea of the concept as an abstract mental construct extremely re mote from all the wealth of concrete reality. From the point of view of formal logic, the development of concepts is subject to the basic law of inverse proportionality between the scope and content of a concept. The broader the scope of a concept, the narrower its content. This means that the greater the number of objects that the given concept can be applied to, the greater the circle of concrete things that it encompasses, the poorer its content, the emptier it proves to be. The process of forming concepts according to formal logic is extremely simple. The points of abstracting and generalizing are internally closely connected with each other from the point of view of one and the same process, but taken from different aspects. In the words of K. Bühler, what logic terms an abstraction and generalization is completely simple and understandable. A concept from which one of the traits is taken away becomes poorer in content, more abstract and augmented in scope, and becomes general.

It is completely clear that if the process of generalizing is considered as a direct result of abstraction of traits, then we will inevitably come to the conclusion that thinking in concepts is removed from reality, that the constant represented in concepts becomes poorer and poorer, scant and narrow. Not without reason are such concepts frequently termed empty abstracts. Others have said that concepts arise in the process of castrating reality. Concrete, diverse phenomena must lose their traits one after the other in order that a concept might be formed. Actually what arises is a dry and empty abstraction in which the diverse, full-blooded reality is narrowed and impoverished by logical thought. This is the source of the celebrated words of Goethe: "Gray is every theory and eternally green is the golden tree of life."

This dry, empty, gray abstraction inevitably strives to reduce content to zero because the more general, the more empty a concept becomes. Impoverishing the content is done from fateful necessity, and for this reason psychology, proceeding to develop the teaching on concepts on the grounds of formal logic, presented thinking in concepts as the system of thinking that was the poorest, scantiest, and emptiest.

Moreover, the true nature of a concept was seriously distorted in the formal presentation. A real concept is an image of an objective thing in its complexity. Only when we recognize the thing in all its connections and relations, only when this diversity is synthesized in a word, in an integral image through a multitude of determinations, do we develop a concept. According to the teaching of dialectical logic, a concept includes not only the general, but also the individual and particular.

In contrast to contemplation, to direct knowledge of an object, a concept is filled with definitions of the object; it is the result of rational processing of our experience, and it is a mediated knowledge of the object. To think of some object with the help of a concept means to include the given object in a complex system of mediating connections and relations disclosed in determinations of the concept. Thus, the concept does not arise from this as a mechanical result of abstraction—it is the result of a long and deep knowledge of the object.

Together with overcoming the formal-logical point of view of the concept, together with exposing the incorrectness of the law of inverse proportionality between scope and content, the new psychology is beginning to grope for a correct position in the study of concepts. Psychological research is disclosing that in a concept, we always have an enrichment and deepening of the content that the concept contains. In this respect, the Marxist equating of the role of abstraction with the power of the microscope is completely correct. In genuine scientific research, with the help of the concept, we are able to penetrate through the external appearance of phenomena, across the external form of their manifestations, and see the hidden connections and relations lying at the base of the phenomena to penetrate into their essence, just as with the aid of a microscope, we disclose in a drop of water a complex and rich life, or the complex internal structure of a cell hidden from our eyes.

According to the well-known definition of Marx, if the form of a manifestation and the essence of things coincided directly, then all science would be superfluous (see K. Marx and E Engels, *Works*, Vol. 25, Part II, p. 384). For this reason, thinking in concepts is the most adequate method of knowing reality because it penetrates into the internal essence of things, for the nature of things is disclosed not in direct contemplation of one single object or another, but in connections and relations that are manifested in movement and in development of the object, and these connect it to all the rest of reality. The internal connection of things is disclosed with the help of thinking in concepts, for to develop a concept of some object means to disclose a series of connections and relations of that object with all the rest of reality, to include it in the complex system of phenomena.

Also, the traditional representation of the intellectual mechanism itself that is the basis for the formation of the concept changes. Formal logic and traditional psychology reduce the concept to a general representation. The concept differs from the concrete representation according to this teaching in the same way that the group photograph of E Galton differs from the individual photographic portrait. Or another comparison is frequently made: it is said that instead of general representations, we think by means of their substitutes—words which play the role of credit cards that substitute for gold coins.

In the most developed form, modern psychological research assumes that if both of these points of view are insupportable, then everything must still exist, as K. Bühler maintained, as some equivalent logical operation—abstraction and generalization—if not directly in a separate representation, then in any case in the course of representation in abstract thinking, since the real course of mental phenomena is closely linked to these operations. In what does Bühler see the psychological equivalent of these logical operations? He finds it in orthoscopic thinking and perception, in the development of invariants, that is, in the fact that our perceptions and other processes of reflection and cognition of reality have a certain constancy (a stability of perceived impressions). In Bühler's opinion, anyone who could indicate more precisely how this happens, how, independently of the changing position of the observer and the changing distances relative to the impressions of form and size, a kind of absolute impression develops, would render a decisive service to the teaching on the formation of concepts.

By referring to orthoscopic or absolute perceptions or to graphic representations, Bühler does not solve the problem that confronts him but moves it to a still earlier stage of development. In this case, it seems to us that he creates a logical circle in the definition, since the problem itself of absolute perception must be solved by means of the reverse influence of concepts on the stability of perception. We will consider this in the following chapter. But the main deficiency of Bühler's theory is that it tries to find a psychological equivalent of logical operations that lead to the development of a concept, in elementary processes that are identically proper to both perception and thinking. From this it is clear that all boundaries, all qualitative difference between elementary and higher forms, between perception and cognition are erased.

The concept seems to be simply a corrected and stable perception; it seems to be not a simple representation, but its diagram. From this it is understandable that specifically the theory of Bühler in its logical development led to the rejection of the qualitative uniqueness of the adolescent's thinking and to admitting that his thinking is, in the main, identical with the thinking of the three-year-old.

Together with the radical change in the logical point of view, the logical view of the concept, there is also a change in the direction of search for the psychological equivalent of the concept. Here again the words of K. Stumpf are confirmed: what is true in logic cannot be false in psychology and vice versa. Comparison of the logical and the psychological in the study of concepts, so characteristic for neo-Kantians, must actually be replaced by the opposite point of view. Logical analysis of the concept, disclosing its essence, provides a key also to its psychological study. It is quite clear that when formal logic imagines the process of formation of a concept as a process of gradual narrowing of content and extending of scope, the process of simple loss by the object of a series of traits, the psychological study directs itself to finding similar processes equivalent to this logical abstraction in the sphere of intellectual operations.

This is the source of the famous comparison with the Galton group photograph, the source of the teaching on general representations. Together with the new understanding of the concept and its essence, psychology is confronted by new problems in its study. The concept begins to be understood not as a thing, but as a process, not as an empty abstraction, but as a thorough and penetrating reflection of an object of reality in all its complexity and diversity, in connections and relations to all the rest of reality. It is natural that psychology will begin to seek an equivalent of the concept in a completely different area.

It has long been noted that the concept in essence represents nothing other than a certain aggregate of judgments, a certain system of acts of thinking. Thus, one of the authors says that the concept considered psychologically, that is, not only from the one aspect of content as it is in logic, but also from the aspect of the form of the concept in reality, in a word, as an activity, is a certain number of judgments and, consequently, not a single act of thinking, but a series of these acts. The logical concept, that is, the simultaneous sum total of traits, different from the aggregate of traits in its form, is a fiction, among other things, completely essential for science. Regardless of its duration, the psychological concept has an internal unity.

Thus, we see that for the psychologist, the concept is an aggregate of acts of judgment, apperception, interpretation, and recognition. The concept taken in action, in movement, in reality, does not. lose unity, but reflects its true nature. According to our hypothesis, we must seek the psychological equivalent of the concept not in general representations, not in absolute perceptions and orthoscopic diagrams, not even in concrete verbal images that replace the general representations—we must seek it in a system of judgments in which the concept is disclosed.

Actually since we have rejected the representation of the concept as a simple aggregate of some number of concrete traits that differs from a simple representation only in that it is poorer in content and more extensive in scope of form, seemingly a large envelope empty of content, we must assume beforehand that the psychological equivalent of the concept can only be a system of acts of thinking and some combination and processing of patterns.

The concept, as has already been said, is an objective reflection of a thing in its essence and diversity; it arises as a result of rational processing of representations, as a result of disclosing connections and relations of the given object with others and, consequently, it includes a long process of thinking and cognition that is seemingly concentrated in it. For this reason, in the definition cited above, it seems completely correct to indicate that from the psychological aspect a concept turns out to be a long activity that includes in itself a series of acts of thinking.

K. Bühler comes close to the truth when he says that an abstract word, for example, "mammal," for us adults, educated people, not only is a representation of all kinds of forms of animals associatively linked, but, what is more important, is a rich complex of judgments, more or less introduced into the system, from which, in conformity with circumstances, one judgment or another is at our service.

A great merit of Bühler is his pointing out that a concept arises not mechanically like a group photograph of the objects in our memory, that functions of judgment take part in the development of a concept, that this thesis is correct even for single forms of concept formation, and that for this reason, concepts cannot be pure products of associations, but have their place in the connections of knowledge, that is, concepts have a natural place in judgments and conclusions, acting as a component part of the latter. From our point of view, only two points are in error. First, Bühler assumes the connection of the concept with the complex of judgments introduced into the system to be an associative connection that arises outside thinking. He erroneously assumes the process of judgment to be a simple reproduction of judgment. None of the representatives of the teaching on general representations as a basis of concepts would take exception to such an associative understanding of the character of the connection between a concept and acts of thinking. Actually, there is almost nothing that a concept can be associated or connected with. The circle of various associations is, of course, absolutely unlimited, and for this reason, the presence of associative connections with judgments still says nothing about the psychological nature of the concept, nothing is changed in its traditional understanding, and it is completely compatible with identifying the concept with a general representation.

Bühler's second error is the representation that concepts have their own natural place in acts of judgment making up their organic part. This point of view seems to be erroneous to us because a concept, as we have seen, makes up not simply a part of judgment, but arises as a result of the complex activity of thinking, that is, as a result of multiple operations of judgment, and is disclosed in a series of acts of thinking. Thus, from our point of view, a concept is not a part of judgment, but a complex system of judgments combined as a certain unit and a special psychological structure in the full and true sense of the word. This means that the system of judgment in which a concept is disclosed is contained in a contracted, abbreviated form, as if in a potential state, in the structure of the concept. This system of judgment, like any structure, has its unique properties that characterize it specifically as a whole system, and only an analysis of this system can bring us to understanding the structure of a concept.

Consequently, from our point of view, the structure of a concept is disclosed in a system of judgments, in a complex of acts of thinking that represent a single whole formation which has its own principles. In this representation, we find the main idea on the unity of form and content as the basis of the concept realized. Actually, the totality of judgments introduced in the system represents a certain content in an ordered and connected form and it is a unit of a series of points of content. Also, the totality of acts of thinking, acting as a single whole, is constructed as a special intellectual mechanism, as a special psychological structure, and is made up of a system or of a complex of judgments. Thus, the unique combination of a series of acts of thinking acting as a certain unit represents a special form of thinking, a certain intellectual method of behavior.

With this we can conclude the review of the changes that occur in the content of an adolescent's thinking. We can assert that all changes in the content, as we have pointed out repeatedly, necessarily also presuppose a change in the form of thinking. Here we come as close as possible to the general psychological law which states that a new content does not mechanically fill an empty form, but content and form are factors in a single process of intellectual development. It is impossible to pour new wine into old skins. This applies completely also to thinking during the transitional age.

## 9

It remains for us to consider the important changes that the form of thinking undergoes during the transitional age. Actually, the response to this question has been determined in the preceding course of discussion. It consists in the theory of the concept that we attempted to develop briefly above. If we accept the outlined view of the concept as a certain system of judgments, then we inevitably will agree also that the unified activity in which a concept is disclosed, the unified sphere of the manifestation of the system, is logical thinking.

From our point of view, logical thinking is not composed of concepts so much as of separate elements; it is not added to concepts as something standing above them and developing after them—it is the concepts themselves in their action, in their functioning. Like a certain expression that defines function as an organ in action, we could define logical thinking as concept in action. From this point of view, in the form of a general premise, we could say that the most important revolution in forms of thinking in the adolescent is the revolution that occurs as a result of the formation of concepts, and mastery of logical thinking represents the second basic consequence of the acquisition of this function.

Only during the transitional age is mastery of logical thinking a real fact, and only owing to this fact are those deep changes in the content of thinking which we mentioned above possible. We have much evidence from investigators who place the development of logical thinking at the transitional age.

In the words of E. Meumann, for example, real logical deduction in the form in which textbooks use it, becomes easy for the child only quite late. Approximately toward the last year in a German school, that is, at 14 years of age, the child appears to be capable of seeing the connection between deductions made and to understand them. True, Meumann's opinion has been disputed many times. It developed that logical thinking appears not long before the. period of sexual maturation, and the attempt to reject Meumann's position has always taken two different directions.

Some authors try simply to lower the age indicated by Meumann, and their common disagreement with Meumann was only a seeming disagreement. Thus, in a recent study, H. Ormian found that mastery of logical thinking begins at age 11. Other authors, as we shall see subsequently, also indicate age 11–12, that is, the age when primary education ends, as the period when the child's prelogical form of thinking ends and the threshold of mastery of logical thinking is crossed.

The opinion that attempts simply to lower by two years the time of appearance of logical thinking indicated by Meumann is not at variance, as we can see, with the position defended by Meumann himself, because he has in mind the final mastery of logical thinking in its developed form. Some authors, who studied the whole process of development of concepts more finely and precisely, indicate its beginning. And all agree that only after primary school age and only with the beginning of the adolescent years is the transition made to logical thinking in the real and true sense of the word.

There are authors who differ radically and decisively with this position. On the basis of serious study of the thinking of the very young child and with almost no reference to the study of the thinking of the adolescent, these authors, as we indicated many times, are inclined to reject all differences between the thinking of the three-year-old and the adolescent. On the basis of purely external data, the investigators ascribe developed logical thinking to the three-year-old, forgetting that logical thinking is impossible without concepts and concepts develop relatively late.

The controversy created by this psychological disagreement can be resolved only if we are able to answer the question, is the very young child capable of abstract thinking and concepts, and how do concepts and logical thinking differ qualitatively from generalization and the thinking of the very young child. Essentially, in all the preceding exposition, we proceeded from a desire to answer this question. Specifically for this reason we did not limit ourselves to a simple statement that the formation of concepts begins at the transitional age, but resorted to the method of genetic sections, and by comparing various stages in the development of thinking, we tried to show how a pseudo concept differs from true concepts,[52] how complex thinking differs qualitatively from thinking in concepts and, consequently, how what is new that makes up the content of the development of thinking in the transitional age is inferred.

Now we would like to reinforce the position arrived at experimentally by a consideration of the results of the studies of other authors especially dedicated to the study of the characteristics of the thinking of the child up to the transitional age. These studies, set up with a completely different goal, seem almost specially directed to refuting the idea that the child of early, preschool, and school age is already capable of logical thinking.

The basic conclusion that can be reached from these studies is the discovery of the fact that the forms of thinking that resemble logical forms externally essentially conceal qualitatively different thinking operations. We have in mind three basic points connected with disclosing the qualitative uniqueness of the thinking of the child and the principal differences between it and logical thinking. Considering again the results of the work of others, we must resort to the method of genetic sections and try to find the uniqueness of thinking in concepts and to compare it with other genetically earlier forms of thinking.

For this reason we must obviously digress from the thinking of the adolescent and concentrate our attention on the thinking of the child. But in essence, we will always keep in mind specifically thinking in the transitional age. We only want to find the path to recognizing its characteristics through comparative-genetic study and comparison with earlier forms of thinking because, as we have already indicated, the argument about whether the formation of concepts is an achievement of the transitional age in its essentially modern formulation is reduced to the question: is a child capable of logical thinking and the formation of concepts?

## 10

As we have already said, we have no other means of understanding that which is new that develops in the thinking of the adolescent in comparison with the thinking of the child than through a comparative study of genetic sections of the developing intellect. Only by comparing the intellect of the adolescent with the intellect of the young child of preschool and school age, only by comparing these four sections made at early stages of development, will we be able to include the thinking of the adolescent in the genetic chain and to understand what is new, what develops in that thinking.

We also said that specifically the erroneous interpretation of early sections in the development of the intellect and interpretation based exclusively on apparent similarity, on external traits, usually led to overestimating the child's capability of logical thinking and, consequently, to an underestimation of that which is new that develops in the thinking of the adolescent.

We formulated the task that confronts us in the following way: we must consider whether the child is capable of logical thinking in the essential sense of the word, whether the child has the function of forming concepts. In order to answer this question, we must turn to a series of newer studies that leave no doubt with respect to the problem that interests us. Recently D. N. Uznadze did special work on this problem; through various experiments, he undertook systematic study of the formation of concepts at the preschool age. The study (D. N. Uznadze, 1929) involved 76 children age two to seven years. The experiments required classification of various objects into groups, then followed experiments with naming a new thing with some kind of unfamiliar name and experiments of generalizing the names given and defining the new words. Thus, the experiments encompassed different functional points in the formation of concepts.

The basic task of these studies, as we have said, was to disclose what are the equivalents to our concepts at the preschool age, what makes a mutual understanding of the adult and the child possible regardless of the fact that the child has not yet mastered the development of concepts, and finally, how these equivalents are unique at the early stage of development.

We cannot consider in detail the course of the study, and will turn directly to the basic results in which we will find the answer to the question that interests us. As a general characterization of three-year-olds, Uznadze assumes that it can be said that words which they use evoke in them visual, whole undifferentiated images of objects that are also the meaning of these words.

Thus, the three-year-old does not apply true concepts, but in the best case uses only certain equivalents of these in the form of undifferentiated whole examples of an idea. The three-year-old takes a significant step forward along the path to the development of concepts, and one of the greatest achievements of Uznadze's research is that he tries to trace step by step, year by year the internal process of change in the structure of the meaning of children's words.

We cannot present the course of development year by year. We are interested only in the final conclusion. Uznadze says that finally in the seven-year-old, the developing forms of thinking attain decisive dominance. In them, 90% of sound combinations form real words in which meaning is not a whole idea, but mainly an appropriate individual trait. This is especially evident in experiments with generalizations in 84% of which the process occurs on the basis of similarity of individual traits. With respect to this, the seven-year-old attains a stage of development that makes him capable for the first time of an adequate understanding and treatment of our thinking processes. Thus, genuine school maturity occurs only with the end of the seventh year of life, only at the time that the child becomes capable of a true understanding and processing of thinking operations; before that he uses only equivalents of our concepts pertaining to the same circle of objects, but with a different meaning. The author does not analyze the uniqueness of children's meaning, but the indication of the whole concrete-like and undifferentiated character of these formations is a basis for bringing them close to the complexes we found in the experiment with complex forms of thinking.

In essence, with the help of the more penetrating research of Uznadze, we were able to show that the characteristics of thinking that former research ascribed to the young child are actually predominant by the eighth year. This is the principal merit of Uznadze's work. He succeeded in showing that where there is an obvious predominance of logical thinking there are only equivalents of our concepts that permit an exchange of thought, but not an adequate application of appropriate operations.

In application to the young child, these equivalents have long been recognized by investigators. Thus, W. Stern (1922, 1926) in a study of children's language, citing W. Ament (1899), establishes that in children's speech from the very beginning there is no differentiation of symbols for individual and generic concepts. The child is more likely to begin from certain pre-concepts from which only gradually both types in which we are interested develop. But, in contrast to Ament, Stern takes a decisive step further and asserts: as long as we speak in general of concepts, we interpret the first verbal meanings logically.

Moreover, this must be decisively rejected. Only according to external form do they seem to be concepts. The process of their psychological development is completely alogical and rests on much more primitive functions than the function of concept formation. These are quasi or pseudo concepts. Analysis of pseudo concepts allows Stern to reach the conclusion that the first words are simply symbols of familiarity, that is, what Groos calls a potential concept. This is the basis on which Stern interprets the change in meaning of words at an early age of which we spoke above. In subsequent analysis the author comes to the conclusion that the first individual concepts that encompass a certain concrete object develop in the child. For a child, a doll is always the same doll that is the child's favorite toy; mama is always the same person that satisfies the child's needs, etc.

It is enough to look at Stern's examples to see that that which we term an individual concept rests exclusively on recognizing the identity of one and the same object—operation, which even animals have and which in no way permits us to speak of concept in the real sense of the word.

As far as generic concepts that encompass a whole group of objects are concerned, according to Stern, they require a somewhat longer period of development. They exist at first only in a preparatory stage in which they encompass a concrete plurality of similar specimens, but not an abstract commonality of traits. Stern calls these plural concepts. As Stern maintains, the child now knows that a horse is not simply a single specimen that appeared once, but that it can be found in many specimens.

However, the statements of the child always refer to only one specimen or another that is at the time the subject of his perception or expectation. He places each new specimen among many others that he perceived previously, but he still does not subordinate all of these specimens to a general concept. On the basis of our experience, we conclude that the child approaches this only in his fourth year.

Our studies convinced us that for the child the initial function of the word is indicating a specific object, and for this reason, we understand these plural concepts as a verbal indicative gesture which he makes each time toward a concrete specimen of one thing or another. Just as with the help of a pointing gesture, attention can be called each time to only some specific, single object, using one of his first words, the child always has in mind a concrete specimen of some general group.

In this case, in what is a real concept manifested? Only in that the child recognizes the similarity or belonging of different specimens to one and the same group, but as we have seen before, this is also proper to animals at the earliest primitive stages of development. As we remember, when the situation requires it, instead of a stick, a monkey uses many very different objects which it classifies in the same group because of a similar trait. Stern's assertion that a child masters general concepts by the fourth year, completely rejected in the studies of Uznadze cited above, seems to us to be a natural consequence of inserting logic into children's speech, of intellectualism, of ascribing to the child, on the basis of external similarity, a developed and logical thinking; this is the most essential deficiency of Stern's important research.

Uznadze's achievement is that he showed how insupportable it is to ascribe the formation of general concepts to such an early age. He increased the period indicated by Stern by three to four years. But it also seems to us that he still makes a substantial error, similar to the error of Stern, which consists in his accepting as true concepts, formations that appear to be similar to concepts. It is true that a child by the age of seven takes a decisive step along the path of developing his concepts. We could say that specifically by this time, he makes a transition from syncretic ideas to complex thinking, from lower forms of complex thinking to pseudo concepts. But, as Uznadze points out, identifying concrete common traits as the single symptom of formation of concepts in the seven-year-old is, as we have seen, nothing other than a potential concept or a pseudo concept. Identifying a common trait by no means constitutes a concept, although it is a very important step along the path to its development. Our studies, which disclosed a complex, genetic diversity of forms in the development of concepts, are a basis for the assertion that Uznadze's analysis is also incomplete, that by the age of seven, the child has not mastered the formation of concepts, although he takes a very important step on the path to this achievement.

11

In this respect, the remarkable studies of J. Piaget on speech and thinking in the child and his judgments and deductions leave no doubt. These studies (1932) undoubtedly constituted an epoch in the study of children's thinking and played the same role in the study of the thinking of the schoolchild as the studies of Stern and other authors played in their time in the study of early childhood.

By means of extremely clever and penetrating studies, Piaget succeeded in showing that the forms of thinking during early school years, regardless of their apparent similarity to logical thinking, are in fact qualitatively different from operations of logical thinking, and in them other patterns are dominant that differ substantially in structural, functional, and genetic relations from abstract logical thinking, which, in the strict sense of the word, begins only after primary school age, that is, at the age of 12.

As Piaget says, Jean Jacques Rousseau liked to repeat that "the child is not a small adult," that he has his own needs and his mind is adapted to those needs. All the studies of Piaget follow this basic line; his studies also try to show that with respect to thinking, the child is not a small adult and that the development of thinking when he makes the transition from primary school age to secondary does not consist exclusively of a quantitative growth, enrichment, and extension of the same forms that were dominant in the first stage.

Analyzing the thinking of the schoolchild and the adolescent, Piaget establishes a number of qualitative differences and shows that all of them represent a unit based on one principal, general cause.

In this respect, it seems to us that E. Claparède, in his foreword to Piaget's work, correctly evaluates its great merit: Piaget posed the problem of the child's thinking and its development as a qualitative problem. Claparède writes that we might have defined the new idea to which Piaget brings us by comparing it to the opinion generally tacitly accepted. While the problem of the child's thinking was usually treated as a quantitative problem, Piaget changed it to a qualitative problem. While in the child's development, what was usually seen was the result of a certain number of additions and subtractions, acquisition of new experience and exclusion of certain errors, we are now shown that the child's intellect changes its character gradually. If the child's mind frequently seems to be quite muddled in comparison with that of the adult, this is not because of his having somewhat more or less of some elements or because it is full of gaps and bumps, but because he depends on a different type of thinking, a type that the adult has long since left behind in his development, as Claparède emphasizes.

Thus, in the problem that interests us, Piaget's studies directly continue the work started by other authors and can be directly connected with the work of Uznadze. Piaget begins where the research of Uznadze ends and seems to reconsider the conclusion that Uznadze reached. Actually, beginning at age seven, a great upward shift occurs in the child's thinking that consists of his moving from subjective, syncretic connections to complex, objective connections that are extremely close to the concepts of the adult. For this reason there may be the impression that a child of seven thinks like an adult, that he is capable of using our thinking operations. But Piaget shows that this is just an illusion.

We cannot discuss in detail the course of his research and must limit ourselves to certain basic conclusions that may have a direct relation to our theme. Piaget's general conclusion is the following: formal thinking develops only at age 11–12. Between 7–8 and 11–12, there is syncretism; contradictions are found almost exclusively in purely verbal thinking not based on direct observations. Only at age approximately 11–12 can we actually speak of the child's logical experience. Nevertheless, age 7–8 represents a serious forward step. Forms of logical thinking appear in the area of visual thinking.

This is how we may present the basic results of Piaget's research. His data show that the thinking of the child passes through three major phases (if we put aside the thinking of the earliest age). During early and preschool age, thinking is egocentric.

The child thinks in whole connected graphic impressions that are usually termed syncretic. Pre-causality dominates his thinking. By age 7–8, the child's thinking is altered significantly: the characteristics of early thinking drop off and are replaced by a structure of the child's thinking that is closer to logic. However, the features that characterized the child's thinking at the early stage do not disappear altogether. They are only transferred to a new area, specifically the area of purely verbal thinking. The child's thinking now is seemingly divided into two large spheres. In the area of visual and effective thinking, the child no longer exhibits the characteristics that he exhibited at an earlier stage of development. But in the area of purely verbal thinking, the child still is subject to syncretism, he still has not mastered the logical forms of thought. This basic law Piaget terms the law of shift or displacement. Using this law, the investigator tries to explain the characteristics of thinking during the first years of school.

The essence of the law is that the child, perceiving his own operations, in this way transfers them from the plane of action to the plane of speech. In the transfer, when the child begins to reproduce his operations verbally, he is again confronted by the difficulties that he overcame in the plane of action. Here a shift will occur between two different methods of mastery. The dates will differ, but the rhythm will remain similar. The shift between thinking and action can be observed continually and has a major potential for understanding the child's logic. It holds the key to elucidating all the phenomena disclosed in our studies.

Thus, as a characteristic of the thinking of the schoolchild, Piaget sees in the transfer to the verbal plane, to the plane of thinking in speech patterns, the same operations that the child has already mastered in the plane of action, and for this reason the whole course of development of thinking is not subordinate to the continuity and gradualness that the associationists, H. Taine and T. Ribot, ascribed to it, but discloses a step backward, interference and transitions of various duration. All the characteristics of the very young child's thinking do not finally disappear. They only disappear from the plane of his concrete thinking, but they move, shift, to the plane of verbal thinking and are manifested there.

We might formulate the law of shift as follows: on the plane of verbal thinking, the schoolchild displays the same characteristics and the same differences from the logic of the adult as the preschooler displayed on the plane of visual and action thinking. The schoolchild thinks just as the preschooler acts and perceives.

With the law of shift, Piaget connects the law of realization established for the intellectual development of the child by E. Claparède, who in a special study attempted to elucidate the development of the child's realization of similarity and difference. It developed that realizing similarity appears much later in the child than realizing difference. In the plane of action, however, the child adapts earlier and more simply to similar than to different situations. Thus, in action, he reacts to similarity earlier than he does to difference. On the other hand, distinguishing objects creates a state of nonadaptation, and specifically this nonadaptation prevents the child from realizing the problem. On this basis, Claparède deduces a general law which states that we realize only to the extent of our unsuccessful adaptation.

The law of shift explains for us why and how the development of thinking occurs during the transition from the preschool to school age and shows that the child begins to realize his operations and his nonadaptation only when he needs to realize them. In particular, using a concrete example, Piaget shows what an enormous role social factors, to use his expression, play in the development of the structure and function of the child's thinking. He shows how logical reflection of the child develops under the direct influence of an argument that arises in the children's group, and only when an external social need arises to prove the rightness of his thinking, to argue for it, to motivate it does the child begin to use the same operations in his own thinking also. Piaget maintains that the logical reflection is a discussion with oneself that reproduces a real argument in an internal aspect. For this reason it is completely natural for the child to master his internal operations, his visual and action thinking, and he becomes capable of directing these earlier and of realizing them sooner than he masters the operations of his verbal thinking. Piaget assumes that it would be no exaggeration to say that because logical thinking does not exist before the age of seven or eight but appears at the age of seven or eight only on the plane of concrete thinking, the child continues to be at the prelogical stage of development on the plane of verbal thinking.

In order for the child to approach logical thinking, an exceptionally interesting psychological mechanism, which Piaget discovered in his studies, is needed. Logical thinking becomes possible only when the child masters his thinking operations, subjects them to himself, begins to control and direct them. According to Piaget's opinion, it is incorrect to equate all thinking without exception to logical thinking. The latter is distinguished by its substantially new character in comparison with other forms of thinking. Piaget says that this is man's experience of controlling himself as a thinking being, experience similar to what a man exercises over himself in controlling his moral behavior. Consequently, this is an effort to realize one's own operations and not just their result, and to establish whether they agree with each other or are in opposition to each other. In this respect, logical thinking is different from all other forms of thinking. Thinking in the ordinary sense is the perception of certain realities and realizing these realities, but, according to Piaget, logical thinking presumes the realization and control of the construction mechanism itself. Thus, logical thinking is characterized most of all by mastery and control. In this sense, Piaget compares mental experience with logical experience in the following way: the need of results of our mental experience is the need of facts. Need resulting from logical experience is mandatory for the operations to agree with each other. This necessity is moral, emanating from the obligation to remain true to oneself. For this reason, the thinking of the child age 8 to 12 exhibits a dual character.

Thinking is connected with actual reality, with direct observation; logical, formal-logical thinking is not yet available to the child. At approximately 11–12 years, on the other hand, the child's method of thinking comes somewhat closer to the thinking of the adult or, in any case, to that of the uneducated adult. Only by the age of 12 does logical thinking appear that assumes an unfailing realization and mastery of thinking operations as such. From the psychological aspect, this is the most essential trait that Piaget identified in the development of logical thinking. He establishes that the new realization is due directly to a social factor and that the incapacity for formal thinking is the result of the child's egocentrism.

At the age of approximately 12, life takes on a new direction, and this brings the child to completely new problems. We see here an exceptionally clear example of how the life around the child elicits ever newer problems that require mental adaptation on his part, how, in the process of solving the problems, the child masters ever newer content of his thinking and how the new content nudges him to the development of new forms.

Better and more graphic evidence of this is the dependence that exists between the development of an argument in a group of children, the need to present evidence and argue, the need to firmly ground and confirm one's own idea, and the development of formal-logical thinking. On the basis of this, Piaget says that specifically owing to the law of shift, the test of the three brothers of Binet-Simon is accessible only to a child age 11, that is, at an age when formal thinking begins. Piaget believes that if this test were performed for the child instead of being told to him, if the personages were presented to him concretely, the child would make no mistakes. But as soon as he begins to consider, he makes mistakes.

Realization of his own operations has a direct and very close relation to language. Piaget notes that this is why speech is such an important factor. It indicates realization. This is why we must study the forms of verbal thinking in the child with such care.

## 12

It remains for us to say something about an essential factor that will explain for us what interferes from the psychological aspect with the development of abstract thinking at this time. Studies have shown that the school-age child realizes his own thinking operations inadequately still, and for this reason he cannot fully master them. He still has little ability for internal observation, for introspection. Piaget's experiments showed this extremely graphically. Only under the pressure of argument and objections does the child begin to try to confirm his idea before the eyes of others and begin to observe his own thinking, that is, look for and differentiate through introspection the motive that drives him and the direction toward which he aims. In trying to confirm his idea in the eyes of others, he begins to confirm it for himself also. In the process of adapting to others, he gets to know himself.

Piaget tries, using special methods, to establish the capacity of the schoolchild for introspection. He assigned the child small problems and when he got an answer, asked: "How did you get this?" or "What did you say to yourself in order to get this?" Most suitable for the experiments were simple arithmetic problems since they make it possible, on the one hand, to trace the path the child took to get the answer and, on the other hand, introspection becomes exceptionally accessible to the child since he can very easily establish the path and trace his thinking.

With the solving of simple arithmetic problems, Piaget studied 50 children ages 7 to 10. He was struck by the difficulty with which the children answered the question as to how they got the answer, regardless of whether it was correct or not. The child was not able to reproduce the path that his thinking took. After reaching a solution, he invents another way. All of this occurs as the child solved the problem in the same way that we solve an empirical problem by manipulation, that is, realizing every result, but not directing or controlling separate operations, and what is most important, not picking up the whole consequence of our thinking with the help of introspection.

The child seemed not to realize his own thoughts or, in any case, seemed incapable of observing them. Let us recall a single example. The child was asked: "When will it be 5 minutes sooner than 50 minutes?" He answered: "In 45 minutes." This showed that the child understood "5 minutes sooner" as "sooner by 5 minutes." When he was asked how he got this result, the child could neither describe the course of his thought, nor even say that he took 5 from 50. He answered: "I looked for it" or "I found 45." If he was asked further how he found it, if they insisted that he describe how he was thinking, the child presented another and some kind of new operation, completely arbitrary, and applied earlier to the response, "45." For example, one boy answered: "I took 10, 10, 10, and 10 and added 5."

Here we have direct evidence of the fact that the child still does not realize his internal operations and consequently, is not capable of controlling them, and this is the source of his incapacity for logical thinking. Introspection, perceiving one's own internal processes, is, therefore, a necessary factor for mastering them.

Let us remember that the whole mechanism of controlling and mastering behavior, beginning with propriocentric irritations that arise with any kind of movement and ending with introspection, is based on self-perception, on reflection on one's own processes of behavior. This is why the development of introspection is such an important step in the development of logical thinking, and logical thinking is certainly conscious and at the same time it is thinking dependent on introspection. But introspection itself develops late and mainly under the influence of social factors, under the influence of the problems that life puts before the child, under the influence of inability to solve problems of increasing complexity.

# 13

We must not in the least be surprised that the schoolchild, seemingly externally managing to deal with devices of logical thinking, nevertheless has not yet mastered logic in the true sense of that word. Here, we observe an extremely interesting parallel to the general law of child development: as a rule, the child always masters external forms earlier than the internal structure of any mental operation. The child begins to count long before he understands what counting is and he applies it intelligently. In speech, the child has such conjunctions as "because," "if" and "although" long before the realization of causality, conditionality, or opposition appears in his thinking. Just as grammatical development in children's speech precedes the development of logical categories corresponding to these language structures, the mastery of external forms of logical thinking, especially as applied to external concrete situations in the process of visual and action thinking, precedes internal mastery of logic. For example, Piaget established in special studies that conjunctions expressing opposition were not completely understood by children be fore the age of 11–12, whereas they appear in children's speech extremely early. Moreover, in some completely concrete situations, the child uses them extremely early and properly.

Special study showed that conjunctions such as "although," "regardless of," "even if," etc. are acquired by the child in their true meaning quite late. A study of sentences requiring completion after these conjunctions showed a positive result on the average in 96% of schoolgirls age 13.

Using a method corresponding to Piaget's, A. N. Leont'ev also developed sentences that the child had to finish after appropriate conjunctions expressing causal relation, opposing relations, etc. The children were given 16 tasks to do.

We will present quantitative data on the study of one group of schoolchildren. The data show that only in class IV did the child finally master the logical categories and relations corresponding to the conjunctions "because" and "although." Thus, in class IV in the school studied; on the average 77.7% of the sentences that included "because" and "although" were logically correctly completed.

As is known, solving any problem is considered feasible for one age or another when 75% of the children solve the problem. True, the children in the group studied ranged in age from 11 to 15. Their average age was between 12 and 13. As we can see, only at this age does the average child finally master relations of causality and opposition in completely concrete situations.

The range of these data is extremely interesting. The minimum number of solutions observed in the children in this group was 20% and the maximum, 100%. Separate examples of unsuccessful solutions show to what degree the child approaches a logical form in the guise of ideas syncretically close to the unsuccessful solutions. Thus, a child who solved 55% of the problems wrote: "Kolya decided to go to the theater because although he did not have any money"; "If an elephant is stuck with a needle it will not hurt him although it hurts all animals because they don't cry"; "The cart fell and broke although they will rebuild it"; "After the bell rang, everyone went to assembly because although there was a meeting." Another child who did 20% of the problems wrote: "If an elephant is stuck with a needle, it will not hurt him although his skin is thick"; "The cart fell and broke although not the whole thing." A child who did 25% of the problems wrote: "Kolya decided to go the theater because he had money"; "The pilot flew an airplane and fell although he did not have enough gas"; "A boy in Class III still counts poorly because he cannot count"; "When you cut your finger, it hurts because you cut it"; "The cart fell and broke although it was broken," etc. A child who did 20% of the problems wrote: "The cart fell and broke although its wheel did not break"; "If an elephant is stuck with a needle, it will not hurt him although he has a thick skin," etc.

From these examples, we see to what degree the child associatively, syncretically, according to impression, matches two ideas that are actually connected: the thick skin of the elephant and the painlessness of the prick and the broken wheel and the breakdown of the cart. But the child finds it difficult to qualify the relation of the two ideas as a logical relation. His "because" and "although" alternate. Frequently both "because" and "although" occur in the same sentence, as the examples above indicate.


# 14

Using a concrete example, we would like to show the characteristic of thinking during the primary school age that is a holdover of the deficiencies of the very young child's thinking which also separates his thinking from the thinking of the adolescent. We have in mind verbal syncretism, a trait that marks the thinking of the schoolchild as described by Piaget. As syncretism, Piaget understands the undifferentiated combination of the most varied impressions that the child takes in simultaneously that comprise the initial nucleus of his perception. For example, when a five-year-old is asked why the sun does not fall, the child responds: "Because it is yellow"; "Why is the sun hot?" "Because it is high" or "Because there are clouds around it." All of these impressions simultaneously perceived by the child are merged into a single syncretic image, and for the child, these initial syncretic connections take the place of developed and differentiated temporal and spatial, causal and logical connections and relations.

The child of primary school age, as we have already said, gradually overcame syncretism in the area of visual and practical thinking but transferred this characteristic to the area of abstract of verbal thinking. To study this characteristic, Piaget presented 10 proverbs and 12 sentences to schoolchildren ages 8 to 11. The child had to select a sentence for each proverb that expressed the same idea as the proverb but in other words. Two sentences of the 12 had no relation in meaning to the proverbs and the child was to remove them. It became clear that the children correlated the proverbs and sentences on the basis not of the objective connection of ideas, not according to the abstract meaning they contained, but according to the syncretic, graphic, or verbal connection. The child matched two different ideas if they had only some kind of common graphic factor, and he constructed a new syncretic pattern in which both ideas were included. Thus for the proverb, "The cat is away and mice are dancing," a child age 8 years 8 months selected the sentence, "Some people bustle a lot, but do nothing." The child understood each of these expressions if they were presented separately, but here he responded as if they meant the same thing. "Why do these sentences mean the same thing?" "Because there are almost the same words." "What does this sentence mean, 'Some people . . .'?" "It means that some people bustle a lot, but then they can't do anything—they are a little tired. There are some people who bustle; and it doesn't make any difference, like cats when they chase chickens and birds.

Then they rest in the shade and sleep. There are also a lot of people who run around a lot and then when they can't run any more, they lie down."

Instead of approaching and generalizing the two ideas according to the objective meaning, the child assimilates or merges them into a syncretic image misrepresenting the objective meaning of both sentences.

Under the direction of A. N. Leont'ev, our colleagues conducted a series of systematic studies involving level I schools for normal children and for mentally retarded children. The studies showed that verbal syncretism when studied under special experimental conditions actually is manifested as a characteristic of children's thinking over the whole course of school age. Leont'ev modified Piaget's test: the sentences presented in the test contained some traps—common words or common images with the proverbs to which they referred in their meaning. Because of this, in the experiment we obtained some seemingly condensed data that show extremely exaggerated expression of the verbal syncretism of the schoolchild. We succeeded in establishing an exceptionally interesting point: verbal syncretism appears in the child only because this test is especially difficult for children's thinking. Piaget indicated that the test is meant for 11 to 16-year-olds, that is, essentially it is feasible only for the adolescent. But specifically by applying it at an earlier age, we were able to produce a genetic section of the intellect in the process of solving the same problem and to consider the new element that appears in the intellect when solving similar problems. The difficulty of the proposed test is that it requires abstract thinking in a concrete form.

If we had given the schoolchild similar problems, but separately for matching sentences concrete in meaning and situations abstract in meaning, he would be able to solve both, as comparative studies have shown. But here the difficulty is that both the proverb and the sentence are constructed graphically, concretely; however, the connection or relation that must be established between the one and the other is abstract. The proverb must be understood symbolically; the symbolic attribution of an idea to another concrete content requires a complex merging of abstract and concrete thinking that is feasible only for the adolescent.

We must say that these experimental data must not be generalized, regarded as absolute and transferred to all thinking of the schoolchild. It would be absurd to maintain that a schoolchild is not capable of matching two ideas or seeing an identical meaning in two different verbal expressions except when guided by the graphic sense of the one and the other. Only under special experimental conditions, by means of a trap, only with especially difficult merging of abstract-concrete thinking does this characteristic appear as a dominant trait of thinking.

Mentally retarded children in the transitional age continue to give the same matches that the normal schoolchild gives at the earliest school age.

Let us give some examples. Thus, the child of 13 (I*–10 years of age) who matched the proverb, "A thread from his village is a shirt to the naked" with the sentence, "Don't try to be a tailor if you never held a thread in your hands" explained this by the fact that thread appears in both. To the proverb, "Don't sit in a sleigh that isn't yours," he matched the sentence, "In the winter people ride in sleighs and in the summer, in carts" and explained it: "Because in the winter people sled and there are sleighs here."

---

* I—Mental age.—Editor's note.

Frequently the child in his justification explains not the process of matching but some single phrase separately. It is very typical for the child to understand correctly each sentence taken separately, but to have great difficulty in understanding the relation between them. Obviously, the graphic thinking that continues to be dominant in the verbal intellect is not suited to establishing relationship. For example, for the proverb, "Not all that glitters is gold," a child of 13 years 10 months selected the sentence, "Gold is heavier than iron," explaining: "Gold glitters, but iron doesn't." For the proverb, "A thread from his village is a shirt to the naked," a child of 12 selected the sentence, "One should not postpone things," explaining: "Because if he doesn't have a shirt, he must not postpone, but must hurry and make one." For the proverb, "Strike while the iron is hot," a child of 13 years 5 months selected the sentence, "A blacksmith who works without hurrying frequently does more work than one who hurries. That's what they say about the blacksmith." The common elements of the subject, the common elements of the images are enough for matching the two sentences that differ in meaning, that state opposing ideas and are in contradiction to each other: one maintains it is necessary to hurry while the other, that it isn't necessary to hurry. The child identifies the one with the other without noticing the cryptic contradiction, being guided exclusively by the common image of the blacksmith which makes them similar.

We see that the difficulties in establishing relations, the insensitivity to contra diction, syncretic matching not according to objective, but according to subjective connections are typical of the verbal thinking of the schoolchild just as visual thinking is of the preschooler. Frequently such associative matching has a simple justification: "Because here and there we are talking about gold"; "Here and there about the sleigh." For the proverb, "The more quietly you go, the farther you'll get," the same child selected the sentence, "A job that is hard for one person to do can be easily done by group effort," explaining: "It's hard for one to do it, but a horse is one. It's hard for it—we have to ride more quietly."

For the proverb, "The more quietly you go, the farther you'll get," a child age 13 years 9 months selected the sentence, "In the winter we ride in sleighs and in the summer, in a cart," explaining: "It's easier for a horse to pull a sleigh and without hurrying, it goes fast." The same child was a good example of how thinking overcomes contradiction, combining different factors of contradictory statements. Matching the proverb we remember [Strike while the iron is hot.] to a sentence pertaining to a blacksmith, the child includes both points of the contradiction in a syncretic pattern and explains: "The blacksmith who works without hurrying and the hotter the iron, the work goes better."

For the proverb, "In for a little, in for a lot," a child of 13 years, 5 months selected the sentence on the blacksmith and explained: "Maybe the horse had a loose shoe and the blacksmith will fix it." Here we see very clearly a fact noted by Piaget that in matching ideas, a child does not distinguish logical justification from factual. Having seen the factual connection between the blacksmith, riding, and the horse, the child is satisfied with this and his thought goes no further. Frequently, the child matches ideas that seem to us to have absolutely no connection to each other. The unique relation appears that Blonsky termed syncretism of incoherent connectedness in children's thinking.

For example, for the proverb, "Don't sit in a sleigh that isn't yours," a child of 14 years 7 months selects the sentence, "If you already got somewhere, then it's too late to turn back from half-way there," explaining: "If you sit in a sleigh that isn't yours, then the owner can throw you out when you're half-way there." Frequently in such cases, the sense of the sentence is twisted to mean the opposite. The child does not feel constrained by the given premises and changes these in order to adapt them to the conclusion.

We will limit ourselves to the following two examples. To the proverb, "Not all that glitters is gold," a child of 13 years 6 months selected the sentence: "Gold is heavier than iron," explaining: "It isn't just gold that glitters, iron does too." Or for the proverb, "A thread from his village is a shirt to the naked," he selected the sentence: "Don't take up trade as a tailor if you have never held a thread in your hands," explaining: "If you didn't pick up a needle, then you must pick it up."

The examples presented, as we have already said, characterize the thinking of a retarded child. Here we see only the manifestation of those characteristics that persist in a cryptic form in the normal schoolchild also at an earlier stage of development.

In this research, A. N. Leont'ev came across a most important fact: when the child is asked to explain why he matches a given proverb with a given sentence, the child frequently reconsiders his decision. The need to justify the match, to express in words and set out the course of his judgment for another leads to completely different results.

When the child, having matched two sentences syncretically, comes to explaining it aloud, he notices his mistake and begins to give a correct response. Observations showed that the child's justification is not simply a representation in words of what he has done—it represents the whole process of the child's thinking on new bases. Speech is never simply attached as a parallel series, it always represents a process.

In order to confirm this, we undertook a special study in which the child was given two pages of tasks constructed according to the same principle, but with different material. In the first instance, the child, in matching a proverb with a sentence, thinks for himself, depending on processes of internal speech; in the second, he is required to think and reason aloud. As we might have expected, the study showed that between the two methods, thinking to oneself and thinking aloud, there is a great difference for the schoolchild. The child matching sentences syncretically while thinking to himself, begins to match similar proverbs according to an objective connection as soon as he makes the transition to explaining it aloud. We will not stop to give examples. We will only say that the whole process of solving changes its character strikingly as soon as the child makes the transition from internal to external speech (A. N. Leont'ev and A. Shein).

In school-age pedology, we tried to establish that internal speech is generally developed only at the beginning of school age. It is a young, weak, unstable form not yet fully functional. For this reason the discrepancy between internal and external speech of the schoolchild is the most characteristic feature of his thinking. In order to think, the schoolchild must speak aloud and to another. We know that external speech, serving as a means of communication, is socialized earlier in the child than internal speech, which he has not yet mastered.

We have already presented the opinion of Piaget on the fact that the child has not yet mastered his own processes of thinking and become conscious of them. A controversy, the need to justify, to prove, to argue—this is one of the basic factors in the development of logical thinking. For this reason, socialized speech is also more intellectual, more logical.

Thus, we see that internal speech does not appear during school age simply as the spoken word transferred inward, ingrown, and having lost its external part. We could not give a more false definition of internal thinking than in that certain formula: "Thought is speech minus the sound." From the fact of divergence between internal and external speech in the schoolchild, we see the degree to which internal and external speech is formed at that age on different bases, how internal speech still retains features of egocentric thinking and moves on a plane of syncretic matching of ideas, and external speech is already quite socialized, recognized, and directed in order to move along a logical plane.

This study had already been conducted when it became clear to us that, strictly speaking, we approached a fact long known in school practice from the other end. Let us recall the proven device of all schoolteachers who make pupils who solve a problem incorrectly solve it aloud. The pupil, in solving this same problem to himself, gives an absurd answer. When he is made to solve the problem aloud, the teacher teaches him to be conscious of his own operations, to follow their course, to correct it sequentially, and to control the course of his thoughts. We might say that in making the child solve the same problem aloud, the teacher transfers the child's thinking from the syncretic plane to the logical plane.

Let us recall Piaget's observation, which we cited, about the relative weakness of introspection that the child exhibits in solving arithmetic problems. We will remember that the child solving a simple arithmetic problem either correctly or incorrectly often cannot say how he solved the problem, which operations he used—up to this point he is not consciousness of the course of his own thinking and does not correct it. In the same way, it is often hard to say why it is difficult to remember one event or another.

At this stage, the child's thinking has an involuntary character. Absence of arbitrariness and of consciousness of his own thinking operations is also exactly the psychological equivalent of absence of logical thinking. As research shows, specifically with the end of the initial school age, the child begins to understand properly and be conscious of his own operations that he carries out with the help of words and the meaning of the word as a certain sign or an auxiliary means for thinking. Before this time, as Piaget's research showed, the child continues to remain at the stage of nominal realism, considering the word as one property among a number of the properties of the object.

Not understanding the arbitrariness of verbal meaning, the child does not distinguish its role in the process of thinking from that of the object, from that of the meaning that is grasped with the help of that word. To the question, "Why is the sun called the sun?" an 11-year-old boy responds: "For no reason. It's a name." "And the moon?" "For no reason too." Any kind of names can be given. Such answers appear only at age 11–12. Before that, the child does not recognize the difference between the name and the thing named and tries to base one name or another on the properties of the thing they represent.

The unconsciousness of one's own operations and the role of the word is retained in the primitive adolescent even at the stage of sexual maturity. We cite several examples from the research of Golyakhovskaya on explaining some representations and the perception of pictures in Kazakh children. A girl of 14, daughter of a poor peasant, is illiterate. The question: "What is a dog?" The answer: "It's not a man, it's unclean, not for eating. And this is why it's not a man, it's unclean and is called a dog." A girl of 14, daughter of a peasant of average means, is slightly literate. Question: "What is a sparrow?" Answer: "Something that flies, with wings. Because it's small, we call it a sparrow. In Kazakh language, it's called an animal." Question: "What is a rabbit?" Answer: 'An animal. Since it's white and small, we call it a rabbit." Question: "What is a dog?" Answer: "It's an animal too. Since it's unclean, and not for eating, we call it a dog."

A boy of 12, son of a rich landowner, semi-literate. Question: "What is a rock?" Answer: "It comes out of the ground as a rock by nature. That's what we call a rock." Question: "What is the steppe?" Answer: "What was created in the beginning. Of course, the steppe was created. Then we called it the steppe." Question: "What is sand?" Answer: "From the very beginning sand was formed from under the earth. Then we called it sand." Question: "What is a dog?" Answer: "From the very beginning there was a dog and now we call it a dog." Question: "What is a marmot?" Answer: "It's a special animal. From the very beginning it was made a marmot. Then he started to dig a den and began to live there. How do I know this? There was some kind of single marmot and he had children. I concluded that he was created a marmot."

Here the characteristic of thinking that the word is considered as an attribute of the thing, as one of the properties of the thing, is clearly evident. Only with progressing socialization of the child's thinking does intellectualization occur. Being conscious of his own and others' thoughts in the process of verbal communication, the child begins to be conscious of his own thoughts and to direct their course. Progressing socialization of internal speech and progressing socialization of thinking are the basic factors in the development of logical thinking during the transitional age, the basic and central fact of all changes that occur in the adolescent's intellect.

## 15

Thus, we see that only concrete thinking of the schoolchild is logical thinking in the true sense of the word, but on the plane of verbal thinking, abstract thinking, the schoolchild is still susceptible to syncretism, is insensitive to contradictions, is not capable of perceiving relations and uses transduction, that is, conclusion from the particular to the particular, as a basic device of thought.

Piaget maintains that the whole structure of children's thinking up to age 7 or 8, and even to a certain extent until deduction in the true sense of the word appears at the age of 11 or 12, can be explained by the fact that the child thinks of particular or special cases and does not establish common relations among them. Piaget demonstrated that this characteristic of children's thinking, which Stern termed transduction when applied to an early age, was retained on the plane of abstract thinking by the schoolchild who had not yet finally mastered the relation of the general to the particular.

As we have said, underdevelopment of logical thinking consists of the child not being conscious of his own process of thinking, not having mastered it. Piaget says that introspection is actually one of the types of consciousness or more precisely, it is consciousness to the second degree. If the thought of the child did not meet with the thoughts of others and did not elicit adaptation of his own thoughts to the thoughts of others, the child would never become conscious of himself. Logical confirmation of any judgment occurs on a completely different plane than the formulation of that judgment. While judgment may be unconscious and may arise from preceding experience, logical confirmation arises from contemplation and searching, in short—it requires a certain constructive self-observation of one's own thoughts and it requires thinking which alone is capable of meeting logical requirements as Piaget assumes.

Applying the conclusions of his research to the formation of concepts, Piaget establishes that up to the age of 11 or 12, a child is not capable of giving an exhaustive definition of concepts. He always makes judgments from some concrete, direct, and egocentric point of view, not yet having mastered the relation of the general to the particular. The concepts of the school-age child include a certain generalization and uniting of various traits, but the generalization is still not realized by the child himself and he does not know the basis for his concept. The absence of a logical hierarchy and synthesis between various elements of one and the same concept is what characterizes the child's concept.

In these equivalents, children's concepts still retain a trace of what Piaget calls serial position, that is, an insufficient synthesis of a number of traits. In his opinion, children's concepts are a serial position, but not a synthesis, that is, a unity related to the unity in which various elements merge in the syncretic image—a subjective unity. From this, in the process of being developed and used, children's concepts display serious contradictions. These are concepts-aggregates, as Piaget terms them. They continue to dominate in the determinations of the child and are evidence that the child has not yet mastered the hierarchy and synthesis of elements contained in the concepts and does not maintain in the field of his attention all of the traits in their entirety, operating with one, then with another of these traits. According to Piaget, the child's concepts resemble a metallic ball that attaches sequentially and randomly to five or six electromagnets and jumps randomly from one to another.

More simply, synthesis and hierarchy of elements that are dominant in a complex concept and the relations between elements comprising the essence of the concept are still inaccessible to the child regardless of the fact that these elements and their combination are already accessible to him. This is manifested in operations with concepts. Piaget shows that the child is not capable of systematic logical addition and logical multiplication. As the research of Piaget shows, the child is not capable of simultaneously fixing his attention on a series of traits that are part of a complex single concept.

In the field of his attention, these traits alternate, and each time his concept is diminished from some one aspect. The hierarchy of concepts is not accessible to him, and for this reason, although his concepts externally resemble our concepts, in essence they are only pseudo concepts. This is the main goal of all of our research in which we are trying to show that the thinking of the child of school age is at a different genetic stage than the thinking of the adolescent and that the formation of concepts appears only during the transitional age.

Subsequently we will return to this central point, but now we must note one of the ideas that Piaget expressed in passing, an idea that, in our opinion, contains the key to understanding all the characteristics of children's thinking that Piaget established. He said that the child never enters into genuine contact with things because he does not work.[58] This connection of the development of higher forms of thinking, particularly thinking in concepts, with work seems to us to be central and basic, capable of disclosing the characteristics of children's thinking and that which is new, which appears in the thinking of the adolescent.

We will be able to return to this problem in one of the following chapters of our course. Now we would like to consider the problem that seems to us to be closely linked to the forms of merging of abstract and concrete thinking in the adolescent.

## 16

In a special study, Graucob considers the formal characteristics of thinking and language during the transitional age. He bases his study on the correct position that not only the scope and content, but also the formal character of thinking at this age is closely connected with the general structure of the personality of the adolescent. This work draws our attention along two lines. First, it shows the same idea that we tried to defend above, but from a different aspect. We tried to show that neither the preschool child nor the schoolchild is capable of thinking in concepts and that, consequently, it appears no earlier than during the transitional age. But a number of studies show that during the transitional age, this form of logical, abstract thinking in concepts is still not the dominant form, but is flesh and young and only just developed and not yet secure.

Wholly conscious and verbally formulated thinking is not at all the dominant form of thinking in the adolescent. As Graucob correctly notes, most often we find forms of thought in which only the results are distinctly formulated in concepts while the processes leading to those results are not consciously realized. In his graphic expression, the thinking of the adolescent at this time resembles a mountain chain, the peaks of which sparkle in the morning light while everything else is hid den in darkness. The thinking is stepwise and if it is reproduced precisely, it sometimes leaves the impression of being disconnected and without an adequate basis.

It is understood that we are speaking only of spontaneous thinking of the adolescent. His thinking connected with school is in a much more systematized and deliberate form.

Second, the new form of thinking during the transitional age is a merging of abstract and concrete thinking—the appearance of metaphors, words used with a figurative meaning. Graucob correctly notes that the thinking of the adolescent still flows partially in a pre-speech form. True, this pre-speech thinking is not directed mainly toward single, visually present objects and toward external, evoked, eidetic, visual images as it is in the child. It differs from the visual thinking of the child, but it seems to us that the author does not formulate the problem quite correctly when he considers this thinking as a type of metaphysical thinking that in the formal respect is similar to the contemplation of mystics and metaphysicians.

We think that pre-speech and some post-speech thinking frequently does not occur entirely with the participation of speech; nevertheless, as we will try to show in a subsequent chapter, it is done on the basis of speech. A. A. Potebnya compares thought without words to a chess game without looking at the board. He says that in a similar way it is possible to think without words, being limited only to more or less clear pointing to them or directly at the content of what is being thought, and such thinking is found much more frequently (for example, in sciences that partially replace words with formulas) specifically as a result of its greater importance and in relation to many aspects of human life. Potebnya adds that we must not, however, forget that knowing how to think humanly but without words is possible only through words and that deaf-mutes without speaking teachers (or trained speakers) would remain almost animals forever.

This reasoning seems to us just about right. To know how to think like a human, but without words is possible only through words.

In the next chapter, we will try to consider in detail the influence that verbal thinking has on visual and concrete thinking, radically restructuring these functions on new bases. For this reason, we think the author correctly indicates that the combination of speech and thinking during the transitional age is much more firm than in the child; this is apparent in the increasing mastery of speech, in enrichment with new concepts, but most of all in the formation of abstract thinking and in the accompanying elimination of eidetic tendencies.

Graucob believes that, except for early childhood, at no stage in human life can one observe with such clarity as in the transitional age that the development of thinking moves forward together with the development of speech; together with verbal formulation of thinking, making newer and sharper distinctions becomes possible. In the expression of Goethe, language in itself is creative.

Investigating the appearance of metaphors and words used in a figurative sense during adolescence, the author quite justifiably indicates that this unique combination of concrete and abstract thinking must be considered as a new achievement of the adolescent. The verbal tissue of the adolescent exhibits a much more complex structure. Connections of coordination and subordination come forward, and this more complex verbal structure is an expression, on the one hand, of increasingly complex but still not fully clarified thinking, and on the other, a means for further development of the intellect.

How does the metaphor or figurative sense of the word differ qualitatively in childhood and in the transitional age? Even in a child's language, there are graphic comparisons that reinforce the tendency of children toward eidetism. But these comparisons do not involve anything abstract. Metaphors in the true sense of the word do not exist for the child. For him, metaphors are an actual matching of impressions. It is not the same for the adolescent. Typical here is a unique relation of the concrete and abstract that is possible only on the basis of highly developed speech.

We see to what degree the usual comparison of the abstract and the concrete is incorrect and how these two forms of thinking actually are not in contradiction but are mutually connected. Graucob says that during adolescence, the abstract is assimilated more easily when it is reflected in some concrete example of a concrete situation. Thus, he says, we come to a seemingly contradictory result that indicates that, regardless of the development of abstract thinking and the gradual disappearance of eidetic contemplation that parallels it, concrete, graphic comparisons in the language of the adolescent increase and reach a peak, after which they begin to decrease, approaching the language of the adult.

The metaphors of the child, the author continues, leave the impression of something objective, natural. In the adolescent, they are the fruit of subjective processing. In the metaphor, objects are matched not organically, but with the aid of the intellect, and metaphors develop not on the basis of synthetic contemplation, but on the basis of a combining introspection. For this reason, the rapprochement of abstract and concrete thinking is the distinguishing trait of the transitional age. Even in lyric poetry, the adolescent is not free of reflection. His fate consists of the fact that where he must be a thinker, he poetizes, and where he performs as a poet, he philosophizes.

Illustrating metaphors in the speech and thinking of the adolescent, Graucob establishes a series of exceptionally unique metaphors in which their original meaning appears as if in inverted form. Remote, abstract concepts must elucidate what is simple, concrete, and close. In these metaphors, the abstract is not elucidated with the help of the concrete, but the concrete is frequently elucidated with the help the abstract.

In the next chapter, we will consider in detail the unique merging of abstract and concrete thinking that is typical for the transitional age. Now we are interested in the fact that factors of the abstract and concrete are contained in the thinking of the adolescent in proportions and qualitative relations that are different from those in the thinking of the schoolchild.

Kroh, noting correctly that the development of thinking is usually underestimated in theories of the transitional age, establishes the fact, decisive for elucidating the development of intellect, that with the end of [primary] school begins the process of differentiation in thinking influenced by external causes.

Never does the influence of the environment on the development of thinking acquire such great significance as specifically at the transitional age. Then as the intellect develops, the city and the village, the boy and the girl, children of various social and class levels are distinguished more and more. Obviously, the process of development of thinking at this age is directly affected by social factors. In this we see the direct confirmation of the fact that the adolescent's main successes in the development of thinking are in the form of cultural development of thinking.

Not biological development of the intellect, but mastery of historically developed synthetic forms of thinking comprises the principal content at this age. This is why the series of monographs that Kroh cites show that the process of intellectual maturation in different social strata presents a very different picture. External factors that form intellectual development assume a decisive significance in the transitional age: the intellect acquires methods of action that are the product of socialization of thinking and not of its biological evolution. Kroh, as we shall see, establishes that subjective and visual images begin to fall away at approximately age 15–16. In the author's opinion, the main reason for this is the adolescent's development of language, socialization of his speech, and development of abstract thinking. The visual bases for speech diminish. Conceptions that are the basis for words lose their specific meaning. In the child, the visual experience determines the content and frequently also the form of the child's expression. In the adult, speech depends much more on its own bases. In words-concepts, it has its material in grammar and syntax, its normal rules of formulation. Language more and more separates from visual conceptions and becomes more autonomous to a significant degree. This process of automatization of speech occurs predominantly during the transitional age, as Kroh assumes.

E. Jaensch, the author of studies on eidetism, correctly indicates that during historical human development also, in the transition from primitive to developed thinking, speech played a decisive role as a means of liberation from visual images.

Remarkable in this respect is the fact, pointed out by Kroh, that in deaf-mute children eidetic images can be found even when they have almost disappeared in their peers. This is indisputable evidence that elimination of eidetic images is influenced by the development of speech.

Connected with this is another trait of thinking during the transitional age—the transfer of attention of the adolescent to his own internal life and transition from the concrete to the abstract. Gradual introduction of abstraction into the thinking of the adolescent is the central factor in the development of the intellect during the transitional age. However, as Kroh points out correctly, isolating separate properties in a complex of things is already available to the young child. While we usually understand attention that isolates as abstraction, we must mention abstraction that isolates, which is also available to animals; to say that this kind of abstraction is an acquisition of the transitional age is not correct.

Abstraction that generalizes must be distinguished from abstraction that isolates. It arises when the child subordinates a number of concrete objects to one general concept. But the child forms and uses even this kind of concept extremely early. Obviously this does not comprise what is new, what engages the thinking of the adolescent. Abstraction that generalizes leads the child to thinking of contents that are not accessible to visual perception. When people say that the adolescent first involves the abstract world for himself, then the statement, in the words of Kroh, must not be understood in the sense that this form of abstraction becomes accessible only at this age.

It is much more important to emphasize something else: as a rule, comprehended mutual relations of similar abstract concepts become accessible to the adolescent. Not so much do separate abstract traits in themselves become accessible at this age as do connections, relations, and interdependencies of traits. The adolescent establishes relations between concepts. By means of judgments, he finds new concepts.

It seems to us that Kroh's mistake was his opinion that the use of proverbs and abstract expressions presented in a visual form is a transitional stage from concrete to abstract thinking. Kroh believes that this form usually was not noted by investigators and, moreover, that it is an end stage of the development of abstract thinking for many people.

As we have said and as we will try to explain in detail subsequently, merging of the abstract and the concrete is not accessible to the child and is not at all a transition from concrete to abstract thinking, but a unique form of changing concrete thinking, a form that already appears on a base of the abstract similarly, as Potebnya says, to knowing how to think without words is determined in the last analysis by the word. The same thing pertains also to logical conclusions.

Although, as Deuchler pointed out, these conclusions are evident as early as in the four-year-old, they are still based completely on a visual or graphic combination of premises and their content. The logical requirement for the result obtained, like the whole path of logical consideration, is still not accessible to the child. The normal child becomes capable of these operations only during the period of sexual maturation. Such an intelligent understanding of logical-grammatical thinking occurs only at that time. In the child, mastery of grammar is based mainly on the feeling for language, on the habits of speech, on the formation of analogies. Kroh justifiably connects these successes in the adolescent's thinking with his successes in the area of mathematics. He asserts that the comprehended course of evidence and independent discovery of mathematical laws and conditions are actually possible only during the transitional age. A serious change in the content of thinking of the adolescent is coupled with these features of formal thinking. The task of self-knowledge, prepared by understanding other people and mastering mental categories, brings the adolescent to directing his attention more and more toward the aspect of external life. For the adolescent, separating the internal from the external world is a necessity related to the needs and the tasks with which development confronts him. Kroh believes that the task of creating a life plan requires greater separation of the essential from the nonessential as time goes on. Without a logical evaluation, this can not be done. For this reason, it is understandable that development of higher forms of intellectual activity is so very important during the transitional age. Genuine, correlated, abstract thinking becomes all the more crucial.

It does not arise at once of course. The child knew previously how to perceive data visually and the relatively complex connection of things, meanings, actions. He was in a state to understand and apply abstractions of various kinds. The transitional age brings with it only the capability of an intelligent correlation of abstract concepts and general content. Real logical capabilities develop together with this. Kroh repeats that the child's environment has a decisive influence over this thinking. According to the author's observations, in a peasant environment, we frequently encounter adults who have not gone beyond the intellectual level of a schoolchild. Over their whole life, their thinking has not moved beyond the sphere of the visual, never made the transition from specifically logical thinking to its abstract forms.

Since soon after finishing school, the adolescent enters the kind of environment in which higher forms of thinking have not been mastered, it is natural that he himself does not reach a higher degree of development, although he displays great ability. It cannot be more decisively confirmed that the formation of concepts is the product of the cultural development of the intellect and depends in the last analysis on the environment.

In various spheres of practical life there are completely different methods of applying intellectual activity which, on the one hand, are determined by the prevailing structure of that sphere of life and on the other, by characteristics of the individual himself.

Kroh's most important conclusion, it seems to us, is the conclusion regarding the central significance of intellectual development for the whole transitional age. The intellect plays a decisive role for the adolescent. Even in selecting one profession or another, processes of a typical intellectual nature are applied to a large degree. Together with E. Lau (1925), Kroh maintains that specifically in the adolescent, the influence of the intellect on will is exceptionally strong. Considered and conscious decisions play a much greater role in his whole development than does the influence of the usually overrated increasing emotionality.

In the next chapter, we will try to elucidate in detail the central significance of intellectual development and its leading role.

Using the method of genetic sections and their comparative study, we were able to establish not only what is lacking during the initial school age, but also a number of mechanisms that aid in developing the central function of the whole age, the formation of concepts.

We saw what a decisive role in this process is played by introspection, realizing one's own processes of behavior and controlling them, transfer of forms of behavior arising in the group life of the adolescent to the internal sphere of the personality, and the gradual growing into new methods of behavior, transferring inward a number of external mechanisms and socialization of internal speech and, finally, work as a central factor of all intellectual development.

Further, we can establish the significance the acquisition of a new function—the formation of concepts—has for all the thinking of the adolescent. We have shown that if objects are represented in thinking in an immovable and isolated form, then a concept actually combines the content of the thinking. However, if we assume that an object is disclosed in connections and mediations, in relations with the rest of reality and in motion, we must conclude that thinking that has concepts at its disposal begins to master the essence of the object and discloses its connections and relations with the other object and begins for the first time to combine and correlate various elements of experience, and then the complicated and comprehended picture of the world as a whole is disclosed.

The concept of number may serve as a simpler example of the changes that concept introduces into the thinking of the adolescent.

## 17

We would like to use a graphic example to show what new material thinking in concepts introduces into the recognition of reality in comparison with concrete or visual thinking. To do this, we need only compare the concept of number that the educated person usually has with the idea of number based on direct perception of number that prevails among primitive peoples. Just as in a very young child, the perception of number is based on number images, on concrete perception of form and size of a given group of objects. With transition to thinking in concepts, the child is liberated from purely concrete numerical thinking. In place of a number image, a number concept appears. If we compare the concept of number with a number image, at first glance it may seem to justify premises of formal logic relative to the extreme poverty in content of the concept in comparison with the riches of the concrete content contained in the image.

Actually, this is not so. The concept not only excludes from its content a number of points proper to the concrete perception, but for the first time, it also discloses in the concrete perception a number of such points that are completely inaccessible to direct perception or contemplation, points that are introduced by thinking and are identified through processing the data of experience and synthesized into a single whole with elements of direct perception.

Thus, all number concepts, for example, the concept "7," are included in a complex number system, occupy a certain place in it, and when this concept is found and processed, then all the complex connections and relations that exist between this concept and the rest of the system of concepts in which it is included are given. The concept not only reflects reality, but also systematizes it, includes data of concrete perception into a complex system of connections and relations, and discloses the connections and relations that are inaccessible to simple comprehension. For this reason many properties of size become clear and perceptible only when we begin to think of them in concepts.*

---

\* In opposition to Kant, Hegel was *essentially* completely correct. Thinking going from the concrete to the abstract does not deviate—if it is *correct . . . from* truth, but approaches it. The abstraction of material, a law of nature, abstraction of *value*, etc., in a word, *all* scientific (correct, serious, not foolish) abstractions reflect nature more deeply, more reliably, more *fully*. From a living contemplation to abstract thinking *and from it to practice*—such is the dialectical path of recognizing *truth*, recognizing objective reality (V. I. Lenin, *Complete Works*, Vol. 29, pp. 152–153).

As a rule, it is pointed out that even a number has some qualitative characteristics. Nine is a square of three, it can be divided by three, it occupies a definite place and can be placed in a definite relation to any other number. All of these are properties of number: its divisibility, its relation to other numbers, its construction from simpler numbers—all this is disclosed only in the concept of number.

Investigators, for example, H. Werner, turn very frequently to number concepts to elucidate the characteristics of primitive thinking; these concepts disclose these characteristics most graphically. M. Wertheimer, when he tries to penetrate primitive thinking using analysis of number images, proceeds in the same way. We have the same, completely satisfactory device available to disclose the reverse qualitative uniqueness of thinking in concepts and to show how concept is infinitely enriched by elements of mediated knowledge of the subject, raising its very content to a new height.

We shall limit ourselves to an analysis of an example that clearly shows what a systematizing and ordering function thinking in concepts fulfills in recognizing reality. If for the school-age child, the word represents a family of things, then for the adolescent, the word represents a concept of things, that is, its essence, laws of its structure, its connection with all other things, and its place in the system of already recognized and ordered reality.

# 18

A number of investigators who use the method of describing a picture to determine the nature of children's visual thinking note the transition to a systematic development of experiment and realization. Piaget indicates the nature of the thinking of the school-age child by the term "serial position," which indicates the weakness of synthesis or combination in the thinking of the child. Just as the child does not simultaneously combine all the traits included in a concept, but thinks alternately of one then another trait as being equivalent to the content of the concept as a whole, precisely so does he not order, not bring into the system the structure of his thoughts, but places them as if in a row, one after another, without combining them.

As Piaget says, in the thinking of the child, logic of action dominates, but not logic of thought. One thought is connected with another, as one movement of the hand elicits another and is connected with it, but not as thoughts are constructed hierarchically subordinate to one main thought. Piaget and R. Rossell recently applied the method of describing pictures to the study of the development of thinking in the child and adolescent. These studies show that only with the beginning of adolescence does the child make the transition from the stage of enumerating separate traits to the stage of interpretation, that is, combining visually perceived material with elements of thinking that the child introduces into the picture on his own. Forms of logical thinking are the basic means for describing pictures. Forms of logical thinking seem to order the material of perceptions. Perceiving, the adolescent begins to think; his perception is turned into concrete thinking and is intellectualized. C. Burns studied concepts in 2000 children, age six to fifteen, using the method of definition. The results of his research are presented in Table 3, which indicates that during this period, the number of purpose-directed and functional definitions decreases by a factor of more than 2.5, yielding to logical definition of concept.

TABLE 3.

| Age, years | Purpose-directed and functional definition of concept, % |
|:---:|:---:|
| 6 | 79 |
| 7 | 63 |
| 8 | 67 |
| 9 | 64 |
| 10 | 57 |
| 11 | 44 |
| 12 | 34 |
| 13 | 38 |
| 14 | 38 |
| 15 | 31 |

M. Vogel (1911) established that the relations the adolescent finds through thinking increase as he approaches the transitional age. Specifically, judgments pertinent to causes and effects increase by more than 11 times with the transition from school age to adolescence. These data are particularly interesting in connection with the pre-causal thinking that Piaget established as a characteristic of the initial school age.

The basis for pre-causal thinking is the egocentric character of the child's intellect, which leads to confusing mechanical causality with psychological causality. According to Piaget, pre-causality is a transitional stage between motivation, the purposeful basis of phenomena, and causal thinking in the true sense of the word. The child frequently confuses the causes of a phenomenon with purpose and, in Piaget's words, it is as if nature were the product or, more accurately, a duplicate of thoughts in which the child tried to find sense and purpose at every moment.

The studies of H. Roloff show that the function of defining a concept increases markedly in the child between ages 10 and 12, the time of the beginning of the transitional age. This is observed in conjunction with the development of logical thinking of the adolescent. We have already cited the opinion of Meumann regarding the late appearance of deduction in the child (approximately age 14). H. Schfissler, disputing the opinion of Meumann, sets the intensification of this process at age 11–12 and 16–17. H. Ormian puts the beginning of formal thinking at about age 11.

No matter what we think of these studies, one thing remains completely clear: in agreement with all of this data, somewhat inconsistent from the external aspect, thinking in concepts and logical thinking develop in the child relatively late: only at the beginning of the transitional age does this development take its principal steps.

E. Monchamps and E. Moritz recently again studied the thinking of the child and the adolescent using description of pictures. In contrast to the usual experiments, which were limited to describing simple pictures accessible to a very young child's understanding, the new studies establish, as the last stage of visual thinking, the stage of precise synthesis that is accessible only to half of adult educated people and which assumes not an average, but a superior intellectual giftedness.

According to these data, the time of sexual maturation was marked by the fact that a typical form of children's thinking at the age that interests us seems to be a partial synthesis, that is, elucidation of the general sense of the picture accessible usually at the sixth stage of development. The same data show to what extent the child's development and his movement along the stages is determined by social-cultural conditions. A comparison between those studying in public schools and those studying in privileged schools discloses substantial differences: whereas 78% of the children from privileged schools reached the sixth stage at the age of 11, approximately the same percentage was reached by those studying in the public schools at the age of 13–14.

The studies of H. Eng (1914), who tried to elucidate the development of concepts using the method of definition, also show that this development has significant success beginning at age 12. By age 14, the number of correct responses increases by a factor of almost four in comparison with the age of ten.

Recently, G. Müller studied the logical capabilities of adolescents using two tests. The adolescents were required to establish the relation between concepts and to find new concepts that are in a certain relation to the given concept. The distribution of the solutions of these problems according to age shows that logical thinking becomes the dominant form in boys at the age of 13 and in girls at the age of 12.

19

In conclusion, it remains to be said that we have spent so much time on the development of thinking because, for the transitional age, we cannot consider it as one of the partial processes of development in a series of other such partial processes. Thinking at this age is not one function in a series of other functions. Development of thinking has a central, key, decisive significance for all the other functions and processes. We cannot express more clearly or tersely the leading role of intellectual development in relation to the whole personality of the adolescent and to all of his mental functions other than to say that acquiring the function of forming concepts is the principal and central link in all the changes that occur in the psychology of the adolescent. All other links in this chain, all other special functions, are intellectualized, reformed, and reconstructed under the influence of these crucial successes that the thinking of the adolescent achieves.

In the following chapter, we will try to show how the lower or elementary functions, being processes that are more primitive, earlier, simpler, and independent of concepts in genetic, functional, and structural relations, are reconstructed on a new basis when influenced by thinking in concepts and how they are included as component parts, as subordinate stages, into new, complex combinations created by thinking on the basis of concepts, and, finally, how, under the influence of thinking, foundations of the personality and world view of the adolescent are laid down.

# 14

# Dynamics and Structure of the Adolescent's Personality

## 1

We are approaching the end of our study. We began with a review of the changes that occur in the structure of the organism and its most important functions during the period of sexual maturation. We were able to trace the complete restructuring of the whole internal and external system of activity of the organism, the radical change in its structure and the new structure of organic activity that is connected with sexual maturation. Tracing many stages, passing from drives to interests, from interests to mental functions, and from these to the content of thinking and to creative imagination, we have seen how the new structure of the adolescent's personality, which differs from the structure of the child's personality, is formed.

Then we considered briefly certain special problems of pedology of the transitional age and were able to trace how the new structure of the personality is manifested in complex, synthetic, vital actions, how the social behavior of the adolescent changes and rises to a higher level, how it arrives internally and externally at one of life's decisive moments—the selection of a vocation or profession, and, finally, how the unique, vital forms, the unique structure of the personality and world view of the adolescent are developed in the three main classes of contemporary society. Many times during our study, we came upon separate elements for constructing a general teaching on the personality of the adolescent. Now it remains for us to correlate what has been said and to try to give a graphic picture of the structure and dynamics of the adolescent's personality.

We deliberately unite these two sections of the study of personality since we believe that traditional pedology of the transitional age has given much attention to purely descriptive representation and study of the adolescent's personality. To do this, it used self-observation, journals, and poetry of adolescents and tried to recreate the structure of the personality on the basis of separate documented experiences. We think that the most plausible path would be the simultaneous study of the adolescent's personality from the aspect of its structure and dynamics. More simply put, in order to answer the question of the unique structure of the personality during the transitional age, it is necessary to determine how this structure develops, how it is constituted, and what the principal laws of its construction and change are. We shall now proceed to do this.

The history of the development of personality can be encompassed by a few basic patterns which have been suggested by all of our foregoing study.

Originally appeared in English as Chapter 5 in *The Collected Works of L.S. Vygotsky, Volume 5: Child Psychology* (Robert W. Rieber, Ed.; Marie J. Hall, Trans.) (pp. 167–184). New York: Kluwer Academic/Plenum Press, 1998.

The first law of the development and structure of higher mental functions which are the basic nucleus of the personality being formed can be called the law of *the transition from direct, innate, natural forms and methods of behavior to mediated, artificial mental functions that develop in the process of cultural development*. This transition during ontogenesis corresponds to the process of the historical development of human behavior, a process, which, as we know, did not consist of acquiring new natural psychophysiological functions, but in a complex combination of elementary functions, in a perfecting of forms and methods of thinking, in the development of new methods of thinking based mainly on speech or on some other system of signs.

The simplest example of the transition from direct to mediated functions may be the transition from involuntary remembering and remembering that is guided by the sign. Primitive man, having first made some kind of external sign in order to remember some event, passed in this way into a new form of memory. He introduced external, artificial means with which he began to manage the process of his own remembering. Study shows that the whole path of historical development of man's behavior consists of a continuous perfecting of such means and of the development of new devices and forms of mastering his own mental operations, and here the internal system of one operation or another also changed and sustained profound changes. We shall not consider the history of behavior in detail. We shall only say that the cultural development of the behavior of the child and the adolescent is basically of the same type.

Thus we see that cultural development of behavior is closely linked to the historical or social development of humanity. This brings us to the second law, which also expresses certain traits common to phylo and ontogenesis. The second law can be formulated thus: considering The History of the Development of Higher Mental Functions that comprise the basic nucleus in the structure of the personality, we find *that the relation between higher mental functions was at one time a concrete relation between people; collective social forms of behavior in the process of development become a method of individual adaptations and forms of behavior and thinking of the personality*. Every complex higher form of behavior discloses specifically this path of development. That which is now united in one person and appears to be a single whole structure of complex higher internal mental functions was at one time made up of separate processes divided among separate persons. Put more simply, higher mental functions arise from collective social forms of behavior.

We might elucidate this basic law with three simple examples. Many authors (J. Baldwin, E. Rignano, and J. Piaget) demonstrated that the logical thinking of children develops in proportion to the way in which argument appears and develops in the children's group.[93] Only in the process of working with other children does the function of the child's logical thinking develop. In a position familiar to us, Piaget says that only cooperation leads to the development of logic in the child. In his work, Piaget was able to trace step by step how in the process of developing cooperation and particularly in connection with the appearance of a real argument, a real discussion, the child is first confronted by the need to form a basis, to prove, confirm, and verify his own idea and the idea of his partner in the discussion. Further, Piaget traced that the argument, the confrontation that arises in a children's group is not only a stimulus for logical thought, but is also the initial form in which thought appears. The dying out of those traits of thinking that were dominant at the early stage of development and are characterized by absence of systematization and connections coincides with the appearance of argument in the children's group. This coincidence is not accidental. It is specifically the development of an argument that leads the child to systematizing his own opinions. P. Janet showed that all deliberation is the result of an internal argument because it is as if a person were repeating to himself the forms and methods of behavior that he applied earlier to others. Piaget concludes that his study fully confirms this point of view.

Thus, we see that the child's logical deliberation is as if an argument transferred to within the personality and, in the process of the child's cultural development, the group form of behavior becomes an internal form of behavior of the personality, the basic method of his thinking. The same might be said of the development of self-control and voluntary direction of one's own actions which develop in the process of children's group games with rules. The child who learns to conform and coordinate his actions with the actions of others, who learns to modify direct impulse and to subordinate his activity to one rule or another of the game, does this initially as a member of a small group within the whole group of playing children. Subordination to the rule, modification of direct impulses, coordination of personal and group actions initially, just like the argument, is a form of behavior that appears among children and only later becomes an individual form of behavior of the child himself.

Finally, in order to avoid multiplying examples, we might point to the central and leading function of cultural development. The fate of this function confirms as clearly as is possible the law of transition from social to individual forms of behavior, which might also be called the law of sociogenesis of higher forms of behavior: speech, being initially the means of communication, the means of association, the means of organization of group behavior, later becomes the basic means of thinking and of all higher mental functions, the basic means of personality formation. The unity of speech as a means of social behavior and as a means of individual thinking cannot be accidental. As we have said above, it indicates the basic fundamental law of the construction of higher mental functions.

As indicated by P. Janet (1930),94 the word was at first a command for others, and then a change in function resulted in separating the word from action and this led to the independent development of the word as a means of command and independent development of action subordinated to the word. At the very beginning the word is connected with action and cannot be separated from it. It is itself only one of the forms of action. This ancient function of the word, which could be called a volitional function, persists to these times. The word is a command. In all its forms, it represents a command and in verbalized behavior, it is always necessary to distinguish the function of command which belongs to the word from the function of subordination. This is a fundamental fact. Specifically because the word fulfilled the function of a command with respect to others, it begins to fulfill the same function with respect to oneself and becomes the basic means for mastering one's own behavior.

This is the source of the volitional function of the word, this is why the word subordinates motor reaction to itself; this is the source of the power of the word over behavior. Behind all of this stands the real function of command. Behind the psychological power of the word over other mental functions stands the former power of the commander and the subordinate. This is the basic idea of Janet's theory. This same general theory may be expressed in the following form: every function in the cultural development of the child appears on the stage twice, in two forms—at first as social, then as psychological; at first as a form of cooperation between people, as a group, an intermental category, then as a means of individual behavior, as an intramental category. This is the general law for the construction of all higher mental functions.

Thus, the structures of higher mental functions represent a cast of collective social relations between people. These structures are nothing other than a transfer into the personality of an inward relation of a social order that constitutes the basis of the social structure of the human personality. The personality is by nature social.

This is why we were able to detect the decisive role that socialization of external and internal speech plays in the process of development of children's thinking. As we have seen, the same process also leads to the development of children's ethics; the laws of construction here are identical to the laws of development of children's logic.

From this point of view, adapting the well-known expression, we might say that the mental nature of man is an aggregate of social relations transferred within and becoming functions of the personality, the dynamic parts of its structure. The transfer inward of external social relations between people is the basis for the structure of the personality, as has long been noted by investigators. K. Marx wrote: "In certain respects man resembles merchandise. Just as he is born without a mirror in his hands and is not a Fichtean philosopher: 'I am I,' man initially sees himself in another person as in a mirror. Only by relating to the man, Paul, as being similar to himself, does the man, Peter, begin to relate to himself as to a man. Also, Paul as such, in all his Paulian corporeality, becomes for him a form of manifestation of the genus 'man'" (K. Marx and E Engels, *Works*, Vol. 23, p. 62).

The third law, connected with the second, may be formulated as the law of *transition of a function from outside inward*.

We understand now why the initial stage of the transfer of social forms of behavior into a system of individual behavior of the personality is necessarily connected with the fact that every higher form of behavior initially has the character of an external operation. In the process of development, the functions of memory and attention are initially constructed as external operations connected with the use of an external sign. And we can understand why. Of course, as we have said, initially, they were a form of group behavior, a form of social connection, but this social connection could not be implemented without the sign, by direct intercourse, and so here the social means becomes the means of individual behavior. For this reason, the sign always appears first as a means of influencing others and only later as a means of affecting oneself. Through others, we become ourselves. From this, we can understand why all internal higher functions were of necessity external. However, in the process of development, every external function is internalized and becomes internal. Having become an individual form of behavior, in the process of a long period of development, it loses the traits of an external operation and is converted into an internal operation.

According to Janet, it is difficult to understand how speech became internal. He believes this to be so difficult a problem that it is the basic problem of thinking and is being solved extremely slowly by people. Eons of evolution were required to implement the transition from external to internal speech, and Janet assumes that if we were to look closely, we would find that even now there are very many people who have not mastered internal speech. Janet calls the idea that internal speech is well developed in all people a great illusion.

We noted the transition to internal speech during childhood in one of the preceding chapters (Vol. 2, pp. 314–331) [Translator's note: this is probably Vol. 1, pp. 71–76 in the current series.] We showed that the child's egocentric speech is a transitional form from external speech to internal, that the child's egocentric speech is speech for himself that fulfills a mental function completely different from that of external speech. In this way, we showed that speech becomes internal mentally sooner than it becomes internal physiologically. Without further attention to the process of transition of speech from external to internal, we can say that this is the common fate of all higher mental functions. We have seen that transition inward is specifically the main content of the development of functions during the transitional age. Through a long process of development, function moves from an external to an internal form, and this process is concluded at this age.

The following point is closely connected to the formation of the internal character of these functions. As we have said repeatedly, the higher mental functions are based on mastery of one's own behavior. We can speak of the formation of the personality only when there is mastery of the person's own behavior. But as a prerequisite, mastery assumes reflection in consciousness, reflection in words of the structure of one's own mental operations because, as we have indicated, freedom in this case also signifies nothing other than recognized necessity. In this respect, we can agree with Janet, who speaks of the metamorphosis of language into will. What is called will is verbal behavior. Without speech, there is no will. Speech enters into volitional action sometimes cryptically and sometimes openly.

Thus, the will, being the basis of the structure of personality, is, in the final analysis, initially a social form of behavior. Janet says that in all voluntary processes there is speech and the will is nothing other than a conversion of speech into implementation, regardless of whether it is for another or for oneself.

The behavior of the individual is identical to social behavior. The higher fundamental law of behavioral psychology is that we conduct ourselves with respect to ourselves just as we conduct ourselves with respect to others. There is social behavior with respect to oneself and if we acquired the function of command with respect to others, applying this function to ourselves is essentially the same process. But subordinating one's actions to one's own authority necessarily requires, as we have already said, a consciousness of these actions as a prerequisite.

We have seen that introspection, consciousness of one's own mental operations, appears relatively late in the child. If we trace the process of development of self-consciousness, we will see that it occurs in the history of development of higher forms of behavior in three basic stages. At first, every higher form of behavior is assimilated by the child exclusively from the external aspect. From the objective aspect, this form of behavior already includes in itself all the elements of the higher functions, but subjectively, for the child himself who has not yet become conscious of it, it is a purely natural, innate method of behavior. It is only due to the fact that other people fill the natural form of behavior with a certain social content, for others rather than for the child himself, that it acquires the significance of a higher function. Finally, in the process of a long development, the child becomes conscious of the structure of this function and begins to control his own internal operations and to direct them.

Using the simplest examples, we can trace the sequence in the development of the child's own functions. Let us take the first pointing gesture of the child. The gesture is nothing other than an unsuccessful grasping movement. The child stretches out his hand toward a distant object and cannot reach it, but his hand remains stretched out toward the object. Here we have a pointing gesture with the objective meaning of a word. The movement of the child is not a grasping movement but a pointing movement. It cannot affect the object. It can affect only the people nearby. From the objective aspect, it is not an action directed toward the external world, but is really a means of social effect on people nearby. But the situation is such only from the objective aspect. The child himself strives for the object. His hand, stretched out in the air, maintains its position only because of the hypnotizing force of the object. This stage in the development of the pointing gesture can be called the stage of the gesture in itself.

Then the following occurs. The mother hands the child the object; for her rather than for the child, the unsuccessful grasping movement is converted into a pointing gesture. Because of the fact that she understands it in this way, this movement objectively turns ever more into a pointing gesture in the true sense of the word. This stage can be called the pointing gesture for others. Only significantly later does the action become a pointing gesture for the self, that is, a conscious and deliberate action of the child himself.

In exactly the same way, the child's first words are nothing other than an affective cry. Objectively, they express one need or another of the child long before the child consciously uses them as a means of expression. Again, as before, others, not the child, fill these affective words with a certain content. Thus, the people nearby create the objective sense of the first words apart from the will of the child. Only later are his words converted into speech for himself used deliberately and consciously.

In the course of our study, we have seen a number of examples of this kind of origin of functions through three basic stages. We have seen how speech and thinking intersect objectively in the child at first, apart from his intention in the practical situation, how at first a connection arises objectively between these two forms of activity, and how only later does it become a deliberate connection for the child himself. In development, every mental function passes through these three stages. Only when it rises to a higher level does it become a function of the personality in the true sense of the word.

We see how complex patterns appear in the dynamic structure of the adolescent's personality. What we have usually called personality is nothing other than man's consciousness of himself that appears specifically at this time: new behavior of man becomes behavior for himself; man himself is conscious of himself as a certain entity. This is the end result and central point of the whole transitional age. In a graphic form, we can express the difference between the personality of the child and the personality of the adolescent using different verbal designations of mental acts. Many investigators have asked: why do we attribute a personal character to mental processes? What should we say: I think or *It seems to me?* Why not consider the processes of behavior as natural processes that occur of themselves due to connections with all the other processes and why not speak of thinking impersonally, just as we say *it's getting dark* or *it's getting light?* To many investigators, such a manner of expression seemed to be solely scientific, and for a certain stage of development, this is actually so. Just as we say *mne snitsya* [the impersonal, idiomatic Russian expression, *it dreams to me*], the child says *it seems to me.* The course of his thought is as involuntary as our dreaming. But, in the well-known expression of L. Feuerbach, it is not thinking that thinks—man thinks.

This can be said for the first time only in application to the adolescent. Mental acts acquire a personal character only on the basis of a personality's self-consciousness and on the basis of their being mastered. It is interesting that this kind of terminological problem could never arise with respect to action.

No one would ever think to say *it* acts to me or doubt the correctness of the expression *I act*. Where we feel ourselves to be the source of a movement, we ascribe a personal character to our actions, but it is to specifically this level of mastery of his internal operations that the adolescent rises.

2

Recently in the pedology of the transitional age, much attention has been given to the problem of development of the personality. As Spranger has indicated, one of the basic features of the age as a whole is the discovery of one's own "I." This expression seems to us to be inaccurate since Spranger has in view the discovery of personality. It seems to us that it would be more correct to speak of the development of personality and of the conclusion of this development during the transitional age. Spranger justifies his formulation by the fact that the child too has his "ego." However, he is not conscious of it: Spranger has in mind the unique transfer of attention and internal reflection, that is, thinking directed toward oneself. Reflection appears in the adolescent; it is impossible in the child.

Recently, A. Busemann did two special studies (1925, 1926) on the development of reflection and the self-consciousness connected with it during the transitional age. We shall briefly consider the results of his studies since they present rich *factual* material for understanding the dynamics and structure of personality during the transitional age. Busemann proceeds from an entirely correct position that self-consciousness is not something original. Lower forms of organisms live in interrelation with the environment, but not with themselves. The development of self-consciousness is accomplished extremely slowly, and we must seek its rudiments even in early animal forms. Engels noted that even in the organization of the nervous system, around which all the rest of the body is constructed, the first rudiment is given for the development of self-consciousness.

We believe that Busemann is fully justified in considering the most primitive forms of interrelations with one's own organism as the biological roots of self-consciousness. When an insect, a beetle for example, smoothes his wings with his feet, his extremities touch, stimulate each other, and are perceived as an external stimulation. Further, through a series of biological forms of development, this process rises to reflection directed toward one's own body, if under this word, we follow Busemann in understanding all transfer of experience from the external world to oneself.

The psychology of reflection, as the author correctly indicates, requires a radical review of a number of theoretical positions. The psychology which considers man as a natural being does not consider the problem of the development of self-consciousness. Only in taking into account the historical development of man and child do we approach a correct formulation of this problem.

Busemann set a goal of studying the development of reflection and the self-consciousness connected with it on the basis of free compositions of the child and the adolescent. The compositions disclosed to what extent the writer had mastered reflection or self-consciousness. The basic result of the study revealed a close connection between the environment and the adolescent's self-consciousness. In complete agreement with what we have said above, Busemann found that the vital form of the adolescent's personality depicted by Spranger refers only to an adolescent from a certain type of environment. Its transfer to other social strata is not borne out by facts. Transferring this structure to proletarian and peasant youth is completely inadmissible. Busemann's first study showed a tremendous difference in the development and structure of self-consciousness and personality of the adolescent depending on the social environment to which he belongs. Children and adolescents wrote compositions on themes such as: "My good and bad qualities," "What kind of person I am and what kind I should be," and "Can I be pleased with myself (am I satisfied with myself)." The author was interested not in the plausibility of the responses, but in their character, which made it possible to judge the extent of the development or lack of development of the adolescent's self-consciousness.

One of the basic facts as expressed in the words of Busemann is the connection between social position and reflection. Another basic fact is that the process of self-consciousness is not some kind of fixed and constant ability that arises instantly in full measure, but one that undergoes a long development through various stages; this makes it possible to separate the stages of development and compare people in this respect. According to Busemann, the function of self-consciousness develops in six different directions which basically constitute the principal factors that characterize the structure of the adolescent's self-consciousness.

The first direction is simply growth and the appearance of a self-image. The adolescent begins to recognize himself more and more. This recognition becomes more firmly grounded and connected. There are many intermediate steps between the completely naive lack of knowledge of oneself and the rich, profound knowledge that is evident at another time toward the end of the period of sexual maturation.

The second direction in the development of self-consciousness takes this process inward from outside. Busemann says that at first children know only their own body. Only at age 12–15 is there a consciousness of the existence of an interior world in other people also. The adolescent's own self-image is transferred inward. At first, it encompasses dreams and feelings. It is important that the development in the second direction does not move in parallel with the increase in self-consciousness in the first direction. Table 4 presents the increase in transition inward at the beginning of the adolescent years and the dependence of this process on the environment. We see to what extent the village child remains at the stage of external self-consciousness for a significantly longer time (see Table 4).

The third direction in the development of self-consciousness is its internalization. The adolescent begins to recognize himself more and more as a single whole. In his consciousness, separate traits increasingly become traits of character. He begins to perceive himself as something whole and every separate development as apart of the whole. Here we can observe a number of stages qualitatively different from each other which the child passes through gradually depending on age and social environment.

TABLE 4. Frequency of Mentioning Ethical Judgments Depending on Age, Sex, and Social Environment, % (According to A. Busemann)

| Age, years | Boys | | | Girls | | |
|---|---|---|---|---|---|---|
| | A | B | C | A | B | C |
| 11 | 0 | 0 | 0 | 10 | 25 | 100 |
| 12 | 5 | 4 | 17 | 40 | 39 | 45 |
| 13 | 13 | 11 | 22 | 51 | 44 | 73 |
| 14 | 6 | 7 | 9 | 53 | 83 | 31 |

Note: A—uneducated workers'; B—educated workers and lower-level employees; C—mid-level employees and officials, independent craftsmen, small farmers, and tradesmen.

The fourth direction in the development of the adolescent's self-consciousness is setting a boundary between his personality and the surrounding world, recognizing the differences and uniqueness of his own personality. Inordinate development of self-consciousness in this direction leads to reticence and to acutely painful alienation, which frequently marks the transitional age.

The fifth line in development consists of the transition to judging oneself on ethical scales,* which a child or adolescent begins to apply to evaluating his own personality; these scales are acquired from objective culture and not simply assimilated biologically. Busemann says that up to the age of 11, the child judges himself on a scale of strong—weak, well—sick, beautiful—ugly. Country adolescents, age 14–15, frequently still remain at this stage of biological self-evaluation. But in complex social relations, development moves forward very rapidly. The center of gravity is transferred to one capability or another. Following the stage of "Siegfried ethics" according to which corporal virtues and beauty are everything, the ethic of skills becomes part of the child's development. Busemann believes that the child takes pride in knowing how to do something which attracts the respect of adults.

Under the influence of adults who continuously repeat the formula, "You must obey us," the child enters the stage of evaluation, which is determined by what the adults require of him. Every so-called well-brought-up child goes through this stage. Many children, especially girls, remain at the stage of ethical obedience.

The next stage in development leads to group ethics and is attained by the adolescents only at the age of approximately seventeen, and not by all of them.

The sixth and last line of development of the adolescent's self-consciousness and personality consists of an increase in differences between individuals and increase in interindividual variation. In this respect, reflection orders the fate of the remaining functions. As instincts become more mature and the influence of the environment continues, people become less and less alike. Up to the age of 10, we find insignificant difference in the self-consciousness of the city and the rural child; at age 11–12, this difference becomes clearer, but only in the transitional age does the difference in environment bring the various types in the structure of the personality to a full expression.

---

* Editor's note: internal, moral criteria.

## 3

The most substantial result of Busemann's study is that he established three factors that characterize reflection during the transitional age.

The first: reflection and the adolescent's self-consciousness based on it are rep resented in development. The appearance of self-consciousness is taken not only as a phenomenon in the life of consciousness, but as a much broader factor bio logically and socially based on the whole preceding history. Rather than approaching this complex problem only phenomenologically, from the aspect of experience, from the aspect of analysis of consciousness, as Spranger had done, we obtain an objective reflection of the real development of the adolescent's self-consciousness.

On a solid base, Busemann says that the roots of reflection must be sought very deeply in the living world and that its biological bases are wherever there is a reflection not only of the external world, but also a self-reflection of the organism and a relation of the organism with itself that results from this. Spranger describes this change in the transitional age as a discovery of one's own "I," as a turning of the gaze inward, as an event of a purely spiritual order. In this way he takes the formation of the adolescent's personality as something primary, independent, and primordial and from this as from a root, he derives all further changes that characterize the age. Actually, what we have before us is not primary, but one of the very last, perhaps even the last link in the chain of the changes which constitute the characteristics of the transitional age.

We pointed out above that the potentials for self-consciousness are established even in the organization of the nervous system. Further, we tried to trace the long path of psychological and social changes that leads to the appearance of self-consciousness. We have seen that there is no instantaneous and unexpected discovery of a purely spiritual order. We have seen how of natural necessity all mental life of the adolescent is reconstructed so that the appearance of consciousness is only the product of the preceding process of development. This is the main thing, this is the essence.

Self-consciousness is only the last and highest of all the restructuring that the adolescent's psychology undergoes. For us, the formation of self-consciousness is nothing other, I repeat, than a certain historical stage in the development of personality that arises inevitably from preceding stages. Thus, self-consciousness is not a primary, but a derivative fact in the adolescent's psychology and appears not through discovery, but through a long development. In this sense, the appearance of self-consciousness is nothing other than a certain moment in the process of development of a consciousness being. This moment is part of all of the processes of development in which consciousness begins to play any perceptible role.

This concept corresponds to the pattern of development that we find in Hegel's philosophy. In contrast to Kant, for whom a thing in itself is a metaphysical entity not subject to development, for Hegel, the concept itself "in oneself" means nothing other than the initial moment or stage of development of the thing. Specifically from this point of view, Hegel considered a seedling as a plant in itself and a child as a man in himself. All things are in themselves from the beginning, Hegel said. A. Deborin (1923) considers it interesting that in formulating the question in this way, Hegel inseparably connects the knowability of a thing with its development or, using a more general expression, with its movement and change. From this point of view, Hegel justifiably pointed to the fact that the "I" serves as the closest example of "life for oneself." "It can be said that the man differs from the animal and, consequently, from nature in general mainly by the fact that he knows himself as 'I.'"

The concept of self-consciousness as developing definitively liberates us from the metaphysical approach to this central fact of the transitional age.

The second factor which facilitates our real approach to this process is Busemann's finding the connection between the development of self-consciousness and the social development of the adolescent. Busemann moves the discovery of the "I," which Spranger places at the beginning of the creation of adolescent psychology, from the heavens to earth and from the beginning of the mental development of the adolescent to the end when he indicates that the picture drawn by Spranger corresponds only to a certain social type of adolescent. Busemann maintains that transferring this image to proletarian and peasant youth would be a big mistake.

Most recently, Busemann conducted a study in which he again tried to elucidate the connection between the environment and the adolescent's self-consciousness. If, as the author himself believes, it was possible on the basis of his former work to elucidate the differences in self-consciousness between the city and the rural child, between pupils of higher, middle, and folk schools, not by the influence of social position, but simply by the educational effect of type of school, then the results of the new study contradict this. The great amount of material collected was processed. The statements of the adolescents were divided into four groups:

1. Representation of the conditions in which the child lives instead of his representation of his own personality. This was accepted as evidence of his own naive relation to the theme "Am I satisfied with myself."
2. Description of his own body, which also was evidence of a primitive understanding of this question.
3. Self-evaluation at the level of ethical knowledge.
4. Self-evaluation of actual ethical character (regardless of whether it referred to ethical compliance or to group ethics).

The author presents the differences in self-consciousness of various social groups in Table 5. These differences cannot be explained exclusively by type of schooling since all the children studied were in the same school.

In itself, the *fact of the close connection* established by Busemann between the adolescent's social position and development of his self-consciousness seems to us to be completely indisputable. The interpretation of the factual data, however, seems to be so *erroneous* that even the simplest analysis would detect this.

If we compare the differences in stage of development of the self-consciousness of adolescents depending on their social position with the same difference depending on sex, we see to what extent sex differentiation exceeds social differentiation (Table 7). For example, while the number of naive responses indicating an undeveloped self-consciousness in boys in group A is only 1.5 times greater than the number of the same responses in group C, compared with

**TABLE 5.** Distribution of Naive Statements (First and Second Category in the Total) According to Sex and Social Groups, % (According to A. Busemann)

| | Social Groups | | |
|---|---|---|---|
| Sex | A | B | C |
| M | 66 | 53 | 43 |
| F | 21 | 15 | 13 |

Note: Designations A, B, C as in Table 6.

responses of girls in the same social group, it is more than 3 times greater. The same thing holds for the rest of the social groups. Can we call this fact accidental? We think not. The difference in development of self-consciousness between the sexes is much more significant than between children of different social strata.

To explain this, Busemann constructs what is in our view an unsustainable theory: he assumes that even in unfavorable socioeconomic circumstances, girls develop a mature ethical self-consciousness while boys require especially favorable conditions in their domestic environment or a strong influence of school to do so. Busemann sees confirmation of this fact in that we have known for a long time that the feminine sector of proletarian youth is psychologically remarkably close to the type of youth found in the best social conditions.

Girls are ahead in the same way in everything that pertains to transfer inward and animation of the personality, and all influences of a particularly favorable environment, for example, attending higher school, only bring boys closer to the feminine type in this respect. Busemann says that a man of the cultured type, especially a man who is highly cultured intellectually, falls on the line of transition from the masculine to the feminine type of self-consciousness. Busemann believes that our culture is masculine according to origin, but strives toward feminization according to psychological direction of development.

It is difficult to imagine a less sustainable explanation dictated by trying to place the facts obtained into some kind of preconceived pattern. Busemann's error lies in the fact that he cannot bring to an end the point of view of development and the point of view of social

**TABLE 6.** Distribution of All Types of Judgments According to Sex and Social Groups, % (According to A. Busemann)

| | Boys | | | Girls | | |
|---|---|---|---|---|---|---|
| Type of Judgment | A | B | C | A | B | C |
| Mentioning circumstances | 40 | 34 | 25 | 18 | 11 | 13 |
| Body | 26 | 19 | 18 | 3 | 4 | 0 |
| Skill | 27 | 40 | 42 | 33 | 41 | 33 |
| Ethical character | 7 | 7 | 15 | 46 | 43 | 53 |

TABLE 7. Mention of One's Own Body in Statements of Rural and
City Children of Different Ages, % (According to A. Busemann)

| Age, years | Rural | City |
|------------|-------|------|
| 9–11       | 63.2  | 15.5 |
| 12–14      | 40.8  | 4.7  |

dependence in questions of the origin of the adolescent's self-consciousness. For this reason he does not take note of two major facts.

First, the girl precedes the boy in sexual maturation and consequently also in mental development. Due to this, it is natural that a greater percentage of girls will attain a higher stage of development earlier than boys. Thus, here we have not superiority of the feminine type over the masculine, but the fact of earlier onset of sexual maturation, a different rate and rhythm of development. In fine agreement with this is the fact that such a quantitative difference in rate and rhythm exists between children of different social strata. Since development of self-consciousness is the result mainly of social-cultural development of the personality, it is understandable that the differences in the cultural environment must also directly affect the rate of development of this higher function of personality in children living in unfavorable social-cultural conditions. It is completely understandable that this difference between children of different social groups is one-half the difference between boys and girls.

However, this does not at all mean that Busemann's position on the internal connection between environment and self-consciousness must be discarded. This is far from the case. But the connection must be sought not where Busemann seeks it. Not in quantitative delay in growth, not in lag in rate of development, not in arrest at an earlier stage, but *this difference lies in a different type, in a different structure of self-consciousness.* The quantitative differences that Busemann found are not the most essential for the required connection between the environment and self-consciousness.

With respect to self-consciousness, the working-class adolescent is not simply arrested at an earlier stage of development in comparison with the bourgeois adolescent, *but is an adolescent with a different type of personality development, with a different structure and dynamics of self-consciousness.* The differences here are not in the same plane as the differences between boys and girls. For this reason, the roots of these differences must be sought in the class to which the adolescent belongs and not in one degree or another of his material well-being. For this reason, putting adolescents who belong to different classes into one group, as Busemann does, seems to us to be wrong.

He makes the same mistake when he considers the effect of social environment in age brackets.

As Tables 9 and 10 show, a corresponding influence of environment begins to show extremely early, but it is insignificant in comparison with the differences that exist between boys and girls. This again convinces us that the differences Busemann found are primarily differences in rate of development in which, as we know, girls precede boys. This is a major fact in the light of which we must understand all of Busemann's results.

However, his basic conclusion seems to us to be correct. He maintains that the development of self-consciousness depends on the cultural content of the environment to an extent greater perhaps than any other aspect of internal life. In Busemann's attempt to deduce the features of self-consciousness of the adolescent from the vital needs of the social group to which this adolescent belongs, there is an enormous omission, but his methodology marks out a completely correct path of research. He believes that the adolescent who has passed all of his life in an atmosphere of physical work and material want, who is not trained to any skill, naturally considers himself from this point of view: body plus external conditions.

Children of educated workers have a different point of view. We should pay attention here to how much the percentage of self-evaluation based on skills increases. In this respect, the children of skilled workers surpass even the children of the next group: for a skilled worker, Busemann believes that skill is the most important. For this reason children assimilate this factor in self-evaluation, transferred from the external inward, from a social criterion it becomes individual, from a group factor it is converted to a factor of self-consciousness. Finally, children of the third group also reflect the ethical level of their own families in their self-evaluations.

In general, Busemann says that the character and method by which the child recognizes his own existence and activity depend to a high degree on how his parents consider and value themselves. Value scales of adults become the value scales of the child himself. Busemann urges that prejudgment be avoided as if everything had to be done consciously and with reflection so that it might be good. He says that it is not just in the area of ethics that the very best happens when the left hand does not know what the right hand is doing. There is the perfection of the unconscious person.

This hymn to limitedness definitely shows the falsity of the basic premise of the author. Instead of giving a qualitative analysis and disclosing qualitative differences between the adolescent's consciousness in different social environments, the author is satisfied with a simple establishment of a delay in the transition from one stage to another. But the matter obviously is *not in stages* but *in types* of self-consciousness and in the course of the process itself of development. In certain respects, for example, in the sense of being conscious of one's own personality from the social-class aspect, the working-class adolescent will, of course, reach a higher stage of self-consciousness than the bourgeois adolescent. In other respects, he is slower. But we cannot say anything in general on the lag and movement forward where the paths of development form completely immeasurable qualitatively different curves.

TABLE 8. Mention of One's Own Feelings in Statements of City and Rural Children of Different Age and Sex, % (According to A. Busemann)

| Age, years | City | | Rural | |
|---|---|---|---|---|
| | M | F | M | F |
| 9–11 | 20 | 16 | 28 | 20 |
| 12–14 | 18 | 29 | 38 | 52 |

TABLE 9. Degree of Internalization of Representations of Oneself (% of Compositions on the Internal World of the Personality, Taking into Account the Total Number of Compositions, according to Busemann)

| | Schools | | | | | | | |
| | | | City | | | | Rural | |
| | Total | | Higher | | Folk | | Folk | |
| Age, years | M | F | M | F | M | F | M | F |
| --- | --- | --- | --- | --- | --- | --- | --- | --- |
| 9 | 30 | — | 36 | 43 | 25 | 80 | 20 | 16 |
| 10 | 41 | 45 | 23 | 50 | 36 | 67 | 30 | 27 |
| 11 | 50 | 52 | 19 | 79 | 37 | 53 | 24 | 22 |
| 12 | 95 | 88 | 26 | 72 | 50 | 69 | 16 | 26 |
| 13 | 89 | 96 | 30 | 100 | 49 | 52 | 19 | 50 |
| 14 | 80 | 92 | 58 | 96 | 42 | 60 | 37 | 69 |
| 15 | 79 | 90 | 50 | 90 | — | — | — | — |
| 16 | 77 | 92 | 60 | 100 | — | — | — | — |
| 17 | 74 | — | 61 | — | — | — | — | — |

4

The third point in the work of Busemann that frees us from the metaphysical approach to self-consciousness is that self-consciousness is not taken as some kind of metaphysical essence that is not subject to analysis. Together with the aspect of development and social dependence, an aspect of empirical analysis of self-consciousness is introduced. The six points listed above that characterize the structure of self-consciousness in the plane of development are the first attempt at such empirical analysis of personality. Figure 1 presents the course of development of self-consciousness (assimilating internal criteria of evaluation). We can easily see the rise in the curve and the sharp rise during the period of sexual maturation.

Busemann's great achievement is that he realized the new point, the new stage in the development of the adolescent as being a qualitatively unique time in his maturation. The investigator was fully justified in calling attention to the fact that reflection on its part can affect the subject in a reconstructive way (self-shaping). This is the great significance of reflection for the psychology of individual differences. Together with the primary conditions of the individual cast of the personality (instincts, heredity) and secondary conditions of its formation (environment, acquired traits), there is a set of *third conditions* (reflection, self-shaping).

Busemann is on firm ground in posing the question: does the principle of convergence established by Stern also apply to relations between the given individuality and its self-shaping by consciousness? In other words, the question concerns the independence of this third group of traits that arise on the basis of the self-consciousness of the personality. Can

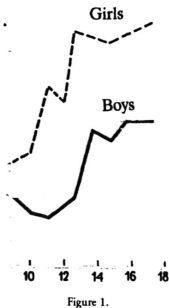

**Girls**

**Boys**

10   12   14   16   18

Figure 1.

we imagine development of this group of traits on the basis of the principle of convergence? In other words, does the process of development in this area follow the same principle as does the formation of secondary traits on the basis of interaction of innate instincts and the effect of the environment? We believe that posing this question is enough to give it a negative answer. Here a new acting persona enters the drama of development, a new, qualitatively unique factor—the personality of the adolescent himself. We have before us the very complex structure of this personality.

Busemann notes six different facets in its development. Each of them can develop at a different rate, and for this reason the personality may present very different forms at each stage of development, depending on the different interrelation and different structure of the basic six facets. For this reason, Busemann says that the most various forms are possible. On the one hand, there are people who know themselves very well, but at the same time, their self-evaluation does not include ethical scales to any significant degree. On the other hand, self-consciousness that is still vague may operate with such scales. For this reason Busemann believes that this matter is much more intricate than it may seem at first glance.

Specifically, it is an understanding of the qualitative self-image to the degree attained by the adolescent approaching self-consciousness that makes it possible for Busemann to evaluate the significance of reflection in the whole cycle of mental development at this age.

If we look at the significance of reflection for mental life as a whole, we will clearly see the profound difference between the structure of the personality that is nonreflecting, naive, on the one hand, and the structure that is reflecting on the other. True, the process of self-consciousness is a continuous process so there is no sharp boundary between naiveté and reflection.

Since the word, "naive," is used in still another sense, Busemann introduces a new term, "sympsychia," to designate a mental life complete, closed within itself and not divided by any kind of reflection. By this term, he understands the single attitude and activity of the primitive mind, an example of which may be the child wholly absorbed in play. An opposite example: the adolescent who reproaches him self in light of his own feelings. The state of this kind of division Busemann terms diapsychia. It is characteristic of reflection of a developed consciousness. The adolescent, according to the ideas of Busemann, is differentiated internally into the acting "I" and into another "I"—the reflecting "I."

The effect of reflection is not exhausted by just the internal change in the personality itself. In connection with the development of self-consciousness, it becomes possible for the adolescent to understand other people immeasurably more profoundly and broadly. The social development that leads to the formation of the personality acquires a support in self-consciousness for its further development.

Here we come in earnest to the last and most difficult and complex of all the questions connected with the structure and dynamics of personality. We have seen that the development of self-consciousness marks the transition to a new principle of development and to the formation of tertiary traits. We recall that the changes we noted above as changes characteristic of the mental development of the adolescent indicate this new type of development. We designated it as the cultural development of behavior and thinking. We saw that development of memory, attention, and thinking in concepts at this age consists not in a simple branching out of inherited instincts in the process of their realization under certain environmental conditions. We saw that the transition to self-consciousness and to mastery of internal control of these processes is the real content of the development of functions during the transitional age. If we were to try to determine more precisely what the new type of development consists of, we would see that it consists primarily of the formation of new connections, new relations, and new structural links between various functions. If the child did not see how others manage memory, he would not be able to master this process.

In the process of sociogenesis of higher mental functions, tertiary functions are formed based on the new type of connections and relations between separate processes. For example, we have seen that the development of memory is made up mainly of the new relation that is created between memory and thinking. We said that if for the child thinking means remembering, then for the adolescent, remembering means thinking. The same task of adaptation is resolved by different methods. The functions enter into new, complex relations with each other. This pertains also to perception, attention, and action.

All of these new types of connections and interrelations of functions presuppose reflection, reflection of his own processes as a substrate in the consciousness of the adolescent. We recall that logical thinking develops only on the basis of such reflection. Characteristic for mental functions in the transitional age is participation of the personality in each separate act. The child [using the idiomatic Russian expressions] would say impersonally, "it seems to me," and "it comes to my mind," but the adolescent would say, "I think" and "I remember." In the true expression of J. Politzer, it is not the muscle, but the man that works. Precisely so we can say that it is not memory that remembers, but man. This means that the functions entered a new connection with each other through the personality. In these new connections, in these tertiary, higher functions, there is nothing mysterious or secret because, as we have seen, the law of their construction consists of the fact that what were at one time relations between people became psychological relations transferred to the personality. This is why this diapsychia, this distinguishing of the acting, reflecting "I," of which Busemann speaks, is nothing other than a projection of social relations to within the personality. Self-consciousness is social consciousness transferred within.

Using a very simple example, we can elucidate how the new tertiary connections of separate functions specific to the personality arise and how specifically in connections of this type, the personality finds its full embodiment, its adequate description, and how in connections of this type, instincts that characterize the personality (primary traits) and acquired experience (secondary traits) become a removed category, a subordinate instance. Connections that characterize the personality at the most primitive stage of development differ qualitatively from connections that are habitual for us to such a degree that their comparative study shows better than anything what the very nature of these connections and the type of their formation is. The study shows that connections of personality habitual to us are characterized by a certain relation between separate functions and, because they are new psychological systems, it is understandable that they are not something constant, everlasting, but are a historical formation characteristic for a certain stage and form of development.

Here is an example borrowed from the book on the primitive mind by L. Lévy-Bruhl (1930). Dreams play a completely different role in the life of primitive man than they do for us. The connection of dreams with other mental processes and, derived from this, their functional significance in the general structure of the personality are completely different. Almost everywhere, dreams were at first a guide which was followed, an infallible companion, and frequently even a master whose commands were not disputed. What could be more natural than an attempt to compel this adviser to speak, to go for help to this master, to learn his commands in difficult situations. Here is a typical example of such a case. Missionaries insist that the leader of a tribe send his son to school, and he responds: "I will dream about it." He explains that the leaders of the Magololo⁑ are very often guided by dreams in their actions. On a solid basis, Lévy-Bruhl maintains that the response of the leader of the primitive tribe expresses completely the state of his psychology. A European would have said, "I'll think about it"; the leader of the Magololo answers, "I'll dream about it."

Thus we see that in this kind of primitive man, dreams fulfill the function that thinking fulfills in our behavior. The laws of dreams are, of course, the same, but the *role* of dreams for the man who believes in them and is guided by them and for the man who does not believe in them is different. This is the source also of the different structures of the personality that are realized in the connections of separate functions with each other. For this reason, where we say, *"I dream,"* a Kafir would say, *"I see a dream."*

The mechanism of behavior that is evident in this example is typical for tertiary traits, and what pertains to dreaming in this example, actually pertains to all functions. Let us take the thinking of modern man. As for Spinoza, for one, thinking is the master of passions, and for others (those described by Freud, people autistically oriented and closed within themselves), thinking is the servant of passions. And autistic thinking differs from philosophical thinking not in its laws, but in its *role*, in its functional significance in the total structure of the personality.

Mental functions change this hierarchy in various spheres of social life. For this reason, diseases of the personality are most often apparent in the change in the role of separate functions and the hierarchy of the whole system of functions. It is not the raving that distinguishes the mentally ill from us, but the fact that the person believes the raving and obeys it while we do not. On the basis of reflection, on the basis of self-consciousness and understanding our own processes, new groups and new connections of these functions with each other develop, and these connections which arise on the basis of self-consciousness and characterize the structure of the personality we call tertiary traits. The prototype of connections of this kind is the connection of the type that we illustrated with the dream of the Kafir. One set of internal convictions or another, one set of ethical standards or another, one set of principles of behavior or another—all of this in the last analysis is embodied in the personality through connections of this type specifically. The man who follows his convictions and does not decide on some complex and doubtful action before he considers it in the light of these convictions essentially sets in motion a mechanism of the same type and structure as the Kafir set in motion before deciding on what was for him the doubtful and complex proposal of the missionary. We call this mechanism a *psychological system.*

The transitional age is also a time of formation of tertiary connections, mechanisms of the type of the Kafir's dream. What is acting here is the law of transition from external to internal processes, which we have noted earlier. According to the determination of Kretschmer, one of the basic laws disclosed by the history of development is the law of transition from external to internal reaction. Kretschmer attaches great importance to the fact that in the higher living beings, reactions that involve selection move more and more inward. They depend less and less on peripheral organs of movement and, on the contrary, more and more on the nervous central organ. A new stimulation over a large area no longer evokes an apparent storm of arousal movements, but evokes an invisible sequence of mental states within the organism, the end result of which is an already prepared purposeful movement. Thus, attempts are now no longer made on the scale of the movements themselves, but only as if on the scale of an embryo of movement. The process of consciousness is connected with these physiological acts of selection in the nervous central organ. We call these volitional processes.

This law is also valid with respect to mechanisms of the new type of which we spoke above. They also develop initially as certain external operations, external forms of behavior, which then become internal forms of thinking and action of the personality.

## 5

E. Spranger was the first to turn his attention to an interesting fact that has substantial significance for understanding the structure and dynamics of the personality during the transitional age. He points out that no period in our life is remembered as are the years of sexual maturation. In recollections, significantly less is retained of the real rhythm of internal life during these years than of internal life at other age levels. This fact is really remarkable. We know that memory is the basis of what psychologists usually call unity and identity of the personality. Memory is the basis of self-consciousness. Disruption of memory usually indicates a transition from one state to another, from one structure of the personality to another. For this reason, it is typical that we do not remember our sickly conditions and our dreams very well.

There may be two explanations for disruption of memory. For example, let us take amnesia that involves early childhood. It can be explained on the one hand by the fact that memory at that stage is not connected with the word, with speech, and for this reason acts in a manner different from our memory. On the other hand, we see that the completely different structure of the infant's personality results in a development which makes nonseparability and heredity impossible in the development of the personality.

We have the same thing, but in a different form, in the transitional age. Here amnesia occurs again. Having lived through the transitional age, we forget it, and this is evidence of our transition to a different structure of personality, to a different system of connections between separate functions—here development is achieved not along a direct, but along a very complex and meandering curve. In the structure of the personality of the adolescent there is nothing stable, final, and immovable. Everything in it is *transition, everything is in flux*. This is the alpha and omega of the structure and dynamics of the adolescent's personality. This is, therefore, the alpha and omega of the pedology of the transitional age.

# 15

---

# The Crisis at Age Seven

School age, like all other age levels, opens with a critical or turning-point period; this was described in the literature as the crisis at age seven before the other age levels were described. It was noted for a long time that in making the transition from preschool to school age, the child changes abruptly and becomes more difficult with respect to rearing than he was previously. This is a kind of transitional stage—he is no longer a preschooler and not yet a school child.

Recently a number of studies on this age have appeared. The results of the studies can be expressed graphically: more than anything, the loss of childlike directness distinguishes the child at seven years of age. The proximate cause of childlike directness is an inadequate differentiation of internal and external life. The experiences of the child, his desires and expressed desires, that is, behavior and activity, usually are an inadequately differentiated whole in the preschooler. In us, this is all very definitely differentiated, and for this reason, the behavior of the adult does not make as direct and naive an impression as the behavior of the child.

When the preschooler enters the crisis, even the most experienced observer is struck by the fact that the child suddenly loses naiveté and directness; in his behavior and in relations with those around him, he becomes less understandable in all aspects than he was formerly.

Everyone knows that the seven-year-old child grows taller rapidly, which indicates a number of changes in the organism. This age is the age during which teeth are replaced and the age of stretching up. Actually the child changes abruptly, and the changes are more profound and more complex than the changes that were observed during the crisis at age three. It would take a long time to enumerate all the symptoms of the crisis under consideration since it is multifaceted. It is sufficient to indicate the general impression that investigators and observers usually convey. I shall elaborate on two traits that are observed in almost all seven-year-olds, especially those who have a difficult childhood and experience the crisis in a concentrated form. The child begins to behave affectedly and capriciously and to behave not as he had previously. Something deliberate, ridiculous, and artificial, some kind of frivolousness, clownishness, and playing the fool appears in his behavior; the child makes himself a jester. Even before the age of seven, the child may play the fool, but at that time, people would not say the same things about him that they would say at this point. Why is this unmotivated clowning so striking? When the child looks at the samovar, on the surface of which he sees a distorted image, or makes faces before a mirror, he is simply playing. But when the child walks into a room with a funny gait, and talks in a squeaky voice, this is not motivated and it is striking. No one is surprised when

---

Originally appeared in English as Chapter 11 in *The Collected Works of L.S. Vygotsky, Volume 5: Child Psychology* (Robert W. Rieber, Ed.; Marie J. Hall, Trans.) (pp. 289–296). New York: Kluwer Academic/Plenum Press, 1998.

a preschool child talks nonsense, jokes, plays, but if the child makes a fool of himself and elicits censure and not laughter, this leaves the impression of unmotivated behavior.

The traits indicated point to a loss of the directness and naiveté which were traits of the preschooler. I think that the impression is correct that the external, distinguishing trait of the seven-year-old is the loss of childlike directness and the appearance of oddities that are hard to understand. He exhibits behavior that is somewhat fanciful, artificial, mannered, and forced.

The most essential trait of the crisis at age seven might be called the beginning of the differentiation of the internal and external aspects of the child's personality. What is concealed behind the impression of naiveté and directness in the child's behavior prior to this crisis? Naiveté and directness indicate that the child is the same inwardly as he is outwardly. The inward quietly makes a transition to the outward, and we regard the one as a disclosure of the other. What kinds of acts do we regard as direct? There is very little childlike naiveté and directness in adults, and if adults exhibit them, they leave a comical impression. For example, the comic actor, Charlie Chaplin, reflects this when, in playing serious people, he begins to behave with unusual childlike naiveté and directness. This is the main point of his comedy.

The loss of directness signifies the introduction of the intellectual factor into our acts, and this wedges itself between experience and the direct act, which is the direct opposite of the naive and direct action proper to the child. This does not mean that the crisis at age seven leads from direct, naive, nondifferentiated experience to the opposite pole, but only that a certain intellectual factor appears in each experience, in each of its manifestations.

One of the most complex problems of contemporary psychology and psychopathology of the personality, which I will try to elucidate with an example, is the problem that might be called experience of meaning.

I will try to approach this problem using the analogy to the problem of external perception. Then it will be clearer. The essential distinction of human perception is its intelligence and its objectivity. We realize the perceived complex of impressions simultaneously and together with external impressions. For example, I see immediately that this is a clock. In order to comprehend the characteristic of human perception, we must compare it with the perception of a patient who has lost this characteristic as a result of a nervous brain disease. If such a patient is shown a clock, he will not recognize it. He sees the clock, but does not know what it is. When you begin to wind the clock, or place it to your ear to see whether it is running, or look at it to see what time it is, the patient will say what it is, that it is a clock. He guesses that what he sees is a clock. For you and for me, what we see and the fact that it is a clock is a single act of realization.

Thus, perception does not occur separately from visual thinking. The process of visual thinking is done in unity with intellectual designation of the thing. When I say: this thing is a clock and then see some other kind of clock on a tower that does not resemble the first clock at all, but is also called a clock, this means that I perceive this thing as a representative of a certain class of things, that is, I generalize them. In short, a generalization is made in each perception. To say that our perception is intellectual perception is to say that all of our perception is generalized perception. This may be elucidated as follows: if I should look at a room without generalizing, that is, look the way an agnostic or an animal might, then the impressions of the things would appear in relation to each other as they appear in the visual field. But since I generalize them, I perceive the clock not only within the structure of the things that are together with it, but also within the structure of what a clock is, within the structure of the generalization in which I see it.

The development of intellectual perception in man may be compared to how a child sees a chessboard or plays on it while just learning, but not knowing how to play. The child, not knowing how to play, may amuse himself with the chess pieces, sort them according to color, etc., but the movement of the pieces will not be structurally determined. The child who learned to play chess will proceed differently. For the first child, the black knight and the white pawn have no connection with each other, but the second child, knowing the moves of the knight, understands that an attacking move by the knight threatens his pawn. For him, the knight and the pawn are a unit. In precisely this way, a good player can be distinguished from a poor player by the fact that he sees the chess field differently.

An essential trait of perception is structural quality, that is, perception is not made up of separate atoms, but represents an image within which there are various parts. Depending on what the position of the pieces on the chessboard is, I see it differently.

We perceive surrounding reality the way a chess player perceives a chessboard: we perceive not only the neighborhood of the objects or their contiguity, but also the whole reality with its intellectual connections and relations. In speech, there are not only names, but also meanings of objects. Quite early, the child develops the ability to express in speech not only the meanings of objects, but also his own actions and the actions of others and his own internal states ("I'm sleepy," "I'm hungry," "I'm cold"). Speech as a means of communication leads to naming and connecting our internal states to words. However, the connection to words never signifies the formation of a simple associative connection, but always signifies a generalization. Every word signifies more than one thing. If we say that it is cold now, and can say the same thing a day later, this means that every single feeling of cold has also been generalized. Thus, a generalization of an internal process is developed.

In an infant, there is no intellectual perception: he perceives a room but does not separately perceive chairs, a table, etc.; he will perceive everything as an undivided whole in contrast to the adult, who sees figures against a background. How does a child perceive his own movements in early childhood? He is happy, unhappy, but does not know that he is happy, just as an infant when he is hungry does not know that he is hungry. There is a great difference between feeling hunger and knowing that I am hungry. In early childhood, the child does not know his own experiences.

At the age level of seven years, we are dealing with the onset of the appearance of a structure of experience in which the child begins to understand what it means when he says: "I'm happy," "I'm unhappy," "I'm angry," "I'm good," "I'm bad," that is, he is developing an intellectual orientation in his own experiences. Precisely as a three-year-old child discovers his relation to other people, a seven-year-old discovers the fact of his own experiences. Because of this, certain features characterizing the crisis at age seven appear.

1. Experiences acquire meaning (an angry child understands that he is angry), and because of this, the child develops new relations to himself that were impossible before the generalization of experiences. As on a chessboard, where completely new connections between the pieces develop with each move, so here also completely new connections appear between experiences when they

acquire a certain sense. Consequently, the whole character of experiences of the child is reconstructed at the seventh year the way the chessboard was when the child learned to play chess.

2. Generalizations of experiences or affective generalization, logic of feelings, appears at the beginning of the crisis at age seven. There are deeply retarded children who experience failure at every step" normal children play, the abnormal child tries to join them, but they reject him and he goes along the street and is laughed at. In a word, he loses at every step. In each separate case, he has a reaction to his own inadequacy, but after a minute, you will see—he is completely satisfied with himself. A thousand separate failures, and there is no general sense of his worthlessness, he does not generalize what happened many times. In a school-age child, there is generalization of feelings, that is, if this kind of situation had happened to him many times, an affective formation would have developed, the character of which would relate to a single experience or affect the way understanding relates to a single perception or recollection. For example, a preschool child has no real self-evaluation, self-love. The level of our demands of ourselves, of our success, of our position, arises specifically in connection with the crisis at age seven.

A child of preschool age likes himself, but self-love as a generalized relation to himself which remains constant in various situations, self-evaluation as such, generalized relations to those around him and understanding his own value, is something a child of this age does not have. Consequently, toward the seventh year, a number of complex formations develop that lead to an abrupt and radical change in the difficulties of behavior that are fundamentally different from the difficulties of the preschool age.

Neoformations such as self-love and self-evaluation remain, but the symptoms of the crisis (affectation, posing) are transitional. In the crisis at age seven, because of the fact that a differentiation of the internal and external develops and intellectual experience first appears, a sharp conflict of experiences also develops. The child who does not know which candy to choose—the bigger or the sweeter—finds himself in a state of internal conflict even as he vacillates. The internal conflict (contradiction of experiences and selection of his own experiences) becomes possible only at this time.

There are typical forms of difficulties in rearing that are never encountered during the preschool age. These include conflicts and contradictory experiences, unresolved contradictions. As a matter of fact, where this internal division of experiences is possible, where first the child understands his experiences, where internal relations arise, there also occurs a change in experiences indispensable for the school-age level. To say that in the crisis at age seven, preschool experiences change to school experiences, is to say that a new unity of environmental and personal factors has appeared that makes the new stage of development possible—school age. For the child, his relation to the environment has changed, and this means that the environment itself has changed, it means that the course of the child's development has changed and that a new period in development has started.

It is necessary to introduce into science a concept, little used in the study of the social development of the child: we have studied inadequately the internal relation of the child to those around him, and we have not considered him as an active participant in the social situation. We admit in words that it is necessary to study the personality and the environment of the child as a unit. But we must not think that the influence of the personality is on one side and the influence of the environment, on the other, that the one and the other act the way external forces do. However, exactly this is actually done frequently: wishing to study the unity, preliminarily investigators break it down, then try to unite one thing with another.

Even in the study of difficult childhood, we cannot go beyond the limits of this formulation of the question: what played the main role, constitution or environmental conditions, psychopathic conditions of a genetic character or conditions of external circumstances of development? This brings us to two basic problems that must be elucidated on the plane of the internal relation of the child to the environment during the periods of crises.

The first principal inadequacy in practical and theoretical study of the environment is that we study the environment in its absolute characteristics. Whoever is involved in practical study of difficult cases knows this very well. You are given a social, life-style investigation report on the child's environment in which the cubic capacity of the living area is explained, whether the child has his own bed, how many times he goes to the bath house, when he changes his underwear, whether the family reads papers, and what the mother's and father's education was. The investigation is always the same, regardless of the child and his age. We study some absolute indicators of the environment as circumstances, trusting that knowing these indicators, we will know their role in the development of the child. Some Soviet scientists have made a principle of this absolute study of the environment. In a textbook edited by A. B. Zalkind, you will find a statement that the social environment of the child remains basically unchanged over the whole course of his development. Keeping in mind the absolute indicators of the environment, we can agree with this to a certain degree. In actual fact, this is completely false from both the practical and theoretical points of view. Of course, the essential difference between the child's environment and that of an animal is that the human environment is a social environment, that the child is a part of a living environment and that the environment never is external to the child. If the child is a social being and his environment is a social environment, then it follows from this that the child himself is a part of this social environment.

Consequently, the most essential turn-around that must be made in the study of the environment is the transition from absolute to relative indicators; the environment of the child must be studied: most of all, we must study what it means for the child, what the child's relation to the separate aspects of this environment is. Let us say that the child does not talk before he is a year old. When he starts to talk, the speech environment of those around him remains unchanged. And for the year before and the year after, in absolute indicators, the speech culture of those around him did not change at all. But I think that everyone will agree that from the minute the child began to understand the first words, when he began to pronounce the first deliberate words, his relation to speech factors in the environment, the role of speech in relation to the child changed a great deal.

Every step in his movement changes the influence of the environment on the child. From the point of view of development, the environment becomes entirely different from the minute the child moves from one age level to another. Consequently, we may say that perception of the environment must change in the most substantial way in comparison with the way we have usually treated it in practice thus far. The environment must be studied not as such, not in its absolute indicators, but in relation to the child. An environment that is the very same in absolute indicators is completely different for a child at age one, three, seven, or twelve. Dynamic change in the environment, its relation, is brought to the forefront. But, naturally, where we speak of relation, another factor develops: the relation is never purely external relation between the child and the environment taken separately. One of the important methodological problems is the problem of how the study of unity is really approached in theory and in research. Unity of personality and environment, unity of mental and physical development, and unity of speech and thinking are spoken of frequently. What does it really mean in theory and in research to approach the study of some unity and all properties that are pertinent to this unity as such? It means finding the principal unity every time, that is, finding the proportions in which the properties of the unity as such are combined. For example, when the relation of speech and thinking is studied, speech is artificially separated from thinking and thinking from speech, and then the question is raised as to what speech does for thinking and thinking for speech. The matter is presented in this way, as if these were two different liquids that could be mixed. If you want to know how a unity developed, how it changes, how it affects the course of the child's development, it is important not to break down the unity into its component parts because when this is done, the essential properties of specifically this unity are lost; the unity, for example, in the relation of speech and thinking, must be taken as a unity. Recently, an attempt has been made to isolate such a unity; take meaning, for example. Meaning of a word is a part of the word, a speech formation, because a word without meaning is not a word. Since all meaning of a word is a generalization, it is a product of the intellectual activity of the child. Thus, the meaning of a word is a unity of speech and thinking that cannot be broken down further.

A unity can be noted in the study of personality and environment. This unity in psychopathology and psychology has been called experience. The child's experience is also this kind of very simple unity about which we must not say that in itself it represents the influence of the environment on the child or the individuality of the child himself; experience is the unity of the personality and the environment as it is represented in development. Thus, in development, the unity of environmental and personality factors is achieved in a series of experiences of the child. Experience must be understood as the external relation of the child as a person to one factor or another of reality. All experience is always experience of something. There is no experience that would not be experience of something just as there is no act of consciousness that would not be an act of being conscious of something. But every experience is my experience. In modern theory, experience is introduced as a unity of consciousness, that is, a unity in which the basic properties of consciousness are given as such, while in attention and in thinking, the connection of consciousness is not given. Attention is not a unity of consciousness, but is an element of consciousness in which there is no series of other elements, while the unity of consciousness as such disappears, and experience is the actual dynamics of the unity of consciousness, that is, the whole which comprises consciousness.

Experience has a biosocial orientation; it is what lies between the personality and the environment that defines the relation of the personality to the environment, that shows what a given factor of the environment is for the personality. Experience is determining from the point of view of how one environmental factor or another affects the child's development. This, in any case, is confirmed at every step in the teaching on difficult childhood. Any analysis of a difficult child shows that what is essential is not the situation in itself taken in its absolute indicators, but how the child experiences the situation. In one and the same family, in one family situation, we find different changes in development in different children because different children experience one and the same situation differently.

Consequently, on the one hand, in experience, environment is given in its relation to me, how I experience this environment; on the other hand, features of the development of my personality have an effect. My experience is affected by the extent to which all my properties and how they came about in the course of development participate here at a given moment.

To state a certain, general, formal position, it would be correct to say that the environment determines the development of the child through experience of the environment. Most essential, therefore, is rejection of absolute indicators of the environment; the child is a part of the social situation, and the relation of the child to the environment and the environment to the child occurs through experience and activity of the child himself; the forces of the environment acquire a controlling significance because the child experiences them. This mandates a penetrating internal analysis of the experiences of the child, that is, a study of the environment which is transferred to a significant degree to within the child himself and is not reduced to a study of the external circumstances of his life.

Analysis becomes very complex, and we are confronted here with tremendous theoretical difficulties. Nevertheless, with respect to separate problems of development of character, critical age levels, and difficult childhood, separate factors connected with the analysis of experiences become somewhat more clear and visible.

Careful study of the critical age levels shows that changes in the child's basic experiences occur in them. The crisis is most of all a turning point that is expressed in the fact that the child passes from one method of experiencing the environment to another. The environment as such does not change for the child at the age of three. The parents continue to earn as much as they did before, and for every mouth there is the same budgeted minimum and maximum as before, there are subscriptions to the same number of papers as before, underwear is changed as frequently as before, the living area is the same, and the parents have not changed their relations to the child. Observers who study the crisis say that without any reason, the child who behaved so well, was obedient and affectionate, is suddenly capricious, bad and stubborn.

All bourgeois investigators emphasize the internal character of the crisis. Most of them explain the internal character of the crisis with biological causes. One of the most widespread theories for explaining the crisis at age thirteen is that there is a parallel between sexual maturation and the crisis, and internally established biological maturation of the child is seen as the basis of the crisis.

Other authors, like A. Busemann, who want to emphasize the significance of the social environment, correctly point to the fact that the crisis may have a completely different course depending on the environment in which it occurs. But Busemann's point of view does not differ essentially from the point of view that considers the crisis as a phenomenon due to purely exogenous causes. Busemann considers the crisis, like all features in the child not established as biological features, as a manifestation of changes in a changed environment. The idea arises that bourgeois research is wholly incorrect, or incorrect to some extent at least. Let us start with the factual aspect. It seems to me that the bourgeois investigators have a very limited range of observations, that is, they always observe the child in conditions of the bourgeois family with a certain type of rearing. Facts show that in other conditions of rearing, the crisis occurs differently.

In children who go from nursery school to kindergarten, the crisis occurs differently than it does in children who go into kindergarten from the family. However, the crisis occurs in all normally proceeding child development; the age of three and the age of seven will always be turning points in development: there will always be a state of things where the internal course of the child's development will conclude a cycle, and the transition to the next cycle will necessarily be a turning point. One age level is reconstructed in some way in order to allow a new stage of development to begin.

The observers' most general, naive impression that the child has somewhat suddenly, unrecognizably changed is correct: over the course of three to six months, the child has become different from what he was before; the crisis passes as a process that is little understood by those around the child since it is not connected with changes that occur around the child. To put it more simply, the crisis is a chain of internal changes of the child with relatively insignificant external changes. For example, when the child enters school, he changes over the course of school age from year to year, and this does not surprise us since the whole situation in which the child grows, all the circumstances of his development, change. When the child moves from nursery school to kindergarten, it does not surprise us that the preschooler changes, and here the changes of the child are connected with the changes that occur in the conditions of his development. But essential to every crisis is the fact that the internal changes occur in a much greater dimension than the changes in the external circumstances, and for this reason they always cause impressions of an internal crisis.

It is my impression that the crises actually have an internal source and consist in changes of an internal nature. There is no precise correspondence here between external and internal changes. The child enters the crisis. What has changed so abruptly outwardly? Nothing. Why has the child changed so abruptly in such a short time?

Our idea is that we must object not to the bourgeois theories of the critical age levels, or the idea that the crisis is a very profound process interwoven into the course of the child's development, but we must object to the understanding of the internal nature itself of the process of development. If, in general, everything that is internal in development is understood as biological, then of necessity, it will be the change in glands of internal secretion. In this sense, I would not call the critical ages the ages of internal development. But I think that internal development always occurs in such a way that there is a unity of personality and environmental factors, that is, every new step in development is directly determined by the preceding step, by all that has already happened and appeared in development at the preceding stage. True, this means that development must be understood as a process where all subsequent change is connected with what went before and with the present in which the features of personality that have developed previously are now manifested and now act. If we understand the nature of the internal process of development correctly, then there will be no theoretical objections to understanding the crisis as an internal crisis.

It seems to me that behind every experience, there is a real, dynamic action of the environment with respect to the child. From this point of view, the essence of every crisis is a reconstruction of the internal experience, a reconstruction that is rooted in the change of the basic factor that determines the relation of the child to the environment, specifically, in the change in needs and motives that control the behavior of the child. Growth and change in needs and motives are the least conscious and least voluntary part of the personality, and in the transition from age level to age level, new incentives and new motives develop in the child; in other words, the motive forces of his activity undergo a reevaluation. That which was essentially important, controlling, for the child becomes relative and unimportant at the subsequent stage.

The restructuring of needs and motives and the reevaluation of values are basic factors in the transition from age level to age level. Here, the environment also changes, that is, the relation of the child to the environment. Other things begin to interest the child, he develops other activity, and his consciousness is restructured, if we understand consciousness as the relation of the child to the environment.

# VI

## Scientific Legacy
### *Tool and Sign in the Development of the Child*

ANNA STETSENKO, *City University of New York*

This section reproduces the first four chapters of Vygotsky's famous work on *Tool and Sign* (in other places, translated as *Tool and Symbol*). There are an infinite number of ways to understand and interpret a scholarly text. However, it is absolutely indispensable to keep one thing in mind when seeking to make sense of an author's ideas: a text, just like any other meaningful creation of the human mind, must be considered to be *alive*. It is alive because it is born out of the author's attempt to make sense of the world and to bring something new to the world, transforming that world and, in the process, simultaneously transforming oneself. A text is alive in another way in that it is always born out of collective, not solitary, efforts of many people who are involved in the process of knowledge creation in multiple roles: as immediate and distant partners in dialogues of ideas, as opponents whose views are critiqued, and more often than not, as colleagues who collaborate shoulder to shoulder in carrying out the scholarly project. A scholarly text is alive in yet another sense: it always needs to be read by someone anew, to be made into a meaningful part of the reader's own life and work, thus continuing that text's existence within the continuously unfolding and creative human pursuits in the world.

On the surface, such a view on the origin and meaning of scholarly texts, and of the production of knowledge in general, might seem to be a rather belletristic description. However, this view is actually solidly grounded in principles inspired by Vygotsky's cultural—historical theory of human development. To illustrate this point, this essay will first briefly discuss how the cultural—historical ideas themselves have been brought to life, in order to show that their creation followed, in a wonderfully explicit way, the general path that marks the production of knowledge as a meaningful, value-laden, and collaborative human endeavor grounded in practical social pursuits in the world and itself aimed at transforming the world. Then we will see how these principles for understanding human knowledge are directly embodied in the major tenets of Vygotsky's cultural—historical theory (drawing from *Tool and Sign*) and how these ideas can be further explored in the service and context of challenges facing psychology today. It should be noted that, although much progress has been recently made in interpreting Vygotsky's theory (e.g., in works by Cole, Scribner, Rogoff, Wertsch, and others), the understanding of Vygotsky's theory of human knowledge and development is still in the early stages. Therefore, new generations of students and scholars who have just begun their acquaintance with Vygotsky can expect to join in and to contribute substantially to the important work of unraveling the full potential and the implications of his approach, which holds great promise for the future of the whole discipline of psychology and neighboring disciplines.

### The Cultural-Historical Origins of Vygotsky's Cultural-Historical Theory

That scholarly works are living creations of humans–part and parcel of their meaningful and practical pursuits in the world–is perhaps especially evident when we read Vygotsky's work, *Tool and Sign in the Development of the Child*. Indeed, he wrote this in dialogue with a number of prominent contemporary researchers: Bühler and Gesell, Piaget and Köhler, Stern and Werner. In fact, it was written in dialogue with, and as a critique of, essentially all the dominant trends in psychology of the time, from Gestalt psychology to behaviorism. It is a distinctive feature of Vygotsky that he criticizes and dialogues with a broad scope of the ideas of others. However, it is not just the scope of reference that uniquely marks Vygotsky's works; what is even more amazing is Vygotsky's ability, as critic, to expose the essential core of each approach; that is, to reveal the sometimes tacit and hidden meanings behind layers of expressed ideas, as he seeks the pivotal assumptions lying at the very heart of each theory or research agenda. This ability to derive the foundational premises of various, often competing, approaches allowed Vygotsky meaningfully to juxtapose and to compare various approaches, to derive important implications from them, and, most importantly, to move beyond these approaches by creatively synthesizing, negating, and advancing their insights in view of Vygotsky's own genuinely new horizons of ideas and pursuits. The new horizons in Vygotsky's research agenda formed truly novel, synthetically whole structures, which assimilated many of the ideas developed by his predecessors while making these ideas acquire new potentialities and meanings. Synthetically whole structures are able to cast new light on the 'old' components that have been drawn into them. This principle was not only a mode of operation that guided Vygotsky's own thinking; it was also a theoretical principle that he reflected upon in many of his writings, including *Tool and Sign*. This peculiar feature of much of Vygotsky's work and writings–that he often describes the very principles that de facto guide his own research–will be illustrated by several examples in this introduction.

Furthermore, note that Vygotsky wrote *Tool and Sign* in close collaboration and in lively discussions with a number of people: A. R. Luria, A. N. Leontiev, R. E. Levina, N. G. Morozova, L. S. Slavina, A. V. Zaporozhets, and others. They formed the so-called Vygotsky Circle, which included several brilliant women, and they carried out research projects collectively. It is quite revealing, in this respect, that even the authorship of Tool and Sign is disputed; there is some reason to believe that Vygotsky wrote it together with Luria. Because the historical records are not completely clear, the work has been published with varying authorship—either under Vygotsky's name or under the names of both Vygotsky and Luria (see Vygotsky, 1999; Vygotsky & Luria, 1994).

Whatever the case of the authorship of this particular work, the ubiquitously collaborative nature of Vygotsky's project in general must be emphasized, especially because it has often been underestimated or even ignored in previous accounts of his heritage. Vygotsky has been portrayed, in line with the old-fashioned "Great Man" version of the history of science (of. Leahy, 2002), as the scholar who "single-handedly" (Kozulin, 1999, p. 2) created the cultural-historical approach in his solitary pursuit of theoretical principles, and his close collaboration with members of his team is, for the most part, only briefly mentioned (e.g. Valsiner and van der Veer, 2000; van der Veer and Valsiner, 1991). However, any attempt to understand the cultural-historical approach is incomplete if one disregards the complex dynamics of how this approach emerged and developed as an essentially *collaborative investigative project* that entailed the truly collective efforts of a number of scholars committed to the same ideals and goals and dedicated to the same agenda: to develop psychology as a science that is capable of making a difference in the real world by contributing to the creation of a just and equality-based society. In that sense, the cultural-historical theory represents an example of a genuine school in psychology, rooted in a shared philosophical background and in a commitment to common ideological, moral, theoretical, and pragmatic ideals and goals. Ignoring the collaborative nature of Vygotsky's work goes against the very spirit of his theory, with its assertion of the deeply social and collaborative nature of the human mind in any of its expressions, including scholarly products such as theoretical ideas and programs of research.

Perhaps even more importantly, Vygotsky wrote his works not out of an ivory tower of purely academic pursuits, but from the midst of a very active engagement with the practical tasks of the turbulent and often violent, but also invigorating and innovative, social life that unfolded after the Russian Revolution, the immediate context of Vygotsky's work. It would be a mistake to imagine that Vygotsky sat in solitude in his armchair, contemplating abstract psychological issues, and then put his solutions on paper, the final destination of his efforts. According to what we know from memoirs and biographies that discuss Vygotsky, he participated in and contributed to the *drama of life*, not just the world of ideas, by himself engaging in practical endeavors and pursuits: reorganizing the whole national system of education and devising special rehabilitation programs for homeless and handicapped children, consulting with these children and other patients, lecturing to teachers and workers, participating in political debates, and otherwise trying to contribute to the growth of the new society of his times.

Vygotsky's ideas and scholarly texts emerged directly out of his practical, passionate, and distinctly collaborative engagements with these real-life problems. His writings are not simply expressions of abstract thinking and insights that emerged and existed separately from his life and practice; they are the very embodiments and vehicles of his practical engagements with his society and the challenges of his time. In this sense, Vygotsky's texts represent the stepping stones–simultaneously products and tools–of his overall pursuit to devise a new psychology for a society built on the ideals of social equality and equal opportunity for all, even for the most disadvantaged ones, such as homeless and disabled children. Thus, Vygotsky's texts are also deeply imbued with clear moral values and commitments, which cannot be ignored in any interpretation of his cultural-historical theory. Of course, Vygotsky and many others who, like him, had enthusiastically welcomed, and contributed to, the new Soviet society later became bitterly disappointed by the tragic failings of this gigantic social experiment, as it gradually turned into a repressive and stifling regime. However, these subsequent failings and related disappointments do not change the initial moral thrust that motivated Vygotsky and his colleagues and formed the basis of their work.

Vygotsky's theories and texts, including *Tool and Sign*, should be seen as both products and vehicles, tools for his deeply passionate and ideologically driven practical engagements with the realities of his turbulent time. His psychological ideas and philosophical principles resulted from, embodied, and simultaneously helped advance his practical engagements and commitments. Thus, the very history of Vygotsky's project in psychology provides a clear alternative to the narrowly mentalistic and individualistic notion of knowledge (as being processes only "in the head") as it reveals that ideas, theories, and knowledge in general are not merely mental constructs, but elements within real-life transformative activities in the world, activities that serve practical purposes and that change the world. This conceptualization challenges dominant theories in psychology that reduce knowledge to the purely intellectual realm and development of knowledge to the dynamics of voices and intellectual dialogues among the scholars. The following discussion will show how this view of Vygotsky's work is consistent with his major stance on the nature of human development, drawing upon several interrelated ideas developed specifically in *Tool and Sign*.

## Central Principles of Human Development in *Tool and Sign*

In this important work Vygotsky elaborates on at least four main ideas about human development. The first major issue, quite consistent with the overall quest of Vygotsky's deeply ideological project in psychology, is the issue of *human freedom,* that is, the human ability to act purposefully according to socially meaningful goals and with the help of socially developed tools, thus overcoming the dictates and constraints of nature and environment. This issue is a common thread that runs through most of Vygotsky's works and reflects his major goal to develop an approach that can address not only abstract principles in psychology but that can advance and put to use knowledge about specific conditions that are necessary for individuals to develop into fully responsible, free, and competent members of a human community.

Vygotsky often discussed the issue of freedom in terms of the differences between lower and higher psychological functions. (See Section IV of the present book.) Couching human freedom in these terms, Vygotsky was dialoguing with and critiquing the prevailing trends in psychology of his times. He aptly summarizes these prevailing trends on the very first pages of *Tool and Sign,* as he describes two metaphors underpinning most of the contemporary theories of child development: the metaphor of a growing plant (derived from botany) and that of animal development (derived from studies of animal behavior or comparative psychology). According to these metaphors, child development can be seen as the simple mechanical growth of capacities that are present in the child right from birth (as in the growth of a plant seed) and that unfold according to predetermined and essentially unchangeable laws of nature (as in the straightforward training of habits in animals).

To counter these views and to reveal what constitutes specifically human development, Vygotsky needed to introduce a concept that would stand in clear contrast to processes in nonhuman nature. The concept of "higher mental functions" was evidently meant to play such a role. That psychological processes in very young children were described by Vygotsky as "lower" or "natural" and not yet belonging to the realm of cultural development was perhaps a rhetorical overstatement of this contrast, inevitable at the early stages of introducing a new concept when sharp contrasts are necessary and useful. The strict opposition between the lower and higher mental processes, however, should not be taken as an absolute principle; indeed, it was often questioned by Vygotsky himself, when he stated, for example, that the "whole history of the child's mental development teaches us that from the first days, his adaptation to the environment is achieved by social means through the people around him;" for this and similar ideas, see Vygotsky's work on child psychology, described in Section V of this book). The idea of a strict dichotomy between lower and higher mental processes was later abandoned by Vygotsky's immediate co-workers and students (e.g., El'konin, Zaporozhets), in favor of seeing all human development, right from the first days of child's life, as an essentially sociocultural and tool-mediated process. As further discussion will show, this interpretation is quite consistent with the gist of Vygotsky's theory that all human psychological processes develop out of collaborative social forms of interaction.

How does psychological development proceed to overcome the natural constraints of environment, thus becoming free? Vygotsky's answer is that this process involves the use of signs, symbols, and other cultural tools (most importantly, language, the tool *par excellence*); humans use these to transform the world rather than passively adapt to the world's conditions. Cultural tools represent humankind's greatest invention, and they arguably form the very basis of a specifically human way of life, creating everything that is human in humans. Cultural tools allow people to embody their collective experiences (e.g., skills, knowledge, beliefs) in external forms such as material objects (e.g., words, pictures, books, houses), patterns of behavior organized in space and time (e.g., rituals), and modes of acting, thinking, and communicating in everyday life. Such external (or reified) forms that embody collective social knowledge and experience constitute a unique dimension of existence—*human culture,* into which each child is born and which he or she has to acquire in order to participate in social life. The existence and continuous exponential growth of human culture, throughout history, tremendously expands the horizons of human development because large amounts of collectively accumulated experience are passed from one generation to another in teaching-and-learning processes, without having to rely on more biologically based and inflexible processes such as instincts.

Because complex cultural signs embody experiences and skills of previous generations, learning to use them brings a dimension of social history and culture into each individual's development. This emerging capacity to use tools and signs, according to Vygotsky, gradually allows humans—in their history as a biological species (phylogeny), as a civilization (social history), and as individuals (ontogeny)—to leap from the constraints of the natural environment, defined by the laws of biological evolution and stimulus—response modes of behavior, into the realm of cultural—historical development with its infinite degrees of freedom.

This freedom, according to Vygotsky's painstaking explanation, is chiefly due to the emancipating role of speech, as children begin to act through that medium while solving practical problems posed by life. The amazingly powerful role of speech would be impossible if speech were simply added to previous, more elementary psychological processes. However, instead of being a mere addition, the use of speech radically changes and even creates *a whole new system of behavior*, allowing the child to plan for future actions, to direct attention to elements of the visual field that are important in view of certain goals and purposes, to select the actions that are most efficient in a given situation, to integrate others into the solution of the problem (for example, by asking adults for help and clarification), and so on. The result is an emerging ability to steer actions in a desired and planned direction, turning those actions into a voluntary, self-regulated, and purposeful complex activity planned over time, according to certain meaningful goals. This ability to consciously plan one's own behavior in advance and then to carry it out according to a preestablished plan constitutes, according to Vygotsky, the essence of specifically human forms of behavior.

A second central principle of *Tool and Sign* is that collaborative forms of behavior lie at the very root of human development. The child never acts alone but is intimately related to and dependent on other people. In this sense, the human infant, according to Vygotsky, is paradoxically the ultimate social being because of its complete dependency on other people. These collaborative behaviors, the primary form of which is the parent—child interaction, always entail tools and symbols carried over from previous generations and introduced by adults to the child to facilitate collective efforts aimed at solving present tasks. The child gradually appropriates these tools, as well as the modes of action embodied in them, through internalization, whereby the tools are converted into the resources of each child's individual behavior. The converted, internalized forms of behavior, nonetheless, retain a social method of functioning and thus always remain essentially social, even when, at the later stages of development, people appear to be acting alone. Thus, Vygotsky discloses the development of human psychological functions as a sociohistorical process. Namely, he reveals development as the process of converting resources of social behavior, discovered by generations of people and reintroduced to each member of a human community through collaborative shared activities with more experienced partners (i.e., adults) into the resources of individual psychological functioning and behavior.

The third, and perhaps the most important, concept in *Tool and Sign* is actually not a separate idea but a logical continuation of the previous two. As Vygotsky points out in several places, there is always a *unity of processes,* such as voluntary attention, logical memory, perception, movement, as well as practical intellect and action. Human development entails the emergence of unified systems that combine symbolic, affective, practical, social, motor, and intellectual processes together–systems that constitute, in Vygotsky's words, "the only actual object of psychology." This conclusion, he claims, is of "great theoretical importance" that needs to be explored, especially because it has been insufficiently emphasized in current interpretations of his theory.

Vygotsky's remarkable statement has often been interpreted as the unity of *mental* processes, for example, as drawing together memory and thinking processes. Indeed, Vygotsky gives many examples of this kind, such as when he shows that memory, in its mature form, includes active conceptualizing and reasoning about what has to be memorized, therefore constituting the complex unified processes of *conceptual memory.* This view indeed indicates a progressive shift away from seeing mental functions as discrete and narrowly focused processes that can be defined and studied separately from each other (compare, for example, information-processing models of cognition).

However, Vygotsky's point is broader than the claim about unity of mental processes. What he essentially states, and this might sound like a paradoxical idea, is that mental processes are always more than simply mental. A mental process is always an element of a larger unity; that is, it is part of a system of processes that goes beyond the mental realm (i.e., of cognition and mind) and unites instead the mental and practical, the internal and external, dimensions of human functioning, essentially blurring the strict demarcation between these dimensions. To illustrate this idea, Vygotsky discusses activities such as playing, reading, writing, counting, and drawing–processes that stretch far beyond the confines of purely mental and solitary activities into the realm of social and collaborative activities in the real world. These activities, according to Vygotsky, are the true objects of psychological analysis; in these realities of human development, mental and physical are blended, because people never merely perceive, memorize, think, etc., outside of larger meaningful activities that relate them to the world and to other people. Such meaningful activities always involve achieving something out there in the world, outside the "mind," for example, establishing and maintaining friendship, becoming a successful learner, or simply eating lunch. Mental processes are not separate faculties that emerge and develop on their own grounds but are parts or versions of very worldly activities that humans pursue during their lives. It is in the service of such activities, and following the logic of their development, that the human mind evolves and develops, always driven by necessities, regularities, constraints, potentialities, and goals of meaningful life pursuits.

This broader view of the unity of processes that constitute human development has tremendous implications for the whole discipline of psychology. Essentially, it overcomes the centuries-old belief that the mental and the physical are two distinct realms, each of which exists on its own and relates to the other through some complex (and as yet unknown) mechanism. This belief, in its various forms (e.g., the dichotomies of mind—body, spirit—flesh, etc.), is entrenched in academic vocabulary, in everyday language, and even in popular culture, continuing to permeate much of our thinking, discourse, and practice. Because this belief is so ubiquitous and deeply entrenched, it is very hard to grasp an alternative view. Vygotsky himself occasionally slips into a more traditional mode of expression, drawing the old-fashioned lines between the two realms and speaking of the unity of "mental processes."* It is not surprising, then, that some Vygotsky-inspired research today remains de facto within the traditionally dichotomous approach.

Some wavering between the older views and his groundbreaking insights notwithstanding, Vygotsky's views on the most vexing problems of human development are amazing and truly revolutionary in their consequences. In place of traditional boundaries and dichotomies, Vygotsky directly asserts that mental and physical (practical) processes do not belong to separate realms but

---

\* Here again one of the principles described by Vygotsky can be seen at work in his own writing. In *Tool and Sign* Vygotsky explains how each new element brought into an older system (of ideas or psychological processes) cannot reveal itself at once with its full force but, instead, is dragged down to lower levels that are defined by older processes of understanding. It takes time for the new idea to overcome the larger set of ideas as a whole and to elevate them to the new level.

are merged to form one unified whole–*the single process of cultural development of a child.* Thus, he establishes the foundation for studying complete systems of meaningful life activities in the real world, systems that allow individuals to transform this world while in the process transforming themselves, and that also entail psychological processes as inherent ingredients and instruments of these activities. The meaning of this approach is best revealed if we consider some specific instances, examples, and implications.

In *Tool and Sign* Vygotsky makes considerable effort to illustrate and substantiate this extremely innovative view, both for his times and for today. These illustrations include, for example, his analysis of the child's evolving ability to speak as representing *a natural continuation of the child's practical contacts with the world.* Thus, Vygotsky notes that, for a child, the first naming of a thing is simultaneously a whole new way of *dealing* with this thing, and is no less practical than touching and otherwise physically handling it. The child initially even believes that names literally belong to things, that the names blend with the things and cannot be taken away, so that the table, for example, must necessarily be named "a table" and be known by no other word. Similarly, changing a thing's name, for a child, practically equals changing the thing itself. Rather than simply reflecting a child's naïveté, these beliefs contain a solid grain of truth. As Vygotsky puts it, children use speech not as an operation that simply accompanies their practical attempts at solving some problem; rather, children solve problems *with and through speech itself,* instead of solving it solely with hands and eyes. Therefore, Vygotsky insisted, the chief problem with previous theories was exactly that the "origin and development of speech and any other symbolic activity was considered as something that had no connection with the practical activity of the child, just as if he were purely a rational subject." Vygotsky, in contrast, regarded the history of speech as "flowing in the process of practical activity" and thus asserted the practical relevance of speech in unity with other forms of social behavior that realize the relations of individuals to themselves, to other people, and to the world around them.

Thus, in Vygotsky's interpretation, speech acts and other 'mental' processes are not fleeting, ephemeral phenomena in the shadow of action, but instead are powerful ways of changing the world. This is what he means by his powerful statement at the very end of *Tool and Sign,* namely that a *word is itself a deed.* This statement stands out in force and crowns this whole masterpiece of Vygotsky's psychology.

The idea that cultural development represents a unified system of processes driven by the logic of real-life tasks and contacts between the child and the world (including, importantly, other people) brings us to the fourth, and pivotal, theme of *Tool and Sign,* namely, that transformations of practical activity constitute the very reality of human development in all of its forms, including the emergence of 'mental' processes. A careful reading reveals an idea (ironically glossed over in previous interpretations of this work) that Vygotsky emphasizes again and again throughout the whole text, namely that development "arises neither through the path along which a complex habit is developed, nor through the path along which the child's discovery or invention arises" (p. 9). The child does not invent new forms of activity as an "intellectual discovery" (here Vygotsky criticizes a famous notion by Karl Bühler, that children discover that objects have names). Neither are these forms of activity a result of simple memorization and training, as in the development of a habit.

How then does such new activity develop? Vygotsky attempts to formulate his answer to this question in several places, as if trying out and de facto developing a solution through his own writing (and, thus, through his own speech), as he thinks in and through words, following through with various implications of his conceptualizations to see how certain ideas work, or do not work, for his purposes.* Vygotsky emphasizes that the child's activity never simply improves, as in the process of mere training in animals, but instead undergoes deep qualitative changes that "must be described as development in the true sense of the word." Development cannot be conceived as emerging from a mere training of skills to solve a certain problem, because even one and the same problem, when presented at different points in time, is never quite the same. The seemingly 'same' problem, in fact, presents a new situation each time, with certain new demands and conditions, as well as new meanings and new contexts of its realization. Therefore, previously developed skills and methods turn out to be insufficient or inadequate in a new situation, thus often becoming obstacles rather than factors contributing to the solution. Furthermore, according to Vygotsky, the formation of a new activity, even an intellectual one, least of all resembles a purely logical transformation, in which the child mentally derives new solutions. The process of development goes beyond training and intellectual discovery and instead involves sequential changes in, and reorganization of, the process of practical activity, giving rise to new forms of it. In other words, it is the flow of activity itself, and the contradictions in activities that arise in life, that engender transformations of activity and constitute the development of its new forms, including 'mental' activities.

A child's activity undergoes transformations, essentially because the child is faced with situations that constantly change their social meaning as the child becomes involved in more and more complex forms of cooperation with other people, including forms of cooperation that demand complex symbolic forms of interaction. It is in this sense, according to Vygotsky, that the sources of development lie in the social environment of the child. Note that the centrality of social environment in development does not mean that the former directly dictates developmental paths and outcomes. Rather, the impact of the social environment is indirect, coming to force only through the child's own activity as the child participates in shared and culturally shaped social collaboration. One could say that the social environment imposes important features and parameters on the child's activity (e.g. through cultural supports provided in social collaboration), but ultimately it is the child's own activity that drives the development, while the child gradually turns into a more and more active participant in this collaboration.

Perhaps the most cogent formulation of what human development is all about comes in Chapter 1, in the section, "Development of higher forms of practical activity in the child," where Vygotsky states: "The child does not invent new forms of behavior and he does not derive them logically, but forms them by the same means as walking displaces crawling and

---

\*   Here, again, Vygotsky's style of writing embodies the very psychological principles that he purported to develop. Thus, looking for solutions to problems in the form of directly thinking *through* speech, Vygotsky illustrates his own idea that thought is never simply expressed in speech but is born in it (see Section I of this book, on "Thinking and Speech").

speech displaces babbling. . . ." Indeed, how does the child acquire the ability to walk? Walking does not emerge through the training of a previously existing skill; neither is it discovered by a child; instead, walking comes about through the unfolding of an increasingly complex activity that serves the goal of freely moving in space, a goal that itself emerges in the course of collaborative shared activities with adults, because moving around on foot is a necessary ingredient of participating in these activities. In the process, the initial forms of this activity (i.e., crawling), as they are carried out in social contacts and joint activities with other people, face growing social demands and an expanding range of mediating support that bring about the change and elevate the initial forms to new levels of complexity, ultimately substituting for them.

This description by Vygotsky indicates that development unfolds in the context of real-life activities, always initially collaborative, as those activities undergo complex transformations, driven by demands of social life (themselves the results of the child's participation in more and more complex forms of social cooperation) and supported by new cultural resources that are introduced to the child in the course of social cooperation. Development is crucially dependent on the mastery of culturally defined modes of action (including modes of speaking, thinking, and even moving), but this mastery can take place only in the ongoing real-life activities of social cooperation, leading to mastery of one's own behavior in such a way as to make this behavior free, that is, able to pursue the goals of human endeavors. Importantly, a specifically psychological development (e.g., of attention, memory, or speech) is not a separate process, but it is an intrinsic part of the overall process of cultural development and is thus subordinate to the goals of participation in collaborative practical forms of social life.

This final theme of *Tool and Sign* is remarkably congruent with the point that was made at the beginning of this essay. Just as Vygotsky described the process of human development in *Tool and Sign,* this work itself was by no means a mere intellectual discovery; neither did it come about as a result of the simple growth of its author's purely mental capacities to develop psychological ideas and concepts. This work, like other creations by Vygotsky, was a product of his activities and collaborative practical engagements within a unique sociohistorical context that presented him with an unprecedented challenge–and opportunity!–to devise a new system of psychology that could help trace the development of human freedom and could be used to promote and realize such a development. This unique challenge became the foundation for Vygotsky's whole life project with its commitment to *social change* in a very clear direction toward justice and equality, in stark contrast to mainstream directions of psychology at the time that, for the most part, were pursuing knowledge that could result in *social control* and in preserving the status quo. Vygotsky's project, importantly, was not limited to mere intellectual tasks but came out of a unique and living system of his activities–a system of social practice–in which practical and intellectual, moral and emotional, and individual and social components all blended into a unified whole.

*Tool and Sign* was a product of these active, and often passionate, practical–intellectual pursuits by Vygotsky and his colleagues, and this work also became an instrument of their further pursuits. Thus, the ideas about conditions and regularities in the development of higher, free forms of human behavior were put to work by Vygotsky himself in his day-to-day practical engagements in the field of education, including, for example, the education of handicapped children. As Vygotsky believed, when provided with adequate mediational (i.e., sign-based) support from adults in organizing their activities in life settings, all children can progress to the highest levels of functioning to become fully competent members of society. Vygotsky's many followers later used the same ideas in highly successful rehabilitation and education programs for severely handicapped children, including deaf-and-blind, and in similar work. In this sense, Vygotsky's own work embodied one of the major metaphors of *Tool and Sign*, namely, that at the beginning of his work there were his deeds, which he turned into words that, in the end, again themselves became deeds.

Thus, Vygotsky's writings can arguably be seen as an essential part—a product as well as an instrument—of a broad collaborative social project that stretched beyond the confines of a merely intellectual enterprise, in its traditional mentalist guise, into the realm of social practice in which intellectual, cognitive, and practical processes are all blended. In this sense, Vygotsky's ideas can be best viewed not merely as ideas (in the traditional connotation of ideas being fleeting and ephemeral reality separate from action and practice) but as just *another form of an active engagement with the world, with the ultimate fundamental purpose of changing something in this world and oneself.* In a similar vein, an understanding of Vygotsky's work is best achieved in the context of a reader's active pursuit of some meaningful socio-practical task. That is, the best way to penetrate Vygotsky's ideas is to turn them into an instrument of one's own social practice, for example, by trying them out in solving some meaningful problems related to social change and human development. This does not mean that one can understand Vygotsky only while literally doing, in parallel, some practical work. Such an extreme view would presuppose a strict demarcation between practical and theoretical dimensions, and thus would go against the very spirit of Vygotsky's approach, in which theory and practice were seen as extensions of each other, as merely different facets of one and the same process, that of meaningfully contributing to practical tasks posed by life. Just as, according to Vygotsky, the mental and material are not separate and mutually exclusive realms, so are theoretical and practical types of work simply different aspects of one and the same reality of human social praxis and the purposeful transformation of the world. Kurt Lewin's famous expression, that there is nothing more practical than a good theory, could be extended, following the gist of Vygotsky's approach, by the mirror expression that there is nothing more theoretically rich than good practice. Vygotsky's works both theoretically stated these principles (although not explicitly in this form) and embodied them in the ways that these works were carried out and implemented in life by him and by his colleagues.

In conclusion, the inherent interdependency among the major themes developed by Vygotsky in *Tool and Sign* should be emphasized. From the foregoing analysis it follows that Vygotsky was pursuing a coherent and multifaceted research project rather than one single idea, such as that of mediation, as has often been presumed in previous interpretations of his work. Thus, the theme of the mediating role of speech and other signs is intricately connected with the idea that psychological processes, such as speech and thinking, form a unified whole of verbal thinking and conceptual speech. This idea is further linked to the broader theme of the unity of mental and practical processes, and, through the latter, to the centrality of child's participation in social collaborative activities as a guiding principle in development. These ideas of Vygotsky shed light on one another and make sense when regarded as a unified whole. Incidentally, these ideas presage much of today's cutting-edge research on child development, research that represents the best antidote to the individualist and mentalist fallacies of mainstream cognitivism. It would be not difficult, space allowing, to address how many avenues of research—such as distributed cognition, collaborative participation, participatory learning, dialogical inquiry, and dynamic systems approach–all bear significant similarities to ideas developed in Vygotsky's school. At the same time, these ideas, with their emancipatory and humanistic potential, in their ability to serve as an instrument of profound social changes in how we educate and treat children, are still in the Zone of Proximal Development of today's psychology. Again, it is perhaps the new generation of psychologists who will take over Vygotsky's passionate words—deeds and turn them into their own novel ideas and programs, which are urgently needed to meet the challenges that face psychology and society today.

## References

Kozulin, A. (1999). *Vygotsky's psychology: A biography of ideas.* Cambridge: Harvard University Press. (Paperback edition, first published in 1990.)

Leahy, T. H. (2002). History without the past. In *Evolving perspectives on the history of psychology* (W. E. Pickern & D. A. Dewsbury, Eds.; pp. 15–20). Washington, DC: American Psychological Association.

Valsiner, J., & van der Veer, R. (2000). *The social mind: Construction of the idea.* Cambridge: Cambridge University Press.

van der Veer, R., & Valsiner, J. (1991). *Understanding Vygotsky: A quest for synthesis.* Oxford: Blackwell.

Vygotsky, L. S., & Luria, A. R. (1994). Tool and symbol in child development. In *The Vygotsky reader* (J. Valsiner & R. van der Veer, Eds.; pp. 99–175). Oxford: Blackwell.

Vygotsky, L. S. (1999). Tool and sign in the development of the child. In *The collected works of L. S. Vygotsky, Volume 6: Scientific Legacy* (R. W. Rieber, Ed.; pp. 3–68). New York: Kluwer Academic/Plenum.

# 16

## The Problem of Practical Intellect in the Psychology of Animals and the Psychology of the Child

At the very beginning of the development of child psychology, as a separate branch of psychological study, K. Stumpf attempted to define the character of the new scientific area, comparing it to botany. He said that C. Linnaeus, as is known, called botany a pleasant science. This is scarcely applicable to modern botany. . . . If any science deserves to be called pleasant, then it is specifically child psychology, the science of what is most dear, loved, and pleasant in the world, what we care for especially and what we are, for this reason, obliged to study and understand.

Behind this beautiful comparison is hidden something much greater than a simple transfer to child psychology of an epithet applied by Linnaeus to botany. Behind it is hidden the whole philosophy of child psychology, a unique conception of child development that emerged silently in all studies from the premise advanced by Stumpf. The botanical, plant-like character of child development was brought to the forefront in this conception and the mental development of the child was understood basically as a phenomenon of growth. In this sense, even contemporary child psychology has not been liberated definitively from a botanical tendency that hangs over it and interferes with its recognizing the uniqueness of the mental development of the child in comparison with the growth of a plant. For this reason, A. Gesell[5] is completely right when he indicates that our ordinary conception of child development thus far is still full of botanical comparisons. We speak of the *growth* of the child's personality and we call the system of education in early childhood a *garden*.

Only in the process of long-term studies that encompass decades has psychology been able to overcome the initial conceptions that the processes of mental development are constructed and occur along the botanical model. In our time, psychology has started to master the idea that the processes of growth do not exhaust the whole complexity of child development and that frequently, especially when we speak of forms of behavior that are most complex and specific to man, growth (in the direct sense of the word) enters into the complement of the processes of development, not as a determining, but as a subordinate, constant. The processes of growth themselves also exhibit complex qualitative conversions of one set of forms into another, and, as Hegel might say, with respect to such transitions of quantity into quality and vice versa, the concept of growth seems quite inapplicable.

Originally appeared in English translation as Chapter 1 in *The Collected Works of L.S. Vygotsky, Volume 6: Scientific Legacy* (Robert W. Rieber, Ed.; Marie J. Hall, Trans.) (pp. 3–25). New York: Kluwer Academic/Plenum Press, 1999.

But if contemporary psychology has parted, as a whole, from a botanical prototype of child psychology, it seems to have ascended the ladder of the sciences and is now full of ideas that child development essentially represents only a more complex and developed variant of the appearance of those forms of behavior that we observe even in the animal world. The botanical enslavement of child psychology was replaced by its zoological enslavement, and many of the strongest trends of our contemporary science are seeking a direct answer to the question of the psychology of child development in experiments with animals. These experiments, with insignificant modifications, are being transferred from the zoopsychological laboratory to the children's room, and it is not without reason that one of the most authoritative investigators in this area has been forced to admit that the most important methodological successes in the study of the child are due to the zoopsychological experiment.

The convergence of child psychology with zoopsychology contributed a great deal to the biological basis of psychological studies. It actually led to the establishment of many important points that bring together the behavior of the child and the animal in the area of lower and elementary mental processes. But, recently, we have come to an exceptionally paradoxical stage of the development of child psychology when a chapter is being written on the development of higher intellectual processes typical specifically to man and consisting of a direct continuation of the corresponding chapter in zoopsychology. Nowhere is this paradoxical attempt to resolve the specifically human in child psychology and its establishment, in the light of analogous forms of behavior of higher animals, so clearly evident as in the teaching on the practical intellect of the child, the most important function of which (of the intellect) is the use of tools.

## Experiments on the Practical Intellect of the Child

A new and fruitful series of studies was started by W. Köhler in his widely recognized work with human-like apes. As we know, Köhler from time to time compared the reactions of a child with the reactions of a chimpanzee in experiments in similar situations. This was fateful for all later studies. A direct comparison of a child's practical intellect with similar actions of apes became the guiding thread of all further experiments in this area.

Thus, at first glance, we can see that all the studies generated by Köhler's work can be regarded as a direct continuation of the ideas developed in his work, which is already a classic. But this seems to be so only at first glance. If we look carefully, it is easy to see that while there is an external and apparent similarity, new studies essentially present a trend that seems to be opposite to that which Köhler followed.

One of Köhler's basic ideas, as Lipmann correctly points out, was the idea of innateness of behavior of anthropoids and man in the area of practical intellect. Over the course of all his work, Köhler was occupied essentially with an effort to show the behavior of the anthropoid to be similar to human behavior. Here, as a silent prerequisite, he is served by the assumption that corresponding behavior of man is known to everyone from direct experience. However, new studies in which an attempt was made to transfer to the child the patterns of practical intellect of the ape discovered by Köhler followed an opposite trend that is beautifully specified in the interpretation of experiments of K. Bühler presented by the author himself. The investigator speaks of his observations of the earliest manifestations of practical intellect of the child. These were actions, in his words, completely similar to the actions of the chimpanzee. For this reason, the indicated phase of the child's life can appropriately be called the chimpanzee-like age. In the child observed, this period encompassed the tenth, eleventh, and twelfth months. At the chimpanzee-like age, the child makes his first inventions, extremely primitive of course, but from the mental aspect, extremely important, according to K. Bühler.

Naturally, as applied to the child, Köhler's methodology must be changed in many respects. But the principle of the study and its basic psychological content remain the same. Bühler used a game of catch with the child to study the child's ability to use alternate ways to achieve a goal and to use primitive tools. Some of the experiments transferred Köhler's experiments directly to the child. These were experiments that could be solved by taking a ring off a rod on which the ring had been placed or experiments with a string tied to a piece of dry bread.

Bühler's experiments led him to a quite important discovery, specifically: the first manifestations of practical intellect by the child, like the action of the chimpanzee, are completely independent of speech. (In subsequent studies by C. Bühler, manifestations of practical intellect on the part of the child were also established, but these studies placed the first rudiments at a still earlier age—the sixth or seventh month of the child's life.) K. Bühler firmly establishes the fact, important from the genetic aspect, that instrumental thinking exists prior to speech, that is, grasping mechanical connections and devising mechanical means for reaching mechanical final goals.

Actually, the child's practical thinking thus precedes the first rudiments of his speech, being, obviously, the most primary phase in the development of the intellect from the genetic aspect. If Köhler tries to disclose the human-like aspects in the actions of higher apes, then Bühler tries to demonstrate similarity to the chimpanzee in the actions of the child.

This tendency remains unchanged with all subsequent investigators with few exceptions. Expressed most clearly in it is the cited danger of zoologizing child psychology, which, as has been said, is the dominant trait of all the studies in this area. In Bühler's studies, however, this danger is presented in the least serious form. Bühler deals with the child before the development of speech, and in this respect, the basic conditions necessary for confirming the psychological parallels between the chimpanzee and the child can be observed, True, Bühler himself underestimates the significance of the similarity between the basic conditions, saying that the actions of the chimpanzee are completely independent of speech and that in the later life of man, technical, instrumental thinking is connected to a much lesser degree with speech and concepts than other forms of thinking.

Thus, Bühler proceeds from the assumption that characteristic for the ten month-old child is a relation between practical thinking and speech—independence of intelligent action from verbal thinking—that is also preserved in the later life of the person, and that development of speech, consequently, essentially changes nothing in the structure of the child's operation based on practical intelligence. As we shall see subsequently, this assumption of Bühler's is not factually confirmed during experimental study directed toward elucidating the connection between verbal thinking in concepts and practical, instrumental thinking. Our experiments show that the independence of practical action from speech typical for the ape has no place in the development of the practical intellect of the child, which basically follows exactly the opposite path, a path in which speech and practical thinking are closely intertwined.

As we have already said, Bühler's incorrect assumption, however, is shared by most of the investigators whose experiments are done with an older child who can already speak. We cannot present any very complete and detailed review of the main studies of this problem. We shall only consider the basic conclusions that may have a real significance for our principal theme, the connection of practical action with the symbolic forms of thinking in the development of the child.

Elegant, systematically conducted investigations of O. Lipmann and H. Bogen brought these authors, as is known, to a conclusion that is not very different from Bühler's position. They used a more complex method of study that made it possible to catch the practical intellect of the school-age child within the net of the experiment and, on the whole, the experimentally confirmed dogma on the chimpanzee like practical actions of the child remains, that is, the dogma of the general similarity of the mental nature of animal and human operation of using tools, and of the principal unity of the path along which the development of practical intellect in the ape and in the child proceeds, moving forward in both cases through a growing complexity of internal factors that determine the operations we are interested in, but not through a radical and basic change in its structure.

Bühler correctly noted that mentally, the child is less stable, less formed biologically, less capable than a four-year-old or seven-year-old almost-adult chimpanzee. Subsequent studies proceed along the same path, developing newer and newer, but not essential, differences between the operations of the child and the operations of the chimpanzee. Lipmann and Bogen see the main difference in the domination of physical structures in the behavior of the child, but not an optical structure that is dominant in the behavior of the ape. If the behavior of the ape in an experimental situation that requires the use of tools is determined, as Köhler demonstrated, mainly by the structure of the visual field, then in the child, a "naive physics," that is, his naive experience pertaining to the physical properties of the objects around him and his own body, takes the forefront as a determining factor.

H. Bogen briefly summarizes the results of a comparison between the actions of children and anthropoids as follows. As long as the physical action is dependent predominantly on optical structural components of the situation, the difference between the child and the ape is only a matter of degree. If the situation requires a reasoned inclusion of physical structural properties of things, then we must admit that the actions of the ape differ from the actions of the child. As long as there are no new interpretations of the behavior of the ape, like Köhler, we can explain the difference by the fact that the actions of the ape are determined predominantly by physical relations.

Thus, we see that the whole difference between the development of the practical intellect of the child and that of the ape can be reduced to replacing optical structures with physical structures, that is, development of practical intellect is determined essentially by purely biological factors rooted in the biological difference between man and the chimpanzee. It is true that the author admits a change in this hypothesis in connection with new studies of the actions of apes, evidently not expecting that specifically the actions of the child, when considered more closely, would be an occasion for reviewing the conclusion reached.

For this reason, it is not surprising that after finishing the experiments, Lipmann and Bogen had to admit that even in Köhler's descriptions referring to the chimpanzee, there is much that is very applicable to the behavior of the child. To a certain degree, the descriptions contradict Köhler, who says that in describing the practical action of man, we are speaking of a *terra incognita*, about an area that has not been studied at all. For this reason, we must not anticipate in advance that a comparison of the actions of the child and the actions of the ape will yield anything substantially new. The authors see the whole significance of their studies in the fact that it allows them to show with greater clarity the similarity and difference already noted by Köhler. Not surprising, therefore, is the authors' conclusive admission that on the basis of the experiments on children, they could not obtain a substantially different picture of training of intelligent action than that which was drawn so elegantly and convincingly by Köhler on the basis of his experiments with apes. For this reason, as their experiments show, they had to conclude that with training, no qualitative difference can be established between the behavior of the child and the behavior of the anthropoid.

Further studies in this area differ little in main respects from corresponding experiments of Bühler and Bogen. Similar experiments done with mentally retarded children and children of low intelligence are closer to the methodology of Köhler. In precisely the same way, applying these experiments to psychotechnical screening and to deaf-mute children, using the experiments as mute tests, and finally, systematically using them for a comparative study of children of different ages—none of these studies revealed anything essentially new from the aspect that interests us.

As an example, we shall give one of the last studies published in 1930. We are speaking of the work of Brainard, who repeated Köhler's experiments very precisely step by step. He came to the conclusion that in all of the children studied, the same general attitudes, devices, and methods of solving the problem are disclosed. He says that older children solve the problem more easily, but use the same processes. A three-year-old child exhibits approximately the same difficulties in solving the problem as does Köhler's ape. The child has an advantage in the form of speech and understanding instruction, while the apes have an advantage in the form of longer arms and more experience in dealing with large objects.

Thus, we see that the reaction of the three-year-old child is approximately comparable to the reaction of the ape, and the participation of speech in the process of solving a practical problem, which, by the way, all the authors noted, is comparable also to one of the two-step, secondary factors that give the advantage to the child in comparison with the longer arms of the ape, which are its advantage over the child. Most of the investigators do not admit at all that, together with speech, the child also acquires an essentially different relation to the whole situation in which solving the practical problem occurs and that, from the psychological aspect, his practical action itself presents a completely different, superior structure.

Summarizing the results of his experiments, Brainard says directly that the three-year-old child displays almost the same reaction with respect to similar problems as do adult apes.

The first attempt to find not only similarity, but also a substantial difference, in the practical intellect of the child and the intellect of the ape was done in the laboratory of M. Ya. Basov. In an introduction to the series of their experiments, S. A. Shapiro and E. D. Gerke note that social experience plays a dominant role in man. Drawing a parallel between the chimpanzee and the child, the authors propose to carry out this comparison mainly from the point of view of that factor. The authors see the influence of social experience in the fact that the child, in imitating and using tools or objects according to a given example, not only develops ready, stereotypically reproduced patterns of action, but in the last analysis, develops mastery of the principle of the given activity. The authors say that repeated actions are sequentially super-imposed one atop the other like a multiple exposure in a photograph with isolation of general traits and suppression of those that do not conform. In the process, the pattern is crystallized, and the principle of the action is mastered. As the child's experience increases, the number of models of concepts that he uses increases. The authors assume that the models are a kind of refined pattern of all past actions of the same type and a theoretical plan of possible forms of future behavior.

We will not speak in detail of the fact that the appearance of such patterns, which resemble F. Galton's group photograph, resurrects, in the theory on the practical intellect, the theory of concept formation or innate representations corresponding to verbal meaning long established in psychology. We will also put aside the question of the extent to which a factor different from intellect, understood as a function of adaptation to new circum-stances, is involved as well as the involvement in the solution of the problem of any patterns that are formed purely mechanically as a result of repetition. We will only point to the fact that the very significance of social experience in this case is understood exclusively from the point of view of the presence of adequate models that the child finds in his environment. Thus, while it does not change anything substantial in the internal structure of the intellec-tual operations of the child, social experience simply fills these operations with a different content, creating a series of ready clichés, a series of stereotypic motor formulas, a series of motor patterns that the child uses in solving the problem.

True, in the process of factual description of their experiments, Shapiro and Gerke, like almost all investigators, are forced to indicate the unique role that speech plays in the practical-action adaptation of the child. This role, however, is indeed unique since speech, in the words of the author, replaces and compensates for authentic adaptation but it does not serve as a bridge for transition to past experience and the purely social form of adaptation that occurs through the mediation of the experimenter.

Thus, speech does not create an essentially new structure of practical activity for the child, and the former dominance of ready patterns in his behavior and the use of ready clichés from the archive of old experience remain in effect. What is new is that speech is a surrogate that replaces unsuccessful action with the word or with the actions of others.

Here we could conclude the review of the most important experimental studies of the problem that interests us. But before forming a general conclusion, we would like to point to still another recently published work that allows us to visually identify the general inadequacy of all the works mentioned and to mark the point of departure for an independent solution to the problem in which we are involved. We have in view the work of Guillaume and Meyerson (1930) to which we will return later. These authors studied the use of tools by apes. Children were not involved in their experiments. However, comparing the general results of the experi-ments with corresponding actions of man, the authors reach the conclusion that the behavior of apes is similar to the behavior of a person suffering from aphasia, that is, the behavior of a person whose speech is switched off.

This indication seems to us to have much significance and to touch on the most central point of the problem we are considering. We are returning, in essence, to what we spoke of at the beginning of our review. If, as Bühler's experiments establish, the practical actions of the child before the development of speech are completely similar to the actions of apes, then, according to the new studies of Guillaume and Meyerson, the actions of a person who has lost speech as a result of a pathological process begin again to be, on the whole, somewhat similar to the actions of the chimpanzee. But is not all of the diversity of forms of practical human activity that lie between the two extreme points, are not all of the practical actions of the child who can speak also, on the whole, similar in structure and in psychological nature to the actions of mute animals? This is the basic question that we must answer. To solve it, we must turn to the experimental studies which we and our colleagues performed that start from main premises that are different in kind from those which are at the base of most of the studies mentioned thus far.

Most of all, we tried to disclose the specifically human in the behavior of the child and the history of the establishment of this behavior. In particular, in the problem of practical intellect, we were interested in the first place in the history of the appearance of those forms of practical activity that could be recognized as specific to man. It seemed to us that this most important element was missing in a number of previous studies that were guided by the basic methodological premise of zoopsychological similarity. All preceding studies undoubtedly have great significance: they disclose the connection between the development of human forms of activity and their biological rudiments in the animal world. But in the behavior of the child, they do not disclose anything except what it contains of the former animal forms of his thinking. The new type of relation to the environment characteristic for man, new forms of activity which led to the development of work as a determining form of relation of man to nature, the connection between use of tools and speech—for previous studies, all of this remained out of reach because of the basic, original points of view. Our further problem is a consideration of this problem in the light of experimental studies directed toward disclosing specifically human forms of practical intellect in the child and the basic lines of their development.

The study of the use of signs by the child and development of this operation brought us, of necessity, to the study of how the symbolic activity of the child arises and what its origin is. Special studies were devoted to this problem which were developed in four series: 1) a study of how symbolic meaning arises in the child's experimentally organized play with objects; 2) analysis of the connection between sign and meaning, between the word and the object it designates for the child of preschool age; 3) a study of motivation that the child gives in explaining why a given object is called by a given word (according to the clinical method of J. Piaget); 4) the same study using a selective test (N. G. Morozova).

If we can generalize their results from the negative aspect, the studies indicated brought us to the conclusion that this activity arises neither through the path along which a complex habit is developed nor through the path along which the child's discovery or invention arises. The symbolic activity of the child is not invented by him and is not memorized. Intellectualistic and mechanistic theories are equally incorrect, although points in the development of habit and points of intellectual discoveries frequently are interwoven into the history of the use of signs by the child; they do not, however, determine the external course of this process, but are included in it as subordinate, auxiliary, secondary structures. The sign arises as a result of a complex process of development—in the full sense of the word. At the beginning of the process, there is a transitional, mixed form that combines in itself the natural and the cultural in the behavior of the child. We call it the stage of the child's primitiveness or the natural history of the sign. In contrast to naturalistic theories of play, our experiments Compel us to reach the conclusion that play is the main channel of cultural development of the child, and specifically of the development of his symbolic activity.

Experiments show that in play and in speech, consciousness of conditionality, of the arbitrariness of uniting sign and meaning, is foreign to the child. In order to be a sign for a thing, a word must be supported by the properties of the thing signified. Not "everything can be anything" in the child's play. In play, real properties of the thing and its symbolic significance exhibit a complex structural interaction. In the same way, for the child, the word is coupled with the thing through its properties and is interwoven in their general structure. For this reason, in our experiments, the child does not agree that the floor might be called a tumbler ("you couldn't walk on it"), but he makes a chair a train, changing its properties in the game, that is, treating it as a train. The child refuses to change meanings of the words "table" and "lamp" because "you could not write on a lamp and a table would burn." For him, to change the name means to change the properties of the thing.

The fact that the child does not discover the connection between the sign and the meaning at the very beginning of the development of speech and does not become conscious of this connection for a long time could not be more clearly expressed. Subsequent experiments show that the *function of the name* does not arise through a single discovery, but also has its own natural history. What appears at the beginning of the child's formation of speech is not the discovery that each thing has its name, but a new method of dealing with things, specifically their names.

Thus, those connections between the sign and the meaning that, according to external traits, begin very early to suggest corresponding connections due to similarity of method of functioning, are, according to their internal nature, psychological formations of an entirely different kind in the adult. To refer the mastery of the connection between sign and meaning to the very beginning of the cultural development of the child is to ignore the most complex history of the internal construction of this connection that stretches over more than a whole decade.

With the turning in, that is, the transition of the function inward, there is a most complex transformation of its whole structure. As experimental analysis shows, the following must be considered as the essential points that characterize the transformation: 1) replacement of function, 2) change in the natural functions (elementary processes that are the basis for the higher function and enter into its composition), and 3) the appearance of new psychological functional systems (or systemic functions) that assume the function in the whole structure of behavior that was fulfilled earlier by particular functions.

For the sake of brevity, we will elucidate all three internally interconnected factors with an example of the change that occurs with the revolution of higher functions of memory. Even with the simplest form of mediated remembering, the fact of replacement of function is most obvious. Not in vain did A. Binet call mnemotechnical remembering of a number series a simulation of number memory. The experiment shows that it is not the power of memory or the level of its development that is the deciding factor in remembering of this type, but the combinative activity, the creation and change in the structure of perceiving relations, thinking in the broad sense of the word, and other processes that replace memory in the given operation and determine the fate of the whole activity. With the transition of the operation inward, substitution of the functions leads to verbalization of memory and remembering in concepts which is connected with this. Due to the substitution of functions, the elementary process of remembering is shifted from its place, but even now is not wholly eliminated from the new operation, but loses central significance and occupies a new position with respect to the whole new system of cooperating functions. Entering into the new system, it begins to function according to the laws of that whole, part of which it now is.

As a result of all the changes, the new function of memory (the internally mediated process) coincides only in name with the elementary processes of remembering; according to internal essence, it is a specific neoformation with its own special laws.

This transfer of a social method of behavior into a system of individual forms of adaptation nevertheless is not purely mechanical and is not accomplished automatically, but is connected with the adaptation of the structure and function of the whole operation, and itself forms a whole stage in the development of higher forms of behavior. The former, complex form of cooperation begins to function according to laws of the primitive whole of which it is now an organic part.

There is a genetic, but not a logical, contradiction between the claim that higher mental functions, an inseparable part of which is the use of signs, arise in the process of cooperation and social intercourse, and the other claim that these functions develop from primitive roots on a base of lower or elementary functions, that is, a contradiction between the sociogenesis of higher functions and their natural history. The transition from a collective form of behavior to the individual form lowers the character of the whole operation in the first stages, includes it in a system of primitive functions, and places it on a level common to all of these functions. Social forms of behavior are more complex and develop earlier in the child; becoming individual, they drop to functioning according to simpler laws. Egocentric speech, for example, is lower than speech but higher as a stage in the development of thinking than the social speech of a child of this age. For this reason, perhaps, Piaget considers it a precursor of socialized speech and not as its derived form.

Thus, we come to the conclusion that the operation of using a sign, which stands at the beginning of the development of each of the higher mental functions, initially has, of necessity, a character of external activity. At first, as a rule, the sign is an external auxiliary stimulus, an external means of autostimulation. This is due to two factors: first, to the origin of this operation from a group form of behavior that always belongs to the sphere of external activity, and, second, to the primitive laws of the individual sphere of behavior, which in its development has still not separated from external activity, still not been emancipated from visual perception and external action (for example, the visual or practical thinking of the child). The laws of primitive behavior state that the child masters external activity earlier and more easily than he does the course of internal processes.

For this reason, the operation, changing from intermental into intramental, does not at once become an internal process of behavior. For a long time, it continues to exist and change as an external form of activity before it finally moves inward. For a number of functions, the stage of the internal sign always remains the last stage of their development. Other functions proceed further in development and gradually become internal functions. They acquire the character of internal processes at the end of a long path of development. Making the transition inward, they again change the laws of their activity and again become part of a new system where new patterns are dominant.

We cannot now consider in any great detail the process of the transition of higher functions from a system of external into a system of internal activity; we omit many pertinent abrupt changes in development, but we will try to present briefly the more important points connected with the transition of higher functions inward.

As experimental material in a careful study of the structure and development of the function of perception, we used the mute tests of S. Kohs, which are usually used for testing combinative activity. In solving the test, the child must produce a more or less complex, varicolored figure by combining cubes with varicolored borders. In this case, we can observe how the child perceives the sample and the material and how he produces the form and color in various combinations, how he compares his construction with the sample, as well as many other points that characterize the activity of his perception. The study involved more than 200 subjects and was carried out from the comparative-genetic aspect. Together with the children (ages four to twelve years), adults were also studied (normal, belonging to various cultural environments and levels, as well as neuropsychiatric patients with hysteria, aphasia, and schizophrenia), as were deaf-mute children and the mentally retarded (L. S. Geshelina).

If we consider the most basic and general results pertaining to the aspect that interests us, the study shows that factual data do not confirm the standard conception of the independence of the processes of perception from speech, of the essential directness of the mental function of perception, or the conception of the possibility of using mute tests to study adequately the nature of the function of perception at all levels of its development and, at the same time, completely independently of speech.

The facts speak for the opposite status of the matter. Just as in our experiments with the transmission of the content of pictures by verbal description and by acting out, by comparing the solution of one and the same problem by a deaf-mute and a hearing child, an aphasic and a normal subject, a child at early and later stages of development, we could establish profound changes introduced by speech into the process of perception, precisely so in this special study we could observe how verbal thinking, whose system increasingly includes processes of perception, transforms its own laws of perception. This is especially easy to observe because the laws of the one function and the other exhibit opposite tendencies at an early stage: integral perception, analytical speech.

In the processes of *direct* perception and transfer of the perceived form, not mediated by speech, the child captures and fixes an impression of the whole (colored spot, basic traits of the form, etc.)—all the same, he does this, as far as we know, reliably and, as far as we know, not primitively. When speech comes into play, his perception is no longer connected with the direct impression of the whole; new centers fixed by words and connections of various points with these centers arise in the visual field; perception stops being "the slave of the visual field" and, independently of the degree of correctness and completeness of resolution, the child perceives and transfers an impression deformed by the word.

Very important conclusions may be reached from this with respect to mute tests: to solve a problem in silence does not yet mean, as our studies show, that it is solved without the help of speech. Knowing how to think as humans do, but without words, is possible only through the word. This hypothesis of psychological linguistics (A. A. Potebnya) is fully confirmed and borne out by the data of genetic psychology.

A study of the function of concept formation, started by our colleague, L. S. Sakharov, who developed a special methodology of experimentation for this purpose, showed that functional use of the sign (word) as a means of guiding attention, abstraction, establishing connection, generalizing, etc. of operations entering into the composition of the given function is a necessary and central part of the whole process of development of a new concept. All the basic, elementary mental functions participate in this process in a unique combination dominated by the operation of using a sign (L. S. Sakharov, Yu. V. Kotelova, E. I. Pashkovskaya).

## The Function of Speech in the Use of Tools: The Problem of Practical and Verbal Intellect

Two processes of exceptional importance which are the subject of this paper—the use of tools and the use of symbols—have been considered thus far in psychology as isolated and independent of each other.

For a long time, there existed in science the opinion that practical intellectual activity connected with the use of tools does not have a substantial relation to the development of sign, or symbolic, operations, for example, speech. In the literature of psychology, almost no attention was given to the problem of the structural and genetic connection of these two functions. On the contrary, all the information that was available to contemporary science was more likely to lead to understanding these mental processes as two completely independent lines of development that might possibly be in contact, but had, on the whole, nothing in common with each other.

In the classical study of the use of tools by apes, W. Köhler observed a form of behavior that might be called a pure culture of practical intellect adequately developed, but not connected with the use of a symbol. Describing the splendid examples of the use of tools by human-like apes, he showed, in subsequent studies, how futile were all attempts to develop in animals even the most elementary sign and symbol operations.

The practical, intellectual behavior of the ape was completely independent of symbolic activity. Further attempts to develop speech in apes (see the work of R. Yerkes and B. Learned) also gave negative results, showing once again that practical *ideational* behavior of the animal occurs completely autonomously and in isolation from speech activity and that speech remains inaccessible to the ape regardless of the similarity of the vocal apparatus of ape and man.

Admitting the fact that the beginnings of practical intellect may be observed in almost full measure in pre-human and pre-speech periods led psychologists to the following hypothesis: the use of tools, appearing as a natural operation, remains the same in the child also. A number of authors, studying practical operations in children of different ages, tried to establish with great precision the time before which the behavior of the child in all respects resembled the behavior of the chimpanzee. The child's adding speech was evaluated by these authors as something completely different in nature, secondary and not connected with practical operations. At best, speech was considered as something that accompanied operations, like an accompaniment that goes with a basic melody. For this reason, it is natural that in studying signs of practical intellect, there was a tendency to ignore speech, and the practical activity of the child was analyzed through simple mechanical subtraction of speech from the whole system of the child's activity.

The tendency toward isolated study of the use of tools and symbolic activity was firmly rooted in the works of authors occupied with the study of the natural history of practical intellect; psychologists studying development of symbolic processes in the child adhered mainly to this line. The origin and development of speech and any other symbolic activity was considered as something that had no connection with the practical activity of the child, just as if he were purely a rational subject. This approach to speech necessarily led to a proclamation of pure intellectualism, and psychologists, inclined to study development of symbolic activity not so much as natural but as mental history of the development of the child, frequently attributed the appearance of this form of activity to the child's spontaneous discovery of the relation between signs and their meaning. This fortunate moment, in the well-known expression of W. Stern,[24] is the greatest discovery in the life of the child. Many authors claim that this occurs at the boundary between the first and second year of life and is considered to be the result of conscious activity of the child. The problem of development of speech and other forms of symbolic activity was thus eliminated, and the matter was presented as a purely logical process that was laid down in early childhood and contained in a finished form all the stages of subsequent development.

From studies of symbolic speech forms of activity, on the one hand, and practical intellect on the other, as isolated phenomena, it not only followed that genetic analysis of these functions led to viewing them as processes that had absolutely different roots, but even their participation in one and the same activity was considered to be an accidental factor that had no major psychological significance. Even when speech and the use of tools were closely intertwined in one and the same activity, they were considered separately as processes that belonged to two completely different classes of independent phenomena and the reason for their joint existence was believed to be external at best.

If the authors who studied practical intellect in its natural history concluded that its natural forms were not in the least degree connected with symbolic activity, then child psychologists who studied speech reached similar conclusions from the opposite aspect. "Tracking the mental development of the child, they established that over the whole period of development of symbolic processes, speech, which accompanied the general activity of the child, exhibits an egocentric character, but existing mainly separately from action, does not interact with it, but proceeds parallel to it. J. Piaget described egocentric speech of the child from this point of view. He did not ascribe to speech any substantial role in the organization of the behavior of the child and did not admit a communicative function for it, but was forced to admit its practical importance.

A series of observations led us to the idea that such isolated study of practical intellect and symbolic activity is absolutely wrong. If one could exist without the other in higher animals, then it follows naturally from this that the combination of the two systems is specifically what must be considered as characteristic for the complex behavior of man. As a result of this, symbolic activity begins to play a specifically organizing role, penetrating into the process of using tools and ensuring the appearance of basically new forms of behavior.

We were led to this conclusion by the intense study of the child and new studies that succeeded in discovering the functional features that distinguish his behavior from the behavior of animals and at the same time the specifics of this behavior as human behavior.

Subsequent studies convince us that nothing can be more false than those two points of view discussed above that consider practical intellect and verbal thinking as two independent lines of development that are isolated from each other. The first, as we have seen, expresses an extreme form of zoological views which, once having found natural roots of human behavior in the behavior of apes, tries to consider the higher forms of human work and thinking as a direct continuation of those roots, ignoring the leaps that exist in the transition of man to a social form of existence. The second point of view, defending the independent origin of higher forms of verbal thinking and considering it as "the greatest discovery in the life of the child," which happens at the threshold of the second year of life and consists in disclosing the relations between the sign and its meaning, expresses, primarily, an extreme form of spiritualism on the part of contemporary psychologists who treat thinking as a purely mental act.

## Speech and Practical Action in the Behavior of the Child

Our studies led us not only to be convinced of the falsity of this approach, but also to a positive conclusion that the greatest genetic point in all intellectual development, from which purely human forms of practical and cognitive intellect arose, consists in uniting the two initially completely independent lines of development.

The child's use of tools resembles the tool activity of apes only while the child is at the pre-speech stage of development. As soon as speech and the use of symbolic signs are included in the manipulation, it is transformed completely, superseding the former natural laws and engendering for the first time properly human forms of using tools. From the moment the child begins, with the help of speech, to master situations, having preliminarily mastered his own behavior, a radically new organization of behavior arises, as well as new relations to the environment. Here, we are present at the birth of specifically human forms of behavior that, having broken away from animal forms of behavior, subsequently create intellect and then become the basis for work—specifically the human form of using tools.

This connection is apparent with absolute clarity in the experimental genetic example taken from our studies. The first observation of the child in an experimental situation, similar to the situation in which Köhler observed practical use of tools by apes, shows that the child does not simply act to achieve his goal, but speaks at the same time. As a rule, speech appears spontaneously in the child and goes on almost continuously over the course of the whole experiment. It is manifested with great persistence and increases whenever the situation becomes more difficult and the goal not so easily attained. Attempts to interfere with the speech (as experiments of our colleague R. E. Levina have shown) either had no effect or stopped the action, freezing the whole behavior of the child.

In this situation it seems natural and necessary for the child to speak as he acts. The experimenters usually get the impression that speech does not simply follow practical activity, but plays some kind of relatively important and specific role in it. The impression we have as a result of similar experiments brings the investigator face to face with the following two facts that are of great significance:

1. The child's speech is an inseparable and internally necessary part of the .process, just as important as the action, for achieving the goal. According to the Impression of the experimenter, the child does not simply speak of what he is doing, but, for him, the discussion and action in this case are a single, complex mental function directed toward solving the problem.
2. The more complex the action required and the less direct the path toward solution, the more important does the role of speech in the whole process become. Sometimes speech becomes so important that without it, the child is definitely not capable of concluding the task.

These observations bring us to the conclusion that the child solves a practical problem not only with his eyes and hands, but also with the help of speech. The unity of perception that has developed, of speech and action, which leads to a reorganization of the signs of the visual field, also makes up a subordinate and very important object of analysis directed toward the study of the origin of specifically human forms of behavior. In experimental study of the child's egocentric speech involved in one activity or another, we also established the following fact, which is very significant for elucidating the mental function and genetic description of this stage in the child's development of speech: the coefficient of egocentric speech, computed according to Piaget, clearly increases as difficulties and interference are introduced into the child's activity. As our experiments have shown, for a certain group of children, the coefficient almost doubles at the moment difficulties arise. This fact forces us to assume that the child's egocentric speech begins very early to fulfill the function of primitive verbal thinking—thinking aloud. Further analysis of the character of this speech and its connection with difficulties fully confirmed our assumption.

On the basis of these experiments, we developed the hypothesis that the child's egocentric speech must be considered as a transitional form between external and internal speech. Egocentric speech, according to the proposed hypothesis, is internal speech psychologically if we take into account its function, but external in its form of expression. From this point of view, we are inclined to ascribe to egocentric speech the function that internal speech fulfills in the developed behavior of the adult, that is, an intellectual function. From the genetic point of view, we are inclined to present the general sequence of the basic stages of development of speech as, for example, J. Watson formulates it: external speech—whispering—internal speech or, in other words, external speech—egocentric speech—internal speech.

What is especially remarkable in the actions of the child who has mastered speech in comparison with the ape's solving of a practical problem?

The first thing that strikes the experimenter is the incomparably greater freedom in operations carried out by children, the children's incomparably greater independence than that of the animal from the structure of the directly presented visual or practical situation. The child forms significantly greater potentials in words than the ape can realize in action. The child can free himself more easily from the vector that directs attention directly to the goal and he can carry out a series of complex additional actions using a comparatively long chain of auxiliary instrumental methods. He is capable of independently introducing objects that are not in the direct or in the peripheral visual field into the process of solving the problem. Creating certain designs with the help of words, the child develops a substantially larger circle of operations, using objects that are not at hand as tools, but he also seeks and prepares those that may become useful for solving the problem and plans further actions.

Among the reorganizations to which practical operations were subjected due to including speech in them, two are striking. First, the practical operations of the child who has mastered speech are significantly less impulsive and direct than in the human-like ape that makes a series of uncontrolled attempts to resolve a given situation. The activity of the child who has mastered speech can be divided into two sequential parts: in the first, the problem is solved on the speech plane with the help of verbal planning, and in the second, in a simple motor realization of the prepared solution. Direct manipulation is replaced by a complex mental process in which internal planning and creation of design, postponed in time, themselves stimulate their own development and realization. These completely new mental structures are not present in any kind of complex form in the ape.

Second, and this is a fact of decisive importance, with the help of speech, in the sphere of things available to the child for transformation, is his own behavior. Words directed toward solving a problem refer not only to the objects of the external world, but also to the child's own behavior, his actions and intentions. With speech, the child is, for the first time, able to control his own behavior, relating to himself as if from the sideline, considering himself as a certain object. Speech helps him master this object by preliminary organization and planning of his own actions and behavior. The objects that were outside the sphere of activity available for practical activity, owing to speech, now become accessible for the child's practical activity.

The fact described cannot be considered only as a special moment in the development of behavior. Here we see cardinal changes in the relation itself of the individual to the external world. With more careful consideration, the changes seem to be exceptionally profound. The behavior of the ape, described by Köhler , is limited to the animal's manipulation in a directly presented visual field, while the child who is able to speak moves away from the natural field to a significant degree. Owing to the planning function of speech directed toward his own activity, the child creates from the environment, in addition to stimuli available to him in the environment, another series of auxiliary stimuli that stand between him and the environment which guide his behavior. Specifically due to the second series of stimuli created with the help of speech, the child's behavior is raised to a higher level and acquires a relative freedom from the immediate attracting situation, and impulsive attempts are transformed into planned, organized behavior.

Auxiliary stimuli (speech in this case) that fulfill a specific function of organization of behavior are nothing other than the symbolic signs that we have been considering here. They serve the child primarily as a means of social contact with the people around him and begin to be used as a means of acting on himself, as a means of autostimulation, engendering in this way a new, higher form of behavior.

An interesting parallel to the facts presented above and pertaining to the role of speech in the acquisition of specifically human forms of behavior can be found in the extremely interesting experiments of R. Guillaume and G. Meyerson and in their analysis of the use of tools by apes. Our attention was drawn to the conclusions in this work in which the intellectual operations of apes were compared to the processes of solving practical problems by aphasics (clinically and experimentally studied by H. Head). The authors find that the methods of carrying out a task by the aphasic and the human-like ape are similar on the whole and coincide in the most essential points. This fact thus confirms our idea that speech plays an important role in the organization of higher mental functions.

If on the genetic plane we saw a combining of practical and speech operations and the birth of a new form of behavior and the transition from lower forms of behavior to higher, then in the disintegration of the unity of speech and action, we note the reverse movement—the transition of the person from higher forms to lower. In a person with disturbed symbolic functions, that is, in the aphasic, intellectual processes lead not simply to a decline of the function of practical intellect or more difficulty in realizing it, but are a manifestation of another more primitive level of behavior of the same genetic formation that we found in the behavior of the ape.

What is lacking in the actions of the aphasic and what, consequently, is due in its origin to speech? It is sufficient to analyze the behavior of an aphasic patient in a practical situation that is new to him to see how much it differs from the behavior of a normal person who can speak in a similar situation. The first thing that strikes the eye in observing an aphasic is his unusual confusion. As a rule, there is not even a hint of the somewhat complex planning for solving the problem. Producing a preliminary intention and its subsequent systematic realization are absolutely inaccessible to such a patient. Every stimulus arising in the situation and attracting the attention of the aphasic evokes an impulsive attempt to answer directly with an appropriate reaction without taking into account the situation and solution as a whole. The complex chain of actions presuming the creation of intention and its systematic sequential realization is inaccessible to the patient and is turned into groups of generalized unorganized trials.

Sometimes the actions are inhibited and take on a rudimentary form, and sometimes they are turned into complex and unorganized bodies of practical actions. If the situation is sufficiently complex and can be carried out only by means of a sequential system of preliminarily planned operations, the aphasic becomes confused and seems completely helpless. In simpler cases, he solves the problem with the help of simple simultaneous combinations within the limits of the visual field and with methods of solving that differ very little essentially from those that Köhler observed in experiments with human-like apes.

Having lost speech, which should have made him free from the visual situation and would have made planning connected with a sequence of actions possible, the aphasic seems to be a slave to the direct situation a hundred times more than a child who is able to speak.

## Development of Higher Forms of Practical Activity in the Child

From what has been said, it follows that both in the behavior of the child and in the behavior of a cultured adult, the practical use of tools and the symbolic form of activity connected with speech are not two parallel chains of reaction. They form a complex psychological unity in which symbolic activity is directed toward the organization of practical operations through the creation of stimuli of the second order and through the subject's planning his own behavior. As a counterpoise to higher animals, in man, a complex functional connection between speech, use of tools, and the natural visual field develops. Without analyzing this connection, the psychology of practical activity of man would always remain incomprehensible. But it would be completely erroneous to think, as some behaviorists do, that the indicated unity is simply the result of training and habit and forms a direct line of natural development proceeding from animals and only accidentally acquiring an intellectual character. It would be just as erroneous to consider the role of speech, following a number of child psychologists, as the result of a random discovery made by the child.

The formation of a complex unity of speech and practical operation is the product of a process of development that goes profoundly inward in which the individual history of the subject is closely tied to his social history.

Due to a lack of space, we are forced to simplify the actual problem and take the phenomena that interest us in their extreme genetics forms, comparing only the beginning and end of the process of development under consideration. The process of development itself with its great variability of phases and manifestation of ever new factors remains outside our consideration. We deliberately take the phenomenon in its most developed form, by-passing the mixed intermediate stages. This allows us to show with maximal clarity the end result of development and, consequently, to evaluate the basic direction of the whole process. A combination of logical and historical approaches in a study such as this one, which voluntarily drops a number of stages of the process studied, has its dangers, which destroyed more than one theory that seemed flawless. The investigator must circumvent the dangers and remember that this is the only way to study the phenomena behind which history lies; he must inevitably turn to an analysis of the history.

We cannot stop to consider all of the sequential changes in the process. Here, we can isolate only the central connecting link; consideration of this will be adequate for making clear the general character and direction of the whole process of development. We must, consequently, turn again to the results of experiments.

We observed the activity of the child in experiments similar in structure, but spread over time and representing a series of situations of increasing difficulty. We established an important point that psychologists overlook, which makes it possible to describe definitively the difference between the behavior of the ape and the behavior of the child on the genetic plane. Previous observations allowed us to attain this with respect to the structure of activity since, as we studied it, the child's activity changed over the course of a number of experiments and did not simply improve, as happens in the process of training, but underwent such deep qualitative changes that they must be described as development in the true sense of the word.

As soon as we made the transition to studying activity from the point of view of the process of its formation (in a series of experiments over a course of time), we immediately were confronted by the fact that we were actually studying not one and the same activity in its concrete expression, but, over the course of a number of experiments, the object itself of the study changed. Thus, we obtained, in the process of development, forms of activity completely different in structure. This was an unpleasant increased complexity for all the psychologists who wanted at any price to preserve the unchanging quality of the activity they were studying, but for us, this immediately became the central fact and we turned all of our attention to its study. It led to the conclusion that the child's activity differs from the behavior of the ape in organization, structure, and methods of action and is not instantly available in ready form, but grows out of sequential changes in psychological structures connected genetically, and thus forms a whole historical process of development of higher mental functions.

This process is the key to understanding the organization, structure, and methods of activity in the child's development that we observed. In it, we are inclined to see from a new point of view the main difference that distinguishes the complex behavior of the child from the behavior of the ape. Actually, the use of tools by apes remains unchanged over a whole series of experiments if we do not take into account the secondary points that are more likely connected with gradual improvement of the function due to training than with changes in their organization. In experiments, neither Köhler nor any other investigator of the behavior of higher animals observed the appearance of qualitatively new operations formed in a genetic series that unfolded over time. The stability of the operations they described and their unchangeability in various situations was one of the remarkable characteristics of all of these studies.

This never occurred in the child. Combining a number of transformations in the experiment and creating in this way a kind of model of development, we never observed constancy, unchangeability of activity (except for extreme cases in children who were mentally retarded). For us the real reorganization of the process of activity was obvious at every new stage of the experiment.

We will describe the process of transformation primarily from the negative aspect.

The first thing that draws our attention and may seem to be paradoxical is the following: the process of forming higher intellectual activity resembles least of all the developed process of logical transformations. This means that the subject forms, interconnects, and divides the operations according to a different law of connection from one that would have to connect them in logical thinking. Very often the mental process of development of children's thinking resembles the process of discovery of methods of logical thinking. Some maintain that the child initially involves the basic principle of thinking, and individual, various, concrete forms are derived subsequently by the deductive method flowing as a logical and not a genetic consequence from this fundamental discovery by the child. The process of development is understood incorrectly here; in fact, confirmed here is Köhler's claim that intellectualism is not wrong anywhere as much as in the theory (and we must add, in the history) of intellect. This is the first and basic conclusion that prompted our study. The child does not invent new forms of behavior and he does not derive them logically, but forms them by the same means as walking displaces crawling and speech displaces babbling, not at all by his being convinced of their advantages.

Another hypothesis that we must reject in light of our studies is the opinion that higher intellectual functions develop in the process of improving complex habits and in the process of teaching the child, and that all qualitative difference of form of behavior is a change of the same type as a change in memorized text when it is repeated. This kind of possibility was excluded from the very beginning because there was a new situation in the experiment each time which required that the child be adequately adapted to new conditions and to a new method for solving the problem. But the matter was not exhausted by this: as the child developed, the problems presented to him made new and qualitatively different demands. The complexity of the structure of solving the problems increased corresponding to the demands so that even a solution that seemed most effective and was most fixed by training was necessarily inadequate to the new demands and became more of an obstacle than a factor helping with the solution of the new problem.

In light of the data that describe the process of development under discussion, it becomes clear that not only from the point of view of facts, but also from the point of view of theory, the two hypotheses we rejected at the beginning were wrong. According to one of them, the essence of the process is considered as a result of intellectual actions; according to the other, it is a product of an automatic process of perfecting a habit that arises as an insight at the very end of the process. Both hypotheses ignore development equally and are clearly unsatisfactory in the face of facts.

## The Path of Development in Light of Facts

As is apparent from our experiments, the actual process of development occurs in a different form.

Our reports show that even at the earliest stages of the child's development, the factor that moves his activity from one level to another is neither repetition nor discovery. The source of development of activity lies in the social environment of the child and is concretely expressed in those specific relations with the experimenter that permeate the whole situation that requires the practical use of tools and that introduce a social aspect into it. In order to express the essence of the forms of the child's behavior characteristic for the earliest stage of development, we must say that the child enters into relations with the situation not directly, but through another person. Thus, we come to the conclusion that the role of speech, which we identified as the basic point in the organization of the practical behavior of the child, is crucial for understanding not only the structure of behavior, but also its genesis: speech stands at the very beginning of development and is its most important and decisive factor.

The child who talks as he solves a practical problem connected with the use of tools and unites speech and action into one structure adds a social element to his action in this way and determines the fate of this action and the future path of development of his behavior. In this way, the behavior of the child is first carried to a completely new plane, it begins to be guided by new factors and results in the appearance of social structures in his mental life. His behavior is socialized. This is the main determining factor in all further development of his practical intellect. A situation in which people begin to act as well as things, acquires for him social significance as a whole. For him, the situation is like a problem set up by the experimenter, and the child feels that a person stands behind it the whole time regardless of whether that person participates directly or not. The child's own activity acquires its own meaning in the system of social behavior and, being directed toward a certain goal, is refracted through the prism of the social forms of his thinking.

The whole history of the child's mental development teaches us that from the first days, his adaptation to the environment is achieved by social means through the people around him.

The path from the thing to the child and from the child to the thing lies through another person.[28] The transition from the biological to the social path of development is the central link in the process of development, a cardinal turning point in the history of the child's behavior. The path through another person is the central track of development of practical intellect, as our experiments demonstrated. We are speaking here of a paramount role.

The following picture opens up before the investigator. The behavior of very small children in the process of solving a problem is a very specific merging of two forms of adaptation—to things and to people, to the environment and to the social situation; these are differentiated only in adults. Reactions to things and to people comprise in children's behavior an elementary, undifferentiated unity from which both actions directed toward the external world and social forms of behavior later evolve. At this time, the child's behavior is an odd mixture of the one with the other—a chaotic (as it seems to adults) mixture of contacts with people and reactions to things. Combination in one activity of the different objects of behavior that can be explained by the preceding history of the child's behavior, beginning with the first days of his existence, can be observed in every experiment. The child left alone by himself and stimulated to action by the situation, begins to act according to principles that developed earlier in his relations with the environment. This means that action and speech, the mental influence and physical influence, are syncretically mixed. This central feature in the child's behavior we term *syncretism of action* in analogy to syncretism of perception and verbal syncretism, which have been so thoroughly studied in contemporary psychology due to the works of E. Claparéde and J. Piaget.

Records of experiments we conducted with children show a similar picture of syncretism of action in their behavior. A small child placed in a situation in which the direct attainment of a result seems impossible exhibits very complex activity which can be described as a random mix of direct attempts to get the desired object, emotional speech, sometimes expressing the wishes of the child and sometimes substituting for the unattainable actual satisfaction with a verbal substitute, attempts to get the object by verbal formulation of methods, turning to the experimenter for help, etc. These manifestations are a confused bundle of actions, and the experimenter at first finds himself in trouble before this rich, frequently grotesque mix of forms of activity that interrupt one another.

With further consideration of the experiments, our attention is drawn to a series of actions that are, at first glance, outside the general plan of activity of the child. After the child carried out a series of sensible and mutually connected actions that should have helped him solve the problem successfully, confronted suddenly by a difficulty in realizing his plan, he abruptly stops his attempts and turns to the experimenter with a request that the object be moved closer so that it would be possible for him to carry out the task.

An obstacle in the child's path breaks up his activity and the verbal turning to another person is an attempt to correct this break. The circumstances that play a psychologically decisive role consist in the following. The child, turning for help to the experimenter at a critical moment, shows in this way that he knows what must be done to attain the goal, but cannot attain it himself and that the plan for solving is basically ready, although inaccessible to the child's own actions. For this reason, the child, having earlier separated the verbal description of the action from the action itself, takes off on a path of cooperation, socializing practical thinking by sharing his activity with another person. Due to this specifically, the child's activity enters into a new relation with speech. The child, consciously including the action of another person in his attempts to solve the problem, begins not only to plan his activity in his head, but also to organize the behavior of an adult according to the requirements of the problem. Owing to this, socialization of practical intellect leads to the need for socialization not only of objects, but also of actions, creating in this way a reliable prerequisite for carrying out the task. Control of the behavior of another person in this case is a necessary part of the whole practical activity of the child.

The new form of activity directed toward control over the behavior of another person is still not separated from the syncretic whole. We have frequently observed that in the process of carrying out a task, the child, grossly mixing the logic of his own activity with the logic of solving the problem cooperatively, introduces into his own activity the action of the other person. It seems that the child unites the two approaches to his own activity, combining them into one syncretic whole.

Sometimes the syncretism of action is exhibited against a background of primitive thinking of the child, and in a number of experiments, we observed how the child, seeing the hopelessness of his attempts, turned directly to the object of his activity, to the goal, asking it to come closer to him or to drop out, depending on the conditions of the task. Here we see a mixture of speech and action of the same person. We are confronted by this kind of mixture when the child, in carrying out an action, talks to the object, dealing with words the same way he does with a stick. In the latter cases, we see an experimental demonstration of how deeply and inseparably speech and action are connected in the activity of the child and how much this connection differs from the connection between them which can frequently be observed in adults.

Thus, the behavior of the small child in the situation described above is an intricate complex in which are mixed direct attempts to attain a goal, the use of tools, and speech directed either toward the person doing the experiment or simply accompanying the action, and, as if augmenting the exertions of the child, directed toward the goal. Sometimes speech, regardless of how paradoxical this sounds, is turned directly toward the object of the activity. The odd merging of speech and action seems to be senseless if we consider it outside the dynamics. However, if we analyze it on the genetic plane, tracing the stages of the child's development, or in a condensed form in a number of sequential experiments, this strange merging of two forms of activity discloses its fully determined function in the history of the development of the child as well as the internal logic of its development.

We shall consider two points of the dynamics of this complex process. They play a decisive role in the appearance in the child of higher forms of control of his own behavior.

## The Function of Socialized and Egocentric Speech

The first process we studied (egocentric speech) is connected with the formation of *speech for oneself*, which, as was noted above, regulates the action of the child and allows him to do the problem set before him in an organized way by means of preliminary control of himself and his activity.

With an attentive study of the records of our experiments with small children, one can note that together with turning to the experimenter for help, the child also exhibits a wealth of egocentric speech. We already know that complicated situations elicit copious egocentric speech and that under conditions of increased difficulty, the coefficient of egocentric speech almost doubles in comparison with situations that are not complicated. In another case, deciding to study more thoroughly the connection between egocentric speech and difficulties that arise before the child, we organized experimental complexities in the child's activities.

We were convinced that the situation requiring the use of tools, the central point of which was the impossibility of direct actions, best presents conditions for the appearance of egocentric speech. Facts confirmed our assumptions. Both psychological factors connected with difficulties—emotional reaction and deautomatization of action, which required including intellect in the process—basically determine the nature of egocentric speech and the situation that interested us. To understand egocentric speech correctly and disclose its genetic function in the process of socialization of practical intellect of the child, it is important to remember the fact, which the experiments bring out and which we emphasized, that egocentric speech is connected with social speech of the child by thousands of transitional stages.

Very often we did not understand the transitional forms well enough to determine to which form of speech one expression of the child or another may belong. The similarity and interdependence of both forms of speech exhibit the close connection of those functions of the child that both of these forms of speech activity fulfill. It is a mistake to think that the child's social speech consists exclusively of turning to the experimenter for help; the child's speech invariably contains emotional-expressive moments, information on what he intends to do, etc. During the experiment, it was enough to inhibit his social speech (for example, the experimenter left the room, ignored the child's questions, etc.) in order for egocentric speech to increase immediately.

If at the earliest stages of the child's development, egocentric speech still does not contain indications of the method for solving the problem, then this is expressed in speech turned to the adult. The child despairs of attaining the goal in a direct way, he turns to the adult and verbally formulates a method which he himself cannot apply. Enormous changes in the child's development occur when speech is socialized, when instead of turning to the experimenter with a plan for solving the problem, he turns to himself. In the latter case, speech that participates in solving the problem is converted from the category of intermental to intramental function. The child, organizing his own behavior according to a social type, applies to himself the same method of behavior that he applied earlier to the other person. The source of intellectual activity and control over his behavior in solving a complex practical problem is, consequently, not the invention of some kind of purely logical act, but applying social relation to himself, a transfer of the social form of behavior to his own mental organization.

The series of observations allows us to note the complex path taken by the child in transition to interiorization of social speech. The cases we described in which the experimenter to whom the child formerly turned for help left the site of the experiment demonstrate this decisive moment most clearly. Specifically under these conditions, the child is deprived of the possibility of turning to an adult, and this socially organized function is switched over to egocentric speech and indications of the path for solving the problem gradually bring him to their independent realization.

The series of sequential experiments carried out over time makes it possible to identify a series of stages of this process, and the formation of the new system of behavior of a social type becomes significantly more understandable. The history of this process is, consequently, the history of socialization of the practical intellect of the child and at the same time the social history of its symbolic functions.

## Change in the Function of Speech in Practical Activity

We would like to identify a second no less important transformation that the child's speech undergoes in our experiments. Disclosing the mutual relation between the speech and actions of the child over time and studying this dynamic structure, we established the following fact: The structure is not constant over the duration of the experiments; speech and action are related to each other and form a mobile system of functions with an unstable type of interconnections.

If we turn away from a number of complex changes that interest us on a different plane, we will be able to identify the basic functional shift in the system that has a decisive influence On its fate and leads it to an internal reconstruction: the child's speech, which formerly accompanied his activity and reflected its essential changeability in an unconnected and chaotic form, shifts more and more to reversing, to initial points of the process, beginning to anticipate action and explaining the action thought about but not yet realized. In the development of practical intellect, we observed a process similar to the process that occurs in another dynamic system of functions—in drawing with the participation of speech. Just as initially, the child draws and only when he sees the results of his work, recognizes and indicates in words the subject of the drawing, in practical activity, at first, he fixes in words the result of the activity or its separate points. At best, he does not name the result, but indicates the preceding moment of the action. Just as the naming of the subject of the drawing in the process of developing the drawing shifts to the beginning of the process, in our experiments, the *plan of action* begins to be formulated by the child in words directly before the beginning of the action, anticipating its further development.

This kind of shift represents not just a temporal shift of speech with respect to action, but also a change in the functional center of the whole system. At the first stage, speech, following action, reflecting it, and augmenting its results, remains subordinate to action in structural relation and is elicited by the action; at the second stage, speech shifts to the initial moment of action, begins to dominate action and direct it, and determines its subject and its course. For this reason, at the second stage, the planning function of speech is born in earnest and in this way, begins to determine the direction of action in the future.

The planning function of speech usually is considered as isolated from its reflecting function and is even opposed to it. Nevertheless, genetic analysis shows that this opposition is based on a purely logical construction of both functions. In experiments, we noted that there are, on the contrary, various forms of internal connection between both functions, and from this fact, it follows that the transition from one function to the other and the development of the planning function of speech from the reflecting function, is the same genetic nodal point that connects the lower functions of speech with the higher and explains their true origin.

Specifically because at first it is a verbal model of an action or a part of it, the child's speech reflects action or augments its results and begins later to shift to the beginning of the action and to predict and direct the action, forming it to correspond to the model of former activity that was previously fixed in speech.

This process of development has nothing in common with the process of logical *deduction*, logical conclusion from a principle of practical application of speech discovered by the child. Studies at each step indicate facts that compel us to assume that this summarizing speech, which creates a model of the path followed, plays an important role in the formation of the process, and due to this, the child acquires the possibility not only of accompanying his actions with speech, but of finding a reliable way of solving a problem with its help. As speech becomes an intramental function, it begins to prepare in verbal form a preliminary solution of the problem which, in the course of our further experiments, is improved and, from the speech model that summarizes what has been completed, it is converted into preliminary verbal planning of future action.

This reflecting function of speech helps us disclose the process of formation of its complex planning function and understand its true genetic roots. We can then see the origin of higher degrees of intellectual activity in all their complexity and with the whole complement of sequential transitions from stage to stage. What was formerly considered to be a process of unexpected *discovery* by the child turns out to be the result of a long and complex development in which the emotional and communicative functions of primary speech and the function of reflecting and creating a model from a situation have their place at a certain step of the genetic ladder. The ladder begins with primitive reactions of the child's glance and concludes with complex activity planned over time.

The history of speech, flowing in the process of practical activity, is connected with profound reconstructions of the whole behavior of the child. In this, there is something greater than the simple point indicating the fact that speech, being at first an intermental process, now becomes an intramental function, and that, at first diverting from the solution of the problem, at the end of the genetic path begins to play an intellectual role and becomes the instrument for an organized solution of the problem. This reconstruction of behavior has an incomparably more profound significance. If at the beginning of the genetic path, the child carried out manipulations in a direct situation, aiming his activity directly at the objects that attracted him, now the situation has become significantly more complex. Between the object that attracts the child as a goal and his behavior, stimuli of a second order appear that are no longer aimed directly at the object, but toward organization and planning of his own behavior. Verbal stimuli directed toward the child himself, being transformed in the process of evolution from a means of stimulating another person to stimulating one's own behavior, radically reconstruct his whole behavior.

The child is in a position to adapt to the situation presented to him by a mediated path through preliminary control over himself and preliminary organization of his own behavior, and this differs essentially from the behavior of animals. The child's behavior contains, as internal necessary factors, social relation to himself and to his actions, which are social activity transferred to within the subject. The child attains this as a result of the path of development passed, ensuring freedom of behavior with respect to the situation and independence from the concrete objects that surround him which the ape does not have, being, in the classical expression of Köhler, "slave to the visual field." Moreover, the child stops acting in a directly given and visual space. Planning his behavior, mobilizing and generalizing his previous experience for organizing future activity, he makes a transition to active operations developed over time.

At the moment when, with the planning aid of speech, a conception of the future is included as an active component in the activity of the child, the whole mental field in which he operates changes radically and his whole behavior is restructured in a radical way. The child's perception begins to be constructed according to new laws different from the laws of the natural visual field.

The merging of sensory and motor fields is overcome, and the direct, impulsive actions with which he reacted to every object that appeared in the visual field and that attracted him are now restrained. His attention begins to work anew and his memory is transformed from passive recording into a function of active selection and active and intellectual remembering.

With the inclusion of the complex mediated level of higher mental functions, there is a radical reconstruction of behavior on a new basis. Having studied the genetic progress that resulted from including methods of using tools and symbolic forms of activity in development, we must now turn to an analysis of the reconstructions that this progress engendered in the development of basic mental functions.

# 17

## The Function of Signs in the Development of Higher Mental Processes

We have considered some of the complex behavior of the child and have concluded that in a situation connected with the use of tools, the behavior of a small child differs substantially and in a major way from the behavior of the human-like ape. We could say that in many ways, it is characterized by an opposite structure and that instead of a complete dependence of the operation with tools on the structure of the visual field (as in the ape), in the child we observe a significant emancipation from it. Due to the participation of speech in the operation, the child acquires an incomparably greater freedom than is observed in the instrumental behavior of the ape; the child has the possibility of resolving the practical situation by using tools that are not in the direct field of his perception; he controls the external situation with the help of preliminarily mastering himself and preliminarily organizing his own behavior. In all of these operations, the very structure of the mental process changes substantially; direct actions on the environment are replaced by complex mediated acts. Speech included in the operation was the system of psychological signs that acquired a very special functional significance and resulted in a complete reorganization of behavior.

A series of observations convinces us that this cultural reorganization is characteristic not just for that form of complex behavior connected with the use of tools that we described. On the contrary, even separate mental processes, more elementary in character, are components of the complex act of practical intellect and are profoundly changed and restructured in the child in comparison with the way they occur in higher animals. In the child, even those functions that are considered most elementary are subject to laws other than those of earlier stages of phylogenetic development, and they are characterized by the same mediated psychological structure that we have just considered using the example of the complex act of using tools. A detailed analysis of the structure of separate mental processes that participate in the act of child behavior that we described convinces us of this and shows that even the teaching on the structure of separate elementary processes of child behavior requires a radical review.

### Development of Higher Forms of Perception

We shall begin with perception, an act that always seemed to be an act wholly subordinate to elementary natural laws, and we shall try to show that, in the child, this developmental process,

Originally appeared in English translation as Chapter 2 in *The Collected Works of L.S. Vygotsky, Volume 6: Scientific Legacy* (Robert W. Rieber, Ed.; Marie J. Hall, Trans.) (pp. 27–38). New York: Kluwer Academic/Plenum Press, 1999.

most dependent on the actual given situation, is reconstructed on a completely new base and, preserving external, *phenotypic* similarity to the same function in the animal, in its internal composition, structure, and method of action, in its whole psychological nature, belongs to higher functions established in the process of historical development and has a special history in ontogenesis. In the higher function of perception, we already encounter patterns completely different from those that were disclosed by psychological analysis for its primitive, or natural, forms. It is understood that the laws that hold in psychophysiology of natural perception are not abolished with the transition to the higher forms that interest us, but move as if to the background and continue to exist in a contracted and subordinate form within the new patterns. In the history of development of perception in the child, we observe a process essentially similar to that which has been well studied in the history of the construction of the nervous apparatus where lower, genetically older systems with their more primitive functions are included in the newer and higher levels and continue to exist as subordinate units within the new whole.

Following the works of Köhler (1930), we know the kind of decisive significance the structure of the visual field has in the process of the practical operations of the ape; the whole course of solving a problem presented, is, from beginning to end, essentially the function of the ape's perception, and Köhler is fully justified in saying that these animals are slaves of the sensory field to a much greater degree than adult humans and that apes are not capable of tracking the available sensory structure through voluntary efforts. Specifically in the subordination to the visual field, Köhler sees what brings the ape close to other animals even as remote in their organization as the crow (experiments of M. Hertz). Actually, we are scarcely in error if, in the slavish dependence on structure of the sensory field, we see a general law that dominates perception in all the multiplicity of its natural forms.

This common trait is part of every perception since it does not go beyond natural psychophysiological forms of organization.

Since the child's perception becomes the adult's perception, it develops not as a direct continuation and a further improvement of those forms that we observed in animals, even those closest to man, but it leaps from the zoological to the historical form of mental evolution.

A special series of experiments that we set up for elucidating this problem disclosed the main patterns that characterize higher forms of perception. We cannot consider this problem in its full extent and complexity here, but will limit ourselves only to an analysis of one point which is truly central in significance. This can be done most conveniently with experiments on the development of the perception of pictures.

Experiments that made it possible for us to describe the specific features of children's perception and its dependence on the involvement of higher mental mechanisms were set up in their essential form by A. Binet and analyzed in detail by W. Stern (1922). Observing the description of a picture by a small child, both established that this process is not the same at different levels of the children's development. If, in describing what he sees in the picture, a two-year-old child usually limits himself to indicating separate, disparate objects, after a time, he makes a transition to describing actions in order later to indicate complex relations between the separate objects pictured. These data moved Stern to establish a certain path of development of children's perception and to describe the stages of perception of separate objects, actions, and relations as stages through which perception passes during childhood.

Now these data, accepted by contemporary psychology as firmly established, aroused very serious doubts in us. Actually, it is enough to consider this material carefully to see that it contradicts everything that we know of the development of children's behavior and its basic psychophysiological mechanisms. A number of incontrovertible facts indicate that the development of psychophysiological processes begins in the child with diffuse, whole forms and only later makes a transition to the more differentiated.

A remarkable number of physiological observations show this for the motor system: the experiments of H. Volkelt, H. Werner, and others convince us that the child's visual perception passes along this same path. Stern's assertion that the stage of perceiving separate objects precedes the stage of perception of the whole situation directly contradicts all of these data. Moreover, taking Stern's idea to its logical conclusion, we are forced to assume that at even earlier phases of development, the child's perception has an even more fragmented and particulate character and that perception of separate objects is preceded by a stage in which the child can perceive their separate parts or qualities and only later unites them into objects and after that unites the objects into actual situations. We have before us a picture of development of children's perception permeated by rationalism and contradicting everything that we know from newer studies.

The contradiction that we see between the basic line of development of psychophysiological processes in the child and facts described by Stern can be explained only by the fact that the process of perceiving and describing a picture is significantly more complex than a simple, natural psychophysiological act and that new factors are involved here that radically reconstruct the process of perception.

Our first task was to show that the process of describing the picture studied by Stern is inadequate to the child's direct perception, the stages of which this author tries to disclose in his experiment. We were able to establish this with a very simple experiment. It was enough to ask a two-year-old to show us by pantomime the content of a picture, eliminating speech, to convince ourselves that the child at the *object* stage, according to Stern, splendidly perceived the whole real situation of the picture and very easily reproduced it.*

Behind the phase of *object perception* was actually hidden a rich and integral perception wholly adequate to the picture presented, which destroyed the hypothesis on the elementary character of perception at that age. What was usually considered a property of the child's natural perception was in fact a feature of his speech, or, in other words, the feature of his verbalized perception.

Observations of children at a very early age showed us that the primary function of the word that the child uses actually can be reduced to pointing, to isolating a given object from all the whole perceived by the child in the integral situation. The fact that the child's first words are accompanied by very expressive gestures as well as a series of test observations convinces us of this. Even at the first steps of the child's development, the word intrudes into his perception, isolating separate elements, surmounting the natural structure of the sensory field, and seemingly forming new, artificially introduced and mobile structural centers. Speech does not simply accompany children's perception—from the very early

---

* For the experiments, we used Stern's original pictures; the dynamics of these pictures made it possible for the child to disclose his perception of the pictures quite adequately by pantomiming the scene.

stages, it begins to assume an active part in it; the child begins to perceive the world not only through his eyes, but also through his speech. The essential point in the development of children's perception can be reduced specifically to this process.

This complex, mediated structure of perception also affects the character of the descriptions that Stern got from the child in the experiments with pictures. The child, giving a response about the picture presented, does not simply verbalize his natural perception of it, expressing it in an incomplete verbal form; speech dissects his perception, isolates definite points from the whole complex, introduces into perception an analyzing moment, and in this way replaces the natural structure of the process under consideration with a complex, psychological, mediated structure.

Only later when intellectual mechanisms connected with speech are transformed, when the isolating function of speech develops into a new synthesizing function, does verbalized perception undergo further changes, overcoming the initial dissecting character and passing into more complex forms of comprehending perception. The natural laws of perception, which can be observed in especially striking forms in receptor processes of higher animals, are restructured in their elements because of the inclusion of speech which dissects, and human perception takes on a completely new character.

The fact that including speech actually has a certain restructuring influence on the laws of natural perception is obvious with special clarity when speech intrudes into the process of reception, impedes and complicates adequate perception, and constructs it according to laws sharply different from the natural laws of reflecting the situation. Most clearly, we can see the child's verbal reconstruction of perception in a specially conducted series of experiments.*

## Division of the Primary Unity of the Sensory-Motor Function

The child's transition to qualitatively new forms of behavior is not at all limited to the changes within the sphere of perception that we described. What is much more important, also changed are the relation of perception to other functions that participate in the whole intellectual operation and its place and role in the dynamic system of behavior that is connected with the use of tools.

Perception of higher animals never acts independently and in isolation, but always forms a part of a more complex whole, and only in connection with this can the laws of this perception be understood. The ape does not passively perceive the visually presented situation, but its whole behavior is directed toward getting an object that attracts it. The complex structure that constitutes a real merging of instinctive, affective, motor, and intellectual factors is the only actual object of psychological study from which only by abstraction and analysis can perception be isolated as a relatively independent system closed within itself. Experimental-genetic studies of perception show that this whole dynamic system of connections and relations among separate functions is restructured in the process of the child's development no less radically than the separate points in the system of perception itself.

---

*    Editor's note: For more details, see Chapter 16.

As to objective significance, of all the changes that play a decisive role in the child's mental development, the special relation, perception—movement, must be placed first.

In psychology, the fact that all perception has its dynamic continuation in movement has long been established, but only in more recent times has the position of the old psychology been refuted according to which perception and movement, as separate, independent elements, can act in an associative connection with each other like two meaningless syllables in experiments on memorizing. Contemporary psychology is increasingly adopting the idea that the initial unity of sensory and motor processes is a hypothesis much more in accordance with the facts than the teaching on their initial isolation. Even in initial reflexes and simplest reactions, we observe a merging of perception and movement which convincingly shows that both these parts are inseparable points of one dynamic whole, one psychophysiological process. The specific adaptation of the structure of the motor response to the character of the stimulation, which was an insoluble problem for the old views, is explained only if an initial unity and wholeness of the sensory-motor structures are assumed.

We find such correspondence of the structure of sensory and motor processes, elucidated by the dynamic character of perception, not only in elementary forms of reactive processes, but also at higher levels of behavior in experiments with intellectual operations and the use of tools by apes: the observation of the experimenter (W. Köhler) shows that objects seemingly acquire vectors and move in the visual field in the direction of the goal when the ape considers the situation it must solve. The self-observation that is inaccessible to the ape is fully replaced here by the beautiful description of its movements which are as if a direct dynamic continuation of its perception. E. Jaensch gives a felicitous experimental commentary (we had the occasion to confirm it in our own laboratory) on experiments with eidetics who resolved the same situation in a purely sensory way in which movement actually carried out by the ape was replaced by moving the object in the visual field. Thus, in this case, the unity of sensory and motor processes in an intellectual operation acts in pure form; movement is included in the sensory field, and the internal mechanisms that elucidate the corresponding sensory and motor parts of the intellectual operation in the ape become completely understandable.

In experiments on the study of the motor system linked to internal affective processes, we demonstrated that the motor reaction is so merged and inseparably participates in the affective process that it can serve as a reflecting mirror in which it is possible to literally read the hidden structure of the affective process that is hidden from direct observation. Specifically this is a fact of major significance that is decisive in using an involuntary, linked motor reflex to produce an elegant symptomatological means for establishing objectively both experiences hidden by the subject (experiments with diagnostics of traces of crimes) and displaced complexes (posthypnotic suggestion, subconscious affective traces, etc.).

The initial natural relation of perception and movement and their being included in a single psychological system, as experimental-genetic study shows, disintegrates in the process of cultural development and is replaced with completely different structural relations as soon as the word or some other sign appears between the initial and final stage of this process, and the whole operation acquires an indirect, mediated character.

Specifically with this fate of psychological structures and with the elimination of the initial relationship between perception and movement, elimination that occurs on the basis of including stimuli-signs (new in the functional sense) in the psychological structure, it becomes possible to overcome the primitive forms of behavior, a necessary prerequisite for the development of all higher mental functions specific to man. In this case, experimental-genetic study also sees the complex and tortuous path of development in the old series of experiments, one of which can serve as an instructive example for us.

In studying the child's movement in a complex selection reaction under experimental conditions, we were able to establish that his movement does not remain completely the same at different stages, but, on the contrary, undergoes evolution, the central turning point of which is a radical change in relations between sensory and motor parts of the reactive process. Up to a certain point, the child's movement is directly merged with the perception of the situation, blindly follows each shift in the field, and in this way reflects the structure of the perception directly in the dynamics of the movement just as in Köhler's experiment, the chick at the garden fence repeats in movement the structure of the field it perceives.

The concrete experimental situation makes it possible to trace this. For example, we ask a child age four or five to press one of five keys in response to a specific stimulus. The task exceeds the natural capabilities of the child and for this reason elicits in him intensive difficulties and even more intensive attempts to solve the problem. We have before us the real process of selection as distinct from the analysis of a learned reaction that always replaced the process of genuine selection with stereotypic functioning of habit. Most remarkable here is that in the child, the whole process of selection is not separated from the motor system, but is moved to the outside and concentrated in the motor sphere: the child selects, directly making possible movements to which the selection situation impels him. The structure of his action does not in the least resemble the action of an adult who makes a preliminary decision and then carries it out in the form of a single effective movement. The child's selection is more likely to resemble a somewhat delayed selection of his own movements; here, fluctuations in the structure of perception are directly reflected in the structure of the movement; a mass of diffuse, probing trials arrested in the very process, interrupting and replacing each other, represents in the child the process of selection itself.

We could not better express the essence of the difference in processes of selection between the child and the adult than to say that in the child, selection is replaced by a series of trial movements. He selects not the stimulus (the required key) as a guide point for subsequent movements but selects the movement, comparing his result with the instruction. Thus, the child solves the problem of selection not in the perception, but in the movement when he fluctuates between two stimuli and his finger moves from one to the other, returning at midpoint; when he turns his attention to a new point, creating in this way a new center in the dynamic structure of perception controlled by the selection, his hand, forming a single merged whole with his eye, obediently goes to the new center. In short, the child's movement is not separated from perception: the dynamic curves of the one process and the other coincide almost completely in the one case and in the other.

However, this primitive-diffuse structure of the reactive process changes radically as soon as a complex mental function is introduced into the process that converts the natural process, fully available to animals, into a higher mental operation characteristic for man.

We suggested that the child, in whom we have just observed a diffused impulsive process of motor selection organically merged with perception, facilitate the task of selection by placing before each of the keys corresponding auxiliary signs to serve as supplementary stimuli to guide and organize the process of selection. A child of five or six years carries out this task very easily using an auxiliary sign to mark the key which he must press when a certain stimulus is presented. The use of an auxiliary device does not, however, remain as a secondary and additional fact that only somewhat complicates the character of the operation of selection; the structure of the mental process is reconstructed radically under the influence of the new ingredient, and the primitive, natural operation is replaced here by a new cultural operation.

The child, resorting to an auxiliary sign in order to find the right key for the given stimulus, no longer produces the hesitantly seeking movements in the air that arise directly with perception of motor impulses, which we observed in the primitive selection reaction. The use of an orienting sign disrupts the fusion of the sensory and the motor fields and introduces a certain *functional barrier* between the beginning and end point of the reaction, replacing the direct outflow of excitation into the motor sphere with preliminary closures with the help of higher mental systems. Earlier, the child solved the problem impulsively, now he solves it by an internal establishment of the connection of the stimulus with a corresponding auxiliary sign, and the movement, which itself carried out the selection earlier, now serves only as a goal of the operation. The symbolic system radically reconstructs the structure of this operation, and the child who can speak controls his movement on a completely new basis.

Including the functional barrier moves the complex reactive processes of the child to another plane: it excludes blind impulsive trials, affective in nature, that distinguish the primitive behavior of an animal from behavior based on preliminary symbolic combinations of intellectual behavior of man. Movement separated from direct perception and subject to symbolic functions included in the reactive act breaks from the natural history of behavior and turns a new page—the page of higher intellectual activity of man.

With special clarity, pathological material convinces us that including speech in behavior, and the higher symbolic functions connected with it, restructures the motor system itself and moves it to a new and higher level. We had the opportunity to observe that in aphasia with cessation of speech, the functional barrier we described arose, and movement again became impulsive, merging into a single whole with perception. In an experimental situation similar to the one described, in a number of aphasics, we observed the characteristic diffuse and premature motor impulses, seeking motor trials, with which the patients made a selection. These trials showed that the movements were no longer subject to preliminary planning in symbolic factors that created genuine intellectual behavior out of the movements of an adult cultured person.

We considered the genesis and fate of two fundamental functions in the behavior of the child. We saw that in a complex operation of using tools and practical intellectual action, these functions, which play a real decisive role, do not persist in the child as one and the same, but, in the process of development, undergo a complex transformation, changing not only their internal structure, but also appearing in new functional relations with other processes. Consequently, according to psychological composition, the use of tools, as we observe it in the behavior of the child, is not a simple repetition or direct continuation of what comparative psychology observed in the ape. Psychological analysis discloses, in this act, substantial and qualitatively new traits, and the inclusion in this act of higher, historically created symbolic functions reconstructs the primitive process of solving a problem on a completely new basis (of these functions, we considered speech and the use of tools here).

True, at first glance, in the use of tools by the ape and by the child, we see a certain external similarity that caused investigators to consider both of these cases as essentially related. The similarity was connected exclusively with the fact that in both cases functions are used that are similar in their final purpose. However, the study shows that these externally similar functions differ from each other no less than the depositions on the Earth's crust in different geological eras. If in the first case, the functions of the biological formation solve the problem presented to the animal, then in the second case, similar functions of the historical formation come forward and begin to play a leading role in solving the problem. From the aspect of phylogenesis, being a product not of biological evolution of behavior but of historical development of the human personality, and from the aspect of ontogenesis, these functions also have their own special developmental history closely connected with the biological formation, but not coinciding with it or with the second line of mental development of the child that is formed together with it. We call these functions higher, having in mind primarily their place in development, but we are inclined to call the history of their formation sociogenesis of higher mental functions, in contrast to biogenesis of lower functions, having in mind, in the first place, the social nature of their origin.

The appearance in the process of the child's development of new historical formations together with comparatively primitive layers of behavior is, thus, the key without which the use of tools and all higher forms of behavior will remain a puzzle for investigators.

## Reconstruction of Memory and Attention

The brief form of a review does not allow us to analyze in detail all the basic mental functions that participate in the operation we studied. We will limit ourselves therefore to the most general reference to the fate of those that are the most important without which the psychological structure of using tools would remain unclear for us. Attention must be first according to degree of participation in this operation. All investigators, beginning with Köhler, note that the appropriate directing of attention or distracting of it is an essential factor in the success or lack of success of a practical operation. This fact, noted by Köhler, retains its significance in the behavior of the child also. However, it is essential that, in contrast to the animal, the child first is in a state of independently and actively shifting his attention, restructuring his perception and, in this way, freeing himself to a large degree from subjection to the structure of the visual field that he is given. At a certain stage of development that connects the use of tools with speech (at first syncretically, and later also synthetically entering into this operation), the child in this way transfers the activity of his attention to a new plane. With the help of the indicative function of words, which we noted above, he begins to control his attention, creating new structural centers of the perceived situation, and in this way, changing, in the fortuitous expression of G. Kafka, not the degree of clarity of one part of the perceived field or another, but its center of gravity, the significance of its separate elements, isolating ever new figures from the background and, in this way, infinitely broadening the possibility of actively controlling his attention.

All of this frees the child's attention from the power of the actual situation that affects him directly. Using speech to create, together with the spatial field, a temporal field of action that is just as visible and real as the optical situation (although perhaps somewhat more vague), the child who can speak has the possibility of dynamically directing his attention, acting in the present from the point of view of a future field, and frequently referring to actively created changes in the present situation from the point of view of his past actions. Specifically owing to the participation of speech and the transition to a free distribution of attention, the future field of action is converted from the old and abstract verbal formula into an actual, optical situation; in it, all of the elements that are part of the plan of future action enter into the basic configuration, eliminating possible actions from the general background in this way. With the help of speech, the fact that the field of attention does not coincide with the field of perception extracts from the latter the elements of an actual *future field* and results in the specific difference between the child's operation and the operation of higher animals. In the child, the field of perception is organized by the verbalized function of attention and if, for the ape, absence of direct optical contact between the object and the goal is enough to make the problem insoluble, the child easily eliminates this difficulty by verbal intervention, reorganizing his sensory field.

Owing to this circumstance, the possibility arises of placing into a single field of attention a figure of a future situation consisting of elements of the past and present sensory fields. And in this way, the field of attention encompasses not one perception, but a whole series of potential perceptions that form a general successive dynamic structure spread over time. The transition from a simultaneous structure of the visual field to a successive structure of a dynamic field of attention is accomplished as a result of a reconstruction—on the basis of including speech—of all the basic connections between separate functions that participate in the operation: the field of attention is separated from the field of perception and develops over time, including the given actual situation as one instance of a dynamic series.

The ape, perceiving a stick at one moment, in one visual field, no longer turns its attention to it in the following moment when its visual field changes. It must see the stick first of all in order to pay attention to it; the child can turn his attention in order to see.

The possibility of placing elements of the past and the present visual fields (for example, the tool and the goal) into a single field of attention leads, in turn, to a major reconstruction of another important function that participates in the operation—memory. Just as the action of attention, in the valid observation of Kafka, has its effect not in augmenting the clarity of one part or another of the sensory field, but in shifting the center of gravity, in its structure and in a dynamic change of this structure, in a change in the figure and background, the role of memory in the operation of the child affects not simply the extension of the segment of the past that actually is merged into a single whole with the present, but results in a new method of combining the elements of past experience with the present. A new method develops on the basis of including into a single focus of attention the speech formulas of past situations and past actions. As we have seen, speech forms the operation along laws different from direct action precisely just as it merges, unites, synthesizes the past and the present in a different way, freeing the action of the child from the power of direct remembering.

## The Voluntary Structure of Higher Mental Functions

Subjecting the mental operation of practical intellect connected with the use of tools to further analysis, we see that the temporal field created for action with the help of speech extends not only backward, but also forward. Anticipation of subsequent moments of the operation in a symbolic form makes it possible to include special stimuli in the present operation; the task of these is reduced to presenting in the situation at hand instances of future action and actually realizing their effect in the organization of behavior in the present moment.

In this case, including symbolic functions in the operation, as we have seen in the example of the operation of memory and attention, does not lead to a simple extension of the operation over time, but creates conditions for a connection of a completely new character, a connection of elements of the present and future (actually perceived elements of the situation at hand are included in one structural system with symbolically represented elements of the future), and a completely new psychological field for action is created that leads to the appearance of the function of formation of intention and of a target action planned in advance.

This transformation in the structure of the child's behavior is connected with changes of a significantly more profound order. In comparing the solving of a problem by deaf-mute children in Köhler-like experiments, even Lindner turned his attention to the fact that stimulating motives that compel the ape and the child to attain a goal must not be considered to be identical. The animal's dominant instinctive motives yield in the child to new motives, social in origin that have no natural analog, but, regardless of this, reach a significant intensity in the child. K. Lewin called these motives, which have a decisive significance in the mechanics of a developed volitional act, quasi-needs,* noting that including them constructs in a new way the affective and volitional systems in the child's behavior, and specifically changes his relation to the organization of future actions. Two principal features make up an original form of this new layer of "motors" of human behavior: the mechanism of implementing an intention at the moment of its appearance, first, is separated from the motor apparatus and, second, contains an impulse to action, the implementation of which is referred to a future field. Neither of these features is present in the action organized by a natural need where the motor system is inseparable from direct perception and all the action is concentrated in a real mental field.

The way in which actions referring to the future develop, thus far inadequately explained, is revealed from the point of view of a study of symbolic functions and their participation in behavior. This functional barrier between perception and the motor system, which we established above and which is forced by its origin to insert a word or other symbol between the beginning and end of action, explains the separation of the impulses from the direct realization of the act,

---

* With the transition to artificially established needs, the emotional center of the situation is transferred from the goal to the solving of the problem. Essentially, the "situation of the problem" in the experiment with the ape exists only in the eyes of the experimenter; only the goal and the obstacle that interferes with achieving it exist for the animal. The child, however, tries most of all to solve the problem that has been presented to him, in this way including in his world completely new relations to the goal. Because of the possibility of forming quasi-needs, the child is in a position to segment the operation, converting each of its separate parts into an independent problem which he formulates for himself with the help of speech.

separation that in turn is a mechanism of preparation for actions postponed for the future. Specifically the inclusion of symbolic operations makes possible the appearance of a psychological field completely new in composition, not based on what is at hand in the present, but presenting a sketch of the future, and in this way creating free action independent of the direct situation.

A study of the mechanisms of symbolic situations, which seemingly extract the action from the three natural primary connections already present due to the biological organization of behavior and transfer it into a completely new psychological system of functions, allows us to understand by which pathways man arrives at the possibility of forming "any intentions"— a fact that thus far has not received adequate attention and which, according to Lewin's correct observation, distinguishes the cultured adult from the child and the primitive.

If we attempt to summarize the results of analysis of how separate mental functions and their structural connections are changed under the influence of including symbols, and to compare on the whole, the non-verbal operation of the ape with the verbalized operation of the child, we will find that one is related to the other the way voluntary action is related to involuntary.

The traditional view refers everything to voluntary actions that are not primary or secondary automatic action (instinct or habit). Moreover, actions of a third order are possible that are neither automatic nor voluntary. As K. Koffka demonstrated, *intellectual actions* of the ape cannot be reduced to ready automatisms, but neither do they have a *voluntary* character. Studies that we rely on explain for us what is lacking in the action of the ape that would make it *voluntary: a voluntary* action begins only where one controls one's own behavior with the help of symbolic stimuli. Rising to this level in the development of behavior, the child makes a leap from the "rational" action of the ape to the rational and free action of man.

Thus, in the light of the historical theory of higher mental functions, the boundaries, standard in contemporary psychology, that separate some and unite other mental processes, shift. What was earlier ascribed to different areas proved to be united into one, and what was placed in one class of phenomena actually proved to belong on completely different rungs of the genetic ladder and was subject to different laws. For this reason, the higher mental functions form a system united in genetic character, but dissimilar in the structures that comprise it. At the same time, this system is constructed on bases completely different from those that underlie elementary mental functions. The decisive factor that cements the whole system, whether or not one mental process or another is related to it, is the unity of the origin of structures and the character of functioning.

Genetically, in terms of phylogenesis, their basic trait is the fact that they were formed as a product not of biological evolution, but of historical development of behavior; they preserve a specific social history. In terms of ontogenesis, from the point of view of structure, their characteristic is that, in contrast to the direct structure of elementary mental processes, they are direct reactions to stimuli and are constructed on a base of utilizing mediating stimuli (signs), and because of this, they have a mediated character. Finally, with respect to function, they are characterized by the fact that they play a new and essentially different role in comparison with elementary functions, and appear as a product of the historical development of behavior.

All of this integrates the given functions into a broad field of genetic study and, instead of being interpreted as lower or higher variants of the same functions consistently manifested parallel to each other, they begin to be considered as different stages of a single process of the cultural formation of personality. From this point of view, we can, on the same basis on which we spoke of logical memory or voluntary attention, speak of logical attention and voluntary or logical forms of perception, which differ sharply from natural forms of these processes that operate according to laws proper to a different genetic stage.

As a logical consequence of admitting into the system of psychological categories the use of signs as being of decisive importance to The History of the Development of Higher Mental Functions, external symbolic forms of activity such as verbal communication, reading, writing, counting, and drawing are also involved. Usually these processes were considered as dissimilar and auxiliary with respect to internal mental processes, but from the new point of view from which we proceed, they are admitted into the system of higher mental functions as equivalent to all other higher mental processes. We are inclined to consider them primarily as special forms of behavior formed in the process of sociocultural development of the child and forming the external line of development of symbolic activity that exists together with the internal line represented by cultural development of such formations as practical intelligence, perception, and memory.

Not only the activity connected with practical intellect, but all other functions, just as primary and frequently even more elementary, that enter into the biologically formulated forms of behavior manifest, in the process of development, those laws that we discovered in the analysis of practical intellect. The path taken by the practical intellect of the child constitutes, in this way, the general line of development of all basic mental functions, each of which, like practical intellect, has its own human-like form in the animal world. This path is similar to the one we considered in preceding pages: it also begins with natural forms of development, soon outgrows them, and results in a radical reconstruction of elementary functions on the basis of using signs as means of organizing behavior.

Thus, as strange as this may seem from the point of view of the traditional approach, the higher functions of perception, memory, and attention, movements internally connected with sign activity of the child, can be understood only on the basis of analysis of their genetic roots and of the reorganization to which they are subjected in the process of their cultural history.

Now we are confronted with a conclusion of enormous theoretical importance. Shortly, we will consider the problem of the unity of higher mental functions based on the substantial similarity that is manifested in their origin and development. Such functions as voluntary attention, logical memory, higher forms of perception and movement, which thus far have been studied in isolation, as separate psychological facts, now, in the light of our experiments, appear essentially as phenomena of one order—united in their genesis and in their psychological structure.

# 18

## Sign Operations and Organization of Mental Processes

### The Problem of the Sign in the Formation of Higher Mental Functions

The material collected leads us to psychological positions whose meaning goes far beyond the limits of an analysis of the narrow and concrete group of phenomena which was thus far the main subject of our study. Upon closer examination, the functional, structural, and genetic patterns disclosed in the study of factual data appear to be patterns of a more general order and compel us to revise altogether the problem of the construction and genesis of higher mental functions. Two paths lead to this review and general conclusion.

On the one hand, a broader study of other forms of symbolic activity of the child shows that not just speech, but all operations connected with the use of signs, with all their differences in concrete forms, display the same patterns of development, construction, and functioning as does speech in its role as considered above. Their psychological nature seems to be the same as the nature of the speech activity we considered in which properties common to all higher mental processes are presented in a full and developed form. Consequently, in the light of what we have learned concerning the functions of speech, we must consider other psychological systems similar to it, whether we are dealing with symbolic processes of a second order (writing, reading, etc.) or with the most basic, such as speech and forms of behavior.

On the other hand, not only the operations connected with practical intellect, but all other functions that are just as primary and frequently even more elementary, functions that belong to the inventory of biologically formed types of activity, display, in the process of development, patterns that we have found in the analysis of practical intellect. The path that the child's practical intellect takes, which we considered above, is, thus, a common path of development of all basic mental functions; these are united with practical intellect by the fact that they have human forms in an animal world. The path is similar to the one we have taken: beginning with the natural forms of development, it soon outgrows them and undergoes a radical reconstruction of those functions on the basis of using a sign as a means for organizing behavior. Thus, no matter how strange it seems from the point of view of traditional teaching, the higher functions of perception, memory, attention, movement, and others are internally connected with the development of the symbolic activity of the child, and

Originally appeared in English translation as Chapter 3 in *The Collected Works of L.S. Vygotsky, Volume 6: Scientific Legacy* (Robert W. Rieber, Ed.; Marie J. Hall, Trans.) (pp. 39–44). New York: Kluwer Academic/Plenum Press, 1999.

they can be understood only on the basis of an analysis of their genetic roots and the reconstruction that they were subjected to in the process of cultural history.

We are confronted by a conclusion of great theoretical significance: opening before us is a unity of higher mental functions based on an essentially identical origin and mechanism of development. Functions such as voluntary attention, logical memory, higher forms of perception, and movement that thus far were considered separately, as specific psychological facts, in the light of our experiments, appear as phenomena of one psychological order, a product of a basically single process of historical development of behavior. By the same token, all of these functions enter into the broad aspect of genetic study and instead of constantly co-existing together with lower and higher varieties of one and the same function, are seen as actually being different stages of a single process of the cultural formation of the personality. From this point of view, we would have the same basis with which we speak of logical memory or voluntary attention to speak of voluntary memory and logical attention, of voluntary or logical forms of perception, which are decidedly different from natural forms.

The logical conclusion from recognizing the paramount importance of using signs in the history of the development of all higher mental functions is to include in the system of psychological concepts the external symbolic forms of activity (speech, reading, writing, counting, drawing) that are usually considered as something peripheral and accessory with respect to internal mental processes and which, from the new point of view that we are defending, enter into the system of higher mental functions on equal footing with all other higher mental processes. We are inclined to consider them first of all as unique forms of behavior constituted during the history of sociocultural development of the child and forming an external line in the development of symbolic activity together with the internal line represented by the cultural development of such functions as practical intellect, perception, memory, etc.

Thus, in the light of the historical theory on higher mental functions that we are developing, the customary boundaries that divide or unite separate processes according to contemporary psychology are shifted: what was formerly placed in different cells of the pattern actually belongs to one area and conversely, what seemed to belong to one class of phenomena actually is placed on completely different rungs of the genetic ladder and is subject to completely different laws.

The higher functions, therefore, are one according to genetic nature although they are different in the constitution of the psychological system constructed on quite different bases from the system of elementary mental functions. The uniting points of the whole system that determine the relation to it of one specific mental process or another is the common quality of their origin, structure, and function. In the genetic respect, they differ in that, on the plane of phylogenesis, they arose as a product not of biological evolution, but of historical development of behavior, and on the plane of ontogenesis, they also have their special social history. With respect to structure, their uniqueness lies in the fact that, as distinct from the direct reactive structure of elementary processes, they are constructed on the basis of using stimuli-means (signs) and because of this, they have an indirect (mediated) character. Finally, with respect to function, they are characterized by the fact that they play a new and essentially different role in behavior from the role of the elementary functions; they carry out an organized adaptation to a situation with preliminary control of the person's own behavior.

## Social Genesis of Higher Mental Functions

Thus, if the sign organization is the most important distinguishing characteristic of all higher mental functions, then, naturally, the first question that arises before the theory of higher functions is the question of the origin of this type of organization.

While traditional psychology was looking for the origin of symbolic activity either in a series of "discoveries" or other intellectual operations of the child or in processes of formation of ordinary conditioned connections, seeing in them only a product of invention or a complicated form of habit, the whole course of our research compelled us to isolate an independent history of sign processes that form a special line in the general history of the mental development of the child.

In this history, both diverse forms of habits connected with the full functioning of any system of signs and complex processes of thinking necessary for rational use of these habits also find their subordinate place. But neither of these can provide an exhaustive explanation for the origin of higher functions, but are themselves explained only in the broader connection with the processes of which they are an ancillary part. The process of the origin of operations connected with the use of signs, however, not only cannot be deduced from the formation of habits or invention, but is, in general, a category that cannot be deduced, a category that remains within the limits of individual psychology. By its very nature, it is a part of the history of the social formation of the child's personality, and only within the structure of this whole can the patterns that control it be disclosed. Human behavior is the product of development of a broader system than just the system of a person's individual functions, specifically, systems of social connections and relations, of collective forms of behavior and social cooperation.

The social nature of every higher mental function has thus far escaped the attention of investigators who did not think to represent the development of logical memory or voluntary activity as part of the social formation of the child because in its biological beginning and in the end of mental development, this function appears as an individual function; only genetic analysis discloses the path that unites the beginning and end points. Analysis shows that every higher mental function was formerly a unique form of psychological cooperation and only later was converted into an individual method of behavior, transferring into the psychological systems of the child the structure that, even in the transfer, retains all the basic traits of symbolic structure, changing only its situation basically.

Thus, the sign initially acts as a means of social connection in the behavior of the child, as an intermental function; subsequently it becomes a means of controlling his own behavior and he just transfers the social relation to a subject inward into his personality. The most important and basic of the genetic laws, to which the study of the higher mental functions leads us, states that every symbolic activity of the child was at one time a social form of cooperation and retains, along the whole path of development to its very highest points, the social method of functioning. The history of higher mental functions is disclosed here as the history of converting means of social behavior into means of individual-psychological organization.

## Basic Rules of Development of Higher Mental Functions

The general positions at the base of the historical theory of higher mental functions that we are developing allow us to reach certain conclusions connected with the most important rules that control the process of development that is of interest to us.

1. The history of development of each of the higher mental functions is not the direct continuation and further improvement of the corresponding elementary functions, but undergoes a radical change of direction in development and a subsequent movement of the process to a completely new plane; each higher mental function is, thus, a specific neoformation.

On the plane of phylogenesis, this position does not present any difficulties because the biological formation and the historical formation of any function are so sharply delimited from each other and so clearly belong to different forms of evolution that they present two processes in pure and isolated form. In ontogenesis both lines of development are complexly interwoven and for this reason frequently led investigators into error, being merged for the observer into an inseparable whole and, as a result of this, the illusion always developed that the higher processes are a simple continuation and development of the lower. We will cite only one factual reason that confirms our position based on the material from more complex mental operations: we shall consider the development of counting and arithmetic processes.

In a series of psychological studies, the view was established that arithmetic operations of the child are, from the very beginning, a complex symbolic activity and grow out of elementary forms of the operation with numbers through continuous development.

Experiments conducted in our laboratory (Kuchurin, N. A. Menchinskaya) convincingly show that there cannot be any talk here of a direct, gradual perfecting of elementary processes but that the change in forms of counting operations is a deep, qualitative change of the mental processes that participate in it. Observations have shown that if in the beginning of development, the operation with numbers is reduced only to direct perception of certain numbers and number groups, and the child cannot count at all but perceives a number, then further development is characterized by a breaking up of this direct form and its replacement by a different process in which a series of mediated auxiliary signs participate, specifically such as analytical speech, the use of fingers and other auxiliary objects that lead the child to the process of counting. Further development of counting operations is again connected with radical reconstructions of the mental functions that participate in them, and counting with the help of complex counting systems again presents a qualitatively special psychological neoformation.

We have come to the conclusion that the development of counting is reduced to the participation in it of basic mental functions, and the transition from preschool arithmetic to school arithmetic is not a simple, continuous process, but a process of surmounting primary elementary patterns and replacing them with new, more complex processes. We shall demonstrate this with a concrete example.

If, for a small child, the process of counting on the whole is determined by perception of forms, then subsequently, this relation is inverted and perception of form itself is determined by the segregating tasks of counting. In our experiments, we asked a small child to count the number of buttons in the figure of a cross made up of them. As a result, we invariably got a mistake: the child perceiving this figure as a whole system of a cross, counted twice the center element, which is part of both systems that cross each other. Only significantly later did he move to a different type of process; from the very beginning, perception was determined by the tasks of counting and was divided into three separate groups of elements that were counted in sequence. In this process, we cannot help but see a replacement of two psychological methods of behavior with the emancipation from a direct connection of sensory and motor fields and with the processing of perception by complex psychological units.

All of these studies convincingly show that evolutionism in the study of development of the child's behavior must yield to more adequate ideas that take into account the completely unique, dialectical character of the process of formation of new mental forms.

2. Higher mental functions are not built up as a second story over elementary processes, but are new psychological systems that include a complex merging of elementary functions that will be included in the new system, and themselves begin to act according to new laws; each higher mental function is, thus, a unit of a higher order determined basically by a unique combination of a series of more elementary functions in the new whole.

In our experiments on the reorganization of perception when speech is included, and more broadly, on the mutual and deep change in the function with the formation of the complex psychological system "speech-practical intellectual operation," we have already traced the aspect that has a decisive significance in the study of the formation and structure of higher mental functions. In these cases, we actually observed the formation of complex psychological systems with new functional relations between separate members of the system and corresponding changes of the functions themselves. If perception connected with speech begins to function not according to laws of the sensory field, but according to laws organized by the system of attention, if the meeting between the symbolic operation and the use of tools produces new forms of mediated control of an object with preliminary organization of the person's own behavior, then we can speak here of a certain general law of mental development and the formation of higher mental functions.

In a series of psychological studies, we became convinced that both the most primitive and the most complex higher mental functions undergo this kind of reconstruction; a psychological study of imitation done in our laboratory (L. I. Bozhovich and L. S. Slavina) showed that primitive forms of reflecting mechanical imitation, being included in the system of sign operations, form a new whole, begin to be constructed according to completely new laws, and acquire a different function. In other experiments, in a psychological study of the process of formation of concepts according to the methods developed by Sakharov, our colleagues, Kotelova and Pashkovskaya, showed that, at higher stages of mental processes as well, the inclusion of complex speech functions is connected with the production of completely new forms of categorical behavior not previously observed at all.

3. With the disintegration of higher mental functions, in disease processes, the connection between symbolic and natural functions is disrupted first of all, and this brings about a detachment of a number of natural processes that begin to act according to primitive laws as more or less independent psychological structures. Thus, the disintegrations of higher mental functions represent a process that, from the qualitative aspect, is the reverse of their construction.

It would be difficult to imagine more clearly than in aphasia the general disintegration of higher mental functions with a disturbance of speech symbolics. Damage to speech is accompanied in this case by the loss (or significant disruption) of sign operations; this loss, however, does not at all occur as an isolated monosymptom, but entails general and deeper disruptions in the activity of all higher mental systems. In a special series of studies, we were able to establish that, in practical actions, the aphasic who has lost higher sign operations is wholly subject to elementary laws of the optical field. In another series, we experimentally established sharp changes characteristic for operating activity of the aphasic that reverts to the primitive immaturity of sensory and motor spheres: direct motor manifestation of impulses and the impossibility of inhibiting action and forming future intentions, an inability to transform an image once developed by shifting attention, and a total inability to move away from understood and habitual structures in reasoning and actions; a return to primitive forms of reflecting imitation—these are the deepest consequences connected with damage to the higher symbolic systems.

Studies of aphasia show with exceptional persuasiveness that higher mental functions do not simply exist alongside the lower or above them; actually, the higher functions permeate the lower and reform all of them, even the deepest layers of behavior, to such an extent that their disintegration, connected with the detachment of lower processes in their elementary forms, radically changes the whole structure of behavior, making it revert to the most primitive, "paleopsychological" type of activity.

# 19

## Analysis of Sign Operations of the Child

We are in a position to close the circle of our discussion and to return to what was indicated at the beginning of this work by the patterns that control the development of the practical intellect of the child, which is only a specific case of the patterns of construction of all higher mental functions. The conclusions we reached confirm this and show that higher mental functions arise as a specific neoformation, as a new structural whole that is characterized by the new functional relations that are being established within it. We have indicated that these functional relations are connected with the operation of using signs as a central and basic factor in the construction of every higher mental function. Thus, this operation appears to be the common trait of all higher mental functions (including the use of tools, which is always our point of departure), a trait that must be taken out of parentheses and subjected in the conclusion of our study to special consideration.

My colleagues and I performed a series of studies on this problem in recent years, and based on the data obtained, we can now sketch the basic patterns that characterize the structure and development of sign operations of the child.

Experimentation is the only path by which we can delve into the patterns of higher processes in sufficient depth; specifically in an experiment, we can elicit in a single, artificially created process the most complex changes separated in time, frequently with years passing latently, which are never accessible to observation in all their real totality in the natural genesis of the child and cannot be comprehended directly in a single glance and correlated with each other. The investigator who is trying to understand the laws of the whole and wants to penetrate beyond the external traits into the causal and genetic connection of these points must go to a special form of experimentation which we describe below from the methodological aspect; the essence of this consists in creating processes that disclose the true course of development of the function that interests the investigator.

The experimental-genetic study also allows us to study the problem from three mutually connected aspects: we will describe the structure, origin, and subsequent fate of sign operations of the child that lead us directly to understanding the internal essence of higher mental processes.

### The Structure of Sign Operations

We will consider the history of child memory, and using an example of its development, we will try to show the general features of sign operations in the sections mentioned

Originally appeared in English translation as Chapter 4 in *The Collected Works of L.S. Vygotsky, Volume 6: Scientific Legacy* (Robert W. Rieber, Ed.; Marie J. Hall, Trans.) (pp. 45–56). New York: Kluwer Academic/Plenum Press, 1999.

above. For a comparative study of the construction and method of action of elementary and higher functions, memory is exceptionally convenient material.

Consideration of human memory on the phylogenetic plane shows that even at the most primitive stages of mental development two methods of its functioning, essentially different from each other, can be clearly distinguished. One of these, dominant in the behavior of primitive man, is characterized by direct impression of material, a simple sequence of actual experience, an imprint of those mnemic traces whose mechanism was tracked in especially clear form by E. Jaensch in the phenomenon of eidetism. This memory is as direct as immediate perception with which it has not yet broken the direct connection, and it arises from direct action of the external impression on the person. From the point of view of structure, the directness is the most important characteristic of the entire process as a whole, a characteristic that connects the person's memory with the memory of the animal; this also accords us the right to call this form of memory, natural memory.

This form of the functioning of memory is not, however, the only form even in the most primitive man; on the contrary, even in him, other forms of remembering are noted together with this form, forms which on closer analysis appear to belong to a completely different genetic order and lead us to a completely different formation of human mentality. Even in such comparatively simple operations as the use of a knot or a notch to aid remembering, the psychological structure of the process changes completely.

Two essential points distinguish this operation from elementary retention in memory: in this case, on the one hand, the process clearly goes beyond the limits of elementary functions directly connected with memory and is replaced by more complex operations, which in themselves may not have anything in common with memory, but which carry out the function of a new operation in the general structure that was previously carried out by the direct impression. On the other hand, here, the operation goes beyond the limits of natural, intracortical processes and includes in the psychological structure elements of the environment that begin to be used as active agents that control the mental process from outside. Both points result in an entirely new type of behavior; analyzing its difference from the natural forms of behavior, we can assume this type of behavior to be cultural.

The essential point in the mnemonic operation is the participation in it of certain external signs. Here, the subject does not solve a problem by direct mobilization of his natural potentials; he approaches certain manipulations anew, organizing himself through organization of things, creating artificial stimuli that differ from others in that they are retrograde: they are directed not toward others but toward himself, and make it possible for the subject to remember with the aid of an external sign. We see an example of such sign operations that organize the memory process very early in cultural history. The use of tallies and knots, rudiments of writing and primitive signs—all of this is the equipment that indicates that at early stages of cultural development, man already went beyond the limits of given natural functions and moved on to a new, cultural organization of his behavior.

It is completely understandable that in a higher symbolic operation such as the use of signs for remembering, we have the product of a most complex historical development; comparative analysis shows that this kind of activity does not exist in any species of animals, even in the highest, and there is every basis for thinking that it is the product of specific conditions of social development. It is clear that this kind of autostimulation could have arisen only after similar stimuli were already created for stimulation of another and that behind it lies a great special history. Evidently, the sign operation follows the same path as speech followed in ontogenesis, being formerly a means of stimulating another person and then becoming an intramental function.

With the transition to sign operations, we not only move on to mental processes of a higher complexity, but actually leave the field of the natural history of the mind and enter into the area of the historical formations of behavior.

The transition to higher mental functions by way of their mediation and construction of a sign operation can be successfully traced in an experiment with a child. For this purpose, we can make the transition from elementary experiments with direct reaction to a problem to those in which the child solves the problem with the help of a number of auxiliary stimuli that organize the psychological operation. In the problem of remembering a certain number of words, we can give the child a number of objects or pictures that do not represent the word presented, but can serve as a conditional sign for it which will then help the child reproduce the required word. The process we studied in this experiment must, consequently, be distinctly different from simple, elementary remembering; in this case, the problem must be solved through a mediated operation, by means of establishing a certain relation between the stimulus and the auxiliary sign; in place of simple remembering, a whole process is involved that assumes a significantly more complex method of organization of behavior than that which is characteristic of elementary mental functions. Actually, if, in the final analysis, each elementary form of behavior assumes a certain direct reaction to the problem placed before the organism and may be expressed in the simple formula S—R, the structure of a sign operation is enormously more complex. Between the stimulus and the reaction, previously united by a direct connection, an intermediate member intervenes and plays a completely special role clearly different from anything that we could see in elementary forms of behavior. This. stimulus of the second order must be involved in the operation with the special function of serving its organization; it must be specially established by the personality and must have a retrograde effect, eliciting specific reactions; consequently, the pattern of a simple reactive process is replaced here by a pattern of a complex, mediated act in which the direct impulse to react is inhibited and the operation proceeds along an indirect path, establishing an auxiliary stimulus that accomplishes a mediated operation.

Careful study shows that in significantly higher forms, as compared to the elementary pattern presented, we see this structure in the higher mental processes. The mediating member, as one might imagine, is simply a method of improving and perfecting the operation; having the specific function of retrograde effect, it transfers the mental operations into higher and qualitatively new forms and allows man to control his own behavior from outside with the aid of external stimuli. The use of the sign, being simultaneously a means of autostimulation, results in a completely new and specific structure of behavior in man, a structure that breaks with the traditions of natural behavior and creates for the first time a new form of cultural-psychological behavior.

Experiments conducted in our laboratory using an external sign for remembering (A. N. Leontev, 1930) showed that this form of mental operations is not only essentially new in comparison with direct remembering, but also helps the child to overcome the boundaries set before memory by natural laws of mnemonics; moreover, it is preeminently the mechanism in memory that is subject to development.

The presence of such higher or indirect paths of remembering, like the possibility of similar indirect operations, is not an unknown thing. Experimental psychology deserves credit for their empirical isolation. Nevertheless, classical studies could not see in them the new, specific, and singular forms of behavior acquired in the process of historical development. Operations of a similar type (for example, mnemotechnical memorization) were presented as nothing other than a simple artificial combination of a series of elementary processes; this fortuitous coincidence itself resulted in a mnemotechnical effect; the device created in practice was not considered by psychology as an essentially new form of memory, as a new method of its activity.

Our experiments led to a completely opposite conclusion. Considering the operation of remembering with the aid of an external sign and analyzing its structure, we are convinced that it is not a simple "psychological focus," but has all the traits and all the properties of an actually new and whole function and represents a unit of a higher order, the separate parts of which are united by relations not reducible either to laws of association or to laws of structure that have been well studied with direct mental operations. We designate these specific functional relations as a sign function of auxiliary stimuli on the basis of which a principally different relation of mental processes that are included in the given operation is established.

We can observe the whole and specific character of sign operations with particular clarity in experiments. Experiments show that if the connections with which the child who tries to remember a given word according to a sign are also formed according to laws of association or structure (we are not now in essence going into solving this problem), then the specificity itself of the sign operation cannot be explained by them. Actually, simple association or a structural connection still is not reversible, and the sign connected with the word does not necessarily bring back the given word that is presented again. We have many cases in which a process occurring according to the usual laws of structural or associative connection did not lead to a mediated operation, and the picture presented repeatedly elicited new associations in the child instead of returning him to a certain word. What is still needed for a specific sign relation to the auxiliary stimulus to develop in the child is for the child to become aware of the goal-directed character of the whole operation, and only then will the structural or associative connection acquire its necessary reversible character, and repeated presentation of the sign will, of necessity, return the subject to the word fixed with the help of this sign.

Subsequently we will consider the roots of these complex mental processes; here we would just like to note that only within the limits of an *instrumental operation* will associative or structural processes begin to play an auxiliary, mediated role. Opening before us is not a random combination of mental functions, but an actually new and special form of behavior.

The process we described is characteristic only for the construction of higher forms of memory. We would be wrong, however, if we thought that such operations introduce only a quantitative improvement into the activity of mental functions. Special experiments show that the plan described is a common principle of construction of higher mental functions and that, with their help, new psychological structures will be created that were not there before and, obviously, are impossible without this kind of sign operation.

We will illustrate this idea using an example from genetic study of the child's voluntary attention activity.

Placing a seven- or eight-year-old child in a situation that requires high and constant application of attention (for example, telling him to name the color of objects mentioned in questions without repeating one and the same color twice and not naming two prohibited colors), we find that the child is completely unable to carry out this task correctly when he tries to solve it directly. However, as soon as the child chooses the mediated organization of the process, using certain auxiliary signs, he solves the problem easily.

In experiments done in our laboratory (A. N. Leontev), we gave the child a number of colored cards and proposed that he use them to make the task easier. When the child did not use these cards in his activity (for example, did not set aside the prohibited colors and did not remove them from the fixed field), the task remained insoluble. However, the child solved it easily if he replaced the direct naming of colors with a complex structure of responses based on auxiliary signs: if he placed the two prohibited colors into a fixed field together with the color that he had already named, forming in this way a group of prohibited stimuli that controlled subsequent responses. Always answering through the mediated auxiliary stimuli, the signs, the child organized his active attention from outside and adapted to the problems that he could not solve by direct, elementary forms of behavior.

## Genetic Analysis of the Sign Operation

We shall consider mediated mental operations as a specific characteristic of the structure of higher mental functions. It would be a great mistake, however, to assume that this process arises through purely logical means, that it is invented or discovered by the child in the form of a lightning guess (an aha! experience), by means of which the child assimilates the relation between the sign and the method of using it for all time so that all further development of this special operation occurs purely through deduction. It would be as much a mistake to think that the symbolic relation to certain stimuli will intuitively be comprehended by the child as if he were retrieving it from the depths of his own soul, that symbolization is primary and not reducible further to the Kantian *a priori* by an ability to create and comprehend symbols that was primordially established in the consciousness.

Both these points of view, the intellectualistic and the intuitive, essentially eliminate metaphysically the question of the genesis of symbolic activity since for one of them, the higher mental functions are preliminarily given prior to any experience, as if implanted in the consciousness and waiting only for the chance to appear with the empirical cognition of an object. This point of view also inevitably leads to the *a priori* conception of higher mental functions. For the other view, in general, the question of origin of higher mental functions is not a problem since it admits that these signs are invented and, subsequently, all corresponding forms of behavior will be derived from them like results of logical prerequisites. Finally, we already mentioned in passing the attempt, insupportable from our point of view, to deduce complex symbolic activity from simple interference and summation of habits.

Observing over the course of several experimental series the different mental functions and studying the path of their development step by step, we came to a conclusion exactly opposite to the two views just presented. The facts disclosed before us the process of deepest significance that we call the natural history of sign operations. We were convinced that sign operations develop in no other way than as a result of a most complex and long process that displays all the typical traits of genuine development and is subject to the basic patterns of mental evolution. This means that sign operations are not simply invented by children or acquired from adults, but arise from something that is not at first a sign operation and that becomes a sign operation only after a series of qualitative transformations of which each promotes the next step, being itself promoted by the preceding step, and connects them as a stage of a single process historical in nature. In this respect, the higher mental functions are not an exception to the general rule and do not differ from other elementary processes: they are, without exception, subject in the same way to the basic law of development; they arise not as something introduced from outside or from inside into the general process of the child's mental development but as a natural result of this process.

True, by including the history of higher mental functions in the general context of mental development and attempting to comprehend their origin from its laws, we must inevitably change the usual conception of this process itself and its laws: even within the general process of development, two basic, qualitatively unique lines are clearly distinguishable—the line of biological forming of elementary processes and the line of sociocultural formation of higher mental functions; these merge and give rise to the real history of child behavior.

Accustomed by the whole course of our observations to distinguishing the two lines indicated, we were confronted, however, by a striking fact that casts light on the question of the origin of the sign function in the ontogenesis of the child: a number of studies established experimentally the existence of a genetic connection between both lines and, by the same token, of the transitional forms between the elementary and higher mental functions. It developed that the earliest maturing of the most complex sign operations is concluded even in the system of purely natural forms of behavior and that the higher functions have in this way their own "intrauterine period" of development connecting them with the natural bases of the child's mind. Objective observation showed that between the purely natural layer of elementary functioning of mental processes and the higher layer of mediated forms of behavior there is an enormous area of transitional psychological systems; in the history of behavior, there is an area of the primitive between the natural and the cultural. These two points—the history of development of higher mental functions and their genetic connection with the natural forms of behavior—we designate as the *natural history of the sign*.

The idea of development seems to be simultaneously the key to the comprehension of the unity of all mental functions and of the origin of higher, qualitatively different forms; we come, therefore, to the position that the most complex mental formations arise from the lower through development.

Experiments studying mediated remembering make it possible for us to track the process of development in its entirety. To a significant degree, a certain primitive quality of all psychological operations is characteristic for the first stage in using a sign. Careful study shows that the sign used here for remembering a certain stimulus is not yet completely separated from it;

together with the stimulus, it enters into a kind of common syncretic structure, encompassing both the object and the sign, and does not yet serve as a means for remembering.

For the child who is at the first stage of development, cognition of a goal-directed operation connected with the use of the sign is still strange; if he turns to the auxiliary picture in order to recall the word he is given, this still does not mean that the reverse path—reproducing the word according to the sign presented—is just as easy for the subject. Experiment with such reproduction shows that the child at this stage usually does not recall the initial stimulus according to the sign presented, but reproduces subsequently the whole syncretic situation toward which the sign nudges him and which may include the basic stimulus among other elements. It must be remembered on the basis of the given sign. The period during which the auxiliary sign is not a specific stimulus that necessarily returns the child to the original situation, but is always only an impulse to further development of the whole syncretic structure of which it is a part, is indisputably typical for the first, primitive stage in the history of the development of sign operations.

A series of facts convinces us that at this stage of development, the sign still acts as a part of the general syncretic situation.

1. Not just any sign is suitable for the child's operation and not just any sign can be linked to any meaning. Limited use of the sign is connected with the need for it to enter into a determined, ready complex that includes both the basic meaning and the sign connected with it. This tendency is especially clearly apparent in children age four to six. Among the signs presented, the child seeks one that has an already established connection with the word to be remembered. For the child of this age, statements that among the presented auxiliary cards "there is nothing like it," for recalling the presented stimulus are typical. While easily remembering the word presented with the help of a card that enters into a ready complex with the word, the child is not in a state to use any sign connecting it with the given word with the help of an auxiliary verbal structure.

2. In experiments in which nonsense figures were used as auxiliary material for remembering (L. V. Zankov), we very frequently got neither a refusal to use them nor an effort to connect them with the given word with a certain artificial method, but an attempt to make the figure a direct reflection of the word, its direct picture. In no case was the auxiliary figure connected with the presented meaning through any mediated connection, but was a kind of direct, nonmediated drawing of the word.

Thus, as we might assume, introducing nonsense sign material into the experiment not only failed to stimulate the child's transition from using ready, prepared connections for creating new connections, but it led to the directly opposite result: to an effort to see directly in the given figure a schematic image of one object or another and to refusing to remember when it was impossible to see such a figure.

3. As a rule, this kind of development was also observed in experiments with small children when sensible pictures, not connected directly with the word presented, served as auxiliary stimuli. The experiments of Yusevich showed that, in a significant number of cases, an auxiliary picture was not really used as a sign either, but the child tried to see in it directly the object that he was supposed to remember. Thus, the child easily remembered the word "sun" with the aid of a picture of a hatchet; he pointed to a small yellow spot and said, "Here, this is the

sun." The complex mediated character of the operation is replaced here by an elementary attempt to create directly an "eidetoid" image of the content presented in the auxiliary sign.

Thus, in both cases, we can speak of the fact that the child, reproducing the required word, also reminds us of how, in glancing at a photograph, we recall the names in the original.

These facts show that at this stage of development, the word is still united with the sign according to completely different laws than in a developed sign operation. Specifically in connection with this, all the mental processes that enter into the composition of mediated operations (for example, choice of the auxiliary sign, the process of remembering and reestablishing the filled-in meaning) occur here in an essentially different way. Precisely this fact is the functional verification and confirmation that the intermediate stage of development between the elementary and the fully mediated processes actually has its own laws of connections and reactions from which the fully developed mediated operation evolves only later.

Special experiments allowed us to study the natural history of the sign in greater detail. In studying the child's use of a sign and development of this activity, we inevitably came to studying how sign activity arises. This problem was the subject of special studies which can be divided into four series.

1.  A study of how the meaning of the sign arises in the child in the process f experimentally organized play with objects.
2.  A study of the connection between sign and meaning, between word and object.
3.  A study of the statements of the child in explaining why a given object is signified by a given word (corresponding to the clinical method of J. Piaget).
4.  Studies done with the method of selection reaction.

If we expound these results negatively, the studies bring us to the conclusion that sign activity arises in the child differently from complex habits, inventions, or discoveries. The child does not devise sign activity, neither does he learn it. Intellectualistic and mechanistic theories are equally wrong. Although instances of development of habits or instances of intellectual "discoveries" are frequently interwoven into the history of the use of a sign by the child, they nevertheless do not determine the internal development of this process and enter into it only as auxiliary, subordinate, secondary components of its structure.

Sign operations are the result of a complex process of development. In the beginning of the process, we can observe transitional, mixed forms that combine both natural and cultural components of the child's behavior. We termed these forms stages of children's primitiveness or the natural history of the sign. As a counterbalance to the naturalistic theories of play, our experiments bring us to the conclusion that play is the basic path of the child's cultural development and specifically the development of his sign activity.

Experiments show that in play and speech, the child is far from recognizing the arbitrariness of the sign operation and is far from recognizing the voluntarily established connection between the sign and the meaning. In order to become a sign of a thing (word), the stimulus must be supported by the qualities of the object itself that is denoted. Not all things are equally important for the child in such play. The real qualities of the object and their sign meaning enter into complex structural interrelations in the play. Thus, for the child, the word is connected with the object through its qualities and included in a common structure with it. For this reason, in our experiments, the child does not agree to call the floor a mirror (he cannot walk on a mirror), but converts a chair into a train, which acquires its qualities in his play, that is, he manipulates it as a train. The child refuses to call a lamp a table, and vice versa, since "one must not write on a lamp and a table cannot be lit." For him, to change the designation means to change the qualities of the thing.

We know of nothing that points more obviously to the fact that at the very beginning of mastery of speech, the child still does not see any connection between sign and meaning and does not recognize this connection for a long time. As further experiments show, the *function of naming* does not arise from a single discovery, but has its own natural history; evidently, at the beginning of speech development, the child does not discover that each object has its own name, but masters new methods of acting with objects.

Thus the relations between sign and meaning, which, because of a similar manner of functioning and because of external similarity, begin at first to remind us of corresponding connections in adults, are, in their internal nature, actually psychological patterns of a completely different kind. To place mastery of this relation at the very beginning of the child's cultural development means to ignore the complex history of the internal formation of a relation, a history that covers more than ten years.

## Further Development of Sign Operations

We have described the structure and genetic roots of sign operations of the child. It would, however, be improper to think that mediation by means of certain external signs is a perpetual form of higher mental functions; careful genetic analysis convinces us of the exact opposite and compels us to think that this form of behavior is only a certain stage in the history of mental development growing out of primitive systems and presupposing a transition at subsequent stages to a significantly more complex psychological formation.

Observations of the development of mediated remembering, which we cited above, point to an extremely unusual fact: if mediated operations occur at first exclusively through external signs, then at later stages of development, external mediation stops being the only operation used by higher psychological mechanisms to resolve the problems that confront them. Experiment shows that not just the forms of using signs change in this case, but the very structure of the operation changes in a radical way. Most essentially, we can express this change by saying that from the externally mediated, it becomes internally mediated. This is expressed by the fact that the child begins to remember the material presented to him according to the method we described above, except that he does not resort to the external signs, which at this point become unnecessary for him.

The whole operation of mediated remembering now occurs as a purely internal process, and we cannot say that it differs in any way in external form from the initial forms of direct remembering. Judging only by external data, it may seem that the child simply began to remember more and better, that somehow he improved and developed his memory, and, what is most important, returned to the method of direct remembering from which our experiment diverted him. But the regression is only a seeming regression: development, as frequently happens, moves not in a circle in this case, but along a spiral, returning on a higher plane to a point that was passed.

We call this withdrawal of the operation inward, this interiorization of higher mental functions connected with new changes in their structure *the processes of revolution,* having in mind mainly the following: the fact that higher mental functions are constructed initially as external forms of behavior and depend on an external sign is not to any extent accidental, but, on the contrary, is determined by the very psychological nature of the higher function, which, as we have said above, does not arise as a direct continuation of elementary processes, but is a social method of behavior applied to one's self.

The transfer of social methods of behavior to the interior of the system of individual forms of adapting is not at all a purely mechanical transfer; it is not done automatically but is connected with a change in structure and function of the whole operation and is a special stage in the development of higher forms of behavior. Complex forms of cooperation transferred into the sphere of individual behavior begin to function according to laws of the primitive whole, of which they now make up an organic part. A genetic, but not a logical, contradiction exists between the position that higher mental functions (an inseparable part of which is the use of signs) arise in the process of cooperation and social interaction and the position that these functions develop from primitive roots on the basis of lower or elementary functions, that is, between sociogenesis of higher functions and their natural history. The transition from a collective to an individual form of behavior initially lowers the level of the whole operation since it is included in a system of primitive functions and assumes qualities common to all functions of this level. Social forms of behavior are more complex and their development goes forward in the child; having already become individual, they *are lowered* and begin to function according to simpler laws. For example, egocentric speech as such is lower in structure than ordinary speech, but as a stage in the development of thinking, it is higher than social speech of a child of the same age and perhaps for this reason Piaget considers it a precursor of socialized speech and not a form derived from it.

Thus we come to the conclusion that every higher mental function inevitably initially has the character of an external activity. As a rule, at first the sign represents an external auxiliary stimulus, an external means of autostimulation. This is due to two factors: first, the roots of this kind of operation lie in the collective forms of behavior that always refer to the sphere of external activity, and, second, this occurs because of the primitive laws of the individual sphere of behavior, laws which are not yet separated from external activity and are not isolated from direct perception and external action, for example, laws of the practical thinking of the child.

The fact of "interiorizing" sign operations was experimentally tracked in two situations: in group experiments with children of various ages and in individual experiments in long-term experimentation with one child. For this purpose, in our laboratory in Leontev's work, a large number of children, beginning with age seven and ending with adolescence, were taken through an experiment in direct and mediated remembering. The change in the number of filled-in elements in both cases yields two lines that disclose the dynamics of sign operations over the course of the whole process of child development. The figure shows the line of development of direct and mediated remembering at different ages.*

A number of points are immediately striking: neither line follows a random path, but each forms a certain pattern. It is completely understandable that the line of direct remembering is lower than the line of mediated remembering and both of them display a certain relation to age. Increase, however, is unequal at different segments of child development: if before age ten to eleven, externally mediated remembering increases sharply and the lower line lags markedly behind this, then specifically during this period, there is a break, and at the upper school age, mediated memory displays a special dynamics. In rate, it out-strips the line of development of the externally mediated operations.

An analysis of this pattern, which we conditionally term *parallelogram of development*, which remains stable in all experiments, shows that the pattern is due to forms that play a primary role in the development of higher mental processes in the child. If it was characteristic for the first stage of development that a child was able to mediate his memory by just turning to certain external devices (this is responsible for the sharp increase in the upper line), abandoning remembering that is not dependent on external signs in a substantial, direct, almost mechanical retention in the memory, then at the second stage of development, a sharp jump occurs: external sign operations reach their limits, but in return the child now begins to reconstruct the internal process of remembering without depending on external signs; the *natural* process is mediated and the child begins to apply certain internal devices—and a sharp increase in the lower curve indicates the break that was made.

The phase of applying external signs plays a decisive role in the development of internal mediated operations. The child makes the transition to internal sign processes because he passed the phase in which these processes were external. The series of individual experiments convinces us of this: having the child's coefficient of natural remembering, over a certain time, we conducted experiments with externally mediated remembering and then again tested operations that did not depend on the use of external signs. The results show that even in the experiment with a mentally retarded child, there is at first a significant increase in externally mediated, and then in *nonmediated* remembering which, after an intervening series of experiments, results in an effect that is two or three times better, transferring, as analysis shows, the devices of the external sign operation to internal processes.

In describing the operations, we are confronted by a twofold process: on the one hand, the natural process undergoes profound reconstruction, being converted into a circuitous, mediated act, and, on the other hand, the sign operation itself is changed, ceasing to be external and being reorganized into most complex internal psychological systems. The double change also is symbolized in our diagram by a break in both curves that coincides at one point and points to the internal dependence of these processes. We are confronted here by a process of greatest psychological importance: what was an external operation with a sign, a certain cultural method of controlling oneself from outside, is converted into a new intrapsychological layer and gives

---

*    Editor's note: The figure is not given. See: Leontev, A. N., *Collected Psychological Works:* in two volumes, Moscow, 1983, Vol. 1, pp. 55, 56, 58.

rise to a new psychological system incomparably higher in composition and cultural-psychological in genesis.

The *process of revolution* of cultural forms of behavior which we have just considered is connected with profound changes in the activity of the most important mental functions and with a radical reconstruction of mental activity on the basis of sign operations. On the one hand, the natural mental processes, as we see them in animals, cease to exist in a pure form, being included in the system of behavior reconstructed on a cultural-psychological base into a new whole. Of necessity, this new whole includes in itself the former elementary functions which, however, continue to exist in it in a derived form, already acting according to new patterns characteristic for the whole system that developed.

On the other hand, the operation itself of using an external sign is radically reconstructed. Being a decisive, important operation for the young child, it is here replaced by substantially different forms; the internally mediated process begins to make use of completely new connections and new devices not similar to those that were characteristic for the external sign operation. In this case, the process undergoes changes similar to those that were observed in the transition of the child from external to internal speech. As a result of the process of revolution of the cultural psychological operation, we obtain a new structure, a new function of devices used formerly, and a completely new composition of complex mental processes.

It would be extremely primitive to think that further reconstruction of higher mental processes under the influence of the use of the sign occurs on the basis of transferring all the ready sign operation inward; it would be just as wrong to think that in a developed system of higher mental processes, there is a simple building of a higher story over the lower and a simultaneous existence of two relatively independent forms of behavior—the natural and the mediated. Actually, as a result of the revolution of the cultural operation, we obtain a qualitatively new interweaving of the systems which sharply distinguishes human psychology from the elementary functions of animal behavior. These most complex interweavings have not been studied thus far, and we can now only indicate several basic points that are characteristic for them.

With the *revolution,* that is, with the transfer of the function inward, a complex reconstruction of its whole structure occurs. As experiment shows, the following are essential points of the reconstruction: 1) replacement of functions; 2) change in natural functions (elementary processes that form the basis for the higher function and make up a part of it); 3) the appearance of new psychological, functional systems (or systemic functions), taking on in the general structure of behavior a role that had been carried out thus far by separate functions.

We might briefly explain these three points, which are internally connected with each other, on the basis of changes that occur in the revolution in higher functions of memory. Even in the simplest forms of mediated remembering, the fact of replacement of the function is completely obvious. Not in vain did Binet call the mnemotechnique of remembering a series of numbers a model of number memory. Experiment shows that in such remembering, the decisive factor is made up not of the strength of memory or the level of its development, but actually in combining, in building a structure, in perceiving relations, thinking in the broad sense, and other processes that replace memory and determine the structure of this activity. In the transition of activity inward, the replacement of functions itself leads to verbalization of memory and, in connection with this, to remembering with the help of concepts. Due to the replacement of function, the elementary process of remembering is shifted from the place it initially occupied, and is still not separated from the new operation, but uses its central position in the whole psychological structure and occupies a new position with respect to the whole new system of jointly acting functions. Entering into this new system, it begins to function according to laws of this whole, part of which it now is.

As a result of all the changes, the new function of memory (which has now become an internal, mediated process) is similar only in name to the elementary process of remembering; in its internal essence, this is a new, specific formation with its own laws.

# Bibliography of Works about Vygotsky in English

*Editors' Note:* Fairly extensive listings of works about Vygotsky are to be found in the bibliographies of Elhammoumi (1997) and Veresov (1999), which also include references in languages other than English, especially Russian. A very large bibliography of works about Vygotsky (mostly Russian) is included at the end of Volume 6 of *Collected Works* (1999), which also gives an extensive bibliography of Vygotsky's writings, though likely incomplete. Much bibliographic scholarship on Vygotsky remains to be done. The list given here is simply meant to be a short, useful guide for the beginner.

Asmolov, A. G. (1998). *Vygotsky today: On the verge of nonclassical psychology.* New York: Nova Science.

Bain, B. (1978). Toward an integration of Piaget and Vygotsky: Bilingual considerations. *Linguistics, 16,* 5–19.

Bakhurst, D. (1991). *Consciousness and revolution in Soviet psychology: From the Bolsheviks to Evald Ilyenkov.* Cambridge: Cambridge University Press.

Bauer, R. (1968). *The new man in Soviet psychology.* Cambridge: Harvard University Press.

Bein, E. S., Vlasova, T. A., Levina, R. E., Morozova, N. G., & Shif, Zh. I. (1993). Afterword. In *Collected works, Volume 2: The fundamentals of defectology (abnormal psychology and learning disabilities)* (R. W. Rieber & A. S. Carton, Eds.; pp. 302–314). New York: Kluwer Academic/Plenum.

Bell, R. Q. (1968). A reinterpretation of the direction of effect in studies of socialization. *Psychological Review, 75,* 81–85.

Bell, R. Q. (1971). Stimulus control of parents or caretaker behavior by offspring. *Developmental Psychology, 4,* 63–72.

Berg, E. E. (1970). L. S. Vygotsky's theory of the social and historical origins of consciousness (Doctoral dissertation. University of Wisconsin).

Berk, E., & Winsler, A. (1995). *Scaffolding children's learning: Vygotsky and early childhood education.* Washington: NAEC.

Bernhardt, R. (Ed.) (1998). *Curriculum leadership: Rethinking schools for the 21st century.* Cresskill, NJ: Hampton Press.

Bickley, E. E. (1977). L. S. Vygotsky's contributions to a dialectical materialist psychology. *Science and Society, 41,* 191–207.

Bozhovich, L. I. (1977). The concepts of the cultural-historical development of mind and its prospects. *Soviet Psychology, 16,* 5–22.

Bronckart, J. P. (1973). The regulating role of speech: A cognitivist approach. *Human Development, 16,* 417–439.

Brown, A. L. (1979). Vygotsky: A man for all seasons. *Contemporary Psychology, 24,* 161–163.

Brozek, J. (1973). Soviet psychology. In *Systems and theories in psychology* (M. H. Marx & W. A. Hillix, Eds.; pp. 529–548). New York: McGraw-Hill.

Brozek, J. (1977). Vygotskii, Lev Semenovich. In *International encyclopedia of psychiatry, psychology, psychoanalysis, neurology* (Vol. 11, B. B. Wolman, Ed.; p. 409). New York: Aesculapius Publishers/Van Nostrand Reinhold Co.

Bruner, J. S. (1962). Introduction. In *Thought and Language* by L. S. Vygotsky (pp. v–x). Cambridge: MIT Press.

Bruner, J. S., (1967). Preface to Vygotsky Memorial Issue. *Soviet Psychology, 5,* 3–5.

Bruner, J. S. (1975). The beginning of intellectual skill: I and II. *New Behavior, 1,* 20–25, 58–61.

Bruner, J. S. (1984). The Zone of Proximal Development: hidden agenda. In *Children's learning in the Zone of Proximal Development* (B. Rogoff & J. V. Wertsch, Eds.). San Francisco: Jossey-Bass.

Buim, N., Runders, J., & Turnure, J. (1974). Early material linguistic environment of normal and Down's syndrome language-learning children. *American Journal of Mental Deficiency, 79,* 52–58.

Cole, M. (1977). Alexander Romanovich Luria: 1902–1977. *American Psychologist, 32*(11), 969–971.

Cole, M. (1977). Introduction. In *Soviet developmental psychology: An anthology* (pp. ix–xxii). White Plains, NY: M. E. Sharpe.

Cole, M. (1979). A portrait of Luria. In *The making of mind: A personal account of Soviet psychology* by A. R. Luria (pp. 181–225). Cambridge, MA: Harvard University Press.

Cole, M. (1980). The unmaking of mind behind the autobiography. *Psychology Today, 14,* 88–89.

Cole, M. (1996). *Cultural psychology: A once and future discipline.* Cambridge: Harvard University Press.

Cole, M., & Bruner, J. (1971). Cultural difference and inferences about psychological process. *American Psychologist, 26*(10), 867–876.

Cole, M., & Maltzman, I. (1969). Introduction. In *A handbook of contemporary Soviet psychology* (pp. 3–38). New York: Basic Books.

Cole, M., & Scribner, S. (1974). *Culture and thought: A psychological introduction.* New York: Wiley.

Cole, M., & Scribner, S. (1978). Introduction. In *Mind in Society: The development of higher psychological processes* by L. S. Vygotsky (pp. 1–15). Cambridge: Harvard University Press.

Cole, M., & Wertsch, J. V. (1996). *Contemporary implications of Vygotsky and Luria.* Worcester, MA: Clark University Press.

Collins, C. (1999). *Language, ideology and social consciousness: Developing a sociohistorical approach.* Aldershot, England: Ashgate.

Cox, B. D., & Lightfoot, C. (Eds.) (1997). *Sociogenetic perspectives on internalization.* Mahwah, NJ: Lawrence Erlbaum.

Cumming, J. (1975). Vygotsky, Lev Semenovich. In *Encyclopedia of psychology* (Vol. 2, H. J. Eysenck, W. J. Arnold, & R. Meili, Eds.; p. 1170). Fontana: Collins.

Daniels, H. (Ed.) (1993). *Charting the agenda: Educational activity after Vygotsky.* London: Routledge.

Daniels, H. (Ed.) (1996). *An introduction to Vygotsky.* London: Routledge.

Das, J. P. (1995). Some thoughts on two aspects of Vygotsky's work. *Educational Psychologist, 30*(2), 93–97.

Davydov, V. V., & Radzikhovskii, L. A. (1985). Vygotsky's theory and the activity- oriented approach in psychology. In *Culture, communication, and cognition: Vygotskian perspectives* (J. V. Wertsch, Ed.; pp. 35–66). Cambridge: Cambridge University Press.

Davydov, V. V., & Zinchenko, V. P. (1989). Vygotsky's contribution to the development of psychology. *Soviet Psychology, 27*(2), 22–36.

Delefosse, M. S., & Delefosse, J. M. O. (2002). Spielrein, Piaget and Vygotsky: Three positions on child thought and language. *Theory and Psychology, 12,* 723–747.

Dixon-Krauss, L. (Ed.) (1996). *Vygotsky in the classroom: Mediated literacy instruction and assessment.* White Plains, NY: Longman.

Elhammoumi, M. (1997). *Socio-historicocultural psychology: Lev Semenovich Vygotsky, 1896–1934: Bibliographical notes.* Lanham, MD: University Press of America.

Elsasser, N., & John-Steiner, V. (1977). An interactionist approach to advancing literacy. *Harvard Educational Review, 47*(3), 355–370.

Emerson, C. (2000). Bakhtin, Lotman, Vygotsky

Emihovich, C., & Lima, E. S. (1995). The many facets of Vygotsky: A cultural-historical voice from the future. *Anthropology and Education, 26*(4), 375–383.

Engestrom, Y., Miettinen, R., & Punamaki, R. (Eds.) (1999). *Perspectives on activity theory.* Cambridge: Cambridge University Press.

Ervin, S. (1962). Incisive ideas from the Soviet Union. *Contemporary Psychology, 7,* 406–407.

Etkind, A. M. (1994). More on L. S. Vygotsky: Forgotten texts and undiscovered contexts. *Journal of Russian and East European Psychology, 32*(6), 22–36.

Fodor, J. (1972). Some reflection on L. S. Vygotsky's *Thought and Language. Cognition, 1*(1), 82–95.

Fosberg, I. (1948). A modification of the Vygotsky block test for the study of the higher thought processes. *American Journal of Psychology, 61,* 558–561.

Fraser, C., & Roberts, N. (1975). Mothers' speech to children of four different ages. *Journal of Psycholinguistic Research, 4,* 9–16.

Frawley, W. (1997). *Vygotsky and cognitive science: Language and the unification of the social and computational mind.* Cambridge: Harvard University Press.

Frederick, S. (1974). Vygotsky on language skills. *The Classical World, 67,* 283–290.

Garai, L., & Kocski, M. (1990). The psychological status of activity and social relationship: On the continuity of the theories of Lev Vygotsky and Alexei Leontyev. *Soviet Psychology, 11*(5), 3–14.

Gellatly, A., Rogers, D., & Sloboda, J. (Eds.) (1989). *Cognition and social world.* Oxford: Oxford University Press.

Glassman, M. (1994). All things being equal: The two roads of Piaget and Vygotsky. *Developmental Review, 14*(2), 186–214.

Glick, J. (1983). Piaget, Vygotsky and Werner. In *Toward a holistic developmental psychology* (S. Wapner & B. Kaplan, Eds.). Hillsdale, NJ: Erlbaum.

Golden, M., Montare, A., & Bridger, W. (1977). Verbal control of delay behavior in two-year-old boys as a function of social class. *Child Development, 48,* 1107–1111.

Guimaraes-Lima, M. (1995). From aesthetics to psychology: Notes on Vygotsky's psychology of art. *Anthropology and Education, 26*(4), 410–424.

Gulutsan, M. (1967). Jean Piaget in Soviet psychology. *Alberta Journal of Educational Research, 13*(3), 239–247.

Hanfmann, E., & Kasanin, J. (1937). A method for the study of concept formation. *Journal of Psychology,* No. 3, 521–540.

Hanfmann, E., & Kasanin, J. (1942). Conceptual thinking in schizophrenia. *Nervous and Mental Disorder Monographs,* No. 67.

Hanfmann, E., & Vakar, G. (1962). Translators' preface. In *Thought and Language* by L. S. Vygotsky (pp. xi–xiii). Cambridge: MIT Press.

Harris, A. (1975). Social dialects and language: Mother and child construct the discourse. In *The development of dialectical operations* (K. Riegel, Ed.; pp. 80–96). Basel: S. Karger.

Hautamäki, A. (1982). *Activity environment, social class and voluntary learning: An interpretation and application of Vygotsky's concepts.* Helsinki: University of Joensuu.

Hedegaard, M. (1992). The Zone of Proximal Development as basis for instruction. In *Vygotsky and education: Instructional implications and applications of sociocultural psychology* (L. C. Moll, Ed.; pp. 349–371). New York: Cambridge University Press.

Hewes, D., & Evans, D. (1978). Three theories of egocentric speech: A contrastive analysis. *Communication Monographs, 45,* 18–32.

Howe, A. C. (1996). Development of scientific concepts within a Vygotskian framework. *Science Education, 80*(1), 35–51.

Jakobson, R. (1971). Anthony's contribution to linguistic theory. In *Selected writings* (Vol. 2, pp. 285–288). The Hague: Mouton.

Jakobson, R. (1978). *Six lectures on sound and meaning.* Cambridge: MIT Press.

John-Steiner, V., & Souberman, E. (1978). Afterword and note. In *Mind in Society: The development of higher psychological processes* by L. S. Vygotsky (pp. 121–140). Cambridge: Harvard University Press.

Joravsky, D. (1987). L. S. Vygotskii: The muffled deity of Soviet psychology. In *Psychology in twentieth-century thought and society* (M. G. Ash & W. R. Woodward, Eds.; pp. 189–211). Cambridge: Cambridge University Press.

Joravsky, D. (1989). *Russian psychology: A critical analysis.* Oxford: Blackwell.

Kim, M. H. (1994). Vygotsky's inner speech and ESL composing processes: A case study of two advanced ESL students (Doctoral dissertation. University of Missouri-Columbia).

Knox, J. E. (1989). The changing face of Soviet defectology: A study in rehabilitating the handicapped. *Studies in Soviet Thought, 37,* 217–236.

Knox, J. E., & Stevens, C. (1993). Vygotsky and Soviet Russian defectology: An introduction. In *Collected works, Volume 2: The fundamentals of defectology (abnormal psychology and learning disabilities)* (R. W. Rieber & A. S. Carton, Eds.; pp. 1–25). New York: Kluwer Academic /Plenum.

Kohlberg, L., Yaeger, J., & Hjerthol, E. (1968). Private speech: Four studies and a review of theories. *Child Development, 39,* 691–736.

Kowal, K. H. (1997). *Rhetorical implications of linguistic relativity: Theory and application to Chinese and Taiwanese interlanguages.* New York: Peter Lang.

Kozulin, A. (1984). *Psychology in Utopia.* Cambridge: MIT Press.

Kozulin, A. (1990). *Vygotsky's psychology: A biography of ideas.* Cambridge, MA: Harvard University Press.

Kozulin, A. (1991). Introduction: Lev Vygotsky and contemporary social thought. *Studies in Soviet Thought, 42,* 71.

Kozulin, A. (1996). The concept of activity in Soviet psychology: Vygotsky, his disciples and critics. In *An introduction to Vygotsky* (H. Daniels, Ed.; pp. 264–274). London: Routledge.

Kozulin, A. (1998). *Psychological tools: A sociocultural approach to education.* Cambridge: Harvard University Press.

Kvale, S. (1975). Memory and dialectic. In *The development of dialectical operations* (K. Riegel, Ed.; pp. 181–193). Basel: S. Karger.

Lantolf, J. P., & Appel, G. (Eds.) (1994). *Vygotskian approaches to second language research.* Norwood, NJ: Ablex.

Lee, B. (1985). Intellectual origins of Vygotsky's semiotic analysis. In *Culture, communication, and cognition: Vygotskian perspectives* (J. V. Wertsch, Ed.). Cambridge: Cambridge University Press.

Lee, C. D., & Smagorinsky, P. (Eds.) (2000). *Vygotskian perspectives on literacy research: Constructing meaning through collaborative inquiry.* Cambridge: Cambridge University Press.

Leontiev, A. N. (1932). The development of voluntary attention in the child. *Journal of Genetic Psychology, 40*(2), 52–81.

Leontiev, A. N. (1974–75). The problem of activity in psychology. *Soviet Psychology, 2*(13), 4–33.

Leontiev, A. N. (1978). *Activity, consciousness and personality.* Engelwood Cliffs, NJ: Prentice-Hall.

Leontiev, A. N. (1981). *Problems in the development of mind.* Moscow: Progress.

Leontiev, A. N. (1981). The problem of activity of psychology. In *The concept of activity in Soviet psychology* (J. V. Wertsch, Ed.). New York: Sharpe, Armonk.

Leontiev, A. N. (1989). The problem of activity in the history of Soviet psychology. *Soviet Psychology, 27*(1), 22–39.

Leontiev, A. N., & Luria A. R. (1968). The psychological ideas of L. S. Vygotsky. In *Historical roots of contemporary psychology* (B. B. Wolman, Ed.). New York: Harper & Row.

Leontiev, A. N., & Luria, A. R. (1972). Some notes concerning Dr. Fodor's " Reflection on L. S. Vygotsky's *Thought and Language.*" *Cognition, 1*(2–3), 311–316.

Levitin, K. (1982). Chapter 1: Ages and Days. In *One is not born a personality: Profiles of Soviet education psychologists* (pp. 16–101). Moscow: Progress.

Linn, M. (1973). The role of intelligence in children's response to instruction. *Psychology in the Schools, 10,* 67–75.

Lloyd, P., & Fernyhough, C. (Eds.) (1999). *Lev Vygotsky: Critical assessments* (Vols. 1–4). New York: Routledge.

London, I. (1949). A historical survey of psychology in the Soviet Union. *Psychological Bulletin, 46,* 241–277.

Luria, A. R. (1928). The problem of the cultural behavior of the child. *Journal of Genetic Psychology, 35,* 493–506.

Luria, A. R. (1928). Psychology in Russia. *Journal of Genetic Psychology, 35,* 347–355.

Luria, A. R. (1930). The new method of expressive motor reactions in studying affective traces. In *Ninth International Congress of Psychology, held at Yale University, New Haven, Connecticut, September 1st to 7th, 1929, Proceedings and Papers* (J. M. Cattell, Ed.). New York: Psychological Review.

Luria, A. R. (1931). Psychological expedition to Central Asia. *Science, 74,* 383–384.

Luria, A. R. (1932). *The nature of human conflicts.* New York: Liveright.

Luria, A. R. (1932). Psychological expedition to Central Asia. *Journal of Genetic Psychology, 40,* 241–242.

Luria, A. R. (1934). The second psychological expedition to Central Asia. *Journal of Genetic Psychology, 44,* 255–259.

Luria, A. R. (1936). The development of mental functions in twins. *Character and Personality, 5,* 35–47.

Luria, A. R. (1939). L. S. Vygotsky: A biographical sketch. *Psychiatry, 2,* 53—54.

Luria, A. R. (1961). *The role of speech in the regulation of normal and abnormal behavior.* New York: Liveright.

Luria, A. R. (1965). L. S. Vygotsky and the problem of localization of functions. *Neuropsychology,* No. 5, 387–392.

Luria, A. R. (1974). Autobiography. In *A history of psychology in autobiography* (G. Lindzey, Ed.; pp. 251–292). Englewood Cliffs, NJ: Prentice-Hall.

Luria, A. R. (1974). Towards the basic problems of neurolinguistics. *Brain and Language,* No. 1, 1–14.

Luria, A. R. (1976). *Cognitive development, its cultural and social foundations* (M. Lopez-Morillas & L. Solotaroff, Trans.). Cambridge: Harvard University Press.

Luria, A. R. (1978). Biographical note on L. S. Vygotsky. In *Mind in Society: The development of higher psychological processes* by L. S. Vygotsky (pp. 15–16). Cambridge, MA: Harvard University Press.

Luria, A. R. (1979). *Higher cortical functions in man.* New York: Basic Books.

Luria, A. R. (1979). *The making of mind: A personal account of Soviet psychology* (S. Cole & M. Cole, Eds.). Cambridge: Harvard University Press.

Luria, A. R., & Majovski, L. V. (1977). Basic approaches used in American and Soviet clinical neuropsychology. *American Psychologist, 32,* 959–968.

Markova, I. (1990). The development of self-consciousness: Baldwin, Mead, and Vygotsky. In *Reconsidering psychology: Perspectives from continental philosophy* (J. E. Faulconer & R. N. Williams, Eds.; pp. 151–174). Pittsburgh: Duquesne University Press.

Mason, J. M. (1992). *Emerging literacy in the early childhood years: Applying a Vygotskian model of learning and development.* Champaign: University of Illinois at Urbana-Champaign.

McCagg, W. O., & Siegelbaum, L. (Eds.) (1989). *The disabled in the Soviet Union: Past and present theory and practice*. Pittsburgh: University of Pittsburgh Press.

Meacham, J. (1972). The development of memory abilities in the individual and in society. *Human Development, 15*, 205–228.

Meece, R., & Rosenblum, R. (1965). Conceptual thinking of sixth-grade children as measured by Vygotsky block test. *Psychological Review, 72*, 195–202.

Meichenbaum, D. (1975). Theoretical and treatment implications of developmental research on verbal control of behavior. *Canadian Psychological Review, 16*, 22–27.

Minick, N. (1987). The development of Vygotsky's thought: An introduction. In *The collected works of L. S. Vygotsky, Volume 1: Problems of general psychology* (R.W. Rieber & A. S. Carton, Eds.; pp. 17–36). New York: Kluwer Academic/Plenum.

Moll, L. C. (Ed.) (1990). *Vygotsky and education: Instructional implications and applications of sociohistorical psychology*. Cambridge: Cambridge University Press.

Moore, T. (1968). Language and intelligence: A longitudinal study of the first eight years; Part II: Environmental correlates of metal growth. *Human Development, 11*, 1–24.

Netchine-Grynberg, G. (1995). The functionality of cognition according to Cassirer, Meyerson, Vygotsky, and Wallon: Toward the roots of the concept of cognitive tool. In *Trends and issues in theoretical psychology* (I. Lubek, R. Van Hezewijk, G. Pheterson & C. Tolman, Eds.; pp. 207–223). New York: Springer.

Newman, F., & Holzman, L. (1993). *Lev Vygotsky: Revolutionary scientist*. London: Routledge.

Papadopoulos, D. D. (1996). Observation on Vygotsky's reception in academic psychology. In *Problems of theoretical psychology* (C. Tolman, F. Cherry, R. V. Hezewijk & I. Lubek, Eds.; pp. 145–155). North York, Canada: Captus.

Penuel, W., & Wertsch, J. V. (1995). Vygotsky and identity formation: A sociocultural approach. *Educational Psychologist, 30*(2), 83–92.

Pesic, J., & Bauca, A. (1996). Vygotsky and psychoanalysis. *Journal of Russian and East European Psychology, 1*(34), 33–39.

Phillips, S. (1977). The contribution of L. S. Vygotsky to cognitive psychology. *Alberta Journal of Educational Research, 23*, 31–42.

Piaget, J. (1962). Comments on Vygotsky's critical remarks concerning "The language and thought of the child and reasoning in the child." In *Thought and Language* by L. S. Vygotsky (pp. 169–183). Cambridge: MIT Press.

Radzikovskii, L. A. (1990). The language of description of holism and L. S. Vygotsky's notion of "units." *Soviet Psychology, 28*(3), 5–22.

Radzikovskii, L. A. (1991). The historical meaning of the crisis in psychology. *Soviet Psychology, 29*(4), 73–99.

Radzikovskii, L. A., & Khomskaya, E. (1981). A. R. Luria and L. S. Vygotsky: Early years of their collaboration. *Soviet Psychology, 20*(1), 3–21.

Rahmani, L. (1966). Studies on the mental development of the child. In *Present-day Russian psychology* (N. O'Connor, Ed.; pp. 152–177). Oxford: Pergamon Press.

Rahmani, L. (1973). *Soviet psychology: Philosophical, theoretical and experimental issues*. New York: International University Press.

Ratner, C. (1991). *Vygotsky's sociohistorical psychology and its contemporary applications*. New York: Plenum.

Ratner, C. (1994). The unconscious: A perspective from sociohistorical psychology. *Journal of Mind and Behavior, 15*, 323–342.

Ratner, C. (1996). Activity as a key concept for cultural psychology. *Culture and Psychology, 2*, 407–434.

Ratner, C. (1997). *Cultural psychology and qualitative methodology: Theoretical and empirical considerations.* New York: Kluwer Academic/Plenum.

Ratner, C. (1999). Three approaches to cultural psychology: A critique. *Cultural Dynamics, 11,* 7–31.

Ratner, C. (2000). A cultural-psychological analysis of emotions. *Culture and Psychology, 6,* 5–39.

Ratner, C. (2002). *Cultural psychology: Theory and method.* New York: Kluwer Academic/Plenum.

Riegel, K. F. (1973). Dialectic operations: The final period of cognitive development. *Human Development, 16,* 346–370.

Riegel, K. F. (1975). Toward a dialectical theory of development. *Human Development, 18,* 50–64.

Riegel, K. F. (1976). Dialectical operations of cognitive development. In *Contributions to human development* (Vol. 2, pp. 60–71). Basel: S. Karger.

Riegel, K. F. (1979). *Foundations of dialectical psychology.* New York: Academic Press.

Rogoff, B. (2003). *The cultural nature of human development.* New York: Oxford University Press.

Rogoff, B., & Wertsch, J. V. (Eds.) (1984). *Children's learning in the Zone of Proximal Development.* San Francisco: Jossey-Bass.

Sahakian, W. S. (1975). *History and systems of psychology.* New York: Wiley.

Sameroff, A. (1975). Transactional models in early social relations. In *The development of dialectical operations* (K. F. Riegel, Ed.; pp. 65–79). Basel: S. Karger.

Scheerer, E. (1980). Gestalt psychology in the Soviet Union; Part 1: The period of enthusiasm. *Psychological Research, 41,* 113–132.

Schneuwly, B. (1994). Contradiction and development: Vygotsky and paedology. *European Journal of Psychology of Education, 9*(4), 181–191.

Schubert, F. C. (1975). Vygotsky test. In *Encyclopedia of psychology* (Vol. 2, H. S. Eysenck, W. J. Arnold, & R. Meili, Eds.; p. 1170). Fontana: Collins.

Scribner, S. (1985). Vygotsky's use of history. In *Culture, communication, and cognition: Vygotskian perspectives* (J. Wertsch, Ed.). Cambridge: Harvard University Press.

Scribner, S., & Cole, M. (1973). Cognitive consequences of formal and informal education. *Science,* No. 182, 553–559.

Scribner, S., & Cole, M. (1981). *The psychology of literacy.* Cambridge: Harvard University Press.

Semeonoff, B., & Laird, A. (1952). The Vygotsky test as a measure of intelligence. *British Journal of Psychology, 43,* 94–102.

Shchedrovitskii, L. P. (1994). L. S. Vygotsky's "Tragedy of Hamlet Prince of Denmark." *Journal of Russian and East European Psychology, 32*(2), 49–65.

Shotter, J. (1993). Vygotsky: The social negotiation of semiotic mediation. *New Ideas in Psychology, 11*(1), 61–75.

Sinclair, H. (1972). Some comments on Fodor's "Reflections on L. S. Vygotsky's *Thought and Language.*" *Cognition, 1,* 317–318.

Smith, L., Dockrell, J., & Tomlinson, P. (Eds.) (1997). *Piaget, Vygotsky and beyond: Future issues for developmental psychology and education.* London: Routledge.

Snow, C. E. (1972). Mothers' speech to children learning language. *Child Development, 43,* 549—565.

Sobkin, A., & Leontiev, D. (1992). The beginning of a new psychology: Vygotsky's psychology of art. In *Emerging visions of the aesthetic process: Psychology, semiology, and philosophy* (G. J. Cupchik & G. Laszlo, Eds.). New York: Cambridge University Press.

Stewin, L., & Martin, J. (1977). The development stages of L. S. Vygotsky and J. Piaget: A comparison. *Alberta Journal of Educational Research, 23,* 31–42.

Still, A., & Costall, A. (1991). The mutual elimination of dualism in Vygotsky and Gibson. In *Against cognitivism: Alternative foundations for cognitive psychology* (A. Still & A. Costall, Eds.; pp. 225–236). London: Harvester Wheatsheaf.

Stutton, A. (1980). Cultural disadvantage and Vygotskii's stages of development. *Educational Studies, 6*(3), 199—209.

Toulmin, S. (1978, September 28). The Mozart of psychology [Review of the book *Mind in Society*]. *New York Review of Books,* 51–57.

Toulmin, S. (2002) Vygotsky's psychology: A biography of ideas. *Common Knowledge, 8,* 209.

Tryphon, A., & Voneche, J. (Eds.) (1996). *Piaget-Vygotsky: The social genesis of thought.* Hove, UK: Psychology Press.

Tudge, J., & Rogoff, B. (1989). Peer influences on cognitive development: Piagetian and Vygotskian perspectives. In *Interaction in human development: Crosscurrents in contemporary psychology* (M. H. Bornstein & J. S. Bruner, Eds.; pp. 17–40).

Hillsdale, NJ: Erlbaum.

Tudge, J., & Winterhoff, P. (1993). Vygotsky, Piaget, and Bandura: Perspectives on the relations between the social world and cognitive development: *Human Development, 36*(2), 61–81.

Valsiner, J. (1988). *Developmental psychology in the Soviet Union.* Bloomington: Indiana University Press.

Valsiner, J., & van der Veer, R. (1988). On the social nature of human cognition: An analysis of the shared intellectual roots of G. H. Mead and L. Vygotsky. *Journal for the Theory of Social Behavior, 18,* 117–136.

Valsiner, J., & van der Veer, R. (1993). The encoding of distance: The concept of the Zone of Proximal Development and its interpretations. In *The development and meaning of psychological distance* (R. Rodney, K. Cocking & A. Renninger, Eds.). Hillsdale, NJ: Erlbaum.

Valsiner, J., & van der Veer, R. (2000). *The social mind: Construction of the idea.* Cambridge: Cambridge University Press.

van der Veer, R. (1987). From language and thought to thinking and speech. *Journal of Mind and Behavior, 8, 175–177.*

van der Veer, R. (1991). *Understanding Vygotsky: A quest for synthesis.* Oxford: Blackwell.

van der Veer, R. (1994). The concept of development and the development of concepts: Education and development in Vygotsky's thinking. *European Journal of Psychology of Education, 9*(4), 293–300.

van der Veer, R., & Valsiner, J. (1991). *Understanding Vygotsky: A quest for synthesis.* Oxford: Blackwell.

van der Veer, R., & Valsiner, J. (Eds.). (1994). *The Vygotsky reader.* Oxford: Blackwell.

Veresov, N. N. (1999). *Undiscovered Vygotsky: Etudes on the pre-history of cultural-historical psychology.* European Studies in the History of Science and Ideas, vol. 8. Frankfurt-am-Main: Peter Lang.

Vygodskaya, G. L., & Lifanova, T. M. (1988). L. S. Vygotsky: Life and work. In *Proceedings of the Seventh European CHEIRON Conference* (pp. 733–739). Budapest: Hungarian Psychological Association.

Weinreich, V. (1963). Review of the book *Thought and Language. American Anthropologist, 65*(6), 1401–1404.

Wells, C. G. (1999). *Dialogic inquiry: Towards a sociocultural practice and theory of education.* Cambridge: Cambridge University Press.

Wertsch, J. V. (Ed.) (1978). *Recent trends in Soviet psycholinguistics.* White Plains, NY: M. E. Sharpe.

Wertsch, J. V. (1979). From social interaction to higher psychological processes: A clarification and application of Vygotsky's theory. *Human Development, 22,* 1–22.

Wertsch, J. V. (1980). The significance of dialogue in Vygotsky's account of social egocentric and inner speech. *Contemporary Educational Psychology, 5,* 150—162.

Wertsch, J. V. (Ed.) (1981). *The concept of activity in Soviet psychology.* Armonk, NY: M. E. Sharpe.

Wertsch, J. V. (1983). The role of semiosis in L. S. Vygotsky's theory of human cognition. In *The sociogenesis of language and human conduct* (B. Bain, Ed.). New York: Plenum.

Wertsch, J. V. (Ed.) (1985). *Culture, communication, and cognition: Vygotskian perspectives.* Cambridge: Cambridge University Press.

Wertsch, J. V. (1985). *Vygotsky and the social formation of mind.* Cambridge: Harvard University Press.

Wertsch, J. V. (1991). *Voices of the mind: A sociocultural approach to mediated action.* Cambridge: Harvard University Press.

Wertsch, J. V. (2002). *Voices of collective remembering.* Cambridge: Cambridge University Press, 2002.

Wertsch, J. V., del Rio, P., & Alvares, A. (Eds.) (1995). *Sociocultural studies of mind.* New York: Cambridge University Press.

Wertsch J. V., & Sohner, R. (1995). Vygotsky on learning and development. *Human Development, 38*(6) 332–337.

Wilson, A., & Weinstein, L. (1992). An investigation into some implications of a Vygotskian perspective on the origins of mind. *Journal of the American Psychoanalytic Association, 40,* 349–380.

Wilson, A., & Weinstein, L. (1996). The transference and the Zone of Proximal Development. *Journal of American Psychoanalytic Association, 44*(1), 167–200.

Wozniak, R. H. (1996). Qu'est-ce que l'intelligence? Piaget, Vygotsky, and the 1920s crisis in psychology. In *Piaget—Vygotsky: The social genesis of thought* (A. Tryphon & J. Vonèche, Eds.; pp. 11–24). Hove, UK: Psychology Press.

Yaroshevsky, M. G. (1994). L. S. Vygotsky–Victim of an "optical illusion." *Journal of Russian and East European Psychology, 32*(6), 35–43.

Yaroshevsky, M. G. (1996). Marxism in Soviet psychology: The social role of Russian science. In *Post-Soviet perspectives on Russian psychology* (V. A. Koltsova, Yu. Oleinik; A. Gilgen, & K. Gilgen, Eds.; pp. 161–186). Westport, CT: Greenwood.

Yoo, Y. (Ed.). (1980). *Soviet education: An annotated bibliography and reader's guide to works in English.* Westport, CT: Greenwood Press.

Zinchenko, V. P. (1985). Vygotsky's ideas about units for the analysis of mind. In *Culture, communication, and cognition: Vygotskian perspectives* (J. V. Wertsch, Ed.; pp. 94–118). Cambridge: Cambridge University Press.

Zinchenko, V. P. (1990). The problems of the "formative" elements of consciousness in the activity theory of mind. *Soviet Psychology, 28*(2), 25–40.

# Index

For fuller indexes, including names and authors, see the six-volume *Collected Works*.

Printed in the United States
203510BV00002BD/1-2/A